D1296519

DeGowin's
Diagnostic Examination

NOTICE

Medicine is an ever-changing science. As new research and clinical experience broaden our knowledge, changes in treatment and drug therapy are required. The authors and the publisher of this work have checked with sources believed to be reliable in their efforts to provide information that is complete and generally in accord with the standards accepted at the time of publication. However, in view of the possibility of human error or changes in medical sciences, neither the authors nor the publisher nor any other party who has been involved in the preparation or publication of this work warrants that the information contained herein is in every respect accurate or complete, and they disclaim all responsibility for any errors or omissions or for the results obtained from use of the information contained in this work. Readers are encouraged to confirm the information contained herein with other sources. For example and in particular, readers are advised to check the product information sheet included in the package of each drug they plan to administer to be certain that the information contained in this work is accurate and that changes have not been made in the recommended dose or in the contraindications for administration. This recommendation is of particular importance in connection with new or infrequently used drugs.

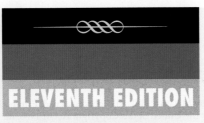

ELEVENTH EDITION

DeGowin's
Diagnostic Examination

Manish Suneja, MD, FACP, FASN
Professor of Internal Medicine
The University of Iowa Carver College of Medicine
Iowa City, Iowa

Joseph F. Szot, MD, FACP
Professor of Internal Medicine
The University of Iowa Carver College of Medicine
Iowa City, Iowa

Richard F. LeBlond, MD, MACP
Professor Emeritus of Internal Medicine
The University of Iowa Carver College of Medicine
Iowa City, Iowa

Donald D. Brown, MD, FACP
Professor of Internal Medicine
The University of Iowa Carver College of Medicine
Iowa City, Iowa

Illustrated by
Elmer DeGowin, MD, Jim Abel, and Shawn Roach

New York   Chicago   San Francisco   Athens   London   Madrid   Mexico City
New Delhi   Milan   Singapore   Sydney   Toronto

DeGowin's Diagnostic Examination, Eleventh Edition

1 2 3 4 5 6 7 8 9 DSS 25 24 23 22 21 20

ISBN 978-1-260-13487-2
MHID 1-260-13487-3

This book was set in Palatino LT Std by MPS Limited.
The editors were Kay Conerly and Kim J. Davis.
The production supervisor was Richard Ruzycka.
Project management was provided by Ishan Chaudhary, MPS Limited.
The cover designer was W2 Design.
Cover image by George Tsartsianidis / iStock / Getty Images.

This book is printed on acid-free paper.

Library of Congress Cataloging-in-Publication Data

Names: LeBlond, Richard F., author. | Suneja, Manish, author. | Szot, Joseph F., author. | Brown, Donald D., 1940- author.
Title: DeGowin's diagnostic examination / Manish Suneja, Joseph F. Szot, Richard F. LeBlond, Donald D. Brown; illustrated by Elmer DeGowin, Jim Abel, and Shawn Roach.
Other titles: Diagnostic examination
Description: Eleventh edition. | New York: McGraw-Hill Education, [2020] | Richard F. LeBlond's name appears first on previous edition. | Includes bibliographical references and index. | Summary: "DeGowin's Diagnostic Examination describes the techniques for obtaining a complete history and performing a thorough physical exam, links symptoms and signs with the pathophysiology of disease, presents an approach to differential diagnosis, based upon the pathophysiology of disease, which can be efficiently tested in the laboratory, and does all of this in a format that can be used as a quick point-of-care reference and as a text to study the principles and practice of history taking and physical examination"– Provided by publisher.
Identifiers: LCCN 2019046392 (print) | LCCN 2019046393 (ebook) | ISBN 9781260134872 (paperback; alk. paper) | ISBN 1260134873 (paperback; alk. paper) | ISBN 9781260134889 (ebook) | ISBN 1260134881 (ebook)
Subjects: MESH: Physical Examination | Diagnosis | Signs and Symptoms
Classification: LCC RC78.7.D53 (print) | LCC RC78.7.D53 (ebook) | NLM WB 200 | DDC 616.07/54–dc23
LC record available at https://lccn.loc.gov/2019046392
LC ebook record available at https://lccn.loc.gov/2019046393

To our patients,
who allow us to practice our art,
encourage us with their confidence,
and humble us with their courage.

— RICHARD F. LEBLOND

It is not easy to give exact and complete details of an operation in writing; but the reader should form an outline of it from the description.

—Hippocrates
"On Joints"

[Studies] perfect nature, and are perfected by experience: for natural abilities are like natural plants, that need pruning, by study; and studies themselves, do give forth directions too much at large, except they be bounded in by experience. Crafty men contemn studies, simple men admire them, and wise men use them; for they teach not their own use; but that is a wisdom without them, and above them, won by observation. Read not to contradict and confute; nor to believe and take for granted; nor to find talk and discourse; but to weigh and consider.

—Francis Bacon
"Of Studies"

A little observation and much reasoning lead to error; many observations and a little reasoning to truth.

—Dr. Alexis Carrel

It is only by persistent intelligent study of disease upon a methodical plan of examination that a man gradually learns to correlate his daily lessons with the facts of his previous experience and that of his fellows, and so acquires clinical wisdom.

— Sir William Osler

Sources for Quotations:

Brecht quotation from: Bertolt Brecht. *Poems, 1913–1956.* London, Methuen London Ltd., 1979.

Eliot quotation from: T.S. Eliot. *The Complete Poems and Plays, 1909–1950.* New York, Harcourt, Brace & World, Inc., 1971.

Frazer quotation from: Sir James George Frazer. *The Golden Bough, A Study in Magic and Religion,* abridged edition. New York, MacMillan Publishing Company, 1922.

Hippocrates quotation from: Jacques Jouanna (M.B. DeBevoise translator). Hippocrates. Baltimore, The Johns Hopkins University Press, 1999.

Osler quotation from: Sir William Osler. *Aequanimitas, with other Addresses to Medical Students, Nurses and Practitioners of Medicine.* Philadelphia, P. Blakiston's Son and Co., 1928.

Roethke quotations from: Theodore Roethke. *On Poetry and Craft.* Port Townsend, Washington Copper Canyon Press, 2001.

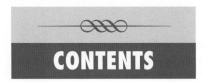

CONTENTS

PREFACE

To The Reader:
Pray thee, take care, that tak'st my book in hand
To read it well: that is, to understand.

—Ben Jonson

The purpose of taking a clinical history and performing the physical exam is to generate diagnostic hypotheses. This was true for Hippocrates and Osler and remains true today. *DeGowin's Diagnostic Examination* encourages a thoughtful, systematic approach to the history, physical exam, and diagnostic process.

The practice of medicine would be simple if each symptom or sign indicated a single disease. There are enormous numbers of symptoms and signs (we cover several hundred) that can occur in a nearly infinite number of combinations and temporal patterns. These symptoms and signs are the raw materials from which the clinician must weave an anatomically and pathophysiologically explicit clinical narrative forming the diagnostic hypotheses. Mastering the diagnostic process requires:

(1) **Knowledge:** Familiarity with the pathophysiology, symptoms, and signs of common and unusual diseases.
(2) **Skill:** The ability to take an accurate and complete history and perform an appropriate physical examination.
(3) **Experience:** From longitudinal exposure to many clinical situations, diseases, and patients, each thoroughly evaluated, the skilled clinician becomes familiar with the presenting symptoms and signs of a wide variety of pathophysiologic processes allowing generation of a probabilistic differential diagnosis for each patient.
(4) **Judgment:** Knowledge of basic medical science and the medical literature, combined with reflective experience, promotes the judgment necessary to efficiently test diagnostic hypotheses in the laboratory or by clinical interventions.

DeGowin's Diagnostic Examination has been used by students and clinicians for over 50 years precisely because of its usefulness in honing this diagnostic process:

(1) It describes the techniques for obtaining a complete history and performing a thorough physical exam.
(2) It links symptoms and signs with the pathophysiology of disease.
(3) It presents an approach to differential diagnosis, based upon the pathophysiology of disease, which can be efficiently tested in the laboratory.
(4) It does all of this in a format that can be used as a quick point-of-care reference and as a text to study the principles and practice of history taking and physical examination.

In undertaking this eleventh edition of a venerable classic, our goal is once again to preserve the unique strengths of previous editions, while adding recent information and references, reducing redundancy, and improving clarity. The reason is that *DeGowin's Diagnostic Examination* emphasizes the unchanging aspects of clinical medicine—the symptoms and signs of disease as related by the patient and discovered by physical examination. We remain true to the original goal of this book which was to encourage a thoughtful systematic approach to diagnosis based on history and physical examination. In this edition at the end of chapter 4 to 16 you will also find examples of clinical vignettes (followed by questions) demonstrating essential concepts used in framing diagnostic hypothesis. The answers to these questions can be found in the Appendix. Along with the factual information stored in long-term memory, these vignettes will help facilitate development and implementation of diagnostic strategies using memory schemes that represent and interrelate clinical problems.

Pathophysiology links the patient's story of their illness (the history), the physical signs of disease, and the changes in biologic structure and function revealed by imaging studies and laboratory testing. Patients describe symptoms, we need to hear pathophysiology; we observe signs, we need to see pathophysiology; the radiologist and laboratories report findings, we need to think pathophysiology. Pathophysiology and pathologic anatomy provide the framework for understanding disease as alterations in normal physiology and anatomy, and illness as the patient's experience of these changes.

A discussion of pathophysiology (highlighted in the second color) occurs after many subject headings. The discussions are brief and included when they assist understanding the symptom or sign. Readers are encouraged to consult physiology texts to have a full understanding of normal and abnormal physiology. In addition, each chapter discusses syndromes associated with that body region to give a sense of the common, and uncommon but serious, disease patterns.

DeGowin's Diagnostic Examination is organized as a useful bedside guide to assist diagnosis. Part 1, Chapter 1 introduces the conceptual framework for the diagnostic process, Chapter 2 the essentials of history taking and documentation, and Chapter 3 the screening physical examination with a short introduction to bedside ultrasound. Every clinician needs a thorough understanding of Part 1 and Part 4, Chapter 17, the latter introducing the principles of diagnostic testing.

Part 2, Chapters 4 through 15, forms the body of the book. Two introductory chapters discuss the vital signs (Chapter 4) and major physiologic systems that do not have a primary representation in a single body region (Chapter 5). Chapters 6 through 14 are organized around the body regions sequentially examined during the physical examination. Each chapter has a common structure outlined in the Introduction and User's Guide. To avoid duplication, the text is heavily cross-referenced. I hope the reader finds this useful and not too cumbersome.

References to articles from the medical literature are sparingly included in the body of the text. We have chosen articles that provide useful diagnostic information including excellent descriptions of diseases and syndromes, thoughtful discussions of the approach to differential diagnosis and evaluation of common and unusual clinical problems, and, in some cases, photographs illustrating key findings. Most references are from the major general medical journals, the *New England Journal of Medicine*, the *Lancet*, the *Annals of Internal Medicine*, and the *Journal of the American Medical Association*. This implies that a clinician who regularly studies these journals will keep abreast of the broad field of medical diagnosis. Some references are dated in their recommendations for laboratory testing and treatment; they are included because they give thorough descriptions of the relevant clinical syndromes, often with excellent discussions of the approach to differential diagnosis. **Tests and treatments come and go, but good thinking has staying power. The reader must always check current resources before initiating a laboratory evaluation or therapeutic program.**

Evidence-based articles on the utility of the physical examination are included, mostly from the Rational Clinical Examination series published in the *Journal of the American Medical Association*. They are included with the caveat that they evaluate the physical examination as a hypothesis-testing tool, *not as a hypothesis generating task.*

Each chapter was independently reviewed by faculty members. Their feedback and assistance are gratefully acknowledged. Reviewers for this edition are Bimal Ashar, MD, MBA, Division of General Internal Medicine, Johns Hopkins University School of Medicine (Chapters 5 and 16), Karolyn Wanat, MD, Department of Dermatology, Medical College of Wisconsin, (Chapter 6), Doug Van Daele, MD, Department of Otolaryngology, University of Iowa Hospitals & Clinics (Chapter 7), Karl Thomas, MD, Department of Internal Medicine, Wake Forest School of Medicine (Chapter 8), Christopher J. Goerdt, MD, MPH, Division of General Internal Medicine, University of Iowa Roy J. and Lucille A. Carver College of Medicine (Chapter 9), Aash Bhatt, MD, Department of Internal Medicine, Western Michigan University, Homer Stryker School of Medicine (Chapter 10), Abby Hardy-Fairbanks, MD, Department of Obstetrics and Gynecology, University of Iowa Roy J. and Lucille A. Carver College of Medicine (Chapter 11), Chad Tracy, MD, Department of Urology, University of Iowa Roy J. and Lucille A. Carver College of Medicine (Chapter 12), Chadwick Johr, MD, University of Pennsylvania Perelman School of Medicine (Chapter 13).

All editors for this edition, Manish Suneja, MD, Joseph Szot, MD, Richard F. LeBlond and Donald D. Brown, MD, have been instrumental in seeing that the eleventh edition maintains the strengths of previous editions while continuing to evolve to meet the reader's needs.

Ms. Kay Conerly is the senior editor at McGraw Hill for the eleventh edition. She has been actively involved in the planning and execution of the eleventh edition. Her encouragement and support are deeply appreciated. The McGraw Hill editorial and publishing staff have been prompt and professional throughout manuscript preparation, editing, and production.

The eleventh edition includes **video segments** demonstrating fundamental physical examination procedures. Complimentary access to these videos is available at: **www.mhprofessional.com/DeGowinsDiagnosticExam**.

Finally, we wish to thank our colleagues who have encouraged us throughout the course of this project. We have incorporated many suggestions from our reviewers/readers and would like to thank those who have taken the time to write recommendations for this edition. Ultimately, you, the reader, will determine the strengths and weaknesses of this edition. We welcome your feedback and suggestions.

Manish Suneja, MD, FACP, FASN
Joseph Szot, MD, FACP
Richard F. LeBlond, MD, MACP
Donald D. Brown, MD, FACP
Iowa City, Iowa

COMMON ABBREVIATIONS

CHF	congestive heart failure
COPD	chronic obstructive pulmonary disease
CLL	chronic lymphocytic leukemia
CML	chronic myelogenous leukemia
CMV	cytomegalovirus
CN	cranial nerve
CNS	central nervous system
CSF	cerebrospinal fluid
CVP	central venous pressure
DDX	differential diagnosis
DIP	distal interphalangeal joint
EBV	Epstein–Barr virus
HIT	heparin-induced thrombocytopenia
HSV	herpes simplex virus
ITP	idiopathic immune thrombocytopenia
LLQ	left lower quadrant
LUQ	left upper quadrant
LV	left ventricle
MCP	metacarpal–phalangeal joint
MI	myocardial infarction
MS	multiple sclerosis
MTP	metatarsal–phalangeal joint
NBTE	nonbacterial thrombotic endocarditis
PE	pulmonary embolism
PIP	proximal interphalangeal joint
RA	rheumatoid arthritis
RLQ	right lower quadrant
RUQ	right upper quadrant
RV	right ventricle
SBE	subacute bacterial endocarditis
SLE	systemic lupus erythematosus
TTP	thrombotic thrombocytopenic purpura

INTRODUCTION AND USER'S GUIDE

> Read with two objectives: first to acquaint yourself with the current knowledge on the subject and the steps by which it has been reached; and secondly, and more important, read to understand and analyze your cases.
>
> —Sir William Osler
> *"The Student Life"*

DeGowin's Diagnostic Examination provides the introductory knowledge base, describes the skills, and encourages the reader to acquire the experience and judgment needed to become a master clinical diagnostician. Despite recent advances in testing and imaging, the clinician's skills in taking a history and performing a physical examination are needed now more than ever.

The history is the patient's story of his or her illness related as the time course of their symptoms; the physical examination reveals the signs of disordered anatomy and physiology. The symptoms and signs of disease form temporal patterns, which the clinician recognizes from experience and knowledge of anatomy, physiology, and diseases. From the history and physical examination, the clinician generates testable pathophysiologic and diagnostic hypotheses—the differential diagnosis. Proficiency and confidence in differential diagnosis should improve with regular use of *DeGowin's Diagnostic Examination*.

The differential diagnosis is subjected to laboratory testing. Proper use of the laboratory and imaging are based upon accurate diagnostic hypotheses generated while taking the history and performing the physical examination. Undisciplined use of both laboratory tests and imaging modalities is a major cause of increasing healthcare costs and leads to further inappropriate testing and patient harm. Over-reliance on technology has contributed to loss of clinical bedside skills.

DeGowin's Diagnostic Examination is intended to assist the student and clinician in making reasonable diagnostic hypotheses from the history and physical examination. Part 1, Chapters 1 to 3, discusses the diagnostic framework in detail. Chapter 1 discusses the importance of diagnosis and the process of forming a differential diagnosis specific to each patient. Chapter 2 discusses the process of history taking and documentation of the findings in the medical record. Chapter 3 outlines the screening physical examination.

The heart of *DeGowin's Diagnostic Examination* is Part 2, Chapters 4 thru 15. It is organized in the sequence in which the clinician traditionally performs the examination. Chapter 4 discusses the vital signs. Chapter 5 introduces some systems to keep in mind throughout the examination since they present with symptoms and signs not easily referable to a specific body region. Chapters 6 thru 13 discuss the diagnostic examination by body region: the skin (Chapter 6), the head and neck (Chapter 7), the chest and breasts (Chapter 8), the abdomen (Chapter 9), the urinary system (Chapter 10), the female genitalia and reproductive system (Chapter 11), the male genitalia and reproductive system (Chapter 12), the spine and extremities (Chapter 13), the neurologic examination (Chapter 14), and the psychiatric and social evaluations (Chapter 15).

Parts 3 and 4 provide supplemental information. Chapter 16 discusses the preoperative examination. The intent is to give the reader a framework for evaluating the medical risks in the perioperative period and an approach to communicating those risks to the patient and surgeon. Chapter 17 introduces the principles of laboratory testing and imaging critical to an efficient use of the laboratory and radiology. Chapter 18 lists many common (not "routine") laboratory tests that provide important information about the patient's condition not accessible from the history or physical examination. More specialized tests used to evaluate specific diagnostic hypotheses are not discussed.

Chapters 6 thru 14 have a uniform organization: (A) each chapter begins with a brief overview of the major organ systems to be considered; (B) next is a discussion of the superficial and deep anatomy of the body region; (C) the physical examination of the region or system is described in detail in the usual order of performance; (D) the symptoms particularly relevant to the body region and systems are presented; (E) the physical signs in the region or system examinations are listed (some findings can be both symptoms and signs; discussion of a finding is in the section where it is most likely to be encountered, then cross-referenced in the other section); and (F) discusses diseases and syndromes commonly in the differential diagnosis of symptoms and signs in the body region and systems under discussion. To avoid duplication, the text is heavily cross-referenced.

Brief discussions of many diseases and clinical syndromes are included so the reader can appreciate the patterns of symptoms and signs they commonly manifest. This will help the clinician determine whether that disease or syndrome should be included in the differential diagnosis of the symptoms and signs in their specific patient. Particularly useful points of differentiation are listed after the **DDX** symbol.

DeGowin's Diagnostic Examination is not a textbook of medicine. The reader must use this with a comprehensive textbook of medicine to fully understand the diseases and syndromes. We strongly recommend *Harrison's Principles of Internal Medicine* as a companion text.

We emphasize the characteristics of diseases because a clinician who knows the manifestations of many diseases will ask the right questions, obtain the key history, and elicit the pertinent signs distinguishing one disease from another. Instructions on how to elicit the specific signs are included in the physical examination section for each region; if the maneuver is not part of the usual examination, it is discussed with the sign itself. Following the descriptions of many symptoms and signs is a highlighted **CLINICAL OCCURRENCE** section. This is a list of diseases often associated with the symptom or sign. The organization of the Clinical Occurrence section is based upon the approach to the differential diagnosis of the symptom or sign felt to be most clinically useful.

Where a broad differential exists, we have introduced an organizational scheme for the **CLINICAL OCCURRENCE** based upon the pathophysiologic mechanisms of disease. The clinician can often narrow their differential diagnosis to one or a few basic mechanisms of disease: congenital, endocrine, degenerative/idiopathic, infectious, inflammatory/immune, mechanical/traumatic, metabolic/toxic, neoplastic, neurologic, psychosocial, or vascular. This facilitates the creation of a limited yet reasonable differential diagnosis.

The categories in this scheme are not mutually exclusive; a congenital syndrome may be metabolic, infections are usually accompanied by inflammation, and a neoplastic process may cause mechanical obstruction. Although not rigid, this is a useful conceptual construct for thinking about the patient's problems.

Symptoms, signs, syndromes, and diseases that may indicate an emergent condition requiring immediate and complete evaluation are noted by the • marginal symbol.

Use your understanding of normal and abnormal anatomy and physiology as the basis for thinking within clinical medicine, you can avoid the trap of "word-space." This is the term one of us (RFL) has given to the common practice of using lists and word association as an approach to diagnosis: associating a word (for instance, cough) with a memorized list of other words (pneumonia, bronchitis, asthma, postnasal drip, gastroesophageal reflux, etc.). The inherent emphasis on memorization in this scheme is the bane of all medical students; fortunately, it is not only unnecessary, it is counterproductive. Cough is a protective reflex arising from sensory phenomena in the upper airway, bronchi, lungs, and esophagus mediated through peripheral and central nervous system pathways and executed by coordinated contraction of the diaphragm, chest wall, and laryngeal muscles. With this physiologic context, and our understanding of the mechanisms of disease, we can hypothesize the irritants most likely to be relevant in each specific patient.

New diseases are being encountered with surprising frequency. They present not with new symptoms and signs, but with new combinations of the old symptoms and signs. It is our hope that the reader will learn to recognize the patterns of known diseases and to be alert for patterns that are unfamiliar (those not yet in their knowledge base) or previously unrecognized (the new diseases). HIV/AIDS was recognized as an unprecedented clinical syndrome with a new pattern of familiar symptoms (weight loss, fever, fatigue, dyspnea, cough) and signs (wasting, generalized lymphadenopathy, mucocutaneous lesions, Kaposi's sarcoma, opportunistic infections) in a unique population (homosexual males and IV drug users). Continuous expansion of our personal knowledge of the known while welcoming the unfamiliar and unknown is the excitement of clinical practice.

The testing of specific diagnostic hypotheses is beyond the scope of this book. It is subject to constant change as new tests are developed and their usefulness evaluated in clinical trials. Part 4 discusses the principles of laboratory testing (Chapter 17) and some common laboratory tests (Chapter 18). The reader should consult *Harrison's Principles of Internal Medicine* and the current literature when selecting specific tests to evaluate their diagnostic hypotheses [Guyatt G, Rennie D, eds. *Users' Guides to the Medical Literature: A Manual for Evidence-Based Clinical Practice.* Chicago, IL: AMA Press; 2002; Guyatt G, Rennie D, Meade MO, Cook DJ, eds. *Users' Guides to the Medical Literature: A Manual for Evidence-Based Clinical Practice.* 2nd ed. New York, NY: McGraw-Hill; 2008].

User's Guide

DeGowin's Diagnostic Examination can be read cover-to-cover with benefit to the student or practitioner; however, most will not, and should not, choose this strategy. As Osler said, read to understand your patients and to answer your questions.

We strongly suggest that all readers start with Chapters 1, 2, 3, and 17, which outline the conceptual basis for the diagnostic examination, including the approach to laboratory testing and imaging. This context is critical to efficiently using time and resources.

If you have questions about the systems being examined consult part A of the relevant chapter and *Harrison's Principles of Internal Medicine*. If your question concerns anatomy, consult part B and an anatomy textbook. If you are uncertain of the techniques of the physical examination, see Chapter 3 and part C of the body region chapters. If you are uncertain what to make of a symptom, see part D of the relevant chapter. If you are wondering how to elicit or interpret a sign, see part E of the relevant chapter. To find out more about the diseases mentioned in the section, consult part F of that chapter or look in the index for the page where it is discussed. Remember, the disease and syndrome discussions in this book are brief and must be complemented with reading in a textbook of medicine, for example, *Harrison's Principles of Internal Medicine*.

The Table of Contents should be scanned to familiarize yourself with the structure and general content of the text. The index locates all the subject matter in the text.

There is no right way to use a book. The key is to use the information to inform your thinking about patients and the problems they present. No text is definitive, and the reader is encouraged to consult other texts and the current and historic literature to develop a full understanding of your patients and their illnesses. The acquisition of clinical skills is a journey without end; this is an intimidating thought for the student but is the source of lifelong stimulation for the practitioner.

After all, what we call truth is only the hypothesis which is found to work best.
——Sir James George Frazer

DeGowin's
Diagnostic Examination

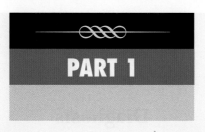

The Diagnostic Framework

To carefully observe the phenomena of life in all its phases,
normal and perverted, to make perfect that most difficult
of all arts, the art of observation, to call to aid the science of
experimentation, to cultivate the reasoning faculty, so as to be
able to know the true from the false—these are our methods.

– Sir William Osler

Don't strain for arrangement. Look and put down and let your
sensibility be the sieve.

– Theodore Roethke
"Poetry and Craft"

. . . the framing of hypotheses is the most difficult part of
scientific work, and the part where great ability is indispensable.
So far, no method has been found which would make it
possible to invent hypotheses by rule. Usually some hypothesis
is a necessary preliminary to the collection of facts, since the
selection of facts demands some way of determining relevance.
Without something of this kind, the multiplicity of facts is
baffling.

– Bertrand Russell
"A History of Western Philosophy"

1

CHAPTER 1

Diagnosis

Accurate Diagnosis Is Imperative: An ill person has three fundamental questions: (1) What is happening to me and why? (2) What does this mean for my future? (3) What can be done about it? Providing answers to these questions are the three timeless tasks of the healing professions: explanation, prognostication, and treatment. This has been true across time and cultures, regardless of the belief system underpinning the culture: magic, faith, rationalism, or science. Accurate explanation, prognostication, and appropriate treatment require precise diagnosis. The history and physical exam are the basis for diagnostic hypothesis generation, the first step in the diagnostic process.

Knowledge, an understanding of clinical epidemiology, and experience are necessary to determine when pursuit of specific symptoms and signs is warranted. For common minor complaints in healthy people without alarm symptoms, a good prognosis can be assumed without knowing the exact cause, as, for instance, an upper respiratory infection (URI). The patient can be reassured that further testing will not change prognosis or treatment. When the diagnosis is not self-evident from the initial symptoms, or the course deviates from what is expected, a more exacting diagnostic evaluation becomes necessary.

Diagnostic Process: In the process of making a diagnosis, the clinician makes a series of inferences about the nature of bodily dysfunction. When making these inferences from clinical data, clinicians use many strategies to combine, integrate, and interpret the data. After collating the data, the next step in the diagnostic process is *generation of one or more diagnostic hypotheses*. A hypothesis is sometimes generated merely from a patient's age, sex, race, appearance, and presenting complaint. On the other hand, hypotheses may emerge exclusively from a physical finding or laboratory data. New hypotheses are triggered as new findings emerge. Diagnostic hypotheses can be general (infection or inflammation) or quite specific (acute right ventricular myocardial infarction). Diagnostic reasoning proceeds by *progressively modifying and refining the hypotheses*. This inferential reasoning process continues until the clinician arrives at *a working diagnosis*, a diagnostic hypothesis sufficient to establish a prognosis and direct therapeutic intervention. The hypothesis should yield accurate predictions of test results and the patient's future clinical course.

Diseases and Syndromes: A diagnostic hypothesis provides entry to the medical literature for current information about etiology, diagnostic findings, prognosis, and treatment. Recurring patterns of disordered bodily structure, function, and mentation suggest a common cause. When a shared pathophysiology and etiology are confirmed, the condition is a *disease*. Combinations of features not clearly related to a single cause are *syndromes*. Diseases and syndromes are intellectual constructs that do not exist independently of the patients who manifest them. These constructs allow aggregation of patients with relatively homogeneous physiologic disorders for study to promote understanding of disease and to evaluate potential treatments. Accurate diagnosis is indispensable for initiating treatment.

THE DIAGNOSTIC PROCESS

An accurate diagnosis requires the clinician to catalog each anatomic, physiologic, and cognitive abnormality. Each disease and syndrome has a temporal sequence of clinical and laboratory features distinguishing it from similar conditions. During the diagnostic examination, the clinician performs two parallel tasks: (1) develops a problem list of the symptoms and signs requiring explanation; and (2) generates physiologic, anatomic, and etiologic hypotheses regarding the diagnoses. A recursive process is used to work toward a diagnosis.

Stories: The patient tells us a story of their illness. The clinician creates an anatomic and pathophysiologic story congruent with the illness narrative. A good medical story has the same elements as a good newspaper story: **who, what, when, where, how, and why**. The first three items come directly from the patient narrative:

WHO: This is a description of *this person*, including their social history (religion, beliefs, priorities, education, sexual preferences, habits, demographics, employment, and leisure activities), family history, past medical and surgical history, and current medications.

WHAT: The patient relates the story of their illness experience describing their symptoms and signs, diagnostic efforts and studies, treatments, and concerns. Encourage a free narrative flow by not interrupting or expecting premature clarity. Ascertain their thoughts about what might be wrong and why. Estimate illness severity by how it has affected their life. Ask why they sought evaluation at this time. No symptom is irrelevant. Often patients dismiss the symptoms that they think are irrelevant, which, in fact, may be a key diagnostic clue. Determine when each symptom began, how long it lasts, how often it occurs, what makes it better or worse, its course over time, and any other associated symptoms.

WHEN: Timing is everything. The sequence, pattern, and duration of symptoms are critical for identifying the etiology of a unique combination of symptoms each common to many diseases. Understanding the *timeline* (intermittent, relapsing, acute, subacute or chronic, etc.) for each symptom is vital as it reflects the dynamic pathophysiologic disease process and is one of the most important clues to diagnosis.

The last three story elements are constructed from the history and physical exam:

WHERE: All disease processes take place somewhere. Your job is to precisely envision the anatomy of the problem (anatomic hypothesis). Envision the precise location of the pathophysiologic processes producing the disease: which systems, organ(s), tissues, and cells. The process can be localized or diffuse. If diffuse, look for a pattern of involved tissues.

HOW: This is the testable pathophysiologic hypothesis. How, by what physiologic mechanism(s), did this illness come about? There are only a limited number of ways people become ill. A useful way of parsing pathophysiology is used in this text. Ask which one or more of the following mechanisms are most likely: congenital, degenerative/idiopathic, endocrine, infectious, inflammatory/immune, mechanical/traumatic, metabolic/toxic, neoplastic, neurological, psychosocial, and/or vascular. The pathophysiologic explanation must precede search for a specific etiology.

WHY: This is the etiologic hypothesis. Strive for an exact diagnosis that explains the illness narrative and each abnormality. An accurate prognosis also requires understanding why the disease is affecting the patient now.

The ability to reproduce a story verbatim is a rare gift, but our brains effortlessly capture and recall the gist and flow of stories even if we retain only a few specific phrases. Similarly, we easily recall visual images and the sensation of what we hear. As the patient tells their story, listen actively. Try to avoid analysis until you have captured the whole story. Just listen, translating the words into a mental recording of your shared experience, as you would for any other story. During the exam, mentally record what is seen, felt, and heard. Do not translate the observations into words until the experience of the exam has been captured. Later it may be a struggle to find the best words, but the words will be trying to describe the remembered experience. By performing the screening physical exam in a structured and relatively stereotypic sequence, each patient is observed in a comparable manner. When the process becomes routine little or no thought is required, so the mind is free to observe. If attention is too sharply focused, as is often the case with beginners, one thing may be seen, whereas much is missed.

Gathering and Processing Information:

Clues to the diagnosis. The diagnostic examination has four components: (1) history taking, where the patient's perceptions are *symptoms*; (2) physical exam, where the examiner observes physical *signs*; (3) laboratory examinations; and (4) special anatomic and physiologic examinations, e.g., imaging studies. DeGowin's diagnostic examination focuses on generating hypotheses from the history and physical exam. Most diagnoses are suggested by the history and to a lesser extent the physical exam. Laboratory testing is for evaluating hypothesis, not hypothesis generation.

The diagnostic examination begins with first patient contact. The patient's age and sex are surrogates for diseases common in that demographic. Ethnicity is important for suggesting genetic diseases like sickle cell anemia. X-linked diseases such as hemophilia are rarely encountered in females. Males do not get pregnant. Although seemingly obvious, it is important to make explicit each categorical probability decision. The correct diagnosis can be unconsciously passed over by such a heuristic.

Each symptom and sign is analyzed for consistency. Assess the level of concern attached to each symptom. Symptoms are only as reliable as the patient's memory and description. Whenever possible, obtain collateral history from family and friends to corroborate the patient's history. Ascertain if each sign was present previously, and, if so, has it changed from previous exams.

The problem list. List every problem identified by history, physical exam, and initial laboratory studies. This is a frequently omitted step in the diagnostic algorithm. Grouping problems into clusters likely to have a common pathophysiology assists hypothesis generation. Only chunk problems when it is certain they are closely linked. Common examples are nausea and vomiting, and fever and chills. Avoid lumping if uncertain.

Problem representation. A problem representation is a brief summary of the patient encounter translating the patient's story into medical terminology. A well-formed problem representation facilitates clinical reasoning and serves as the backbone for how clinicians communicate with one another. By summarizing the most salient features and minimizing distractors, effective problem representations reduce cognitive load and facilitate clinical problem-solving. Problem representation generally includes semantic qualifiers which are paired opposing descriptors that can be used systematically to compare and contrast diagnostic considerations: sharp/dull, acute/chronic, tender/nontender, productive/nonproductive, insidious/abrupt, proximal/distal. A problem representation is iteratively updated as further data is gathered.

Translating lay language into abstractions (problem representation with semantic qualifiers) using medical terminology enables easier access and retrieval of knowledge stored as *illness scripts*, mental representations of potential diagnoses within the clinician's memory (see below). The clinician develops a prioritized differential diagnosis based on the degree of match between the patient's problem representation and previous illness scripts and disease prototypes.

A thorough problem representation answers three questions:

1. Who is the patient, including pertinent demographics and risk factors?
2. What is the temporal pattern of illness, including acuity (hyperacute, acute, subacute, chronic) and tempo (stable, progressive, resolving, intermittent, waxing, and waning)?
3. What is the clinical syndrome integrating key signs and symptoms?

It is easy to get lost in the problems and miss a unifying synthesis, missing the forest for the trees. Avoid this error by creating an explicit problem statement that, in one or two sentences, reassembles the problems into a concise summary of the big picture.

Illness scripts. An illness script is a narrative structure for recalling the key attributes of a typical case presentation of a condition or diagnosis. These are packets of stored knowledge that are retrieved by specific presentations. Classically, the components of a thorough illness script fall into three main categories: the predisposing conditions, the pathophysiological insult, and the clinical consequences. Within these categories, illness scripts often include a disease's pathophysiology, epidemiology, time course, salient symptoms and signs, diagnostics, and treatment.

Differential Diagnosis:
Hypothesis generation. The process by which skilled clinicians form hypotheses has attracted the attention of physicians, mathematicians, and psychologists. As the Bertrand Russell quote at the beginning of this section indicates,

this is still a mysterious cognitive process, even to the clinician performing the task.

Pattern recognition. The whole of the patient's illness is greater than the sum of its parts. Mechanical application of likelihood ratios is far less accurate than the patterns that emerge in a skilled examiner's mind from the totality of observations. For example, it is easy to identify hundreds of faces at a glance, but identification is much more difficult if observations are limited to one or two features in isolation. The persistent unity of the whole allows recognition of familiar faces even when much of the face is covered. Pattern recognition is one of the most powerful properties of the human brain.

   Create an anatomic and physiologic story matching the patient's narrative in time and tempo indicating where and by what pathophysiologic mechanism(s) the illness is being produced. Then identify diseases known to have this pathophysiology producing these or similar symptoms and signs. Listing all possible diagnoses is rarely helpful. For isolated symptoms and signs a list of potential diagnoses is possible, but there is no means to differentiate their probabilities. Rather, use this specific patient's findings to estimate the probability of each diagnosis. This is the **differential diagnosis**, each with a *pretest probability*. Because the clues distinguishing diseases of high and low probability are *unique to this patient*, differential diagnosis is only possible for an individual patient, not a problem.

Probability. The clinician must know the incidence and prevalence of diseases in the population represented by the patient. This is the starting place for determining the probability of each disease *for this patient*, but never the actual probability. If the incidence and prevalence were the whole story, rare diseases would almost never be considered. The population statistics are adjusted for a hypothetical population of the patient's same age, gender, ethnicity, history, and concurrent conditions.

Anatomic and Pathophysiologic Diagnostic Hypotheses:

Anatomic hypotheses. All disease processes take place somewhere in the patient. Predict the likely sites of disease pathology. Be precise; visualize which systems, organs, tissues, and cells within each organ are involved. For example, jaundice results from prehepatic hemolysis, hepatocellular damage, intrahepatic biliary obstruction (canicular or larger ducts), or extrahepatic obstruction. If the latter, find clues suggesting the location relative to the cystic duct, pancreatic ducts, and duodenum. Many disease processes involve multiple organs. The tissues involved in each organ may suggest a pattern, e.g., multiple enlarged organs with few effects on function is the pattern of deposition diseases like amyloidosis.

Pathophysiologic hypotheses. There are a limited number of physiologic mechanisms by which disease is produced. Any classification scheme is somewhat arbitrary with significant overlaps since one mechanism often triggers a second, e.g., autoimmune thyroid disease produces the metabolic changes of hypothyroidism or hyperthyroidism. The scheme presented below is a guide to critical thinking assuring that all mechanisms are considered. Fuzzy boundaries between categories, with many ways to get to the same place, are a strength making it less likely to overlook something.

Congenital	Degenerative/Idiopathic
Endocrine	Infectious (includes infestations)
Immune/Inflammatory	Mechanical/Traumatic
Metabolic (includes toxins)	Neoplastic
Neurologic	Psychosocial
Vascular	

Congenital. This is not a physiologic mechanism but rather a reminder that each specific mechanism may result from an abnormality present at birth (congenital) in the hardware (developmental anomalies) or software (genome). This category includes developmental anomalies, familial genetic disease (germline mutations), somatic mutations during embryonic growth, and inborn errors of metabolism. Genetic abnormalities usually present in infancy and childhood but also appear in adults at any age, e.g., adrenoleuko-dystrophy, atrial septal defect, anomalous vasculature, hypertrophic cardio-myopathy, and multiple endocrine neoplasia, to name a few.

Degenerative/Idiopathic. Again, not a mechanism, rather a loose collection of diseases and structural abnormalities whose precise mechanism is uncertain but the incidence of which generally increases with age and/or increased exposure to specific structural or metabolic stresses. Aging itself, though quite normal, falls into this category. Other examples are the dementias, osteoar-thritis, osteoporosis, emphysema, and atherosclerosis.

Endocrine. This includes functional and structural abnormalities of the duct-less glands: pituitary, thyroid, parathyroid, pancreatic islets, testes, ovaries, adrenal, and neuroendocrine tissues. Onset of endocrine disorders is often indolent, delaying recognition. Symptoms are systemic without localization. Signs may be few and missed if not specifically sought by directed exam, e.g., goiter, lid lag, tremor, lagging reflexes, tetany, change in testicle size, and con-sistency. Acute endocrine disorders are not common but are often life threat-ening if not treated promptly, e.g., thyroid storm, pituitary apoplexy, adrenal hemorrhage, and pheochromocytoma.

Infectious (including infestations). Humans are susceptible to attack by innumerable viruses, bacteria, fungi, and parasites. Congenital or acquired defects in the innate or adaptive immune systems and disruption of surface barriers (skin, intestinal mucosa) increase the risk of infection. Infection is com-monly, but not always, associated with signs of inflammation. Organisms can also cause illness by release of toxins, e.g., toxic shock syndrome and tetanus. Intracellular organisms have adapted to life within host cells. These unique organisms shield themselves from the immune response so signs of inflam-mation may be minimal or absent. They always require specific consideration.

Immune/Inflammatory. When present, fever and/or inflammation indicate an immune response. Though they frequently coexist, do not equate inflam-mation with infection. Many immunologically mediated diseases do not cause clinical inflammation, e.g., Hashimoto thyroiditis and celiac disease. Autoimmune diseases may or may not incite an inflammatory response and can be limited to one organ, e.g., thyroiditis, or systemic involving multiple organs, e.g., vasculitis and systemic lupus. Specific cytokines induce systemic responses manifest as fever, fatigue, malaise, and loss of appetite.

Mechanical/Traumatic. Obstructions within the genitourinary and gastro-intestinal systems are examples of mechanical problems, often associated with severe colic pain. Similarly, obstruction within the vascular system produces symptoms depending on the site of obstruction. Arterial obstruction produces pallor and ischemic pain while venous obstruction produces tissue engorgement, cyanosis, and less severe pain. Congenital and acquired mechanical problems of the heart and great vessels are common, e.g., aortic stenosis, mitral insufficiency, pericardial tamponade, and coarctation of the aorta. Impingement by a mass, large or small, can compress and displace adjacent structures, e.g., extruded intravertebral disk and common bile duct obstruction by pancreas cancer. Fractures are mechanical failure of bone. Visualization helps formulate mechanical hypotheses.

Metabolic/Toxic. Metabolism is highly complex and finely regulated. Inborn errors of metabolism usually present in infancy or childhood, but not always. Metabolic disturbances have systemic effects with symptoms and signs according to the pathway affected, but inflammation is absent. Inability to properly metabolize specific substrates underlies storage diseases often leading to organ enlargement and dysfunction, e.g., amyloidosis and nonalcoholic fatty liver disease. Ingested or injected toxins and drugs are examples of metabolic disturbances, e.g., cyanide uncouples mitochondrial electron transport.

Neoplastic. Neoplasms, benign and malignant, present at all ages with peaks in childhood and later adult life. Symptoms may be local, e.g., pain, or systemic, e.g., anorexia and weight loss. Benign neoplasms usually present with mechanical mass effects, except for endocrine neoplasms presenting with unregulated hormone production, e.g., parathyroid adenoma producing the metabolic effects of hypercalcemia. Some neoplasms produce systemic effects by immune mechanisms, e.g., paraneoplastic neurologic disorders associated with certain hematopoietic neoplasms. Others secrete hormones or hormone mimics, so the presentations suggest a primary endocrine or metabolic problem, e.g., parathyroid-related-peptide and hypercalcemia, and antidiuretic hormone from small cell lung cancer.

Neurologic. Though not a pathophysiologic mechanism, damage to the central or peripheral nervous systems by another mechanism is a common cause of pain and altered perceptions in many body regions. Examples are complex regional pain syndrome, tabes dorsalis, diabetic polyradiculopathy, and postherpetic neuralgia. The initial inciting pathophysiology (in the examples two infections, one metabolic derangement, and previous injury) is rarely relevant to the current presentation. Recognition that the symptom, most often pain, arises in the damaged nerves themselves, rather than the nerve transmitting pain from another source, is the key to making the correct diagnosis.

Psychosocial. Anorexia nervosa can lead to weight loss and depression to weight loss or gain. Poverty and illiteracy are prevalent in adults and children, limiting access to proper nutrition or ability to obtain and correctly take medications. Poor response to a medication may indicate lack of financial resources or nonadherence. The living environment may contribute to incontinence by impeding access to bathroom facilities, e.g., use of a wheelchair or walker, or inability to use the facilities due to cognitive impairment. Physical and emotional violence produce protean effects and should always be considered when a presentation is ambiguous. Take a thorough family and social history asking about literacy and the living environment.

Vascular. Vascular disorders can be acute, e.g., embolism or thrombus, or chronic, e.g., peripheral vascular disease. They are local, e.g., aortic coarctation, or systemic, e.g., atherosclerosis and vasculitis. Arterial obstruction (mechanical) due to atherosclerosis (metabolic) leads to tissue ischemia with symptoms and signs corresponding to the affected organ, e.g., myocardial infarction or stroke. Vasculitis is classified by the size of the affected vessels so visualize which arteries are affected. Atherosclerosis is a generalized process of large and small arteries. When only the aorta and its major branches are affected, think Takayasu or giant cell arteritis. Venous disorders are usually mechanical, either obstruction or valvular insufficiency of leg veins. The latter produces secondary skin and subcutaneous inflammation, which is often mistaken for cellulitis. Bleeding is mechanical disruption of the vessel or a failure of hemostasis.

Evaluate each hypothesis with laboratory tests and imaging studies having appropriate likelihood ratios. The results change the probability of each hypothesis to a *posttest probability*: some are now much more probable, whereas others are much less probable. To reach a new, refined differential diagnosis, return to the patient, review the history, and repeat specific parts of the physical exam. This process is repeated until a diagnosis that fully explains the illness is confirmed.

In this book, under many symptoms and signs, there is a list of CLINICAL OCCURRENCES. It is up to the clinician using this list as an organizational tool to generate a meaningful differential diagnosis which is pertinent to their patient. Specific clues that will help refine the differential diagnosis are listed after the *DDX:* symbol.

Many patients develop an acute problem on the background of two or more chronic disorders. The new problem may result from an exacerbation of a known disease or by a new superimposed disorder.

Verifying diagnoses. Verification of a working diagnosis, the current diagnostic hypothesis, tests its validity. Since the diagnostic process is inferential, all diagnostic hypotheses reflect a belief or a conviction by the physician regarding the underlying condition from which the patient suffers. Accepting a diagnostic hypothesis before it is fully verified is known as *premature closure*. Inappropriate and premature acceptance of a diagnostic hypothesis can be avoided if physicians insist that all data is considered before accepting a diagnostic hypothesis as verified. Adequacy, coherency, and parsimony are cognitive aids that help to avoid making a premature or incorrect diagnosis. These three tests are useful for deciding whether a diagnostic hypothesis qualifies as a working diagnosis.

1. **Coherency.** Is the working diagnosis pathophysiologically consistent with all the clinical findings, i.e., are all physiologic linkages,

predisposing factors, and complications consistent with the hypothesis in this patient? Causal reasoning is based on cause-and-effect relations between clinical variables or chain of variables. It is a function of normal anatomic, physiologic, and biochemical mechanisms and their consistent pathophysiology in disease.

2. **Adequacy.** Does the working diagnosis explain all the patient's findings, normal and abnormal? A hypothesis is more likely to be correct if it accounts for every symptom and sign.

3. **Parsimony.** Does the working diagnosis offer a simple explanation of all the patient's findings? This is Occam's razor: the simplest solution is likely to be correct. When one diagnosis does not explain all the findings, those that are able to account for the greatest proportion of the patient's signs and symptoms are more likely to be correct. Parsimony is most applicable to the previously well patient with an acute or subacute disease, the most common clinical challenge faced by Sir William Osler who introduced Occam's razor to medicine. However, sometimes multiple diagnoses become necessary for a physiologically and causally consistent explanation of the patient's findings and clinical features. As we care for more patients with one or more chronic diseases, bear in mind that more than one pathologic process may be occurring.

Cognitive Tests of Diagnostic Hypotheses: When prioritizing the list of possible diagnoses, the following tools help identify the most likely diagnosis.

Chronology. It is possible to have a perfect match of attributes between patient and disease, but if the epidemiology, onset, tempo, and course of illness are not congruent, the hypothesis is probably wrong.

Severity of illness. The global severity assessment made by an experienced clinician includes many intangibles, often based upon prior knowledge and experience with the patient. Experience-based emotional cues are essential to this assessment. An inexperienced clinician may diagnose a URI, whereas a more experienced clinician hypothesizes pneumonia because the patient looks too sick for just a URI. Severity of illness is valid and diagnostically useful.

Prognosis: *At presentation, it is more important not to miss a serious condition than to make the correct final diagnosis.* The clinician should proceed first to lower the probability of life and function-threatening conditions to below a reasonable probability, then proceed with evaluation of the other hypotheses. For instance, acute severe pelvic pain in fertile women is an ectopic pregnancy until proven otherwise; all other diagnoses can wait.

Therapeutic trial. If the uncertainty is between an untreatable morbid disease and one with potentially successful therapy, consider a therapeutic trial. Each trial must have a protocol that explicitly states the intervention and duration, the objective and subjective end points for interpretation at a specified time, and the planned response to a successful outcome or treatment failure. Experience shows that such trials are often inconclusive if they fail to adhere to these parameters, exposing patients to prolonged and hazardous treatments of little or no benefit. Doing something is not necessarily better than observation and close follow-up.

Selecting Diagnostic Tests: Select diagnostic investigations to test the hypotheses generated from the history and physical exam. Unfocused testing or an uncritical search for unlikely diagnoses frequently leads to more testing, without leading to an explanatory diagnosis. This cascade effect heightens the patient's anxiety, is hazardous, expensive, and often delays treatment. See Chapter 17 for a discussion of an appropriate testing strategy. Tests are performed to answer specific diagnostic, prognostic, or therapeutic questions, and should not be a response to curiosity.

Rare Diseases: Some physicians, especially the inexperienced, tend to search and test for rare diseases. It is good to recall that rare diseases occur rarely. The proverb "when you hear hoofbeats think horses, not zebras" works in America, but not in Africa. It is necessary to know the epidemiology of a population of patients like yours to really know what is common and what is rare in each clinical setting.

Certainty and Diagnosis: How certain should the clinician be that a diagnosis is correct before it is accepted? There is no accepted scale for degrees of certainty. A diagnosis may be defined by an image, laboratory test, culture, or the biopsy result. A fractured tibia is diagnosed by X-ray with assurance. Many types of neoplasia and inflammatory diseases are diagnosed by biopsy. Culture, serology, or polymerase chain reaction identify specific organisms establishing the diagnosis of an infectious disease. Laboratory tests are specific for endocrine and metabolic diseases. On the other hand, for many diseases and syndromes, there are no definitive diagnostic tests. For each clinical scenario the clinician must establish a *stopping rule*, the level of certainty required to stop further investigation. This decision is based upon the severity of illness, an estimate of the prognosis, and whether a specific diagnosis is needed to guide a decision between mutually exclusive interventions which would harm the patient if applied to the wrong disease. When a satisfactory diagnosis has not been established, the following steps should be considered, in addition to close follow-up.

Consultation. Obtaining consultation from an excellent generalist or appropriate subspecialist may produce a diagnosis, but even if not, the patient and physician are reassured. It is better to offer this option than to wait for the patient to insist out of frustration. However, avoid excessive consultation or visits to multiple physicians. Like excessive laboratory testing, this is more likely to add confusion than clarity.

Repeat the history and physical exam. The patient or a family member may recall additional information stimulated by the first inquiry. Talk to more relatives and attendants to confirm or deny the original story and to add details. Obtain copies of patient records from all previous caregivers. Carefully repeat the physical exam to confirm your previous evaluation and to search for signs that were originally overlooked.

Repeat selected laboratory tests. Specimens may have been mixed up on the initial evaluation, or an error in the first test may be uncovered. As always, each test should provide the answer to a specific question; do not search for diagnostic ideas in the laboratory.

Defer diagnosis. Carefully explaining the uncertainty helps to secure the patient's confidence so that follow-up occurs. Time, study, and reflection often lend perspective to the case. Present the case to colleagues as an unknown for their suggestions. Retain the problem list marking the record "Diagnosis Deferred." Do not let medical records rules, or an insurance company, force a premature diagnosis. *Remember, when a diagnosis is made, thinking often stops.*

Make a provisional diagnosis. It may be appropriate to make a provisional diagnosis understanding that it is difficult to avoid diagnosis creep: over time a provisional diagnosis becomes an assumed diagnosis. Even though the meticulous physician qualified the diagnosis as probable or provisional, these modifiers get dropped as the patient passes through several visits with different physicians. Always review the original information to confirm that each diagnosis has been confirmed.

Prognostic Uncertainty: If two hypotheses with widely differing prognoses seem equally probable and neither can be proved nor disproved immediately, inform the patient and review the diagnostic and prognostic possibilities. Encourage discussion with the patient and family. It is best to help the patient prepare for the bad prognosis, while maintaining hope for a better outcome. Regular follow-up and frequent reevaluation are mandatory.

Summary of the Diagnostic Process:
Step 1:   **Take a History.** Elicit symptoms and a timeline; begin a problem list.
Step 2:   **Develop Hypotheses.** Generate a mental list of anatomic sites of disease, pathophysiologic processes, and diseases that might produce the symptoms.
Step 3:   **Perform a Physical Exam.** Look for signs of the physiologic processes and diseases suggested by the history while identifying new findings for the problem list.
Step 4:   **Make a Problem List.** List all the problems found during the history and physical exam that require explanation.
Step 5:   **Create an Accurate Problem Representation.** Briefly summarize the patient encounter translating the patient's story into appropriate medical terminology.
Step 6:   **Generate a Differential Diagnosis.** List the most probable diagnostic hypotheses with an estimate of their pretest probabilities.
Step 7:   **Test the Hypotheses.** Select laboratory tests, imaging studies, and other procedures with appropriate likelihood ratios to evaluate your hypotheses.
Step 8:   **Modify Your Differential Diagnosis.** Use the test results to reevaluate your hypotheses, eliminating some, adding others, then adjust the probabilities.
Step 9:   **Repeat Steps 1 to 7.** Reiterate your process until you have reached a working diagnosis or decided that a definite diagnosis is neither likely nor necessary.

Step 10: Make the Working Diagnosis or Diagnoses. When the tests of your hypotheses are of sufficient certainty that they meet your stopping rule, you have reached a diagnosis. If uncertain, consider a provisional diagnosis or watchful waiting. Decide whether more investigation (return to Step 1), consultation, treatment, or watchful observation is the best course based upon the severity of illness, the prognosis, and comorbidities. If the diagnosis remains obscure, retain a problem list of the unexplained symptoms and signs, as well as laboratory and imaging findings, assess the urgency for further evaluation and schedule regular follow-up visits.

Caveat: The complex process presented here is best suited to the complex undifferentiated presentations encountered in internal medicine and pediatrics. The majority of patients seen by most physicians do not require such a comprehensive process. Although the principles hold for all patients, variations from the described process may be appropriate for a given patient's condition and the medical or surgical specialty involved. A dermatologist can make many diagnoses by visual inspection before hearing about symptoms. On the other hand, the psychiatrist relies exclusively on the history given by the patient, friends, relatives, and attendants. It follows that the scope of the history and the extent of physical exam vary greatly among medical specialties and with the patient's presenting complaints.

An Example of the Diagnostic Process: The objective of the diagnostic examination is to discover the physiologic cause of the patient's complaint, identify the specific disease, and determine its severity and prognosis. These are the data needed to counsel a patient regarding treatment.

A 21-year-old woman presents with a painless lump in her neck (symptom). You consider her age and select hypotheses including lymphoma, infection, and collagen vascular disease. She denies fever, itching, weight loss, exposure to pets, tuberculosis, arthralgias, and Raynaud phenomenon. Exam reveals a single, firm, 3-cm nontender lymph node in the right anterior cervical chain (sign); the spleen is not palpable and there are no other signs of disease. The patient's blood counts are normal (laboratory), and a biopsy of the enlarged node (supplemental test) discloses Hodgkin disease. Bone marrow biopsy and imaging studies of the chest and abdomen fail to reveal more disease (supplemental tests for staging and prognosis).

The diagnosis is stage I Hodgkin disease. The diagnosis is explained to the patient and the prognosis with and without treatment is discussed with the patient and her family. Treatment with radiotherapy and/or chemotherapy is discussed and oncology consultation is requested. Follow-up is scheduled for shortly after the consultation to provide an opportunity for questions and more discussion as needed.

CHAPTER 2

History Taking and the Medical Record

> . . . [T]here is no more difficult art to acquire than the art of observation, and for some men it is quite as difficult to record an observation in brief and plain language.
>
> – SIR WILLIAM OSLER

Safe high-quality medical care requires a medical record documenting the observations and data needed for the patients' care. Ideally, this record will be accessible to all providers at any site at any time, a goal that electronic medical records make feasible. A standard format is used to record: demographics; active and past medical problems; surgical history; medications, allergies, and drug intolerances; family, social, and sexual history; personal habits; and preventive care services. A standard format facilitates rapid review and updating of pertinent information at each visit. It is important to enter information so that it is always current; for example, record the first names of children and siblings with their year of birth (rather than age).

OUTLINE OF THE MEDICAL RECORD

The medical history is recorded in a standard sequence. The following sequence is suggested for adults.

1. Identification
2. Informant
3. Chief complaints (CCs)
4. History of present illness (HPI)
5. Past medical and surgical history (PMH)
   a. General health
   b. Chronic illnesses and conditions
   c. Operations and injuries
   d. Hospitalizations
6. Family history (FH)
7. Social history (SH)
8. Review of systems (ROSs)
9. Medications
10. Allergies and medication intolerances
11. Preventive services, including immunizations
12. Physical examination (PE)
13. Laboratory and imaging studies
14. Assessment/Problem list
15. Plan

The medical history is the history of this person. The current illness cannot be fully understood without knowing the unique history of the person, not just as patient, but as a person in society. The details of their family and social history provide context for their medical care. All serious illnesses including surgeries, injuries, and hospitalizations are recorded. The status of preventative care is also established. Verification of these events by review of the previous medical records is advised.

A medical history is more than a list of facts. It is a unique literary form in which the physician writes an account of perceptions and events *as related by the patient*. The history may be given spontaneously, or may require some probing, returning to areas of uncertainty for clarification. The history should record key statements in the patient's words. A history is usually incomplete at the first telling; repeat questioning after an interval of hours or days will yield additional information. Take particular care to establish the sequence of events. Neither the patient in the telling nor the physician in the recording should introduce medical terms or jargon; be sure that the story is told in everyday language. *The history is the patient's story of their illness, not the physician's interpretation of the patient's history*. The challenge is to understand the patient's experience and interpretation of their illness.

Scope of the History: The literature on history taking discusses the extended history, which is complicated and demands maximal skill. However, it would be folly to insist on an extended history for every patient; in many situations, it is unnecessary, and unnecessarily time consuming. The experienced clinician adjusts their technique to the setting and the patient's problem. When seeking care for dermatitis, the necessary diagnostic history is brief, possibly only a few sentences. For a fractured tibia, a long history is unnecessary and even inhumane. In contrast, a chronic, obscure disease may require a long, careful history, perhaps repeated and expanded, with supplementation as the results of studies open new diagnostic possibilities.

How to Take a History: The patient–physician encounter is a ritual invested with many layers of meaning; do not take it for granted. Accurate histories are obtained by empathetic clinicians who inspire confidence so that the patient feels free to relate their symptoms, fears, and uncertainties. Communication is much more than words; it is also inflection, facial expression, and body language. Patient listening, respecting pauses and silences, and avoiding the appearance of impatience will put the patient at ease so that they feel safe relating their story. As you learn more about the patient you will be better prepared to draw out details of their history. You cannot learn to take a good history from a book, this one included; proficiency is only obtained by interviewing patients. Your confidence and skill will improve as more is learned of people, life, and disease.

Clinical experience and reflection upon your experience are necessary to link your knowledge of diseases with the history being obtained from the patient. With this knowledge and experience, you can face the patient confidently and adapt your questioning to the evolving history. There are only a few principles to keep in mind: (1) listen actively; (2) do not interrupt; (3) ask open-ended questions; and (4) be patient, give the patient time to think and speak. It is most important to be a real person yourself; have a conversation.

Do Not Make Assumptions

Language. The English vocabulary is vast and formidable, even to the scholar, so ask your questions in simple, nontechnical terms. Gauge the meaning attached to the patient's words; words have different meanings for each person. Even lay words can be misunderstood. For example, when a patient complains of "heartburn," ask them to describe their symptoms. Repeating to the patient what you heard, will help to assure accuracy. Have the patient read-back your explanations so you can check their comprehension.

Belief systems. Physicians are trained in the scientific method and in science-based rules of evidence. It is essential to understand how the patient views cause and effect, and to what sources they attribute disease and illness. Their belief systems may include magic, faith, and rationalism. The clinician's task is to understand the patient; it is not the patient's task to understand the clinician. Educating each other to reach a mutual understanding becomes an important part of providing proper care for chronic diseases.

Patient's motivation. The utility of the history for diagnosis assumes that the patient's history and descriptions of their symptoms are complete and truthful. Never doubt the veracity of the patient's story and actively acknowledge your trust in the honesty of their full disclosure. Only compelling evidence should alter this commitment to the patient's story. The physician must ascertain whether the patient is motivated by potential secondary gain. Patients with substance use disorders may present symptoms calculated to obtain drugs.

Conducting the interview. The following describes taking an extended interview in the clinic, with these caveats: the patient is not in acute distress, time limitations are not critical, and the presentation is relatively obscure. Circumstances often vary greatly from these stipulations.

Arrangement. The room should be comfortable and soundproof to outside distractions. The patient and interviewer should sit at eye level without a desk between the two; do not assume a dominating position. The conversation should not be overhead. Limit the interview to the patient and one other informant; the presence of the patient's spouse or a relative is often helpful. The interview is a conversation between two parties, not a discussion among a group.

Physician's manner. Address patients formally, do not use their first name unless they request it. Present yourself as unhurried, interested, and empathetic. In no way should you express a moral judgment on the patient's actions or beliefs. Permit patients to begin their story in their own way; listen for several minutes before gradually injecting questions to guide the interview. Gently, but firmly, keep the discussion centered on the patient's problems.

Note taking. Use of standardized forms for recording the past medical history, FH, and SH (which the patient can fill out before the interview) decreases the need to take notes. While the patient is speaking, write sparingly. Avoid writing the story verbatim; it is usually too lengthy and poorly organized. Remember that the patient is telling you a story; try to understand the story while jotting down key words and phrases to assist recall.

Procedure. Patients often have several issues on their visit agenda. Obtain a complete list of their concerns for this visit before the illness narrative. Ask them for anything else until the full agenda is ascertained. This will prevent the "Oh, by the way, ..." questions at the visit's end. Long or complicated agendas will need to be negotiated.

After recording the routine data, sit back and listen to the narrative, interjecting only a few questions. Ask the patient to "Please tell me about your problem," or "Please tell me what's happening to you." Do not ask for conclusions ("What is the matter with you?" or "What is troubling you?"). Listen for several minutes without interruption; use open-ended questions to probe areas that aren't clear. After the general outline becomes apparent, you may need to ask direct questions. Ask about symptoms not mentioned but that are relevant to the systems and sites likely involved with the illness. You may pause periodically to write notes, including key words and phrases.

Check for completeness. Finally, review what you have obtained and ask for any remaining information to complete the history. Briefly summarize the story highlighting key phrases and events; ask the patient to correct you if anything has been missed or misinterpreted.

COMPLETION OF THE MEDICAL RECORD

It is the clinician's responsibility to see that the medical record is complete and accurate. Your signature attests to the accuracy of the information and that you have verified it to your satisfaction. *Once entered and signed, the information in the medical record cannot be altered*, although addendums and corrections can be added.

Identification: These data are frequently provided for the clinician, but should be checked for accuracy.

Patient's name. Record the complete name, including the family and given names, being careful to obtain correct spelling and birth date. When a married woman who has taken her husband's name, place her husband's given names in parentheses, as Brown, Mary Elizabeth (Mrs. Edward Charles), since she may sign her name as Mrs. Edward C. Brown in correspondence. Determine whether she wishes to be addressed as Ms. or Mrs.

Sex and gender. Sex is determined by genetics, gender is the patient's sexual identity. Usually, this is obvious, but specific questions asked sensitively may be required.

Referral source. Confirm the reason for referral and the name, address, telephone, and FAX numbers of the referring clinician.

The Informant
Sources of the history. The history is best obtained from the patient with supportive information from others. Record your impression of the historian's accuracy.

Interpreters. Do not use untrained interpreters. Telephonic interpreters are available for most languages. The following is a frequent experience with a lay interpreter, especially a family member. You ask, "Do you have pain?" The interpreter and patient have an animated conversation for a minute or two after which the interpreter says, "No, she doesn't have any pain." It is reasonable to assume that there is uncertainty about the content of the discussion between interpreter and patient. You cannot evaluate the patient's story or answers unless you know how the questions were asked. Your only recourse is to ask short concrete questions and insist that the resulting conversation be no longer than you judge necessary.

Chief Complaints: Begin the record with CC, the symptom that precipitated the visit. Complaints should be listed as single words or short phrases with the approximate length of time they have been present: for example, nausea for 2 months; vomiting for 1 week. Use the patient's own words free of interpretation. Do not accept a previous diagnosis as a CC; probing may be needed before the patient relates their symptoms rather than their diagnoses or those of previous providers and family members.

The CC is the starting place for making a differential diagnosis; the details of the symptoms should always be fully elucidated. Since these are the symptoms for which the patient sought care, they will require therapy or an explanation of why therapy is not given. The patient's CC should be the first problem on your problem list. This would seem obvious, but occasionally the physician finds an interesting disease, unrelated to the CC; the medically attractive condition receives all the attention, and the CC is ignored.

Do not press the patient for a CC too early in the interview. After they have told some of their story, they may be better able to articulate their complaints and concerns. Occasionally, when asked for their symptoms, the patient produces a long detailed list of notes. The French label this *la maladie de petit papier*, which may signal an inappropriate level of concern or obsession with their symptoms.

History of present illness. The HPI is the patient's story of their illness experience; *it is the most important part of the diagnostic examination*. It should be recorded in complete sentences as a lucid, succinct, and chronologic narrative. Ideally, the HPI should be brief, so that it is easily read and digested, but this is only possible if the history is relatively straightforward. Some stories are complex and the diagnostic possibilities broad, requiring inclusion of more detail since you can't be certain what is pertinent and what is superfluous. You must avoid premature interpretation such as replacing their words with medical terminology or failing to record seemingly irrelevant symptoms or events.

Searching for diagnostic clues. The chief purpose of the history is to help you form diagnostic hypotheses. As the narrative unfolds, you should be simultaneously performing three operations: (1) accumulating data (obtaining the history), (2) evaluating the data (assessing the meaning of symptoms, seeking more details of time and quantity), and (3) preparing three sets of hypotheses. The hypotheses are anatomic (where is the problem?), physiologic (what is the pathophysiology?), and diagnostic (what diseases could account for this pathophysiology in that place?).

Symptoms. A symptom is an abnormal sensation perceived by the patient. Insist that the patient describes their symptoms; do not accept diagnoses or medical jargon as a substitute. Record the symptoms using the patient's words. Evaluation of a symptom can be straightforward, as when the patient says, "I've found a lump in my neck" (symptom), and the examiner can palpate a mass (physical sign). However, when the patient complains of a nonspecific symptom, such as chest pain, more information is required. The acronym PQRST is a useful mnemonic; ask about *P*rovocative or *P*alliative maneuvers, symptom *Q*uality, the *R*egion involved, the *S*everity, and *T*emporal pattern of the symptom (see the discussion of pain, Chapter 4, page 74).

Question the patient about other symptoms specific for processes and diseases you are considering, either to support or undermine a hypothesis. For example, when the patient complains of chest pain, ask if it is related to respiratory movements. A positive answer prompts questions about inflamed muscles, fractured ribs, and pleurisy. If the answer is negative, ask for an association with exertion or radiation suggestive of angina pectoris. Thus, each step leads to another, resulting in refinement of your hypotheses.

Clarification. Question the patient until sufficient details are obtained to categorize the symptom. Do not accept vague complaints such as "I don't feel well." If the patient complains of weakness, ascertain if she is weak in one or more muscle groups or if she experiences lassitude, malaise, or myalgia. When a patient says she is dizzy, have her describe the experience without using the word "dizzy." Determine whether shortness of breath occurs at rest or with exertion.

Quantification. It is good to have the patient quantify the symptoms. For instance, pain cannot be measured, but the severity can be estimated by how it affects the patient. A patient may have a "terrible pain," but if the pain has never interfered with work, sleep, or other activities, "terrible" acquires a clearer meaning. Shortness of breath can be assessed by the amount of exertion required to produce it; for example, ask, "Can you climb a flight of stairs? Can you walk two blocks without stopping?" Neither you nor your reader can interpret what "heavy smoker" means. Heavy varies from one person to another, but smoking 20 cigarettes daily everyone understands. The patient with hemoptysis should estimate the amount of blood lost in household measures, such as teaspoonfuls or cupfuls.

Chronology. The duration of a symptom and the time of its appearance in the course of illness are important for diagnosis. When the disease is chronic and the course complicated, the patient may have difficulty placing events in order. A timeline can assist in clarifying the details: draw a vertical line demarcated in appropriate units of time, days, weeks, months, or years. Indicate on the timeline the certain dates supplied by the patient, as well as anchoring dates such as birthdays, New Years, and holidays. Seeing the chart, the patient frequently recalls further details and can place the symptoms more accurately. The sequence and doses of medication can also be recorded.

Current activity. Include this in the HPI. Determine how the illness has diminished the patient's quality of life and whether therapy has improved it. You should evaluate the severity of disease, the patient's adjustments to illness, and response to therapy by obtaining a detailed picture of the patient's average work and weekend day, before and after the onset of illness.

Summary. Review your understanding of the history and ask the patient for corrections and confirmation. Test the completeness of your history by asking whether your summary conveys a clear picture of the patient's experience of their illness, that is, how the illness has affected them and their family, how it has interfered with their work, and how the symptoms have progressed.

Past Medical and Surgical History: The past history helps you understand the person you are evaluating and the preconditions that may substantially alter current and future risks for specific health conditions. When relevant, specific facts may be included in the HPI, but they must be recorded again in this section. The significance of past illnesses may only be appreciated after future developments in the patient's condition or as newly recognized disease associations are reported.

General health. The patient's lifetime health, before the present illness, is sometimes revealing. Factors to consider include body weight (present, maximum, and minimum, with dates of each), previous PEs (dates and findings), and any periods of medical disability.

Chronic and episodic illnesses
Chronic medical illness. List all illnesses, diseases, or conditions for which the patient receives, or has received, chronic medical treatment.

Infectious diseases. Infectious diseases have had an important history in medicine. Knowledge of past infections is important to understand current and future infection risk. List dates and complications of these illnesses with particular attention to hepatitis, rheumatic fever, tuberculosis, sexually transmitted diseases, and HIV. Give dates and duration of antibiotic treatment.

Operations and injuries. Give dates and nature of injuries, operations, operative diagnoses, and infection, hemorrhage, blood transfusions, or other complications.

Previous hospitalizations. Record each hospitalization, including the dates, names, and location of hospitals. If the hospital records are available, summarize the dates and diagnoses for each admission.

Family History: A FH is essential for all patients receiving more than the most cursory care. This should include four generations, when available: grandparents, parents, aunts and uncles, siblings, and children. For parents and grandparents, record the birth year and current health or age at death and causes. For aunts, uncles, siblings, and children, record the birth year, first name, and current health or cause of death and age at death. Make note of any FH of hypertension, heart disease, diabetes, kidney disease, autoimmune diseases, gout, atopy, asthma, obesity, endocrine disorders, osteoporosis, cancer (particularly breast, colon, ovarian, and endocrine cancers), hemophilia or other bleeding diseases, venous thromboembolism, stroke, migraine, neurologic or muscular disorders, mental or emotional disturbances, substance abuse, and epilepsy.

Social History

Place of birth. This information may be useful in assessing prevalence of diseases.

Nationality, ethnicity, and language. It is important to record the patient and family's country of origin and first language(s). English as a second language (ESL) is common in North America and Europe. Ethnic and genetic backgrounds are important in diagnosis of diseases such as hemoglobinopathies and familial Mediterranean fever.

Marital status. Note whether the patient is single, married, divorced, or widowed, and the duration of marriages or long-term relationships and how they ended.

Occupations. Some diseases produce symptoms years after exposure, so tabulate past occupations as well as current work. Precise knowledge of the patient's work history sheds light on education, social status, physical exertion, psychologic trauma, exposure to noxious agents, and a variety of conditions that may cause disease. You must ask specifically what work is actually done to assess risk for exposures. Ask if an illness is connected with their surroundings and if coworkers have similar symptoms. Always ask about part-time work. For agricultural workers ask about contacts with agricultural chemicals and animals. Determine how much stress accompanies the job, the attitudes of superiors, and the degree of work fatigue.

Military History: Note military service by branch, geographic locations, discharge (honorable or dishonorable), and eligibility for veteran's benefits.

Gender preference. Labels, such as heterosexual, homosexual, and bisexual, are often more confusing than helpful. Ask each patient if they have had sex with anyone of the same sex. For example, ask men, "Have you ever had sex with men?" If the patient answers "yes," you should ask further questions about sex with women and the patient's past and current practices and preference. Nonjudgmental inquiry about exchange of sex for drugs, money, or services can disclose high-risk behaviors.

Social and economic status. Record the patient's years of formal education, vocational training, current living arrangements, and any financial problems.

Habits. Determine the patient's former and current use of tobacco, coffee, alcohol, sedatives, illicit drugs (especially injection drug use), tattoos, and body piercing.

Violence and safety. Record the patient's use of vehicle restraints, bicycle and motorcycle helmets, and the presence of home smoke and carbon monoxide alarms. Domestic, child, and elder abuse are common problems that go unidentified unless they are asked about explicitly and discreetly. In complete privacy, inquire whether the patient has ever been in a relationship in which she felt unsafe. If the answer is "yes," ask if she feels safe in her current situation. If she answers "no," ask if she wishes help to find a safe environment.

Never try to explicitly identify the individual whom the patient finds threatening, though this information may be volunteered by the patient.

Prostheses and in-home assistance. Record the patient's use of eyeglasses, dentures and dental appliances, hearing aides, ambulation assistance devices (cane, walker, scooter, wheelchair), braces, prosthetic footwear, and any aide or assistance received in the home (visiting nurse, physical therapy, homemaker services).

Review of Systems: The following outline can help inquire for symptoms associated with each system or anatomic region. Symptoms related to the patient's current problem, discovered during your ROS inquiry, should be recorded in the HPI. Become familiar with these symptoms and learn their diagnostic significance: record positive answers and negative responses when they are pertinent to the differential diagnosis. It is efficient to ask the questions while examining the body to which the questions pertain. Use of a standardized check in questionnaire will facilitate a thorough review and save time.

Constitutional. Weight loss or gain, fatigue, fevers, chills, or sweats.

Skin, hair, and nails. *Skin:* Color, pigmentation, temperature, moisture, eruptions, pruritus, scaling, bruising, bleeding. *Hair:* Color, texture, abnormal loss or growth, distribution. *Nails:* Color changes, brittleness, ridging, pitting, curvature.

Lymph nodes. Enlargement, pain, tenderness, suppuration, draining sinuses, location.

Bones, joints, and muscles. Fractures, dislocations, sprains, arthritis, myositis, pain, swelling, stiffness, degree of disability, muscular weakness, wasting or atrophy, night cramps.

Hemopoietic system. Anemia (type, therapy, and response), lymphadenopathy, bleeding, or clotting (spontaneous, traumatic, familial).

Endocrine system. History of growth, body configuration, and weight; size of hands, feet, and head, especially changes during adulthood; hair distribution; skin pigmentation; goiter, exophthalmos, dryness of skin and hair, intolerance to heat or cold, tremor; polyphagia, polydipsia, polyuria; libido, secondary sex characteristics, impotence, sterility.

Allergic and immunologic history. Dermatitis, urticaria, angioedema, eczema, hay fever, rhinitis, asthma, conjunctivitis; known sensitivity to pollens, foods, danders, X-ray contrast agents, bee stings; previous skin tests and their results; results of tuberculin tests and others; desensitization, serum injections, vaccinations, and immunizations.

Head. Headaches, migraine, trauma, syncope, convulsive seizures.

Eyes. Loss of vision or color blindness, diplopia, hemianopsia, trauma, inflammation, glasses (date of refraction), discharge, excessive tearing.

Ears. Deafness, tinnitus, vertigo, discharge from the ears, pain, mastoiditis, operations.

Nose. Coryza, rhinitis, sinusitis, discharge, obstruction, epistaxis.

Mouth. Soreness of mouth or tongue, symptoms referable to teeth and gums.

Throat. Hoarseness, sore throats, tonsillitis, voice changes, dysphagia, odynophagia.

Neck. Swelling, suppurative lesions, enlargement of lymph nodes, goiter, stiffness, and limitation of motion.

Breasts. Development, lactation, trauma, lumps, pains, discharge from nipples, gynecomastia, changes in nipples, skin changes.

Respiratory system. Pain, shortness of breath, wheezing, cough, sputum, hemoptysis, night sweats, pleurisy, bronchitis, tuberculosis (history of contacts), pneumonia, asthma, other respiratory infections.

Cardiovascular system. Palpitation, tachycardia, irregularities of rhythm, pain in the chest, exertional dyspnea, paroxysmal nocturnal dyspnea, orthopnea, cough, cyanosis, edema; intermittent claudication, cold extremities, postural or permanent changes in skin color; hypertension, rheumatic fever, chorea, syphilis, diphtheria; drugs such as digitalis, quinidine, nitroglycerin, diuretics, anticoagulants, antiplatelet agents, and other medications.

Gastrointestinal system. Appetite, dysphagia, nausea, eructation, flatulence, abdominal pain or colic, vomiting, hematemesis, jaundice (pain, fever, intensity, duration, color of urine and stools), ascites, stools (color, frequency, incontinence, consistency, odor, gas, cathartics, pain or difficulty with passage, urge to stool), hemorrhoids, change in bowel habits.

Genitourinary system. Color of urine, polyuria, oliguria, nocturia, dysuria, hematuria, pyuria, urinary retention, urinary frequency, incontinence, pain or colic, passage of stones.

Gynecologic History: Age of menarche, frequency of periods, regularity, duration, amount of flow, leukorrhea, dysmenorrhea, date of last normal and preceding periods, date and character of menopause, postmenopausal bleeding; pregnancies (number, abortions, miscarriages, stillbirths, chronologic sequence), complications of pregnancy; birth control practices (oral contraceptive medications, barrier methods, etc.).

Male History: Erectile dysfunction, premature ejaculation, blood in the semen, contraceptive methods, and condom use.

Venereal Disease History: Sexual activity (sex of partners and practices), chancre, bubo, urethral discharge, treatment of venereal diseases.

Nervous system

General. Headache, loss of consciousness, unsteadiness, vertigo, falls, sleep disorders (insomnia, nonrestful sleep, leg movements of sleep, sleep walking), restless legs.

Cranial nerves (CNs). Disturbances of smell (CN I), visual disturbances (CN II, III, IV, VI), orofacial paresthesias and difficulty in chewing (CN V), facial weakness and taste disturbances (CN VII), disturbances in hearing and equilibrium (CN VIII), difficulties in speech, swallowing, and taste (CN IX, X, XII), limitation in motion of neck (CN XII).

Motor system. Paralyses, weakness, muscle wasting, involuntary movements, convulsions, gait, incoordination.

Sensory system. Pain, lightning pain, girdle pain, paresthesia, hypesthesia, anesthesia, allodynia.

Autonomic system. Control of urination and defecation, sweating, erythema, cyanosis, pallor, reaction to heat and cold, postural faintness.

Psychiatric history. Describe difficulties with interpersonal relationships (with parents, siblings, spouse, children, friends and associates), sexual adjustments, school and employment success and difficulties, impulse control, sleep disorders, mood swings, difficulty with concentration, thought, or the presence of hallucinations.

Medications: Keep a list of current medications by name, dose, effect, indication, and duration of use. Ask the patient to bring the original containers with the labels. If the labels are absent, call the pharmacy where they were dispensed. Be sure to list all nonprescription drugs, herbal remedies, supplements, and vitamins.

Allergies and Medication Intolerances: Untoward drug reactions should be as explicit as possible. Ask for the type of reaction or intolerance experienced. Common side effects may be incorrectly identified as allergies: for example, stomach upset with codeine or erythromycin. Identify known or suspected causes of anaphylaxis (drugs, stings, and foods, e.g., peanuts). This summary of allergies and medication intolerances must be consulted when drugs are being prescribed.

Preventive Care Services: Record the patient's history of preventive care services. List the dates and results of screening tests (e.g., mammograms, Pap smears, colorectal cancer screening, tuberculin tests), and immunizations using age- and sex-specific national guidelines as your standard.

Advance Directives: Each adult should be asked if they have a living will and/or durable power of attorney for health care and, if so, who is their surrogate decision maker. Each adult should be given information about advance directives and be given an opportunity to record their wishes concerning resuscitation, mechanical ventilation, and prolonged life support. Although these discussions are more likely to be particularly relevant to the frail older adults, you should initiate this discussion with all adults more than 50 years of age, before the anticipated time of need.

Physical Examination: Record the observations from your PE in the following sequence:

1. Vital signs
2. General appearance
3. Head, eyes, ears, nose, and throat
4. Neck and spine
5. Chest: breasts
6. Chest: chest wall and lungs
7. Chest: heart, major arteries, and neck veins
8. Abdomen
9. Genitourinary examination, including inguinal hernias
10. Rectal examination
11. Extremities
12. Lymph nodes
13. Neurologic examination, including the mental status examination
14. Skin

Laboratory: Record the laboratory results used in developing your differential diagnosis.

Assessment
Case summary. It is sometimes useful to write a brief abstract of the history and significant observations.

The problem list and assessment. A working problem list should be maintained with notes and dates indicating their status. The problem list records each of the diagnostic and management problems needing attention. A problem may be a symptom, a sign, a laboratory finding, or a cluster of several associated items. A previously confirmed disease may be listed as a problem. It is important to update and revise the problem list.

Generate a *differential diagnosis* for each problem. As discussed in Chapter 1, the differential diagnosis can be pathophysiologic, diagnostic, or both. It is a good practice to keep the patient's CC as the first problem. Beyond that, attempts to number the problem list in a prioritized or numerically consistent fashion are not useful; priorities change as the evaluation and treatment proceed and problems disappear or consolidate as more information is acquired.

Diagnostic problem solving is much like putting together a jigsaw puzzle without the picture and with only a few pieces provided at a time. To eventually solve the puzzle, you place the pieces on the table and, as new pieces appear, keep trying different arrangements until the pattern emerges. The problem list is your table full of pieces; your hypotheses are attempts to explain the pattern. It is often the odd piece that does not seem to fit anywhere that is the key to the puzzle. When the diagnosis is obscure, beware of lumping problems together prematurely; this may serve to obscure rather than to clarify the diagnosis.

The Plan: For each problem, and the patient as a whole, you need to develop a management plan. The plan for each problem has three parts: (1) plans for testing your hypothesis, (2) therapy to be considered or given, and (3) education for the patient and family.

A plan is only as good as the diagnostic hypotheses that generated it. Our emphasis in this text is to help you think about the information acquired in the history and physical exam so that you can generate sound, testable hypotheses. Once you have generated a concise differential diagnosis, you can consult textbooks and/or search the medical literature to find an efficient method for testing your hypotheses.

THE ORAL PRESENTATION

The optimal oral presentation holds your listener's attention for 5 to 7 minutes while you identify your patient and briefly summarize the case. Summarize the history, review the vital signs, pertinent physical findings and lab results, state the problems and diagnostic hypotheses, and then recommend a diagnostic and therapeutic plan. Excellent presentations require that you edit and organize the information, to tell the story of the illness as it appears to you. If you regurgitate all of the extensive information that you place in the medical record, you will quickly lose your audience.

The oral presentation is not simply an academic exercise. Brief, accurate presentations benefit patients by clearly communicating their problems to other participants in their care, including nurses, your teachers, fellow house officers, sign-out partners in practice, and consultants.

OTHER CLINICAL NOTES

Inpatient Progress Notes: Progress notes are made daily and additionally whenever necessary. Each note should be dated and the time of day recorded. Each note has four subheads. Use the mnemonic SOAP to remember them: *S*ubjective data (symptoms and changes in symptoms, their appearance and disappearance, and their response to therapy); *O*bjective data (changes in or new physical signs and laboratory findings and response to therapy); *A*ssessments (updates to your problem list and hypotheses); and *P*lans (diagnostic tests, therapeutic interventions, and instructions to the patient and nursing staff). When a problem is resolved by inclusion in another diagnosis, or by cure or disappearance, it should be so noted in the progress note and in the working problem list. The full and legible name of the writer is appended to each progress note.

Discharge Summary: When the patient leaves the hospital, a discharge summary is created containing the principal diagnosis and all problems addressed during the hospitalization, an abstract of the history and hospital course, future plans, and each medication by dose and schedule, noting new, discontinued, or changed medications. Note the patient's condition and functional status at discharge and any information or instructions given to the patient and attendants for home and follow-up care.

Clinic Notes: Clinic notes follow the same SOAP format described for progress notes in the hospital. If the chart contains standardized forms as part of the medical record, the note may refer to those forms to avoid repetition. Clinic notes should state the expected response to therapy, when that response is anticipated and when the patient is to be seen in follow-up.

CHAPTER 3

Physical Examination

A systematic history and physical exam is the foundation of the diagnostic process. Likewise, the screening physical exam is foundational to the clinician–patient relationship. Laying on of hands is symbolic of the trusting, respectful relationship between clinician and patient necessary for good care. The hands-on physical examination by an experienced clinician is frequently undervalued.

The exam imprints an image of the person in their nonidealized normal state while screening for signs of unsuspected disease or developmental abnormalities. All four senses are used during the physical exam: *inspection* uses sight and smell, *palpation* is systematic touch and feel, *percussion* uses hearing and feel, and *auscultation* uses hearing. Each physical exam is an opportunity to further train these senses. Deliberate practice, study, and experience improve the ability to detect structural and functional changes overlooked by inexperienced examiners. Skill is achieved by routinely comparing exam findings to laboratory and imaging studies. If discrepancies are observed, repeat the exam. Experts have refined their senses and skills through repetition and reflection and learned from experience.

METHODS FOR PHYSICAL EXAMINATION

Inspection: Observation using sight and smell is both simple and difficult. Simple because sight and smell are continuous during wakefulness; hard because learning to *see* actively, rather than passively, is a skill acquired by deliberate practice. Attention is unconsciously selective so that what we *see* and consciously remember is biased toward what is expected and known. The ability to *see* the unexpected or unknown is acquired by *deliberate practice*, not just by doing many exams; remember, *sight is a faculty, seeing is an art*. Consequently, inspection depends entirely on the observer's knowledge, expectations, and training. This is epitomized in maxims such as "We see what's behind the eyes" (Wintrobe), "The examination does not wait the removal of the shirt" (Waring), and "Was Man Weiss, Man sieht" (Goethe: "What one knows, one sees"). The layperson sees someone who looks peculiar. The expert physician sees enlarged supraorbital ridges, widely spaced teeth, large tongue, and wide hands and feet; he sees acromegaly.

Smells are impossible to describe, only experience provides a context for interpretation. The body odors of poor hygiene, the fetor of advanced liver disease, the putrid smell of anaerobic infections, the smell of alcohol or acetone on the breath, and many others are useful diagnostic clues to a trained observer.

General visual inspection. The physical exam begins by inspecting the whole person at first contact. If possible, watch how the patient walks into the exam room. Note how he is dressed and groomed, whether eye contact is established, the tone and pattern of speech, how he moves and changes position, his facial expression, skin type, overall body form and proportions, deformities or asymmetry of face, limbs, or trunk, nutrition, specific behaviors, presence of tremor, and signs of pain. Bear in mind that the patient will be inspecting you at the same time.

Close visual inspection. Close or focused inspection concentrates on a single anatomic region; the closer you look, the more you see. The art is in seeing all that is there and distinguishing what is important from what is not. Proper inspection requires uniform white light to avoid color distortion. Use a hand-held lens, otoscope, or ophthalmoscope for magnification. Oblique lighting emphasizes subtle changes in surface contours and motion that may be invisible with direct lighting, e.g., the apical impulse on the chest.

Olfactory inspection—smell. Odors provide valuable clues; experience is required to properly identify even common odors. Odors on the breath may indicate acetone or alcohol. Foul-smelling sputum suggests bronchiectasis or lung abscess. Stomach contents may emit the odors of alcohol, phenol, or other poisons, or the sour smell of fermenting food. A fecal odor may indicate intestinal obstruction. Particularly foul-smelling stool is common in pancreatic insufficiency. An ammonia odor in the urine suggests fermentation in the bladder. Pus with a nauseatingly sweet odor, like the smell of rotting apples, is indicative of gas gangrene while a fecal odor is typical of anaerobic infection.

Palpation: The hands are incredibly sensitive to a variety of stimuli: tactile, thermal, and the kinesthetic senses of position and vibration. All normal persons possess these senses, but training and practice are required to hone their use as diagnostic tools, just as a blind person practices using braille to acquire reading proficiency. The fingertips are most sensitive for *fine tactile discrimination* such as shape, surface regularity, crepitus, texture, movement, and moisture. The thin skin on the back of the hand and fingers can detect subtle *temperature differences*. Bone is more sensitive to *vibration* than the fingertips. To probe for thrills and especially fremitus, rather than use the fingertips, press the palmar aspects of the metacarpophalangeal joints or the ulnar side of the hand (fifth metacarpal and fifth phalanges) to the surface. Test this for yourself by touching a vibrating tuning fork to a fingertip and then to the base of the finger on the palm.

Specific qualities elicited by palpation
Texture. Note the surface characteristics of the skin and hair. Are they brittle, coarse, thick, thin, roughened, or smooth?

Moisture. Assess the moisture content of the skin, hair, and mucous membranes. Are they moist and supple or dry and cracked?

Skin temperature. Palpate the head, face, trunk, arms, hands, legs, and feet assessing the local skin temperature and the distribution of heat.

Characteristics of masses. When a mass or enlarged organ is discovered, record its size, shape, consistency, mobility, surface regularity, and the presence or absence of expansile or transmitted pulsation.

Precordial cardiac thrust. Palpate the precordium for signs of heart action.

Crepitus. Feel for crepitation when examining bones, joints, tendon sheaths, pleura, and subcutaneous tissue.

Tenderness. Note discomfort or pain on palpation of accessible tissues and over major organs. How much pressure is required to induce the uncomfortable sensation?

Thrills. Palpate the precordium for thrills. If bruits are heard in the major arteries, palpate them for thrills.

Vocal fremitus. Palpating vocal vibrations through the chest wall provides important information about the underlying pleura and lung.

Sensitive parts of the hand
Tactile sense. The fingertips are the most sensitive for fine tactile discrimination.

Temperature sense. Use the dorsa of the hands or fingers; the skin is much thinner than elsewhere on the hand.

Vibratory sense. Palpate to detect vibrations with the palmar aspects of the metacarpophalangeal joints or the ulnar side of the hand (fifth metacarpal and fifth phalanges) rather than with the fingertips. Test this for yourself by touching first the fingertip and then the palmar base of your finger with a vibrating tuning fork.

Sense of position and consistency. Use the grasping fingers perceiving with sensations from your joints and muscles.

Methods of palpation
Light palpation. Always begin palpation with a light touch. Your sense of touch is most acute when lightly applied, and the patient is put at ease. Gently sliding the fingertips over the skin surface may detect subtle or mobile masses missed by forceful palpation. This also locates tender areas for later examination.

Deep palpation. Firm pressure displaces superficial tissues allowing palpation for deeper structures. Though especially useful in the abdomen, deep palpation is also used in the neck, breasts, and large muscle masses. Whenever possible, avoid firm palpation over nerves and other tender structures.

Bimanual palpation. The tissue is examined between the fingers of both hands. It is useful for abdominal, pelvic, muscle, and joint examinations and soft tissues such as breasts and intraoral structures.

Percussion: In percussion the body surface is struck generating a sound wave that vibrates the underlying tissues producing percussion notes of frequencies that vary with the density of the tissues and structures being percussed.

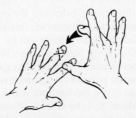

FIG. 3-1 Method of Indirect (Bimanual) Percussion. The terminal digit of the left long finger is firmly applied to an interspace, or other body surface, as a pleximeter. The distal interphalangeal joint of that finger is struck a sharp blow with the tip of the flexed right long finger. To furnish blows of equal intensity, the fingers of the right hand are held partly flexed and the wrist is loose so that the striking hand pivots exclusively at the relaxed wrist. To avoid dampening the vibrations after striking the blow, withdraw the plexor hand rapidly from the pleximeter.

Bimanual, mediate, or indirect method of percussion. The tool used to strike is a *pleximeter*. The body surface is struck directly or an object, a *plexor*, applied to the body surface is struck. The latter is *indirect or mediate percussion*. Most commonly, the distal phalanx of the nondominant long finger is firmly pressed onto the body surface and struck by the partly flexed and rigid dominant long fingertip by bending the wrist, the hand's momentum ensuring repetitive blows of equal force (Fig. 3-1). The wrist is relaxed and neither the elbow nor the shoulder move. To avoid damping the vibrations, the plexor must rebound quickly from the pleximeter. To compare notes at two sites, two or three staccato blows are struck in one place before moving the pleximeter to percuss the second site. Reflex hammers are excellent easy to use plexors.

Direct percussion. Striking the body surface directly by a finger, hand, or reflex hammer is *direct or immediate percussion*. Be careful not to strike too firmly.

Sonorous percussion. Percussing a low-density air-filled lung produces one sound while a dense fluid-filled lung produces quite another. This principle is used to estimate the density of the lungs, pleura, pleural space, and abdominal viscera. In the chest, it requires a blow strong enough to vibrate tissue to a radius of 6 cm. The sounds correlating with different densities have specific names. Percussing air in the stomach yields *tympany*. The note from air-filled normal lung, filled with small air sacs and septa, has a different pitch and timbre termed *resonance*. Percussing over emphysematous lung produces *hyperresonance*, intermediate between resonance and tympany. *Dullness* is elicited by percussion over the heart when not covered by inflated lung. The note from percussion of the thigh muscles is *flatness*. Language cannot describe these sounds and attempts to do so are futile and confusing. The sounds' pitch and timbre are learned by listening. In a nontechnical sense, the percussion sounds are notes on a scale progressing from high-density tissues to those of low-density in the sequence flat, dull, resonant, hyperresonant, and tympanitic. The duration of sound varies inversely with the density. Flatness is very short, and, as the density decreases, each succeeding note is longer. With practice, changes in resonance can be felt by lightly placing the index and ring finger on either side of the middle finger plexor.

Definitive percussion. When the density of an organ is invariable and different from the surrounding tissue's density, the organ's borders are at the transition point from one sound to the other; this is *definitive percussion*. For example, normally, the lateral heart border can be identified by percussion where it lies against air-filled lung. Strike a lighter blow for definitive percussion than for sonorous percussion. Estimate an organ's size by mapping the density boundary. Definitive percussion locates the lung bases, diaphragm movement, a pleural fluid level, mediastinal width, heart size, the size and shape of the liver and spleen, and the size of a distended gallbladder or urinary bladder. Caveat: definitive percussion is not definitive. At best it generates a hypothesis.

Auscultation: Use a stethoscope to *listen* to sounds arising within the body, particularly from the lungs, heart, abdomen, and great vessels. This is *auscultation*. The ear can be trained to distinguish sounds quite accurately. Each person recognizes familiar voices by rhythm and patterns of pitch and overtones. Similarly, with *deliberate practice,* auscultatory skill is developed as initial impressions are compared to findings from investigations testing the examiner's hypotheses, e.g., comparing the auscultatory impression of a heart murmur to the findings from an echocardiogram. By listening as often as possible to known lesions of different types and severity, both the ear's discrimination and the examiner's interpretations improve.

The stethoscope. The stethoscope encloses a vibrating air column connecting the body wall to the ears. All stethoscopes modify sound to some extent, so use the same instrument whenever possible. The basic stethoscope excludes extraneous sounds but does not amplify sound. Electronic stethoscopes amplify, record, and project sounds making them particularly useful for teaching. Binaural instruments have a chest piece, thick-walled tubing, and two earpieces connected by a spring. Two chest pieces are needed to detect the full range of frequencies. The bell's hollow cone transmits all chest sounds particularly the low-frequency sounds, e.g., mitral stenosis murmurs and fetal heart sounds may only be heard with the bell. A wide bell transmits lower-pitched sounds than a narrow-diameter bell. The diaphragm is a flat cup covered with a semirigid diaphragm that filters out low-pitched sounds making the isolated high-pitched sounds seem louder. The diaphragm is best suited for breath sounds and high-pitched heart sounds, e.g., aortic regurgitation. For optimal acoustics, the tubing should not exceed 30 cm. The earpiece should close the external auditory meatus without discomfort.

Technique for Auscultation. The diaphragm is pressed firmly against the skin while the bell's rim should lightly touch the skin with just enough pressure to form a seal. Heavy pressure with the bell stretches the skin creating a diaphragm effect that excludes low pitches. Learn to ignore extraneous ambient noise. This subconscious editing can lead to missing important findings. To avoid this, listen actively, searching the full frequency spectrum. Breathing on the tubing produces a recognizable noise. Skin or hair rubbing on the chest piece produces sounds like crackles. Eliminate this by wetting the hair or using a rubber rim on the bell. Muscle, joint, and tendon movements sound like friction rubs; learn to recognize them. Use the bell for narrow spaces such as the supraclavicular fossae. Keep the stethoscope clean and free of cerumen. Regularly inspect the instrument replacing damaged parts promptly.

THE SCREENING PHYSICAL EXAMINATION

A screening physical exam is performed periodically for children and most adults. The *screening exam* is standardized for patients of the same age and gender. Every clinician must become proficient at a structured screening exam that will identify significant abnormalities. The exam is sequenced for efficiency and patient comfort. Examine the body by regions. *Examine regions; think systems.* This requires deliberate practice, reflection, and experience. A novice may identify all the signs but have trouble integrating those findings into a complete anatomic and physiologic picture. This integration is critical for generating unifying diagnostic hypotheses (see Problem Lists and Hypothesis Generation, Chapter 1 pages 5-6). Abnormalities encountered focus attention on possible anatomic or physiologic problems needing more detailed evaluation, including a detailed *diagnostic exam.*

Efficiency requires a well-organized exam room with easily accessible instruments familiar to the examiner. Examining each patient from head to foot in the same sequence avoids missing signs and develops an appreciation of normal variations. Avoid excessive changes of position by the examiner or patient. Each change takes time and may be uncomfortable for both. The screening exam outlined below can be performed in 15 minutes or less. Keep the following points in mind:

1. Respect the patient's modesty.
2. Maintain professional demeanor throughout.
3. Performed properly and professionally, the screening exam supports a professional relationship and reassures the patient.

Preparing the Screening Examination: This multisystem screening exam is performed with the patient in four or five positions (Fig. 3-2). It should take no more than 15 minutes to complete. The following sections describe the exam sequence. The methods for each regional examination are detailed in their respective chapters.

Preparation

Equipment. The following equipment must be easily accessible: stethoscope, sphygmomanometer, otoscope, ophthalmoscope, penlight, tongue blades, reflex hammer, tuning fork, calibrated monofilament, tape measure, gloves, lubricant, sterile swabs, and materials for specimen collection during the female pelvic exam. Wear gloves when examining the anus, rectum, genitalia, infected skin, oral cavity, and when contact with body fluids may occur.

Patient. The patient undresses in private, puts on a gown, and sits on the end of the exam table with a sheet draped over the lap and the legs.

Clinician. The clinician must be modestly and neatly dressed. To assure privacy and avoid problems, always leave the room while the patient prepares for the exam. If the patient requires assistance, ask a nurse or family member to assist. Always address patients as Mr., Mrs., Miss or Ms. and by his or her last name, unless otherwise directed by the patient. The clinician must be comfortable with the form of address; excessive informality may lead to problems. As you proceed, keep the patient informed about the plan and sequence of the examination so they can anticipate the next steps. Always have a chaperone

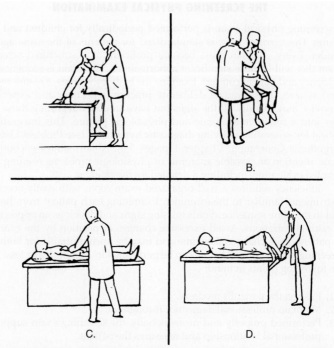

FIG. 3-2 The Office Screening Physical Examination. A. Patient draped and seated (physician facing). **B.** Patient draped and seated (physician to right and back). **C.** Patient draped and supine (physician to right). The patient placed in the left lateral decubitus position to listen at the cardiac apex. **D.** Female pelvic exam: patient draped and supine, knees and hips flexed (physician at foot).

present for opposite gender genital and female breast exams; avoid delays by alerting staff of the need for their presence before entering the room. Preserve and protect the patient's modesty keeping genitalia and female breasts covered when not being directly examined. Always observe first without comment and control facial and body language throughout the exam. Remember, patients observe clinicians as closely as clinicians observe patients. Be sure communications, both verbal and nonverbal, convey professionalism and inspire confidence.

Performing the Screening Examination

Phase A. Vital signs; inspection, general and close; palpation of the head, ears, eyes, nose, and throat.

Patient and examiner positions. The patient is seated on the exam table, draped and facing the examiner.

The clinician cleans their hands in view of the patient.

Vital signs. Obtain the vital signs or, if previously obtained, review them rechecking abnormal findings.

General inspection. Note the patient's general appearance. Inspect the head and face, sclera and conjunctivae, external ears, scalp, skin of the head and neck, the hands and fingernails, and the skin of the arms. To expose the scalp, brush hair back moving against the grain.

Close inspection. Examine the ears with the otoscope, check hearing, test visual fields by confrontation, elicit extraocular movements, observe pupil size and reactions, examine the fundi, and inspect the oral cavity and oropharynx using a tongue blade to expose the posterior pharynx, lateral tongue, and gums.

Palpation. Palpate any concerning areas of head, face, or mouth using gloved bimanual palpation for intraoral lesions. Palpate any hand, wrist, and elbow joint deformity for synovitis or effusion. Palpate all skin rashes.

Phase B. Inspection of the back of the head, neck, back, and shoulders; palpation of the neck, shoulders, and back; percussion of the spine and lungs; auscultation of the lungs.

Patient and examiner positions. Patient seated and draped; examiner stands and/or sits on the exam table behind and to the patient's right.

Inspection. Expose the patient's back inspecting the skin; inspect the neck from back and side; check range of neck motion.

Palpation. Palpate the anterior neck noting carotid pulsations, thyroid, and position of the trachea; search each lymph node bed for adenopathy; identify the thoracic and lumbar vertebral spines by inspection and palpation, note scoliosis or excessive kyphosis or lordosis; palpate any deformity or swelling of the neck, back, shoulders, or scapulae.

Percussion. Use direct fist percussion to check for spinal or costovertebral angle tenderness; percuss the chest front and back comparing right to left and apices to bases; percuss in inspiration and expiration to ascertain movement of the diaphragm.

Auscultation. Auscultate the chest posteriorly, laterally, and anteriorly under the gown, comparing right to left and apices to bases.

Phase C (female patients). The seated breast examination.

Patient and examiner position. Patient draped and seated facing the examiner. After proper explanation, expose the breasts while the patient sits with the arms relaxed.

Inspection. Inspect for symmetry, skin dimpling, and nipple retraction; have the patient press her hands to her waist then raise her hands over her head, each time repeating the inspection.

Palpation. Pendulous breasts are most easily examined bimanually in this position.

Phase D. Examination of the anterior neck and chest, breasts, axillae, abdomen, legs, and feet.

Patient and examiner positions. Patient is draped lying supine with examiner standing on the patient's right, even if left-handed. Starting at the neck, work toward the feet exposing one area at a time: the neck, anterior chest, each breast separately, abdomen, groin, and legs.

Neck

Inspection. Observe the neck veins for fullness and pulsations.

Chest and precordium

Inspection. Inspect for deformities of the sternum and ribs then identify the apical impulse.

Palpation. Palpate the apical impulse then search for lifts, heaves, and other palpable cardiac signs.

Percussion. Percuss the lung fields anteriorly identifying the border of cardiac dullness.

Auscultation. Starting at the apical impulse, identify the first heart sound. Listen at the apex, the lower and upper left sternal borders, in the second right intercostal space, and at the carotid bifurcation. Next auscultate lung sounds on the anterior chest and in supraclavicular fossae.

Breasts. Expose each breast separately.

Inspection. Inspect the breasts for symmetry, skin dimpling, or nipple retraction.

Palpation. Palpate the breasts and nipples.

Axillae

Inspection. Lift the arms exposing the axilla to inspection.

Palpation. With patient's arms at their sides, palpate for axillary and infraclavicular lymph nodes.

Abdomen. Reposition the drape over the chest and expose the abdomen from below the breasts to the symphysis pubis. Relax the abdominal wall muscles by having the patient flex the hips and knees.

Inspection. Observe the symmetry and shape of the abdomen while noting scars and skin lesions. Tensing the abdominal muscles will reveal an abdominal wall hernia (Fig. 3-3).

Auscultation. Listen over the epigastrium, both flanks, and both femoral triangles.

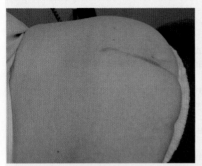 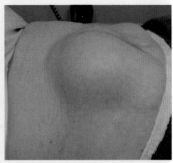

FIG. 3-3 Abdominal Wall Hernia. This hernia is not evident when the patient is at rest on the exam table. Straining forces the abdominal contents into the hernia as the abdominal wall muscles contract.

Percussion. Percuss the abdomen noting areas of tympany or tenderness. Identify the liver by definitive percussion. Percuss above the left costal margin for splenomegaly.

Palpation. Perform superficial and deep palpation of the abdomen. Palpate deeply to identify the aorta then palpate both femoral pulses and the inguinal lymph nodes.

Legs and feet. Cover the abdomen then expose the legs and feet.

Inspection. Inspect skin, muscles, and joints. Keep genitalia covered with a tucked sheet when examining the inner thighs. Flex each hip to 90° and perform internal and external rotation.

Palpation. Palpate dorsalis pedis and posterior tibial pulses. Palpate for edema and any areas of asymmetry, deformity, or joint enlargement.

Return the patient to the sitting position. This is the time to do further neurologic examination as indicated by the history and exam to this point.

Phase E. Supplementary neurological exam, sitting.
Patient and examiner positions. Patient is draped and seated facing the examiner.

Screening neurologic exam. Test cranial nerves, muscle tone and strength in the arms, reflexes, and sensation (position, vibration, touch, and 10-g monofilament), followed by stance, gait, and leg strength in Phase F.

Phase F. Supplemental neurologic and spine exams, standing. Done only if the history or exam suggests neurologic disease or back problems.

Patient and examiner positions. Patient is standing facing the examiner.

Inspection. Observe the stance, then perform the Romberg maneuver. Check the range of spinal motion. The patient walks away from the examiner, then turns and walks back; repeat on tip toes and heels. Have the patient hop on the balls of both feet, and then, if possible, on one foot at a time.

Phase G. The urogenital exams
Patient and examiner positions. Female patients should be in the lithotomy position, male patients standing; examiner at the foot of the table.

Females. With the help of an assistant, the patient assumes the lithotomy position. Perform the pelvic and rectal exams, see page 34.

Males. The patient stands facing the examiner.

Inspection. Inspect the penis, scrotum, and inguinal areas.

Palpation. Palpate the testes and evaluate for inguinal hernias.
     Next, have the patient turn and bend over the exam table, or lie on the table in the left lateral decubitus position.

Inspection. Examine the perineum and anus.

Palpation. Perform the rectal and prostate exams.
     Provide tissues for the patient to clean themselves and repeat hand hygiene in view of the patient. Excuse yourself and exit the room.

Phase H. Concluding the visit. The patient dresses while alone in the exam room. When you return, make sure the patient is comfortable. Review the exam findings, problem list, and recommendations for diagnostic tests, treatment, and follow-up. Conclude by asking if there are any questions. Arrange a follow-up appointment appropriate for the patient and the problems.
     The preceding routine has served the senior author well for many years. Remember, the screening examination's purpose is to detect significant abnormalities in any body region or system, establish a baseline against which future findings are compared, and continually hone the clinician's exam skills. Truncating the exam in the interest of false efficiency leads to overlooking important findings and loss of valuable clinical experience.

ULTRASOUND IN BEDSIDE DIAGNOSIS

Ultrasound is a versatile diagnostic modality permitting real-time bedside visualization of dynamic anatomy synergizing naturally with the physical exam. If ultrasound is being considered to confirm or exclude a disease process, then an initial bedside ultrasound could prove useful increasing efficiency.

Technical Considerations: A basic understanding of the physics of ultrasonography is essential for proper use of this tool. Ultrasound imaging detects ultrasound waves reflecting from the body's tissues. The intensity of the reflected wave is directly proportional to the tissue density. The exceptions are gas-filled structures which do not transmit the ultrasound wave and therefore block penetration to deeper structures, and, at the other extreme, bone so dense that ultrasound cannot penetrate. The boundaries between tissues of different density are seen most clearly. This is an important consideration in deciding which probe to use and how to obtain the best image.

B-mode. Basic gray scale two-dimensional images refer to the standard black and white image on the ultrasound monitor.

Machine presets. Most machines have settings that will adjust an image based on the anatomy being scanned.

Depth. The depth controls how much distance into the body the image displays in the far field.

Gain. This adjusts the signal amplification, essentially how hard the machine "listens" for returning echoes. As the gain is increased, all returning echoes are amplified producing a brighter image. The correct gain is that which balances the desired signal against the background noise.

Zoom. This function allows magnification of one area on the screen.

M-mode. This is the mode to visualize moving structures. The motion occurring in a one-dimensional scan line is displayed on the vertical axis over time on the horizontal axis. It is used in conjunction with B-mode scanning. The M-mode cursor is placed over the moving object on the B-mode image, and the M-mode button is pressed. This is very helpful in measuring the respiratory variability of the inferior vena cava (to assess volume status) and in evaluating the chest for pneumothorax.

Probe selection. Ultrasound probes are described by the size and shape of their face (footprint). High-frequency probes provide better resolution at the expense of decreased penetration compared with low-frequency probes which provide better penetration with less resolution. Three basic probes are used for a goal-directed ultrasound.

Linear (frequency 5–13 MHz). High frequency and better for imaging superficial structures and vessels.

Curvilinear (frequency 1–8 MHz). Wider footprint and lower frequency for transabdominal imaging.

Phased array probe (frequency 2–8 MHz). Smaller footprint which allows maneuvering between ribs which is ideal for echocardiography.

Ultrasound orientation. Orientation is a key to understanding what is seen on the display screen. The two main aspects of orientation are: (1) how the indicator is oriented relative to the screen, and (2) how the probe and the indicator are oriented relative to the patient. Ultrasound orientation can be challenging because it involves understanding how a two-dimensional plane cuts through a three-dimensional object not just in the three standard planes (sagittal, transverse, or coronal), but at any orientation.

Indicator–screen orientation. The "indicator" on the probe may differ between manufacturers but is typically a bump or a groove. There are two rules for this orientation: (1) the left side of the screen corresponds to the side of the probe marked with the indicator, and (2) the top of the screen displays structures closer to the probe and the bottom of the screen those farthest away from the probe.

Indicator–patient orientation. Once indicator–screen orientation is verified, the probe is placed on the patient, and images are viewed on the screen. Most diagnostic ultrasounds are performed using the standard orientation where the indicator (screen left) is toward the patient's right, patients head, or in the arc between these directions.

Anatomic planes. There are three standard anatomic planes scanned in diagnostic ultrasonography.

Transverse plane. The transverse plane is obtained by placing the probe on the anterior surface of the patient with indicator directed toward the patient's right. In this orientation, anterior structures will be toward the top of the screen, and right-sided structures will be on the left side of the screen as viewed.

Sagittal plane. The sagittal plane is obtained by placing the probe on the anterior of the patient with the indicator toward the patient's head. In this orientation, anterior structures will be toward the top of the screen, and the patient's head (cephalad structures) is to the left of the screen and feet (caudal structures) to the right.

Coronal plane. The coronal plane is obtained by placing the probe on the right or left flank with the indicator to the patient's head. If the probe is on the right flank, the top of the screen will be right and the bottom left. If the probe is on the left, the top of the screen will be left and the bottom right. In both the cases, the indicator should be directed to the patient's head, and thus the cephalad structures will be on the left of the screen and caudal structures will be on right.

Scope of Ultrasound in Diagnostic Examination

Symptom- or sign-based ultrasound. This uses specific algorithms that delineate which organ system should be examined based on patient's primary complaints, e.g., shortness of breath, chest pain, undifferentiated hypotension, or undifferentiated abdominal pain. *Bedside ultrasound should be limited and goal-directed*, which means that the purpose of the examination must be clearly specified and goal-directed to impact the clinical decision-making of the physician performing the exam. If there is suspicion of a particular disease, the study should be limited to a specific organ system that can be expeditiously evaluated. After formulating a diagnostic hypothesis and differential diagnosis based on the patient's presenting symptoms and signs, a quick focused ultrasound may identify the correct diagnosis and hasten treatment. These are some examples where ultrasound can be a useful adjunct to physical examination:

Abdominal pain. A quick bedside ultrasound can be used to identify free fluid, abdominal aortic aneurysm, acute cholecystitis, or hydronephrosis.

Chest pain and shortness of breath. The chest can be evaluated for pleural effusion and the lung for interstitial pulmonary edema. The heart can be assessed for systolic function, pericardial effusion, and signs of right ventricular strain.

Hypotension. Bedside ultrasound can quickly evaluate for free fluid and abdominal aortic aneurysm. Volume status is ascertained from inferior vena cava dimensions. Focused echocardiography identifies cardiac dysfunction and pericardial effusion.

Diagnostic ultrasound for an emergent condition. Ultrasound is used to diagnose an emergent condition at the bedside, e.g., to assess for pneumothorax in a patient presenting shortness of breath or a ruptured aneurysm in a patient presenting with abdominal pain. Ultrasound can assist in the evaluation of an unstable patient who cannot give a good history and/or cannot be safely transported for definitive imaging.

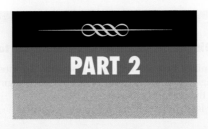

PART 2

The Diagnostic Examination

In order to observe one must learn to compare. In order to
compare one must have observed. By means of observation
knowledge is generated; on the other hand knowledge is
needed for observation. And he observes badly who does
not know how to use what he has observed. The fruit grower
inspects the apple tree with a keener eye than the walker but
no one can see man exactly unless he knows it is man who is
the measure of man.

    The art of observation applied to men is but a branch of
the art of dealing with men.

–BERTHOLD BRECHT
*"Speech to Danish Working Class Actors on the Art of
Improvisation"*

Early learn to appreciate the differences between the
descriptions of disease and the manifestations of that disease in
an individual—the difference between the composite portrait
and one of the component pictures.

–SIR WILLIAM OSLER

Not only to perceive the thing sharply, but to perceive the
relationships between many things sharply perceived.

–THEODORE ROETHKE
"Poetry and Craft"

The Diagnostic Examination: Chapters 4 to 15

This section, organized by body region, explains the diagnostic utility of the symptoms and signs commonly associated with each region, often with a brief summary of the relevant physiology.

Each chapter is organized in the following sequence:

- A brief review of the *Major Systems* examined, including relevant physiology, and anatomic landmarks.
- The *Physical Exam* of the region.
- The *Symptoms* commonly associated with region.
- The *Signs* commonly encountered during examination of this region.
- The *Diseases and Syndromes* associated with symptoms and signs in the region.

The **symptoms** and **signs** are set in boldface type as paragraph heads. These are clues to the pathophysiology of each disease which is important for accurate diagnostic hypotheses. The *key symptoms* are commonly chief complaints. The clinician should be familiar with the diseases and syndromes summarized in the last subsection.

Symptoms, signs, and syndromes marked with the icon • signal the need for urgent evaluation to avoid delaying diagnosis of a life-threatening condition.

The signs are placed in approximate order as they are encountered during the head-to-foot physical exam.

When particular symptoms and signs are useful in differentiating between the various etiologies, they are discussed after the *DDX:* notation.

Some findings are both a symptom and a sign. For instance, severe jaundice can be both the patient's symptom and a clinical sign. In these instances, the finding is discussed where it most commonly occurs: vomiting is most often a symptom, though it can be witnessed; tenderness, although noted by the patient, is a sign elicited by the examiner.

Diseases and syndromes associated with each symptom and sign are listed under **CLINICAL OCCURRENCE.**

CHAPTER 4

Vital Signs, Anthropometric Data, and Pain

This chapter discusses the vital signs (temperature, pulse, respirations, and blood pressure [BP]), followed by measures of body size (height, weight, and body-mass-index [BMI]), and finishes with pain assessment.

VITAL SIGNS

Why are temperature, pulse, respirations, and BP called *vital* signs? These are the signs of life (L. *vitalis*, from *vita*: life); their presence confirms life and their absence confirms death. The more abnormal these parameters become, singly, but especially in combination, the greater the life is threatened. Since ancient times, practitioners have used skin temperature, pulse, and respirations as prognostic signs. More recently, the BP was found to have similar predictive value. Entire texts were written on the interpretation of pulse, fever, and respiratory patterns. It is now apparent that these signs are insufficient for establishing a specific diagnosis. On the other hand, they are sensitive indicators of disordered physiology and are useful in forming pathophysiologic hypotheses and differential diagnoses. They are strongly correlated with severity of illness and outcome.

Body Temperature: Internal body temperature is tightly regulated to maintain vital organ function, particularly the brain. Temperature deviation of more than 4°C above or below normal can produce life-threatening cellular dysfunction. Internal temperature is regulated by the hypothalamus, which maintains a temperature set point. The autonomic nervous system maintains body temperature by regulating blood flow, conducting heat from the internal organs to the skin, and innervating sweat glands. Increasing flow and dilating cutaneous capillaries radiate heat away by conductive loss whereas sweat increases evaporative heat loss. Behavioral adaptations are also important. In hot conditions, people become less active seeking shade or a cooler environment. Decreased body temperature is countered by shivering, which generates heat, and by behavioral adaptations such as putting on clothes and seeking a warmer environment. Sustained temperature deviation indicates a change in the set point, increased heat production, decreased heat dissipation, failure of the regulatory systems, or any combination of those.

Record the patient's temperature at each visit to establish a baseline for future reference. Deviations from this baseline are either fever or hypothermia. Scales on clinical thermometers are either Fahrenheit or Celsius. Conveniently remembered clinical equivalents are 35°C = 95°F, 37°C = 98.6°F, and 40°C = 104°F.

Normal temperature.
Normal body temperature. Internal body temperature is maintained within a narrow range, $\pm0.6°C$ (1.0°F). The population range of this set point varies from 36.0°C to 37.5°C (96.5–99.5°F), making it necessary to establish a baseline for each patient. Without a baseline, an oral temperature above 37.5°C (99.5°F) and a rectal temperature over 38.0°C (100.5°F) is considered fever.

Diurnal variation. Daytime workers, who sleep at night, have minimum temperatures between 3 and 4 AM, rising slowly to a maximum between 8 and 10 PM. This pattern is reversed in nightshift workers. Transitioning from one pattern to the other requires several days.

Regional temperature variation. Heat is produced by cellular metabolism. The temperature is highest in the liver and lowest at the skin surface. Customarily, body temperature is measured in the rectum, mouth, ear, axilla, or groin. Among these sites, rectal temperature is ~0.3°C (0.6°F) higher than that of the oral or groin reading; the axillary temperature is ~0.5°C (1.0°F) less than the oral value.

Elevated temperature. Increased temperature results from excessive heat production or impaired heat dissipation. Each mechanism may be a normal response to physiologic challenge or be due to damage to the thermoregulatory pathways. *Fever* is a physiologic elevation of the set point for body temperature by the hypothalamus. Pathologic elevations of body temperature, *hyperthermia*, results from unregulated heat generation and/or impaired heat exchange with the environment.

Fever. Release of endogenous pyrogens, particularly interleukin (IL-1), triggered by tissue necrosis, infection, inflammation, and some tumors, elevates the hypothalamic set point leading to increased body temperature. Fevers often begin with a chill and shivering, which generates heat, accompanied by cutaneous vasoconstriction reducing heat loss; *rigors* are particularly severe chills. Be aware that the skin temperature may be low or normal, while the core temperature is markedly elevated. The skin becomes warm again when the new set point is reached. Fever is accompanied by tachycardia in proportion to the temperature elevation. The body returns to normal temperature through dissipation of heat by flushing and sweating. *Night sweats* are an exaggeration of the normal diurnal temperature variation, the sweat marking nocturnal temperature decline. They occur in many chronic infections, inflammatory diseases, and some malignancies, particularly lymphomas. Fever requires special consideration in immunocompromised, HIV-infected, and hospitalized patients. Some patients cannot mount a febrile response to infection, particularly those with renal failure, on high doses of corticosteroids, and the elderly.
   CLINICAL OCCURRENCE: *Congenital:* Familial Mediterranean fever, other familial periodic fevers, porphyrias; *Endocrine:* Hyperthyroidism, pheochromocytoma; *Degenerative/Idiopathic:* Seizures; *Infectious:* Bacterial, viral, rickettsial, fungal, and parasitic infections either localized (e.g., SBE) or systemic (occult abscess is common); *Inflammatory/Immune:* Systemic lupus erythematosus (SLE), acute rheumatic fever, Still disease, vasculitis, serum

sickness, any severe local or systemic inflammatory process (e.g., sarcoidosis, bullous dermatosis); *Mechanical/Traumatic:* Tissue necrosis (e.g., myocardial infarction, pulmonary infarction, stroke), exercise; *Metabolic/Toxic:* Drug reactions, gout; *Neoplastic:* Leukemia, lymphomas, and solid tumors; *Psychosocial:* Factitious; *Vascular:* Thrombophlebitis, tissue ischemia and infarction, vasculitis, subarachnoid hemorrhage.

Fever patterns. The pattern of temperature fluctuations may be a useful diagnostic clue.

Continuous fever. The diurnal temperature fluctuation is 0.5°C to 1.0°C (1.0°F to 1.5°F).

Remittent fever. The diurnal fluctuation is more than 1.1°C (2.0°F) without normal readings.

Intermittent fever. Fever episodes are separated by days. Examples include tertian fever of *Plasmodium vivax*, quartan fever of *Plasmodium malariae*.

Relapsing fever. Fevers occur every 5 to 7 days in borreliosis and Colorado tick fever.

Episodic fever. Typical of the familial periodic fevers, fever lasts for days or longer followed by a remission of at least 2 weeks. [Drenth PPH, van der Meer JWM. Hereditary periodic fever. *N Engl J Med*. 2001;345:1748–1757].

Pel–Epstein fever. Characteristic of Hodgkin disease, several days of continuous or remittent fever are followed by afebrile remissions lasting an irregular number of days.

Fever of unknown origin (FUO). Three conditions define an FUO: (1) the illness has lasted >3 weeks; (2) the temperature is repeatedly >38.3°C (100.9°F); and (3) more than three outpatient visits or ≥3 days in the hospital have not yielded a diagnosis. In the modern era the most common causes of FUO in immunocompetent patients are noninfectious inflammatory diseases, infections, and malignancies, especially hematologic malignancies. However, fever remains unexplained in almost 50% of patients, especially those with episodic.

CLINICAL OCCURRENCE: *Noninfectious Inflammatory Diseases:* Polymyalgia rheumatica, Still disease, SLE, sarcoidosis, Crohn disease, vasculitis (giant cell arteritis, Wegener disease, polyarteritis nodosa); *Infections:* Endocarditis, tuberculosis, urinary tract infection, cytomegalovirus, Epstein–Barr virus, HIV, subphrenic abscess, cholangitis and cholecystitis; *Neoplasms:* Non-Hodgkin lymphoma, Hodgkin disease, leukemia, adenocarcinoma; *Miscellaneous:* Habitual hyperthermia, subacute thyroiditis, Addison disease, drug fever.

Rheumatic fever. See Chapter 13, page 586.

Pathologic overproduction and impaired dissipation of heat.

- **Hyperthermia.** Unregulated heat production or damage to heat dissipation systems leads to rapid and severe uncompensated temperature elevation. Common causes of fever rarely produce hyperthermia. More commonly, the environment, impaired judgment, or toxin exposure is the direct cause.

CLINICAL OCCURRENCE: *Impaired Heat Loss:* High environmental temperature and humidity, moderately hot weather for a person with congenital absence of sweat glands, congestive heart failure, heat stroke, anticholinergic drugs and toxins. Poverty, homelessness, and psychosis all inhibit the ability to adapt to environmental challenges. *Increased Heat Generation:* Malignant hyperthermia, neuroleptic malignant syndrome, heavy exertion in hot and humid environment.

- *Neuroleptic malignant syndrome.* Medications disrupt central dopamine pathways leading to uncontrolled hyperthermia. One to two days after exposure to a neuroleptic (antipsychotic) drug, the patient develops hyperthermia, rigidity, altered mental status, labile BP, tachycardia, tachypnea, and progressive metabolic acidosis. Myoglobinuria and acute renal failure can occur. It can be confused with worsening of the psychotic state leading to delayed diagnosis and administration of more neuroleptics.

- *Malignant hyperthermia.* An inherited disorder of muscle sarcoplasmic reticulum calcium release produces sustained muscle contraction on exposure to inhalational anesthetics or succinylcholine. The patient develops rigidity, hyperthermia, rhabdomyolysis, metabolic acidosis, and hemodynamic instability. Prompt recognition and treatment is lifesaving.

- *Heat stroke.* Failure of the thermoregulatory system leads to decreased sweating and rapid increases in core body temperature. Cardiovascular disease increases risk by restricting the increased cardiac output necessary for skin perfusion. Diuretics and anticholinergic drugs also increase the risk. The typical victim is a chronically ill adult confined in a hot, humid environment during heat waves. The patient is often delirious or comatose; the diagnostic clue is the hot dry skin.

Heat exhaustion (heat prostration). Exertion in a hot, usually humid, environment leads to loss of fluid and electrolytes and decreased ability to dissipate body heat. This is classically seen in younger individuals participating in athletic events or working in hot, humid environments. Symptoms are palpitations, faintness, lassitude, headache, nausea, vomiting, and cramps. Patients have tachycardia, diminished BP, diaphoresis, ashen, cool, moist skin, and dilated pupils. The core body temperature is elevated, but <40°C (104°F). Untreated it can lead to heat stroke.

Factitious fever. Common in malingering and Munchausen syndrome, clues are unexpectedly high temperatures with unusual fluctuation, and fever without other signs of acute illness.

Infections presenting as fever. Fever accompanies many infections and inflammatory diseases. The following are diseases that often present with fever without localizing symptoms or signs.

Tuberculosis. Infection with *Mycobacterium tuberculosis* may be limited to the lung or spread via the lymph nodes or bloodstream to affect any organ. *Primary infection* is in the lung and may leave a calcified middle or lower lobe nodule and hilar lymph nodes (Ghon complex). *Progressive primary tuberculosis* is seen commonly in HIV-infected patients but may occur in otherwise healthy people. It presents as progressive lung infection (usually in the lower lung zones), pleural effusion, and lymphadenopathy. Immunosuppressed hosts and dark-skinned races have increased risk for early hematogenous dissemination. *Miliary tuberculosis* presents with fever, anorexia, and weight loss and may have hepatomegaly, splenomegaly, and/or lymphadenopathy. *Reactivation tuberculosis* most commonly occurs in the lung apices. Patients present with fever, malaise, night sweats, cough with sputum production, and lung consolidation and/or cavity formation. Reactivation can also occur in bones, especially the spine (Pott disease), the peritoneum, meninges, kidneys and urinary tract, lymph nodes, intestine, and pericardium [Tanoue LT, Mark EJ. Case records of the Massachusetts General Hospital. Case 1–2003. *N Engl J Med*. 2003;348:151–161].

Endemic North American fever syndromes. Several infections, presenting as an undifferentiated febrile illness, are found exclusively or with increased frequency in certain regions of the United States. In the first days of illness, they cannot be clinically differentiated, so travel history is essential for timely recognition and treatment.
  CLINICAL OCCURRENCE: Rocky Mountain spotted fever (RMSF), other rickettsial infections, babesiosis, ehrlichiosis and anaplasmosis, Lyme disease, Q fever, leptospirosis, relapsing fever, Colorado tick fever, and other viral exanthems.

Rickettsial spotted fever syndromes. Rickettsia are transmitted by arthropod bites and usually present as systemic disease with headache and rash without localizing symptoms or signs. Travel and exposure history are essential for an accurate differential and evaluation. Prompt treatment can be lifesaving. *DDX:* RMSF is described below; it produces the archetypical syndrome. The other rickettsial diseases present in a similar fashion with severe headache, fever, myalgias, and malaise. Careful history and exam minimize confusion with babesiosis, Lyme disease, or Ehrlichiosis and anaplasmosis.

Rocky Mountain spotted fever. *Rickettsia rickettsii* are transmitted by the bite of an infected tick. The obligate intracellular parasites infect endothelial cells producing acute systemic illness. The disease is highly endemic to the Atlantic coastal states. The onset is nonspecific with headache, fever, chills, myalgias, and asthenia frequently accompanied by nausea, vomiting, and abdominal pain. An erythematous macular rash spreading centrally from the wrists and ankles may be seen after the third day; the palms and soles may be affected, and dorsal edema of the hands and feet is characteristic. The lesions are initially blanching but progress to papules which become non-blanching purpura. Systemic involvement leads to widespread organ damage and death in 25% of untreated patients.

Louse-borne typhus (epidemic typhus, trench fever), endemic typhus (murine typhus), and rickettsialpox. All are endemic to the United States and are also imported. Rickettsialpox, seen in the Northeastern United States, has a papular erythematous rash at the mite bite site that becomes a necrotic eschar with regional lymphadenopathy. Nausea and vomiting are highly characteristic of murine typhus.

Babesiosis. Babesia are intracellular protozoa transmitted by infected Ixodes ticks. Babesiosis is a worldwide zoonotic infection in which humans are infected incidentally. They parasitize red blood cells and can be identified on blood smears. It is highly endemic in the Atlantic coastal regions of New York, Connecticut, Rhode Island, and Massachusetts. It has been reported from other locales and imported cases are seen. There is gradual onset of fever, headache, myalgias, and fatigue. There may be hepatosplenomegaly and hemolysis. A rash does not occur. Coincident infection with other tick-borne diseases (Lyme and anaplasmosis) should be considered.

Lyme disease. Infection with *Borrelia burgdorferi* is transmitted by bites of Ixodes ticks. Initially infection is in the skin with a characteristic rash, but it disseminates to virtually all organs and tissues within days. If the characteristic erythema migrans rash is missed or ignored, the patient presents with fever, headache, myalgias, neck stiffness, arthralgias, and striking fatigue and malaise. These symptoms may persist for weeks, gradually resolving or being replaced with neurologic symptoms and signs (peripheral neuropathy, mononeuritis multiplex, cranial neuropathy, aseptic meningitis, or chorea); Bell palsy is quite common at this stage. Cardiac conduction block with symptomatic bradycardia may be seen. The most common late manifestation is an inflammatory large joint oligoarthritis, commonly affecting the knee.

Ehrlichiosis and anaplasmosis. Ehrlichia and anaplasma are intracellular parasites that reproduce in either mononuclear phagocytic cells in the blood and tissues *(Ehrlichia chaffeensis)* or granulocytes *(Ehrlichia ewingii and Anaplasma phagocytophilia) forming vacuolar inclusions (morula) visible on light microscopy.* Human monocytotropic ehrlichiosis and *ehrlichiosis ewingii* are transmitted by the Lone Star tick *(Amblyomma americanum)* and are most prevalent in the south-central, southeastern, and Mid-Atlantic States. Onset of both diseases is nonspecific with fever, headache, malaise, and myalgia often accompanied by nausea, vomiting, and diarrhea. Rash, cough, and confusion may be seen. *A. phagocytophilia* is transmitted by bites of the Ixodes ticks with high concentrations in the northeastern and upper Midwestern states. A high index of suspicion is required to make these diagnoses promptly.

Cat-scratch disease. Gram-negative bacilli *(Bartonella henselae)* are inoculated by the scratch, lick, or bite of a healthy cat. The organisms travel to the regional lymph nodes then disseminate. Symptoms are nonspecific with malaise and headache. Signs include fever, an inoculation site papule or pustule, followed by painful fluctuant regional lymphadenopathy with overlying erythema. In immunocompromised hosts dissemination can lead to hepatitis (peliosis hepatitis), osteomyelitis, or meningoencephalitis. Conjunctival infection produces preauricular lymphadenopathy (Parinaud oculoglandular syndrome).

Leptospirosis. Leptospirosis is a worldwide zoonosis transmitted by ingestion of contaminated water or contact with urine or tissues of infected animals. The onset is abrupt with fever, headache, myalgias, and malaise often accompanied by conjunctival suffusion. There may be muscle tenderness, lymphadenopathy, hepatosplenomegaly, or rashes. History of contact with contaminated water in the summer or fall is a key to making the diagnosis. Men are more often exposed than women. If not initially recognized and treated symptoms may subside or disappear for a week only to recur. Severe disease causes multiorgan failure known as Weil syndrome with jaundice, renal insufficiency, and hemorrhage.

Relapsing fever. *Borrellia* spp. infects humans from louse or tick bites. The organisms can change their antigenic coating of variable major proteins causing escape from an initially effective immune response producing a relapsing illness. Tick-borne relapsing fever is a zoonotic infection. The patient presents with fever, myalgias, chills, nausea, vomiting, and arthralgias. Abdominal pain, cough, photophobia, neck stiffness, and rash are less common. Delirium can accompany the high fever. The illness reaches a crisis in 3 to 5 days when the fever peaks with chills followed by lysis of fever, diaphoresis, and hypotension. Relapse occurs with the next antigenic variant after 7 to 9 days. Each crisis is equivalent to a Jarisch–Herxheimer reaction. *DDX:* Louse-borne relapsing fever is transmitted by the human body louse. The symptoms are similar. It is endemic to portions of Ethiopia but has caused major epidemics in wartime Europe.

Q fever. This is a zoonotic infection with *Coxiella burnetii* transmitted by infected cattle, goats, and sheep, especially via products of conception during delivery, and infected milk. Both inhalation and ingestion of organisms produce infection. The illness has protean manifestations. Common symptoms are fever, severe fatigue and headache, cough, nausea, and vomiting. Diarrhea and rash may be present. Presentations include an influenza-like illness, pneumonia, hepatitis, meningoencephalitis, and culture negative endocarditis. Chronic disease with hepatosplenomegaly implies persistent endocardial infection. Diagnosis is difficult, requiring a high index of suspicion, and usually made by serology.

Colorado tick fever. Colorado tick fever virus is transmitted by infected wood ticks (*Dermacentor andersoni*) in the northern Rocky mountain states from late spring to fall. It causes a biphasic illness manifest as fever, myalgia, headache, and occasionally meningoencephalitis and rash. It is self-limited.

Fever in returning travelers. This frequent problem is associated with rapid global air travel. Patients present with fever and a history of travel to exotic, usually tropical, locations. In addition to common illnesses, a host of unusual infections are possible.

Dengue. The four dengue viruses are transmitted by Aedes mosquitoes well adapted to tropical and subtropical urban environments worldwide. Common in travelers returning from the Caribbean, patients present with fever, headache, back pain, and severe myalgias (break-bone fever). Dengue hemorrhagic fever is potentially fatal.

Chikungunya. Extensively distributed in the tropics and subtropics, it is transmitted by Aedes mosquitoes. Key features include polyarthralgia, myalgias, rash, and thrombocytopenia. Polyarthralgia begins 2 to 5 days after onset of fever and commonly involves multiple joints. Rash is usually macular or maculopapular often starting on the limbs and trunk.

Zika virus. Found mostly in South and Central America, the Caribbean, sub-Saharan Africa, and South and Southeast Asia, it is transmitted by Aedes mosquitoes. Key features include myalgia, pruritic rash, arthralgia, nonpurulent conjunctivitis, and thrombocytopenia.

Malaria. *P. vivax, Plasmodium ovale, P. malariae P. knowlesi, and Plasmodium falciparum* are transmitted by Anopheles mosquitoes. Initial hepatocyte infection is followed by invasion of erythrocytes. Cyclical release of mature merozoites from ruptured erythrocytes produces cyclical fever. *Plasmodium falciparum* infection can produce severe hemolysis, hypoglycemia, and obstruction of cerebral capillaries (cerebral malaria). *P. vivax* and *P. ovale* can persist in the liver causing relapsing infections. Patients present with fever, headache, malaise, and myalgias. Nausea, vomiting, and abdominal pain may be present, and progression to delirium and coma can occur. Prompt diagnosis relies on the travel history and examination of blood smears by trained personnel. *DDX:* Dengue fever may present a similar clinical picture, but blood smears are negative.

Typhoid Fever. Disseminated *Salmonella typhi* or *Salmonella paratyphi* infection follows ingestion of contaminated food or water. The incubation period is 3 days to as much as 60 days. Symptoms are chills and prolonged, persistent fever, prostration, cough, epistaxis, and constipation or diarrhea. There is slowly progressing lassitude, abdominal distention and tenderness, splenomegaly, and rose spots on the trunk and chest. Delirium may occur. Complications include localized infections (gallbladder, bone, liver, spleen, endocarditis, pneumonia, meningitis, and orchitis), gastrointestinal bleeding and bowel perforation with peritonitis.

Brucellosis. Systemic infection with *Brucella abortus* (cattle), *suis* (pigs), *melitensis* (goats), or *canis* (dogs) is acquired by exposure to unpasteurized milk, and contaminated meat or other animal tissues. Lassitude and weight loss accompany recurrent fever and sweating, *undulant fever*. Back and joint pains are common. Physical findings include splenomegaly, lymphadenopathy, and tender bones or joints. The disease may be acute or chronic [Drapkin MS, Kamath RS, Kim JY. Case 26–2012: a 70-year-old woman with fever and back pain. *NEJM.* 2012;367:754; Vogt T, Hasler P. A woman with panic attacks and double vision who liked cheese. *Lancet.* 1999;354:300].

Rickettsiosis. Rickettsial infections endemic to other countries, as well as those endemic to North America, may be imported. Fever, headache, myalgias, and rash are characteristic of the *spotted fever syndromes* (e.g., Boutonneuse fever). In addition, cough is a prominent symptom in *scrub typhus* imported from Australia, the southern Pacific region and southern and southeast Asia. An inoculation eschar from the mite bite and regional lymphadenopathy typical of *ulceroglandular syndromes* may be present (Chapter 6, page 142). Because the mite vector frequently bites in moist areas of the body that are usually covered, such as the genitalia, the perineum, and the area beneath the breasts, the eschar of scrub typhus is often missed. An eschar should be specifically sought. In travelers returning from southern Africa, one or more eschars may point to the relatively benign African tick typhus (caused by *Rickettsia africae*). In those returning from South or Southeast Asia, an eschar suggests scrub typhus (*Orientia tsutsugamushi* infection), a potentially fatal disease

Lowered body temperature.
Hypothermia. Decreased hypothalamic set point, insufficient heat genera-tion, and excessive heat loss due to behaviors and environmental conditions all lead to a sustained decline in core temperature. Low body temperature impairs cellular metabolism and brain function, particularly judgment, and the combination prevents protection from continued exposure leading to fatal hypothermia. Hypothermia protects tissues from ischemic injury, so complete recovery is possible from rapid and sustained cooling, even when the patient appears clinically dead. This is especially true for cold-water im-mersion (drowning). Relative or absolute hypothermia in situations where fever would be expected, e.g., severe infection, is a poor prognostic sign. Core temperature is usually lower in older adults making them particularly sus-ceptible to decreased environmental temperatures.

CLINICAL OCCURRENCE: *Endocrine:* Hypothyroidism; *Degenerative/Idiopathic:* Advanced age, seizures; *Infectious:* Sepsis; *Mechanical/Traumatic:* Exposure and immersion, hypothalamic injury from trauma or hemorrhage, burns; *Metabolic/Toxic:* Hypoglycemia, drug overdoses; *Neoplastic:* Brain tumors; *Psychosocial:* Poverty, homelessness, and psychosis impair the abil-ity to adapt to environmental challenges; *Vascular:* Stroke.

The Pulse: Rate, Volume, and Rhythm. The heart's normal pacemaker is the sinoatrial (SA) node in the right atrial wall near the superior vena cava (Fig. 4-1). It generates regular depolarization waves that spread rapidly through both atria. The atrioventricular (AV) node, located in the posterior interatrial septum, delays the impulse during atrial systole prior to its entering the His bundle. The His bundle divides into right and left branches on either side of the interventricular septum exciting the right and left ventricular myocar-dium nearly simultaneously. Changes in atrial or ventricular excitation or AV conduction alter the cardiac rate and/or rhythm. Left ventricular contraction ejects blood into the aorta producing a pulse wave through the arteries whose speed varies with the ejection force and elasticity of the arteries. The pulse's rate and rhythm are functions of the active pacemaker and depolarization pattern in the conduction system and myocardium.

Examining the pulse.
Palpation. Palpate the carotid, radial, femoral, posterior tibial, and dorsalis pedis arteries (Fig. 4-2). Assess rate and rhythm in the radial, carotid, or femo-ral artery. Pulse contour and volume are discussed in Chapter 8, page 334, and Fig. 8-42.

Normal rate and rhythm. Normal sinus rhythm (NSR) is regular at a pulse rate between 55 and 100 beats per minute (bpm). Infants and children have higher rates; consult pediatric references for normal ranges. Well-conditioned

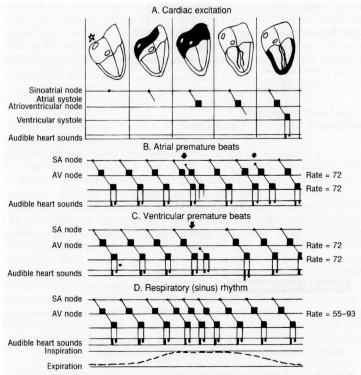

FIG. 4-1 Disturbances of Cardiac Rate and Rhythm I. A. Diagram illustrating the spread of excitation over the heart. The stimulus starts in the SA node and spreads throughout the walls of the atria, finally reaching the AV node, where there is a short delay. The stimulus then proceeds down the His bundle by its two branches along the right and left wall of the interventricular septum to the apex, spreading from there to the muscle of the right and left ventricles. The atria contract before the impulse the leaves the AV node; ventricular systole occurs when the impulse has spread over the ventricles. Note that the heart sounds resulting from ventricular systole are the only physical signs of this process. **B. Atrial premature beat originating outside the SA node, an ectopic beat.** This is followed by a short compensatory pause that cannot ordinarily be detected. **C. An ectopic ventricular beat with a detectable compensatory pause. D. Respiratory or sinus arrhythmia.** The heart rate accelerates near the height of inspiration; this acceleration originates in the SA node. In any dysrhythmia, the heart sounds of a beat following a shortened interval are often fainter than normal; beats following an abnormally long pause are louder than normal. **E. Ventricular rates.**

athletes have resting rates into the low forties. Deconditioned adults may have rates approaching 100 bpm. Ventricular diastole is longer than systole at rates <100 bpm. They become equal at about 100 bpm and, at >100 bpm, systole is longer. Rates <55 bpm are *bradycardias* and those >100 bpm, *tachycardias*. Exertion accelerates the rate to a maximum of 200 bpm in young, healthy adults. The maximum achievable heart rate declines predictably with age. The pulse rhythm is normally regular with slight respiratory variation. Vagus stimulation by breath holding, Valsalva, or carotid sinus massage slows the rate.

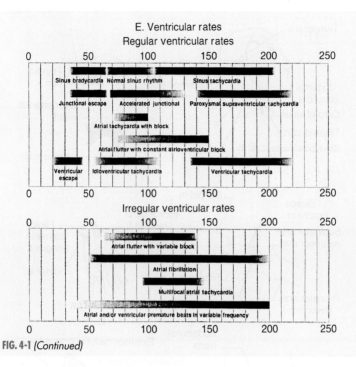

E. Ventricular rates
Regular ventricular rates

Sinus bradycardia — Normal sinus rhythm — Sinus tachycardia

Junctional escape — Accelerated junctional — Paroxysmal supraventricular tachycardia

Atrial tachycardia with block

Atrial flutter with constant atrioventricular block

Ventricular escape — Idioventricular tachycardia — Ventricular tachycardia

Irregular ventricular rates

Atrial flutter with variable block

Atrial fibrillation

Multifocal atrial tachycardia

Atrial and/or ventricular premature beats in variable frequency

FIG. 4-1 *(Continued)*

Variations in rate and rhythm. The signs of heart action are practically all ventricular (Fig. 4-1E); the atria produce only the atrial components of neck vein pulsations, the fourth heart sound, the variably loud first heart sound accompanying AV dissociation, and ventricular filling sounds associated with atrial contraction sometimes heard with AV block. Rhythm disorder hypotheses are grouped by heart rate (slow, normal, fast) and pattern (regular, irregular in consistent pattern—regularly irregular, or irregular without pattern—irregularly irregular). *All rhythm disorders suspected by physical exam must be confirmed or refuted by an ECG.*

Slow regular rhythms. Rates <55 bpm suggest sinus bradycardia, second-degree AV block (Fig. 4-3A), and third-degree AV block with junctional or ventricular escape rhythms (Fig. 4-3B).

Regular rhythms with rates >120 bpm. Sinus tachycardia, atrial flutter with 2:1 AV block, paroxysmal supraventricular tachycardia (PSVT) (Fig. 4-3C), and ventricular tachycardia (VT) are possibilities. *DDX:* The response to vagal stimulation is a clue to the rhythm. In flutter, the rate slows stepwise. Paroxysmal atrial tachycardia (PAT) does not slow but can convert to a normal rate. Sinus rhythm gradually slows and VT does not change.

Regular rhythms with rates of 60 to 120 bpm. These include sinus rhythm, accelerated junctional rhythm (non-paroxysmal junctional tachycardia), atrial

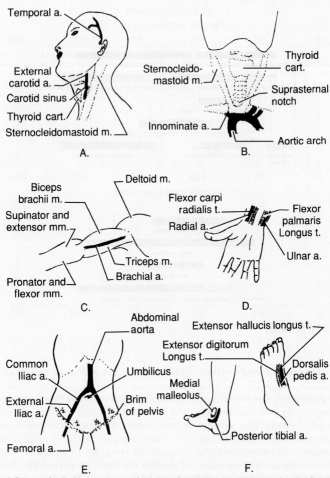

FIG. 4-2 Sites of Palpable Arteries. A. The temporal artery is anterior to the ear and overlies the temporal bone, one of the few normally tortuous arteries. **The common carotid** is deep in the neck near the anterior border of the sternocleidomastoid muscle. The bifurcation of this artery is opposite the superior border of the thyroid cartilage. The carotid sinus is at the bifurcation. **B. Elongation or dilation of the ascending aorta and arch** makes this vessel accessible to palpation in the suprasternal notch. With slight shifting to the right or left, the innominate or left carotid arteries may also be felt in the notch. **C. The brachial artery** lies deep in the biceps-triceps furrow on the medial side of the arm near the elbow. It courses toward the midline of the antecubital fossa, where it is usually just medial to the biceps tendon. **The radial artery** is just medial to the outer border of the radius and lateral to the tendon of the flexor carpi radialis, where the finger can press it against the bone. **The ulnar artery** is in a similar position to the ulna, but it is buried deeper, so it often cannot be felt. **E. The abdominal aorta and parts of the iliac arteries** can usually be felt as generalized pulsations through the abdominal wall. **The femoral artery** is palpable at the inguinal ligament midway between the anterior superior iliac spine and the pubic tubercle. **F. The posterior tibial artery** is palpable as it curves forward below and around the medial malleolus of the tibia. **The dorsalis pedis artery** is felt usually in the groove between the first two tendons on the medial side of the dorsum of the foot.

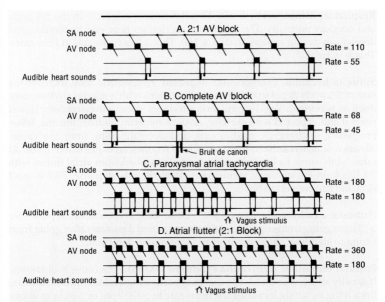

FIG. 4-3 Disturbances of Cardiac Rate and Rhythm II. In all diagrams, the audible heart sounds are the only physical signs indicating the mechanism. **A. Second-degree AV block with a 2:1 ratio.** Alternate stimuli from the atria are blocked in the AV node, so the ventricles beat only half as fast as the atria. The only physical sign is a slow regular heartbeat with first sounds of equal intensity. **B. Complete AV block.** The ventricles beat independently of the atria, usually with a rate <50/min accelerating minimally with exertion. A louder-than-common first sound occurs when ventricular filling is augmented by an atrial contraction occurring by chance at the optimal time; this is called by the French—the "bruit de canon." **C and D.** When ventricular beats are regular with rates between 160 and 220/min, two conditions must be distinguished. **C. Paroxysmal atrial tachycardia. D. Atrial flutter.** Vagal stimulation may convert paroxysmal atrial tachycardia to normal rhythm, but there is no temporary slowing. In contrast, the only response of flutter to vagus stimulus is slowing for a few beats.

tachycardia with block, idioventricular tachycardia (accelerated ventricular rhythm and slow or benign VT), and atrial flutter (Fig. 4-3D) with 3:1 or 4:1 AV block.

Irregular rhythms without pattern. Consider atrial flutter with variable AV block, atrial fibrillation, multifocal atrial tachycardia (MAT), and frequent atrial or ventricular premature beats occurring without a consistent pattern. These rhythms produce rates of 50–200 bpm. Atrial flutter with variable AV block rarely exceeds 150 bpm and MAT is usually 100–150 bpm.

Regularly irregular rhythms. Consider atrial or ventricular premature beats occurring at regular intervals (i.e., bigeminal, trigeminal, and quadrigeminal premature beats) or Mobitz I (Wenckebach) AV block producing grouped beats. An ECG is necessary for definitive diagnosis.

Common dysrhythmias and their physical signs. *Only an electrocardiogram can diagnose specific rhythms.*

Respiratory (sinus) arrhythmia. Depolarizations originate in the SA node and conduct normally. The heart rate accelerates near end-inspiration and decelerates during expiration (Fig. 4-1D). This is less noticeable at slow rates. This is normal.

Sinus tachycardia. Exertion and increased sympathetic tone increase the rate of SA node depolarizations to 100–160 bpm with a regular rhythm; conduction is normal. Vagal stimulation produces smooth deceleration. This is normal and expected with exercise, anxiety, hyperthyroidism, anemia, fever, pregnancy, β-adrenergic medications, and deconditioning from any cause. Absence of tachycardia in these situations requires an explanation. *DDX:* At rates >140, sinus tachycardia must be distinguished from atrial flutter with 2:1 block. In flutter, vagal stimulation slows the rate stepwise; PAT doesn't slow but can convert to NSR.

Orthostatic tachycardia. See page 67, Orthostatic Hypotension. A pulse rise >15 bpm going from supine to sitting or measured 2 minutes after going from sitting to standing, suggests intravascular volume depletion.

Postural orthostatic tachycardia syndrome (POTS). The cause is unknown. It usually affects women 15–50 years of age following a minor illness. Standing from lying or sitting increases the heart rate to >120 bpm or >30 bpm above baseline. Tachycardia is often associated with tremor, palpitations, and nausea (signs of autonomic hyperactivity) or light headedness, weakness, and visual changes (signs presyncope). *Sinus bradycardia.* The slow rate is due to vagal stimulation or a SA node disorder. The rhythm is regular, and conduction is normal. Rates are rarely <40 bpm. This is expected in well-conditioned athletes. Severe hypothyroidism and sick sinus syndrome (SSS) are other causes. *DDX:* The rate accelerates smoothly with exertion.

Sinus rhythm with second-degree AV block. In Mobitz I (Wenckebach) AV block, there is decremental conduction in the AV node so that, after a series of conducted beats, one beat is dropped. This produces grouped beats with a P to QRS ratio of *n:n*–1 (e.g., 3:2, 5:4). In Mobitz II block, SA impulses are regularly blocked in the His bundle or below; complete heart block may occur. The atrial rate is a multiple of the ventricular rate, 2:1, 3:1, 4:1, or higher, e.g., when every third atrial impulse is transmitted, it is 3:1 block. Mobitz I is the most common AV block. The ventricular complexes appear in groups followed by a pause. The beat-to-beat interval shortens until a beat is dropped producing a longer pause, then the cycle repeats. The shortening R-R interval is only apparent on ECG. In Mobitz II block, ventricular systoles occur at regular intervals with a rate dependent upon the sinus rate and degree of block (Fig. 4-3A). Each beat has the same intensity. In 2:1 block, two A-waves may be seen in the jugular vein for each ventricular contraction. Although 2:1 block is relatively common, 3:1 block is rare. *DDX:* In sinus bradycardia and second-degree block the rate increases with exertion.

CLINICAL OCCURRENCE: Acute infections (especially rheumatic fever, Lyme disease, and diphtheria), valvular heart disease, digitalis intoxication, hyperkalemia, drugs (diltiazem, verapamil, β-blockers), coronary artery disease.

- **Third-degree (complete) AV block.** The atria beat regularly, but there is no conduction from the atria to the ventricles. Block may occur in the AV node or ventricular conduction system (His bundle or both bundle branches). Junctional pacemakers establish an escape rhythm at 25–60 bpm; the higher the pacemaker, the faster the escape rate. Ventricular contractions are regular. When an atrial systole precedes ventricular contraction, the intensity of the heart sounds increases (Fig. 4-3B). When ventricular contraction and atrial contraction nearly coincide, there is a booming sound, *bruit de canon*; it comes infrequently, so listen for >60 seconds. The causes are the same as second-degree AV block with the addition of degenerative and granulomatous diseases such as sarcoidosis. *DDX:* Exertion does not accelerate the ventricular rate. The variation in intensity of the first sounds is distinctive.

Premature beats. A depolarization arises from an ectopic focus in the atrium or ventricle producing a premature beat. An atrial premature beat occurs before its expected time (Fig. 4-1B) with a shorter compensatory pause than with ventricular premature beats. If the premature beat occurs shortly after a normal ventricular systole, ventricular filling is minimal, the heart sounds are less intense, and the stroke volume may be insufficient to produce a palpable arterial pulse. Very frequent premature beats are a diagnostic problem (Fig. 4-4A).

Coupled rhythm: bigeminy, trigeminy. One or two normal beats are followed regularly by a premature beat arising from reentry or an ectopic focus in the atrium or ventricle. The ventricular beats are grouped in pairs (bigeminy) or triplets (trigeminy), the last a premature beat; the compensatory pause after the premature beat separates one group from its successor (Fig. 4-4C). Bigeminy has a regular rhythm. Since the premature beat may not be palpable, a regular rhythm at half the true ventricular rate may be suspected if only the peripheral pulse is examined; heart auscultation reveals the bigeminy. As with other premature beats, exercise may restore the normal rhythm. Coupled premature ventricular contractions (PVCs) occur in normal hearts, all forms of organic heart disease and digitalis intoxication. *DDX:* A similar pulse pattern is produced by Mobitz type I second-degree AV block (Wenckebach) with 3:2 Wenckebach simulating bigeminy and 4:3 simulating trigeminy.

Grouped beats and dropped beats. The causes include sinus pauses, SA exit block, second-degree AV block (Mobitz type I or II), or regular premature atrial beats in a trigeminal or quadrigeminal pattern that are blocked in the AV node. A series of two, three, four, or more beats is followed by a pause. The pattern may recur regularly. The rhythm is unchanged by increases in the heart rate. Electrocardiography is essential to distinguish between these rhythms.

Atrial fibrillation. The risk for atrial fibrillation increases with increasing atrial volume. The atria do not contract synchronously. Stimuli arrive randomly at the AV node. Most are blocked but some conduct to the ventricles

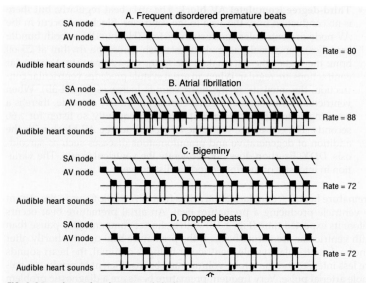

FIG. 4-4 Disturbance of Cardiac Rate and Rhythm III. As in previous diagrams, only the audible heart sounds are physical signs of these disorders. **A. Normal rhythm is interspersed with two random premature beats.** If such beats are very frequent, the ear may not be able to distinguish them from atrial fibrillation. The rhythm seems regular as the rate reaches ~120 bpm. **B. Atrial fibrillation.** The ventricular rhythm is grossly irregular and continues to be irregular as the rate accelerates to >120/min. **C. Bigeminy.** A normal beat is followed by a premature beat, this pattern repeating many times. The premature beats tend to extinguish when exercise accelerates the rate to >120/min. **D. Dropped beats in second-degree AV block.** Each successive impulse going through the AV node is delayed longer until one fails to conduct. In contrast to premature beats, exercise tends to increase the number of dropped beats.

at irregular intervals (Fig. 4-4B). The pulse is irregularly irregular without pattern. Rapid irregular ventricular contractions are difficult to identify by palpation. At ventricular rate >70 bpm, the rhythm may seem regular with premature beats. At rates <60 or >120 bpm, the irregularity may be difficult to detect. Because ventricular contractions occur at all stages of chamber filling, the heart sounds and pulse volume vary in intensity. The pulse volume is greater after longer R–R intervals. The ventricular rate is accelerated by exertion. Atrial fibrillation can only be diagnosed by ECG with accurate measuring of the intervals. *DDX:* In flutter with variable AV block, exercise increases the rate by large increments.

CLINICAL OCCURRENCE: Organic heart disease (especially mitral and tricuspid valve disease and congestive heart failure), hyperthyroidism, acute infections including rheumatic fever, postoperative (especially chest surgery), electrolyte imbalances, hypoxia, and hypercarbia. Lone atrial fibrillation, occurring without structural or metabolic abnormalities, increases in frequency with age >70.

Atrial flutter. Atrial reentry circuits incite atrial contraction 220–360 times per minute (Fig. 4-3D). The AV node cannot transmit such rapid stimuli, so block develops, at 2:1, 3:1, 4:1, or higher; the block may be highly variable. Digitalis, verapamil, diltiazem, and β-adrenergic blocking drugs increase the AV block. Vagal maneuvers may suddenly increase block, the atrial rate remaining unchanged. Ventricular contractions are regular with consistent beat-to-beat intensity of heart sounds. Variable block produces irregular ventricular contractions, mimicking atrial fibrillation. Flutter is seen with almost any organic heart disease and is especially common after heart surgery. *DDX:* In sinus tachycardia, vagal stimulation causes smooth slowing; PSVT will not slow but may convert.

Paroxysmal supraventricular (atrial) tachycardia (PSVT, PAT, SVT). The mechanism is most often reentry or reciprocating tachycardia involving the AV node. True ectopic atrial tachycardia does occur. Attacks last minutes to days, beginning and ending suddenly. The rhythm is regular at 150–225 bpm. All beats have the same intensity. PSVT occurs in normal hearts and with AV bypass pathways (Wolf–Parkinson–White syndrome). *DDX:* Vagal stimulation and adenosine do not slow the rate. There is either no response or the attack is abruptly terminated (Fig. 4-3C). Sinus tachycardia slows smoothly; atrial flutter slows with varying AV block.

- **Ventricular tachycardia (VT).** *The mechanism is usually reentry triggered by a PVC and sustained by dispersion of conduction and repolarization in damaged ventricular muscle.* Urgent treatment is needed since ventricular fibrillation (VF) may supervene leading to sudden death. There is usually complete AV dissociation, the ventricles beating faster than the atria. The onset and, when self-limited, the ending are abrupt. The ventricular rate usually is 150–250 bpm, but can be <150 bpm. The rhythm is regular and unaffected by vagal stimulation; it must be distinguished from atrial flutter and PSVT. The variable relationship of atrial to ventricular systole produces variation in the intensity of the first sound. Some sounds are especially loud cannon sounds resulting from superimposition of atrial systole with ventricular systole. The cannon sounds are absent when the atria are fibrillating. Only the first heart sound may be audible.

  CLINICAL OCCURRENCE: *Acquired heart diseases:* Acute myocardial ischemia and infarction, coronary artery disease, drugs (digitalis, quinidine, procaine amide), heart trauma from surgery or catheterization. *Congenital heart diseases:* Right ventricular dysplasia, long QT syndrome, hypertrophic cardiomyopathies and Brugada syndrome.

- **Ventricular fibrillation (VF).** Chaotic depolarization of ventricular muscle fibers does not produce effective ventricular contraction. No ventricular emptying occurs, so there are no heart sounds. The diagnosis is made by ECG. Unless terminated by prompt electrical defibrillation, death follows rapidly.

Abnormal pulse contour and volume. See Chapter 8, page 334.

Respiratory Rate and Pattern.
Normal respirations. The normal newborn respiratory rate is ~44 breaths per minute gradually decreasing to 14–18 bpm in adults, women having slightly higher rates than men. Breathing tends to be faster when it's being observed, so count unobtrusively.

Increased respiratory rate—tachypnea. Increased respiratory rate occurs with central nervous system (CNS) stimulation and as compensation for metabolic acidosis. Hypoxia, increased oxygen demand, and increased CO_2 generation, and increased $PaCO_2$ increase respiratory rate and tidal volume. In restrictive lung disease, minute ventilation is maintained by increasing the respiratory rate to compensate for reduced tidal volume. Tachypnea occurs with exertion, fear, fever, cardiac insufficiency, pain, pulmonary embolism, pleurisy, anemia, hyperthyroidism, and acute respiratory distress of any cause. Breathing is faster with respiratory muscle weakness, emphysema, pneumothorax, and obesity. An arterial blood gas (ABG) distinguishes pathological from compensatory tachypnea.

Decreased respiratory rate—bradypnea. Minute ventilation is preserved when slowing rates are accompanied by increasing tidal volumes *(hyperpnea)*. Slow rates without increased tidal volume indicate an abnormality of the medullary respiratory center and result in alveolar hypoventilation. A slow respiratory rate is not abnormal if gas exchange is preserved. Alveolar hypoventilation ($PaCO_2$ > 45 mm Hg) is often the result of CNS depressant drugs (e.g., opiates, benzodiazepines, barbiturates, alcohol), uremia, or structural intracranial lesions, especially with increased intracranial pressure.

Deep breathing—hyperpnea (Kussmaul breathing). Increasing tidal volume increases CO_2 excretion by increasing alveolar ventilation *(hyperventilation)*, the appropriate compensatory response to metabolic acidosis. It is also seen with hypoxia and is a direct toxic effect of salicylates. The key observation is deep, regular breaths. Triggers are metabolic acidosis (diabetic ketoacidosis, uremia), and decreased oxygen delivery from severe anemia. Hypernea is not synonymous with hyperventilation which can only be diagnosed by ABG.

Shallow breathing—hypopnea. Decreased medullary respiratory drive, respiratory muscle weakness, airway obstruction, and restrictive disease limit tidal volume. Muscular weakness results from myasthenia gravis, amyotrophic lateral sclerosis, Guillain–Barré, drugs (e.g., paralyzing agents, rarely amino-glycosides), and exhaustion from prolonged increased work of breathing accompanying decreased chest wall and/or lung compliance. Decreased effective lung volume results from alveolar filling disorders (pulmonary edema, acute lung injury, alveolar hemorrhage, pneumonia, etc.), severe restrictive lung or chest wall disease, or severe airways obstruction (asthma, emphysema). Hypopnea associated with obstructive sleep apnea is particularly common.

Periodic breathing—Cheyne–Stokes respiration. Cyclic hyperventilation followed by compensatory apnea is caused by phase delay in the feedback controls attempting to maintain a constant $PaCO_2$. This is the most common periodic breathing pattern. In each cycle, the rate and amplitude of successive breaths increase to a maximum, then progressively diminish into the next apneic period. Pallor may accompany the apnea. The patient is frequently unaware of the irregular breathing. Patients may be somnolent during the apneic periods and then arouse and become restless during the hyperpneic phase.

    CLINICAL OCCURRENCE: It is seen during sleep in normal children and the aged. *Disorders of Cerebral Circulation:* Stroke, atherosclerosis; *Heart*

Failure: Low cardiac output of any cause; *Increased Intracranial Pressure:* Meningitis, hydrocephalus, brain tumor, subarachnoid hemorrhage, intracerebral hemorrhage; *Brain Injury:* Stroke, head injury; *Drugs:* Opiates, barbiturates, alcohol; *High Altitude:* During sleep before acclimatization.

Irregular breathing—Biot breathing. An uncommon variant of Cheyne-Stokes respiration, periods of apnea alternate irregularly with a series of equal depth breaths that terminate abruptly. It is most often seen in meningitis.

Irregular breathing—painful respiration. Painful chest movements interrupt normal breathing. Causes are pleurisy, injured or inflamed muscles, fractured ribs or cartilage, or upper abdominal inflammation, e.g., liver and subdiaphragmatic abscess, acute cholecystitis, and peritonitis.

Irregular breathing—sleep apnea. *Obstructive sleep apnea (OSA)* results from extra-thoracic airway obstruction caused by pharyngeal muscle and/or tongue relaxation. Ineffective inspiratory efforts often terminate with a loud snort or snore. *Central apnea* results from decreased or absent medullary respiratory drive. Hypoxia, acidosis, and cardiac dysrhythmias accompany the apneic periods. Arousals associated with apneas lasting >10 seconds lead to deep sleep deprivation and daytime somnolence. The classic patient is a morbidly obese male with daytime somnolence, polycythemia, alveolar hypoventilation, and pulmonary hypertension producing right ventricular failure. Early symptoms include early morning headaches, depression, irritability, and systemic hypertension. Physical exam findings predictive of OSA are oropharyngeal narrowing (Mallampati grade ≥3, Chapter 7, page 231), tonsil size, neck circumference, and BMI.

Irregular breathing—sighing. Occasionally a long, deep sigh interrupts resting respirations. The patient may sense shortness of breath, but without limitation of aerobic exercise. This is commonly encountered in anxious individuals.

Blood Pressure (BP) and Pulse Pressure: Every patient's BP should be checked at each visit to detect hypertension and establish a benchmark for future comparisons. At the first visit, take the BP in both arms and again in both arms if there are new cardiovascular or neurologic complaints. Elevated arm pressures in a young person mandates taking pressures in both legs. Many circumstances temporarily raise BP, for example, anxiety, the white-coat syndrome, rushing to make the appointment on time, bladder distention, chronic alcoholism, amphetamines, cocaine, recent caffeine intake, and cigarette smoking. Frequent BP checks are encouraged.

BP measurement. The pressure necessary to occlude an artery, measured in millimeters of mercury, is assumed to be the intraarterial pressure. The arm cuff should ≥10 cm wide, the thigh cuff ≥18 cm. Unless a wide cuff is used, pressures from a thick arm are 10–15 mm Hg higher than the actual pressure.

- In some situations, the BP measured by the arm cuff may be higher than the actual intraaortic pressure; this can lead to further efforts to lower an already low BP with tragic consequences. It is important for the clinician caring for critically ill patients to understand this possibility.

- When using a sphygmomanometer, intense peripheral vasoconstriction accompanying hypotensive states, as in shock, can lead to serious underestimation of intraarterial pressure. With less vasoconstriction the Korotkoff sounds underestimate the systolic pressure and overestimate diastolic pressure.

Measuring brachial artery pressure. Measure the BP after a 5–10 minutes rest. If sitting, support the back and feet. Apply the cuff snugly to a bare arm with the distal cuff margin ≥3 cm above the antecubital fossa, approximately at heart level. While palpating the brachial artery, inflate the cuff to ≥30 mm Hg above where the pulse disappears. While listening with the bell pressed lightly over the artery, drop the pressure at ≤2 mm Hg per second. Arterial vibrations, Korotkoff sounds, determine the BP. The pressure at which sounds first appear is the systolic pressure. Continuing to deflate the cuff, the sounds become louder, maintain a maximum, then become muffled, and finally disappear. Note the pressures at muffling and disappearance. Record the readings, e.g., 130/80/75. The highest value is the systolic pressure, but it is unclear whether the second or third value is the best estimate of diastolic pressure. The American Heart Association recommends the point of disappearance for the diastolic pressure. If, as sometimes occurs with., hyperthyroidism and aortic regurgitation, the sounds persist to zero pressure accept the second value, since zero diastolic pressure is impossible. To check the auscultation result, and when Korotkoff sounds are imperceptible, palpate the brachial or radial artery recording the pressure at which the pulse first appears. A Doppler ultrasound device identifies the pulse and systolic pressure. Sometimes the Korotkoff sounds appear, disappear, then reappear as the cuff pressure is lowered, producing an *auscultatory gap*. This is observed in older individuals with hypertension and may indicate increased arterial stiffness. To avoid a falsely low systolic pressure, inflate the cuff to well above the putative systolic pressure. The *pulse pressure* is the difference between systolic and diastolic pressures. The normal mean value is 50 mm Hg in men and women.

Wrist BP. If it is difficult to get an accurate brachial BP, the wrist BP should be recorded. With the cuff around the forearm, listen over the radial artery.

Femoral artery BP. With the patient lying prone, wrap a wide cuff around the thigh, with the lower margin several centimeters above the popliteal fossa. Inflate the cuff and auscultate the popliteal artery. Even compression is difficult on a conical thigh.

Ankle BP. With the patient supine, the cuff just above the malleolus, place the bell on the posterior tibial artery behind the medial malleolus or over the dorsalis pedis artery at the ankle's extensor retinaculum. With unobstructed arteries, BP by this method is comparable to brachial artery BP.

Detection of variable pulse waves. Differing pulse wave volumes, too subtle to be detected by palpation, can be observed on the monometer in atrial fibrillation, pulsus paradoxus (tamponade), chronic obstructive pulmonary disease (COPD), and pulsus alternans.

Normal arterial pressure. The definitions of normal BP and hypertension continue to evolve (Table 4-1). There is normally a circadian variation in the BP, highest midmorning, and falling during the day, reaching a low point at ~3 AM. Systolic pressure increases with age and cardiovascular risk increases with pressures >115/75 and doubles for each additional 20/10 mm Hg. BP is a continuous biologic variable not allowing a clear normal-abnormal dichotomy. It should be thought of as one of many risk factors for cardiovascular disease, especially stroke and heart failure, the importance of which must be interpreted in the context of the patient's gender, age, and other cardiovascular risk factors. Many guidelines are published and continuously revised, each eliciting new controversies. It is generally agreed that pressures reproducibly >140 systolic and >90 diastolic are undesirable and treatment should be considered. Also, systolic pressure >180 and diastolic pressure >120 present imminent risk and should be treated. Severe BP elevation associated with new or progressive end-organ damage is a true emergency requiring immediate BP control, usually over the course of minutes to hours. Table 4-1A presents the classification from Joint National Committee (JNC) which remains a reasonable starting point for discussion of BP issues with patients. Table 4.1B presents the recent changes to this classification by ACC/AHA (American College of Cardiology and American Heart Association).

Inequality of arm BPs. Arm BPs normally differ by <10 mm Hg. Greater inequality is frequent and sometimes cannot be explained. Consider subclavian artery obstruction, thoracic outlet syndrome, and aortic dissection

TABLE 4-1A JNC-7 BP Classification

Classification	Systolic Pressure (mm Hg)	Diastolic Pressure (mm Hg)
Normal	<120	<80
Prehypertension	120–139	80–89
Hypertension		
Stage 1	140–159	90–99
Stage 2	>159	>100

TABLE 4-1B ACC/AHA BP Classification

BP Category	SBP		DBP
Normal	<120 mmHg	and	<80 mmHg
Elevated	120–129 mmHg	and	<80 mmHg
Hypertension			
Stage 1	130–139 mmHg	or	80–90 mmHg
Stage 2	≥140 mmHg	or	≥90 mmHg

High blood pressure.
Hypertension. The cause of most hypertension is unknown, i.e., *essential hypertension.* The primary lesion is suspected to be in the kidney. Increased stroke volume and decreased aortic compliance increase systolic pressure. Vasoconstriction and intimal thickening increase peripheral vascular resistance and diastolic pressure. *Isolated systolic hypertension* is elevated systolic pressure with normal diastolic pressure, often seen in the elderly. More commonly, both systolic and diastolic pressures are elevated. Mean arterial pressure is largely a function of diastolic pressure, the minimal continuous load on the vascular tree. Elevated diastolic with normal systolic pressure lowers the pulse pressure suggesting reduced cardiac output. Hypertension is a major risk factor for stroke, heart failure, left ventricular hypertrophy, and chronic kidney failure. Over age 50, systolic pressure contributes more to risk than diastolic. With sustained hypertension, search for hypertensive retinopathy, left ventricular hypertrophy, and renal insufficiency.

CLINICAL OCCURRENCE: Essential hypertension is a diagnosis of exclusion, so alternative explanations need to always be considered. *Congenital:* Coarctation of the aorta, congenital adrenal hyperplasia (early or late onset), polycystic kidney disease; *Degenerative/Idiopathic:* Essential hypertension, toxemia of pregnancy; *Endocrine:* Pheochromocytoma, aldosteronoma, adrenal hyperplasia, hypercortisolism (Cushing disease and syndrome), hyperthyroidism, hypothyroidism, hyperparathyroidism, acromegaly; *Inflammatory/Immune:* Atherosclerosis, vasculitis; *Mechanical/Traumatic:* Obstructive sleep apnea, acute spinal cord injury; *Metabolic/Toxic:* Renal insufficiency, medications (NSAIDs, estrogens, oral contraceptives, cyclosporine), drug abuse (cocaine, amphetamines, etc.), porphyria, lead poisoning, hypercalcemia; *Neoplastic:* Adrenal adenoma, pheochromocytoma, pituitary adenoma, brain tumors; *Neurologic:* Stroke, diencephalic syndrome, increased intracranial pressure; *Psychosocial:* Substance abuse (cocaine, amphetamines, alcohol); *Vascular:* Renal artery stenosis (atherosclerosis, fibromuscular dysplasia).

Isolated systolic hypertension (ISH). The increased systolic pressure results from increased stroke volume and/or decreased compliance of the aorta and its branches. Causes of increased stroke volume include hyperthyroidism, anemia, arteriovenous fistulas, aortic regurgitation, and anxiety. Atherosclerosis decreases aortic compliance. ISH increases risk for stroke, left ventricular hypertrophy, and heart failure.

White coat syndrome. BP is elevated in clinical settings but normal at home and by ambulatory BP monitoring. Cardiovascular risk is less than with sustained hypertension.

- *Malignant hypertension.* Severely elevated BP causes end-organ dysfunction that further elevates the BP. Diastolic pressure is >120 mm Hg and systolic pressure usually >200 mm Hg. Patients present with headache, confusion, dyspnea, seizures, angina, or rapidly progressive renal insufficiency. Rapid moderation of pressure prevents irreversible brain, heart, eye, and kidney damage.

- *Paroxysmal hypertension: pheochromocytoma*. Benign adrenal or sympathetic chain tumors secrete epinephrine or norepinephrine. In one-third of the patients, secretion is intermittent. Episodic hypertension is associated with pallor, anxiety, sweating, palpitation, nausea, and vomiting. Most patients have sustained hypertension. Intravascular volume depletion leads to orthostatic hypotension, an early clinical sign. Pheochromocytoma must be distinguished from panic attacks and the white-coat syndrome.

Low blood pressure.

Hypotension. Hypotension results from blood loss, decreased vascular tone, and/or decreased cardiac output. Systolic and diastolic pressures are low. In usually hypertensive patients, normal BPs are concerning. Cool skin, decreased urine output, and decreased alertness are signs of hypoperfusion. Peripheral vasoconstriction and tachycardia, signs of compensatory cardiovascular responses indicate pathologically low BP.

CLINICAL OCCURRENCE: *Loss of Blood Volume:* Bleeding, capillary leak syndrome (anaphylaxis, sepsis, IL-2, idiopathic), third-spacing (ascites, burns, secretory diarrheas), polyuria (diabetes mellitus, diabetes insipidus, diuretics), inadequate fluid intake, excessive sweating (heat prostration and heat stroke), adrenal insufficiency; *Loss of Vascular Tone:* Sepsis, drugs (vasodilators, tricyclic antidepressants, ganglionic blockers), fever, autonomic insufficiency (multisystem atrophy), acute spinal cord injury (spinal shock), arteriovenous malformations; *Decreased Cardiac Output:* Acute myocardial infarction, ischemic cardiomyopathy, idiopathic dilated cardiomyopathy, aortic stenosis, saddle pulmonary embolism, pericardial tamponade, and severe mitral insufficiency.

Orthostatic (postural) hypotension. Causes are hypovolemia, decreased sympathetic drive to the heart and vasculature, and decreased venous return. Supine BP is normal but falls, within 3 minutes of standing, by ≥20 mm Hg systolic or ≥10 mm Hg diastolic, and/or the pulse rate rises by ≥15 bpm. This is an early sign of intravascular volume loss. A BP drop not accompanied by a rise in pulse rate suggests autonomic insufficiency. Patients with chronic orthostatic hypotension frequently have postprandial hypotension and reversal of the normal circadian BP pattern, i.e., higher BP at night than during the day.

CLINICAL OCCURRENCE: *Loss of Blood Volume:* See Hypotension above; *Loss of Vascular Tone:* Deconditioning after long illnesses, autonomic insufficiency (multisystem atrophy), peripheral neuropathies (diabetes, tabes dorsalis, alcoholism), drugs (vasodilators, tricyclic antidepressants, ganglionic blockers); *Impaired Venous Return:* Ascites, pregnancy, venous insufficiency, inferior vena cava obstruction and hemangiomas in the legs.

Postprandial hypotension. In some individuals, especially older adults on vasoactive medications, the BP drops by ≥20 mm Hg following meals. The exact mechanisms are unclear, but the result is increased risk for falls, syncope, dizziness, and fatigue. Question carefully about the relation of symptoms to meals.

- *Anaphylactic shock.* IgE-mediated mast cell degranulation releases histamine and other vasoactive substances producing vasodilatation and opening endothelial tight junctions with loss of plasma volume. This fulminant life-threatening hypersensitivity reaction occurs on exposure to specific allergens. Sudden vascular collapse is preceded or accompanied by malaise, pruritus, pallor, stridor, cyanosis, syncope, vomiting, diarrhea, tachypnea, tachycardia, and distant heart sounds. Angioedema and urticaria may be present but are often absent.

  CLINICAL OCCURRENCE: Hymenoptera stings, drugs (e.g., penicillin and other antibiotics), peanut ingestion, and many others. Anaphylaxis may occur with exercise, cold exposure, heat exposure, or without evident cause (idiopathic anaphylaxis). Clinically identical *anaphylactoid* reactions occur when mast cell release is stimulated by non-IgE-mediated mechanisms such as radiographic contrast agents.

- *Septic shock.* This is a complex physiologic reaction to circulating endotoxin activating inflammatory and thrombotic pathways. Patients present with hypotension, often, but not always, accompanied by fever and prostration. Initially, the skin is warm and flushed, despite the low BP, followed by peripheral vasoconstriction, decreased urine output, confusion, progressive hypotension and acidosis. Prompt recognition and treatment are essential.

- *Toxic shock syndrome.* Toxins produced by strains of *Staphylococcus aureus* produce hypotension with high cardiac output and generalized erythroderma. Though initially described in association with highly absorbent vaginal tampons, surgical wound infections containing foreign bodies (sutures) and sinusitis are now common sites of infection. The patient suddenly develops high fever, myalgia, nausea, vomiting, and diarrhea. Diffuse erythroderma is followed by confusion, acute lung injury, hypotension, and shock. Exfoliation of the palms and soles may occur in convalescence.

Pulse pressure.
Wide pulse pressure. Pulse pressure increases with increased systolic pressure (increased stroke volume, increased rate of ventricular contraction, decreased aortic elasticity) and/or decreased diastolic pressure (decreased peripheral resistance, arteriovenous shunts, aortic insufficiency). Pulse pressure ≥65 mm Hg is abnormal. With large stroke volumes, the pulse is bounding or, in aortic regurgitation, collapsing. Suggestive signs include head bobbing with each heartbeat and thrills and audible murmurs over AV shunts. When vasodilation decreases vascular resistance, the skin is warm and flushed. Widened pulse pressure is a major risk factor for cardiovascular morbidity and mortality, including atrial fibrillation.

CLINICAL OCCURRENCE: *Increased Systolic Pressure:* Systolic hypertension, atherosclerosis, increased stroke volume (aortic regurgitation, hyperthyroidism, anxiety, bradycardia, heart block, post-PVC, after a long pause in atrial fibrillation, pregnancy, fever, systemic arteriovenous fistulas); *Increased Diastolic Runoff:* Aortic regurgitation, sepsis, vasodilators, patent ductus arteriosus, hyperthyroidism, arteriovenous fistulas, beriberi.

Narrow pulse pressure. Pulse pressure narrows with decreased stroke volume and decreased rate of ventricular ejection. Pulse pressures less than 30 mm Hg may occur with tachycardia and conditions associated with a low stroke volume.

CLINICAL OCCURRENCE: *Decreased Stroke Volume:* Severe aortic stenosis, dilated cardiomyopathy, restrictive heart disease, constrictive pericarditis, pericardial tamponade, intravascular volume depletion, venous vasodilatation; *Decreased Rate of Ventricular Contraction:* Ischemic and dilated cardiomyopathy, aortic stenosis, myocarditis.

ANTHROPOMETRIC DATA

Height: Linear growth occurs throughout infancy, childhood, and adolescence, ending with closure of the long bone epiphyses. Mature height is determined by both genetic and environmental factors, especially nutrition. Linear growth requires growth hormone, adequate nutrition (protein, calories, vitamin D, calcium, and phosphorus) and a skeleton able to respond to these signals. Height should not change throughout the years of maturity. With aging, there is a hormone-independent loss of bone mineral density, particularly of trabecular bone, leading to a slow and gradual loss of height often aggravated decreased muscle tone and strength affecting posture. Pathology such as osteoporosis and spinal compression fractures sometimes produce dramatic height loss.

Throughout infancy and childhood height is recorded regularly at well-child visits. Standardized charts visually display growth over time. Once stable height is reached, it is measured once every ~5 years until age 60, when annual measurement resumes.

Measuring height. Height is best measured standing erect against a wall without shoes, the head in neutral position (the occiput does not touch the wall), with heels, buttocks, and scapulae touching the wall. The vertical distance between the floor and the highest point of the scalp is recorded in inches or centimeters. Compress the hair to avoid overestimating height; separate especially thick hair.

Short stature. Short stature indicates a failure of growth hormone production, decreased tissue receptivity, or impaired nutrition. Expected stature is estimated from standard tables or by adding 6.5 cm (2.6 in.) for boys and subtracting 6.5 cm (2.6 in.) for girls from the mid-parental height. Consult pediatric textbooks for the evaluation of short stature in children.

CLINICAL OCCURRENCE: *Congenital:* Intrauterine growth retardation, pseudohypoparathyroidism, vitamin D-resistant rickets, familial short stature, Turner syndrome, achondroplasia, Noonan syndrome, Prader–Willi syndrome; *Endocrine:* Growth hormone deficiency, hypothyroidism, hyperthyroidism, diabetes mellitus, Cushing disease, hypogonadism; *Degenerative/Idiopathic:* Constitutional delay in growth; *Infectious:* Any chronic debilitating infection; *Inflammatory/Immune:* Juvenile rheumatoid arthritis (RA), SLE, chronic glomerulonephritis; *Mechanical/Traumatic:* Brain injury; *Metabolic/Toxic:* Chronic glucocorticoid use, malnutrition; *Neoplastic:* suprasellar masses, cancer treatment during childhood, including brain irradiation; *Psychosocial:* Chronic emotional deprivation, mistaken paternity; *Vascular:* Pituitary infarction.

Accelerated growth: gigantism and acromegaly. A pituitary adenoma secreting growth hormone accelerates linear growth until the epiphyses close in late adolescence. Secretion starting or continuing after epiphyseal closure enlarges hands, feet skull, and mandible disproportionately and thickens soft tissue. Linear growth normally goes through early and late growth accelerations. Growth charts will readily identify deviations from expected growth. Excessive growth hormone production beginning after epiphyseal closure results in acromegaly (enlarged hands, feet, skull, mandible, and soft-tissue thickening) without increasing height. See Chapter 13, page 581.

Abnormal body proportions: Marfan syndrome. Chapter 13, page 570. Affected individuals are tall, extremely slender, and have arm span exceeding height.

Loss of height. Decreasing height after skeletal maturity results from shortening of long bones in the legs, cartilage loss in the hips/or and knees, decreased vertebral and/or intervertebral disc-space height (especially lumbar), or spinal curvature. History and physical exam plus a minimal radiographic investigation quickly identifies the cause(s). Measuring regularly detects slow height loss before disability occurs.

> **CLINICAL OCCURRENCE:** *Long Bones:* Trauma, surgery, osteomalacia; *Cartilage:* osteoarthritis, RA; *Intervertebral Discs:* Herniated discs, desiccated disks, disk infection; *Vertebrae:* Osteoporosis, osteomalacia, Paget disease, traumatic compression fracture, multiple myeloma; *Spinal Curvature:* Scoliosis, pregnancy, abdominal muscle weakness, myositis, polio.

Weight: Body mass is distributed in muscle, bone, adipose tissue, organs, viscera, and intercellular tissue. Weight loss or gain occurs in one or more of these compartments. The organs, viscera, and skeleton vary little in mass. The extracellular fluid, skeletal muscle, and fat compartments are more labile. Inappropriate or unexpected weight changes are the combined changes in body water, muscle, and fat. Physiologic and etiologic hypotheses vary with the compartment(s) involved. A two-compartment scheme divides body mass into water and everything else, water is ~60% of the mass in men, slightly less in women, and decreases with age in both sexes. Fat is low in water so higher body fat lowers the proportion of water. Body water is divided into two compartments, the intracellular water (66%) and the extracellular water (34%). The extracellular compartment is divided into extravascular (75%) and intravascular fluid (25%). Extracellular water is essentially saline with an approximate sodium concentration of 140 mEq/L. Intracellular water is rich in potassium and relatively low in sodium.

Measuring weight. Weight is measured in pounds or kilograms at each visit establishing a baseline range.

Body mass index (BMI). The BMI is a function of weight and height and is a risk factor for adverse events. The BMI is calculated by dividing the weight in kilograms by the (height in meters)^2; the units are kg/m^2. The upper limit of normal is the point at which the risk for adverse health outcomes begins to rise; the lower limit was similarly determined (Table 4-2). The BMI does

TABLE 4-2 Interpretation of BMI

BMI	Description
<18.5	Underweight
18.5–25	Normal
>25–30	Overweight
>30–35	Class I: obese
>35–40	Class II: very obese
>40	Class III: extremely obese

not distinguish increases in lean body mass from increases in fat mass. BMI growth charts are increasingly used in well-child care. BMI is useful in setting weight loss goals enabling patients to compare the population risks associated with their current and target BMI.

Waist–hip ratio. Women more than men put more fat stores subcutaneously. Men, especially with weight gain in mid-life, develop adiposity in the organs and omentum. Visceral adipose tissue is metabolically distinct from subcutaneous fat and appears to contribute to hyperlipidemia and insulin resistance. The waist-hip ratio (the ratio of the body circumference at the hip and waist) is an indicator of visceral adiposity. Waist–hip ratio >0.9 for women and >1.0 for men is abnormal. Waist circumference >40 in. (90 cm) for men or >35 in. (80 cm) for women is another indicator. Increased waist–hip ratio and waist circumference are risk factors for adverse health events and appear to be better predictors than BMI.

Growth retardation—cystic fibrosis. Several autosomal recessive epithelial chloride channel gene mutations lead to production of viscous mucus by the exocrine glands resulting in chronic progressive pulmonary and pancreatic dysfunction. Though most are diagnosed in childhood, mild mutations may escape detection until adulthood. Symptoms include bulky, foul-smelling stools, cough, and dyspnea. Pancreatic obstruction leads to maldigestion and growth retardation. Lung involvement produces cough and recurrent pulmonary infections, often leading to chronic infection with *Pseudomonas aeruginosa* and bronchiectasis. Sweat gland involvement increases susceptibility to salt and water loss in warm environments. Complications include fecal impaction, intussusception, volvulus, and chronic bronchitis. With advanced pulmonary disease cardiomegaly and finger clubbing are seen.

Weight loss. Weight is lost when energy utilization or loss exceeds caloric intake. Decreased effective intake (net of ingestion, emesis and stool losses), maldigestion, malabsorption, increased metabolic utilization, and increased losses of calories are all possible. Failure to gain weight and grow appropriately in childhood and adolescence has the same significance as weight loss in the adult. The history is most useful for hypothesizing a probable pathophysiology. Have the patient estimate the weight lost over a specific time; obtain weight records to validate the history. Ask whether the patient's clothes fit differently or if family or friends have noted a change in appearance. Review the daily intake of food and drink and identify any change in physical activity. Examine the patient's belt for a change in wear pattern. Search for striae and loose skin over the abdomen and upper arms. Often more than one mechanism is implicated. *DDX:* Weight loss with no change of intake suggests impaired nutrient assimilation (maldigestion, malabsorption), glucosuria (diabetes mellitus), or increased metabolic rate (hyperthyroidism, pheochromocytoma). Cancer and psychosocial problems, especially depression, are the two most prevalent explanations.

CLINICAL OCCURRENCE: *Endocrine:* Hyperthyroidism, adrenal insufficiency, diabetes (especially type 1), hypothalamic disorders; *Degenerative/ Idiopathic:* Advanced age (normal adults lose weight gradually after age 60 years), any debilitating disease; *Infectious:* Chronic disseminated infection or advanced local infection, for example, tuberculosis, chronic active hepatitis, AIDS, intestinal parasites; *Inflammatory/Immune:* Any systemic inflammatory disease, for example, SLE, RA, vasculitis; *Mechanical/Traumatic:* Bowel obstruction, dysphagia, odynophagia, dental and chewing problems, decreased mobility, paralysis, apraxia; *Metabolic/Toxic:* Organ failure (uremia, advanced liver disease, emphysema, congestive heart failure), increased physical activity, maldigestion and malabsorption, dieting, decreased intake and starvation; *Neoplastic:* Cancers decrease appetite and increase utilization, especially when disseminated or involving the liver; *Psychosocial:* Dieting, dementia, depression, anorexia nervosa, bulimia, abuse, isolation, poverty; *Vascular:* Vasculitis, multiinfarct dementia.

Cachexia. Cytokines released with chronic infections and malignancies lead to wasting of muscle protein and increased metabolic demands resulting in profound weight loss and redistribution. Cachexia is physiologically distinct from starvation and cannot be reversed by refeeding. Cachexia is classically seen in chronic tuberculosis ("consumption") and slow growing visceral malignancies (e.g., advanced pancreatic and colon cancers), but any chronic disease with persistent activation of the immune system may produce the syndrome.

CLINICAL OCCURRENCE: Common associations are HIV-AIDS, CHF, advanced liver and renal disease, RA, Addison disease, chronic obstructive pulmonary disease, and advanced age.

Weight gain. Weight increases whenever the intake of calories exceeds metabolic demands or when calorie-free salt and water are retained in advanced heart, kidney, and liver disease. Weight gain continues after linear growth stops as skeletal muscle mass increases to adult size, especially in men. After reaching adult body mass, any further weight increase indicates a pathologic condition, a decrease in physical exercise, an increase in caloric intake, or an intense body building program. Fats and alcohol have the highest energy content, 9 and 7.5 kcal/g, respectively; the energy content of carbohydrates and protein is 4.5 kcal/g. A careful history with attention to diet, exercise, appetite, libido, skin, hair, and bowel habits is essential. On physical exam evaluate possible extracellular fluid retention (edema, ascites), adiposity, and muscle mass.

CLINICAL OCCURRENCE: *Increased Intake:* Overeating, mild hyperthyroidism, insulinoma, hypothalamic injury, treatment of diabetes, anabolic steroids; *Decreased Demand:* Hypothyroidism, hypogonadism, inactivity, confinement; *Salt and Water Retention:* Congestive heart failure, kidney failure, nephrotic syndrome, hepatic insufficiency, hypothyroidism, portal hypertension with ascites, idiopathic edema, diuretic rebound, venous insufficiency with dependent edema.

Obesity. Genetics and lifestyle each are important in the development of obesity. Calorie intake in excess of expenditures leads to weight gain, but obesity requires failure of feedback to limit intake; the cause(s) of this failure are unknown. Obesity is epidemic; a third or more of the adult population is obese. Obesity causes insulin resistance and increases risk for hypertension, diabetes, heart disease, cancer, and overall mortality. Obesity is readily recognized and diagnosed, but is very difficult to treat, especially if onset is in childhood or adolescence. Commonly the exact factors leading to the marked weight gain, beyond dietary and exercise habits, are obscure. *DDX:* The *distribution of adipose tissue* assists diagnosis. Truncal obesity with thin limbs, round faces and a prominent hump of fat over the upper back are characteristic of Cushing disease, iatrogenic steroid use, and use of protease inhibitors for treatment of HIV-AIDS. Localized accumulations of fat are seen at sites of repetitive insulin injection (*lipodystrophy*). *Abdominal obesity* is common in men with mid-life weight gain ("beer belly").

Metabolic syndrome. The metabolic syndrome is the association of several conditions with increased risk for diabetes and cardiovascular disease. The cause is unknown, but obesity and insulin resistance play large roles. A consensus definition was published in 2005. Diagnosis is based on increased waist circumference (ethnically specific, Table 4-3), plus any two of the following: elevated triglycerides (>150 mg/dL) or treatment of hypertriglyceridemia; reduced HDL-cholesterol (men <40 mg/dL, women <50 mg/dL) or treatment for low HDL; elevated BP (systolic ≥130 mm Hg, diastolic ≥85 mm Hg) or treatment of hypertension; elevated fasting plasma glucose (≥100 mg/dL) or previously diagnosed type 2 diabetes.

TABLE 4-3 Waist Circumference Norms by Ethnic Group.

Ethnic Group	Waist Circumference (cm)	
	Men	*Women*
European descent	≥94	≥80
South Asians	≥90	≥80
Chinese	≥90	≥80
Japanese	≥85	≥90
Ethnic South and Central Americans	Use South Asian recommendations	
Sub-Saharan Africans	Use European recommendations	

Based upon Alberti KG, Zimmet P, Shaw J. The metabolic syndrome—a new worldwide definition. *Lancet*. 2005;366: 1059–1062.

PAIN

Pain is a complex subject beyond the scope of this text. The reader is encouraged to explore pain texts to understand pain pathways and the pathophysiology of acute and chronic pain, which are distinct entities requiring different diagnostic and management strategies.

Pain can be roughly classified as acute or chronic. *Acute pain* is an *event*. Most acute pain is caused by direct tissue injury, ischemia, or inflammation. Adequate treatment of acute pain decreases the likelihood of progression to chronic pain. Unremitting pain remodels central pain pathways facilitating persistent pain as a chronic pain syndrome. *Chronic pain* is a persistent *experience* frequently accompanied by functional impairment and depression.

Diagnostic Attributes of Pain, PQRST: Pain directs attention to a specific anatomic region and often, although not always, indicates tissue injury. Use of the PQRST mnemonic improves diagnostic precision. The same questioning strategy is useful for other symptoms.

P: provocative and palliative factors. Pain with movement implicates mechanical mechanisms involving moving or displaced structures. The location is confirmed by pressure eliciting tenderness. Conversely, if resting a part relieves pain, those tissues are likely the source of pain. Therapeutic interventions can be used diagnostically: chest pain relieved by nitroglycerin suggests angina pectoris while relief by antacids suggests acid-peptic disease.

Q: quality. Pain quality also assists diagnosis. *Somatic pain*, arising from the skin, skeletal muscles, bones, ligaments, tendons, and soft tissues, is described as sharp or stabbing and is well localized; the patient can point with one finger to the site of maximal pain. *Visceral pain*, arising from ischemia; inflammation; or other injury to the body cavities is poorly localized; the patient can only indicate a general area or areas of pain, often described as deep or inside. It is aching, pressing, or squeezing in quality, and often accompanied by autonomic symptoms such as nausea, vomiting, diaphoresis, and intestinal ileus. *Neuropathic pain* arises from damage to the nerve cells themselves; it is described as burning in the distribution of the affected nerve or nerves. These distinctions are far from exact but are clinically useful. Shooting pain usually results from irritation of a nerve trunk. Displacement of inflamed tissues surrounding a pulsating artery causes throbbing pain.

R: region and referral. Pain is usually located in the anatomic region indicated by the patient. Pain is also referred following developmental and neurological organizational principles. Nerve injury will refer pain, and often cause paresthesias, in the dermatomal distribution subserved by the sensory components of the nerve (Chapter 14, page 643). Muscular pain is referred toward muscles innervated by or derived from the same spinal segments (the *myotome*). Similarly, skeletal pain radiates to structures innervated by or derived from the same spinal segments (the *sclerotome*).

S: severity. Individuals have remarkably similar thresholds for pain. However, they vary greatly in their reactions to pain, and fear may aggravate pain. Assessment of pain severity is mandated by Medicare at each visit. Pain is a subjective sensation, so the patient's statement should be accepted without debate. It is useful to calibrate pain on a 0 to 10 scale: with 0 being no pain and 10 being the worst possible pain. Pain scores are used to follow progression and response to management. Always communicate the goals for pain relief: "We should be able to reduce your pain to a 3/10." Intense pain is usually accompanied by physiologic signs such as apprehension, postures (protecting a limb, abdominal guarding), sweating, pallor, pupil dilatation, hypertension, tachycardia, nausea, and vomiting.

T: timing. Timing and duration of pain often indicate its cause. Pain that is insidious in onset and relentlessly progressive without palliative features suggests cancer pain or increasing pressure in a closed space (e.g., intracranial pressure, toothache). Intermittent episodic pain suggests a predisposition to specific episodic events, e.g., kidney stones, intermittent intestinal obstruction. A single episode may be short or prolonged, steady, worsening, or relenting in waves. Daytime pain is common when movement causes pain; daytime relief suggests muscle or joint stiffening improving with motion. Nighttime pain occurs when muscle relaxation stops splinting tender tissues or the absence of competing sensory inputs allows the persistent pain of an unremitting process to become predominant, typical of bone pain.

Pain Syndromes:. Site-specific pain is discussed in the chapters dealing with each body region.

Complex regional pain syndrome (CRPS)—reflex sympathetic dystrophy, causalgia. Minor injury initiates a complex series of spinal and CNS responses resulting in altered autonomic function and pain perception. CRPS occurs after surgery or injury to an extremity, especially the hands or feet. The pain may involve an entire anatomic region and can occur days to weeks after the injury. The pain is disproportionate to the injury and usually described as constant, burning, aching, and/or throbbing. Examination may reveal hyperalgesia, hyperesthesia, edema, erythema, and skin temperature changes. Progression leads to vascular changes (cyanosis and mottling), altered sweating, atrophic skin, muscle and subcutaneous tissue, and contractures. Two forms are recognized: CRPS type 1 occurs without nerve injury and CRPS type 2 (*causalgia*) is associated with major nerve injury. Early recognition and treatment is necessary.

Postherpetic neuralgia. Reactivation of latent varicella-zoster virus in the dorsal root ganglia produces clinical herpes zoster and can result in a subacute or chronic painful neuropathy. Most patients with acute herpes zoster have intense pain which abates over a period of weeks to months. The pain is burning in quality, sometimes very severe, and associated with *allodynia* where the slightest skin disturbance induces lancinating pain. Older adults are at increased risk for persistent postherpetic neuralgia.

CLINICAL VIGNETTES AND QUESTIONS

Case 4-1

A 34-year-old male presents with confusion and increasing muscle stiffness. He recently started treatment for paranoid schizophrenia. His physical examination is notable for temperature 38.6°C, heart rate 115, blood pressure 148/94, and respiratory rate of 22. He is diaphoretic, tremulous and has "lead pipe rigidity."

QUESTIONS:
1. What is the differential diagnosis of this presentation?
2. What is the most likely diagnosis?
3. What physical examination findings differentiate serotonin syndrome from this diagnosis?

Case 4-2

You have been asked to evaluate an 18-year-old man in the emergency room with a first episode of diabetic ketoacidosis. The arterial pH is 7.14.

QUESTIONS:
1. Describe the expected respiratory pattern of this patient. What is it called?
2. What other conditions can also cause this respiratory pattern?
3. How does this respiratory pattern differ from Cheyne–Stokes respirations?
4. Describe the physiology of Cheyne–Stokes respirations.
5. What underlying conditions cause Cheyne–Stokes respirations?

Case 4-3

A 63-year-old man complains of lightheadedness when getting out of bed in the morning and when standing from a seated position. One year ago he was diagnosed with Parkinson disease without tremor. He has not improved on carbidopa/levodopa. He also has urinary incontinence and erectile dysfunction. His recumbent blood pressure and pulse are 128/84 and 72; his standing blood pressure and pulse are 105/72 and 75.

QUESTIONS:
1. What is notable about the BP and pulse changes and what does this indicate?
2. What are causes of orthostatic (postural) hypotension?
3. What is the most likely diagnosis?
4. Name some subtypes of this diagnosis.

Case 4-4

A 72-year-old man presents to a walk-in clinic with a laceration. Before interviewing the patient you review his vital signs noting a blood pressure of 155/65 and heart rate of 94.

QUESTIONS:
1. What is notable about the blood pressure?
2. What is the physiology of a widened pulse pressure?
3. What are possible causes of the widened pulse pressure?
4. What heart valve condition is associated with a widened pulse pressure and what physical examination findings are associated with this condition?

CHAPTER 5

Nonregional Systems and Diseases

Several physiologic systems are located within multiple body regions and are assessed continuously during the exam. Diseases of these systems most commonly present with nonspecific constitutional symptoms and recognition depends on integrating all exam findings. This concept is captured by the saying "he who knows syphilis knows medicine."

CONSTITUTIONAL SYMPTOMS

Constitutional symptoms are those that relate to the body or a person as a whole. They are combined with physical exam and laboratory findings to make 1–3 general physiologic hypotheses. For example, a middle-aged patient presenting with anorexia, weight loss, and night sweats suggests neoplasm, chronic infectious or inflammatory disease, or possibly Addison disease.

Fatigue: Fatigue results from serious organic disease, mood disorders, or deconditioning. Patients describe decreased energy and endurance during usual activities. Clinical fatigue incorporates three components, present to variable degrees in individual patients: inability to initiate activity (perception of generalized weakness in the absence of objective findings); reduced capacity to maintain activity (easy fatigability); and difficulty with concentration, memory, and emotional stability (mental fatigue). It is important to distinguish fatigue from shortness of breath, muscle weakness, and sleepiness. Fatigue can complicate any chronic disease, e.g., anemia, hypothyroidism, hyperthyroidism, and autoimmune or neurologic disorders. *DDX:* History should determine the severity and temporal pattern of fatigue as follows: *Onset*—abrupt or gradual and relationship to an event or illness. *Course*—stable, improving or worsening, duration and daily pattern, factors that alleviate or exacerbate symptoms, and impact on daily life. Symptoms suggesting underlying occult medical illness should be explored in a detailed review of systems, including presence of weight loss or night sweats. The history should include screening questions for psychiatric disorders (particularly depression, anxiety disorders, somatoform disorders, and substance abuse). When a complete history, physical examination, and screening laboratory evaluation do not find a specific explanation, consider deconditioning, depression, sleep disorders, and myalgic encephalomyelitis/chronic fatigue syndrome (ME/CFS).

CLINICAL OCCURRENCE: These are examples only and not meant to be all-encompassing. *Congenital:* Muscular dystrophies, mitochondrial myopathy; *Endocrine:* Hypothyroidism, hyperthyroidism, Addison disease, hypopituitarism, hypoparathyroidism, hypogonadism; *Degenerative/Idiopathic:* ME/CFS, inclusion body myositis, amyotrophic lateral sclerosis, multiple sclerosis, dementia; *Infectious:* Tuberculosis, infectious mononucleosis, hepatitis, following other viral illnesses, hookworm infestation, HIV infection; *Inflammatory/Immune:* Systemic lupus erythematosus (SLE), rheumatoid arthritis (RA), polymyositis, dermatomyositis, vasculitis, myasthenia gravis; *Metabolic/Toxic:* Hypokalemia, hypocalcemia, hypomagnesemia, hyponatremia, anemia, uremia, hypoglycemia, congestive heart failure, drugs (e.g., β-blockers, sedatives, opioids, anticholinergics), alcohol; *Neoplastic:* Acute and chronic leukemia, myelodysplastic syndromes, myeloproliferative syndromes, solid tumors, lymphomas; *Psychosocial:* Disordered sleep, depression, deconditioning, overwork and overtraining, insomnia, chronic anxiety; *Vascular:* Claudication, strokes.

Appetite Disturbance: Appetite is controlled by the hypothalamus under the influence of multiple hormones, metabolites, neural afferents (especially vagal visceral afferents), and cortical inputs reflecting emotional and cognitive state. Disturbances in any of these systems change appetite.

Anorexia. Lack of appetite is anorexia. Appetite loss is nonspecific but a sensitive indicator of disease and mood disorders. When caloric expenditure is unchanged, anorexia results in weight loss.

CLINICAL OCCURRENCE: *Endocrine:* Adrenal insufficiency, hypothyroidism, hypopituitarism; *Degenerative/Idiopathic:* Dementia, anosmia; *Infectious:* Hepatitis, any acute or chronic systemic infection; *Inflammatory/Immune:* Inflammatory cytokines (interleukin-1, tumor necrosis factor) suppress appetite, so any systemic inflammatory process can lead to anorexia; *Mechanical/Traumatic:* Gastrointestinal obstruction, dysphagia,; *Metabolic/Toxic:* Advanced kidney disease, advanced liver disease, drugs (e.g., amphetamines, and stimulants); *Neoplastic:* Malignancy, especially when metastatic or regionally advanced; *Psychosocial:* Depression, delirium, poverty, social isolation, abuse, school problems, anorexia, and bulimia nervosa; *Vascular:* Vasculitis, stroke.

Polyphagia. Increased or insatiable appetite is uncommon. If calorie intake exceeds expenditure weight is gained, if not weight is unchanged or lost. Balance includes calories expended doing muscle work, ingested calories wasted from vomiting, maldigestion/malabsorption, and calories absorbed but subsequently lost, e.g., glucosuria and proteinuria.

CLINICAL OCCURRENCE: *Endocrine:* Diabetes, hyperthyroidism, insulinoma, hypothalamic disorders; *Genetic*: Prader-Willi; *Metabolic/Toxic:* Malnutrition (protein, essential fatty acids), drugs (e.g., corticosteroids, cannabinoids), iron deficiency; *Neoplastic:* Insulinoma; *Psychosocial:* Bulimia, binge eating syndrome, night eating syndrome.

Abnormal eating behaviors. Behaviors associated with selection, acquisition, preparation, serving, and eating of food are culturally determined and socially important. Changes in food-related behaviors suggest medical, psychiatric, and social problems. See Chapter 15, page 726.

CLINICAL OCCURRENCE: *Endocrine:* Pregnancy; *Degenerative/Idiopathic:* Anosmia; *Infectious:* Hookworm infestation; *Metabolic/Toxic:* Iron deficiency, trace metal deficiency; *Neoplastic:* Food preferences and taste are frequently disturbed by malignant disease, especially with liver involvement; *Psychosocial:* Psychosis, delusions.

Pica. An unusual craving leads to ingestion of clay, paint chips, plaster, laundry starch, and ice chips. Old paint ingestion causes lead poisoning and laundry starch contributes to obesity and hypochromic anemia.

Thirst Disturbance: Water depletion (increased osmolarity and serum sodium) triggers thirst as does moderate to severe extracellular volume depletion. Antidiuretic hormone (ADH) is released increasing water intake and water reabsorption in renal collecting ducts. A defect in the production of ADH or the response of the renal collecting duct to ADH leads to water loss and persistent thirst.

Increased thirst—polydipsia. Thirst indicates a water deficit and/or intravascular volume depletion. Distinguish between isolated water loss (increased osmolarity with normal extracellular volume), loss of extracellular volume alone (normal osmolarity, but decreased volume), and combined losses of extracellular volume and water (increased osmolarity and decreased volume). Most common considerations are diabetes insipidus (central or nephrogenic), diabetes mellitus, hemorrhage, hypotension of any cause, diuretic overuse, dry mouth, psychogenic polydipsia.

Decreased thirst—hypodipsia. A defect in thirst with or without concomitant diabetes insipidus is seen with congenital or acquired hypothalamic structural lesions or hypothalamic stroke.

Constitutional Syndromes and Diseases

Myalgic encephalomyelitis/Chronic fatigue syndrome. The cause is unknown. It usually occurs after a viral illness in young to middle-aged adults. The case definition requires new onset of fatigue not related to exertion and not relieved by rest, resulting in substantial limitation of previous occupational, educational, social, or personal activities. The fatigue must have been present for more than 6 months and should be able to be alleviated by rest. Additionally, postexertional malaise lasting >24 hours and unrefreshing sleep are required to make the diagnosis. Either cognitive impairment or orthostatic intolerance should also be present. Other symptoms like short-term memory loss, sore throat, tender cervical or axillary nodes, muscle pain, polyarthralgias without arthritis, and gastrointestinal impairment may be present.

Diabetes insipidus. Central diabetes insipidus (decreased ADH/vasopressin production) and nephrogenic diabetes insipidus (renal unresponsiveness to ADH) result in an excessive, constant water diuresis. Patients present with an unquenchable thirst, polydipsia, and polyuria with a low urine-specific gravity.

Adipsic diabetes insipidus. Both thirst and ADH secretion are impaired making patients vulnerable to recurrent hypernatremia. Once called essential hypernatremia, this disorder is now called adipsic diabetes insipidus or central diabetes insipidus with deficient thirst. Causes are congenital and acquired central nervous system lesions, the most common being septo-optic dysplasia, germinoma, clipping or rupture of anterior communicating artery aneurysms, craniopharyngioma, and central nervous system sarcoidosis.

THE IMMUNE SYSTEM

Understanding immune system disorders and how they present requires understanding normal immune system physiology. For practical purposes, the immune system has innate, nonspecific, and adaptive components. The latter has evolved more recently. Disorders of innate immunity are often quantitative or qualitative disorders of neutrophils and macrophages. These are discussed with the hematopoietic system. Disorders of adaptive immunity are described below.

Serious congenital immune system disorders present in infancy or childhood and are beyond our scope. Acquired immunologic deficiencies present at any age and are divided into defects of antibody production (humoral immunity) and defects of cell-mediated immunity. Because humoral immunity requires functioning T-cells for proper regulation, defects in cell-mediated immunity are often accompanied by impaired humoral immunity.

Patients with an altered immune system present with a variety of illnesses, most commonly infections, neoplasms, autoimmune disorders, or a combination. This can be the result of a common primary problem (e.g., immunosuppressive drugs), or the presence of a neoplastic disease (e.g., multiple myeloma), severe autoimmune disease (e.g., SLE), chronic infections (e.g., HIV/AIDS, tuberculosis) and chronic systemic illnesses (advanced renal and liver disease). Treatments of neoplastic and autoimmune disorders are often highly immunosuppressive. Iatrogenic immunosuppression is the most commonly encountered immunodeficiency.

Defects in humoral immunity commonly present with infections by encapsulated bacteria (*Streptococcus pneumonia, Haemophilus influenzae, Neisseria meningitidis*, and *Neisseria gonorrhoeae*) that require opsonizing antibodies for control. Since the spleen is needed to clear the blood of opsonized bacteria, rapidly overwhelming infection may occur post-splenectomy. All patients contemplating splenectomy should receive immunization for *Streptococcus pneumonia, Haemophilus influenzae, and Neisseria meningitidis*. Patients with defects in cellular immunity have an increased risk for neoplasms and infections by intracellular pathogens (e.g., tuberculosis) and opportunistic bacterial, viral, and fungal organisms.

The major autoimmune diseases (SLE, RA, vasculitis syndromes, Addison disease, etc.) are discussed elsewhere. Isolated autoimmune hormone deficiencies are common (thyroid, ovary, adrenal, pituitary, islet cells), less common is autoimmune polyglandular syndrome with multiple hormone deficiencies.

Common Immunodeficiency Syndromes

HIV infection and acquired immunodeficiency syndrome (AIDS). HIV infection progressively destroys CD4 cells impairing cellular and humoral immunity. AIDS is defined as <200 CD4 cells/mm³ or an AIDS-defining illness, opportunistic infection, or AIDS-associated neoplasm. Infection is acquired by unprotected sexual intercourse (male homosexuals and heterosexuals of both sexes) intravenous drug use, contact with infected body fluids, and vertical transmission from mother to newborn. Opportunistic infections include parasites (*Pneumocystis jeroveci, Toxoplasmosis encephalitis*, and *Cryptosporidium enteritis*), viruses (cytomegalovirus, Epstein–Barr virus, herpes simplex, herpes zoster, and human herpes virus-8), fungi (candidiasis, cryptococcal meningitis, coccidioidomycosis, histoplasmosis, aspergillosis), bacteria (*salmonella, Strep. pneumoniae, H. influenzae*), mycobacteria (*Mycobacterium tuberculosis, M. avium* complex), *listeria, Treponema pallidum*, and *nocardia*. Symptoms and Signs. Acute HIV infection is a nonspecific viral syndrome, often with exanthem, easily mistaken for Ebstein–Barr virus infection. After a latent period of several years, the patient develops an immunosuppressive syndrome manifest as lymphadenopathy, weight loss, dermatitis, opportunistic infections, and malignancies (e.g., Kaposi sarcoma, central nervous system lymphoma, human papillomavirus-associated anal, and cervical carcinomas).

Common variable immunodeficiency. An acquired defect of B-cell maturation decreases immunoglobulin production and circulating levels of IgG, IgM, and/or IgA. It presents with chronic or recurrent sinusitis and pneumonia. Risk of non-Hodgkin lymphomas is increased.

THE LYMPHATIC SYSTEM

The normal lymphatic system is essential for recognition and response to foreign antigens. Lymphocytes circulate out of capillary blood into tissue, then to lymph nodes, and back to blood via the thoracic duct which empties into the left subclavian vein. Macrophages and Langerhans cells (antigen-presenting cells) migrate from peripheral sites with processed antigen, which they present to T-cells and B-cells in the lymph nodes. T-cells circulate from the capillary circulation to the lymphatics and nodes and then back into the circulation until presented with an antigen specific to their T-cell receptor; recognition leads to activation and proliferation, generating an immune response. Disorders of the lymphatics produce only three physical signs: palpable lymph nodes, red streaks in the skin from superficial lymphangitis, and lymphedema.

Lymph Node Examination: Examination is primarily by palpation though enlarged nodes may be visible by inspection, especially with oblique light. Record these characteristics of palpable lymph nodes: number, size, consistency, mobility, tenderness, warmth, and whether they are discrete or matted together. Procedures for examining the major lymph node beds are described below. All lymph node–bearing areas should be palpated when searching for generalized lymphadenopathy. The spleen should always be examined as part of the lymphatic system examination.

Palpating cervical lymph nodes. With the patient sitting, palpate from behind with the fingertips. Use this sequence for exam: (1) *submental*, midline under the chin and both sides; (2) *submandibular*, under the jaw near its angle; (3) *jugular* (anterior triangle), along the sternocleidomastoid's anterior border; (4) *supraclavicular*, behind the middle of the clavicle; (5) *posterior triangle*, posterior and behind the upper half of the sternocleidomastoid; (6) *postauricular*, behind the ear over the mastoid; (7) *preauricular*, in front of the tragus; (8) *suboccipital*, under the occiput and to either side; and (9) *pre-trapezius*, in front of the upper border of the trapezius (Fig. 5-1). Examine the drainage region of an enlarged node, e.g., anterior cervical triangle—the anterior third

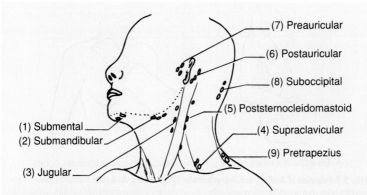

FIG. 5-1 Superficial Lymph Nodes of the Neck. Neck palpation reliably detects lymphadenopathy when each group of nodes is examined systematically. The drawing contains a numbered scheme for examining nine node groups in sequence.

of the scalp and face, posterior cervical triangle, and occiput—the posterior two-thirds of the scalp.

Palpating axillary, infraclavicular, and supraclavicular lymph nodes. With the patient sitting, the right hand palpates the left axilla and the left hand the right axilla (Fig. 5-2A). Relax the arm and axillary muscles by holding the wrist with the other hand, elevating the arm toward the chest. Examine with the palm toward the chest wall, the fingers pointing obliquely toward the axillary apex. Next, rest their hand on the examining arm, while the examiner's other hand supports their shoulder. The central node group on the thoracic wall (Fig. 5-3) is examined by firmly raking the fingers along the chest wall feeling for enlarged nodes. With the arm elevated examine the lateral axillary nodes along the axillary vein medial to the proximal humerus. With the arm still elevated, palpate the pectoral group under the lateral edge of the pectoralis major muscle. From behind with the arm raised, palpate the subscapular nodes under the anterior edge of the latissimus dorsi muscle. Palpate the infraclavicular group under the clavicle. Enlargement in the supraclavicular group is sought by feeling the soft tissues above and behind the clavicle (Fig. 5-2B). Repeat on the other side using the opposite hand for the exam.

Palpating inguinal lymph nodes. Palpate at and just below the inguinal ligament and distally along the course of the greater saphenous vein.

Diseases and Syndromes of Lymphocytes, Lymph Nodes, and Plasma Cells.
Lymphadenopathy. Lymph node enlargement results from a stimulated regional or systemic immune response, direct infection of the node, which can lead to suppuration, deposition of intracellular or extracellular material, or infiltration with neoplastic cells. Describe their distribution, location and number, size, mobility, consistency (fluctuant, soft, firm, hard), surface (smooth, irregular), and any tenderness, warmth, and/or sinus tracts. Perform

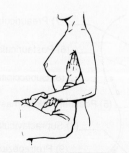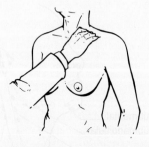

A. Search for axillary nodes   B. Search for supraclavicular nodes

FIG. 5-2 Palpation of Axillary and Supraclavicular Lymph Nodes. A. Axilla: Position the patient's upper arm close to the chest to relax the axillary muscles. Rest the patient's arm on the examining right arm while supporting the shoulder with the left hand. Palpate the left axilla by sliding the right hand toward the axillary apex with palm toward the chest wall. The approximated fingers are extended so the pulps feel the ribs and chest wall. Rake the examining fingertips from apex down the chest wall. Enlarged nodes will slide under the fingertips. The positions are reversed to examine the right side. **B. Supraclavicular fossa.**

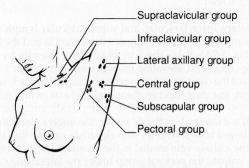

Supraclavicular group
Infraclavicular group
Lateral axillary group
Central group
Subscapular group
Pectoral group

FIG. 5-3 Axillary Lymph Node Groups. Note that the **lateral axillary group** is on the inner aspect of the upper arm, near the axillary vein. The **subscapular group** lies deep to the anterior edge of the latissimus dorsi muscle. The **pectoral group** is behind the lateral edge of the pectoralis major muscle.

a meticulous skin and soft tissue exam of the involved region looking for inflammation, infection, or neoplasm. Pain and tenderness suggest inflammation and/or infection; painless lymphadenopathy is more likely neoplastic. Fluctuant nodes suggest suppurating bacterial, mycobacterial, or fungal infection. Fixation of the nodes to underlying tissue is most common with metastatic carcinoma and chronic inflammation. Matting together of nodes suggests lymphoma or chronic inflammation.

Generalized lymphadenopathy. Lymphadenopathy occurring simultaneously in multiple lymphatic beds, especially above and below the diaphragm, suggests a systemic process, usually infectious, inflammatory or neoplastic.

CLINICAL OCCURRENCE: *Congenital:* Niemann–Pick disease, Gaucher disease; *Degenerative/Idiopathic:* Sarcoidosis, sinus histiocytosis with massive lymphadenopathy (Rosai–Dorfman disease); *Infectious:* Bacteria- Scarlet fever, brucellosis, Lyme disease, secondary syphilis, tularemia, bubonic plague, cat-scratch fever, Whipple disease, melioidosis, scrub typhus; Mycobacteria- Tuberculosis, atypical mycobacteria; Viruses- Rubella, rubeola, infectious mononucleosis, HIV; Protozoa- African trypanosomiasis, Chagas disease, kala-azar, toxoplasmosis; Fungi- Sporotrichosis; Helminths-Filariasis; Ectoparasites- Scabies; *Inflammatory/Immune:* RA, Still disease, dermatomyositis, SLE, amyloidosis, serum sickness, drug allergy, graft-vs-host disease, hyper IgM syndrome; *Metabolic/Toxic:* Drugs (e.g., diphenylhydantoin), berylliosis, silicosis; *Neoplastic:* Hodgkin disease, non-Hodgkin lymphoma, chronic lymphocytic leukemia, systemic mastocytosis, metastatic carcinomas.

Lymphedema. Lymphatic obstruction drainage by whatever cause leads to distal edema from accumulation of interstitial fluid with a high protein content. Patients present with progressive painless swelling of a body part, which can be massive. Initially the edema may pit, but over time fibrosis leads to woody thickening without pitting. Lymphatic injury can result from surgery, irradiation, trauma, and neoplastic obstruction. Longstanding lymphedema is associated with an increased risk for lymphangiosarcoma. *DDX:* The edema may pit at first, but characteristically is not pitting.

Filariasis (wuchereriasis). Lymphatic infestation with *Wuchereria bancrofti* or *Brugia malayi* larvae follows the bite of an infected mosquito. There is inflammation and later scarring with lymphatic obstruction and lymphedema. Headache, photophobia, vertigo, fatigue, low-grade fever, and myalgia are common symptoms. Acute signs include conjunctivitis, orchitis, lymphangitis, and lymphadenopathy; later, obstruction of lymphatic and venous drainage produces edema, hydrocele, and elephantiasis of breasts, scrotum, vulva, or legs.

Inoculation lesion with regional lymphadenopathy. Infectious agents are inoculated into the skin and subcutaneous tissue by trauma, contamination of broken skin, and bites of arthropods and larger animals including humans. The extent of inoculation site inflammation varies with the infecting organism. Local reactions may progress to ulceration and/or necrosis with eschar formation. Spread through subcutaneous lymphatics toward regional lymph nodes is marked by cutaneous inflammation, streaking, and induration.
CLINICAL OCCURRENCE: *Infectious:* Bacterial- Streptococcal infections, syphilitic chancre, anthrax, erysipeloid, ulceroglandular tularemia, bubonic plague, rat-bite fever, cat-scratch disease, nocardia, actinomycosis, glanders; Mycobacteria- Inoculation tuberculosis, atypical mycobacteria; Rickettsia-Scrub typhus, boutonneuse fever, South African tick fever, Kenya typhus, rickettsialpox; Fungi- Sporotrichosis; Viruses- Herpes simplex; Helminths-Filariasis, trypanosomiasis, leishmaniasis; *Neoplastic:* Melanoma, squamous cell carcinoma, lymphangioleiomyomas.

Suppurative lymphadenopathy. Lymph node suppuration is caused by streptococci, staphylococci, bovine tuberculosis, actinomyces, lymphogranuloma venereum, coccidioidomycosis, anthrax, *bartonella henselae*, sporotrichosis, plague, and tularemia.

Ulceroglandular syndromes. See also, Chapter 6, page 142.

Nodular lymphangitis. See Chapter 6, page 142.

HIV infection. See page 81.

B-cell and plasma cell disorders

Non-Hodgkin lymphoma (NHL). NHLs are clonal proliferations, usually of B-lymphocytes, at specific stages of maturation identified by surface markers. Patients present with fever, weight loss, and night sweats, with abdominal pain or fullness, or with palpable lymphadenopathy. They involve multiple sites including non-lymphoid tissue, e.g., lung, stomach, intestine, and central nervous system. They are classified as high-grade disease that is rapidly progressive but potentially curable, and low-grade disease for which curative therapy is generally not available.

Hodgkin disease. This malignant disease of B-cells spreads to contiguous lymph node beds, the spleen, liver, and bone marrow. There are age peaks in the third and eighth decades. Symptoms include pruritus, painless lymph node enlargement, abdominal pain, and occasionally periodic or continuous fever (Pel–Epstein fever, Chapter 4, page 47) and cachexia. Frequently only a single lymph node group is affected, most often in the neck (Fig. 5-4A). The lymph nodes enlarge rapidly over 1–3 weeks or slowly over months and are large, resilient or rubbery. Hepatomegaly and splenomegaly may be present. Nephrotic syndrome may accompany or precede the diagnosis. A thorough examination of all accessible nodes is required. *DDX:* Rarely, drinking alcohol precipitates pain in the nodes so severe and predictable that patients abstain from alcohol. Lymphadenopathy in non-Hodgkin lymphoma is usually generalized and rarely confined to the neck.

Chronic lymphocytic leukemia (CLL). Lymph nodes and bone marrow are infiltrated by a clonal proliferation of mature lymphocytes (90% B-cell, 10%

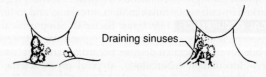

Draining sinuses

A. Cervical lymphadenopathy
of Hodgkin disease

B. Cervical lymphadenopathy
of tuberculosis

FIG. 5-4 Cervical Lymphadenopathy. A. Hodgkin disease. There is no specific pattern of node involvement. The neck is frequently affected first, often unilaterally. The nodes are large, firm, discrete, nontender, and nonsuppurative. **B. Tuberculosis.** One finds a matted mass of nontender lymph nodes. The nodes are firm and some have suppurated forming draining sinuses.

T-cell) with progressive cytopenias and impaired humoral and/or cellular immunity. CLL typically affects older adults, with the average age of diagnosis being about 70. Patients are often asymptomatic until relatively late in the disease. They present with lymphadenopathy and progress to anemia, neutropenia, and thrombocytopenia with recurrent infections. Death usually results from infection or hemorrhage.

Waldenström macroglobulinemia. Proliferation and infiltration of bone marrow, spleen, and liver by proliferating plasmacytoid lymphocytes producing monoclonal IgM (macroglobulin). Elevated circulating IgM leads to hemolytic anemia, immune thrombocytopenia, and increased blood viscosity. Symptoms are insidious onset of anorexia, malaise, weakness, nasal/gingival bleeding, and exertional dyspnea. Signs include any combination of pallor, petechiae, ecchymoses, retinal hemorrhages, lymphadenopathy, hepatosplenomegaly, edema, and heart failure.

Multiple myeloma. A clonal proliferation of plasma cells produces intact immunoglobulins and/or light chains detectable in the serum and urine. Humoral activation of osteoclasts leads to bone resorption without healing, hypercalcemia, and pathologic fractures. Symptoms include bone and muscle pain, backache, weakness, weight loss, and fatigue. There are no specific signs. Bone pain may indicate a pathologic fracture.

Amyloidosis. Deposition of fibrillar amyloid proteins leads to organ enlargement and dysfunction. Several types are identified by the protein deposited. AL amyloidosis results from immunoglobulin light chain deposition. AA amyloidosis occurs in chronic inflammatory diseases. The hereditary amyloidoses have specific fibrillar proteins. Deposition of amyloid proteins can be asymptomatic or cause organ dysfunction. Symptoms are weakness and fatigue. Symptoms vary with the organ system involved: diarrhea, dysphagia, and weight loss (GI involvement); paresthesia (peripheral nerves); dyspnea, orthopnea, and pleural effusions (restrictive cardiomyopathy). Signs also vary with the organs involved: macroglossia, eyelid plaques, hypertension, lymphadenopathy, hepatomegaly, splenomegaly, purpura, nephrotic syndrome, edema, shoulder-pad sign, joint and muscle pain, neuropathy, and fluid in serous cavities.
   CLINICAL OCCURRENCE: AL Amyloidosis: Multiple myeloma, monoclonal gammopathies, primary idiopathic amyloidosis; AA amyloidosis: Chronic inflammatory diseases (e.g., osteomyelitis, tuberculosis, leprosy), familial Mediterranean fever, other familial periodic fevers.

Diseases and Syndromes of Specific Regional Lymph Nodes: Some infectious, inflammatory, or neoplastic lesions in the lymphatic drainage area cause regional lymphadenopathy. Each cause of generalized lymphadenopathy can cause regional adenopathy. Here we list entities more specific to a region.

Lymph node beds of the head and jaw
Suboccipital nodes. Location: Midway between the external occipital protuberance and the mastoid process (Fig. 5-1), near the great occipital nerve. *Drainage:* Afferents from back of scalp and head; efferents to deep cervical

nodes. *Symptoms:* Headache resulting from great occipital nerve impingement by large nodes. *Clinical associations:* Commonly associated with ringworm, pediculosis capitis, seborrheic dermatitis, secondary syphilis, Kikuchi
disease, and metastatic cancer.

Postauricular nodes. Location: On mastoid process and at sternocleidomastoid insertion behind pinna (Fig. 5-1). *Drainage:* Afferents from external
acoustic meatus, back of pinna, temporal scalp; efferents to superior cervical nodes. *Symptoms:* Mastoid tenderness simulating mastoiditis. Common
causes are bacterial or herpetic infection of the acoustic meatus, rubella (not
rubeola), leishmaniasis.

Preauricular nodes. Location: In front of the tragus of the external ear (see
Fig. 5-1). *Drainage:* Afferents from lateral eyelids and palpebral conjunctivae, skin of temporal region, external acoustic meatus, and anterior pinna.
Clinical associations: Consider noninfectious causes like ulcerating basal cell
carcinoma and epithelioma. Infections associated with preauricular nodes are
erysipelas, ophthalmic herpes zoster, rubella, trachoma, ocular-glandular
syndromes, gonorrheal ophthalmia, tuberculosis, syphilis, sporotrichosis,
glanders, chancroid, epidemic keratoconjunctivitis, adenoidal-pharyngeal-
conjunctival virus, Leptothrix infection, lymphogranuloma venereum, tularemia, cat-scratch fever, and Chagas disease.

Mandibular nodes. Location: Under the mandible (Fig. 5-1). *Drainage:* Afferents from tongue, submandibular gland, submental nodes, medial conjunctivae, mucosa of lips and mouth; efferents to superficial and deep jugular
nodes.

Submental nodes. Location: In midline under apex of the mandibular junction (Fig. 5-1). *Drainage:* Afferents from central lower lip, floor of mouth, tip
of tongue, skin of cheek; efferents to mandibular nodes, deep jugular nodes.

Lymph node beds of the neck.
Jugular nodes. Location: Anterior border of the sternocleidomastoid, from
angle of mandible to clavicle (Fig. 5-1). *Drainage:* Afferents from tongue
except apex, tonsil, pinna, parotid gland; efferents to deep jugular nodes.
Clinical associations: Infection or neoplasm of the tonsils and oral cavity and
cancer, especially thyroid cancer are causes.

Posterior sternocleidomastoid nodes. Location: Posterior border of the sternocleidomastoid muscle (Fig. 5-1). *Drainage:* Afferents from the scalp and
neck, upper cervical nodes, axillary nodes, skin of arms and pectoral region,
surface of the thorax. *Clinical associations:* Malignancy, infections (e.g., EBV,
tuberculosis, toxoplasmosis, African trypanosomiasis). In trypanosomiasis,
these nodes are Winterbottom sign.

Scalene nodes. Although not palpable, they are easily biopsied. *Location:* Inferior deep cervical nodes lying deep in the supraclavicular fossa behind the
sternocleidomastoid. *Drainage:* Afferents from the thorax. *Clinical associations:* Intrathoracic granulomatous disease and neoplasms are serious causes.

Important syndromes associated with cervical and supraclavicular lymphadenopathy
Acute cervical lymphadenopathy—localized lymphadenitis. Infections of the scalp, face, mouth, teeth, pharynx, or ear cause localized lymphadenitis of the nodes draining the involved region. Included is chancre with regional lymphadenitis. Cervical adenopathy is common in erythema nodosum, although the subcutaneous lesions are almost always limited to the legs. In a toxic patient with severe tenderness, consider Lemierre syndrome (Chapter 7, page 236).

Subacute localized cervical lymphadenopathy: metastatic carcinoma. Asymptomatic head and neck cancers frequently present with cervical lymph node metastases. The nodes are stony hard, nontender, and nonsuppurative. Epidermoid carcinoma predominates. With anterior triangle involvement, primary malignancies are in the upper aerodigestive tract, including the maxillary sinus, oral cavity, tongue, tonsil, hypopharynx, and larynx. In the submental region, metastases are from a primary neoplasms in the lower lip, anterior tongue, or floor of the mouth. In the posterior triangle, the nasopharynx and scalp are common sites. *Never surgically biopsy a solitary cervical lymph node suspicious for metastatic cancer.* Violation of the neck's tissue planes may preclude surgical cure. Always refer patients for direct exam of the aerodigestive tract by an experienced observer.

Sentinel node (Virchow node). Metastasis via the thoracic duct from a primary carcinoma in the upper abdomen enlarge a single lymph node, usually in the left supraclavicular group, frequently behind the clavicular head of the left sternocleidomastoid. It often escapes casual examination. Examine behind the muscle head from in front, while the patient sits erect. The node may be better appreciated with a Valsalva. Breast, lung, pelvic, and testicular cancers can also spread to the supraclavicular fossa.

Chronic localized cervical lymphadenopathy: tuberculosis (scrofula). This is usually caused by *M. bovis*. Nodes are large, multiple, nontender, and classically matted; this is often difficult to determine by palpation (Fig. 5-4B). The nodes frequently suppurate forming indolent sinus tracts. Extensive scarring often results.

Kikuchi lymphadenitis. Cervical lymphadenopathy in a young woman is characteristic. It is benign, but often confused with other entities.

Actinomycosis. Actinomyces bacteria from the oral flora infect the mouth, face, and cervical lymph nodes crossing tissue planes. The nodes are prone to suppurate, forming sinuses with a bright-red hue. The pus contains sulfur granules 1 to 2 mm in diameter.

Lymph node beds of the chest, axilla, and arms
Supraclavicular nodes. Location: Part of the inferior deep cervical chain behind the origin of the sternocleidomastoid muscle (Fig. 5-1). *Drainage:* Afferents from head, arm, chest wall, breast. *Clinical associations:* Granulomatous diseases, lung and esophageal neoplasms; on the left, abdominal neoplasms.

Axillary nodes. *Location:* Five groups lie on the medial humerus, the axillary border of the scapula, and the lateral border of the pectoralis major (Fig. 5-3). *Drainage:* Afferents from the arm, thoracic wall, and breast. *DDX:* In women, enlarged axillary nodes on the chest wall must be distinguished from the axillary tail of the breast. Small mobile axillary nodes are common and normal.

Epitrochlear nodes. *Location:* In the groove between the biceps and triceps ~3 cm proximal to the medial humeral epicondyle. *Drainage:* Afferents from ulnar aspect of forearm and hand, and entire little and ring fingers, the ulnar half of the long finger. *Clinical associations:* The hands and arms are a common inoculation site of systemic infections, e.g., cat-scratch disease. Epitrochlear nodes are common in secondary syphilis (father-in-law sign).

Mediastinal nodes. *Location:* Chest x-ray shows mediastinal widening, anterior mediastinal mass, and/or an enlarged hilum. *Clinical associations:* Tuberculosis, coccidioidomycosis, histoplasmosis, anthrax, sarcoidosis, silicosis, beryllium poisoning, erythema nodosum, Hodgkin disease, non-Hodgkin lymphoma (lymphoblastic lymphoma), chronic lymphocytic leukemia, testicular cancer.

Abdominal and inguinal lymph node beds.
Abdominal nodes. *Location:* No clinical distinction made between intraabdominal and retroperitoneal nodes. Large nodes may be palpated as intraabdominal masses. Calcified nodes are seen radiographically. *Clinical associations:* Primary lymphoma and metastases from testicular cancers should be considered.

Inguinal nodes. *Location:* Lying horizontally along the inguinal ligament and vertically along the great saphenous vein. *Drainage:* Afferents of the horizontal group from the lower abdominal skin, retroperitoneum, penis, scrotum, vulva, vagina, perineum, buttocks, and lower anal canal; afferents of the vertical group from the leg, penis, scrotum, and buttocks. *Clinical associations:* Palpable inguinal nodes are common without active disease. Testicular tumors metastasize directly to paraaortic nodes not the inguinal nodes; scrotal cancer spreads to inguinal nodes.

Genital lesion with satellite nodes. *Clinical associations:* Consider syphilis, gonorrhea, chancroid, herpes simplex, lymphogranuloma venereum, tuberculosis, and cancer of penis.

THE HEMATOPOIETIC SYSTEM AND HEMOSTASIS

The hematopoietic and immune systems are interlinked through production of B-cells, T-cells, and innate immune system cells (monocytes, macrophages, neutrophils, eosinophils, and basophils). Practically, hematopoietic disorders affect red blood cells, neutrophils, and platelets either quantitatively, an increase or decrease in the specific cell type, and/or qualitatively, a disorder of function with, usually, a normal numbers of cells. Presentations vary with the affected cell.

Red Blood Cell (RBC, Erythrocyte) Disorders

Anemia. Anemia means a persistently low hemoglobin and hematocrit. It results from decreased effective erythrocyte (red blood cell—RBC) production, blood loss, increased RBC destruction (hemolysis), and/or sequestration of erythrocytes in an enlarged spleen. Decreased effective RBC production can be due to decreased erythropoietin (EPO) stimulus for RBC production (e.g., chronic kidney disease), inability to respond appropriately to EPO due to nutritional deficiency (e.g., iron deficiency) or *ineffective erythropoiesis* resulting from defects in normoblast maturation. Patients present with fatigue, dyspnea, decreased exercise tolerance, and weakness. Pallor is notable in the conjunctivae and palmar skin creases when the hemoglobin is <10 g/dL. On exam search for jaundice, lymphadenopathy, splenomegaly, hepatomegaly, and signs of hemorrhage. *DDX:* Unlike congestive heart failure, dyspnea on exertion from anemia is not accompanied by orthopnea.

CLINICAL OCCURRENCE: *Hypoproliferative:* Iron deficiency, anemia of chronic disease, hypothyroidism, kidney failure, marrow damage (tumor infiltration, granulomatous disease, myelofibrosis); *Ineffective erythropoiesis:* Thalassemias, sickle cell disease, vitamin B_{12} and folate deficiency, myelodysplastic syndrome; *Hemolysis:* Congenital erythrocyte disorders (hereditary spherocytosis, hereditary elliptocytosis, glucose-6-phosphate dehydrogenase deficiency, pyruvate kinase deficiency), autoimmune hemolytic anemias (warm-reacting, IgG; cold-reacting, IgM), paroxysmal nocturnal hemoglobinuria (PNH), microangiopathic states (thrombotic thrombocytopenic purpura, hemolytic–uremic syndrome, malignant hypertension), infections, hemophagocytic syndromes, hypersplenism; *Sequestration:* Massive splenomegaly (chronic myelogenous leukemia—CML, portal hypertension); *Hemorrhage:* Overt external bleeding, bleeding into body cavities and muscle, or occult. Occult gastrointestinal hemorrhage is particularly common.

Iron deficiency. Iron is the key element in hemoglobin, myoglobin, and the cytochromes necessary for energy production. The most common cause of anemia worldwide, it results from decreased iron ingestion (rare since iron is ubiquitous in the environment and all but the most restrictive diets), chronic blood loss (menses, occult GI bleeding, phlebotomy), or rarely from iron binding by phytates in the diet. Iron deficiency in infants delays intellectual development. Symptoms are weakness and lassitude often out of proportion to the hemoglobin level.

Sickle cell disease. Patients are homozygous for autosomal recessive hemoglobin-S (HbS), which is unstable at low-oxygen tension. Aggregated HbS produces RBC sickling. Sickled RBCs obstruct the microcirculation causing ischemia and hemolysis. Persons of African ancestry are most commonly affected. Compound heterozygotes with other hemoglobinopathies may present with milder symptoms. Presentation is in childhood with painful crises associated with fever, malaise, headache, epistaxis, and pains in legs and abdomen associated with hemolysis. Growth abnormalities include tower skull, short trunk, thoracic kyphosis, and small stature. Additional signs are abdominal and bone tenderness, pallor, yellow–green sclerae, cardiomegaly, hepatomegaly, splenomegaly, and ulcers on shins.

β-Thalassemia major. A homozygous β-chain gene mutation limits hemoglobin synthesis leading to hemolysis and ineffective erythropoiesis. There is bone marrow expansion, extramedullary hematopoiesis, and increased hemoglobin-F production. The disease is evident in childhood with mongoloid facies, prominent frontal bosses, hepatomegaly, splenomegaly, pallor, cardiac dilatation, and growth retardation.

β-Thalassemia minor. A heterozygous β-globulin gene mutation leads to mild hypochromic, microcytic anemia. Patients are asymptomatic or have mild fatigue and are often misdiagnosed with iron deficiency because of the hypochromic microcytic anemia. Iron overload occurs if iron is given inappropriately. Clue to diagnosis may be mild microcytic anemia with a high-normal or elevated RBC count.

Paroxysmal nocturnal hemoglobinuria (PNH). RBCs are susceptible to complement mediated lysis due to acquired loss or a cell surface anchor protein. Symptoms include abdominal, retrosternal, or lumbar pain. There may be chronic anemia, venous thrombosis, and hemoglobinuria at night. There is an increased risk for acute leukemia.

Pernicious anemia and vitamin B_{12} deficiency. In pernicious anemia, autoimmune gastritis decreases intrinsic factor production resulting in B_{12} malabsorption. Other causes of B_{12} malabsorption (e.g., food-cobalamin malabsorption) are more common. Patients present with fatigue, glossitis, proprioception deficits caused by posterior column disease, and/or dementia. A high index of suspicion is required. Up to 5% of persons >75 years of age are B_{12}-deficient. Other causes of B_{12} deficiency include postgastrectomy, celiac disease, small bowel bacterial overgrowth, intestinal parasites, distal ileum resection, and dietary deficiency.

Erythrocytosis—polycythemia. Increased RBC production results from an abnormally proliferating clone (polycythemia vera) or is secondary to hypoxemia, abnormal hemoglobins, renal tumors, or drugs (testosterone, erythropoietin). Patients present with plethora and dyspnea. In secondary polycythemia, there may be signs of advanced chronic lung disease. Congestive heart failure with edema occurs with hematocrits >60%. Hyperviscosity produces signs of organ dysfunction, stroke, and thrombosis. *DDX:* With polycythemia vera there is splenomegaly and increased plasma and red blood cell volumes, usually with leukocytosis and thrombocythemia.

Neutrophil Disorders
Neutropenia. Decreased neutrophil production (granulocytes, segmented polymorphonuclear leukocytes-PMNs) results from aplastic anemia, a myeloproliferative syndrome, leukemia, infection, or drug toxicity. Hypersplenism reduces the circulating PMNs. The patient is asymptomatic until the neutrophil count is <500 per mm^3 when infection with normal flora, especially *Staphylococcus aureus, Streptococcus pyogenes,* and gram-negative GI flora are greatly increased. Patients often initially present with fever and septicemia. Febrile neutropenia accompanying cancer chemotherapy is a diagnostic and therapeutic challenge.

Leukocytosis. Increased neutrophil production is a normal response to infection and hemorrhage. An increase in bands is most consistent with infection. Epinephrine and corticosteroids cause neutrophils adherent to vessel walls (marginated pool) to demarginate increasing the neutrophil count by 50% to 100%. Increases in mature leukocyte counts are asymptomatic, even at levels >200,000 per mm^3. Diagnostic keys are symptoms and signs of underlying disease. Persistent neutrophilia without evident cause suggests a myeloproliferative disorder such as polycythemia vera or CML. Many circulating immature forms suggests CML.

Myeloproliferative Disorders and Acute Leukemia

Chronic myelogenous leukemia. An acquired balanced genetic translocation of the bcr gene on chromosome 22 and the abl gene on chromosome 9 leads to a functional fusion bcr–abl tyrosine kinase. Symptoms begin gradually with fatigue, malaise, loss of appetite, and abdominal fullness. There is usually palpable splenomegaly which may become massive. With progression, anemia and thrombocytopenia occur. Progression terminates with transformation to a relatively refractory acute leukemia, the blast crisis.

Polycythemia vera (PV). Clonal proliferation of erythrocytes, neutrophils, and platelets increases red cell mass and plasma volume leading to increased blood volume, increased hematocrit, and decreased capillary blood flow from increased blood viscosity. Patients present with fatigue, neurologic symptoms, aquagenic pruritus, and thromboses. Spontaneous hepatic vein thrombosis (Budd–Chiari syndrome) and portal or mesenteric vein thrombosis should trigger an evaluation for PV, even in the absence of elevated hematocrit. Physical findings are plethora and splenomegaly.

Essential thrombocytosis. There is unregulated proliferation of platelets leading to platelet counts >500,000 and often >1,000,000 per mm^3. Patients are asymptomatic until presenting with bleeding or thrombosis, headache, transient ischemic attacks, or hemorrhage.

Myelofibrosis (myeloid metaplasia). Fibrosis obliterates the marrow space leading to extramedullary hematopoiesis in the spleen and liver, and progressive pancytopenia. The cause is unknown. Patients complain of weakness, increased fatigability, weight loss, pallor, and fullness in the left upper quadrant. Splenomegaly and hepatomegaly are usually evident. Dependent edema, bone pain, and fever may be present.

Acute leukemia. Several forms occur, all presenting with clonal proliferation of immature myeloid or lymphoid precursors leading to marrow replacement, neutropenia, and thrombocytopenia. The onset and progression are acute and rapid. Symptoms may be fever, bleeding, or malaise. Prompt recognition and treatment are required. Prevention of disseminated intravascular coagulation associated with acute promyelocytic leukemia requires pretreatment with all-trans retinoic acid.

Platelet Disorders

Thrombocytopenia. Decreased platelet production, increased platelet consumption, immune-mediated platelet destruction, or hypersplenism are the common causes. Patients present with defective hemostasis manifest as bleeding gums, bruising, epistaxis, or bleeding following minor trauma or surgical procedures. Signs include purpura from petechiae to large ecchymoses. Examine for splenomegaly, hepatomegaly, and lymphadenopathy. Spontaneous intracranial hemorrhage is a significant risk with platelet counts <10,000 per mm³.

CLINICAL OCCURRENCE: *Decreased production:* Cytotoxic chemotherapy, other drugs (e.g., heparin, thiazides, ethanol, quinine); *Increased consumption:* Massive hemorrhage, hypertransfusion syndrome, thrombotic thrombocytopenic purpura, disseminated intravascular coagulation; *Immune destruction:* Immune thrombocytopenic purpura, lymphomas, monoclonal gammopathy of unknown significance (MGUS), SLE, HIV infection, heparin-induced thrombocytopenia (HIT); *Hypersplenism:* Portal hypertension, lymphoma.

Immune thrombocytopenic purpura (ITP). Antibodies to platelets lead to their destruction in the spleen. Very low platelet counts persist despite increased platelet production. ITP presents at any age and is especially common in women with other autoimmune diseases especially SLE. Monoclonal gammopathies of unknown significance (MGUS) may be associated. It is asymptomatic, and the signs are those of purpura. Large platelets are seen on peripheral smear.

Heparin-induced thrombocytopenia. Antibodies to platelet factor 4–heparin complex lead to rapid platelet agglutination either directly (HIT-I) or secondary to immune mechanisms (HIT-II). Patients receiving heparin for several days develop acute or worsening thrombosis, often of major arteries, in association with thrombocytopenia. Persons previously exposed to heparin can have onset within hours of starting heparin. The symptoms and signs vary with the sites of thrombosis and infarction.

Thrombocytosis. Increased platelet production occurs with myeloproliferative diseases, iron deficiency, chronic inflammatory disorders, and hemorrhage. This is usually asymptomatic until the platelet count is >750,000 per mm³. Hemorrhage is the most common complication, although thrombosis also occurs. See Essential Thrombocytosis, page 93.

Disorders of platelet function. See Intradermal Hemorrhage, Chapter 6, page 129.

Coagulation Disorders: Coagulation disorders are congenital or acquired. Congenital abnormalities are usually a factor deficiency or decreased factor function. Acquired disorders may be factor deficiencies or functional inhibition of coagulation. In either case, patients present with delayed bleeding from sites of trauma, spontaneous hemorrhage into joints, and severe hemorrhage following surgical procedures.

Hypoprothrombinemia. Warfarin administration, vitamin K deficiency, or hepatic insufficiency lead to deficiencies of vitamin K-dependent coagulation factors (II, VII, IX, X) and proteins S and C. Patients present with visceral bleeding including epistaxis, bleeding from gums, easy bruising, ecchymoses, hematuria, melena, and/or menorrhagia. Symptoms and signs of malabsorption may be present if the cause is malabsorption of fat-soluble vitamins (A, D, E, and K).

Hemophilias: factor VIII deficiency (hemophilia A and antibodies to factor VIII) and factor IX deficiency (hemophilia B). The hemophilias are clinically indistinguishable X-linked disorders with decreased synthesis of physiologically active factor VIII or IX. Symptoms and signs begin in childhood with spontaneous bleeding or excessive hemorrhage following dental extractions and surgery. Hemarthroses lead to joint deformities and contractures. Antibodies to factor VIII are acquired in older adults, postpartum, with drugs, and in SLE.

von Willebrand disease. von Willebrand disease (vWD) is a group of autosomal dominant defects in factor VIII von Willebrand factor production or function. Patients present with signs of bruising and bleeding due to ineffective platelet adhesion. Aspirin use augments the hemostatic defect. The partial thromboplastin time (PTT) is prolonged. Many affected people are never diagnosed.

Thrombophilia. Congenital or acquired disorders of coagulation and fibrinolytic pathways lead to increased risk for thromboembolism. Patients present with venous and, less commonly arterial, thromboembolism. Often there is no identifiable risk factor (e.g., trauma, surgery, immobility) other than a family history of thromboembolic disease. Common causes are factor V Leiden, deficiencies of antithrombin III, proteins C and S, prothrombin gene mutations, and antiphospholipid syndrome. Arterial thromboembolism suggests antiphospholipid syndrome, nonbacterial thrombotic endocarditis (NBTE), or Trousseau syndrome.

Antiphospholipid syndrome. Antiphospholipid antibodies inappropriately activate the clotting system leading to arterial and venous thrombosis. Patients present with in-situ arterial thrombosis, venous thromboembolic disease, livedo reticularis, cardiac valve abnormalities, and/or frequent miscarriage. There is greatly increased risk of end organ damage and death. Though frequently seen in association with SLE, primary antiphospholipid syndrome rarely progresses to SLE.

THE ENDOCRINE SYSTEM

Endocrine disorders are common. Clinicians should think of endocrine disorders when patients present with systemic symptoms (fatigue, weakness, anorexia, change in weight, and malaise) without fever or localizing symptoms and signs.

Diabetes and Hypoglycemia

Diabetes mellitus type-1. Immune destruction of β-cells in pancreatic islets produces absolute insulin deficiency resulting in hyperglycemia, osmotic diuresis, impaired energy metabolism, and reliance on fatty acid oxidation for energy, leading to ketosis and ketoacidosis. With chronic disease there is progressive microvasculature injury in the eyes, glomeruli, nerves, and large vessel atherosclerosis. Symptoms include polydipsia, polyuria, polyphagia, weight loss, and weakness. Physical findings are dryness of the skin and acetone on the breath. After ≥15 years, symptoms and signs of peripheral neuropathy, atherosclerosis, renal insufficiency, and retinopathy may be seen.

Diabetes mellitus type-2. Insulin resistance is the primary disorder. Hyperglycemia results from persistent hepatic gluconeogenesis despite elevated circulating insulin levels. Patients are usually obese adults, although it is seen increasingly in children. There is a strong familial predisposition and an increased risk in some ethnic groups (e.g., Hispanics and Pima Indians). The metabolic abnormalities are like those of type-1 diabetes, but less acute, so many patients escape detection until complications (e.g., myocardial infarction, neuropathy, retinopathy, or renal insufficiency) bring them to medical attention. Polyuria and polydipsia are gradual in onset and less pronounced than in type-1.

Hypoglycemia. Low blood glucose results from increased insulin effects or decreased hepatic glucose production. Hypoglycemia is a common self-misdiagnosis associated with nonspecific complaints related to autonomic activity, e.g., sweating, shakiness, flushing, anxiety, or nausea. True symptoms of hypoglycemia are *neuroglycopenic*, e.g., dizziness, confusion, tiredness, dysarthria, headache, and difficulty thinking, resulting from brain dysfunction. Inadvertent or surreptitious use of insulin or hypoglycemia-inducing medications is the most common cause of hypoglycemia, usually in patients with known diabetes. Insulinoma is rare and reactive hypoglycemia (alimentary hypoglycemia) is an unproven concept.

Disorders of Thyroid Function: Changes in thyroid size and consistency are frequently associated with disturbances of function. Thyroid hormone excess or deficiency alters physiology producing physical signs. Determine thyroid size and morbid anatomy, assess thyroid function, and estimate the likelihood of cancer. Thyroid mass is assessed by history, inspection, and palpation. Thyroid function is assessed by symptoms and signs of hypo- or hyperthyroidism, paying attention to the pulse, pulse pressure, eyes and face, voice, skin and hair, stretch reflexes, affect, and mood. Clinical hypotheses are tested in the lab. The presence or absence of malignancy can only be determined by obtaining tissue. See Chapter 7, pages 256 and 258 for discussion of goiter and thyroid nodules.

Abnormalities of thyroid function. L-Thyroxine (T4) production is controlled by thyrotropin (thyroid stimulating hormone, TSH) released from the anterior pituitary under the control of hypothalamic thyrotropin-releasing hormone (TRH). T4 and triiodothyronine (T3) are released from the thyroid follicles in a ratio of 20:1. In peripheral tissues T4 is converted to the active hormone T3, at a rate specific to each tissue. T4 and T3 inhibit TRH release from the hypothalamus and pituitary TSH release. Thyroid hormones bind to thyroid hormone receptors in the nucleus. Binding of this complex to thyroid response elements of multiple genes affects gene transcription and cellular metabolism.

Hypothyroidism. Underproduction of thyroid hormone slows the metabolism of all tissues producing cellular, organ, and whole-body hypofunction. Myxedema, the most severe form, manifests as soft-tissue thickening consequent to interstitial mucopolysaccharide accumulation. *Symptoms:* Patients complain of fatigue, loss of energy, decreased concentration, coldness, constipation, and weight gain despite decreased food intake. The onset is often gradual and overlooked. *Signs:* The face is rounded, relaxed, and puffy without edema. The expression is placid and good-natured. Responses are slow. Speech is slow, and the voice is hoarse from vocal cord thickening. There is a paucity of motion (*hypokinesia*); movements are slow and deliberate. There is generalized weakness, but muscle wasting, and paralysis are absent. Slow muscle relaxation is seen and felt when testing knee and ankle reflexes; it is as if the part were "hung up." The tongue may be large and awkward. The skin is cool, dry, and thick, often with scaling difficult to distinguish from ichthyosis. The palms and circumoral skin may be yellow from carotenemia. The hair is dry, coarse, and easily broken. The nails are also dry and brittle. The only ocular sign is periorbital edema. Cardiovascular signs include reduced strength of myocardial contraction manifest as a reduced apical impulse and pulse contour. Angina and heart failure may be present at diagnosis or be manifest with thyroid hormone replacement. Pericardial effusion (ECG with low-voltage QRS complexes), ascites, and ankle edema occur without heart failure. The ventricular rate is normal or slow. Dysrhythmias are rare. The blood pressure is normal or there is moderate elevation of both systolic and diastolic pressure. Constipation is common resulting in tympanites suggesting ileus. Menorrhagia is common. Thinking is slowed (*bradyphrenia*), patients are irritable and emotionally labile, and may develop depression. Myxedema coma is a rare but grave condition that paradoxically does not require the patient to be comatose.

Hyperthyroidism. Overproduction or ingestion of thyroid hormone increases the metabolic rate producing changes in all organ systems. Sympathetic nervous system stimulation accounts for many symptoms and signs. *Symptoms:* Patients initially feel energetic and are often happy to be losing weight. They progressively develop tremor, sweaty skin, frequent defecation, and weight loss despite increasing food intake. *Signs:* Patients are alert and vigilant, responses to questions are quick and the emotions are labile. The face is thin with sharp features. Spontaneous movement is increased (*hyperkinesia*). The voice is normal, but speech cadence is accelerated. There is often quadriceps weakness; the patient pushes with the arms to rise from a chair. Reflexes are normal or hyperactive with unsustained clonus; in patients taking β-blockers this may be the only sign of hyperthyroidism. There is almost always a fine tremor. The skin is thin, moist, and sweaty; the hair is fine and oily. The fingernails may separate from the matrix (*onycholysis*); usually only one or two pairs of nails are involved. Lid lag is frequent. Cardiovascular signs include tachycardia and increased strength of myocardial contraction manifest by an accentuated apex beat and sharp heart sounds. Angina and congestive failure may be precipitated in patients with coronary artery disease. The systolic blood pressure is slightly elevated, the diastolic diminished, so the pulse pressure is widened. There is a high incidence of atrial fibrillation. Defecation may be more frequent; the onset of true diarrhea is a grave prognostic sign. Extracellular fluid does not accumulate unless cardiac failure occurs.

Menses are usually normal; occasionally there is oligomenorrhea. Mental status changes include irritability, emotional lability, and depression; occasionally, a manic state develops.

Graves disease (diffuse toxic goiter). Autoantibodies activate the TSH receptor producing TSH-independent hyperplasia and increased T4 release. Myxomatous infiltration of the extraocular muscles produces exophthalmos and abnormalities of gaze. The thyroid is diffusely enlarged, usually ≤2x normal. A thyroid bruit results from increased blood flow through the tortuous thyroid arteries. The eye signs occur at any time and initially can be unilateral. The signs are lid lag, lid spasm, lacrimation, chemosis, periorbital edema, periorbital infiltration with mucopolysaccharides, and exophthalmos (*proptosis*; Chapter 7, page 196, Fig. 7-29). Often there is paresis of extraocular muscles, usually involving one or two symmetrical pairs; isolated weakness of the two superior recti is common. Firm, nontender, pink, well circumscribed areas of elevated skin over the shins known as *pretibial myxedema* usually occurs in association with the ophthalmopathy. Similar skin thickening on the dorsal fingers or toes is *thyroid acropachy*.

Hashimoto thyroiditis. Lymphocytic thyroid inflammation produces induration and gradual loss of function. This is the most common cause of hypothyroidism; it occurs most commonly in women after the fifth decade. The gland is firm, only slightly enlarged, nontender, and nodules may be present.

Postpartum thyroiditis. Painless inflammation of the thyroid gland is common following normal pregnancy. Onset is usually 3–6 months postpartum signaled by signs of either hyper- or hypothyroidism. The latter is often confused with the fatigue and stress of caring for a newborn. The gland is diffusely enlarged and nontender. It usually resolves over a period of months.

De Quervain thyroiditis, viral thyroiditis. Acute inflammation of the thyroid from viral infection or postinfectious inflammation releases thyroid hormone from damaged follicles producing hyperthyroidism with depressed TSH and low iodine uptake. The patient may complain of pain with swallowing which is frequently referred to the ear. The gland is unusually firm and rather small with one or more, often tender, nodules. In the acute phase the patient may be euthyroid or hyperthyroid.

Adrenal Disorders

Corticosteroid excess—Cushing syndrome. Hypercortisolism results from adenoma or adenocarcinoma of the adrenal cortex, excess adrenocorticotropic hormone (ACTH) from a pituitary adenoma, corticosteroids treatment, or ectopic ACTH production. Patients present with weakness, weight gain, amenorrhea, and/or back pain. Physical findings include hypertension, moon face, acne, thoracic kyphosis, supraclavicular fat pads, hypertrichosis, wide purple striae on the abdomen and thighs, and peripheral edema.

Primary adrenal insufficiency—Addison disease. Primary adrenal failure results from autoimmune, ischemic, or hemorrhagic destruction of the gland resulting in cortisol and mineralocorticoid (aldosterone) deficiency and increased circulating ACTH. Increased stimulation of pituitary proopiomelanocortin synthesis and ACTH release causes a secondary increase in melanocyte-stimulating hormone. Symptoms include weakness, fatigue, lethargy, nausea and vomiting, diarrhea, weight loss, abdominal pain, and salt craving. Physical exam may reveal reduced hair growth, hypotension (especially orthostatic), dehydration, mottled skin pigmentation, and pigmented buccal mucosa, lips, vagina, and rectum. Cause to be considered include tuberculosis, fungal infection, other granulomatous processes, amyloidosis, hemochromatosis, tumor metastases, antiphospholipid antibody syndrome, or autoimmune destruction.

Secondary adrenocortical insufficiency. Pituitary insufficiency with decreased ACTH production or inadequate recovery of ACTH responsiveness following prolonged corticosteroid administration leads to inadequate cortisol levels. Symptoms and signs are less prominent than with primary adrenal failure because the mineralocorticoid axis remains intact. Symptoms are often precipitated when relative cortisol deficiency appears in a setting of increased cortisol demand, e.g., infection, trauma, or surgery.

Disorders of Parathyroid Function

Hyperparathyroidism. An adenoma, hyperplasia, or neoplasia of a parathyroid gland leads to excessive secretion of parathyroid hormones (PTH) causing bone resorption and inhibition of renal tubular phosphate reabsorption. Hyperparathyroidism may be primary or secondary to hypocalcemia (renal insufficiency, hypercalciuria) activating the parathyroid glands. In some cases of secondary hyperparathyroidism, the gland becomes autonomous, tertiary hyperparathyroidism. Primary hyperparathyroidism is most common in women in the third to fifth decades. Onset is insidious and often detected by abnormal calcium on serum chemistries drawn for another reason. The clinical triad of peptic ulcer, urinary calculi, and pancreatitis suggests the diagnosis. Symptoms can include muscle weakness or stiffness, anorexia, nausea, constipation, polyuria, polydipsia, weight loss, deafness, paresthesias, bone pain, and renal colic. Signs include band (calcific) keratitis, hypotonia and weakness, fragility fractures, and skeletal deformities.

Hypoparathyroidism. This occurs spontaneously or from removal or damage to the parathyroid glands during thyroidectomy. Inadequate parathyroid hormone secretion leads to hypocalcemia and hyperphosphatemia. Symptoms are nervousness, weakness, paresthesias, muscle stiffness and cramps, headaches, and abdominal pain. Tetany with spontaneous carpopedal spasm may be seen or is induced by inflation of a blood pressure cuff on the arm (*Trousseau sign*). A facial twitch on light percussion over the facial nerve is *Chvostek sign*. Other signs are hair loss, cataracts, and papilledema.

Vitamin D deficiency. Vitamin D_3 is synthesized in the skin under the influence of sunlight. It is converted to the active 1,25-dihydoxycholecalciferol form sequentially in the liver (25-hydorxylation) and kidney (1-hydroxylation). Vitamin D deficiency is common especially in older and/or chronically ill persons in northern latitudes. African Americans and darkly pigmented individuals of other ethnic backgrounds are especially at risk.

Diets low in milk products supplemented with vitamin D are another risk factor. In addition to osteomalacia manifest as low bone density and leading to secondary hyperparathyroidism, patients frequently complain of diffuse persistent musculoskeletal pain. Anyone presenting with these risk factors or complaints should be evaluated for vitamin D.

Disorders of Pituitary Function.

Acromegaly and gigantism. See Chapter 13, page 581.

Cushing disease. See Cushing Syndrome, page 98.

Prolactinoma. Increased prolactin secretion by a functioning pituitary micro-adenoma or macroadenoma suppresses FSH and LH secretion and induces lactation. Women present with galactorrhea and amenorrhea, men with decreased libido and hypogonadotropic hypogonadism. Headache suggests a macroadenoma.

Hypopituitarism. The pituitary gland is destroyed by tumor, injury, infarct, or granuloma leading to progressive pituitary insufficiency with decreased thyroid, adrenal cortex and gonadal function. Symptoms are those of multiple endocrine failure; hypogonadal symptoms are a common early indication. Cold intolerance, weakness, nausea, vomiting, impotence, and amenorrhea are characteristic. Signs include hypothermia, bradycardia, hypotension, skin atrophy, pallor, hypotonia, areolar depigmentation, loss of axillary and pubic hair, and atrophy of sex organs.

Sheehan syndrome. Hemorrhage and shock during obstetrical delivery causes hypopituitarism secondary to pituitary necrosis. Symptoms include failure of lactation, amenorrhea, lethargy, sensitivity to cold, and diminished sweating. There is fine wrinkling of the skin, hair loss, depigmentation of the skin and areola, and mammary and genital atrophy.

CLINICAL VIGNETTES AND QUESTIONS

Case 5-1

A 32-year-old man presents with 2 weeks of fever, fatigue, anorexia, sore throat, and headache. He has multiple sexual partners and used intravenous drugs on and off in the last 2 years. On examination he has generalized lymphadenopathy and a widespread maculopapular rash.

QUESTIONS:
1. What is the most likely diagnosis?
2. What is the differential diagnosis of generalized lymphadenopathy?

Case 5-2

You are examining a 23-year-old man with high fever, pharyngitis, and lymphadenopathy. He has prominent cervical lymphadenopathy (posterior cervical lymph nodes are more pronounced compared to anterior). You also notice some lymphadenopathy in the axillary and inguinal areas.

QUESTIONS:
1. What is the differential diagnosis of cervical lymphadenopathy?
2. Describe some characteristics of mycobacterial cervical node infection (scrofula).
3. What is the most likely diagnosis?

Case 5-3

A 26-year-old man is brought to the emergency room after becoming confused at work while preparing his lunch. He started an exercise program this morning to lose weight. He remembers getting sweaty, shaky, extremely hungry, and seeing double. He appeared confused to coworkers and seemed to be struggling to focus on things around him. He has had similar episodes for 6 months if he skips breakfast, but never this severe. Eating a snack resolves the symptoms; today he improved with orange juice. He does not take any medications and denies any illicit substances. Vital signs are normal and his BMI is 30.

QUESTIONS:
1. What is the most likely etiology for this patient's symptoms?
2. What is Whipple's triad and what does it indicate?
3. What is the most likely diagnosis in this patient?
4. What is the most common cause for this presentation?

Case 5-4

A 55-year-old woman is found to have multiple hard nontender right axillary lymph nodes during a routine screening examination. No upper extremity lesion or source of infection is found.

QUESTIONS:
1. What is the drainage area for axillar lymph nodes?
2. What is the differential diagnosis for axillary lymphadenopathy?
3. What is the most likely cause?

Case 5-5

You are planning a lymph node examination on a 70-year-old man with unexplained weight loss.

QUESTION:
1. When examining lymph nodes, which features of the lymph nodes are essential to forming your differential diagnosis?

CHAPTER 6

The Skin and Nails

Every clinician should be able to characterize skin lesions, identify common conditions, and recognize cutaneous signs of systemic disease.

PHYSIOLOGY OF THE SKIN AND NAILS

Skin protects the body from injury, infection, heat, and fluid loss and is a major intermediary for sensing the outside world. It is continuous with the mucous membranes at body orifices. The dermis is rich in blood vessels that constrict to conserve heat or dilate dissipating heat via radiation, conduction, and convection aided by sweating. Dermal and subcutaneous fat provide insulation assisting heat conservation. Impermeability is maintained with tight junctions formed by intercellular adhesion molecules. Integrity of the dermis depends upon interlacing collagen bundles and elastic tissue.

The skin contains specialized structures including hair follicles, sebaceous and sweat glands, and location specific special sensory structures. The skin is also an immunologic organ. Intradermal *Langerhans cells*, reproducing within the epidermis, are activated by foreign antigens. They then migrate to regional lymph nodes presenting antigens to T-lymphocytes initiating an immune response.

FUNCTIONAL ANATOMY OF THE SKIN AND NAILS

Skin Layers: The layers of the skin are the epidermis, dermis, and subcutaneous tissue.

Epidermis. The avascular epidermis (Fig. 6-1) is the most superficial layer; it has four layers. The keratinized nonliving cells of the outer keratin layer (*stratum corneum*) are stratified and overlapping, the outermost cells sloughing regularly (*desquamation*). Underlying the stratum corneum are the granular layer (*stratum granulosum*), spinous layer (*stratum spinosum*), and basal layer (*stratum basale*). The living cells in these layers, mostly keratinocytes, get nourishment from the dermis and are held together by proteins, including desmosomes. Melanocytes in the lower epidermis contain melanin, whose concentration is determined by genetics, sunlight, injury repair, and hormones. The epidermis contains a visible network of furrows that are exaggerated over joints. The epidermis thickens in areas of high friction such as palms and soles. A basement membrane separates the epidermis from the dermis. The epidermis attaches to the basement membrane by *hemidesmosomes*.

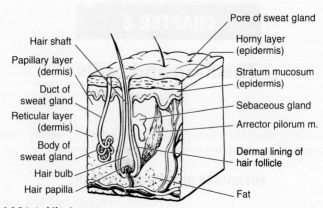

FIG. 6-1 Principal Skin Structures.

Dermis and subcutaneous tissue. The superficial *papillary dermis* forms papillary extensions surrounded by epidermis and containing rich capillary and nerve networks. The deeper *reticular dermis* contains blood vessels, lymphatics, nerves, and fat cells surrounded by collagen bundles mixed with elastic fibers. The dermal appendages, including hair follicles, apocrine glands, eccrine sweat glands, and holocrine sebaceous glands, extend into this layer. The deep reticular dermis merges with the *subcutaneous layer*. In general, the dermis is thicker over dorsal and lateral than over ventral and medial surfaces. It is thickest over the back and extremely thin over the eyelids, scrotum, and penis.

Skin Associated Structures.

Fingernails. Fingernails frequently show signs of systemic disease. The nails grow throughout life, providing a record of nutritional disturbances. Changes in the visible nailfold capillaries are signs of systemic disease. The *nail plate* is a hard, semitransparent convex rectangle, transverse radius of curvature of which is shorter than its longitudinal radius (Fig. 6-2). The nail plate adheres to the *nail bed*, a layer of modified skin studded with narrow longitudinal ridges containing a rich capillary network giving the nail plate its pink color. The proximal third of the nail bed is the *matrix* composed of partially cornified cells containing *keratohyalin* granules. This is where new nail is added to the nail plate forcing it distally. The matrix as seen through the nail plate is the white *lunula*. The proximal root of the nail plate is buried in a dermal pouch. The lip of the pouch is the *mantle* terminating in the *cuticle*. The distal nail plate not adherent to the bed is the *free edge*; the *body* is the intervening portion. The sides of the nail plate are buried in lateral *nail folds* of skin and cuticle. The nail plate elongates continuously from the root and thickens from the matrix. The time for growing a new fingernail is ~6 months, faster in youth than in old age.

Toenails. Toenails undergo the same changes as fingernails, but most are less pronounced. It takes 12–18 months for a toenail to regrow.

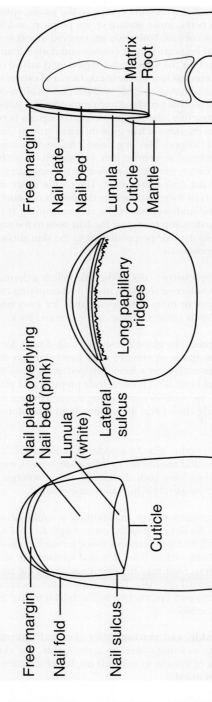

FIG. 6-2 Fingernail Anatomy. The nail plate is formed by the cells of the matrix and extruded distally to the free margin where the plate separates from the nail bed. The lunula marks the extent of the matrix under the nail plate.

Free margin
Nail plate
Nail bed
Lunula
Cuticle
Mantle

Matrix
Root

Long papillary ridges

Nail plate overlying
Nail bed (pink)
Lunula
(white)
Lateral
sulcus

Free margin
Nail fold
Nail sulcus
Cuticle

Hair. The skin is covered with hairs except on the palms, soles, dorsal distal phalanges, glans penis, inner surface of the prepuce, and labia minora. Adults have two types of hair. Both sexes are covered in soft, colorless, short vellus hairs. Terminal hairs are longer, coarser, and darker than vellus hairs. Terminal hair is found on the scalp, pubic region, and axillae of both sexes. Males often exhibit terminal hair on the trunk, face, and extremities. The hair follicle is a tubular invagination of epidermis and dermis often extending into the subcutaneous tissue. The proximal *root* terminates in a hollow bulb that fits over a dermal structure, the *papilla*. Molecular signals between papilla and follicle determine the stage of hair growth: active growth (*anagen*), regression (*catagen*), or rest (*telogen*). The long slender *hair shaft* is round or oval in straight hairs and flattened in a curled hair. The shaft has a *medulla*, which is frequently absent, a *cortex*, containing *pigment* in colored hairs, and a superficial single layer of flat scales, the *cuticle*. The root is softer and lighter in color than the shaft. Hair follicles penetrate the dermis obliquely forming an obtuse angle with the undersurface of the skin containing the involuntary *arrector pili* muscles extending from near the hair bulb to the superficial dermis. Contraction pulls the hair perpendicular to the skin surface producing "goosebumps" or "gooseflesh."

Sebaceous glands. Specialized cells in the hair follicle's dermal lining produce sebum through holocrine secretion into a duct emptying into the follicle near its distal end; one or more sebaceous glands are associated with each follicle. Sebaceous glands are most dense on the face and back.

Eccrine (Sweat) glands. The gland's body is a coiled tube deep in the dermis or subcutaneous tissue. A straight duct leads through the epidermis emerging on the skin surface in a funnel-shaped pore. Only the vermilion border of the lips, nail beds, labia minora, male prepuce, and glans penis lack eccrine glands. They are necessary for cooling through evaporation of sweat. They receive primarily cholinergic innervation from the autonomic nervous system.

Apocrine glands. Apocrine glands associated with hair follicles become active during puberty and are limited to the axillae, breasts, eyelids, genital, and perianal skin. They have both cholinergic and adrenergic innervation. The function of apocrine glands in humans is uncertain.

Nerves. The skin contains nerves transmitting a multiplicity of stimuli. *Meissner corpuscles* in the dermal papillae convey light touch. *Pacinian corpuscles* in the deep dermis and subcutaneous tissue transmit pressure and vibration. Noxious sensations such as pain, itch, and temperature are transmitted by unmyelinated fibers. Skin may become insensate as the result of injury, disease, or developmental anomaly. The density of nerves varies greatly by location. The fingertips and lips are two of the most sensitive areas, and the back one of the least sensitive.

Circulation of the skin and mucosa. Most skin and mucous membrane disorders involve the vascular system to some extent. The skin has a rich anastomotic network of vessels, so ischemia implies obstruction of the larger proximal arterioles or arteries.

Cutaneous wound healing and repair. Healing occurs in three phases: inflammation, proliferation, and maturation. In the inflammatory phase, platelets provide hemostasis and release proinflammatory cytokines. Neutrophils are the first immune cells to infiltrate the wound. Macrophages derived from circulating monocytes arrive later but contribute more to wound healing. Along with neutrophils they debride the wound helping prevent infection. In addition, by releasing growth factors and cytokines, they affect tissue remodeling. The skin has a remarkable ability to repair injury. Injury into the dermis heals with scarring, whereas epidermal wounds typically heal without scarring. Two weeks after injury and appropriate wound closure, skin strength is ~10% of normal. Collagen in the scar remodels for up to a year after injury approaching 80% of normal strength. Multiple factors adversely affect wound healing Chief among these is infection, which delays or halts healing. Well-vascularized tissue heals faster and better than less vascular tissues evident by the rapid healing of richly vascularized scalp and facial injuries compared to slower healing of less well-vascularized lower leg wounds. Some patients are genetically prone to slow healing and/or poor scar formation. Both oral and topical corticosteroids inhibit collagen synthesis dramatically impeding wound healing. Finally, the wound care regimen affects the speed and quality of healing.

EXAMINING THE SKIN AND NAILS

The skin is examined by inspection and palpation. Magnification with dermoscopy can provide details of individual lesions. Palpate for nodularity and induration. Note the morphology and distribution of individual lesions and the pattern of grouped lesions.

Evaluating Skin Turgor and Elasticity: Pinch and release a fold of skin (Fig. 6-3). Normal skin rapidly flattens into place. A persistent fold indicates loss of turgor (indicative of extracellular volume depletion) or elasticity (common in sun exposed skin and the elderly).

Examining Nailfold Capillaries: Use an ophthalmoscope, dermatoscope, or magnifying glass at 15–40x magnification. Select a finger without recent trauma, placing a drop of immersion oil or lubricating jelly on the nail fold. Normal capillary arcs are parallel narrow loops extending from the base of the nail fold toward the nail and returning. Dilation, irregularity, and dropout

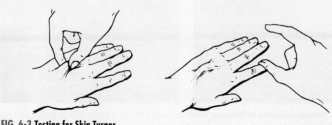

FIG. 6-3 Testing for Skin Turgor.

of loops are abnormal. Abnormal capillaroscopy in a patient with Raynaud phenomenon suggests dermatomyositis, systemic lupus erythematosus (SLE), scleroderma, or another connective tissue disease.

SUPPLEMENTAL AIDS TO DERMATOLOGIC DIAGNOSIS

Magnification: Use a magnifying glass, otoscope, dermatoscope, or ophthalmoscope to closely inspect lesions. Otoscopes and ophthalmoscopes provide illumination and magnification.

Diascopy: Compress red lesions with a magnifying glass or a glass slide. Blanching is indicative of dilated vessels; extravasated blood does not blanch. See Fig. 6-4.

KOH Preparation: KOH preparations visualize dermatophyte hyphae, *Candida* pseudohyphae, budding yeasts, and the spores and fragmented hyphae of tinea versicolor. Scrape skin scales from the lesion onto a glass slide. Adding two drops of a 10% to 20% KOH solution dissolves keratin allowing fungal elements to be more easily seen. Gentle heating catalyzes this process but avoid boiling the solution. Alternatively, KOH with Dimethyl Sulfoxide (DMSO) can be used to help catalyze the process without having to be heated. Start at scanning magnification then move to 10–20x higher power. Hyphae appear as thin, elongated filaments extending beyond cell walls, often best seen slightly out of the plane in which the keratinocytes are in focus. Hyphae may be difficult to distinguish from the outline of a keratinocyte. Other confounders include hair and clothing fibers.

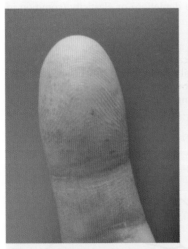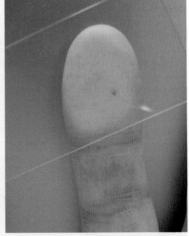

FIG. 6-4 Petechia Confirmed by Diascopy. Several red vascular markings are seen on the index fingertip. Diascopy discloses that the lesions do not blanch and are therefore extravasated blood.

Tzanck Smear: To identify herpes simplex or varicella-zoster viruses in vesicular lesions, firmly scrape the base of an unroofed early vesicle with a scalpel and air dry the specimen on a glass slide. Stain it with Wright or Giemsa stain and examine microscopically for characteristic cytopathic changes such as multinucleated giant cells or ballooning keratinocytes. Perform PCR (polymerase chain reaction) or DFA (direct fluorescent antibody) test on a fresh specimen for virus identification.

Wood Light: Ultraviolet illumination (360 nm) fluoresces scalp infections caused by some dermatophytes, e.g., *Microsporum canis* (yellow), *Pseudomonas* abscesses (pale blue), and intertriginous infections with *Corynebacterium minutissimum* (coral red). Bathing removes some fluorescent material leading to a falsely negative result. Wood light also can be helpful in evaluating depigmented skin conditions (vitiligo) and differentiating them from hypopigmented lesions.

Skin Biopsy: Skin is biopsied using a skin punch, shaving with a scalpel or razor blade, and by sharp excision.

SKIN AND NAIL SYMPTOMS

Itching (Pruritus): Itching is a common symptom and optimal treatment requires a specific diagnosis. Describe the onset, location, severity, and course whether constant or progressive. Determine aggravating and ameliorating factors. Ask about new medications. Excoriations and lichenification indicate scratching.

    CLINICAL OCCURRENCE: *Local Causes:* Contact dermatitis (e.g., poison ivy), insect bites, chigger bites (red larva of Trombiculidae mites), scabies, tinea, candidiasis, trichomoniasis, atopic dermatitis, neurodermatitis, seborrheic dermatitis, lichen simplex, urticaria, pruritus ani, pruritus vulvae, stasis dermatitis, dermatitis herpetiformis, miliaria (heat rash), nostalgia paresthetica; *Systemic Causes:* Asteatosis ("winter itch"), pruritus of pregnancy, pityriasis rosea, psoriasis, medication reactions, uremia, obstructive jaundice, biliary cirrhosis, myxedema, polycythemia vera (aquagenic pruritus), Hodgkin disease, cutaneous and other lymphomas, diffuse cutaneous mastocytosis, pediculosis (body lice), hook worm, onchocerciasis, filariasis.

SKIN AND NAIL SIGNS

Learning to accurately and completely describe observations using precise terminology facilitates use of reference materials and provides accurate information for dermatologic referral or pathology requisition. Each sign is followed by examples of conditions associated with the lesion.

Distribution of Lesions: Many skin diseases have characteristic distributions, some determined by regional skin features and others by exposure to noxious agents. The explanation for many distributions is unknown. Some examples follow (Fig. 6-5).

Head and neck. *Acne:* Face, neck, and shoulders; *Actinic Keratoses:* Face, scalp; *Amyloidosis:* Eyelids; *Atopic Dermatitis:* Face, neck; *Cancer:* Face, nose, ears, lips; *Contact Dermatitis:* Eyelids, face; *Discoid Lupus*

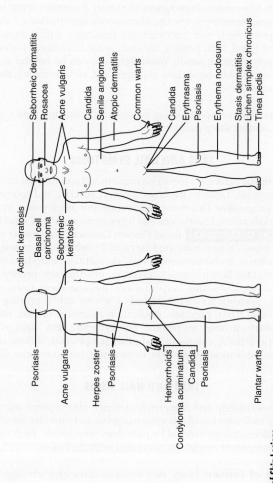

FIG. 6-5 Distribution of Skin Lesions.

Seborrheic dermatitis
Rosacea
Acne vulgaris
Candida
Senile angioma
Atopic dermatitis
Common warts
Candida
Erythrasma
Psoriasis
Erythema nodosum
Stasis dermatitis
Lichen simplex chronicus
Tinea pedis

Actinic keratosis
Basal cell carcinoma
Seborrheic keratosis

Psoriasis
Acne vulgaris
Herpes zoster
Psoriasis
Hemorrhoids
Condyloma acuminatum
Candida
Psoriasis
Plantar warts

Erythematosus: Nose, cheeks; *Herpes Zoster:* Trigeminal nerve distribution; *Psoriasis:* Scalp; *Rosacea:* Mid-face; *Seborrhea:* Scalp, eyebrows, eyelids, nasal alae; *Secondary Syphilis:* Face; *Spider Angiomas:* Cheeks, neck; *Tinea Capitis:* Scalp; *Xanthelasma:* Eyelids; *Varicella (chickenpox):* Face.

Trunk. *Candidiasis:* Under breasts, axillae, inguinal and gluteal folds; *Dermatitis Herpetiformis:* Scapulae, sacrum, buttocks; *Drug Eruption:* Front and back of thorax and abdomen; *Petechiae:* Abdomen; *Pityriasis Rosea:* Front and back of trunk; *Secondary Syphilis:* Thorax and abdomen; *Spider Angiomas:* Chest, shoulders, abdomen; *Varicella (chickenpox):* Trunk and face.

Extremities. *Actinic Keratoses and Cancer:* Backs of the hands; *Atopic Dermatitis:* Antecubital fossae; *Contact Dermatitis:* Arms, hands, legs; *Erythema Multiforme:* Arms, hands, legs, feet, palms, soles; *Erythema Nodosum:* Legs, shins; *Granuloma Annulare:* Backs of hands and fingers; *Onychomycosis:* Fingernails, toenails; *Petechiae:* Forearms, hands, legs, feet; *Pityriasis Rosea:* Upper arms, upper legs; *Plantar Warts:* Soles; *Psoriasis:* Elbows, knees, hands, fingernails; *Secondary Syphilis:* Palms, soles.

Pattern of Lesions: Single lesions may have distinctive shapes and patterns. Sometimes individual lesions appear in distinctive configurations (e.g., herpes zoster). Multiple individual lesions often coalesce into larger less-distinctive patterns, so the evolution of lesions is critical.

Annular, arciform, and polycyclic pattern. The individual lesions are arranged in circles, arcs, or irregular combinations of the two. **Examples:** Drug eruptions, erythema multiforme, urticaria, psoriasis, granuloma annulare, tinea, subacute cutaneous lupus.

Serpiginous pattern. The lesions occur in wavy lines or have wavy, indented margins. **Examples:** Larva migrans.

Target (Iris) pattern. A bull's-eye pattern with an encircled round spot; more than one ring may be present. **Examples:** Erythema multiforme, erythema migrans.

Irregular pattern. Groups of individual lesions have no distinct pattern. **Examples:** Urticaria and insect bites.

Dermatomal pattern. Lesions follow the spinal root sensory dermatome so do not cross the midline. **Examples:** Herpes zoster.

Linear pattern. Lesions follow linear cutaneous and subcutaneous structures (e.g., nerves, lymphatics, or blood vessels), or contact with a linear irritant. **Examples:** Lymphangitis, superficial phlebitis, contact dermatitis (e.g., poison ivy), jellyfish envenomation, trauma, or other infections (sporotrichosis).

Lines of Blaschko. Many skin eruptions, including psoriasis and pityriasis rosea, follow lines of fetal epidermal migration and proliferation.

Retiform pattern. Lesions reflect the deep dermal and medium vessel arterial or venous anatomy. The venous pattern is a lacey network; arteriolar occlusion results in infarcts with angulated or finger-like borders. **Examples:** *Venous Pattern:* Livedo reticularis; *Arterial Pattern:* Necrotizing vasculitis, calciphylaxis, cutaneous emboli, arteriolar thrombosis.

Extrinsic pattern. The lesions follow no anatomic pattern often having relatively straight borders and/or shapes suggesting the pattern is impressed on patient from outside. **Examples:** Radiation injury, including sunburn and radiation dermatitis, contact dermatitis.

Morphology of Individual Lesions: After noting distribution and pattern, examine and characterize several individual lesions. Identify new, mature, and resolving lesions. Palpate to identify papules, nodules, plaques, and infiltration. Use diascopy to disclose lesions obscured by erythema and to distinguish vasodilation from extravasated blood.

Macules and patches. These are nonpalpable changes in skin color or appearance (Fig. 6-6A). Macules are <1 cm and patches are ≥1 cm. The borders can be sharp or indistinct. There may be desquamation or scaling. **Examples:** Freckles, exanthems (rubeola, rubella, secondary syphilis, rose spots of typhoid fever), drug eruptions, petechiae, first-degree burns, SLE, pityriasis rosea, café-au-lait spots, vitiligo.

Papules. Papules are <1 cm lesions that are raised (Fig. 6-6B). The borders and tops may be distinctive. **Examples:** *Acuminate or Pointed:* Bites, acne, physiologic gooseflesh; *Flat-topped:* Lichen planus, molluscum contagiosum, condyloma latum; *Round or Irregular:* Angiomas, melanoma, eczematous dermatitis, papular secondary syphilis; *Filiform:* Condyloma acuminatum; *Pedunculated:* Skin tags, neurofibromas.

Plaques. A diffusely elevated area ≥1 cm in diameter is a plaque, often formed from confluent papules. Plaques are characteristically flat topped and broader than high, like a plateau. **Examples:** Cutaneous lymphomas (mycosis fungoides); *Red, Scaling:* Psoriasis, discoid lupus erythematosus (with

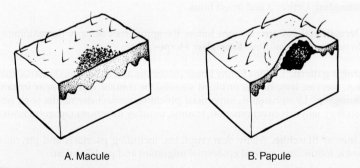

A. Macule   B. Papule

FIG. 6-6 Macules and Papules. A. Macules are visible but not palpable. B. Papules are palpable and <5 mm in diameter.

atrophy); *Yellow:* Xanthomas; *Brown:* Seborrheic keratoses; *Hyperkeratotic:* Plantar warts; *Lichenified:* Atopic dermatitis.

Nodules. Nodules are usually >1 cm in diameter, distinguished from papules by extension into the dermis or subcutaneous tissue (Fig. 6-7A). The skin slides over nodules below the dermis; lesions within the dermis move with the skin. **Examples:** Rheumatoid nodules, lipomas, cysts, cancer, gouty tophi, erythema nodosum, panniculitis.

Wheals. Cutaneous edema produces circumscribed, irregular, and relatively transient plaques (Fig. 6-7B), varying from red to pale depending on the amount of fluid in the skin. Hives (urticaria) often itch. **Examples:** Urticaria, insect bites.

Vesicles. Fluid dissects the epidermis producing an elevation covered by translucent epithelium that is easily punctured releasing the fluid (Fig. 6-8A). Vesicles are <1 cm in diameter. **Examples:** Acute contact dermatitis, second-degree burns, varicella, herpes simplex and zoster, smallpox.

Bullae. Bullae are fluid accumulations >1 cm in diameter dissecting within or under the epidermis (Fig. 6-8A). Tense bullae indicate dissection below the basal layer. Dissection superficial to the basal layer results in flaccid, more easily ruptured bullae, often presenting as superficial erosions without intact bullae. **Examples:** Contact dermatitis, pemphigus, pemphigoid, erythema multiforme (rarely), diabetic bullae, edema bullae.

Pustules. Pustules are pus-filled vesicles or bullae (Fig. 6-8A). The contents are milky, orange, yellow, or green. Pustules frequently arise from hair follicles or sweat glands. **Examples:** Folliculitis, acne, furuncles, pustular psoriasis, bromide and iodide eruptions.

Cysts. Cysts are papules or nodules containing fluid or viscous material enclosed by an epithelium (Fig. 6-8B). *Pseudocysts* are similar lesions without

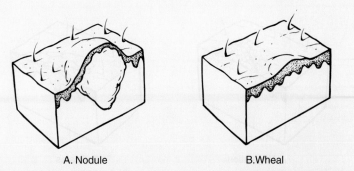

A. Nodule   B. Wheal

FIG. 6-7 Nodules and Wheals. A. Nodules are discrete and firm lesions in the skin or subcutaneous tissue often without any epidermal changes. **B. Wheals** (hives) are transient, discrete areas of edema in the epidermis and dermis.

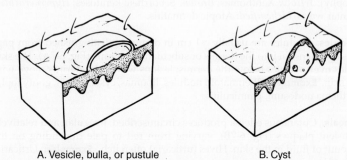

A. Vesicle, bulla, or pustule   B. Cyst

FIG. 6-8 Fluctuant Skin Lesions. A. Vesicle, bullae, and pustules involve the epidermis. **B. Cysts** are subepidermal and may extend into the subcutaneous tissues.

an epithelial lining, a histological distinction. **Examples:** Epidermal inclusion and pilar (trichilemmal) cysts; *Pseudocysts:* Cystic acne.

Vegetations. Elevated irregular growths are called vegetations (Fig. 6-9A). *Verrucous* lesions have keratotic or dried surfaces. *Papillomatous* lesions are covered by normal epidermis. **Examples:** *Verrucous:* Verruca vulgaris (common wart), seborrheic keratosis; *Papilloma:* Condyloma acuminatum.

Scales. Scales are thin plates of partly separated dried cornified epithelium adherent to the epidermis (Fig. 6-9B). **Examples:** *Large Scales:* Psoriasis, exfoliative dermatitis; *Small Scales:* Pityriasis rosea, seborrheic dermatitis.

Hyperkeratosis. Keratotic cells do not slough normally, but pile up producing thick elevated skin. **Examples:** Calluses, seborrheic, and actinic keratoses. Arsenic produces punctate keratoses of the palms and soles.

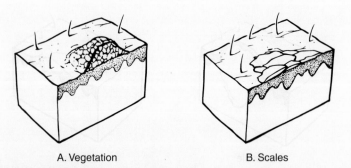

A. Vegetation   B. Scales

FIG. 6-9 Vegetations and Scales. A. Vegetations are irregular growths above the skin surface. **B. Scales** are small or large flakes of cornified epithelium loosely adherent to the skin surface.

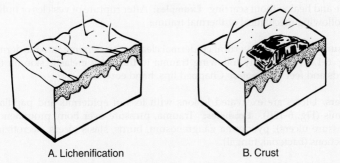

FIG. 6-10 **Lichenification and Crusts. A. Lichenification** is a leathery thickening of all skin layers with prominent furrows. **B. Crusts** form from dried blood, serum, pus or other secretions from the skin.

Lichenification. Repeated rubbing promotes hyperplasia of all layers (Fig. 6-10A) appearing as a dry plaque with accentuated skin lines. **Examples:** Atopic dermatitis, lichen simplex chronicus.

Crusts. A superficial plate of dried serum, blood, pus, or sebum accumulates on a ruptured vesicle or pustule (Fig. 6-10B) or on chronically inflamed skin. **Examples:** Impetigo.

Atrophy. The skin is thinned lacking normal skin lines (Fig. 6-11A). **Examples:** Actinic atrophy, striae, discoid lupus erythematosus, effect from potent topical steroids, steroid injections, and insulin lipodystrophy.

Sclerosis. Collagen are deposited in cutaneous and subcutaneous tissues, often a consequence of chronic inflammation. **Examples:** Stasis dermatitis, scleroderma (systemic and localized) and variants, morphea, nephrogenic fibrosing dermopathy.

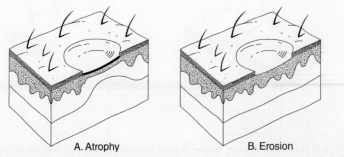

FIG. 6-11 **Atrophy and Erosion. A. Atrophy** is thinning of all skin layers. **B. Erosions** represent traumatic loss of the stratum corneum.

Erosions. Erosions are partial thickness loss of epidermis (Fig. 6-11B) that ooze and heal without scarring. **Examples:** After rupture of vesicles or bullae or following mechanical or thermal trauma.

Fissures. Fissures are vertical epidermal cleavages extending into the dermis (Fig. 6-12A) commonly following trauma to thick dry inelastic skin on the hands and feet. **Examples:** Chapped lips, hand eczema.

Ulcers. Ulcers are excavated lesions with loss of epidermis and papillary dermis (Fig. 6-12B). **Examples:** Trauma, pressure over bony prominences (pressure ulcers), pyoderma gangrenosum, burns, stasis ulcers, necrotizing infections (bacterial, fungal).

Generalized Skin Signs.
Petechiae and purpura. See page 129. Disrupted dermal vessels extravasate blood into the skin producing nonblanching red macules and patches.

Telangiectasia. Telangiectasia are dilated small blood vessels that blanch with pressure. **Examples:** Spider angiomas, hereditary hemorrhagic telangiectasia, rosacea, sun and irradiation damage.

Gangrene. Ischemic skin and subcutaneous tissue necrosis creates a black eschar. In arterial insufficiency, the lesions are atrophic and dry (dry gangrene). Other necrotizing processes may produce an edematous weeping, lesion, moist gangrene. **Examples:** *Dry Gangrene:* Arterial insufficiency, vasculitis. *Moist Gangrene:* Aspergillosis, pyoderma gangrenosum, necrotizing fasciitis.

Urticaria. Inflammatory mediators produce local capillary dilation and leak leading to dermal and epidermal erythema and edema. The lesions are discrete raised erythematous papules and plaques often intensely pruritic. Precipitating factors are allergic, mechanical, or physical. Individual lesions

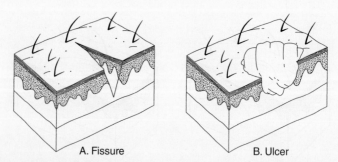

A. Fissure　　　　　　　　　　B. Ulcer

FIG. 6-12 Fissures and Ulcers. A. Fissures are vertical splits extending through the epidermis into the dermis. **B. Ulcers** are actual loss of epidermal and dermal tissues that may extend into the subcutaneous tissue and muscle down to bone.

are present <24 hours distinguishing urticaria from persistent lesions with a similar appearance, e.g., erythema multiforme. Urticarial lesions lasting >24 hours suggest urticarial vasculitis. Chronic urticaria may last for years. **Examples:** *Allergic:* Drug eruptions, topical sensitivity; *Physical:* Cold, exercise, dermatographia; *Systemic Diseases:* SLE.

Dermatographia. Dermatographia is urticaria caused by stroking the skin. Normally, a light scratch produces linear macular blanching limited to the scratched skin. Urtication produces a bright-red macular line becoming more purple with time. In more severe responses, a red mottled flare develops lateral to the red line and a wheal may develop.

Mastocytosis. Mast cells infiltrate the skin producing brown macules that urticate when stroked (*Darier sign*). Mastocytosis may be limited to the skin (*urticaria pigmentosa*) or produce systemic disease with hepatosplenomegaly and signs of systemic histamine release (abdominal pain, diarrhea, peptic ulcer, hypotension, flushing).

Angioedema. Localized interstitial edema in the dermis and subcutaneous tissues may be caused by IgE-mediated allergy, complement activation, nonimmunologic mast cell activation, or it may be idiopathic. Single or multiple pruritic nonpitting swellings appear on the face, tongue, larynx, hands, feet, and/or genitalia that subside with or without treatment. Nausea, vomiting, and diarrhea are indicative of gastrointestinal involvement. Laryngeal angioedema can cause fatal airway obstruction.
CLINICAL OCCURRENCE: *IgE-mediated:* Hymenoptera (bee) stings, drugs (e.g., penicillin and other antibiotics), food allergens (e.g., peanuts, shellfish), foreign proteins used therapeutically, many others; *Non-IgE-mediated*: Angiotensin-converting enzyme inhibitors, radiologic contrast agents, cold exposure; *Complement Mediated:* Hereditary angioedema (C1-esterase deficiency), serum sickness, vasculitis.

Dry skin—xerosis and anhydrosis. Loss of sebaceous and/or sweat gland function leads to excessive drying. The skin is dry, often cracked, and leathery. Lacking normal oils, xerotic skin is more permeable to water. Aging results in progressively more xerotic skin. Causes of dry skin include ichthyosis, anticholinergic drugs, denervation in peripheral neuropathies such as diabetes, and removal of skin oils by frequent bathing with soap.

Decreased skin turgor—extracellular fluid deficit. Loss of extracellular fluid increases viscosity of interstitial fluid. Not to be confused with decreased cutaneous elastic tissue. Check the lying, sitting, and standing BP and pulse for postural changes; check skin turgor and look for longitudinal furrowing of the tongue. Loss of total body water (*dehydration*) does not change skin turgor.

Decreased skin elasticity. Destruction or disruption of the dermal elastic fibers results in decreased elasticity. Decreased elasticity is evident as wrinkling and redundancy of the skin. It is a normal consequence of aging accelerated by sun exposure (solar elastosis), stretching (pregnancy, obesity), and glucocorticoid excess (Cushing syndrome and iatrogenic). Pseudoxanthoma elasticum is an uncommon cause.

Scars. Epidermal injuries heal without scar but may alter pigmentation. Injury to dermal elastic and collagen fibers results in scarring. Deeper injury to the subcutaneous fat and muscle results in visible depressions or masses. All cutaneous scars are initially raised and red, fading over months to years to a pallid hue as the vascularity diminishes. Sutured wounds healing without infection or tension produce thin scars with minimal bridging fibrosis. Wounds healing by secondary intention leave wide inelastic scars. The pattern of scarring reflects the mechanism (sharp trauma, burn, excessive tension, scarification, etc.) and etiology.

Surgical and traumatic scars. Identify each scar relating it to surgery or trauma. Without a history, the cause may only be inferred by its size, pattern, location, and contour (smooth or jagged). Suture marks indicate surgical repair but not the depth of incision or injury. Full thickness burns heal with deep, irregular, broad, inelastic scars.

Hypertrophic scars and keloids. In some individuals, cutaneous injury variably produces persistent raised, red, hypertrophic scars. Scars extending beyond the boundary of the inciting wounds are called keloids. Keloids may progressively thicken over time. Keloids are more prevalent in dark-skinned persons and after complicated wounds. They can occur after minor injury anywhere on the body.

Striae. Stretching normal skin ruptures elastic fibers in the reticular dermis. In adrenal hypercorticism, the epidermis itself becomes fragile and easily tears under normal tension. Striae are permanent. Multiple 1–6 cm scars run axially under the epidermis in regions under chronic tension. When recent, they are pink or blue; older striae are white. Although most common on the abdomen, they are also found on the shoulders, thighs, and breasts. Striae are different from traumatic and therapeutic scarring. Precipitating conditions include abdominal distention (pregnancy, obesity, ascites, tumors), subcutaneous edema, Cushing syndrome (usually fresh-appearing purple striae).

Crepitus. Gas in subcutaneous tissues or muscle produces a peculiar sensation when pressure is applied caused by bubbles sliding under the fingers, often accompanied by a crackling sound. Bubbles feel like small nontender fluctuant nodules moving freely with palpation. *DDX:* Subcutaneous crepitus is pathognomonic of subcutaneous emphysema or gas gangrene. In subcutaneous emphysema, the bubbles contain air that entered the tissues through operative wounds or trauma, e.g., fractured rib piercing the lung. Infection with some anaerobic and microaerophilic organisms produces gas by fermentation. Severe local infection and systemic toxicity distinguish it from subcutaneous emphysema.

Changes in Skin Color.
Constitutive diffuse brown skin—normal melanin pigmentation. This is the inherited constitutive skin color. Persons of African descent have the greatest melanin density. Lesser amounts occur, in order, from South Asians, Native Americans, Indonesians, Oriental Asians (Chinese and Japanese), to Western Europeans who have the least. There is also variation within ethnic groups of related genetic background. For example, natives of India are often

very dark, and inhabitants of the Mediterranean region are darker than the Northern Europeans. Individual variation within a family is also large.

Tattoos. Tattoos are common and may indicate increased risk for blood-borne disease. Determine where and by whom tattoos were placed and the sterility and any instrument sharing. Ask about high-risk behaviors, e.g., intravenous drug use or high-risk sexual behaviors.

Malignant melanoma. See page 155.

Nevi—moles. See page 154.

Acquired diffuse brown skin—melanism. Mechanisms stimulating melanin production include secretion of ACTH and/or MSH and iron deposition in the skin. Melanism is skin darkening from augmented melanin production in facultative pigment deposits. The brown color is diffuse and accentuated in palmar creases, recent scars, and pressure points at elbow, knee, and knuckles. Pigmentation of the oral mucosa is abnormal in whites. Melanism should prompt a search for underlying disease.

CLINICAL OCCURRENCE: *Congenital:* Hemochromatosis, porphyria, alkaptonuria; *Endocrine:* Addison disease, Nelson syndrome, Graves disease, hypothyroidism, pregnancy (melasma—primarily on the face), contraceptive hormones; *Infectious:* Whipple disease; *Inflammatory/Immunologic:* Scleroderma; *Metabolic/Toxic:* Cirrhosis, pernicious anemia, B_{12} and folic acid deficiency, drugs (busulfan, arsenicals, dibromomannitol); *Neoplastic:* Hormone-secreting neoplasms; *Psychosocial:* Tanning.

Hemochromatosis. See Chapter 9, page 457.

Blue-gray color. Deposition of foreign substances discolors the skin. Increased concentrations of unsaturated or abnormal hemoglobin in the cutaneous vessels gives cyanosis (page 127) that blanches with pressure. Consider as etiology use of amiodarone or minocycline; silver deposition of silver (*argyria*), gold, or bismuth salts; hemochromatosis, cyanosis, sulfhemoglobinemia, methemoglobinemia, arsenic poisoning.

Silver (Argyria). Silver salts from ingestion or intranasal absorption are deposited in the skin producing a blue-gray or slate color accentuated in sun exposed areas. The mucosa and nail lunulae may be deposition sites. The pigmentation may appear years after exposure and is typically permanent. It is easily differentiated from cyanosis by not blanching with pressure.

Arsenic. Arsenic ingestion produces a diffuse gray coloration with superimposed 2–10 mm dark macules, often accompanied by punctate hyperkeratoses of the palms and soles. The skin manifestations appear 1–10 years after arsenic ingestion.

Alkaptonuria (ochronosis). An inherited deficiency of homogentisic acid oxidase results in accumulation of black homogentisic acid polymers in the connective tissues and urine. The accumulations give a faint blue-gray color to the skin, especially over the pinnae, tip of the nose, and sclerae. Blackened extensor tendons in the hands may be seen through the skin. Often a dark butterfly pattern appears on the face and the axillae genitalia are pigmented. Exogenous ochronosis (*pseudoochronosis*) results from prolonged use of topical medications, notably hydroquinone used for bleaching skin. Treated areas develop the blue-gray appearance of ochronosis.

Acquired diffuse yellow skin. Yellow discoloration results from pigment deposition in the skin. The most common causes are jaundice and carotenemia, which are easily distinguished on clinical grounds by their different distributions and presentations.

Jaundice. See, Chapter 9, page 414.

Carotenemia. Fat-soluble carotene concentrates in the stratum corneum of the palms and soles and is excreted in sebum. The liver converts carotene to vitamin A with the assistance of thyroid hormone. The liver fails to metabolize carotene in myxedema and diabetes. Carotene deposition appears as yellow skin especially on the forehead, nasolabial folds, behind the ears, and on the palms and soles. Carotenemia results from chronically ingesting copious quantities of carrots, squash, oranges, peaches, apricots, and leafy vegetables. *DDX:* Water-soluble bilirubin pigments are more uniformly distributed including discoloration of sclerae and thin skin.

Erythema. Erythema is skin reddening caused by dilation of the cutaneous vasculature that blanches with pressure, and is often accompanied by increased skin temperature. **Examples:** Local inflammatory lesions, local infection (e.g., cellulitis, lymphangitis), scarlet fever, scarlatiniform drug eruptions, polycythemia, porphyria, pellagra, lupus erythematosus, first-degree burns. Transient erythema occurs in blushing and in some cases of metastatic carcinoid.

Hypopigmentation and depigmentation. Loss of skin pigmentation is patchy or diffuse, usually with discrete borders. The distribution and pattern are important for identifying a specific etiology. **Examples:** *Depigmentation:* Vitiligo, albinism; *Hypopigmentation:* Tinea versicolor, scars, stria, and sites of subcutaneous steroid injection or topical steroid application on ethnically dark skin.

Hyperpigmentation. Increased cutaneous melanin deposition results from local or systemic factors. **Examples:** Addison disease, hemochromatosis, porphyria, arsenic poisoning, progressive systemic sclerosis (scleroderma), sun exposure, post-inflammatory hyperpigmentation, chronic local irritation from burning or scratching.

Acanthosis nigricans. Asymptomatic hyperpigmented velvety plaques are seen on the neck, axillae groin, and other body folds.
   CLINICAL OCCURRENCE: *Congenital:* Hereditary benign; *Endocrine:* Diabetes, increased androgens, acromegaly, Cushing syndrome, Addison disease, insulin resistance syndromes, hypothyroidism; *Metabolic/Toxic:* Obesity, drug induced, for example, nicotinic acid, glucocorticoids; *Neoplastic:* Paraneoplastic.

Hair Changes.

Hirsutism and hypertrichosis. *Hirsutism is excess terminal hair growth from androgen-sensitive pilosebaceous units because of excess androgen secretion or genetically determined increased androgen sensitivity.* In *hirsutism* hair grows in a masculine pattern on the face, shoulders, back, chest, abdomen, thighs, and buttocks. Hirsutism is especially distressing to women. Distinguishing normal variants from androgen excess can be difficult. *Hypertrichosis* is excess vellus hair growth, evenly covering the body. Less hair than normal is *hypotrichosis*.

CLINICAL OCCURRENCE: *Hirsutism:* androgen-secreting tumors, polycystic ovary, late-onset congenital adrenal hyperplasia, glucocorticoid excess, prolactinemia, carcinoma, drugs (e.g., certain oral contraceptives, testosterone, anabolic steroids); *Hypertrichosis:* congenital, anorexia nervosa, hypothyroidism, dermatomyositis, malnutrition, drugs (minoxidil, phenytoin, hydrocortisone, cyclosporine, penicillamine, and streptomycin).

Alopecia. Alopecia is congenital or acquired hair loss. History and hair loss pattern assist diagnosis. Hormonal hair loss is *androgenic alopecia*. Local trauma and traction on hairs or obsessive pulling or twisting hair (*trichotillomania*) also cause alopecia. The most frequently encountered causes are androgenic alopecia (male or female pattern baldness), alopecia areata, telogen effluvium, anagen effluvium, hypothyroidism, and drugs.

Alopecia areata. *The hair loss is an autoimmune condition.* There is complete or patchy loss of hair follicles without other skin changes. It is associated with other autoimmune disorders.

Telogen effluvium. Physiologic stressors such as pregnancy, illness, or emotional distress shift the growth cycle from anagen to telogen which may last for a few months. When the growth phase begins again the new shafts extrude the old hairs, resulting in diffuse hair shedding.

Anagen effluvium. Antimetabolites such as chemotherapeutic agents cause arrest of the growth phase and diffuse hair loss which resolves when the drugs are withdrawn.

Graying. Loss of hair pigmentation is normal with age. The age of onset is familial to some extent. **Examples:** Normal aging, premature aging syndromes, pernicious anemia, chloroquine therapy; localized graying occurs in vitiligo lesions.

Fingernail Signs.

Transverse nail plate furrow—Beau line. *An acute illness decreases nail growth seen as a transverse furrow whose width reflects the duration of illness.* As the nail elongates, the furrow becomes visible from beneath the mantle, progresses distally, and is finally pared off (Fig. 6-13F).

Transverse white banded nail plates—Mees lines. The transverse white bands are laid down during a systemic illness or poisoning. With recovery, normal nail growth resumes, producing a white band moving distally as the nail plate grows (Fig. 6-13N; Fig. 6-14). The bands probably result from minor

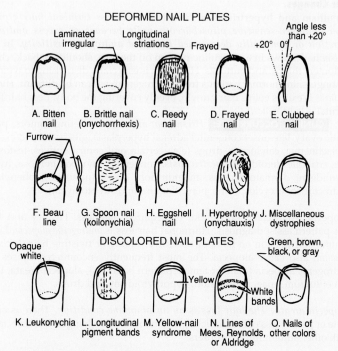

DEFORMED NAIL PLATES

Laminated irregular — Longitudinal striations — Frayed — +20° 0° Angle less than +20°

A. Bitten nail
B. Brittle nail (onychorrhexis)
C. Reedy nail
D. Frayed nail
E. Clubbed nail

Furrow —

F. Beau line
G. Spoon nail (koilonychia)
H. Eggshell nail
I. Hypertrophy (onychauxis)
J. Miscellaneous dystrophies

DISCOLORED NAIL PLATES

Opaque white —
Yellow
White bands
Green, brown, black, or gray

K. Leukonychia
L. Longitudinal pigment bands
M. Yellow-nail syndrome
N. Lines of Mees, Reynolds, or Aldridge
O. Nails of other colors

FIG. 6-13 Diagnosis of Fingernail Lesions I. Many nail lesions are depicted. It is necessary to know whether the lesion is in the nail plate or in the nail bed. The distinction can usually be made by noting if the abnormal color is changed by pressure on the nail plate, indicating a lesion of the nail bed. See text for descriptions.

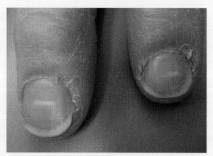

FIG. 6-14 Mees Lines. White transverse lines form in the nails at the time of an acute illness. With very severe illness grooves appear called Beau's lines.

injury, less than Beau lines. **Examples:** Heavily associated with poisoning (arsenic, thallium, fluoride), but also can be seen with chemotherapy, infectious febrile illnesses, renal insufficiency, cardiac failure, myocardial infarction, Hodgkin disease, sickle cell disease, and many others.

Nail pitting. Occasional nail pits are normal. Large numbers are seen in psoriasis, especially psoriatic arthritis. Other skin signs of psoriasis may be subtle or absent. These also can be seen with eczema. Nail pitting in transverse bands is associated with alopecia areata.

Splinter hemorrhage. Minor capillary bleeding, confined within ridges under the nail plate, appear as longitudinal red lines. They are asymptomatic (Fig. 6-15J). **Examples:** Trauma is most common. Consider systemic thrombotic and embolic illness (e.g., endocarditis, antiphospholipid syndrome, vasculitis).

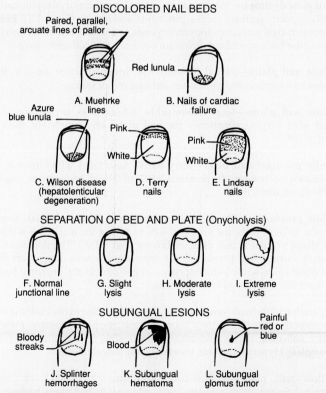

FIG. 6-15 Diagnosis of Fingernail Lesions II. Many nail lesions are depicted. It is necessary to know whether the lesion is in the nail plate or in the nail bed. The distinction can usually be made by noting if the abnormal color is changed by pressure on the nail plate, indicating a lesion of the nail bed. See text for descriptions.

Subungual hematoma. Bleeding into the closed space between the nail bed and plate is intensely painful. Relief of pressure and pain occurs when this is drained or bleeding dissects out from under the nail (Fig. 6-15K).

Nail fold inflammation—paronychia. Nail fold infection produces pain, redness, fluctuance and purulent drainage. Chronic infection of the nail base damages the matrix causing permanent nail deformity. Staphylococci are most common bacterial cause and seen in acute paronychia. *Candida* infection is prevalent in hands frequently immersed in warm water or in persons who bite their cuticles and is the leading infectious cause of chronic paronychia. The cuticle is rounded, erythematous, thickened, retracted from the plate but not tender. Several nails can be involved.

Subungual pigmentation—ungual melanoma. A single nail with a brown or black longitudinal streak that is larger than 3–4 mm and enlarging may be the only sign. Melanin can leach into the nail fold, which is known as the Hutchinson side.

Nail plate dystrophy. Abnormal nail growth produces dystrophic nails manifest as opacity, furrows, ridges, pits, splits, and fraying (Fig. 6-13J). **Examples:** Chronic fungal infections (onychomycosis), psoriasis, lesions of nerves supplying the limb, vascular deficits, amyloidosis, and collagen diseases.

White nail plates—partial leukonychia. Irregular white areas in the nail plates are common and most often indicate minor trauma.

White nail plates—total leukonychia. Inherited as an autosomal dominant with varying penetrance the nail plates are completely chalk white (Fig. 6-13K).

White proximal nail beds—Terry nails. Associated with cirrhosis, but of unknown mechanism, the proximal ≥80% of the nail bed is white (Fig. 6-15D) with a pink distal band.

White proximal nail beds—half-and-half nail (Lindsay nails). Somewhat similar to Terry nails, the proximal 40% to 80% of the nail bed is white while the distal portion is red, pink, or brown (Fig. 6-15E). The demarcation is a sharply curved line parallel to the free edge. Venous congestion deepens the distal color, while inducing only a slight pink in the proximal bed. Most patients have advanced kidney disease.

Separation of the nail—onycholysis. The normal line of plate adhesion to bed is a smooth curve (Fig. 6-15F). In onycholysis, the plate separates more proximally, collecting debris underneath, inaccessible to cleaning (Fig. 6-15G–I). **Examples:** Hyperthyroidism, psoriasis, and fungal infection.

Yellow nail plates—yellow-nail syndrome. Associated with impaired lymph drainage, it can antedate lymphedema. The nail plates become yellow or yellow-green, thicken, and grow slowly with more transverse curvature (Fig. 6-13M). Absence of the cuticle is characteristic. Ridging and onycholysis may occur.

Brittle nail plates—onychorrhexis. Keratin layers delaminating at the cut edge present a stepped appearance with frayed and torn borders (Fig. 6-13B). **Examples:** Aging, malnutrition, iron deficiency, thyrotoxicosis, or calcium deficiency.

Longitudinal brown-banded nail plates (melanonychia). This is a normal variant in black-skinned persons. Most commonly more than one nail is affected (Fig. 6-13L). Similar longitudinal bands occur with some antiretroviral medications. Consider melanoma if a single band affects a single nail.

Discolored nail plates. Drugs, infections, and stains color the nail plates (Fig. 6-13O). The color is a clue to etiology: blue-green = *Pseudomonas* infection; brown or black or yellow = fungal infections, fluorosis, quinacrine; and blue-gray = argyria.

White-banded nail beds—Muehrcke lines. Paired, narrow, arcuate pale bands, parallel to the lunulas, appear in the nail beds (Fig. 6-15A) during hypoalbuminemia (<2.0 g/dL), resolving with normalization of albumin. They are not in the nail plates, so do not move distally with nail growth.

Red lunula. Red lunulas (Fig. 6-15B) are associated with heart failure, rheumatoid arthritis, SLE, hepatic cirrhosis, pulmonary disease, carbon monoxide poisoning, and dermatologic diseases including psoriasis.

Azure lunula—hepatolenticular degeneration (Wilson disease). The lunulas are light blue (Fig. 6-15C). Examine the corneas for Kayser–Fleischer rings.

Painful red or violet subungual spot—glomus tumor. Exquisitely painful sensory glomus body tumors are common in the nail bed, appearing as a round red or violet spot (Fig. 6-15L) resembling a hemangioma, but the latter is not tender. This also could represent skin cancers including squamous cell carcinoma.

Concave nail plate—spoon nails (koilonychia). The nails are concave, saucer nails (Fig. 6-13G) with a thin nail plate. **Examples:** Iron deficiency; rare in rheumatic fever, lichen planus, and syphilis.

Nail plate hypertrophy. Piling up of irregular keratin layers thickens the nail plate (Fig. 6-13I). It may be familial or the result of chronic fungus infection.

Absence of nails. The nails may be congenitally absent, sometimes in association with ichthyosis. A traumatized nail may be shed, matrix damage preventing regrowth.

Malnourished nails. The nails, growing slowly or not at all and thickening over time, are dry, brittle, and have transverse ridges.

Irregular, short nails—bitten nails. The free edge may be absent from nail biting (Fig. 6-13A).

Square, round nail plates. In acromegaly and congenital hypothyroidism disproportionate lateral growth produces nail plates wider than long.

Long, narrow nail plates. In eunuchoidism and hypopituitarism the nails are long and narrow resembling those in Marfan syndrome.

Longitudinal ridging in nail plate—reedy nail. An exaggeration of normal, there is no diagnostic significance (Fig. 6-13C).

Friable nail plates. With radiation injury, growth is stunted, the nail plate is soft, and the edges frayed (Fig. 6-13D).

Foot and Toenail Signs.

Callus. Well circumscribed areas of thickened epidermal keratin develop at points of repeated pressure or friction. Callus normally underlies the first and fifth metatarsal heads and heel. Callus elsewhere, usually accompanying smaller normal calluses, indicates unusual weight distribution or pressure from footwear. Calluses, infrequently painful in themselves, cause pain when hard callus transmits pressure to tissues impinged between callus and underlying bone. Unlike warts, calluses preserve skin lines.

Hard corn. Tight footwear puts pressure on skin overlying bone between toes producing a conical callus pointing into the dermis. Pressure produces pain. The central core is seen when the top is pared away.

Soft corn. This is an interdigital corn macerated by moisture and infection. It is quite painful.

Plantar wart. Warts are caused by human papilloma virus infection. Skin lines are disrupted and black dots from hemorrhage are common. Weight bearing causes pain.

Neuropathic ulcer. Normal pressure and pain sensation protect the foot from excessive and prolonged pressure over boney prominences. In the insensitive foot (e.g., diabetic neuropathy) pressure leads to painless ischemic soft tissue necrosis, infection, and/or ulceration. A punched-out, indolent, painless ulcer develops under a metatarsal head, at the tip of a toe, over the proximal inter-phalangeal joint of a hammertoe, or on the heel. Test pressure sensation with graded monofilament (Chapter 14, page 645). If bone is exposed or reached by probing, osteomyelitis is likely.

Ingrown toenail. Excessive transverse nail plate growth folds the lateral edge pinching the nail fold. Most commonly the lateral great toe nail fold is affected. An ulcer forms by repeated trauma and infection. Weight bearing is painless, but nail plate pressure is tender. Exuberant granulation tissue may form in the nail fold.

Subungual pain—subungual exostosis. An exostosis arising from the dorsal distal phalanx penetrates the distal nail bed and nail plate. The great toe is usually involved. Early, a painless discoloration is visible under the nail. Later, the nail is pushed up and splits.

Toenail overgrowth—Ram's horn nail. The nail is thickened, conical, and curved like a Ram's horn.

Vascular Signs.

Pallor. Normal skin and mucous membranes are pink due to the dense network of subcutaneous capillaries containing red blood. Pallor is the absence of normal pink color of skin and mucous membranes, regardless of the cause. Inspect the conjunctivae, oral mucosa, palmar creases, and nail beds. Pallor occurs with edema surrounding superficial blood vessels, vasoconstriction, anemia, and any combination. **CLINICAL OCCURRENCE:** *Localized Pallor:* Cold exposure, vasoconstriction (e.g., Raynaud phenomenon), arterial insufficiency, edema; *Generalized Pallor:* Generalized vasoconstriction—cold exposure, severe pain, hypoglycemia, volume depletion, or low cardiac output; *Chronic Pallor:* Normal in some persons, anemia, renal failure; *Paroxysmal Pallor:* Apneic periods in periodic breathing, hypertensive periods from pheochromocytoma, vertiginous periods in Ménière disease, migraine; *Obscuration of Skin Vessels:* Edema, myxedema, scleroderma.

Cyanosis. Cyanosis, the blue skin and mucous membrane color, becomes evident when capillary blood reduced hemoglobin concentration is >4.0–5.0 g/dL, or contains >0.5–1.5 g of methemoglobin, or >0.5 g of sulfhemoglobin. The oxyhemoglobin content does not affect color. Local cyanosis occurs when venous blood is deoxygenated in vessels from stasis or in tissues following extravasation. Generalized cyanosis is seen in the lips, nail beds, ears, and malar regions. *DDX:* Central cyanosis becomes more prominent with exertion or in warm environments. Pressure, by emptying venules, capillaries, and arterioles, blanches cyanosis distinguishing cyanosis from argyria. **CLINICAL OCCURRENCE:** *Local Cyanosis:* Localized venous stasis or arterial obstruction, Raynaud phenomenon, blood extravasations into superficial tissue; *Central Cyanosis:* Hypoxemia (right-to-left shunt, impaired oxygenation from lung disorders), abnormal hemoglobins (methemoglobin or sulfhemoglobin); *Peripheral Cyanosis* (normal arterial oxygen content but increased local oxygen extraction because of sluggish capillary flow): Cutaneous vasoconstriction secondary to cold exposure, reflex response to decreased cardiac output.

Abnormal nailfold capillaries—scleroderma. Episodic digital vasospasm is common in scleroderma (*Raynaud phenomena*) and in otherwise normal persons (*Raynaud disease*). Abnormal nailfold capillaries are strongly associated with later appearance of scleroderma. They also can be seen in dermatomyositis and polymyositis.

Arterial circulation signs. Normal skin temperature indicates adequate arterial flow. Normal nail beds are red or pink. If warm feet have blue nail beds, heat has been applied to feet with inadequate arterial flow. Signs of poor arterial flow must be distinguished from those of impaired venous return. Arterial deficits cause dermal pallor, coldness, and tissue atrophy. Small-vessel disturbances are recognizable as specific patterns in the skin. Diseases of larger arteries cause regional hypoperfusion. Conditions which affect smaller vessels, such as vasculitis, tend to be more diffuse.

Skin pallor and coldness—chronic arterial obstruction. See Chapter 8, page 338. Pallid cool skin suggests regional hypoperfusion. Though normal in cold environments, it should rapidly resolve on warming.

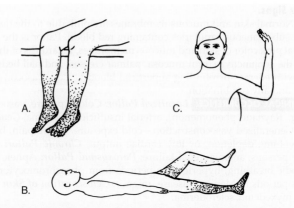

FIG. 6-16 Circulation of the Skin in the Extremities. A. Dependent rubor. The legs are dependent to observe the color of the skin and nail beds. Arterial deficit produces a violaceous color from pooling of the blood in the venules. **B. Elevation produces blanching.** While the patient is supine, the foot is elevated above the level of venous pressure (15 cm [6 in.] above the right heart or 25 cm [10 in.] above the table when the patient is supine). Elevation drains the foot of venous blood, so the skin color reflects only the presence of arterial blood. Compare elevated leg with the opposite extremity. **C. Elevating the hand to asses arterial flow.** The hand is raised above heart level so that skin color is produced exclusively by arterial blood.

Dependent rubor and coldness—chronic arterial insufficiency. The skin and nail beds are blue or purple because arterial flow is not displacing deoxygenated blood from venous capillaries. Raise the part above heart level draining away blue venous blood unmasking pallor of arterial insufficiency (Fig. 6-16). When the part is lowered, the pink color returns in ≤20 seconds. Color return in ≥45–60 seconds confirms arterial insufficiency. See Chapter 8, page 339.

Acute pain, pallor, and coldness. Acute occlusion of a major peripheral artery causes skin and nailbed pallor, decreased temperature, and ischemic pain. See Chapter 8, page 339.

Malnourished skin. The thin skin appears shiny with finely textured wrinkles when pinched. Normal epidermal furrows are absent. Lanugo hair is absent from the backs of hands, feet, and toes.

Skin scars. Skin on the arms and legs contains atraumatic round scars covered with atrophic skin (Fig. 6-17A) resulting from obstruction of small arteries.

Malnourished nails. The nails grow slowly or not at all. They are dry, brittle, and contain transverse ridges. Later, they become thickened (Fig. 6-17B).

Skin ulcers. Ischemic ulcers occur over the tips of the toes, malleoli, heels, metatarsal heads, and dorsal arches. Called cold ulcers, they lack the warm, red coloration that are characteristic of ulcers caused by infection. The borders

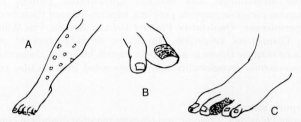

FIG. 6-17 Dermal Lesions from Arterial Deficit. A. Atrophy. The skin over the legs contains round areas of dermal atrophy, with or without pigmentation resulting from small superficial infarctions. **B. Dystrophic nails.** The toenails grow more slowly than normal, and the nail plates become thickened and laminated, the layers forming transverse ridges. **C. Necrosis.** Gangrene of the distal parts may develop from arterial deficit. The sketch shows a round spot of gangrene on the tip of the great toe, and the middle toe blackened from dry gangrene.

frequently appear punched out. They are also seen in sickle cell disease and diabetes mellitus with severe neuropathy.

Retiform necrosis. Necrotic skin in an angulated, stellate (retiform) pattern suggests obstruction of a dermal arteriole; suspect vasculitis.

Skin gangrene. Initial lesions are round, <1 mm in diameter, with pitted centers of black skin (Fig. 6-17C). Gangrene may spread to involve an entire foot. When the skin is black, wrinkled, and dry, the term is *dry gangrene*. Infection is associated with swelling oozing of fluid, *wet gangrene*.

Nodular vessels. —polyarteritis nodosa. See Chapter 8, page 362.

Purpura, intradermal hemorrhage. In general, mucocutaneous bleeding occurs with platelet abnormalities (number or function) or vessel wall problems (e.g., scurvy). Bleeding into joints or viscera is likely related to clotting factor deficiencies or inhibitors. Blood extravasating into the skin is first red, then blue. Within days, hemoglobin degrades changing the color to green or yellow before fading. Pressure does not blanch the area. Petechiae are discrete round hemorrhagic areas <2 mm in diameter. Larger spots are *ecchymoses*. When occurring in groups the term is *purpura*. Purpuric lesions can become confluent, usually without elevating the skin or mucosa (macules and patches). Spontaneous purpura is most common on the lower legs. Minor trauma can induce it elsewhere. A *hematoma* is a hemorrhagic nodule causing skin or mucosa elevation. Extravasated blood dissects along tissue planes. DDX: Infectious purpura may predominate on the thorax and abdomen. *Palpable purpura* suggests vasculitis. Larger nodules may be palpable in polyarteritis nodosa. In subacute bacterial endocarditis septic emboli cause petechiae anywhere. Petechiae can be distinguished from small angiomas by not blanching under pressure.

CLINICAL OCCURRENCE: *Vascular Abnormalities:* Eroded or traumatized large vessels, hereditary hemorrhagic telangiectasia, vasculitis, infections (Rocky Mountain spotted fever), scurvy, Schamberg disease, Cushing syndrome; *Hematologic Abnormalities—Quantitative Platelet Defects:* Autoimmune thrombocytopenic purpura, heparin-induced thrombocytopenia, hypersplenism; *Qualitative Platelet Defects:* Aspirin, von Willebrand disease, Glanzmann syndrome, thrombotic thrombocytopenic purpura (TTP), bone marrow failure (e.g., aplastic anemia, leukemia, chemotherapy), meningococcemia, cryoglobulinemia, disseminated intravascular coagulation (DIC).

Nonpurpuric vascular lesions.
Flushing and blushing. Episodic and often paroxysmal dilation of cutaneous arterioles floods the capillaries causing reddening of the involved skin. *Flushing* is more generalized than *blushing* which is limited to the head, neck, and upper chest. *DDX:* Blushing is usually very situational and transient. Flushing may or may not have a trigger and is more sustained. Generalized erythroderma does not have a trigger and is persistent.

CLINICAL OCCURRENCE: *Flushing: Rosacea*, carcinoid syndrome, pheochromocytoma, fever, hot environments, generalized erythrodermas (toxic shock syndrome, drug eruptions, SLE); *Blushing:* Emotional triggers, for example, embarrassment, shame, fear.

Arterial spider (spider angioma, spider telangiectasia). A coiled arteriole arising perpendicularly from a deeper artery ends in horizontally radiating branches in the plane of the skin. The fiery red vascular figure has a central area, varying from a pinpoint to a papule from which radiate arterialized capillaries forming the spider legs (Fig. 6-18D). The vessels may dip into the tissue to reappear further on, forming short, visible segments. An area of erythema surrounds the body and extends several millimeters beyond the radicular tips. Rarely, the body is visibly pulsatile, and pulsation may be felt. Pressure over the body with a glass slide shows the blood emerging from the punctum in pulses. Pressing the body with a pencil tip fades the radicles which fill centrifugally when pressure is released. Spiders commonly occur on the face and neck and, in diminishing frequency, on the shoulders, anterior chest, back, arms, forearms, and backs of the hands and fingers. Spiders are rare below the umbilicus. In liver disease and pregnancy, they are frequently accompanied by palmar erythema. The most common causes of arterial spiders include high esterogen states including chronic liver disease with cirrhosis, hyperestrinism, pregnancy (disappearing after delivery) and, occasionally, following significant cumulative sun exposure.

Reticular pattern—livedo reticularis. Skin on the arms and legs is mottled with circinate bands of cyanosis surrounding patches of normal skin (Fig. 6-18E, Fig. 6-19). Three types are described. In *cutis marmorata* the mottling appears on exposure to cold and disappears with warming. *Livedo reticularis idiopathica*, which is not associated with other disease, and also can improve with rewarming, whereas *livedo reticularis symptomatica* persists, and is a frequent accompaniment of the antiphospholipid syndrome, cryoglobulinemia, and polyarteritis nodosa. Ulceration sometimes complicates those that persist with warming. Livedo reticularis is seen with atheroemboli (page 153).

Palmar erythema. Fixed, diffuse erythema involves the hypothenar eminence and, with less intensity, the thenar prominence (Fig. 6-18F). In severe

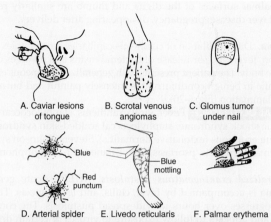

FIG. 6-18 Some Named Superficial Vascular Lesions. A. Caviar Lesions of the Tongue. Varicose veins under the tongue form bluish masses that appear as bunches of caviar. **B. Scrotal venous angiomas.** When the scrotum is spread, multiple dark red or blue papules, 3–4 mm in diameter, are seen. **C. Glomus tumor under the nail.** An elevated nodule, 2–10 mm in diameter, may occur any place in the skin, frequently under the nail plate. It is extremely painful. **D. Venous stars and arterial spiders.** One form of venous star is depicted; the lesions may also appear as cascades, flares, rockets, comets, or tangles. A typical form of arterial spider, with punctum and radicles, is presented. While venous stars are bluish, spiders are fiery red. Both lesions fade with pressure. Pressing the center with a pencil tip will not blanch the branches of a star; the radicles of the spiders will fade with pressure on the punctum. The star always overlies a large vein; the spider is not associated with a visible large vessel. As seen through a pressing glass slide, the venous star does not pulsate; the arterial spider fills from the center with pulsatile spurts. **E. Livedo reticularis.** Seen most often on the legs, the skin is mottled, with deeply cyanosed areas interspersed with round pale spots. In one type, the discoloration disappears with warming; in others, it does not. **F. Palmar erythema.** There is intense diffuse erythema which is deepest over the hypothenar eminence and less pronounced on the thenar eminence and distal fingers. The erythema is not mottled.

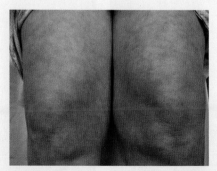

FIG. 6-19 Livedo Reticularis. The netlike pattern of dilated cutaneous veins is readily apparent on both thighs.

cases, the palmar surfaces of the digits and thumb are similarly reddened.
Examples: Liver disease; pregnancy, disappearing after delivery.

Erythroderma. Diffuse dilation of cutaneous capillaries accompanies systemic inflammation, fever, and/or release of bacterial toxins and involves over 80% to 90% of the body. The patient presents with generalized cutaneous erythema. Asymptomatic in benign conditions, it is intensely painful and burning with systemic inflammation (Fig. 6-20).
CLINICAL OCCURRENCE: Fever, viral exanthems, staphylococcal or streptococcal toxic shock syndrome, staphylococcal scalded-skin syndrome, scarlet fever, drug eruptions (exfoliative dermatitis), Stevens–Johnson syndrome, toxic epidermal necrolysis, psoriasis, SLE, cutaneous T-cell lymphoma.

Acute generalized exanthematous pustulosis (AGEP). Acute generalized erythroderma is accompanied by fever, chills, and leukocytosis. The erythroderma progresses over hours to widespread pustulosis. The condition is self-limited and appears to follow exposure to viruses or certain drugs, e.g., NSAIDs.

Pink papules—rose spots of typhoid fever. Rose spots are erythematous papules 2–4 mm in diameter that blanch with pressure. They appear in the second week, usually in crops, commonly on the upper abdomen and lower thorax. Each lesion persists for 2–3 days, then disappears leaving a faint brown stain.

Red macule or papule—cherry angioma (papillary angioma). Usually <3 mm in diameter and often no larger than a pinhead, the cherry angioma is bright red, discrete, and irregularly round, surrounded by a narrow halo of pallid skin. Larger lesions may be slightly elevated. Occasionally they are pedunculated.

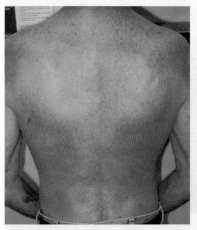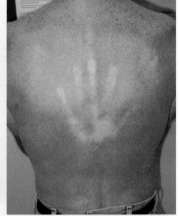

FIG. 6-20 Erythroderma. There is diffuse, generalized cutaneous capillary dilation which blanches with hand pressure. This patient's erythroderma is due to systemic lupus erythematosus.

Pressure causes little or no blanching. Small lesions may be distinguished from petechiae only by their permanence when observed for several days. Angiomas occur more often on the thorax and arms than the face and abdomen; they are less frequent on forearms and on legs. With advancing age, some fade and become atrophic. Everyone has a few, the number increases after age 30 years. They have no clinical significance.

Blue papule—venous lakes. Thin-walled papules fill with venous blood. Gentle pressure empties them leaving lax indentations beneath skin level. They rarely occur before age 35 and increase with age. Associated with sun exposure they are much more common in men than women. Lakes are more frequent on ears and facethan on the lips and neck; they are uncommon elsewhere.

Blue papules—scrotal venous angioma (Fordyce lesion). Figure 6-18B and Chapter 12, page 518.

Blue nodule—rubber-bleb nevi of skin and gastrointestinal tract. There are three types of lesions: a large disfiguring angioma, a fluctuant thin-skinned bleb containing blood that leaves a rumpled sac when compressed, and an irregular blue area gradually merging with surrounding skin and only partially fading with pressure. Similar lesions in the gut are a risk for serious hemorrhage. The skin lesions may be few or many scattered over the body. The condition is not hereditary.

Painful red or blue nodule—glomus tumor. Glomus tumors are more common in the hands and fingers, especially beneath a nail (Fig. 6-18C). The tumor is a red or blue elevated nodule 2–10 mm in diameter. It is exquisitely painful, completely disproportionate to its size. The pain may occur in paroxysms. Relief may require surgical excision.

Irregular spongy tumor—cavernous hemangioma. The tumor occurs in any tissues and varies in size from microscopic to involvement of an entire arm or leg. Usually present at birth and enlarging with age, it can involve skin, subcutaneous tissue, muscle, and even bone. The surface is irregular, nodular, frequently bluish, and fluctuant. Raising the involved limb may cause partial emptying. Hemangiomas can consume platelets and coagulation factors producing a DIC picture (*Kasabach–Merritt syndrome*).

Stellate figure—venous star. Occurring with aging or arising from venous obstruction, small superficial veins radiate from a central point (Fig. 6-18D). Patterns include stars, angular Vs, cascades, flares, rockets, and tangles varying from a few millimeters to several centimeters in diameter. Venous stars are more common in women. Common sites are the top of the foot, leg, medial aspect of the thigh above the knee, and back of the neck. *DDX:* It is easy to distinguish venous stars from arterial spiders. Like spider angiomas, the branches fade with pressure refilling from the center after pressure is released, but the vessels are blue-purple, whereas arterial spiders are bright red. In contrast to arterial spiders, pressure on the central point does not blanch the radicles. Stars always overlie a larger vein; spiders are not associated with another vessel.

Reticular pattern—costal fringe. Usually seen with aging in older men, superficial veins near the anterior ribs and xiphoid form networks, sometimes in bands with rough correspondence to the diaphragm attachments.

Reticular pattern—facial telangiectasis. Vessels on the nose and face dilate from exposure to wind and cold, and with aging in some persons. They also occur with rosacea and liver disease.

Reticular pattern—radiation telangiectasis. Therapeutic irradiation produces skin changes months after exposure. The chief signs are pigmentation, atrophy, and telangiectasias which are the most conspicuous. Fine red or blue vessels form a disordered network.

Signs of Systemic Lipid Disorders.

Xanthomas. Systemic disorders of lipid metabolism lead to lipid deposition in cutaneous and subcutaneous structures including tendons. The asymptomatic lesions are macules, papules, plaques, or nodules, often brown to orange in color. Their distribution is highly suggestive of the underlying disorder.

Xanthelasma. There are soft, usually symmetrical, often coalescent elevated yellow to beige-colored plaques on the eyelids, increasingly common after age 60. It may occur in otherwise normal people and with elevated low-density lipoprotein cholesterol.

Eruptive xanthomas. Hypertriglyceridemia leads to rather sudden appearance of multiple closely packed yellow to red-to-brown cutaneous papules and nodules. Most common on the elbows and buttocks, they may occur anywhere.

Palmar xanthomas. The infiltration of the hand's creases producing yellowish ridges is pathognomonic for familial dysbetalipoproteinemia.

Tendon xanthomas. Relatively large nodules are palpable along tendons and ligaments, particularly the Achilles and hand tendons, associated with markedly elevated serum cholesterol.

SKIN AND NAIL SYNDROMES

Common Skin Disorders:.

Acne vulgaris. Androgens promote sebaceous gland obstruction, and *Propionibacterium acnes* proliferate within the pilosebaceous unit. Lesions are distributed with sebaceous glands on face, chest, and upper back. Uninflamed *comedones* are either open to air oxidizing sebum in orifice (a blackhead) or closed producing a white papule. Rupture of the obstructed pilosebaceous unit leads to inflammatory papules, pustules, and nodules.

Rosacea. Patients develop inflamed papules and telangiectasia on the forehead, cheeks, and chin progressing to chronic edema and thickened skin. Women are more affected than men, although *rhinophyma* is more common in men.

Eczema—Dermatitis. Dermatitis literally means skin inflammation, in practice it is synonymous with eczema a specific class of epidermal inflammation. Several types are distinguished by their etiology, pattern, and appearance.

Atopic dermatitis. Common in first-degree relatives, it is often associated with seasonal allergies, asthma, or atopic dermatitis. Atopy begins in infancy or childhood and may be lifelong. Lesions are erythematous intensely pruritic papules or plaques usually on flexor surfaces of elbows, neck, and wrists, and face, feet, and hands. Scratching temporarily relieves the itch, but increasing inflammation and pruritus producing lichenification.

Lichen simplex chronicus. Chronic rubbing or scratching produces intensely pruritic hyperkeratotic plaques. Nodular lesions, *prurigo nodularis*, occur with persistent picking.

Dyshidrotic eczema. Deep pruritic vesicles coalesce on hands and feet, especially intertriginous areas, palms, and soles. Scratching produces lichenification. *DDX:* Consider contact allergens and autosensitization dermatitis from dermatophyte infection of the feet (*id reaction*).

Asteatotic eczema. Dry skin is cracked into irregular rhomboidal plates, like a drying lakebed, with erythematous margins and commonly marginal scaling. Intensely pruritic, it is common on extremities and trunk in cold dry climates and exacerbated by use of soap and water.

Papular eczema. The lesions are pruritic erythematous papules on the extremities. *DDX:* Guttate psoriasis is similar but has superficial scale.

Nummular eczema. The nummular (coin-like) lesions are 1–3 cm plaques with sharp borders and a raised edge, most common on the legs and trunk of older men. They may weep, especially with excoriation.

Stasis dermatitis. Increased venous and capillary pressure produces inflammation, edema, subcutaneous fibrosis, and skin atrophy with hemosiderin staining. Pitting edema, erythema, and warmth, often with tenderness, are prominent. Chronically, subcutaneous tissues become fibrotic and the edema no longer pits (brawny edema or *lipodermatosclerosis*). The skin thins and is easily injured leading to ulcers and secondary infection. *DDX:* When erythema and warmth are present it can be confused with cellulitis.

Contact dermatitis. This is either a cell-mediated response to prior sensitization or an inflammatory response to skin irritants. Irritant contact dermatitis can occur in anyone, e.g., chemical burns. Allergic contact dermatitis requires prior exposure with sensitization. The lesions are erythematous intensely pruritic plaques. The distribution lesions and exposure history are critical for correct diagnosis (Fig. 6-21). *DDX:* Irritant disease often has early vesiculation (but so does rhus dermatitis) and evolves more rapidly than allergic disease. **CLINICAL OCCURRENCE:** *Allergic:* rhus dermatitis (poison ivy and oak), many other plant and animal sources, drugs (neomycin, sulfonamides), chromate, solvents, latex, metals especially nickel (common in earrings, buckles, snaps), cosmetics, clothing dyes, industrial oils, and many others; *Irritants:* acids and alkali, cement, solvents, cutting oils, detergents, etc.

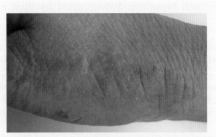

FIG. 6-21 Contact Dermatitis. This lesion on the side of the thumb resulted from latex allergy in a nurse. The skin is erythematous, itchy, thickened and fissured (lichenoid) due to scratching.

Autosensitization dermatitis. Sensitization to antigens from a primary, often infectious or infected, dermatitis leads to distant lesions. The classic example is the id reaction, a vesicular eruption on the hands or distant areas in patients with chronic tinea pedis infection. Secondary lesions heal only after treatment of the primary infection or inflammation.

Seborrheic dermatitis. This very common disorder that produces erythema and scaling in the distribution of sebaceous glands: scalp (dandruff, cradle cap), eyebrows, nasolabial folds, external acoustic meatus, and chest (Fig. 6-22). The skin may be mildly pruritic. It occurs frequently with Parkinson disease; sudden severe disease may be a sign of HIV infection.

Photodermatitis. Skin sensitization to topical or systemic chemicals leads to dermatitis triggered by sunlight. Erythema appears hours to a couple days after exposure and only on sun-exposed skin. It has a burning quality and can blister. *Polymorphic light eruption* refers to a delayed sensitivity reaction to sunlight exposure. Examples are antibiotics (tetracyclines, sulfonamides), antidepressants, antihypertensives, diuretics (thiazides especially), NSAIDs, sunscreens. *DDX:* Consider polymorphic light eruption and porphyria.

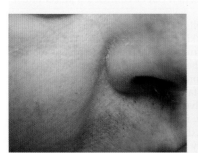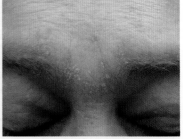

FIG. 6-22 Seborrheic Dermatitis. Erythema and scaling in the nasolabial fold, eyebrows and glabella.

Intertrigo. Skin folds between the buttocks, under the breasts, and in skin creases become inflamed from persistent warmth, moisture, and occlusion. Secondary infection with streptococci, *Pseudomonas aeruginosa, Candida albicans*, and other fungi is common. *DDX:* Cellulitis and psoriasis, especially inverse psoriasis, are confused with intertrigo.

Psoriasis. Increased epithelial cell division with associated inflammation, and reduced surface desquamation produce thickened skin. Psoriasis occurs in 1% to 3% of the population varying from mild to severe. Individual lesions vary from papules to huge plaques with a characteristically adherent scale; the surface bleeds on removing the scales. The nails are frequently pitted and dystrophic. Lesions are bilateral, symmetrical, involve the extensor (e.g., elbows, knees) more than flexor surfaces, and frequently the scalp and gluteal crease. Trunk and extremities are involved in any combination. *Inverse psoriasis* is a pattern opposite to that expected. Skin trauma can precipitate a new lesion (*Koebner phenomena*). A severe mutilating arthritis of the axial skeleton (*spondyloarthropathy*) and distal interphalangeal joints may accompany or occur independently of skin and nail disease.

Guttate psoriasis. Following an infection, often streptococcal pharyngitis, 2-10-mm pink papules appear diffusely on the trunk and extremities. The face and scalp are relatively spared, and palm and sole involvement is rare. The lesions resolve spontaneously over weeks. Classic plaque psoriasis may occur several years after remission of guttate psoriasis. The lesions resemble papular eczema.

Pustular psoriasis. Sudden onset of intense painful erythema is followed within 24 hours by deep pustular dermal lesions which rupture forming erosions. The patient has fever and leukocytosis. Patients may be severely ill. This frequently follows withdrawal of systemic corticosteroid therapy.

Palmoplantar pustulosis. Pustules appear sporadically on the palms and soles associated with burning pain and heal with crusting. The cause is unknown. It may be a localized form of pustular psoriasis. It has been seen with metal allergies and as a reaction to TNF-inhibitors.

Infectious exanthems. *Exanthems* are diffuse skin eruptions associated with bacterial or viral illness (see Erythroderma, page 132). Viral exanthems are often accompanied by mucosal involvement, an *enanthem*. Individual lesions take many forms: diffuse erythroderma (*scarlatiniform*), maculopapules (*morbilliform*, measles-like), or vesicles that may evolve to pustules. The diffuse erythrodermas often heal with desquamation.

   CLINICAL OCCURRENCE: *Viral: (most common)* Rubella, rubeola, parvovirus B19, adenoviruses, cytomegalovirus, Epstein-Barr virus, herpes simplex viruses 6 and 7 (exanthem subitum and roseola infantum, respectively), enteroviruses, HIV, Colorado tick fever, and many others; *Bacterial:* Group A streptococcus (scarlet fever), staphylococcus (toxic shock syndrome), leptospirosis, meningococcemia; *Rickettsial:* Rocky Mountain spotted fever, rickettsialpox, typhus.

Scarlet fever. A Group-A streptococcal exotoxin causes generalized cutaneous erythema. Streptococcal pharyngitis (Chapter 7, page 250) is accompanied by a maculopapular erythematous blanching eruption initially on the neck, axillae, and groin later becoming generalized. The skin feels slightly rough, like fine sandpaper. The rash heals with desquamation beginning around the nails.

Toxic shock syndrome. See Chapter 4, page 68.

Ichthyosis. These are hereditary keratinocyte diseases. The skin is thickened and dry, cracking hexagonally when severe. Hair follicle hyperkeratosis produces pointed follicular papules, *keratosis pilaris*, a common skin condition.

Granuloma annulare. Asymptomatic papules and plaques with sharply demarcated annular or arcuate borders on the hands, feet, elbows, knees, and distal extremities, usually bilaterally. The lesions are pink, purple, or skin colored, and typically self-limited.

Lichen planus. Purple, flat-topped, sharply demarcated pruritic papules appear on the wrists, ankles, eyelids, and shins. Other forms include hypertrophic and bullous lichen planus. Mucous membrane involvement is common, appearing as white linear lesions in the mouth or genital mucosa (*Wickham striae*). Erosions, papules, and plaques can occur in the oral mucosa. Erosive lichen planus is associated with hepatitis C.

Genital white patches—lichen sclerosis. White atrophic lesions with sharp borders appear most often on the vulva, perianal skin, and penis. The skin is thin, and erosions may occur. Pruritus and dyspareunia are common.

Verrucous papules—warts. Skin or mucous membrane infection with human papilloma virus leads to verrucous hyperplasia; uterine cervix infection with specific strains causes cervical cancer. The common wart is a well-demarcated papule with a verrucous surface, commonly on the fingers. Genital involvement is particularly troublesome. Flat confluent lesions without the verrucous surface are *flat warts*. Problematic areas are the sole of the foot, *plantar warts*, and around the nails, *periungual warts*.

Pityriasis rosea. This common disorder primarily affects adolescents and young adults in the fall. The eruption is asymptomatic to mildly pruritic involving the trunk and proximal extremities. An inverse form occurs in the axillae and groin. The general eruption is often preceded by a larger single lesion, the *herald patch*. Lesions are oval, with the long axis in the skin folds, classically creating a Christmas tree pattern on the back. Lesions are 0.5 to 3 cm in diameter and have a slightly raised border with a collar of fine superficial scales on an erythematous base. Resolution is spontaneous over weeks.

Actinic keratosis. Mildly erythematous macules with adherent hyperkeratotic scale appear in sun-exposed areas. They are premalignant and squamous cell carcinoma may arise in chronic lesions.

Seborrheic keratosis. These are begin lesions that appear in midlife as brown macules gradually enlarging to 1–3 cm plaques with a raised adherent hyperkeratotic surface. They appear stuck-on to the skin (Fig. 6-23).

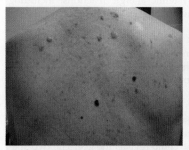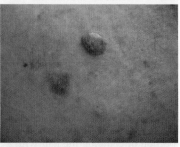

FIG. 6-23 Seborrheic Keratoses and Lipoma. *Left:* Multiple "stuck on" lesions on the upper back with great variation in color. A subcutaneous lipoma is faintly visible superior and medial to the upper border of the right scapular spine. *Right:* Close up of two seborrheic keratoses showing variation in coloration and degree of elevation.

DDX: Pigmented lesions are confused with malignant melanoma and macular lesions with moles or lentigines.

Dermatofibroma. The lesions are 3- to 8-mm firm, variably colored intradermal papules usually on the arms and legs. When pinched the lesion retracts rather than elevates, the *dimple sign. DDX:* May be confused with melanoma and pilomatricoma.

Skin tags (acrochordons). These insensate dermal polyps are most prevalent on the neck, axillary folds, and perineum and are more common with obesity. They are of no clinical significance but can be irritated by clothing or jewelry and are often a cosmetic concern. *DDX:* Nevi, and large skin tags may be confused with neurofibromas.

Vitiligo. Autoimmune destruction of melanocytes results in complete loss of pigmentation in affected areas. The macular lesions are symmetrical with sharp borders. They cause significant cosmetic discomfort in dark-skinned individuals. *DDX:* Vitiligo is confused with hypopigmented lesions (e.g., discoid lupus erythematosus, leprosy), depigmentation from burns or scars, or ash leaf spots of tuberous sclerosis. Vitiligo is more common in families with other autoimmune disorders, e.g., diabetes, Addison disease, Hashimoto thyroiditis.

Body piercing. Piercing has a long and rich cultural history. Western societies saw a dramatic increase in piercing in the late 20th century. Piercing is done for many reasons. Medical professionals must attend to the risks associated with piercing, the types of piercing and their significance, and the personality issues that may be involved in caring for these individuals.

Skin Infections and Infestations.
Mosquito and other insect bites. Insect bites present as painful or pruritic papules with erythema and variable cutaneous edema. Closely inspect early lesions for the central punctum. Most bites are minor and self-limited but extensive bites can cause systemic toxicity. Hymenoptera stings (bees, hornets, and wasps) cause severe local reactions with expansive erythema and

edema. Sensitized individuals have systemic allergic reactions, including anaphylaxis, to hymenoptera and some ant species. *Black flies* leave a 1- to 2-mm hemorrhagic mark.

Bedbugs. Bedbugs are 3 to 5 mm brown insects living in crevices of bedding and clothing and feeding on blood, typically at night. The bite is painless and in a sequence producing linear grouped lesions ("breakfast, lunch, and dinner").

Pediculosis—lice. Lice are wingless insects that feed on skin scales. *Nits* are egg sacs cemented to hair shafts. Patients complain of itching and close inspection or combing the hair with a fine comb reveals the lice. The two species are *Pediculosis humanus* inhabiting the head (*Pediculosis capitis*) or body (*Pediculosis corporis*) and *Phthirus pubis* living in pubic hair (*Pediculosis pubis*).

Myiasis. When being bitten by insects, eggs may be deposited on skin or in wounds. The larvae invade and grow in subcutaneous tissue. Since they breath air, a skin opening is always present. The patient complains of movement under the skin.

Spider bites. Most are benign and no cause for concern. The *common aggressive house spider* attacks while a person is sleeping, so bites are usually on the exposed face, hands, arms, or feet. Bites cause moderate skin necrosis and scarring. The *brown recluse spider* is common but not aggressive. It bites in defense when disturbed in old buildings, woodpiles, and similar habitats. The bite is initially painless, but the site becomes intensely painful with severe necrosis and scarring. The *black widow spider* bite is a minor lesion with minimal erythema; the adverse effects are caused by a systemic neurotoxin.

Mites. Mites, arthropods related to ticks, occupy innumerable habitats bringing them in contact with humans. They feed on skin and cutaneous debris. Exposure history and lesion pattern are the best guides to diagnosis.

Scabies. *Sarcoptes scabiei* burrows through the epidermis laying eggs and depositing feces, which incite inflammation. The infestation is contagious and passes between persons. The intensely pruritic lesions are erythematous papules; linear burrows may be seen. The mite favors thin skin with few hair follicles, especially intertriginous areas of hands, wrists, elbows, and genitalia. A KOH preparation reveals mites, eggs, or feces.

Chiggers. Chiggers are the <1 mm larval form of a mite living in warm grassy or woodland environments. They feed on skin cells by injecting digestive enzymes into the skin. The lesions, commonly around the feet and ankles, are intensely pruritic red papules, usually multiple depending on the length of exposure.

Swimmer's eruption. Larvae of many organisms for which humans are not the primary host (bird schistosome, jellyfish or sea urchin larvae, etc.), penetrate the skin inciting a cutaneous reaction. Patients present with an intensely pruritic rash hours after emerging from the water. Salt water bathers often shower with freshwater in their bathing suits. Freshwater exposure triggers stings by some free-swimming larvae. The rash may be diffuse or restricted to an area where wet clothing held the parasites next to the skin.

Larval migrations—cutaneous larval migrans. Dog and cat hookworm eggs laid in soil hatch into motile larvae that penetrate the skin then migrate through the skin and subcutaneous tissues to their final destinations. The lesions are linear, red, serpiginous, raised and migrate over time. **Examples:** *Ancylostoma braziliense, A. caninum*. There also can be migratory findings with strongyloidiasis (larva currens), fascioliasis, dracunculiasis, and others.

Bacterial infections.
Impetigo. Superficial infection with staphylococcus and streptococcus produces erythematous erosions with amber crusts. Common on children's faces it can occur wherever there is a skin break. Bullae form in severe cases, *bullous impetigo*. Localized painful ulcerations, *ecthyma*, occurs with poor hygiene. Secondarily infected skin lesions are *secondary impetiginization*. Impetigo commonly complicates eczema.

Folliculitis. Pustular infection of hair follicles is common in men's beard area, but also occurs on the scalp, trunk, legs, and buttocks. Organisms include *Staphylococcus aureus, P. aeruginosa* (hot tub folliculitis), herpes simplex, and several fungi. *DDX: Pseudofolliculitis barbae* occurs in men with tightly curled hair who shave. Papules are caused by retained hairs; pustules indicate secondary infection.

Cellulitis. Infection with streptococci or staphylococci spreads radially within the skin and subcutaneous structures. The lesions are warm, raised, and tender with indistinct borders. Any break in the skin can be an entry site. Cellulitis is most common on legs and arms. Fever may or may not be present. *DDX:* Less-common causes of cellulitis are nocardia, mycobacteria, *P. aeruginosa, Haemophilus influenzae*, and vibrios (especially in cirrhotic patients). *Pasteurella multocida* is common following cat and dog bites and has a propensity to cause osteomyelitis. *Erysipeloid* is caused by *Erysipelothrix rhusiopathiae. Erythema chronicum migrans* is caused by Lyme borreliosis (see Chapter 4, page 50). Common causes of noninfectious inflammation often confused with cellulitis are stasis dermatitis, superficial and deep thrombophlebitis, panniculitis, erythema nodosum, and nephrogenic fibrosing dermopathy.

Erysipelas. Streptococcal infection of the dermal lymphatics produces intense dermal and epidermal edema and inflammation. The lesion is intensely erythematous with a sharp, raised border. It is common on the face, often without an evident break in the skin.

Skin abscess—furuncle, carbuncle. Skin infections with S. aureus produce collections of pus and necrotic debris in patterns determined by local skin structure. *Furuncles* (boils) are relatively superficial single collections. *Carbuncles* extend into the subcutaneous tissues involving the deep hair follicles producing interconnected abscesses. Carbuncles arise in areas of especially thick fibrotic skin such as the posterior neck.

Hidradenitis suppurative. Inflammation of areas containing apocrine glands is associated with chronic, painful draining lesions healing with scarring. Infection can occur secondarily. Most commonly seen in obese women involving the axilla or perineum, and rarely the scalp. It can coincide in people with cystic acne.

Erythema migrans—Lyme disease. See Chapter 4, page 50. Asymptomatic erythema at the inoculation site expands, often with an annular configuration, reaching several centimeters in size. Vesicles are uncommon. More than one lesion may be present. Bell palsy, heart block, and arthritis of large joints are late manifestations.

Ulceroglandular syndromes. An often minimally symptomatic ulcer develops at the inoculation site. Lymphatic dissemination produces regional lymphadenopathy. On finding regional lymphadenopathy always search for an inoculation lesion. The nature and location of exposure are key to accurate diagnosis.

CLINICAL OCCURRENCE: Tularemia, plague, syphilis, rat-bite fever, rickettsial pox, cat-scratch disease, anthrax, Mycobacterium marinum, scrub typhus, sporotrichiosis, nocardia, lymphogranuloma venereum, herpes simples, cowpox, trypanosomiasis.

Syphilis. The primary lesion (*chancre*) is a painless shallow ulcer at the inoculation site (penis, glans, vulva, lip, tongue, pharynx, finger, etc.). The discoid underlying induration feels like a small coin. Painless, nonsuppurating regional lymphadenopathy follows.

Tularemia. *Francisella tularensis* is inoculated by fly or tick bites or skin contact with an infected rabbit. Following an incubation period of 1–10 days lassitude, headache, chills, nausea and vomiting, and myalgia accompany a benign inoculation site ulcer with surrounding erythema and little pain. Regional fluctuant painful lymphadenopathy develops which may suppurate. Splenomegaly may be present. Inoculation into the eye causes an *oculoglandular syndrome* with lacrimation, photophobia, lid edema, and preauricular and cervical lymphadenopathy.

Anthrax. *Bacillus anthracis* infection is transmitted from wild or domestic animals by contact with hides or ingestion or inhalation of spores. The painless "malignant pustule" begins as an erythematous papule which then vesiculates and ulcerates surrounded by brawny edema. A black eschar may form. Regional lymphadenopathy is occasionally present. Inhalational exposure leads to rapidly progressive pneumonia with hilar adenopathy and mediastinal widening.

Nodular lymphangitis. Nodular lymphangitis without an inoculation lesion manifests as erythema, induration and nodular thickening of cutaneous and subcutaneous lymphatics. Regional lymphadenopathy may be found. A complete travel and exposure history is key. This is misdiagnosed as cellulitis. **Examples:** *Mycobacteria marinum, Nocardia,* sporotrichosis, leishmaniasis, tularemia, coccidioidosis, histoplasmosis, blastomycosis, cryptococosis, *Psuedomonas psuedomallei,* and anthrax.

Cat-scratch disease. *Bartonella henselae inoculated by the scratch, lick, or bite of a healthy cat travel to regional lymph nodes, then disseminate.* Symptoms are nonspecific with malaise and headache. Signs include fever, an inoculation site papule, or pustule followed by painful fluctuant regional lymphadenopathy with overlying erythema. Dissemination in immuno-compromised hosts leads to hepatitis (peliosis hepatitis), osteomyelitis, or meningoencephalitis. Conjunctival infection produces preauricular lymph-adenopathy (Parinaud oculoglandular syndrome) [Koehler JE, Duncan LM. Case 30-2005: A 56-year-old man with fever and axillary lymphadenopathy. *N Engl J Med.* 2005;353:1387–1394; Pael UD, Hollander H, Saint S. Index of suspicion. *N Engl J Med.* 2004;350:1990–1995].

Rickettsial spotted fever syndromes. See Chapter 4, page 49. These syn-dromes present with an inoculation eschar, high fever, myalgias, and malaise. A thorough travel and residential history is key to accurate diagnosis.

Necrotizing soft-tissue infections. Anaerobic or microaerophilic organisms are inoculated deeply into a puncture wound or ascend via lymphatics. Infec-tion spreads longitudinally along adipose tissue septa and muscle fascia and vertically into deeper structures along neurovascular bundles penetrating tissue planes. The patient complains of severe pain disproportionate to the injury or cutaneous erythema, which is initially minimal. The soft tissues are edematous, indurated, and very tender. Infection progresses rapidly causing extensive tissue necrosis, edema, hypoperfusion, compartment syndromes, systemic hypotension, and death. Rapid diagnosis and surgical debridement are essential to save life and limb. The most common organisms are group A or microaerophilic streptococci. Less common are gas-forming organisms, e.g., *Clostridium perfringens (gas gangrene).*

Erysipeloid. Caused by *Erysipelothrix rhusiopathiae*, it is acquired by han-dling infected mammals and fish. A localized dermal infection of the fingers or hands, rarely extending above the wrist, it presents as swollen, slightly tender, violaceous skin with sharp borders. The inflammation resolves in a few days leaving pigmentation.

Mycobacterial infections. Infection with tuberculous or nontuberculous mycobacterium present as progressive skin infections with negative cul-tures and unresponsive to antibiotics. A high index of suspicion and selec-tive media for culture are required. Fungal infections are mimics, e.g., cryptococcus.

Digital infection—tuberculosis verrucosa cutis. *Mycobacterium tuberculosis* is inoculated into the skin. A bluish-red patch appears, later becoming papil-lomatous and warty; it may exude pus. Pathologists are infected at the au-topsy; butchers and packinghouse workers handle infected meat. The lesions are indolent with no constitutional symptoms.

Fish-tank granuloma—M. marinum. A small nodule or nodules develop on the fingers after exposure to contaminated aquariums. The lesions may ulcerate or form small abscesses. Lymphatic spread resembles sporotri-chosis.

Tropical ulcer—buruli ulcer. Mycobacterium ulcerans is endemic in some tropical countries. A pruritic nodule breaks down forming a chronic, shallow, nonhealing ulcer.

Viral infections.
Human papilloma virus (HPV)—Warts. See page 138.

Herpes simplex virus (HSV). Herpes simplex viruses spread person-to-person by intimate contact. Genital ulceration is more commonly caused by type-2 (genital herpes strain) than type-1 which is more commonly associated with oral infections. Initial type-1 infection produces severe stomatitis with gingival involvement. Initial type-2 genital infection causes a painful vesicular eruption on the genital skin or mucosa. Regional lymphadenopathy and aseptic meningitis can occur. Recurrences manifest grouped vesicles on an erythematous base, commonly on the lips (*herpes labialis*) and buttocks but can be elsewhere (Fig. 6-24). Recurrent lesions are preceded by 1–3 days of discomfort at the site of subsequent lesions.

Varicella-zoster (VZV). VZV infection in childhood causes chickenpox. Before being controlled by a humoral immune response VZV disseminates to spinal and cranial nerve sensory ganglia establishing lifelong latency checked by cell mediated immunity. Latent virus reactivates with waning cell-mediated immunity due to age, immunosuppression, concurrent illness, or immunosuppressive drugs producing herpes zoster (shingles) and, rarely, disseminated infection.

Chickenpox. Initial varicella infection is a mild systemic disease with rash and fever beginning simultaneously. The initial skin lesions are red papules on the trunk more than face, arms, and legs. They evolve to superficial vesicles on erythematous bases (dew drop on a rose petal) that rapidly become pustules. Healing is by crusting leaving little or no scar. Vesicles occur in successive crops, so lesions are at various stages of development.

Herpes zoster (shingles). Severe burning pain and dysesthesia is followed in 1–3 days by clustered vesicles on an intensely erythematous base within a

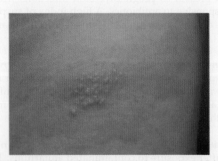

FIG. 6-24 Herpes Simplex. A painful crop of vesicles and pustules has erupted on a well demarcated erythematous base in this patient's left groin.

spinal or cranial sensory dermatome. Unless dissemination occurs, lesions are unilateral not crossing the midline. The vesicles burst, crust, and slowly heal. Pain, *postherpetic neuralgia,* subsides in days, weeks, or months. Diagnosis is uncertain until the rash appears.

Variola—smallpox. Variola infection is a severe systemic illness with a pustular skin eruption predominately on the face and extremities. The rash is preceded by 2–3 days of fever, myalgias, and arthralgias. Unlike varicella, the skin lesions are synchronous, progressing from vesicles to tense deep pustules that break, crust, and heal with scarring. The mortality rate is high.

Monkeypox. This African monkey infection was imported to North America in the spring of 2003. It was transmitted to humans from infected prairie dogs. The illness is acute with fever and malaise, followed by a macular rash with vesicles, which may be umbilicated. The lesions may be asynchronous.

HIV and AIDS. HIV/AIDS has many cutaneous clues to diagnosis. Acute infection is associated with a morbilliform or papular exanthem and enanthem. Herpes zoster occurs early in the chronic course of HIV infection. Severe seborrheic dermatitis is common. *Candida* skin and vulvovaginal infections occur frequently. Dermatophyte infections are more common and difficult to treat. An eosinophilic folliculitis is associated with HIV infection and its treatment. AIDS patients often have pruritic dermatitis with dry skin. HPV-associated cervical dysplasia and cancer are more common in HIV-infected than non-HIV-infected women. In advanced disease, Kaposi sarcoma (KS) presents on the skin and oral and genital mucous membranes. Hairy leukoplakia is a characteristic oral lesion. Abnormal subcutaneous fat distribution, lipodystrophy, is associated with protease inhibitor treatment of HIV/AIDS.

Human herpes virus 8—Kaposi Sarcoma. See page 156.

Superficial fungal infections—dermatophytes, tinea. Dermatophytes infect the dead keratin layer of skin, nails, and hair. Though specific fungus can be cultured, infection is clinically classified by location. Presentation usually involves skin thickening, scaling, and mild erythema. Secondary bacterial infection occurs in macerated chronically moist areas. *DDX:* Chronic noninfectious dermatitis is often confused with tinea.

Tinea pedis—athlete's foot. Infection is a white raised patch with fissures that may ulcerate. It is painful or asymptomatic. Usually between lateral toes, it may involve the entire sole being sharply demarcated at the edge of the sole. Vesicular forms occur especially on the instep.

Tinea manuum. Infection of the palm of one or both hands often occurs in association with tinea pedis.

Tinea unguium. Dermatophyte infection is in the nail plate. See onychomycosis.

Tinea capitis. This involves the scalp and hair. The hair is brittle. The circular areas may become inflamed and ulcerate, leading to permanent loss of hair.

Tinea barbae. This involves the beard area of men; the hair shafts are infected. The lesions are inflammatory papules or pustular folliculitis.

Tinea corporis—ringworm. The erythematous lesions are circular or arcuate, slowly spreading with a raised scaling border and central clearing. Large plaques may form.

Tinea cruris—Jock itch. This is an often-chronic infection in the groin, proximal thighs, and pubis. The tan or reddish scaling lesion is well demarcated and may be asymptomatic.

Tinea versicolor—pityriasis versicolor. Infection with *Pityrosporum ovale* (*Malassezia furfur*) causes a very superficial mildly scaling rash, usually on the trunk or arms. Some patients have hypopigmented scaling macules and patches. Hyperpigmented scaling macules and patches occur in others. The lesions are asymptomatic but cosmetically bothersome.

Candidiasis. Skin infection is common in moist areas, especially the mouth (thrush), vagina and vulva, under pendulous breasts, and on the perineum and groin of incontinent patients. Lesions are raised, intensely erythematous, and coalesce into plaques with smaller satellite lesions. *C. albicans* is the most commonly identified species.

Sporotrichosis. This is a slowly progressive infection with *Sporothrix schenckii*, a soil fungus implanted under the skin by trauma or abrasion. An inoculation site ulcer is followed by nodular cutaneous or subcutaneous lesions that suppurate, ulcerate, and drain through multiple sinuses. Regional lymphadenopathy is expected and dissemination to viscera or bone can occur.

Deep fungal infections. Fungi most commonly associated with deep tissue infections can cause skin disease. The lesions may be papules, nodules, ulcers, or confluent masses. Travel history and places of residence are critical to hypothesizing the most likely organism. Reactivation of latent infection shortly after initiating anti-TNF therapy for rheumatic diseases is not uncommon. Biopsy and culture are required for diagnosis. Cryptococcosis, histoplasmosis, blastomycosis, aspergillosis, coccidioidomycosis are most commonly encountered.

Bullous Skin Diseases.
Hereditary epidermolysis bullosa. These are inherited disorders of epidermal cohesion resulting in blistering following minor trauma. Large superficial blisters develop and break leaving shallow erosions. Severity varies with the specific genetic defect and depth of blistering.

Pemphigus vulgaris. Acquired IgG antibodies to epidermal desmosomes leads to loss of epidermal cell adhesion. The first lesions are often in the oral mucosa, cutaneous bullae appearing later. Vesicles and flaccid bullae rupture easily leaking serous fluid. Slight skin shear causes blistering and a subsequent erosion (*Nikolsky sign*). *Paraneoplastic pemphigus* has histologic findings of pemphigus and pemphigoid.

Bullous pemphigoid. Antibodies against hemidesmosomes in the basal layer of the epidermis activate complement leading to separation of the basal layer from the dermis. The entire body can be affected but predilection for lower legs, axillae, abdomen, legs, and groin exists. Mucous membranes can be involved. Early lesions may be erythematous papules or appear urticarial. Tense bullae develop that may be serous or hemorrhagic; they rupture or heal by drying and crusting.

Dermatitis herpetiformis. This is common in celiac disease (gluten-sensitive enteropathy). The pathophysiology is uncertain. Symmetrically distributed vesicles, papules, excoriations, and/or urticaria appear on the extensor surfaces of the arms and trunk. Pruritus is severe. Symptoms may precede the skin lesions by several hours. *DDX:* Linear IgA dermatosis has a similar histopathologic appearance but is immunopathologically distinct.

Bullous diabetic dermopathy. The lesions are sterile noninflamed bullae appearing without trauma on the lateral aspects of the fingers in patients with poorly controlled diabetes. The blisters are tense and nontender.

Skin Manifestations of Systemic Diseases.

Paroxysmal flushing, blanching, and cyanosis—carcinoid syndrome. Circulating serotonin causes paroxysms of cutaneous erythema intermixed with areas of pallor and cyanosis. A given area of skin may exhibit all three colors in rapid succession. Though most pronounced on the face and neck, it may extend to the chest and abdomen.

Red burning extremities—erythromelalgia. This is an autosomal dominant or acquired syndrome associated with drugs (e.g., nifedipine, bromocriptine) or myeloproliferative diseases; it may antedate polycythemia vera or essential thrombocytosis by years. The patient complains of painful erythema on the extremities, especially the feet and hands, aggravated by dependency. Ambient temperatures above 31°C (87.8°F) usually initiate the attacks; they are relieved by cold exposure. During a paroxysm, the limbs are red, warm, swollen, and painful. The arterial pulses are present and normal. *DDX:* Similar lesions occur with atherosclerosis, hypertension, frostbite, immersion foot, trench foot, peripheral neuritis, disseminated sclerosis, hemiplegia, chronic heavy metal poisoning and gout.

Erythema multiforme. Target lesions appear on the palms and soles, feet, forearms, and face; mucous membranes may be involved. The lesions evolve over days and may be painful or pruritic. They may progress to bullae (*erythema multiforme bullosa*). **Inciting causes:** Herpes simplex, mycoplasma pneumonia drug reactions (sulfonamides, anticonvulsants, penicillin), idiopathic. *DDX:* Psoriasis, secondary syphilis, urticaria.

Panniculitis. Sterile inflammation of subcutaneous fat takes two forms: *lobular*, in which the fat lobule is primarily involved, and *septal*, in which the vascular and fibrous septa separating lobules is involved. Patients present with tender erythematous skin and subcutaneous swellings, usually over areas of abundant subcutaneous fat. The epidermis is intact, and the lesions are not fluctuant. *DDX:* Angioedema is similar, but lesions are transient and not restricted to adipose tissue. Pyomyositis looks similar but lesions are within muscle rather than fat.

CLINICAL OCCURRENCE: *Septal Panniculitis:* Erythema nodosum, eosinophilic fasciitis, eosinophilia myalgia syndrome, scleroderma (localized and diffuse), polyarteritis nodosa; *Lobular Panniculitis:* Trauma, cold injury, steroid induced, idiopathic lobular panniculitis, acinar pancreatic carcinoma, SLE, sarcoidosis, vasculitis.

Erythema nodosum. *EN is a localized panniculitis.* Tender subcutaneous nodules appear on the anterior shins. They are violaceous and slightly warm.

CLINICAL OCCURRENCE: *Infections:* Mycobacteria (tuberculosis, leprosy), bacteria (cat-scratch disease, leptospirosis, tularemia, salmonellosis, yersiniosis), deep fungal infections, viruses (Epstein–Barr virus, lymphogranuloma venereum, hepatitis B); *Noninfectious:* Pregnancy, drug reactions, inflammatory bowel disease, sarcoidosis, paraneoplastic, Sweet syndrome, Behçet syndrome.

Adiposis dolorosa (Dercum disease). In this rare form of obesity, symmetrical adipose tissue masses on the trunk and limbs are painful and tender. If inflammation is present, consider panniculitis [Campen RB, Sang CN, Duncan LM. Case 25–2006: a 41-year-old woman with painful subcutaneous nodules. *N Engl J Med.* 2006;355:714–722].

Serum sickness. See Serum sickness, Chapter 8, page 363.

Scleroderma. The skin and underlying tissues become fibrotic and contracted limiting movement of fingers without joint swelling or ankylosis. The distribution and the pattern of organ involvement identifies each syndrome.

CLINICAL OCCURRENCE: Diffuse cutaneous scleroderma, limited cutaneous scleroderma (CREST syndrome), morphea, toxic oil syndrome, arthralgia–myalgia syndrome, graft-vs-host disease, polyvinyl chloride exposure.

Diffuse cutaneous scleroderma. Tight shiny skin on the distal extremities and face progresses to involve the proximal extremities and, to a lesser extent, the trunk. Raynaud phenomena is common. Cutaneous sclerosis leads to joint immobility, limited mouth opening, and poorly healing ulcers following trauma. Dysphagia, hypertension, acute renal failure, and, less commonly, pulmonary fibrosis complicates the course.

Limited cutaneous scleroderma. The skin lesions are less extensive and favor the trunk. Severe pulmonary involvement with refractory pulmonary hypertension and respiratory failure are common, but kidney disease is less common. *(CREST syndrome.* CREST stands for the first letters of its cardinal features: Calcinosis cutis, Raynaud phenomenon, Esophageal dysfunction, Sclerodactyly, and Telangiectasia.)

Morphea. Localized erythema and induration that can occur anywhere on the body and become sclerotic plaques. They may be linear on the extremities. Women are more affected than men. Visceral sclerosis does not occur. This can be confused with *lipodermatosclerosis* from chronic stasis dermatitis.

Nephrogenic systemic fibrosis (nephrogenic fibrosing dermopathy). Exposure to gadolinium contrast for MRI imaging in the setting of chronic kidney disease is the cause. Patients on dialysis for end-stage renal disease develop diffuse cutaneous and subcutaneous fibrosis most prominent on the legs. Systemic involvement is common with fibrosis of muscles, including the myocardium, and lung. The course is progressive with loss of joint mobility. The face is spared.

Scleromyxedema. Usually associated with a monoclonal gammopathy, the skin is thickened, indurated, tight, and thrown into prominent folds. There is decreased mouth and joint mobility.

Dermatomyositis. There is atrophy, edema, or fibrosis of the skin and non-suppurative inflammation of skin and striated muscle; the cause is unknown. Malaise, weight loss, muscle stiffness, and dysphagia are presenting symptoms; pruritus is especially characteristic. Classic signs are heliotrope discoloration of upper lids and nasal bridge and flat-topped violaceous papules (*Gottron papules*) over the dorsal interphalangeal joints. Erythematous rashes or exfoliative dermatitis may be seen. Proximal muscle weakness and stiffness indicate muscle involvement. Tendon friction rubs, lymphadenopathy, and splenomegaly may be found. Dermatomyositis can be a paraneoplastic syndrome. *Amyopathic dermatomyositis* presents with skin signs and symptoms without proximal muscle weakness.

Lupus erythematosus. This group of inflammatory disorders share similar autoimmune pathophysiology.

Acute cutaneous lupus. Several lesions occur: an acute malar or generalized rash, precipitated by sunlight exposure; erythematous scaling papules and plaques on the extensor surface of the fingers sparing the interphalangeal joints; urticaria with purpura; and, hypersensitivity vasculitis.

Subacute cutaneous lupus. The skin lesions are psoriasiform plaques or annular erythematous lesions on the trunk, shoulders, extensor surfaces of the arms, or other sun-exposed areas. Systemic involvement is uncommon.

Chronic cutaneous lupus—discoid lupus. Sharply defined plaques with adherent scale gradually expand in circles or ovals with central atrophy. The lesions may occur on the face, scalp, forearms, and phalanges. The trunk is less commonly involved. Follicular plugging is characteristic. *DDX:* Psoriasis, lichen planus, confluent actinic keratoses, and polymorphic light eruptions may be confused.

Systemic lupus erythematosus. See Chapter 13, page 586. This systemic disease has prominent, life-threatening involvement of other organs, including the brain and kidneys. The skin findings are those of acute cutaneous lupus, subacute cutaneous lupus, and chronic cutaneous lupus, among other nonspecific skin manfestations (urticaria, vasculitis)

Pyoderma gangrenosum. Painful skin nodules progressing to necrotic ulcers with undermined, violaceous edges most commonly on the legs, buttocks, and abdomen; the face may be involved. The wound base does not granulate, the ulcers healing with thin scars. *DDX:* Ecthyma gangrenosum, necrotic soft-tissue infections, granulomatous angiitis, stasis ulcers.

CLINICAL OCCURRENCE: Most often idiopathic; when an association is identified, inflammatory bowel disease (ulcerative colitis, Crohn disease) is most common. Other associations are paraproteinemia (myeloma, monoclonal gammopathy of unknown significance [MGUS]), leukemia, rheumatologic diseases, and chronic active hepatitis.

Sweet syndrome. This is a sterile neutrophilic dermatosis. Painful papules and nodules most commonly on the arms and face rapidly coalesce forming large plaques infiltrated with neutrophils. Lesions heal with minimal scarring. It may be chronic and recurrent.

CLINICAL OCCURRENCE: Hematologic malignancies, myelodysplasia, MGUS, Granulocyte-macrophage colony-stimulating factor (GMCSF) administration, *Yersinia* infections, idiopathic.

Porphyrias. Inherited or acquired enzyme defects in the metabolism of aminolevulinic acid to heme result in tissue accumulation of specific porphyrins. Photosensitivity is the hallmark of cutaneous porphyrias. Severe mutilating photosensitivity and hypertrichosis occur in *hereditary erythropoietic protoporphyria. Porphyria cutanea tarda* is acquired or inherited. The acquired form is associated with liver disease (cirrhosis, hepatitis-C, hemochromatosis) and chemical exposures. It presents as burning erythematous vesicles or blisters on sun-exposed areas, often the backs of the hands or wrists, which heal with atrophic hypopigmented scars. *Variegate porphyria* is inherited. The skin signs are like porphyria cutanea tarda, but systemic disease is resembles acute intermittent porphyria. *Acute intermittent porphyria* presents with abdominal pain, neuropathy, and altered mental status without skin lesions.

Paraneoplastic skin disease. Several skin diseases are seen in association with known or occult malignant neoplasms. Consider an underlying cancer in association with the following conditions: neutrophilic dermatosis (Sweet syndrome, pyoderma gangrenosum); reactive erythemas (erythroderma, exfoliative dermatitis); vascular dermatoses (vasculitis, erythromelalgia); papulosquamous disorders (ichthyosis); and vesiculobullous diseases (pemphigus, pemphigoid).

Sarcoidosis. Granulomatous skin lesions present as purple or brown asymptomatic papules or plaques on the torso and extremities; nodules may be more common on the face and eyelids. They do not completely blanch with pressure. See Chapter 8, page 346.

Diabetes. Diabetes is associated with a variety of skin lesions. *Necrobiosis lipoidica* is most often seen in diabetics. It begins as a brownish-red papule on the shin that enlarges to a plaque, which spreads with a raised rolled border surrounding a depressed atrophic center commonly with a yellowish coloration. Lesions may be single or multiple and merge by expansion. Diabetic hand syndrome (*diabetic cheiropathy*) is thickening of subcutaneous tissue in the palm and fingers limiting finger extension, demonstrated by the *prayer sign. Diabetic dermopathy* is a chronic condition with crops of erythematous papules appearing on the shins and forearms that heal with atrophic scars. *Diabetic bullous dermopathy* presents with painless bland bullae often on the sides of the fingers; it is associated with poor diabetes control. *Mucocutaneous candidiasis* is much more common in diabetics with poor blood sugar control.

Calciphylaxis. It is believed to be an ischemic injury resulting from calcium deposition in the small arterioles of patients with advanced renal insufficiency and secondary hyperparathyroidism with abnormal calcium-phosphate metabolism. This uncommon disorder presents with painful indurated plaques with vascular mottling or retiform purpura which progress to infarction and ulceration. The lesions gradually enlarge circumferentially. It has high morbidity and mortality.

Pseudoxanthoma elasticum. *This is an inherited disorder of elastic tissue.* There is poor elastic tissue in skin, eye, cardiovascular system, and GI tract. Small, soft, yellow-orange cutaneous papules run parallel to the natural skin folds of the neck, axillae, groin, and abdomen. Angioid streaks are seen in retina. The skin bruises easily. Disintegration of arteries in the GI tract causes hemorrhage.

Tuberous sclerosis. This is an autosomal dominant disorder of ectodermal and mesodermal tissues with hamartoma formation in the skin, brain, and kidneys. The skin signs are hypopigmented spots that may be multiple and small or larger elongated macules, *ash-leaf spots*. Pink, fleshy nodules up to 5 mm in size appear on the central face. Similar lesions are common around the nails. Plaques on the back or buttock, *Shagreen patches,* represent connective tissue nevi.

Neurofibromatosis (NF). Two forms, NF-1 and NF-2, are inherited as autosomal dominant disorders affecting the skin, bones, nervous system, and endocrine organs. *Café au lait* (coffee with milk) spots occur in childhood as uniform pigmented macules from a few millimeters to several centimeters in size. *Neurofibromas* are brown, rounded, raised, often pedunculated, masses that can be reduced below the skin surface with finger pressure (*button-hole sign*). *Plexiform neuromas* are larger, soft, sagging, subcutaneous protrusions from the skin surface; they may become huge. The lesions are often innumerable and particularly common in the axilla.

Vascular Disorders.
Raynaud disease and phenomenon. See Chapter 8, page 375 for a complete discussion.

Warfarin skin necrosis—deficiency of proteins C and S. With congenital protein-C or protein-S deficiency exposure to warfarin leads to intravascular coagulation and skin necrosis. One or two days after starting warfarin, painful indurated lesions appear which progress to necrosis. Areas of adipose tissue are primarily involved, e.g., breast, abdomen, buttocks, and thighs.

- **Meningococcemia.** Patients with meningococcal meningitis and meningococcemia develop petechial hemorrhages, bright-pink tender maculopapules 2–10 mm in diameter involving the trunk and extremities, some developing hemorrhagic centers. Large ecchymoses and hemorrhagic vesicles may form. Gangrene, especially fingers and toes, may occur. Livedo reticularis may be present.

- **Disseminated intravascular coagulation (DIC, consumption coagulopathy).** Platelet-fibrin thrombi form in multiple vessels consuming platelets and clotting factors and activating fibrinolysis leading to hemorrhage. Usually complicating preexisting multisystem disease, onset is characterized by shock, purpura with ecchymoses and petechiae, fever, and bleeding from multiple sites.

CLINICAL OCCURRENCE: Septicemia, malignancy (especially acute promyelocytic leukemia, some adenocarcinomas and sarcomas), surgery, trauma, complications of pregnancy (dead fetus, amniotic fluid embolism, abruptio placenta, septic abortion, preeclampsia, and eclampsia), envenomation, and liver failure.

Thrombotic Thrombocytopenic Purpura (TTP) and Hemolytic Uremic Syndrome (HUS). In TTP inhibition of ADAMTS-13, a metalloproteinase enzyme that cleaves von Willebrand factor (VWF), allows circulation of large VWF multimers. Platelet-rich arteriolar thrombi fragment erythrocytes and cause ischemic infarcts in vital organs. The mechanism of HUS is not understood. Most patients with TTP are young adults, more often women, with a history of recent viral infection. Other risk factors are pregnancy, bee sting, AIDS, SLE, mitomycin C, and recent organ transplantation. Petechiae are a key sign. The classic TTP pentad is: (1) thrombocytopenia, (2) microangiopathic hemolytic anemia, (3) renal insufficiency, (4) nonfocal neurologic deficits, and (5) fever. Headache, confusion, delirium, seizures, and other mental status changes develop in 90% of fatal cases. Rapid diagnosis and treatment are necessary. Finding schistocytes on a peripheral blood smear rapidly establishes the diagnosis. Mortality is >90% without treatment. Relapses of TTP following successful treatment are common. HUS in children produces the same arteriolar lesions and laboratory findings without CNS involvement. HUS occurs sporadically and in epidemics associated with *Escherichia coli* 0157:H7 gastroenteritis.

Immune thrombocytopenic purpura (ITP). Immune-mediated platelet destruction leads to thrombocytopenia, large circulating platelets, and megakaryocyte hyperplasia. Easy bruising, petechiae, menorrhagia, epistaxis, or other mucocutaneous bleeding signals ITP onset. The spleen is not palpable. Children with acute ITP frequently recover without treatment. Adults with very low platelet counts are at risk for intracranial hemorrhage and are more likely to develop chronic thrombocytopenia. *DDX:* The history, physical exam, and selected tests should exclude SLE, HIV infection, cytomegalovirus, Epstein–Barr virus, drug-induced thrombocytopenia, hypersplenism, malignant lymphoma, and other disorders.

Purpura, abdominal pain and arthralgia—Schönlein–Henoch purpura (anaphylactoid purpura). See Chapter 8, page 364.

Scurvy. Punctate cutaneous perifollicular hemorrhages occur most commonly on the legs. Petechiae surround hair follicles containing tightly coiled *corkscrew* hairs. Mucous membrane bleeding and loose teeth are characteristic.

Rickettsial spotted fever syndromes. See Chapter 4, page 49.

Schamberg disease—pigmented purpuric dermatosis. A benign chronic disorder with repeated crops of petechiae and orange to fawn-colored macules on feet and legs.

Atheroembolism (cholesterol emboli). Rupture of an atherosclerotic plaque embolizes its cholesterol-rich contents producing ischemic infarction with hemorrhage in downstream skin and organs. Embolization frequently follows endovascular procedures that mechanically disrupt vessel wall plaque. Hours to 1–2 days postprocedure, pain and erythema are followed by retiform ecchymoses and purpura, which can progress to frank infarction. The lesions, which may be palpable, range from 1 mm to 2 cm in size; toes and fingertips may become necrotic (Fig. 6-25). Livedo reticularis is common. This most commonly follows passage of intravascular catheters during diagnostic or therapeutic procedures, or initiation of warfarin.

Palpable purpura—vasculitis. See Chapter 8, page 360.

Hereditary hemorrhagic telangiectasia (HHT, Osler–Weber–Rendu disease). HHT is a Mendelian dominant trait with extensive arteriovenous malformations (AVM) developing in all organs. AVMs vary from small to quite large. The skin is spotted with dull red lesions (telangiectasias), most developing after puberty. Epistaxis is frequent before appearance of diagnostic skin and mucous membrane lesions. The usual lesion is punctate, 1–2 mm in diameter, usually not elevated, some appearing slightly depressed. Diascopy pressure causes fading and the spots may pulsate. One or two fine superficial vessels may radiate from the punctum. The mucosa is practically always involved, especially the tip and dorsal tongue. Anterior nasal septal lesions cause frequent epistaxis. The most frequent sites of skin involvement are palms and fingers, nail beds, lips, ears, face, arms, and toes. The trunk is least involved. Spontaneous epistaxis, hemoptysis, hematemesis, melena, or hematuria are seen. Pulmonary AVMs are common leading to polycythemia and clubbing. Hepatic AVMs manifest as a RUQ abdominal bruit. Anemia and iron deficiency

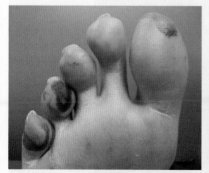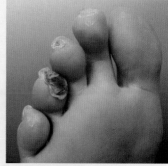

FIG. 6-25 Atheroemboli (Blue Toes Syndrome). *Left:* Multiple sharply demarcated hemorrhagic blisters with surrounding erythema and edema. The foot is intensely painful. *Right:* The same foot six weeks later.

are common due to constant gastrointestinal blood loss. *DDX:* Arterial spiders have more numerous radicles, smaller centers, and are less widely distributed.

Skin Neoplasms: A high index of suspicion is required to diagnose early-stage skin cancers. They are often noticed at a visit for another problem. Periodic complete skin exam should be performed on all patients.

Lipomas. Benign tumors of mature adipose tissue arise in any adipose tissue. They are multiple and appear to be hereditary. Lipomas are common mostly on the trunk and proximal extremities. They can be tender on first appearance and if traumatized. They are smooth or lobular, soft, and not attached to the epidermis so mobile within the subcutaneous tissue. Most are 1–3 cm in size but can be very large causing functional and cosmetic problems. Larger size increases risk of liposarcoma. Multiple lipomas are associated with several rare diseases: Cowden disease, Proteus syndrome, MEN type-1, and NF-1. *DDX:* Epidermal inclusion cysts are attached to the epidermis.

Cutaneous nevi—moles. Nevi are benign proliferations of melanocytes within the epidermis or at the dermal-epidermal junction; genetics determines the number and type of moles. Moles may be congenital, but more commonly they begin appearing during puberty and adolescence. Congenital *hairy nevi* are large pigmented plaques with prominent hairs. *Junctional nevi* are brown to black macules a few millimeters in diameter. *Dermal nevi* are skin colored to reddish domed papules or nodules <1 cm in size. *Compound nevi* have features of both junctional and dermal nevi (Fig. 6-26). *Halo nevi*

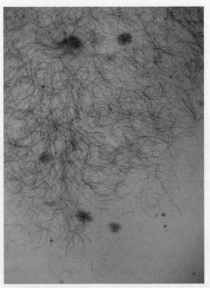

FIG. 6-26 Cutaneous Nevi (Moles). Several benign nevi on the chest with different patterns of pigmentation.

are surrounded by a depigmented halo; they may undergo complete regression. *Blue nevi* are dark blue to deep purple to almost black macules and papules; the blue color results from the Tindel effect in being deep in the dermis. *Atypical moles* have unusual features (asymmetry, irregular border, mixed colors, >6 mm in diameter) raising suspicion for melanoma. Abnormal histologic features on biopsy makes them *dysplastic nevi*. Serial photos are the best way to follow multiple moles; dermatology referral is advised.

Malignant melanoma. Malignant melanocyte proliferation, initially within the epidermis, invades the reticular and papillary dermis. Prognosis is inversely related to depth of invasion. Melanomas are usually pigmented but amelanotic melanoma can occur. The lesions are macules or papules that can become nodules which may ulcerate in advanced disease. Melanoma may arise from preexisting nevi or appear on otherwise normal skin. Risk factors include a personal or family history of malignant melanoma, blond or red hair, marked freckling on the upper back, and three or more blistering sunburns before the age of 20 years. The American Cancer Society uses the mnemonic ABCDE to help distinguish between melanoma and benign moles. Melanomas have *A*symmetry, *B*order irregularity, *C*olor variegation, a *D*iameter >6 mm, and *E*volution of the lesion. Ask about changes in color, shape, elevation, texture, surrounding skin, sensation, and consistency. Any suspicious lesion should be referred to a dermatologist. *Never do a partial shave biopsy for possible melanoma; a full thickness biopsy is required for staging.*

Basal cell carcinoma. This most common skin cancer arises on sun-exposed skin, usually on the face or upper back, without a precursor lesion. The lesions are pearly papules, often with surface telangiectasias. They slowly enlarge and may ulcerate. They can have considerable local extension and tissue destruction, but do not metastasize. *Superficial basal cell cancers* are often shiny pink patches or thin plaques with telangiectasias and a slightly rolled border. Uncommonly basal cell cancer presents as areas of sclerosing skin atrophy, termed *morpheaform basal cell carcinomas*. When advanced, they are erosive with elevated borders.

Actinic keratosis. Abnormal keratinocytes arising in sun-damaged skin can transform into squamous cell carcinoma. Actinic keratoses start as erythematous macules or patches typically with sharp adherent scale. They are asymptomatic or associated with tingling or burning.

Squamous cell carcinoma. These cancers arise in sun-damaged skin from preexisting actinic keratoses or in the genital region from human papilloma virus infection. When limited to the epidermis (*squamous cell carcinoma in situ, Bowen disease*) they present as sharply demarcated plaques with slight scaling up to several centimeters in diameter. Invasive squamous cell carcinoma presents as ulcerated indurated skin (common on the lip) or as an eroded exophytic growth. They invade the dermis metastasizing to regional lymph nodes.

Keratoacanthoma. Often considered subtype of squamous cell cancer, it is a solitary lesion growing rapidly to become an exophytic nodule with a central keratin plug. Some spontaneously regress over weeks to months.

Kaposi sarcoma. Human herpes virus type-8 infection is the cause. *Endemic disease* in the Mediterranean and Africa can present with thickened scaling skin, enlargement of the extremity, and ulceration. HIV infection greatly increases the risk of developing KS in a pattern distinct from endemic disease. *HIV-associated Kaposi sarcoma* frequently involves the skin, mucous membranes (hard palate) and viscera (lungs and gut). The initial lesions are nonblanching, red-blue or bluish-brown papules, plaques, and nodules anywhere on the skin. Some lesions become spongy or compressible tumors moving centripetally from the extremities. Lymphadenopathy and lymphedema are late findings. Iatrogenic immunosuppression in the setting of solid organ transplant also can be a risk factor for the development of Kaposi sarcoma.

Cutaneous T-cell lymphoma—mycosis fungoides, Sézary syndrome. These are proliferations of malignant T-cells within the dermis and epidermis. *Mycosis fungoides* lesions are indurated, often scaly and atrophic patches and plaques reaching several centimeters in size. They are brown or pink and may appear eczematous. The papules and plaques progress to nodules or large masses, the tumor stage of disease. The disease is limited to the skin and may be confused with eczema and psoriasis. *Sézary syndrome* is a systemic disease with leukocytosis, lymphadenopathy, and skin infiltration producing erythematous indurated thickening of the dermis prominently of the face and brows (*leonine facies*).

Metastatic cancer. The skin is the site of metastases from carcinomas or lymphomas. Breast, lung, and colon cancers, B-cell lymphomas, and metastatic melanomas are particularly common in the skin. Any suspicious cutaneous nodule or plaque should be biopsied.

CLINICAL VIGNETTES AND QUESTIONS

Case 6-1

A 54-year-old man presents with generalized erythroderma.

QUESTIONS:
1. What is the pathophysiology of generalized erythroderma?
2. What is the differential diagnosis of an adult with generalized erythroderma?
3. What is erythema multiforme?
4. What are common causes of erythema multiforme?

Case 6-2

A 70-year-old man presents with tense bullae on his arms.

QUESTIONS:
1. What is the most likely diagnosis?
2. What condition may be confused with the correct diagnosis?
3. What is a Nikolsky sign?

Case 6-3

A 33-year-old patient comes in with recurrent painful vesicles on the lips. Each is umbilicated on an erythematous base.

QUESTIONS:
1. What is the most likely diagnosis?
2. What is the differential diagnosis for vesicular skin lesions?

Case 6-4

You just finished examining a 60-year-old man with history of chronic kidney disease stage 4 and severe hypoalbuminemia (secondary to nephrotic syndrome from his recent diagnosis of multiple myeloma). As you are walking out of the patients room you realize that you forgot to examine his nails. You go back to the patients room to examine his nails as they can give you some important clues regarding his condition.

QUESTION:
1. Describe Terry nails, Lindsay's nails, Beau's lines, Muehrcke's lines, and Mees' lines and the significance of each.

Case 6-5

You are examining a 50-year-old man with a 70-pack-year smoking history and Chronic obstructive Pulmonary disease (COPD). You notice that he has clubbing. On further questioning he states that he has lost 10 pounds in the last 3 months.

QUESTIONS:
1. What condition should you be most concerned about in this patient?
2. What is the differential diagnosis of new onset clubbing in adults?

Case 6-6

QUESTIONS:
1. What is the differential diagnosis of one or more cutaneous ulcers associated with regional lymphadenopathy (the ulceroglandular syndrome)?
2. What is the most essential investigation to narrow this broad differential?
3. Describe the clinical findings for syphilis, tularemia, and anthrax.

Case 6-7

A 76-year-old man presents with a skin lesion on his face. You find a 2-cm flat indurated pink plaque with a rolled border.

QUESTIONS:
1. What is the most likely diagnosis?
2. Describe the key features of nonmelanoma skin cancers?

Case 6-8

While examining a 46-year-old man suspected of having infective endocarditis, you remember that subacute bacterial endocarditis (SBE) can be associated with Janeway lesions and Osler nodes.

QUESTIONS:
1. What are Olser nodes? Describe the pathophysiology.
2. What are Janeway lesions? Describe the pathophysiology.

CHAPTER 7

The Head and Neck

This chapter discusses symptoms, signs, and syndromes related to the head and neck; *trauma is not covered*. At least nine specialties focus on the head and neck, each developing detailed exams often utilizing specialized instruments. The exams described here are made with resources available to the general clinician. Symptoms, signs, and syndromes primarily of neurologic significance are discussed in Chapter 14. By necessity, these distinctions are somewhat arbitrary. During the head and neck examination the examiner identifies significant abnormalities and identifies signs of systemic disease. As always, knowing the limits of one's expertize and the indications for specialty referral are imperative.

MAJOR SYSTEMS OF THE HEAD AND NECK

The skull, facial bones, and scalp provide *protection and insulation* for deeper organs. The scalp and face have a rich vasculature that vasodilates on cold exposure to maintain normal temperature within vital organs. The head contains the *organs of special sense*: the eyes, ears, olfactory nerve, and taste buds. Special senses are impaired by problems in the sensory organs, cranial nerves, or brain. The tongue, pharynx, and larynx are *organs of speech* so structural or functional problems alter articulation. The nose, mouth, pharynx, larynx, and trachea form *the upper airways*. Compromised upper airways affect breathing and voice tone and/or volume. The mouth, teeth, mandible, maxilla, tongue, salivary glands, pharynx, and upper esophagus are the *upper alimentary tract* necessary for mastication and swallowing. Together the upper airways and digestive tract are the *upper aerodigestive tract*. The head and neck are highly vascular. The external carotid has rich anastomoses supplying superficial structures so ischemia is unusual. The internal carotid and vertebral arteries supply blood to the brain. The head and neck *lymphatic network* drains to regional lymph node beds. The tonsils and adenoids are lymphatic organs surrounding the upper aerodigestive tract. The neck contains the thyroid and parathyroid glands, major structures of the *endocrine system*.

FUNCTIONAL ANATOMY OF THE HEAD AND NECK

The Scalp and Skull. The scalp has five layers: the skin, subcutaneous connective tissue, epicranius, a subfascial cleft with loose connective tissue, and the pericranium (Fig. 7-1). The outer three are a single thick, tough, and vascular layer, whose strength is supplied by the epicranius. The *epicranius* is formed by the *frontalis muscle* attaching to the occiput by a large central aponeurosis, the *galea aponeurotica*. The skin and subcutaneous tissue are tightly bound to the galea by fibrous bands that sharply limit the spread of blood or pus. The

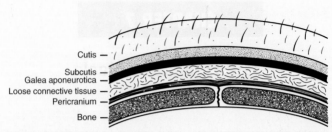

FIG. 7-1 Layers of the Scalp. For practical purposes, the cutis, subcutis, and galea aponeurotica constitute a single, thick, tough layer with fibrous bands compartmentalizing the more superficial tissue and binding it to the galea. Between the galea and the pericranium is a potential space with a little areolar tissue. Fluid and infection spread slowly through the compartments above the galea but spread easily through the space beneath the galea and its attached muscles (the epicranium). The pericranium is the periosteal layer that covers the bones of the skull and dips inward at the suture lines. Subperiosteal fluid is limited to the area over a single bone.

pericranium, the periosteum of the skull, dips into the sutures limiting spread of subperiosteal blood or pus to the surface of a single bone. The subfascial cleft between the pericranium and galea allows the scalp to be lifted off the skull with minimal effort, allowing blood or pus to spreads widely beneath it. A useful mnemonic is SCALP: Skin, Connective tissue, Aponeurosis, Loose connective tissue, Periosteum.

The scalp has three *lymphatic drainage* areas. The forehead and anterior parietal region drain to *preauricular lymph nodes*. The mid-parietal region drains first to postauricular nodes and then to nodes in the *posterior cervical triangle*. The occipital area drains first into nodes at the origin of the trapezius and then into the *posterior cervical triangle*.

The Face and Neck: Facial contour is determined by the *frontal bone* (forming the forehead and the brows), the *maxilla* and *zygomatic arch* (forming the cheeks and inferior orbital rim), the bony and cartilaginous nose, external ears, and mandible. The *mandibles* articulate with the *temporal bone* anterior to the acoustic canal. Each ramus drops inferiorly to the angle of the jaw where the mandible turns anteriorly and medially, the two halves meet in the midline forming the chin. The upper and lower teeth contribute to the vertical facial proportions. The bony superstructure is overlaid with muscles and soft tissues, including the lips, giving the face its rounded contours. Mild facial asymmetry is common. The anterior neck is dominated by the thyroid cartilage, which is more prominent in men (the Adam's apple), the cervical trachea, and the two sternocleidomastoid muscles arising on the mastoid process and inserting on the clavicle and manubrium. The posterior neck is enveloped in thick longitudinal muscles covering the cervical spine from the occiput to the upper back, and the fan-shaped trapezius forming the neck's posterior lateral contour.

The Ear: The pinna, or auricle, and the external acoustic canal compose the *external ear; the middle ear* consists of the tympanic membrane (TM) and tympanic cavity with its three ossicles. The *internal ear*, or bony labyrinth, is composed of the cochlea (the organ of hearing) and semicircular canals (the organ for balance).

External ear. The *pinna or auricle* is a flattened funnel with crinkled walls of yellow fibroelastic cartilage. It has a wide external brim narrowing internally to the *external acoustic meatus*. Several prominent folds have considerable individual variation (Fig. 7-2A). The *helix* originates as the *crus* coursing anteriorly and then winding up, back, and down posteriorly forming the funnel's brim. Above the midpoint of its posterior vertical portion, a fusiform swelling occasionally develops, the *Darwinian tubercle*. An inner concentric fold, the *antihelix*, partially surrounding an ovoid cavity, the *concha*, is divided into an upper and lower portion by the transverse *helical crus*. From the anterior brim of the funnel, below the crus a small eminence, the *tragus,* points back toward the lower concha. From the lower portion of the antihelix, another eminence, the *antitragus,* points forward to the tragus across the *intertragal notch*. The deep lower concha forms the *external acoustic meatus*. At the junction of the inferior limbs of the helix and antihelix is a pendant lobule of adipose and areolar tissue without cartilage, the *earlobe*.

The external acoustic meatus or canal is ~2.5 cm long, extending from the concha to the TM (Fig. 7-2B). The canal's lateral third is walled by cartilage, the medial two-thirds runs through the temporal bone. From the concha, the canal forms a gentle S, tending inward, forward, and upward. Approximately 20 mm inside is a bony constriction, the *isthmus*. Ear wax produced in the cartilaginous canal acidifies and protects the epithelium by suppressing bacterial growth and capturing particles. The wax is moved to the concha by the outward migration of the canal's epithelium.

Middle ear. The acoustic canal widens within the temporal bone's petrous portion forming the tympanic cavity. Separating the *tympanic cavity* from the external canal is the *TM*, an ovoid biconcave disk slanting across the canal in a plane 35 degrees from vertical, its posterior superior portion is more superficial than the anterior inferior attachment (Fig. 7-2B). The *manubrium of the malleus* is firmly attached to the inner TM. Viewed from outside, the attached

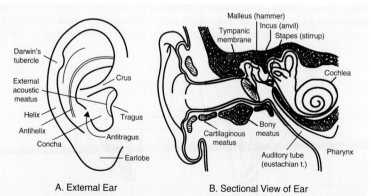

A. External Ear   B. Sectional View of Ear

FIG. 7-2 Pinna and Middle Ear Anatomy. A. Surface of pinna: The main features are depicted, but there are many individual variations. Darwin tubercle is only occasionally present. **B. Middle ear:** A vertical section through the ear. Note the flexible cartilaginous and fixed bony segment of the external acoustic meatus. The plane of the TM slants outward ~35 degrees from vertical; the conical apex points inward and upward.

portion appears as a smooth ridge forming a radius of the membrane, slant-ing upward and slightly anterior.

Inner ear. The inner ear, or *labyrinth*, is within the temporal bone adjacent to the middle ear. It consists of the spiral *cochlea* (the organ of hearing), the *semi-circular canals, ampullae, utricle,* and *saccule* (organs of balance and position sense of the head), and the acoustic nerve endings of CN-VIII. Two windows connect the middle and inner ear: the *oval window* contains the footplate of the stapes communicating mechanical vibrations to the inner ear via the *scala vestibuli*; the *round window* covers the origin of the *scala tympani*.

The Eyes: The structural and functional anatomy of the eyes is complex, but a basic understanding facilitates interpretation of visual signs.

Orbits. The bony *orbits* are quadrilateral pyramids with bases facing anteriorly and apices pointing backward and medially. Their medial sides are parallel, whereas the lateral walls form a 90-degree angle (Fig. 7-3). Seven bones form each orbit. The frontal bone and lesser sphenoid wing form the orbital roof. Portions of the ethmoid, maxillary, lacrimal, and sphenoid bones form the medial wall containing the lacrimal groove for the lacrimal sac anteriorly. The zygomatic bone and greater sphenoid wing form the lateral wall. The orbital floor contains the maxillary, palatine, and zygomatic bones. Several *foramens* open into the orbit. At the posterior apex within the lesser sphenoid wing is the *optic foramen* leading into the optic canal containing the optic nerve (CN-II), ophthalmic artery, and sympathetic nerves. The *superior orbital fissure* between the sphenoid wings separates the roof from the lateral wall. It carries orbital branches of the middle meningeal artery, the superior ophthalmic vein, and four cranial nerves: the oculomotor (CN-III), the trochlear (CN-IV), the first (ophthalmic) division of the trigeminal (CN-V-1), and the abducens (CN-VI).

Eyelids. The *palpebral fissure* is the space between the opened lids. The two angles where the lids meet are the *lateral* (temporal) and *medial* (nasal) *canthi*. The *caruncle*, a small protuberance of modified skin, lies in the medial canthus anterior to a tissue fold, the *plica semilunaris*. On each lid's nasal margin is a *punctum* opening into the superior or inferior canaliculi which meet to form

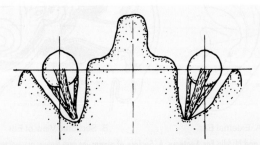

FIG. 7-3 Relationship of the Orbits and Globes. A horizontal section through the orbits. The medial orbital walls are parallel. When the globes are in the primary position, the parallel optic axes are parallel with the medial orbital walls. Because the orbital apices and origins of the ocular muscles are medial to the optic axes in the primary position, the lateral rectus muscles are longer than the medial and the superior and inferior recti pull medially.

the common canaliculus draining into the lacrimal sac. The *upper lid* extends to the superior rim of the bony orbit merging there with the periosteum. The skin covering the lids is the body's thinnest skin and is readily moved and picked up. During elevation the upper eyelid invaginates between the globe and upper orbital border. The shorter lower lid extends inferiorly from the lid margin to merge with the periosteum of the inferior orbital rim. It does not infold. The lids' tight orbital rim attachments limit fluid movement into or out of the orbit. The lids contain circular fibers of the *orbicularis oculi muscle* innervated by the facial nerve (CN-VII). The upper lid also contains vertical tendons of the *levator palpebrae superioris* muscle, which originates in the optic foramen and inserts into the tarsal plate. The levator palpebrae is innervated by the oculomotor nerve (CN-III). In the upper lid posterior to the levator is *Müller muscle* innervated from the cervical sympathetic chain. The lids are stiffened by dense transverse connective tissue plaques, the *tarsal* plates, which adhere posteriorly to the palpebral conjunctiva. The lids contain *meibomian glands* emptying through pinpoint openings in the lid margins. On the lid margins where the conjunctiva and skin meet is a double row of deeply pigmented *eyelashes* curving outward. Deep to the temporal side of the upper lid, beneath the frontal bone, lies the tear-producing *lacrimal gland*. Numerous *accessory lacrimal glands* within the conjunctiva provide baseline tear production. The *epicanthal fold* is a vertical semicircular skin fold over the nasal lids that partially covers the medial canthus. It is present in ~20% of white newborns but disappears in 97% by the age of 10 years. The epicanthus must be distinguished from the horizontal skin fold in Asian patients that originates in the upper lid and variably overhangs the superior lid (Fig. 7-4).

Conjunctiva. The *palpebral conjunctiva* follows the inner lid from the lid margin into the *superior* and *inferior* fornices. In the fornices the conjunctiva reflects covering the sclera as the *bulbar conjunctiva*. The conjunctiva is firmly attached to the tarsal plates but is quite loose in the fornices permitting globe movement. The larger peripheral *episcleral vessels* are visible through the bulbar conjunctiva and slide over the sclera with the conjunctiva. The conjunctiva attaches firmly to the sclera at the corneal limbus. Arising from limbal stem cells the corneal epithelium differs from the conjunctiva. The superficial vessels of the bulbar conjunctiva are radial and tortuous (Fig. 7-33A). The deeper vessels radiate near the limbus and are not normally visible. On either

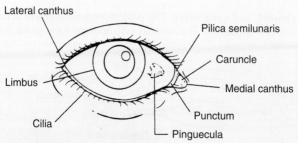

FIG. 7-4 **External Landmarks of the Normal Right Eye.**

side of the limbus is commonly found a raised horizontal yellow plaque, the *pinguecula*, caused by sun damage to conjunctival elastic tissue.

Cornea. The clear convex *cornea* has five transparent avascular layers through which the anterior chamber, iris, pupil, and lens are inspected. The cornea joins the sclera at the *limbus*. The *anterior chamber* between the endothelial surface of the cornea and the iris fills with aqueous fluid produced by the *ciliary body*. The fluid drains peripherally through the *anterior chamber angle* at the circumferential junction of the iris and cornea. The cornea and anterior eye are best examined by slit lamp which allows visualization of individual cell layers.

Sclera. Beneath the bulbar conjunctiva the globe is covered by a tough, dense, avascular fibrous coat, the *sclera*. It is china-white except for brown melanin spots varying in number with complexion and race. Piercing the sclera is the *scleral foramen* for the optic nerve, *long ciliary arteries* and *nerves*, *short ciliary nerves*, and venae vorticosae. The ocular muscle tendons insert into the sclera.

Iris and pupil. The iris is a muscular diaphragm of radial dilating muscle, the *dilator pupillae*, and a central circumferential muscle, the *sphincter pupillae*, surrounding the aperture for light, *the pupil*. These muscles control the pupil's size regulating the amount of light passing through the lens to the retina.

Lens. Behind the iris, the flexible transparent crystalline lens focuses light on the retina. The convex anterior and posterior surfaces join at *the equator*. The lens is suspended from its equator by the *zonula ciliaris* inserting into the *ciliary body* (Fig. 7-5). For distant vision the eye is at rest, the *ciliary muscle* relaxing increases tension on zonula flattening the central lens and decreasing its refractive power. The lens *accommodates* to near focus by contracting the ciliary muscle which decreases tension on the zonules allowing the elastic lens to become more spherical increasing its refractive power.

Vitreous body. The *vitreous* is the clear gelatinous tissue behind the lens attaching circumferentially to the peripheral *pars plana* and retina (vitreous base) and posteriorly to the optic nerve head, vessels, and macula. The vitreous partially liquefies with age. Traction at the vitreous base can tear the retina, allowing liquid vitreous into the subretinal space causing a retinal detachment. In ischemic retinal disease the vitreous is a scaffold for fibrous tissue and proliferating blood vessels which can contract tearing the retina.

Retina, choroid, and optic nerve. The posterior ocular segment is best considered from the inside out. The *retina* loosely lines the inner globe, attaching

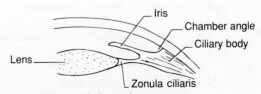

FIG. 7-5 Cross-Section of the Lens and Ciliary Body.

anteriorly to the peripheral ciliary body at the pars plana. The retinal *nerve fiber layer* coalesces to form the *optic nerve* which exits the globe through a lattice-like opening in the posterior sclera, the *lamina cribrosa*. The *central retinal artery and vein* course within the optic nerve branching onto the retina to form superior and inferior temporal arcs around the macula. The center of the macula, the *fovea*, is for detailed vision. The nasal retina, supplied by the nasal vascular arcades, provides indistinct temporal peripheral vision. The *retinal pigment epithelium* shuttles nourishment and waste between the overlying retinal ganglion cells and underlying *choroid* containing net-like blood vessels. External to the choroid is the fibrous sclera.

The Nose: The external nose is a pyramid joined to the face on one side (Fig. 7-6). The *root* connects to the forehead and the sides join in the midline forming the *dorsum nasi* whose superior portion is the *bridge* of the nose. The tip of the nose is the pyramid's apex. The triangular base is pierced on both sides by an elliptic orifice, the *naris* (plural *nares*), separated in the midline by the *columella*, an extension of the *nasal septum*. Still hairs, the *vibrissae*, line the margins of the nares inhibiting foreign body inhalation. Each lateral surface ends inferiorly in a rounded eminence, the *ala nasi* (plural, *alae nasi*). The upper third of the lateral nasal walls are supported medially by the *nasal bone* and laterally by the nasal process of the maxilla. The lower two-thirds is supported by *the greater alar cartilage* and several lesser alar cartilages. The nasal passages are separated anteriorly by the cartilaginous *nasal septum* and posteriorly by bone, the *vomer*.

The nasal septum divides the *nasal cavity* into symmetrical air passages that begin anteriorly at the naris (Fig. 7-7), widen into a *vestibule*, then become a high, narrow passage ending posteriorly at an oval orifice opening into the nasopharynx, the *choana*. A vascular network on the anterior nasal septum, *Kiesselbach plexus*, is the site of most nosebleeds. The central septum is a vertical plane. The lateral walls contain three horizontal, parallel, downward curving bony plates, the *superior*, *middle*, and *inferior turbinates* or *conchae*. The inferior turbinate's mucous membranes are highly vascular and semi-tumescent. Vasoconstrictor drugs reduce blood flow thereby decreasing tumescence. Under each turbinate is a groove, the *superior, middle*, and *inferior meatus*. The *olfactory* nerve (CN-I) endings are above the superior turbinate. Superior and posterior to the superior turbinate is the opening of the *sphenoid sinus*. The superior meatus contains the orifices of the *posterior ethmoid*

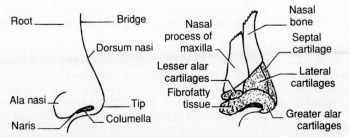

FIG. 7-6 The External Nose. These diagrams show the topographic features and the skeleton. Note that the proximal half of the nose is bone and the distal half (stippled) is cartilage.

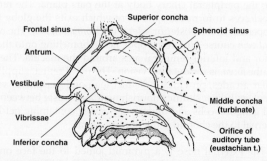

FIG. 7-7 Lateral Nasal Wall. This parasagittal section shows the superior, middle, and inferior conchae; under each is its corresponding meatus. Posterior to the inferior meatus is the orifice of the auditory (Eustachian) tube.

cells. The middle meatus receives drainage from the *maxillary sinus, frontal sinus,* and *anterior ethmoid cells*. The inferior meatus contains the *nasolacrimal duct* orifice. The *auditory (Eustachian) tube* opens into the nasopharynx just behind and lateral to the choana at the level of the middle meatus. The *pharyngeal tonsils,* or *adenoids,* are aggregations of lymphoid tissue in the posterior nasopharynx.

Mouth and Oral Cavity: The mouth is surrounded by two fleshy *lips,* their *vermillion borders* marking transition from cornified epithelium to non-cornified squamous epithelium in the mouth. The *philtrum* is a vertical groove from the columella to vermilion border. The lips are closed and protruded by contraction of the circular *orbicularis oris* muscle surrounding the mouth and innervated by the facial nerve (CN-VII). Each lip is anchored to the gum by a mucosal fold, the *labial frenulum*. A shallow *vestibule* separates the lips and teeth. The *oral cavity* is a short tunnel with an arched *roof* formed by the *hard and soft palate*. The hard palate, composed of maxilla and palatine bones covered by mucosa with a *median raphe,* is the roof's anterior two-thirds. The *soft palate,* a fold of mucosa and muscle, continues the roof posteriorly. The cheeks and teeth form the walls and the tongue is the floor. The tunnel ends in the *isthmus faucium* between the *faucial pillars* opening into the vertical *oropharynx* continuous superiorly with the *nasopharynx*. The conical or bulbous *uvula* is suspended from the free border of the soft palate. The lateral borders split into two vertical folds, the *tonsillar pillars*. Between the anterior and posterior pillars lies the *palatine tonsil,* a mass of lymphoid tissue containing deep crypts or clefts. Similar lymphoid tissue lies in the base of the tongue, the *lingual tonsil*.

Teeth. Upper and lower semicircles of *teeth* are set in the maxilla and mandible. The bony *dental ridges* and necks of the teeth are covered by tough fibrous tissue and mucosa, the *gums*. The gum borders are called the *gingival margins*. A child develops 20 *deciduous teeth*: from the upper and lower midline on each side there are two *incisors,* one *canine,* and a first and second *molar*. These teeth are gradually lost and replaced by *permanent teeth* adding a first and second *premolar,* or bicuspid, and a third molar making a total of 32 (Table 7-1). Dentists use a universal numbering system starting with the right upper third molar as 1 and counting left to the opposite upper third molar as 16, then

TABLE 7-1 Age at Tooth Eruption

	Deciduous (mo)	Permanent (y)
First molars	15–21	6
Central incisors	6–9	7
Lateral incisors	15–21	8
First premolars		9
Second premolars		10
Canines	16–20	12
Second molars	20–24	12–13
Third molars		17–25

continuing down to the left lower third molar as 17 and counting right to 32 at the mandibular third molar. The eruption times of the various teeth are shown in Table 7-1.

Tongue. The *tongue* lies within the mandible's horseshoe curve, its dorsal surface forming the floor of the oral cavity. The thin and narrow *tip* rests against the lingual surface of the lower incisors. The posterior and inferior *root* is composed of muscles and their bony attachments. The tip and dorsal surface are visible portions of a much larger muscular mass. Contracting the *extrinsic muscles* connecting the *symphysis mentis* of the mandible, *hyoid bone,* and *styloid process* of the temporal bone causes protrusion and retraction of the tip, convex and concave curving of the dorsum, and moves the root upward and downward. The *intrinsic muscles* alter the length, width, and curvature of the dorsal surface. The lingual muscles are innervated by the hypoglossal nerve (CN-XII). The tongue is free at its tip, dorsum, sides, and anteroinferior surface (Fig. 7-8). A midline fold of mucosa, the *lingual frenulum,* attaches the tongue to the floor of the mouth and the lingual surface of the lower gum. Near its base the frenulum swells forming twin eminences, the *caruncula sublingualis,* each containing the orifice of a *submandibular duct* (Wharton duct). Running from the caruncula laterally and posteriorly around the tongue base is a ridge of mucosa, the *plica sublingualis,* punctured at intervals by duct orifices from the *sublingual gland* lying deep to the ridges. The *dorsum* of the tongue extends from its tip to the epiglottis. It is bisected by the *median sulcus* from the tip to the posterior third, ending in a depression, the *foramen cecum,* marking the orifice of the embryonic *thyroglossal duct* prior to closure. A *sulcus terminalis* extends forward and laterally from either side of the foramen cecum forming a V. Slightly anterior and parallel is another V formed by 8-12 discrete round eminences with concentric fossae, the *vallate papillae.* The dorsum's anterior two-thirds has a velvet texture from microscopic *filiform papillae* which catch desquamated cells, bacteria, and food particles. Scattered among the filiform papillae at the tip and sides are less numerous large, raised, rounded, and deeper red *fungiform papillae.* Microscopic *taste buds* are numerous in vallate and fungiform papillae, on the tongue's sides and back, in the soft palate, and on the posterior surface of the epiglottis. The sensory root of the facial nerve (CN-VII) supplies the taste buds in the

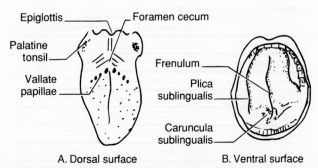

Epiglottis

Foramen cecum

Palatine tonsil

Vallate papillae

Frenulum

Plica sublingualis

Caruncula sublingualis

A. Dorsal surface   B. Ventral surface

FIG. 7-8 Tongue Surfaces. A. The dorsal surface from the tip of the epiglottis is depicted, showing the position of the palatine tonsils. **B. The ventral surface** is viewed from the outside of the mouth. The caruncula sublingualis is at the base of the frenulum; it contains the orifices of the submaxillary salivary ducts. In the plica sublingualis are some sublingual salivary gland orifices.

anterior two-thirds of the tongue via the *chorda tympani*. The posterior third is innervated by the glossopharyngeal nerve (CN-IX).

Larynx: The larynx lies immediately behind and below the oral cavity. The tip of the epiglottis is often visible through the mouth. Because the larynx is on the anterior wall of the pharynx with the plane of its rim sloping posteriorly it is easily viewed using a laryngeal mirror (Fig. 7-9). Visualize the laryngeal apparatus as three stacked incomplete rings, one atop the other, held together by ligaments. Topmost is the arched *hyoid bone* opening posteriorly. Suspended below are the arched *thyroid cartilage*, also opening posteriorly, and the *cricoid cartilage*, a complete ring fixed to the tracheal rings below. Though these structures are practically subcutaneous and easily palpable in the neck, their openings are posterior and well protected.

Phonation depends on the shape, position, and movement of two *arytenoid cartilages* (Fig. 7-10), each a three-sided pyramid with a triangular slightly concave base. The *cricoarytenoid joint*, a synovial joint surrounded by a capsule, allows the arytenoids to glide on the convex surface of the cricoid's posterior rim. The two erect pyramids stand on either side of the cricoid's midline. Muscles pull on the pyramid's faces rotating their bases at the joints. Each pyramid's apex is surmounted by a horizontal crescent of small cartilages and ligaments pointing medially toward its opposite and curving anteriorly. From the curve of each crescent, a tough fibroelastic band, the true *vocal cord* (vocal fold), extends forward to the midline of the thyroid cartilage. The two vocal cords form the opening into the trachea, the *rima glottidis*. When open, the rima is an isosceles triangle, with apex anterior, beneath the epiglottis and base posterior, formed by the tissue bridge between the two arytenoid crescents. As the arytenoids rotate the triangle's legs come together posteriorly approximating the cords over their entire length and closing the airway. Above the true cords is a pair of tissue folds, the *false vocal cords* (ventricular folds). A membrane covering the epiglottis and continuing posteriorly to envelope the arytenoids forms the *aryepiglottic folds*. The protrusion of the larynx from the anterior pharyngeal wall forms

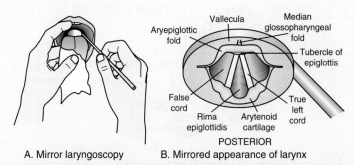

A. Mirror laryngoscopy   B. Mirrored appearance of larynx

FIG. 7-9 Mirror Laryngoscopy. A. Hand and instrument position for laryngoscopy. B. Appearance of the larynx in the mirror. This is the appearance with the cords abducted.

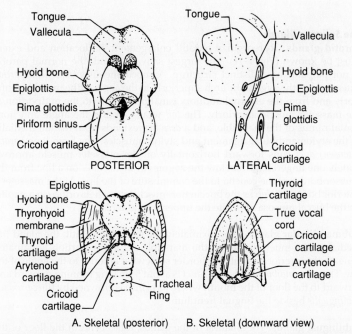

A. Skeletal (posterior)   B. Skeletal (downward view)

FIG. 7-10 Anatomy of the Larynx. The larynx faces posteriorly; it is seen with the mirror behind the plane of the vocal cords. The arytenoid cartilages are small pyramids perched on the cricoid cartilage, to which they are connected by true joints. The arytenoid cartilages twist on their bases to vary vocal cord tension.

pockets, two *valleculae* between the epiglottis and tongue base and two *piri-form sinuses*, one on either side of the cricoid. The intrinsic muscles of the larynx are largely innervated by the *recurrent laryngeal nerve*, a branch of the vagus nerve (CN-X).

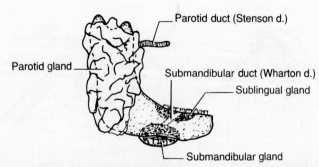

FIG. 7-11 Anatomic Relations of the Salivary Glands to the Mandible. Note that the parotid gland lies on the lateral surface of the mandibular ramus, curling behind its posterior margin. The submaxillary gland is on the medial surface of the mandible with its lower margin protruding below the bone. The sublingual gland is behind the medial mandibular surface near its superior margin. Using the jaw for a landmark, the glands can be accurately located by palpation.

The Salivary Glands

Parotid glands. To recognize parotid enlargement, its location and extent must be known (Fig. 7-11). The largest salivary gland, the normal parotid is not palpable as a distinct structure. A subcutaneously *superficial portion* extends from the zygomatic arch superiorly to the angle of the mandible inferiorly and from the external auditory canal posteriorly to the midportion of the masseter muscle anteriorly. The *tail* wraps around the angle and horizontal ramus of the mandible, and a *deep lobe* extends from the tail medially to the stylomandibular ligament and styloid muscles. The 5 cm long *parotid (Stensen) duct* runs forward horizontally on the masseter muscle approximately one fingerbreadth below the zygomatic arch. It lies on a line from the inferior border of the concha to the commissure of the lips. At the masseter's anterior border it pierces the buccinator muscle to reach its orifice in a papilla on the buccal mucosa opposite the upper second molar.

Submandibular glands. Approximately the size of a walnut, the gland lies medial to the inner surface of the mandible. Its lower portion is palpated beneath the inferior mandibular border somewhat anterior to the angle of the jaw. The *submandibular (Wharton) duct* is about 5 cm long running upward and forward to the floor of the mouth where its orifice is crowned by the *caruncula sublingualis* beside the lingual frenulum.

Sublingual glands. The smallest of the glands, it lies beneath the floor of the mouth, near the symphysis mentis. It empties through several short ducts, some with orifices in the plica sublingualis, some entering the submandibular duct.

The Thyroid Gland: Knowledge of thyroid embryology is necessary for understanding thyroid disorders. A median diverticulum invaginating from the ventral pharyngeal wall (the future *foramen cecum* in the tongue), goes down and back anterior to the trachea as a tubular duct, the *thyroglossal duct*. It bifurcates and further divides into cords that later fuse forming the

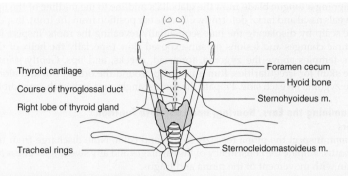

FIG. 7-12 Anatomic Relations of the Thyroid Gland, Anterior View. The blue structures are the thyroid gland and the course of the obliterated thyroglossal duct.

thyroid isthmus and lateral lobes. Normally, the thyroglossal duct is obliterated but remnants may persist forming thyroglossal sinuses or cysts. At the duct's superior end, a normally functioning *lingual thyroid gland* may form. Inferiorly, ductal tissue frequently forms a *pyramidal lobe* arising from the isthmus or a lateral lobe, usually the left. The pyramidal lobe may ascend anterior to the thyroid cartilage as high as the hyoid bone. Occasionally, the isthmus or a lateral lobe may fail to develop. Rarely, a lingual thyroid is the only active thyroid tissue.

The thyroid is the largest endocrine gland. It consists of two lateral lobes whose upper halves lie on either side of the projecting prow of the thyroid cartilage. The lower halves are beside the trachea (Fig. 7-12). The isthmus passes in front of the upper tracheal rings joining the lateral lobes at their lower thirds. The gland is roughly trapezoidal, the top and bottom parallel and the sides converging downward. The normal adult gland weighs ~25–30 g slightly larger in females than males. Each lateral lobe is an irregular cone ~5 cm long, ~3 cm wide, and ~2 cm thick. The right lobe is usually one-fourth larger than the left. The lateral posterior borders touch the common carotid arteries. Usually, the *parathyroid glands* lie on the posterior lateral surfaces. The *recurrent laryngeal nerves* lie close to the medial deep surface. Each lobe is covered anteriorly by the respective sternocleidomastoid, whereas the isthmus lying on the tracheal rings is practically subcutaneous. Paired *superior and inferior thyroid arteries* supply the exceedingly vascular parenchyma. The gland is firmly fixed to the trachea and larynx, ascending with them during swallowing, distinguishing the thyroid from other neck masses. Consider the thyroid as part of the upper anterior mediastinum. Enlargement downward extends behind the sternum, a retrosternal goiter. The *thymus gland* also occupies the anterior mediastinum. Thus, a tumor of the anterior mediastinum can arise from either gland.

PHYSICAL EXAMINATION OF THE HEAD AND NECK

Examining the Scalp, Face, and Skull: Examine by inspection and palpation. *Inspect* for asymmetry of the skull, ears, eyes, nose, mouth, jaw, and cheeks.

Aligning a tongue blade from the glabella's midline to the midline of the lips reveals nasal and facial deformity. Observe ear position from the front. Inspect the scalp by displacing the hair sequentially revealing the roots. Inspect for actinic changes and lesions on sun-exposed skin, especially the helix of the ear, temples above the zygoma, forehead, cheeks, and lips. Gently *palpate* the skull for irregularities. Run a fingertip around the orbital rim and along the zygoma on each side. Palpate the ramus, angle, and arch of the mandible.

Examining the Ears, Hearing, and Labyrinth Function

Ears

Pinna. Inspect the pinna for size, shape, and color. Note discharge from the meatus. Palpate the consistency of the cartilages and any swellings. Assess for pain with movement of the pinna and tragus.

External acoustic meatus. Clean the canal for inspection. Remove liquid material with a cotton applicator. Remove solids under direct vision through an ear speculum with either a cotton applicator or a cerumen spoon. Use a speculum attached to an otoscope or a speculum and a headlamp. Select the largest speculum that will fit the cartilaginous canal. Tip the head toward the opposite shoulder making the canal horizontal. Insert the speculum while retracting the pinna up and back aligning the flexible cartilaginous canal with the bony canal. Use downward traction for infants and young children (Fig. 7-13). The lining epithelium of the bony canal is very sensitive, so be gentle.

TM and middle ear. Light shining on the TM reflects a brilliant wedge of light, the *light reflex*, whose apex is at the center or *umbo* with its legs extending radially in the anterior inferior quadrant of the TM, at approximately a right angle to the manubrium. Examine the normal landmarks of the drumhead. The *manubrium of the malleus* forms a smooth ridge from the umbo running radially upward and forward ending in the knob of the *short process*. The two *mallear folds* diverge from the knob to the periphery. The *shadow of the incus* often shows through the membrane in the upper posterior quadrant. Finally inspect the entire circumference of the annulus for perforations just inside its border. Note the *color and sheen* of the membrane, which should be shiny and pearly gray. Serum in the middle ear colors the TM amber or yellow

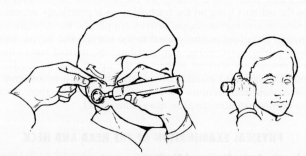

FIG. 7-13 Use of the Otoscope. Insert the ear speculum by pulling the upper edge of the pinna upward and backward to straighten the cartilaginous meatus so that it coincides with the axis of the bony canal.

and air bubbles may be seen. Pus shows as a chalky white membrane and blood appears blue. Note changes in the *definition of the manubrium*. When the TM bulges it makes the landmarks indistinct or obscures them completely. Inadequate auditory (Eustachian) tube function produces TM retraction sharpening the outline of the manubrium and mallear folds. With either bulging or retraction the light reflex is distorted or absent. When the incus is visible, the middle ear is normal.

Testing hearing. *Rough quantitative test for hearing loss.* Difficulty understanding spoken questions signals potential hearing loss. Test with the whispered voice at the patient's side ~ 60 cm (2 ft) from each ear while covering the far ear. The patient repeats whispered numbers, or questions that cannot be answered yes or no. Test with loud, medium, and soft tones. Alternatively, using the same intensity for all tests, find the maximum distance at which the whisper is understood. Hearing acuity is tested with a 256 or 1024 cycles per second tuning fork. The 128-cycle fork for testing vibratory sense is too low pitched.

Distinguishing neurosensory and conductive hearing loss. Use a tuning fork having a frequency of 256 or 1024 cycles per second. Tap the fork on the base of the other hand. The *Weber test* (Fig. 7-14A) places the handle of the vibrating fork against the skull's midline asking whether the sound is louder in one ear than the other. With normal neurosensory hearing and no conductive loss the sounds are equal in both ears. The *Rinne test* (Fig. 7-14B) is done in each ear sequentially. First, press the vibrating tuning fork against the mastoid process (*bone conduction*) and then place the tines near the ear canal (*air conduction*). Ask which is louder. When air conduction is louder than bone conduction, the test is arbitrarily said to be Rinne-positive, a normal result. The test is Rinne-negative when bone conduction is louder than air conduction. Have the patient indicate when the sound is no longer heard by air conduction. See if you can hear the vibrating fork to compare their hearing to yours.

Testing vestibular function. *The Dix–Hallpike maneuver for positional vertigo.* With the patient sitting on the exam table, inspect the eyes carefully for

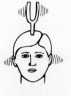
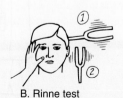

A. Weber test   B. Rinne test

FIG. 7-14 Tests of Hearing Perception and Conduction. A. Weber test: The vibrating tuning fork is on the midline of the skull. Lateralization of the sound to one ear indicates a conductive loss on that side, or a perceptive loss on the other side. **B. Rinne test:** The handle of the tuning fork is first placed against the mastoid process then near the external ear. Each time the patient indicates when the sound ceases. Normally, duration of air conduction is twice that of bone conduction.

spontaneous nystagmus. Then, keeping the eyes open, have the patient lie supine with the head extending beyond the end of the table, the chin elevated ~30 degrees and the head turned 45 degrees to the right. Observe the eyes for 30 seconds looking for nystagmus. Return the patient to the sitting position inspecting the eyes for another 30 seconds. Repeat the test with the head turning to the left. A positive test induces nystagmus, often accompanied by intense nausea. The slow component of the nystagmus is in the direction of endolymph flow; nystagmus is named for its fast component.

Test for Past Pointing. The patient sits with her eyes closed while pointing her forefingers toward the examiner (Fig. 7-15). The examiner's forefingers are lightly placed and held under hers. Ask the patient to raise her arms and hands and then return them to the starting position. Normally, this maneuver can be performed accurately. Past pointing indicates either loss of positional sense or labyrinth stimulation.

Romberg Test. The patient stands with heels and toes close together (Fig. 7-16). Assure the patient that you will not let her fall, being prepared to catch her should she fall. Have her close her eyes and observe for several seconds.

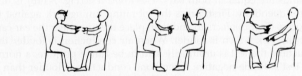

FIG. 7-15 Past Pointing Test for Labyrinthine Disorders.

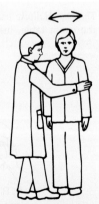

FIG. 7-16 Falling Test for Labyrinthine Disorders (Romberg Sign). Normally, the patient will waver somewhat, but not fall. With labyrinthine stimulation, the patient tends to fall in the direction of the flow of endolymph. Falling may also indicate loss of positional sense as in cerebellar deficits.

Normally, patients will be steady, even with gentle, forewarned, pushes on the trunk. Falling during the test means the *Romberg sign* is present.

Examining the Eyes, Visual Fields, and Visual Acuity

Palpebral fissures and globe position. From a distance, note the width and symmetry of the palpebral fissures. Look for protrusion or recession of one or both globes by inspecting the eyes from the front, profile, and above (looking downward over the forehead), or from below (looking up over the cheekbones). If proptosis (protrusion) is suspected, use a Hertel exophthalmometer to measure the distance from the outer edge of the bony orbit to the anterior surface of the cornea. There are familial and racial degrees of proptosis, and individual variation is great. Progressive anterior displacement on repeated exams is pathologic.

Inspecting for inflammation. Inspect for redness and/or swelling and involvement of one or both eyes and/or eyelids.

Testing for lid lag, lid retraction, and scleral show. Use a finger or penlight as a target ~50 cm (20 inch) away. Starting above eye level, repeatedly move the target slowly up and down in the midline (Fig. 7-17). Lid-lag is present when white sclera appears between the lid margin and limbus. *Lid retraction* is dynamic upper lid elevation while fixing gaze on a spot. *Scleral show* is more constant exposure of the sclera. The inferior sclera shows below the limbus in some normal individuals.

Testing for Strabismus (Heterotropia). First confirm functional vision in each eye.

Cover–uncover test. With the gaze fixed on a target, cover one eye while watching the uncovered eye (Fig. 7-18) seeing if it moves to take up fixation. Allow the patient to look with both eyes, then cover the other eye again watching the uncovered eye seeing if it moves to fixation. If there is fixation movement, the patient has *heterotropia* (strabismus, squint). Constant misalignment of this type is *manifest deviation* or *tropia*.

Alternate cover test. While the patient holds visual fixation, repeatedly cover one eye then the other. If there was not a manifest deviation by cover-uncover testing, but now, when uncovered, each eye moves to pick up fixation, *latent*

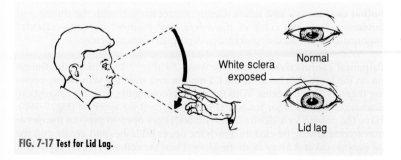

FIG. 7-17 Test for Lid Lag.

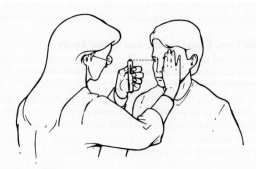

FIG. 7-18 Testing for Strabismus.

deviation or *phoria* is present. The cover-uncover test has shown that the brain can fuse images by aligning the visual axes, but alternating cover breaks that fusion. A phoria is also demonstrated by fixing focus on an object with both eyes then covering one eye for a few seconds. If the covered eye moves to reestablish fixation when uncovered, the eye has *heterophoria*.

Naming the deviation. If the eye swings inward to pick up fixation, it was initially deviated outward (*exotropia* or *exophoria*). If the eye swings outward, it was initially deviated inward (*esotropia, esophoria*). To determine if the heterotropia is comitant or incomitant, have the patient follow a target in the six cardinal directions of gaze. If the eyes move equally without restriction, the deviation is *comitant*. If one eye over-shoots and the other fails to move the entire distance in one or more directions, the deviation is *incomitant*, either a paralytic or restrictive misalignment. A *paralytic misalignment* is pathological and could indicate ischemia (stroke) or compression (tumor); *restrictive misalignments* are caused by scarring or fibrosis, as in thyroid eye disease.

Eyelids. Look for swelling of the lids, and above, below, and near the canthi. Note inversion or eversion of the lid margins. Examine the margins for scaling, normal secretions, exudate, papules, or pustules. Look for lashes turned inward (*trichiasis*). If pressing the lacrimal sac expresses fluid through the punctum, the tear duct is obstructed.

Bulbar conjunctiva and sclera. Gently retract the lids with the thumb and forefinger. Note the color of the sclera, any pigment deposits, vascular engorgement, or vascular pterygium. A pinguecula is avascular.

Palpebral conjunctiva. To *evert the lower lid* (Fig. 7-19A) place the thumb tip on the loose skin beneath the lid margin and slide the skin down, pressing it gently into the orbit. With the patient looking up, look for congestion, discharge, and/or other lesions. If indicated, *evert the upper lid* (Fig. 7-19B). Have the patient look downward with both eyes open to prevent the elevation accompanying lid closure. Pinch the upper lid lashes and gently pull the lid downward and away from the globe. Press the cotton tip of an applicator

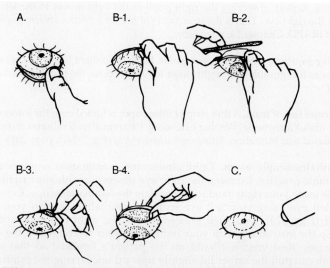

FIG. 7-19 Examination of the Eyelids. A. Eversion of the lower lid. B. Eversion of the upper lid: Tell the patient to look downward and proceed with four steps: (1) with the right thumb and forefinger, grasp a few cilia of the upper lid and pull the lid away from the globe; (2) lay an applicator along the crease made by the superior edge of the tarsal plate and the soft adjacent tissue; (3) quickly fold the lid over the applicator so the tarsal plate turns over and its upper edge faces downward; and (4) replace the right thumb and finger by the corresponding left ones to hold the lid. **C. Testing pupillary reaction to light**.

against the upper lid just above the tarsal plate. Using this as a fulcrum, pull the eyelid quickly upward everting the tarsal plate. Stabilize the everted lid with your fingers. To return the lid to its normal position have the patient glance upward.

Cornea. To search for scars, abrasions, or ulcers, shine a light obliquely on the cornea. The *corneal light reflex* should be smooth and regular as the light is played over the surface. Abrasions are readily demonstrated by *fluorescein staining*. Place the tip of a moistened fluorescein strip in the inferior fornix. After removing it, have the patient blink. Corneal abrasions are green under blue light. The cornea may also be examined with a lens.

Iris, pupils, and lens. Observe the clarity of the iris, noting whether it is distinct or muddy. Look for new vessels and deposits. Note pupil size, shape, and equality. Shining light obliquely through the lens reveals deposits on the lens surface and opacities in the matrix such as cataracts.

Testing the pupil's reaction to light. Have the patient fix focus on an object >3 m (>10 ft) away. Shine light into the right pupil from the side (Fig. 7-19C) while observing the *direct pupillary reaction*. Repeat on the left eye. Next, while continuing to observe the left pupil, swing the light back to the right eye. Normally, as the light swings toward the right eye from the left, there is minimal dilatation followed by constriction of the left pupil, the normal *consensual reaction*. Repeat, observing the right pupil as the light moves to the left eye from the right eye. This is the *swinging light test* for a *relative afferent pupillary defect* (RAPD, Chapter 14, page 665).

Testing pupillary reaction to near point. Have the patient fix on his/her own finger as it is gradually brought closer to his/her nose; the pupil should constrict.

Schirmer test of tears. A thin strip of filter paper is folded over the lower eyelid without anesthesia. Wetting extending <10 mm after 5 minutes indicates decreased tear formation, *keratoconjunctivitis sicca* (Fig. 7-34D, page 201).

Ophthalmoscopic exam. Ophthalmoscopic examination requires considerable practice. Examine the right eye observing with your right eye while using your right hand to manipulate the ophthalmoscope. Examine the left eye using your left eye with the ophthalmoscope in your left hand (Fig. 7-20). Undilated examination of the right eye is described. Grasp the instrument with your right hand, your forefinger on the disk of lenses. Rest your left hand on the patient's forehead so that your thumb can pull the upper lid slightly upward uncovering the pupil and preventing excessive blinking. Have the patient fix vision straight ahead on a distant object.

Media. Place the +8 or +10 diopter lens in the sight hole. Bring it close to your eye or glasses and move forward to ~30 cm (12 inch) in front of the patient's eye. Shine the light into the pupil to see the *red retinal reflex*. A dull red or black reflex is produced by diffuse dense opacities. Look for black spots showing against the red. These shadows of lens or vitreous opacities are made by light reflecting from the retina. Move forward or backward until the spots are clearly focused. While watching the opacities, ask the patient to elevate the eyes slightly; if the spots move upward, they are on the cornea or anterior lens; little movement occurs when located near the lenticular center; downward movement indicates location in the posterior lens or vitreous. Vitreous opacities are more distinct when viewed obliquely with the white optic disk as background.

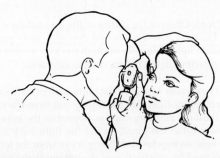

FIG. 7-20 Ophthalmoscopic Examination.

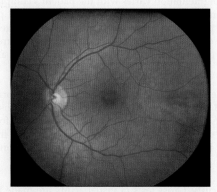

FIG. 7-21 Normal Fundus. Normal left retinal vessels, macula, periphery and disc. (Image used with permission from Brice Critser, CRA.)

Fundus **(Fig. 7-21).** Hold the instrument ~5 cm (2 inch) from the patient's eye with your forehead near or touching the hand on the patient's forehead. Adjust the lenses to find the optimal focus for viewing the retina, the setting varies with the refractive error and degree of accommodation in both patient and examiner. Absent both factors, the best view should be at zero. Minus lenses correct for involuntary accommodation. After cataract extraction without intraocular lens placement, about +10 is needed for correction. High astigmatism cannot be corrected with the spherical ophthalmoscope lenses, so examine through the patient's glasses. When the correct setting is found, examine the following (Fig. 7-21 and Fig. 7-39A, page 206).

Optic disk. The optic disc lies 10 degrees nasal and slightly inferior to the visual axis. Therefore, angle the ophthalmoscope 10 degrees nasally from the line of sight to locate the optic disc. Note the disk's shape and color. Normally, it's round or oval vertically. Most of the disk is red-orange, the color coming from capillaries around nerve fibers. The *physiologic cup* is a pale area at the center of the disk devoid of nerve fibers and forming a depression whose base is the avascular *lamina cribrosa*. The size and shape of the cup vary greatly in normal eyes. Estimate the cup-to-disk *ratio*. If the cup is not circular, use the vertical ratio. Vessels enter and exit at the pale and white *vessel funnel*, which also lacks nerve fibers. The disk borders may merge gradually into the surrounding retina, or they may be sharply demarcated by a white scleral ring. On the temporal side outside the ring, a crescent of pigment may be present.

Retinal vessels. Arteries are bright red with a *light reflex*, the central stripe. Note the width of the reflex stripe. Normally, veins are wider than the arteries in a ratio of ~4:3 and they are darker red and lack a stripe. The vessel branching pattern shows great individual variation. Emerging from the disk, the afferent vessels are true arteries; branches beyond the second bifurcation, ~1 disk diameter from the disk margin, are arterioles. Look for sheathing of the arteries. Observe the veins carefully at the arteriovenous crossings for nicking, deviation, humping, tapering, sausaging, or banking. Retinal veins are normally pulsatile; retinal arteries are not.

Retina. Retinal pigmentation varies with the patient's complexion and race. The retina is thinner and therefore more pale in the nasal periphery. Note areas of white or pigment from scarring. Look for hemorrhages and exudates. Express the size of abnormalities in disk diameters. Measure depression or elevation by the diopters of correction required to focus on an arterial reflex in the area.

Macula. Examine the macula last. It is slightly below the horizontal plane of the disk and 2–3 disk diameters temporal of its margin. Observation of the macula is usually fleeting because the light causes discomfort. The *fovea* in the center of the macula is a small darker red area set apart from visible vessels. In its center is a small even darker spot, the *foveola*, giving off a speck of reflected light.

Testing visual acuity. Gross tests of visual acuity are made without special equipment. Test one eye at a time. Have the patient read a newspaper or magazine, testing first with the fine print and following with larger print if needed. If the patient fails large letters, ask him to count several fingers held 1 m (3 ft) away. If he cannot count them, ask if he can see hand movements. Failing this, flash light into the eye, asking for an indication of when it appears. Ask whether he can tell the direction of the light source. When gross acuity is fair, standard *Snellen* chart testing when done with adequate illumination at the appropriate distance provides greater accuracy. Determine the smallest line of letters the patient can read without error with each eye, and then with both eyes together. Acuity is expressed as the ratio of the distance at which the patient read the line to the distance at which the line is read by normal eyes. The distance is expressed in feet or meters; 20/20 ft and 6/6 m are normal, respectively. If the patient could only read the line for 40 ft, his/her acuity is expressed as 20/40. Record whether glasses or contact lens were used. If the visual acuity is abnormal, the potential acuity from improving optical correction is estimated by the *pinhole test*. A 1-mm hole, or series of holes, is made in a card. The patient is asked to read a Snellen chart through the pinhole(s) providing a close approximation to best-corrected visual acuity.

Testing color vision. Perceived colors are mixture of red, blue, and green. Ask the patient to identify the colors of objects immediately available. Use a book of Ishihara plates for greater accuracy.

Slit-lamp microscopy. Slit-lamp exam is reserved for vision professionals and those with extensive experience. A narrow slit of powerful light is focused on the layers of the cornea, anterior chamber, lens, and anterior third of the vitreous chamber looking for opacities and foci of inflammation.

Examining the Nose and Sinuses: Routinely *inspect* the nose's profile, contour, and symmetry. Test patency of each naris by closing the other while the patient inhales with the mouth closed. *Transilluminate* the nasal septum by pushing the nasal tip upward and illuminating one naris (Fig. 7-22A) while viewing the transilluminated septum through the opposite nares for deviations, perforations, and masses. Palpate the cheeks and supraorbital ridges and over the maxillary and frontal sinuses for tenderness.

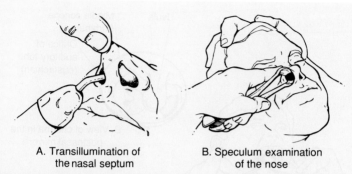

A. Transillumination of   B. Speculum examination
   the nasal septum   of the nose

FIG. 7-22 Examination of the Nasal Septum and Nares. A. Transillumination of the nasal septum. B. Speculum examination of the nose.

Examining with a nasal speculum. Examine the anterior nasal chambers with a nasal speculum and a head mirror or head lamp. Holding the speculum in the left hand (Fig. 7-22B) leaves the right hand free to position the head and/or hold instruments. Insert the closed blades ~1 cm into the vestibule before opening the blades in the plane of the septum. Anchor the ala nasi against the superior blade with the left forefinger to avoid pressure on the septum. Reposition the speculum and head to see each structure. Examine the *vestibule* for folliculitis and fissures. Note the color of the *mucosa* and any swelling. Inspect the nasal septum for deviation, ulcer, or hemorrhage. Examine the *inferior turbinate* on the lateral wall for swelling, increased redness, pallor, or blueness. Identify the *middle turbinate* and inspect the *middle meatus* for purulent discharge from frontal, maxillary, and anterior ethmoid sinuses.

Nasopharynx. A head mirror or headlamp is required for illumination. Warm a No. 0 (small) postnasal mirror in warm water to avoid condensation; check its temperature on your wrist. Depress the tongue, as described for the oropharyngeal examination, inserting it from the corner of the mouth (Fig. 7-23A). Hold the mirror like a pencil, steadying your hand against the patient's cheek. Insert the mirror from the side opposite the tongue blade, keeping the mirror upright to avoid touching the tongue, palate, and uvula. Position it behind the uvula near the posterior pharyngeal wall. Turn the mirror upward to view the *choana* (Figs. 7-23B and C) locating, in the midline, the *vomer*, the posterior end of the nasal septum. Identify the *middle meatus*. Pus draining posteriorly from the meatus comes only from the maxillary sinus. The *inferior meatus* is not well visualized posteriorly. The pale or yellow ~5 mm diameter orifices of the *auditory (Eustachian) tubes* are behind and lateral to the middle meatus. The tubes are closed except during swallowing or yawning. Look for the *pharyngeal tonsil (adenoids)* hanging from the roof into the fossa. Examine the nasopharynx for inflammation, exudate, polyps, and neoplasms. If available, a fiberoptic instrument simplifies the exam.

Sinus Transillumination. Use a cool light in a fully darkened room. For the maxillary sinuses, press a cool light against each maxilla while observing the

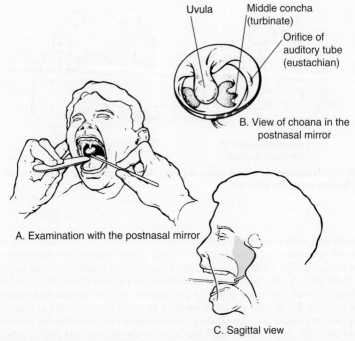

Uvula

Middle concha (turbinate)

Orifice of auditory tube (eustachian)

B. View of choana in the postnasal mirror

A. Examination with the postnasal mirror

C. Sagittal view

FIG. 7-23 Examination of the Nasopharynx. A. Examination with the postnasal mirror. In the drawing, all deep spaces are heavily stippled. **B. View of the choana in the postnasal mirror. C. Sagittal view.**

hard palate through the mouth for transmitted light. For the frontal sinuses, place the light under the nasal half of the supraorbital ridge while shielding the orbit to the eyebrows. Look for bright areas in the forehead. Asymmetry of transillumination is most significant.

Examining the Lips, Mouth, Teeth, Tongue, and Pharynx: Inspect using a tongue blade and light. Using a headlamp or mirror frees one hand for instruments. Completely inspect the oral cavity before beginning palpation.

Lips. Look for congenital and acquired defects. Note the lip color and look for angular stomatitis, rhagades, ulcers, granulomas, and neoplasms. Having the patient attempt to whistle reveals weak face muscles that are innervated by the facial nerve (CN-VII). Inspect the inner surface of the lips by retracting them with a tongue blade while the teeth are approximated.

Teeth. Note the absence of teeth and the presence of caries, discoloration, fillings, and bridges. Note abnormal shapes, such as notching. Tap each tooth for tenderness.

Gums. Have the patient remove any dental appliances. Look for retraction of the gingival margins, pus in the margins, gum inflammation, spongy or bleeding gums, lead or bismuth lines, or localized gingival swelling.

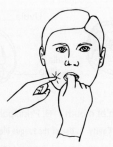

FIG. 7-24 Palpation of the Roof of the Tongue.

Breath. Smell the breath for acetone, ammonia, or fetor.

Tongue. Have the patient protrude the tongue for *inspection*. Assess its size noting deviation from the midline or restricted protrusion. Examine the dorsal surface coat for color, thickness, and adhesiveness. Have the patient raise the tongue tip to the roof of the mouth to inspect the undersurface, including *frenulum* and *carunculae sublingualis*. To relax the muscles for *palpation*, have the tongue inside the teeth for palpation. Wear gloves and with the mouth widely open, push a fold of cheek between the teeth to lessen the chance of being bitten. Insert a forefinger to the back of the mouth and palpate the roof of the tongue, valleculae, and tonsillar fossae (Fig. 7-24) for tenderness and masses. Palpate the sublingual salivary glands and submandibular ducts for calculi. Spraying the throat with a topical anesthetic reduces an overactive gag but is usually unnecessary.

Examining a lingual ulcer. Always wear gloves. Using a cotton sponge, gently dry the ulcer and then inspect it carefully. Palpate the surrounding and underlying tissue. Pain from lingual lesions may be referred to the ear.

Buccal mucosa. Retract the cheek with a tongue blade looking for melanin deposits, vesicles, petechiae, *Candida*, Koplik spots, ulcers, and neoplasms. Examine the orifice of the parotid duct opposite the upper second molar.

Oropharynx. Hold a tongue blade with the thumb underneath and the index finger and long finger on top at the midpoint. Have the patient breathe steadily through the nose keeping the mouth open. Relax the tongue with the tip behind the lower incisors. Using the blade's tip, press the tongue's midpoint downward and forward by pushing down with the two fingers while the thumb pushes upward on the end (Fig. 7-25A). Pressing farther back causes gagging, while pressing anteriorly leads to posterior bulging. Steady the light in the other hand with the ring and little fingers on the patient's cheek. An optimal view may require several blade placements transversely at the midpoint. Test for vagal nerve (CN-X) paralysis by noting whether the uvula is drawn upward in the midline when the patient says "e-e-e."

Tonsils. Use a tongue blade in each hand. Depress the tongue with one while retracting the anterior faucial pillar laterally with the other, disclosing the

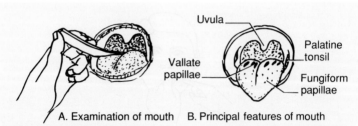

FIG. 7-25 **Examination of the Oral Cavity. A. Use of the tongue blade. B. Principal anatomic features seen in the oral cavity.**

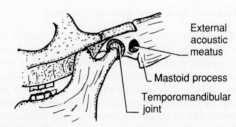

FIG. 7-26 **Anatomy of the TMJ.** Note the nearness of the joint to the external acoustic meatus, so the joint may be palpated by a finger in the meatus (Fig. 7-66).

anterior tonsillar surface. Normally, it's the same color as the surrounding mucosa. Look for hyperplasia, ulcers, membrane, masses, and small, submerged tonsils.

Examining the Temporomandibular Joint: Palpate over the temporomandibular joint (TMJ), anterior to the tragus, while the patient opens and closes the mouth, feeling for clicking or crepitus (Fig. 7-26). Corresponding noises are heard by placing the stethoscope bell over the joint during movement. Search for tenderness by placing the index finger tips in each external acoustic meatus and press forward while the mouth is opened and closed.

Examining the Larynx
Mirror laryngoscopy. *This technique is being largely replaced by use of flexible fiberoptic instruments.* Use a head mirror or head lamp leaving both hands free. To use a mirror, seat the patient with a bright light source immediately behind and to one side of the head. Reflect this light into the oropharynx with the head mirror; practice is required. The patient sits erect with the chin somewhat forward. The examiner sits in front of the patient with the knees outside the patient's knees. Explain each step of the procedure before beginning. Have the patient concentrate on breathing softly and regularly through the mouth (Fig. 7-9A, page 169). Have the tongue protrude maximally over the lower teeth. After rapping a piece of gauze over the tongue, grasp the wrapped portion between thumb and middle finger of the left hand while

bracing with the forefinger against the upper teeth. Pull the tongue gently to the side. Hold a No. 5 (large) laryngeal mirror like a pencil at the handle's midpoint. To avoid condensation, warm the mirror in warm water checking its temperature on your wrist. Brace your fourth and fifth fingers against the patient's cheek. Insert the mirror from the side, with the face downward and parallel to the tongue surface. Move it posteriorly until its back rests against the anterior surface of the uvula. Press the uvula and soft palate steadily upward. To prevent gagging, avoid touching the back of the tongue. Have the patient breathe steadily while you inspect the larynx. While still viewing the vocal cords, ask the patient to say "e-e-e" or "he-e-e" in a high-pitched voice. Sing along with him in the desired pitch and for the proper duration. When viewing in the mirror, remember that upward is anterior, downward is posterior. Examine the *vallate papillae, lingual tonsils, valleculae,* and *epiglottis* (Fig. 7-9B, page 169). Next, look at the *false cords, true vocal cords, arytenoids,* and *piriform sinuses*. Finally, observe the true vocal cords during quiet respiration when the rima is tent-shaped. During phonation, watch the cords meet in the midline.

Examining the Salivary Glands

Parotid glands. When fullness is present anterior to the tragus, ascertain whether it is continuous with an inferior mass, as in parotid swelling, or discontinuous, as in swelling of a preauricular lymph node. Swelling from the parotid gland is seen in front of the tragus and earlobe and behind the lower ear, pushing the pinna outward. Have the patient clench his teeth tensing the masseter muscles. Palpate against the hard muscle to determine the mass's extent, consistency, and tenderness. Feel for swelling behind the mandibular ramus, which is always present in parotid enlargement. Palpate for calculus in the parotid duct. The normal duct is thick enough to be felt when rolled against the tensed masseter. Inspect the parotid duct orifice. While watching the orifice, press the cheek looking for discharge from the duct. With a gloved finger, palpate the orifice and posteriorly for calculus or other mass.

Submandibular glands. Do bimanual palpation with a gloved finger in the floor of the mouth and the opposite hand under the jaw. The gland is felt as a finely lobulated swelling under the mandible slightly anterior to the angle of the jaw. To test for secretion, place cotton gauze under the tongue, have the patient sip lemon juice, and then remove the gauze watching for saliva flowing from each orifice.

Examining the Neck

Cervical muscles and bones. *In trauma cases or if cervical fracture is suspected, immobilize the patient and obtain X-rays before trying to elicit physical signs.* Have the patient's neck and shoulders uncovered. Face the patient looking for swelling and noting any asymmetry of shoulder height and clavicles, or fixed neck posture. Check range of motion on neck flexion, extension, lateral bending, and rotation. Palpate the cervical vertebrae and muscles for tenderness, tightness, and masses.

Thyroid gland. The normal adult thyroid is often not palpable. In a thin neck, the normal isthmus is felt as a tissue band just obliterating the surface of the tracheal rings. A goiter is any enlarged thyroid gland.

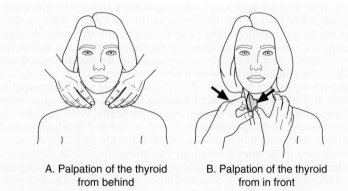

A. Palpation of the thyroid
from behind

B. Palpation of the thyroid
from in front

FIG. 7-27 Palpation of the Thyroid Gland and Adjacent Structures. A. Palpation from behind. B. Frontal palpation.

Inspection. With the patient seated in a good cross-light, inspect the anterior triangles in the lower half of the neck. Have the patient swallow looking for a mass ascending in the midline or behind the sternocleidomastoid. With obesity or a short neck, have the patient swallow with the neck tilted back while supporting the occiput with clasped hands.

Palpation from behind. The examiner is behind the seated patient who lowers their chin relaxing the neck muscles. The thumbs are placed behind the neck curling the fingers anteriorly so long and ring finger tips just touch over the upper tracheal rings (Fig. 7-27A). The patient holds water in the mouth swallowing when asked. Locate the thyroid and cricoid cartilages and tracheal rings. The lateral lobes are on either side of the trachea rising under the fingers during a swallow. Feel for tissue overlying the tracheal rings; it is likely a hyperplastic thyroid isthmus. Palpate systematically the lower poles of both lateral lobes. During the exam, shift the inclination of the patient's head to relax the neck muscles, and have the patient swallow to test the adherence of palpated masses to the trachea. Palpate the anterior surface of each lateral lobe through the sternocleidomastoid with the patient's head slightly inclined toward the side being examined to relax the muscles. Occasionally, the thyroid is more easily felt when the neck is dorsiflexed.

Palpation from the front. Place the fingers of one hand behind the neck with the thumb on the base of the thyroid cartilage (Fig. 7-27B) pushing the trachea gently away from the midline. The fingers of the other hand palpate the posterior aspect of the lateral lobe behind the sternocleidomastoid while the thumb palpates the anterior surface medial to the muscle. Having the patient swallow or depress the chin may further assist the examination. Palpate the other lateral lobe in the same manner with the tasks of the two hands reversed.

Auscultating a goiter. Auscultate goiters for a bruit using the stethoscope's bell.

Examining the Lymph Nodes: See Chapter 5, page 82.

Examining the Vascular System: See Chapter 8, page 287.

HEAD AND NECK SYMPTOMS

General Symptom
Headache. See Chapter 14, page 651.

Skull, Scalp, and Face Symptoms
Blushing and flushing. Transient dilation of superficial blood vessels of the head, face, and neck occurs with emotional, pharmacological, or physical stimulation. Flushing is a normal response to exercise, hot environments, and ingestion of vasoactive substances such as alcohol or capsaicin in hot peppers. Flushing is common in patients with rosacea or carcinoid syndrome, and in women at the menopause. *Blushing* is a term usually reserved for flushing associated with embarrassment or self-consciousness.

Face Pain. Facial pain is usually well localized, indicating the structure involved. Uncommonly, it is a difficult diagnostic problem.
CLINICAL OCCURRENCE: Use an anatomic approach for identifying the cause, sorting the likely causes by the structure involved. *Nerves:* Trigeminal neuralgia, postherpetic neuralgia; *Blood Vessels:* Temporal arteritis, cavernous sinus thrombosis; *Teeth:* Periapical abscess, periodontitis, unerupted teeth; *Bones:* Sinusitis, osteomyelitis; *Joints:* Temporomandibular arthritis; *Salivary Glands:* Parotitis.

Trigeminal neuralgia (tic douloureux). See Chapter 14, page 654.

Herpes zoster. See Chapter 6, page 144. Unilateral sharp burning pain in the distribution of one trigeminal nerve branch develops 2–3 days before vesicles appear. Persistent pain after resolution of the skin lesions is *postherpetic neuralgia.*

Acute suppurative sinusitis, orbital cellulitis. See pages 248 and 241.

Spasms of jaw muscles—trismus. See page 193.

Pain with chewing—masseter claudication. Ischemia of the masseter and/or temporalis muscles is induced by chewing, especially tough meats, and relieved by rest. Patients alter their diet to avoid the pain. Giant cell arteritis should be suspected.

TMJ pain. Symptoms include pain, felt in the ear or temple, clicking, and occasionally locking. Trauma causes joint injury and crepitation. See page 240.

Numb chin syndrome. Invasion of the mental or inferior alveolar nerve causes chin numbness. Patients complain of persistent chin numbness without other symptoms or signs. If a thorough oral exam does not identify a local cause of nerve injury, a search for neoplastic disease is indicated.

Ear Symptoms

Tinnitus. Ringing in the ears, *tinnitus*, is often sufficiently distressing for a patient to seek care. Unilateral tinnitus may be the first symptom of an acoustic neuroma.

CLINICAL OCCURRENCE: *Outer Ear:* Cerumen, foreign body or polyp in the external meatus; *Middle Ear:* Inflammation, otosclerosis, polychondritis; *Inner Ear:* Meniere disease, syphilis, fevers, labyrinth suppuration, basilar skull fracture, acoustic neuroma, trauma; *Drugs:* Quinine, salicylates, aminoglycoside antibiotics.

Temporary altered hearing. Eustachian tube dysfunction causes mild intermittent pain, ear fullness, and altered hearing. Patients hear a popping sound with swallowing or yawning. The eardrum may be retracted (Fig. 7-28B).

Earache. The middle ear arises from the first and second pharyngeal pouches. Pain is caused by inflammation of ear structures or is referred from pharyngeal sites, including the thyroid. Although the cause of acute ear pain is usually readily identified, chronic earache may offer a considerable diagnostic challenge.

CLINICAL OCCURRENCE: *Auricle:* Trauma, hematoma, frostbite, burn, epithelioma, perichondritis, gout, eczema, impetigo, insect bites, carcinoma, herpes zoster; *Meatus:* External otitis, malignant external otitis, carbuncle, meatitis, eczema, hard cerumen, foreign body, injury, epithelioma, carcinoma, insect invasion, herpes zoster, trigeminal neuralgia (CN-V3); *Middle*

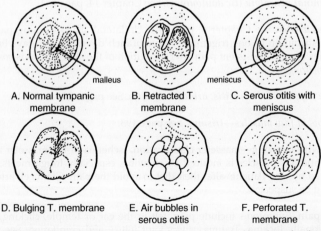

FIG. 7-28 Lesions of the TM. A. Normal: The normal TM is slanted downward and forward; its surface glistens and contains a brilliant triangle, the light reflex, with its apex at the center, or umbo, and its base at the annuals. The handle of the malleus makes an impression on the disk from the umbo upward and forward. **B. The retracted eardrum:** The light reflex is bent, and the malleus stands out in sharper relief than normally. **C. Serous middle ear fluid:** Hairline menisci curve from the handle of the malleus to the annulus. **D. Bulging drumhead:** The curves in the membrane obscure the normal landmarks of the malleus and distort the light reflex. **E. Serous fluid mixed with air:** Bubbles may be seen through the drumhead. **F. Perforations** of the membrane appear as oval holes with a dark shadow behind.

Ear: Acute otitis media, acute mastoiditis, cholesteatoma, malignant disease; *Referred Pain* through CNs-V, IX, and X and the second and third cervical nerves: Unerupted lower third molar, carious teeth, TMJ arthritis, tonsillitis, carcinoma or sarcoma of pharynx, ulcer of epiglottis or larynx, cervical lymphadenitis, subacute thyroiditis, trigeminal neuralgia.

Dizziness and vertigo. See page 245.

Eye Symptoms

Double vision—diplopia. Perception of two visual images results from refraction abnormalities or, less commonly, nonconjugative gaze. Determine the symptom pattern (e.g., vertical or horizontal), precipitating activities, visual axis where diplopia occurs, and head position or gaze giving relief. If the patient reports *monocular diplopia* or diplopia when one eye is covered, the cause is nearly always refractive. *Binocular diplopia*: see Chapter 14, page 653.

Dry eyes. See Keratoconjunctivitis sicca, page 241.

Blurred vision. Inability to sharply focus light on the retina is caused by failure of accommodation, i.e., altering lens shape for near and far vision, or light scattering by cornea, lens, or vitreous opacities. History is the key to identifying the etiology. Eye pain suggests inflammation (keratitis, iritis, and uveitis) or acute angle closure glaucoma. Abnormality of the oils in the tear film is a frequent cause of visual aberration. Use of topical and systemic drugs, especially anticholinergics, dilate the pupil and decreases accommodation. Unilateral vision loss may also be described as "blurred vision," meaning vision is less distinct than normal without binocular sight. The pinhole test (page 180) is used to determine if the blurred vision is refractive.

Eye pain. Eye pain is caused by inflammation, infection, trauma, and increased intraocular pressure. Inspect the lids, conjunctivae, and sclera for lesions. Careful examination of the cornea, anterior chamber, iris, and retina are mandatory. Always assess visual acuity in each eye. Optimal examination requires an ophthalmologist.

CLINICAL OCCURRENCE: *Degenerative/Idiopathic:* Cluster headache; *Infectious:* Infective keratitis (herpes simplex, zoster, and others), sinusitis (ethmoid, frontal, sphenoid); *Inflammatory/Immune:* Hordeolum (sty), chalazion, interstitial keratitis, iritis, iridocyclitis, episcleritis, scleritis, band keratopathy, optic neuritis; *Mechanical/Traumatic:* Foreign body, corneal abrasion, entropion, glaucoma, eye strain.

Vision loss. Injury or impairment to any portion of the visual pathways causes vision loss. Acute vision loss is a medical emergency (see page 243). Chronic progressive vision loss is common with diseases of the cornea, lens, or retina. Standard tests of visual acuity will quantitate the impairment and formal visual field testing is required. Ophthalmology referral is indicated.

Nose Symptoms

Loss of smell—anosmia. See page 218.

Abnormal smell or taste—dysgeusia. This is a common complaint in patients who have loss of smell (*anosmia*). If it is paroxysmal and associated with behavioral symptoms, it suggests complex partial seizures.

Lip, Mouth, Tongue, Teeth, and Pharynx Symptoms
Sore throat. See syndromes, pharyngitis, page 250.

Tongue or mouth soreness. Pain or tenderness in the tongue or mouth is evaluated by inspection and palpation.

CLINICAL OCCURRENCE: *No Lesions:* Tobacco smoking, early glossitis from all causes, menopausal symptom, heavy metal poisoning; *Deep Lesions:* Calculus in duct of submaxillary or sublingual gland, foreign body, myositis of lingual muscles, trichinosis, periostitis of hyoid bone, neoplasm of lingual muscles; *Localized Superficial Lesions:* Tongue biting, trauma to lingual frenulum, dental ulcer, injury while under anesthesia, foreign body (e.g., fish bone), epithelioma or carcinoma, ranula, tuberculous ulcer, herpes, Vincent stomatitis, leukoplakia, thrush; *Generalized Disease:* Irradiation, pellagra, riboflavin deficiency, scurvy, pernicious anemia, atrophic glossitis, leukemia, exanthematous disorders, collagen diseases, pemphigus, cicatricial pemphigoid, lichen planus, heavy-metal poisoning, phenytoin, uremia, cancer chemotherapy, drug sensitivity, systemic fungal infections, e.g., histoplasmosis.

Irradiation injury. Therapeutic irradiation for head and neck malignancy causes temporary or permanent loss of saliva production. Within 2–4 weeks of the beginning of treatment, and lasting 6 or more weeks, patients experience increasing dryness and generalized soreness of the mouth and throat.

Difficult or painful swallowing—dysphagia and odynophagia. Swallowing disorders are *dysphagias*. With *oropharyngeal dysphagia*, the patient describes difficulty initiating a swallow or choking and coughing with swallowing. With *esophageal dysphagia*, the patient experiences a sense of obstruction at a definite level when fluid or a food bolus is swallowed. *Neurogenic dysphagia* is accompanied by regurgitation through the nose. Some dysphagias cause localized pain (*odynophagia*); others are painless. Deglutition involves muscles in the oropharynx and esophagus. Pain from the oropharynx is accurately localized, but esophageal pain is dispersed in the thoracic six-dermatome band, presenting as chest pain (see Chapter 8, page 292 and Chapter 9, page 411).

CLINICAL OCCURRENCE: *Oropharynx—Painful Intrinsic Lesions:* Glossitis, tonsillitis, stomatitis, pharyngitis, laryngitis, lingual ulcer, carcinoma, pemphigus, erythema multiforme, Ludwig angina, mumps, bee sting on the tongue, angioedema, candidiasis, Plummer–Vinson syndrome; *Painful Local Extrinsic Lesions:* Cervical adenitis, subacute thyroiditis, carotid arteritis, infected thyroglossal cysts or sinuses, pharyngeal cysts or sinuses, carotid body tumor, spur in cervical spine, pericarditis; *Painful Systemic Conditions:* Rabies, tetanus; *Painless Intrinsic Lesions:* Cleft palate, neck flexion from cervical osteoporosis, xerostomia in Sjögren syndrome, magnesium deficiency; *Painless Neurogenic Lesions:* CN-IX or CN-X damage, globus hystericus, postdiphtheritic paralysis, bulbar paralysis, West Nile virus, myasthenia gravis, amyotrophic lateral sclerosis, Wilson disease, syphilis, parkinsonism, botulism, poisoning (lead, alcohol, fluoride); *Esophagus—Painful Intrinsic Lesions: (see Chapter 8 pages 292–293 and Chapter 9 page 411)* Foreign body, carcinoma, esophagitis, diverticulum, hiatal hernia; *Painless Intrinsic Lesions:* Achalasia, congenital stricture, stricture, scleroderma, dermatomyositis; Sjögren syndrome, amyloidosis, thyrotoxicosis; *Painless Extrinsic Lesions:* Aortic aneurysm, aberrant right subclavian artery (page 252), vertebral spurs, enlarged left atrium.

Larynx Symptoms
Hoarseness. See page 232.

Salivary Gland Symptoms
Dry mouth—xerostomia. See page 255.

Neck Symptoms
Neck pain. Neck pain is often readily diagnosed by a careful history, neck palpation, and oropharyngeal exam. Posttraumatic and postural cervical strain are most common. Palpate each anatomic structure systematically. Pain increasing with specific movements helps to localize the pain's source.

CLINICAL OCCURRENCE: *Neck Pain Increased by Swallowing—Pharynx:* Pharyngitis, Ludwig angina, inflamed thyroglossal duct or cyst; *Tonsils:* Tonsillitis, neoplasm; *Tongue:* Ulcers, neoplasm; *Larynx:* Laryngitis, neoplasm, ulcer, foreign body; *Esophagus:* Inflamed diverticulum, esophagitis; *Thyroid:* Suppurative or subacute thyroiditis, hemorrhage; *Carotid artery:* Carotodynia, carotid body tumor; *Salivary glands:* Mumps, suppurative parotitis; *Neck Pain Increased by Chewing—Mandible:* Fracture, osteomyelitis, periodontitis; *Salivary Glands:* Mumps, suppurative parotitis; *Neck Pain Increased by Head Movements—Sternocleidomastoid:* Torticollis, hematoma; *Neck Muscles:* Viral myalgia, muscle tension; *Cervical Spine:* Herniated intervertebral disk, spinal arthritis, meningitis, meningismus, craniovertebral junction abnormalities; *Neck Pain Increased by Shoulder Movement—Superior Thoracic Aperture:* Cervical rib, scalenus anticus syndrome, costoclavicular syndrome; *Neck Pain Not Increased by Movement—Skin and Subcutaneous Tissues:* Furuncle, carbuncle, erysipelas; *Lymph Nodes:* Acute adenitis. *Deep Veins:* Septic thrombophlebitis of the internal jugular vein (Lemmiere syndrome); *Branchial Cleft Remnants:* Inflamed pharyngeal cyst; *Salivary Glands:* Duct calculus; *Subclavian Artery:* aneurysm; *Nervous System:* Poliomyelitis, West Nile virus, herpes zoster, epidural abscess, spinal cord neoplasm; *Spinal Vertebrae:* Herniated intervertebral disk, metastatic carcinoma; *Referred Pain:* Pancoast syndrome, angina pectoris, and other conditions in the six-dermatome band.

Carotodynia. Constant or throbbing pain in the anterior lateral neck intensifies with swallowing. It may radiate to the mandible or ear. Symptoms frequently follow viral pharyngitis with fever. Some patients have profound lassitude. Several relapses may occur within a few months. The carotid bulb is exquisitely tender and may seem enlarged with exaggerated pulsations; the common carotid may be tender as well. Carotid compression causes radiating pain along external carotid branches to the jaw, ear, and temple (*Fay sign*). One or both common carotid arteries is/are involved. The pharynx and larynx are normal or have slight hyperemia and edema. Carotid artery tenderness is diagnostic.

Neck fullness. Goiters cause a sense of constriction or fullness in the neck. See page 256.

HEAD AND NECK SIGNS

Scalp, Face, Skull, and Jaw Signs

Scalp wounds. The scalp is extremely vascular so scalp wounds bleed profusely. Gaping wounds have penetrated the galea aponeurotica and may contain an open skill fracture.

Fluctuant scalp mass—hematoma, abscess, fracture. Blood or pus accumulating in the skin or subcutaneously form a discreet soft mass sliding readily over the skull. Blood or pus under an adult aponeurosis forms a boggy, fluctuant mass covering the entire scalp. A fluctuant mass bounded by the skull suture lines indicates subperiosteal blood or pus or a depressed fracture. A subperiosteal hematoma usually has a soft plastic center and firm edges, feeling much like a depressed fracture.

Scalp cellulitis. The scalp is tender, soft, and boggy. Infection expands rapidly causing edema of the eyelids and pinnae. Regional lymph nodes are swollen and tender.

Sebaceous cyst (wen). Arising from the skin, single or multiple cysts slide easily over the skull. Each is firm, nontender, and often hemispheric. Infected cysts bleed easily and may be mistaken for squamous cell carcinoma.

Scalp mass—lipoma. A smooth, soft, mobile, discreet subcutaneous mass, the finger slides easily around its edges. When beneath the pericranium, movement is limited, but palpation detects the smooth, rounded border.

Parotid enlargement. See page 234.

Preauricular abscess. A suppurating preauricular lymph node produces an abscess that may ulcerate. The swelling is localized, tender, and sometimes warm. The source of infection is in the side of the face, pinna, anterior wall of the external acoustic meatus, anterior third of the scalp, eyebrows, or eyelids.

Masseter muscle hypertrophy. Spontaneous hypertrophy of one or both masseter muscles produces facial swelling mimicking parotid gland swelling. If the entire mass hardens when the patient clenches his teeth, it is muscular.

Cheek erythema. Erythema, scaling, pustules, and tenderness in a malar distribution occur with sunburn, cellulitis, rosacea, seborrheic dermatitis, discoid or systemic lupus erythematosus (SLE), or acne vulgaris.

Forehead wrinkles. Absence of normal transverse furrowing with upward gaze is a sign of hyperthyroidism. Deep wrinkling, with longitudinal furrowing and prominence of intervening tissue is the *bulldog skin* of pachydermatosis. Unilateral loss of wrinkling results from paralysis of muscles innervated by the facial nerve (CN-VII).

Enlarged adult skull—Paget disease. See Chapter 13, page 590. In addition to bone pain, the patient complains of hats becoming too small. The calvarium is large compared with the facial bones. A bruit is sometimes heard in the skull.

Mastoid pain and tenderness—mastoiditis. See page 244.

Skull masses—neoplasms. Osteomas, frequent in the skull's outer table, produce a hard, sessile bony eminence. Pericranial sarcoma, metastatic carcinoma, lymphoma, leukemia, or multiple myeloma can present as a hard or soft cranial bone mass.

Trismus. Trismus is tight jaw closure from spasm of the masticatory muscles. Trismus, common with tetanus, has many other more common causes.
    CLINICAL OCCURRENCE: *Local Disorders:* Impacted third molar, TMJ arthritis, malignant external otitis, lymphadenitis, trigeminal neuralgia, scleroderma, dermatomyositis; *Disorders with Widespread Muscle Spasm:* Trichinosis, rabies, tetany, tetanus, strychnine poisoning, typhoid fever, cholera, septicemia; *Cerebral Disorders:* Encephalitis, epilepsy (transient), catalepsy, hysteria, malingering.

Inability to close the jaw—TMJ dislocation. Because the TMJ is a shallow biconcave surface, it easily partially subluxes or completely dislocates. The jaw won't close after a yawn or receipt of an upward blow on the chin with the mouth wide open. The mandible protrudes, the lower teeth overriding the uppers. There is a depression or pit anterior to the tragus that is more obvious when bilateral. In unilateral dislocation, the pretragal depression occurs only on the affected side. No movement of the mandibular head is felt when palpating through the external acoustic meatus on the affected side.

External Ear Signs

Earlobe crease. A visible crease extending at least one-third of the distance from tragus to posterior pinna is associated with a higher rate of cardiac events in hospital admissions with suspected coronary heart disease.

Earlobe nodule: gouty tophus. In long-standing gout, sodium urate crystals accumulate in the helix and antihelix, the olecranon bursa, tendon sheaths, and aponeuroses of the extremities. The nodules are painless, hard, and irregular. They may open discharging chalky contents.

Darwin tubercle. This is a harmless developmental eminence in the upper third of the posterior helix that must be distinguished from acquired nodules, such as tophi.

Other nodules. Nontender nodules may be basal cell carcinomas, rheumatoid nodules, or leprosy. Cartilage calcification is a rare complication of Addison disease.

Hematoma. Trauma or a hemostatic defect results in blood accumulating between the cartilage and the perichondrium as a tender, blue, doughy mass, usually without spontaneous pain. Prompt incision and drainage avoid suppuration or cauliflower ear.

Recurring inflammation—relapsing polychondritis. There is inflammation and degeneration of cartilage especially of the pinna, nasal septum, laryngeal cartilages, tracheal and bronchial rings; joint cartilages may be affected. The ear is painful, swollen, and reddened, except over the lobule. Hoarseness indicates laryngeal involvement and blindness results from involvement of the sclerae, and tinnitus and deafness from middle ear involvement. Rarely, aortic or mitral valve ring degeneration produces valvular regurgitation or aortic aneurysm.

Dermoid cyst. A favorite site is just behind the pinna. It is soft and slightly fluctuant.

External Acoustic Meatus Signs

Cerumen impaction. The wax of Native Americans and East Asians is often dry and flakey, and more yellow than amber. Excessive wax production or a narrow meatus leads to impacted cerumen and partial or complete canal obstruction. Complete obstruction causes partial deafness; tinnitus or dizziness may occur. Partial obstructions can suddenly become complete when water enters the meatus during bathing or swimming. The obstructing wax is easily seen in the external meatus.

Ear discharge—otorrhea. Ear discharge has many causes, the type suggesting the diagnosis: *Yellow Discharge:* Melting cerumen; *Serous Discharge:* Eczema, early ruptured acute otitis media; *Bloody Discharge:* External canal trauma or longitudinal temporal bone fracture with TM and external canal laceration; *Purulent Discharge:* Chronic external otitis, perforating acute suppurative otitis media, chronic suppurative or tuberculous otitis media with or without cholesteatoma.

External otitis. See page 243.

Dermatitis. Seborrheic dermatitis commonly causes scaling and pruritus of the choana and meatus. Medicated eardrops can cause contact dermatitis.

Carcinoma. Either squamous cell or basal cell carcinoma can involve the meatal epithelium. Pain and discharge are presenting symptoms, with deafness and facial paralysis occurring in advanced disease.

Foreign body. Children often place objects in their ears. A purulent discharge from the canal or an earache may be the first indication.

Polyps. A bulbous, reddened, pedunculated mass arising from the canal wall or middle ear is associated with a foul purulent discharge. Moving it with forceps may reveal the origin.

Exostoses and chondromas. Exostoses form nodules in the osseous canal near the TM. They rarely produce obstruction, although the TM may be partially obscured. A single bony osteoma may occur. Rarely, chondromas arise from the cartilaginous canal, usually without obstruction.

Furuncle. A red, tender prominence with or without a pustule forms in the cartilaginous canal producing extreme pain.

Vesicles. Pain in the ear with vesicles in the canal and facial weakness is caused by herpes zoster of CN-VII (Ramsey–Hunt Syndrome), Chapter 14, Facial Weakness and Paralysis, pages 665–666.

TM Signs

Retracted TM. See Otitis Media with Effusion, page 244.

Red or bulging TM. See Acute Suppurative Otitis Media, page 244.

Vesicles on the TM. *Mycoplasma pneumoniae* infection causes severe ear pain and an inflamed TM often with hemorrhagic vesicles (*bullous myringitis*).

Perforated TM. A healed suppurative middle ear infection eroded through the TM leaving an oval hole through which the middle ear cavity is seen. Chronic perforations are asymptomatic other than mildly decreased auditory acuity.

Hearing Signs

Lateralizing Weber test—ipsilateral conductive hearing loss or contra-lateral neurosensory loss. When neurosensory hearing is intact bilaterally, sound lateralizes to the side of conductive loss that has lost the masking effect of background noise. Neurosensory loss on one side results in a *louder* sound on the opposite side. Therefore, lateralization of sound to the right ear means conductive loss on the right or perceptive loss on the left.

Bone conduction greater than air conduction (Rinne-negative test)—conductive hearing loss. When amplification of sound by the TM and ossicles is impaired, direct transmission of vibrations to the cochlea through bone appears louder than sound transmitted through air. Conductive hearing loss results from auditory canal obstruction, TM damage, middle ear fluid, and destruction or ankylosis of the ossicles.

Balance and position sense signs. See Chapter 14, page 671.

Eye Lid Signs

Lacrimation, tearing. Although strictly speaking an overproduction of tears, lacrimation usually refers to any condition resulting in tears. *Epiphora* means an overflow of tears from any cause.
CLINICAL OCCURRENCE: *Increased Secretion:* Weeping from emotion, foreign body irritation, corneal ulcer, conjunctivitis, coryza, measles, hay fever, poisoning (iodide, bromide, arsenic); *Lacrimal Duct Obstruction:* Congenital, cicatrix, eyelid edema, lacrimal calculus, dacryocystitis; *Puncta Separation from the Globe:* Facial paralysis, aging, chronic marginal blepharitis, ectropion, proptosis.

Widened palpebral fissures. The fissures are widened by lid retraction (contraction of Mueller muscle) or protrusion of the globe. Normally, with eyes in the primary position, the upper lid covers the limbus and a white scleral strip usually shows between limbus and lower lid. Widening of the palpebral fissure uncovers the upper border of the limbus exposing white sclera superiorly. When there is no actual proptosis, widened fissures produce the optical illusion of global protrusion. A few normal persons have widened palpebral fissures.

Exophthalmos, ocular proptosis. Proptosis is diagnosed by measurement. If both eyes seem equally prominent, inspect them in profile (Fig. 7-29). Unilateral proptosis is recognized by comparing the two eyes and suggests orbital tumor or inflammation. Displacement medially suggests lacrimal gland disease, upwards suggests maxillary sinus disease, and laterally implies ethmoid or sphenoid sinus disease. Graves disease is the most common cause of bilateral proptosis.
CLINICAL OCCURRENCE: *Unilateral Exophthalmos:* Graves disease, mucocele, orbital cellulitis and abscess, cavernous sinus thrombosis, orbital periostitis, myxedema, orbital fracture, hemangioma, orbital neoplasm, arteriovenous aneurysm, fungal infection, histiocytosis; *Bilateral Exophthalmos:* Graves disease, myxedema, acromegaly, cavernous sinus thrombosis, empyema of the sinuses, lymphoma, leukemia, histiocytosis.

Lid lag. Thyrotoxicosis increases sympathetic stimulation producing contraction of Mueller muscle in the upper lid. Lid lag indicates increased tone, even without widened fissures in the primary position. It is usually bilateral and occasionally one fissure is much wider than the other.

Other lid signs of hyperthyroidism. Stellwag Sign: Infrequent blinking; *Rosenbach Sign:* Tremor of the closed eyelids; *Mean Sign:* Globe lags during elevation; *Griffith Sign:* Lower lids lag during globe elevation; *Boston Sign:* Jerking of the lagging lid; *Joffroy Sign:* Absence of forehead wrinkling with upward gaze, the head tilting down.

Narrowed palpebral fissures—enophthalmos. The globe is recessed in the orbit. When bilateral, it is usually caused by decreased orbital fat or congenital microphthalmos. Unilateral enophthalmos results from trauma or inflammation. The drooping eyelid in *Horner syndrome* produces an optical illusion of globe recession.

Failure of lid closure—paralysis of orbicularis muscle. Damage to the facial nerve (CN-VII) supplying the orbicularis oculi muscle, as in Bell

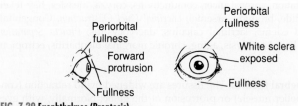

FIG. 7-29 Exophthalmos (Proptosis).

palsy, causes partial or complete orbicularis paralysis. When complete, both upper and lower lids remain retracted, so the eye is unprotected, and tears drain onto the face. *Bell phenomenon* is elevation of the globe while attempting lid closure. Severe exophthalmos also prevents complete lid closure.

Failure of lid opening—lid ptosis. Congenital ptosis is usually bilateral from either paralysis of or failure to develop the levator palpebrae superioris. Acute acquired ptosis usually results from oculomotor nerve (CN-III) disease. In congenital ptosis there is lid lag as the child looks down. With CN-III lesion, paralysis of other eye muscles may be present.

CLINICAL OCCURRENCE: Supranuclear lesions (e.g., encephalitis), Horner syndrome, levator paralysis, levator dehiscence, thinning of levator tendon (the lid droops but has normal excursion, 15–18 mm).

Blepharospasm. Unilateral or bilateral spasmodic lid closure, a focal dystonia, may interfere with function. Unilateral blepharospasm may follow Bell palsy.

Epicanthal fold—Down syndrome. See page 242.

Shortened palpebral fissures—fetal alcohol syndrome. Shortened palpebral fissures, epicanthic folds, shortened nose with anteverted nostrils, hypoplastic upper lip with thinned vermilion and flattened or absent philtrum, together with mental retardation, are stigmata of fetal alcohol syndrome.

Lid inversion—entropion. Structural changes or muscular contraction turns the eyelashes inward to impinge upon the globe. Spastic entropion, caused by increased orbicularis oculi tone, occurs only in the lower lids. The lid turns in only when forcibly closed (Fig. 7-30A). Cicatricial entropion occurs in either lid from contracture of scar tissue, as in trachoma. Irritation from the inverted eyelashes may cause blepharospasm.

Lid eversion—ectropion. The lid turns outward (Fig. 7-30B). Both lids can be affected by spastic or cicatricial ectropion, but paralytic ectropion only involves the lower lid. Senile tissue atrophy sometimes results in ectropion rather than entropion.

Violaceous lids. Heliotrope or violaceous discoloration of the periorbital skin occurs in dermatomyositis.

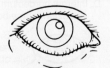 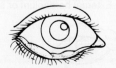

A. Entropion   B. Ectropion

FIG. 7-30 Pathologic Inversion and Eversion of the Eyelids.

Lid erythema. Generalized reddening of the lids is nonspecific. Erythema of the nasal half of the upper lid suggests frontal sinus inflammation. Lacrimal sac disease causes erythema of the medial lower lid. Hyperemia of the temporal upper lid suggests dacryoadenitis. The lid is frequently red over a sty.

Lid cyanosis. Blueness of the eyelid is caused by orbital vein thrombosis, orbital tumors, and orbital arteriovenous malformations.

Lid hemorrhage. Blood extravasating into surrounding tissue after lid trauma is colloquially known as a "black eye." A palpebral hematoma results from a nasal fracture. The appearance of hematoma many hours after head trauma suggests a skull fracture; the greater the time interval, the more remote the fracture site. Basal skull fractures produce a lid hematoma several days after the event. Involvement of both eyes is *raccoon sign*.

Lid edema. Noninflammatory edema is frequent in acute nephritis, but uncommon in chronic nephritis and cardiac failure (Fig. 7-31A). Lid edema is an early sign of myxedema and Graves ophthalmopathy. Lid edema is frequent in angioedema and trichinosis. Contact dermatitis frequently involves the lids. The skin on the hands may not react to the allergen, but when transferred to the lids swelling occurs. Local infections cause inflammatory lid edema, readily identified by redness, warmth, and pain. Sagittal sinus and cavernous sinus thrombosis are less common but serious causes of lid edema.

Xanthelasma. Xanthelasma are raised yellow, painless, and nonpruritic plaques on the upper and lower lids near the inner canthi frequently associated with elevated cholesterol (Fig. 7-31B). They grow slowly and may disappear spontaneously.

Blepharitis. Seborrheic blepharitis is an oily inflammation of the lid margins producing greasy flakes of dried secretion on the eyelashes and reddening

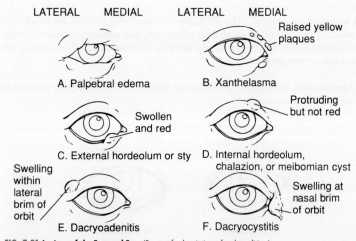

LATERAL   MEDIAL   LATERAL   MEDIAL

A. Palpebral edema   B. Xanthelasma — Raised yellow plaques

C. External hordeolum or sty — Swollen and red   D. Internal hordeolum, chalazion, or meibomian cyst — Protruding but not red

E. Dacryoadenitis — Swelling within lateral brim of orbit   F. Dacryocystitis — Swelling at nasal brim of orbit

FIG. 7-31 Lesions of the External Eye. (See text for descriptions of each condition.)

of the lid margins. Ulceration of the lid margin is usually *staphylococcal blepharitis*. In *angular blepharitis*, caused by the diplococcus of Morax–Axenfeld (*Moraxella lacunata*), the lid margins near the temporal canthi are inflamed.

External hordeolum (sty). An eyelash follicle sebaceous gland is inflamed forming a pustule on the lid margin (Fig. 7-31C). It may be surrounded by hyperemia and swelling. Many rupture and heal spontaneously.

Internal hordeolum and meibomian cyst (chalazion). An internal hordeolum or internal sty is acute inflammation of a meibomian (tarsal) gland. A chalazion or meibomian cyst is a granuloma of the gland (Fig. 7-31D). These internal sebaceous gland lesions produce localized swelling frequently causing a protrusion on the lid. Everting the lid reveals hyperemia, a localized cyst, or enlarged gland.

Dacryoadenitis. Lacrimal duct obstruction leads to acute lacrimal gland inflammation with pain and tenderness at the temporal edge of the orbit. It must be distinguished from orbital cellulitis and upper lid hordeolum (Fig. 7-31E).

Dacryocystitis. Nasolacrimal duct obstruction leads to inflammation and infection presenting as pain and overflow of tears onto the cheek (*epiphora*). Symptoms are increased by irritants such as wind, dust, or smoke. Tenderness, swelling, and redness are present near the medial canthus beside the nose (Fig. 7-31F). Swelling anterior to the eyelid distinguishes it from hordeolum. Fluid can be expressed with pressure on the duct. Conjunctivitis, blepharitis, and lid edema may be present.

Eye Movement Signs: Eye movement abnormalities are caused by either primary extraocular muscle disease or disease of the central nervous system and cranial nerves. Because distinguishing neurologic from primary muscle disease is critical, these signs are discussed with the neurologic examination in Chapter 14, Eye Movement Signs, page 657.

Restricted motion. Globe movement is restricted in all directions by tumors in the orbit or increased orbital contents with Graves disease.

Glaucoma. See page 242.

Conjunctiva Signs

Subconjunctival vessels. The scleral vessels are prominent in some normal individuals, running in from the sides (Fig. 7-32A).

Subconjunctival hemorrhage. Bleeding under the conjunctiva is obvious and harmless (Fig. 7-32B). It can be induced by coughing, sneezing, weight lifting, or defecation. Frequently, the cause is not apparent.

Conjunctival injection. Mild diffuse capillary hyperemia of the scleral and palpebral conjunctivae, without hemorrhage, is common in the coryza phase of respiratory infections and from exposure to direct sunlight or

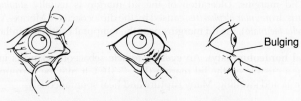

A. Scleral vessels   B. Subconjunctival   C. Chemosis
                          hemorrhage

FIG. 7-32 Vascular Disorders of the External Eye. A. Scleral vessels: These are the most prominent vessels seen normally. **B. Subconjunctival hemorrhage:** Bright-red superficial blotches show through the sclera. They appear suddenly and painlessly. **C. Chemosis:** The conjunctival edema may be demonstrated by pressing the lower lid against the globe, producing a bulge in the boggy global conjunctiva above the point of compression.

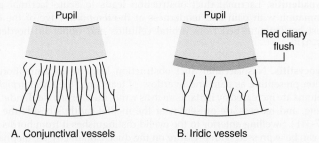

A. Conjunctival vessels   B. Iridic vessels

FIG. 7-33 Hyperemia and Congestion of the Globe. A. Hyperemic scleral vessels are superficial, coursing radially from the periphery to the limbus in tortuous branches. **B. Iritis:** The vessels of the iris are deeper; when congested, individual vessels are not visible, but they produce a pink or red band around the limbus, the ciliary flush.

environmental irritants. It may be mildly uncomfortable. Significant pruritus, pain, or discharge suggests another disorder, e.g., allergic conjunctivitis.

Conjunctival edema—chemosis. The conjunctiva is swollen and transparent, usually in association with lid edema. The edema is demonstrated by inspecting the globe in profile while pressing the lower lid against the bulbar conjunctiva; the lid edge pushes up a wave of edematous bulbar conjunctiva (Fig. 7-32C). This is frequent in Graves ophthalmopathy.

Globe hyperemia and ciliary flush. Dilation of the radial conjunctival vessels and their branches, running from the fornices toward the center of the cornea, causes bulbar conjunctival injection (Fig. 7-33A). Dilation of the deeper, net-like episcleral vessels produces more violaceous injection, noted as ciliary flush at the corneal limbus (Fig. 7-33B). Conjunctival suffusion blanches with pressure; the ciliary flush does not blanch. Ciliary flush indicates uveal tract inflammation (see page 242).

Conjunctivitis. Inflammation of the conjunctiva, regardless of cause, is conjunctivitis. The patient may awaken with eyelids stuck shut and a gritty or

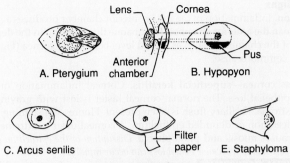

FIG. 7-34 Lesions of the Cornea and Iris. A. Pterygium: This abnormal growth of the pinguecula appears as a raised, subconjunctival fatty structure, growing in a horizontal band toward a position over the pupil. **B. Hypopyon:** A collection of pus in the lowest part of the anterior chamber between the cornea and the iris. **C. Arcus senilis:** A gray, opaque, circular band in the cornea, separated from the limbus by a narrow, clear zone. **D. Assessment of lacrimation:** The Schirmer test, see page 178. **E. Staphyloma:** Anterior protrusion of the cornea or sclera.

burning sensation with excessive lacrimation. There is marked hyperemia of the palpebral and peripheral global conjunctival vessels in one or both eyes. The many causes include viral and bacterial infections, foreign–body reaction, allergies, and blepharitis. *DDX:* Purulent discharge increases the probability for bacterial infection; itching suggests a nonbacterial etiology.

Hyperemic conjunctiva with calcification. Lesions appear when the serum calcium–phosphorus product exceeds 70 in renal failure and sarcoidosis. *Conjunctiva lesions:* The segments from limbus to canthus at 7 to 10 o'clock and at 2 to 5 o'clock show hyperemic reddening, calcified plaques, and pingueculae. The eyes are painful or feel gritty. The affected areas contain calcium deposits, visible to the unaided eye or through the slit lamp. *Cornea lesions:* White material is visible in limbal arcs at 2 to 5 o'clock and 7 to 10 o'clock. This *band keratopathy* occurs with hypercalcemia and in renal disease with conjunctival calcification. The slit lamp reveals calcium deposits.

Pterygium. Chronic irritation from wind and dust stimulates growth of the pinguecula resulting in extension of a vascular membrane over the limbus toward the center of the cornea. Usually bilateral, the resulting pterygium is a raised, subconjunctival fatty structure, growing horizontally toward and over the pupil (Fig. 7-34A), possibly obstructing vision. Its firm attachment to the bulbar surface is strictly horizontal. A *pseudopterygium* is a band of scar tissue extending in any direction and only partially adhering to the bulbar conjunctiva, so a probe can pass beneath it.

Pigmented pingueculae. Brownish pigmentation of the pingueculae is a sign of Gaucher disease. Others are hepatosplenomegaly, thrombocytopenic purpura, and patchy brown pigmentation on the face and the legs.

Cornea Signs

Hypopyon. Inflammation in the iris or anterior chamber produces a purulent discharge in the anterior chamber. The opaque fluid settling in the dependent portion of the chamber is seen as a fluid level behind the cornea (Fig. 7-34B). Iritis is a common cause.

Lusterless cornea—superficial keratitis. Corneal inflammation or drying causes epithelial loss. The normal corneal luster is lost with graying of the anterior stroma. A ciliary flush is often present. Fluorescein staining demonstrates ulceration or denuded epithelium. A corneal ulcer is extremely painful and causes miosis and photophobia. *Disruption of the epithelium demands urgent expert therapy, because visual loss can occur rapidly.*
     CLINICAL OCCURRENCE: Among the many causes of superficial keratitis are contact lens-related ulcers, infected abrasions, herpes simplex and zoster, corneal exposure, trigeminal nerve (CN-V) injury, amiodarone deposits, and infection spreading from the conjunctiva.

Cloudy cornea—interstitial keratitis. Interstitial keratitis, deafness, and notched teeth constitute the *Hutchinson triad* of congenital syphilis. Between ages 5 and 15 years, faint central zone opacity is accompanied by a ciliary flush, pain and lacrimation. Later, the cornea becomes diffusely clouded, obscuring the iris. Blood vessels grow into the cornea. Corneal opacity is permanent. Acquired syphilis and tuberculosis are occasional causes.

Arcus senilis. A gray opaque band, 1.0–1.5-mm wide, is separated from the limbus by a narrow clear zone (Fig. 7-34C). Initially, only a segment of the circumference is affected, later the circle is completed. It is present bilaterally in many persons >60 years of age. If seen before age 40, suspect hyperlipidemia.

Keratoconjunctivitis sicca—Sjögren syndrome. Lymphocytes infiltrate lacrimal and salivary exocrine glands reducing tear flow leading to dry inflamed eyes. Sjögren syndrome is likely if persistent dry eyes, dry mouth, and a positive Schirmer test (page 178 and Fig. 7-34D) are present without obvious cause. HIV infection and sarcoidosis can produce similar findings.

Kayser–Fleischer ring—Wilson disease. Copper deposited in the basement membrane of the cornea's endothelium is seen as a 2-mm-wide golden-brown circular band in the peripheral cornea near the limbus. Beginning superiorly, it spreads inferiorly. The neurologic manifestations of Wilson disease occur simultaneously. A slit lamp is often required to see the ring.

Central corneal opacity. This results from trauma or infection and is seen in 75% of patients with Hurler syndrome.

Dots in the cornea—Fanconi syndrome. Cysteine crystals are deposited throughout the stroma without an inflammatory reaction.

Sclera Signs

Yellow sclera—icterus and fat. In obstructive jaundice (Chapter 9, page 414) conjugated bilirubin colors the sclera evenly. The thicker conjunctiva in the fornices is usually deeper yellow. Fat deposits beneath the conjunctiva commonly impart a yellow color to the periphery, leaving the perilimbal area relatively white. This is more obvious with advancing age and anemia.

Red sclera—scleritis and episcleritis. Inflammation of the sclera and/or Tenon capsule reduces scleral integrity. *Scleritis,* diffuse or nodular, is frequently associated with autoimmune diseases. Patients have severe, deep, boring pain. In sunlight, lesions appear red–purple. Suppurative scleritis is rare and usually metastatic. Tuberculosis, sarcoidosis, and syphilis cause granulomatous scleritis with localized scleral elevation and nodules. Scleral thinning may be non-necrotizing or necrotizing (*scleromalacia perforans*) with acute inflammation surrounding an area of ischemia which may ulcerate. *Episcleritis* is milder inflammation involving the globe's fascial sheath (*Tenon capsule*) appearing clinically as diffuse or nodular violaceous injection (Fig. 7-35).

Blue sclera—osteogenesis imperfecta. Light reflecting off the pigmented choroid appears blue through the thinned sclera. This finding is classic for osteogenesis imperfecta. It may be mimicked by minocycline deposits, scleral thinning after scleritis, or age-related calcification of the horizontal rectus muscle insertions.

Brown sclera—melanin or homogentisic acid. Patches of melanin are commonly seen on the conjunctiva of dark-complexioned people, especially blacks. In alkaptonuria with ochronosis, wedge-shaped areas of homogentisic acid, with their apices toward the limbus, color the sclera brown near the ocular muscles attachments.

Scleral protrusion—staphyloma. Injury to the sclera and/or increased intraocular pressure lead to a protrusion from the surface of the globe. An anterior staphyloma forming near the cornea creates a characteristic profile (Fig. 7-34E).

Pupil Signs: See Chapter 14, The Neurologic Examination, page 624.

Lens Signs
Cataract. Discoloration or disruption of the layers of the lens produces focal or diffuse opacities that obstruct and/or scatter light before it reaches the retina. Because nearly all adults have some lens opacity, a clinical definition of

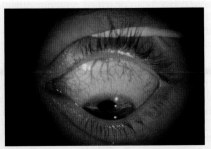

FIG. 7-35 Episcleritis. Because the episcleral vessels lie below the conjunctival vessels, the dilated episcleral arterioles in episcleritis and uveitis has a violet hue.

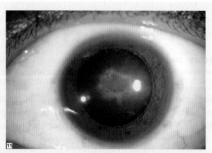

FIG. 7-36 Posterior Subcapsular Cataract. This cataract is just inside the posterior lens capsule. The melanosis of the sclera is a normal variant in African Americans.

cataract implies interference with vision. Some cataracts are seen by shining a light beam obliquely through the lens (*focal illumination*), by ophthalmoscopic inspection against the red retinal reflex with 0 diopter magnification from ~40 cm (15.7 inch), or by using + 10 diopter magnification with close inspection (*direct illumination*). Many are only identified by slit lamp. Centrally placed cataracts are seen without pupillary dilatation; those in the periphery are only visualized with dilation. *This discussion is limited to cataracts detectable without mydriatics or a slit lamp.*

Anterior and posterior polar cataract. A small congenital white plaque is seen in the center of the pupil resulting from a congenital defect in the anterior or posterior capsule.

Nuclear cataract. Yellow to brown discoloration, appearing first in the central lens, gradually becomes diffuse throughout the lens. A central black spot is seen against the red retinal reflex.

Cortical cataract. Wedge-shaped anterior or posterior cortical opacities, arranged radially and extending in from the periphery, appear gray with the penlight and black against the red retinal reflex.

Secondary cataract. Posterior capsule fibrosis, a common sequela of cataract surgery, is more correctly an opacified posterior capsule, the lens being absent. The peripheral lens epithelial cells migrate across the capsular bag left to support the intraocular lens implant. It appears as dense tissue folds and clusters of clear vesicles.

Diabetic cataract. Older diabetic patients have an increased tendency to develop nuclear or cortical cataracts with no distinctive character. Juvenile diabetic patients acquire distinctive snowflake cataracts containing chalky white deposits, the entire lens subsequently becoming milky.

Posterior subcapsular cataract. This lesion is commonly seen after long-term use of corticosteroids, with diabetes, and after trauma or uveitis (Fig. 7-36).

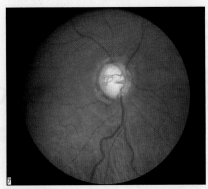

FIG. 7-37 Glaucoma: Optic Atrophy. The right eye of this darkly pigmented patient shows a deeply excavated cup with a cup-to-disk ratio of 0.7–0.8. There is a large notch in inferior rim of the optic nerve, thinning of the rim elsewhere, and a disc hemorrhage nasally all consistent with advanced glaucoma. The remaining rim is pink. The cribriform plate can be seen in the base of the cup superiorly. Note the normal variation in the choroidal pattern of dark pigment and choroidal vessels.

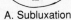

A. Subluxation   B. Dislocation

FIG. 7-38 Displacement of the Lens. A. Subluxation. B. Anterior chamber dislocation.

Lens subluxation and dislocation. Rupture of the zonula ciliaris (zonule of Zinn) permits the lens to move from its fixed position behind the pupil. Slight displacement, with the lens still backing the pupillary aperture, is *subluxation* (Fig. 7-38A), manifested by tremulousness of the iris (*iridodonesis*) when the eye moves horizontally. Viewed through the ophthalmoscope, the equator of the lens may show as a dark, curved line crossing the pupil; a double image of the retina with different magnifications may be seen, one through the lens, the other without the lens. A completely displaced lens is a *dislocation*. It is easily seen if it enters the anterior chamber (Fig. 7-38B). Lens displacement is usually caused by trauma. Nontraumatic dislocation occurs in several hereditary conditions including Marfan disease, homocystinuria, and hereditary spherophakia.

Intraocular pressure changes. Increased tension occurs in glaucoma; decreased tension is seen with myotonic dystrophy, globe rupture, and extreme dehydration. Accurate pressures are obtained with a tonometer.

Retina Signs

Increased cup-to-disk ratio—glaucoma. See page 242 and Fig. 7-37.

Myelinated nerve fibers. Optic nerve fiber myelination usually ends at the lamina cribrosa. Infrequently myelin sheaths continue into the retinal nerve fiber layer (Fig. 7-39B). Semi-opaque white patches emerging from the optic disk spread into one or two retinal quadrants. The disk margin appears

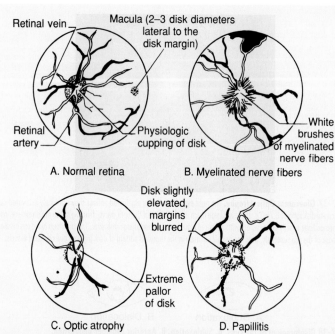

FIG. 7-39 Retinal Abnormalities I. A. Normal left retina: The background of the retina is red-orange; it contains a variable amount of black pigments, depending on race and complexion. Diverging blood vessels emerge from the optic disk to spread over the retina, usually in pairs of an artery and a vein. The veins are solid and dark red, and they may pulsate normally. The arteries are brighter red, contain central white stripes, and are pulseless. The width of an artery is usually approximately four-fifths that of the adjacent vein. The optic disk is lighter red, with sharp borders, often outlined by a strip of black pigment in the adjacent retina. The physiologic cup is white or pale yellow. The macula lies in the horizontal plane of the disk and from 2–3 disk diameters to the temporal side. The macular area is pale red with a central white or shining dot. **B. Myelinated nerve fibers:** White brushes of myelinated nerves emerge from the disk, obscuring segments of vessels and disk margins. **C. Optic atrophy:** The disk is chalk white with sharply defined borders. The blood vessels are normal. **D. Papillitis:** The disk is hyperemic, and its borders are blurred.

frayed and the underlying vessels are partially or completely obscured. It is a normal variation of no clinical significance. Patches of myelinated nerves may occur remote from the disc.

Disk pallor—optic atrophy. Optic nerve damage (compression, ischemia, inflammation, or increased intracranial pressure) leads to nerve fiber atrophy and loss of normal vascularity (Figs. 7-39C and 7-40). The disk is pale pink, yellow, or white; the margins may be less distinct and the physiologic cup and lamina cribrosa are variably seen. The emerging vessels may be surrounded by perivascular glial sheathing, seen as white lines. *DDX:* Pigmented high-water marks or residual exudate around the nerve suggest previous disc edema and increased intracranial pressure producing the optic atrophy. *It is important to recognize that an atrophic nerve can no longer swell, so it cannot be used to monitor increased intracranial pressure.* Brain tumor is a common cause of incidentally found optic atrophy, thus all *optic atrophy should be*

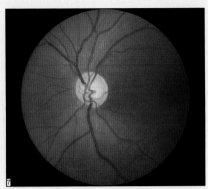

FIG. 7-40 Optic Atrophy. This left optic nerve demonstrates pallor of the rim, making the distinction of the cup difficult. There is a small area of pink rim superonasally, but the remainder of the rim is atrophic. (Image used with permission from Andrew Lee, MD.)

evaluated promptly by an ophthalmologist. In optic atrophy from chorioretinitis, the disk may have a yellow cast, and the surrounding retina may contain hemorrhages, areas of atrophy, and pigment. The distinction between optic atrophy resulting from intrinsic optic nerve lesions versus increased intracranial pressure cannot be made reliably from the physical findings. Disc pallor does not occur in glaucoma until very late in its course.

CLINICAL OCCURRENCE: *Intrinsic Optic Nerve Lesions:* Multiple sclerosis, syphilis; optic nerve compression without increased intracranial pressure. *Increased Intracranial Pressure:* Idiopathic intracranial hypertension, brain tumors.

Disk edema—papillitis, optic neuritis. Optic neuritis involving the optic nerve within the globe, produces papillitis with loss of vision (Fig. 7-39D) and disk edema indistinguishable from papilledema. Visual loss occurs earlier in optic neuritis than with papilledema. The disk is hyperemic, and its margins may be indistinct from edema in the peripapillary nerve fiber layer. The disk surface may be elevated above the surrounding retina (a + 1 or + 2 lens correction is required to focus on the disk).

CLINICAL OCCURRENCE: Ocular inflammation (e.g., uveitis, retinitis, sympathetic ophthalmia), intrinsic optic nerve inflammation (e.g., demyelinating optic neuritis in multiple sclerosis, neuromyelitis optica—Devic syndrome), intracranial inflammation (e.g., meningitis, venous sinus thrombosis), infections (e.g., syphilis, tuberculosis, influenza, measles, malaria, mumps), and intoxications (e.g., methyl alcohol).

Anterior ischemic optic neuropathy (AION). Infarction of the optic nerve head results from inadequate perfusion of the posterior ciliary arteries. AION occurs in two forms, the arteritic, related to giant cell arteritis, and the nonarteritic in patients with vasculopathies, e.g., hypertension or diabetes mellitus and intercurrent hypotension. Onset is usually sudden and painless, with profound visual loss, typically altitudinal, involving the upper and lower fields. The optic nerve is edematous with scant hemorrhage and more pallor than typical for papilledema. *DDX:* In patients aged >55 years, it is imperative to search for giant cell arteritis. The nonarteritic form commonly follows a period of systemic hypotension and is accompanied by a small to absent optic cup in the uninvolved eye.

Papilledema. Increased cerebrospinal fluid (CSF) pressure within the optic nerve sheath compresses the nerve resulting in axoplasmic flow stasis and ischemia (Fig. 7-41A). Early papilledema causes a C-shaped halo of nerve fiber layer edema that surrounds the disc with a gap temporally (Fig. 7-42). With more advanced papilledema, the halo becomes circumferential. Next there is obscuration of major vessels leaving the disc, and later there is obscuration of vessels on the optic disc. The emerging vessels bend sharply in

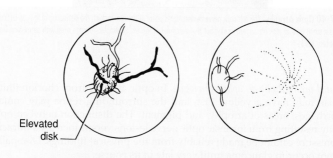

Elevated disk

A. Papilledema, choked disk   B. Star figure of macula

FIG. 7-41 Retinal Abnormalities II. A. Papilledema (choked disk): The disk surface is elevated, the nasal borders blurred. The vessels curve downward over the borders. The veins are distended and pulseless. Both arteries and veins in the disk may be obscured by the swollen structure. **B. Star figure of the macula:** Edema throws the retina into traction folds that radiate from the macula as white lines.

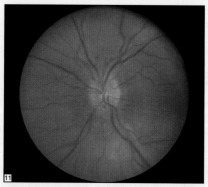

FIG. 7-42 Disc Edema, Early. This left optic nerve head (disc) is hyperemic and the nerve fiber layer shows some edema, obscuring the details of the disc margin. There is a hemorrhage inferiorly on the disc head, dilation of some smaller disc vessels, and obscuration of some of the vessels as they cross within the edematous nerve fiber layer. (Image used with permission from Andrew Lee, MD.)

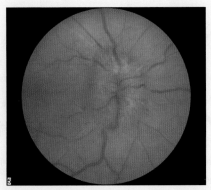

FIG. 7-43 Disc Edema, Late. This right eye shows marked disc edema with hyperemia, nerve fiber layer edema obscuring the disc margins and disc vessels, and small flame hemorrhages. The disc is elevated, evidenced by the different focal plane of the disc head and the retina. The retinal veins are engorged and tortuous, and there is dilation of the smaller vessels on the disc head. (Image used with permission from Andrew Lee, MD.)

passing over the elevated disk edge (Fig. 7-43). Macular retinal edema creates traction folds (*choroidal folds*), seen as white lines radiating from the macula (Fig. 7-41B). Patients with papilledema have an enlarged physiologic blind spot documented by formal visual field testing. The principal causes are brain tumor and idiopathic intracranial hypertension. Less common causes are hydrocephalus, malignant hypertension, subarachnoid hemorrhage, meningitis, and salicylate poisoning. *DDX:* In contrast to papillitis, central vision is unimpaired, but, like glaucoma, there is usually peripheral visual loss.

Pseudopapilledema—drusen bodies. These granular deposits in the optic disk cause pseudopapilledema. Distinguishing early papilledema and from drusen bodies is best done by an ophthalmologist.

Venous engorgement. Distented retinal veins suggest retinal vein occlusion, polycythemia vera, cyanotic congenital heart disease, leukemia, and macroglobulinemia.

Retinal hemorrhage. Hemorrhage occurs in all layers of the retina. The hemorrhage's shape reflects its depth. A large, deep hemorrhage in the choriocapillaris produces a dark, elevated area looking like a melanotic tumor (Fig. 7-44A); suspect a *subretinal vascular membrane* seen in macular degeneration. Smaller, more superficial hemorrhage appears as a round red spot, with blurred margins, called a *blot hemorrhage* (Fig. 7-44B). *Microaneurysms* are also round red spots, but with sharp borders. Unlike hemorrhages, they are not reabsorbed and may occur in clusters about vascular sprigs (Fig. 7-44C). Striated red flame-shaped *hemorrhages* are in the nerve fiber layer (Figs. 7-44D and 7-45). In a *subhyaloid or preretinal hemorrhage*, blood pooling between the retina and hyaloid membrane is seen as a turned-up half-moon; the straight upper border is a fluid level (Fig. 7-44E). A small hemorrhagic spot with a central white area is a *Roth spot*, (Fig. 7-44F), classically seen in subacute

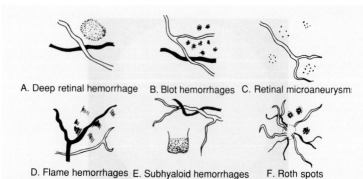

A. Deep retinal hemorrhage   B. Blot hemorrhages   C. Retinal microaneurysms

D. Flame hemorrhages   E. Subhyaloid hemorrhages   F. Roth spots

FIG. 7-44 Hemorrhages and Similar Lesions in the Retina.

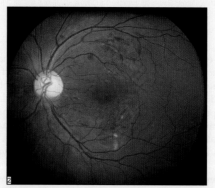

FIG. 7-45 Hypertensive Retinopathy: Flame Hemorrhages. The left eye of this poorly controlled, hypertensive African American patient has a darkly pigmented choroid, a normal variant, which darkens the entire photograph. There are multiple flame hemorrhages within the plane of the nerve fiber layer. There are several cotton wool spots (nerve fiber layer infarctions). The nerve pallor is an artifact, but the enlarged cup-disc ratio of 0.6–0.7 suggests glaucoma.

bacterial endocarditis and leukemia. Many conditions produce retinal hemorrhages, examples are hypertension, diabetes mellitus, papilledema, retinal vein occlusion, SBE, HIV, SLE, Takayasu arteritis, macroglobulinemia, thiamine deficiency, leukemia, polycythemia, sickle cell disease, and sarcoidosis.

Diabetic retinopathy. Diabetic retinopathy leads to blindness by damaging the macula. Microaneurysms occurring around the macula need to be distinguished from blot hemorrhages. With advanced diabetic retinopathy there are white or yellow waxy exudates having distinct, often serrated, borders (Fig. 7-46). The exudates gradually coalesce forming a broken circle around the macula. *Neovascularization* of the disk or elsewhere in the retina is an indication for laser phototherapy (Figs. 7-47 and 7-48). Signs of atherosclerosis and hypertension are sometimes superimposed. **DDX:** Although microaneurysms around the macula are characteristic of diabetes, retinal microvasculopathy

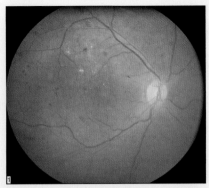

FIG. 7-46 Diabetic Retinopathy: Non-Proliferative Retinopathy. This right eye shows diffuse, scattered dot and blot hemorrhages and microaneurysms. There is a small flame hemorrhage in the inferior macula. There is evidence of old superior macular focal photocoagulation for diabetic macular edema, as well as peripheral panretinal photocoagulation (PRP) for proliferative diabetic retinopathy (small, dull grey spots). There is recurrent neovascularization of the disc supero-temporally. The central macula is dull and the landmarks indistinct suggesting persistent macular edema. The arterial caliber is narrow and the reflex increased, and there are several areas of arteriovenous nicking along the superior temporal arcade suggesting coexisting hypertension.

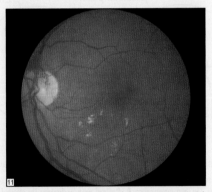

FIG. 7-47 Diabetic Retinopathy: Neovascularization of the Disc (NVD). This left eye shows a superior area of NVD, as well as scattered and inferior macular exudate around background microaneurysms and dot-blot hemorrhages. The disc pallor is an artifact due to manipulating this photo to better demonstrate the diabetic findings.

with cotton–wool spots, intraretinal hemorrhages, and microaneurysms also occur in radiation retinopathy and HIV-AIDS.

Retinal artery occlusion. Sudden loss of vision occurs when the central retinal artery is occluded, usually from thrombosis or embolism. Initially, the retina is pale from ischemic edema, the arteries are narrowed, the smaller arteries being invisible (Figs. 7-49A and 7-50). The veins are full but pulseless. The absence of circulation is demonstrated by failure to induce pulsation in arties or veins with pressure on the eyeball. Retinal edema and pallor are less dense over the fovea because it lacks a nerve fiber layer. The fovea becomes

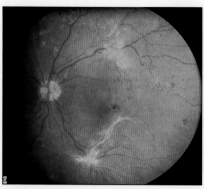

FIG. 7-48 Diabetic Retinopathy: Proliferative Neovascularization. This left eye shows multifocal areas of proliferative fibrovascular diabetic neovascularization elsewhere (NVE), with traction between the superior and inferior vascular arcades. There are multiple omega loops in the veins, with venous beading and irregularity. There are several vessels on the disc head suspicious for neovascularization of the disc (NVD), and evidence peripherally of old incomplete pan retinal photocoagulation. There are multiple areas of dot blot hemorrhages and microaneurysms.

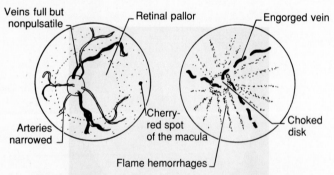

FIG. 7-49 Retinal Vascular Occlusions. A. Retinal artery occlusion: The retinal background is white, and the arteries are much narrowed. The veins are pulseless. **B. Retinal vein occlusion:** The affected veins are engorged and tortuous. Hemorrhages occur near the veins.

a *cherry red spot* due to visualizing choroidal blood flow within the macular edema. It disappears as the edema resolves over weeks. Branch artery occlusion causes findings limited to its distribution area. Common causes of retinal artery occlusion are vascular disease, cardiac valve disease or vegetations, rheumatic fever, and vasculitis, most commonly temporal arteritis. Rarely, it complicates SLE, sickle cell disease, cryoglobulinemia, syphilis, or thromboangiitis obliterans.

Retinal vein occlusion. Central retinal vein thrombosis produces engorgement and tortuosity of all retinal veins (Fig. 7-49B). Nerve fiber layer and blot hemorrhages appear throughout the retina. Macular and disk edema

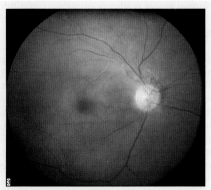

FIG. 7-50 Central Retinal Artery Occlusion (CRAO). This right eye shows a CRAO from cholesterol emboli, fragments of which are lodged in the superior and inferior temporal arteries (Hollenhorst plaques). There is diffuse macular edema, a central cherry red spot, and thready residual arterial flow.

TABLE 7-2 Grades of Retinal Arteriolar Sclerosis

Grade 1	Thickening of vessels with slight depression of veins at arteriolar–venular (AV) crossings
Grade 2	Definitive AV crossing changes and moderate local sclerosis
Grade 3	Venule beneath the arteriole is invisible; severe local sclerosis and segmentation
Grade 4	To the preceding signs are added venous obstruction and arteriolar obliteration

Kirkendall WM, Armstrong ML. Vascular changes in the eye of the treated and untreated patient with hypertension. *Am J Cardiol.* 1962;9:663.

are commonly present. Findings of branch vein occlusion are limited to its drainage area. Vein occlusion is associated with hypertension, the stiffened arterioles compressing the more compliant retinal veins as they cross in their common sheath. Hypercoagulable states also cause venous occlusion from sluggish blood flow as in polycythemia, multiple myeloma, macroglobulinemia, and leukemia. In sickle cell disease, neovascularization accompanies multiple retinal vein thromboses.

Arteriolar sclerosis. Table 7-2 presents the Kirkendall and Armstrong modification of the Scheie classification for scoring retinal artery sclerosis. The retinal changes do not necessarily parallel atherosclerotic disease elsewhere in the body.

Artery stripe. Normal retinal arteries have a bright central stripe caused by light reflecting off the curved vessel. Increased wall thickness produces a wider and brighter stripe. In moderate disease, the walls look like burnished copper (*copper wire reflex*); in advanced disease, the entire width of the artery reflects as a white stripe (*silver wire reflex*).

Vessel sheaths. Normal vessel walls are invisible. Lipid infiltration thickens the walls producing a milky white streak on either side of the blood column called *pipestem sheathing*.

Arteriovenous crossings. As the arterial and arteriolar walls become less compliant, arteriovenous crossing signs are produced (Fig. 7-51A). Arteriovenous *nicking* (Fig. 7-51B) occurs when the thickened arterial sheath obscures a short segment of the more compliant vein, seen as a notch on either side of the artery at their crossing. The vein deviates when the stiffened artery causes it to make a 90-degree crossing angle (Fig. 7-51C); the normal angle is acute. Elevation of a vein by a thickened artery is called *humping* (Fig. 7-51D). When the artery compresses the vein, tapering is seen (Fig. 7-51E). Partial obstruction of venous flow dilates the vein upstream from the artery. This is *banking* (Fig. 7-51F), and may lead to retinal vein occlusion.

Hypertensive retinopathy. Arterial hypertension produces distinctive retinal signs that often coexist with the signs of arteriolar sclerosis (Figs. 7-45 and 7-52). For example, the retina may be classified as "grade 3 arteriolosclerosis, grade 4 hypertension." The signs attributed to hypertension may also be graded by using the Kirkendall and Armstrong classification (Table 7-3). Most ophthalmologists describe the retinal and vascular finding without the use of these scales.

Retina spots. Many diseases and processes leave scars, deposits, pigmentation, etc., in the retina. Active retinal disease and systemic diseases with retinal manifestations cause unifocal or multifocal spots against the normal retina. Carefully examining the retina in patients with confusing systemic disease presentations may assist diagnosis. A challenge is to distinguish active disease from residuae of past events.

Cholesterol emboli. Ulcerated atherosclerotic plaques in the ascending aorta or carotid artery shed cholesterol crystals that lodge at the retinal artery bifurcations.

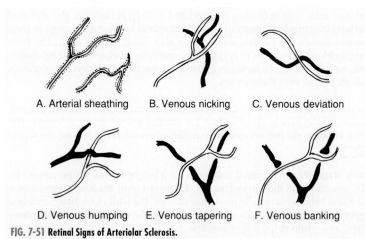

A. Arterial sheathing   B. Venous nicking   C. Venous deviation

D. Venous humping   E. Venous tapering   F. Venous banking

FIG. 7-51 Retinal Signs of Arteriolar Sclerosis.

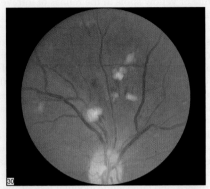

FIG. 7-52 Hypertensive Retinopathy: Cotton Wool Spots and Arteriolar Changes. The superior aspect of this right eye and has multiple cotton wool spots (nerve fiber layer infarctions). There is increased arteriolar light reflex, arteriolar narrowing, and arteriovenous crossing changes consistent with hypertensive retinopathy.

TABLE 7-3 Grades of Retinal Hypertension

Signs	
Grade 1	Narrowing in terminal branches of vessels
Grade 2	General narrowing of vessels with severe local constriction
Grade 3	To the preceding signs are added striate hemorrhages and soft exudates
Grade 4	Papilledema is added to the preceding signs

Patients may be asymptomatic or present with transient monocular visual loss, *amaurosis fugax*, or transient ischemic neurologic attacks (TIA) in the carotid distribution. Finding cholesterol emboli proves plaque rupture with embolization. It is difficult, if not impossible, to differentiate cholesterol emboli from calcific emboli from diseased heart valves.

Cotton-wool patches. Infarcts produce thickening and swelling of the terminal retinal nerve fibers. Gray to white areas with ill-defined fluffy borders in the posterior pole of the retina (Fig. 7-52) are often accompanied by microaneurysms which can rupture producing small striate flame hemorrhages. Cotton-wool patches are found with hypertension, diabetes, SLE, HIV, central retinal vein occlusion, and papilledema.

Hard exudates. Lipids deposited by leaking capillaries are left behind after the retinal pigment epithelium resorbs the associated serous fluid. These are small white spots with sharply defined edges. They are deeper than the retinal vessels and cotton wool patches.

Pigmented spots. Old inflammation or scarring produces a pigmented region in the retina.

Talc deposits. White or yellow spots in the retinas of intravenous drug users result from injecting ground-up tablets containing talc.

Cytomegalovirus (CMV) retinitis. Advanced immunosuppression from HIV infection is accompanied by cytomegalovirus infection of the retina. Patients describe visual loss, blurring, floaters, and flashes of light. Look for whitening of the retina, cotton-wool spots, and intraretinal hemorrhages. Although less common, consider varicella zoster infection, toxoplasmosis, and syphilis. CMV retinitis is uncommon with the advent of highly active antiviral therapy.

Candida endophthalmitis. Systemic Candida infection associated with immunosuppression and indwelling venous catheters is difficult to diagnose. Patients have fever, but blood cultures are often negative. Small white patches on the retina may be the only sign of disease. With advancing disease, there is pain, visual disturbance, and large white globular lesions invade the vitreous.

Macular degeneration. Vision is much reduced, but the only visible sign may be a few spots of pigment near the macula and blurring of the macular borders. In other cases, subretinal hemorrhages, patches of atrophy, yellow drusen, and pigmented areas are seen.

Retinitis pigmentosa. Inherited singly or as a component of several syndromes, retinitis pigmentosa manifests arteriolar narrowing, waxy pallor of the optic disc, and perivascular retinal pigmentation. Night blindness is the earliest symptom, but all types of vision become impaired as the retina degenerates progressively from the periphery to the posterior retina. Spidery strands of pigmented spots form a girdle about the global equator (Fig. 7-53A).

Angioid streaks. Probably the result of elastic tissue degeneration, broad lines of pigment radiate from the optic disk, branching like blood vessels (Fig. 7-53B). They occur in Paget disease and in pseudoxanthoma elasticum.

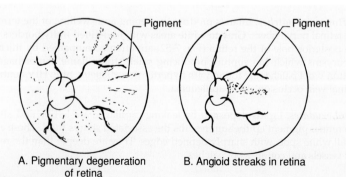

A. Pigmentary degeneration of retina   B. Angioid streaks in retina

FIG. 7-53 Retinal Pigmentation.

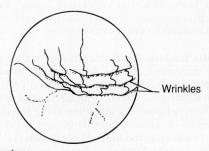

FIG. 7-54 **Retinal Detachment.**

Retinal detachment. Retinal detachments are symptomatic or asymptomatic. Patients complain of flashing lights followed by floaters and then a curtain crossing their vision. The earliest sign is elevation of an area of retina placing it out of focus with surrounding structures. The arteries and veins in the separated membrane appear elevated (Fig. 7-54). When markedly detached, the retina becomes a folded gray sheet. Underlying inflammation produces areas of choroiditis and vitreous opacities. The edge of a tear is horseshoe shaped. The cause of detachment is often undetermined.

Nose and Sinus Signs

Epistaxis (nosebleed). The most common bleeding site is Kiesselbach plexus, a vascular network on the anterior nasal septum. Posterior hemorrhage frequently occurs at the back third of the inferior meatus from large vessels supplied by the external carotid artery. In some cases, there are multiple oozing points in the mucosa. A Nosebleed can be spontaneous and trivial or a sign of serious local or generalized disease. Hemorrhage from the external nares is obvious, but bleeding from the choana needs to be distinguished from hemoptysis and hematemesis. In approaching epistaxis, the first challenges are to identify the bleeding site and determine whether trauma or a predisposing condition is present. Observe universal precautions with gloves, gown, and face protection. Remove clots by suction or by having the patient clear the nose by blowing. Inspect the anterior nasal chambers, especially the septum. If profuse hemorrhage obscures the site, advance the suction tip backward in small increments until the point where the passage immediately fills after clearing; this is the bleeding site. Blood-tinged fluid suggests a CSF leak. Consult textbooks for methods of arresting hemorrhage.

CLINICAL OCCURRENCE: *Local Causes:* Coughing, sneezing, nose picking, fractures, lacerations, foreign bodies, adenoid growth, nasopharyngeal fibroma, angioma, rhinitis sicca. *Generalized Causes: Congenital:* Hereditary hemorrhagic telangiectasia; *Infectious:* Viral rhinitis, typhoid fever, scarlet fever, influenza, measles, infectious mononucleosis, diphtheria, pertussis, psittacosis, Rocky Mountain spotted fever, erysipelas, mucosal leishmaniasis; *Inflammatory/Immune:* Granulomatosis with polyangiitis (Wegener), lethal midline granuloma; *Mechanical/Traumatic:* (see local causes) Changes in atmospheric pressure (mountain climbing, caisson disease, flying) exertion; *Metabolic/Toxic:* Pernicious anemia, aspirin, scurvy; *Neoplastic:* Nasopharyngeal carcinoma, squamous cell carcinomas, leukemia; *Vascular:* Coagulopathy, cirrhosis, uremia, hemophilia, von Willebrand disease, thrombocytopenia, hypertension, aortic coarctation; *Elevated venous pressure:* Cor pulmonale, congestive heart failure, superior vena cava syndrome.

Nasal and maxilla fracture. Nasal fractures are simple or comminuted; seldom are they compound. A blow from the side displaces both nasal bones to the opposite side, producing an S-shaped curve in the dorsum nasi. The septum is fractured with or without nasal bone fracture. Frontal blows depress the nasal bones. If palpation along the inferior border of the orbit discloses an irregularity, maxilla fracture is present; a fragment may displace downward into the sinus. Malocclusion of the teeth indicates displacement of the maxilla. Fracture of the zygoma produces flattening of the cheek.

Anosmia. Nasal obstruction and CN-I injury, often by traumatic shearing of nerve endings passing through the cribriform plate, produce loss of smell. Anosmia is invariably accompanied by a perceived change in taste with food seeming bland and unpalatable. The most common identified cause is closed head trauma. This can be an early sign of Parkinson diseases or Alzheimer dementia.

Congenital nasal deformities. Disturbances in nasal development are myriad. The most common is cleft nose from incomplete fusion at the tip and dorsum (Fig. 7-55B).

Acquired nose deformities. Acquired deformities are the result of trauma, infection, or neoplasms. *Rhinophyma* is an erythematous bulbous enlargement of the distal two-thirds of the nose from multiple sebaceous adenomas (Fig. 7-55A). It may follow long-standing rosacea. *Saddle nose* has a sunken bridge (Fig. 7-55C) resulting from loss of cartilage; common causes are septal hematoma or abscess. Rarely, it is caused by relapsing polychondritis, granulomatosis and polyangiitis (Wegener), or congenital or acquired syphilis. A crooked nose results from fracture.

Vestibule folliculitis. Mild inflammation around the hair follicles is evident on inspection.

Vestibule furunculosis. A small superficial abscess forms in the skin or mucous membrane. The area is extremely tender, swollen, and reddened.

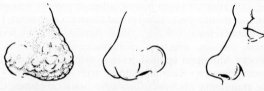

A. Rhinophyma   B. Cleft nose   C. Saddle nose

FIG. 7-55 External Nasal Deformities. A. Rhinophyma. B. Cleft nose. C. Saddle nose: Note the sinking of the dorsum with relative prominence of the lower third.

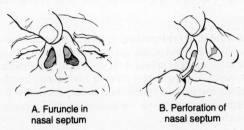

A. Furuncle in nasal septum

B. Perforation of nasal septum

FIG. 7-56 Lesions in the Nasal Vestibule. A. Furuncle: Avoid trauma that might spread infection to the cavernous sinus. **B. Perforation of nasal septum:** Transillumination of the septum discloses a hole.

Swelling may involve the nasal tip, alae nasi, and upper lip (Fig. 7-56A). Avoid instrumentation or other trauma to pyogenic lesions within the triangle anterior to a line from the corners of the mouth to the glabella as it may spread infection directly to the cavernous sinus.

Fissure. Fissures developing at the mucocutaneous junction become overlaid with crusts covering the tender surfaces.

Deviated septum. The nasal septum is seldom precisely a midline structure. The cartilaginous and bony septum may deviate as a hump, spur, or shelf encroaching on one chamber, occasionally causing obstruction.

Perforated septum. The cartilaginous septal perforation is caused by chronic infection, repeated trauma in picking off crusts, nasal or transphenoidal pituitary surgery, or cocaine abuse. Perforation is discovered by looking in one naris while shining a light in the other (Fig. 7-56B).

Septum hematoma. Even slight nasal trauma produces bleeding under the mucoperichondrium, often causing bilateral hematomas. Nasal obstruction necessitates breathing through the mouth. The hematoma is a violaceous, compressible, obstructive mass. The columella may be widened and the nasal tip pales from stretching of the skin. Pressure from the hematoma on the anterior ethmoidal nerve may cause anesthesia of the tip. Hematomas may compromise the septum's blood supply resulting in slow cartilage necrosis and saddle nose deformity.

Septal abscess. The edematous septum swells into both nasal chambers. Infected septal hematomas invariably result in loss of cartilage. Immediate incision and drainage plus appropriate antibiotics lowers risk for progression through the angular veins to produce cavernous sinus thrombosis.

Foreign body. Children frequently put objects into the nose that, remaining for extended periods, produce foul, purulent unilateral discharge.

Neoplasm. Sinus carcinomas cause obstruction, bloodstained discharge, constant boring pain, and they invade bone. Invasion of the orbit causes ocular disturbances, of the maxillary antral floor loosening upper teeth and/or leading to an ill-fitting denture. The hard palate may bulge and become soft.

Cerebrospinal fluid (CSF) rhinorrhea. A traumatic fistula is created between the subarachnoid space and nasal cavity. After head injury or surgery, a unilateral discharge of clear spinal fluid develops. The fluid may be blood tinged but is easily distinguished from a nosebleed. Jugular vein compression increases the flow. If spinal fluid is suspected, test a specimen for beta-2-transferrin. Substantial risk for meningitis and recurrent meningitis demands a search for CSF leak.

Nasal discharge—acute suppurative sinusitis. See page 248.

Nasal discharge—chronic suppurative sinusitis. See page 249.

Sinusitis and periorbital edema—periorbital abscess. See page 241.

Sinusitis and periorbital edema—orbital cellulitis. See page 241.

Sinusitis and ocular palsies—cavernous sinus thrombosis. See page 249 and Figure 7-57A.

Nasal polyps. Nasal polyps are sessile or pedunculated mucosal overgrowths developing after recurrent episodes of mucosal edema. They are frequently seen in long-standing allergic rhinitis, aspirin-sensitive asthma, and cystic fibrosis. Polyps are commonly multiple, most frequently protruding from the middle meatus as smooth, pale, spheric mucosal masses (Fig. 7-57B). Polyps may enlarge obstructing the air passages; they frequently recur after removal. *DDX:* Polyps are mobile and insensitive, distinguishing them from swollen turbinates.

Periorbital masses—mucocele and pyocele. Permanent obstruction of the frontal or ethmoid sinus orifices causes mucus secreted by their mucosae to accumulate. The resulting sac, or mucocele, slowly enlarges, the pent-up mucus exerts pressure on surrounding structures and erodes bone, behaving like a neoplasm. The sac may eventually erode into the frontal sinus or lateral ethmoid wall producing painless swelling beneath the supraorbital ridge, medial to the globe (Fig. 7-58). The painless mass feels rubbery and slightly compressible. The globe is pushed downward and laterally, causing diplopia; proptosis may also occur. Upward and medial eye motions are restricted. Intranasal examination may be negative. An infected mucocele is a *pyocele*. *DDX:* Swelling from a mucocele is above the inner canthus; dacryocystitis causes swelling below the canthus.

Papillomas. Benign *papillomas*, often in the vestibule, are slow-growing sinus neoplasms, usually *osteomas* or *chondromas*. They are asymptomatic until air passages or a sinus orifice is obstructed. *Inverted papillomas* grow downward into the underlying tissues so are difficult to resect.

Granulomatosis and polyangiitis (Wegener). See Chapter 8, page 362.

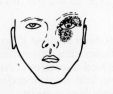
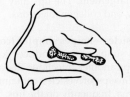

A. Cavernous sinus thrombosis   B. Nasal polyps

FIG. 7-57 Lesions About the Nose. A. Cavernous sinus thrombosis: Early there is paralysis of a single ocular muscle, with the development of edema and proptosis (shown). **B. Nasal polyps:** The parasagittal section shows the lateral wall with three polyps emerging from the middle meatus.

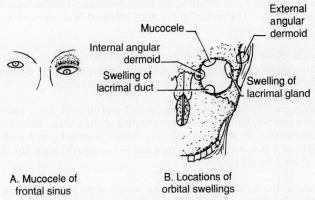

External angular dermoid

Mucocele

Internal angular dermoid

Swelling of lacrimal duct

Swelling of lacrimal gland

A. Mucocele of frontal sinus

B. Locations of orbital swellings

FIG. 7-58 Some Masses About the Orbit. A. Mucocele of frontal sinus: An example of a mucocele, this occurring in the floor of the supraorbital ridge and presenting medially. **B. Locations of masses** about the eye.

Breath Signs

Breath odor. There is great variation in olfactory acuteness, and description of odors is meaningless; experience is necessary. A foul breath odor, *fetor oris*, is common in infection (dental, tonsillar), atrophic rhinitis, putrefaction of food (achalasia, esophageal diverticula, pyloric obstruction), and infected sputum (bronchiectasis, lung abscess). *Acetone* on the breath indicates ketonemia in diabetic or starvation acidosis. In some uremic patients, *ammonia* is detected. A curious *musty odor* occasionally is smelled with severe liver disease. Inhalation or ingestion of *volatile hydrocarbons* produces detectable odor in exhaled air. *Alcohol* on the breath indicates recent ingestion, but medical illness, trauma, or ingestion of other drugs must be excluded as comorbid conditions. A few comatose patients don't have alcohol breath odor, but aspirated gastric contents smell strongly of alcohol. The chronic alcoholic may smell of *acetaldehyde* instead of alcohol. The methyl mercaptan causing garlic's odor is excreted from the lungs for >24 hours.

Lip Signs

Cleft lip. Incomplete fusion of the frontonasal process with the two maxillary processes leaves a persistent cleft in one or both sides of the upper lip, sometimes accompanied by cleft palate.

Lip enlargement. The lips may appear large in cretinism, myxedema, acromegaly, and collagen injections.

Lip vesicles—herpes simplex (cold sores, fever blisters). Reactivating latent herpes simplex virus induces local inflammation, often when the carrier develops another infectious disease, has local trauma, or is exposed to sunlight. Groups of vesicles containing clear fluid are surrounded by areas of erythema, frequently on the lips. The lesions burn or smart.

Cheilosis (angular stomatitis). Maculopapular and vesicular lesions are grouped at the corners of the mouth and the mucocutaneous junction (Fig. 7-59A). Skin irritation leads to crusting and fissuring. Often accompanying profuse salivation from any cause, it is specifically associated with riboflavin deficiency and ill-fitting dentures. Secondary *Candida* infection is common (*perlèche*). The entire lip becomes inflamed from overexposure to sunlight, *actinic cheilosis*.

Carbuncle. Painful localized swelling with erythema and increased skin warmth suggests early cellulitis or carbuncle. On the upper lip, it is exceedingly dangerous, the veins draining into the cavernous sinus.

Lip carcinoma. Early lesions are indurated and discoid, later, becoming warty and crusted, forming a slowly extending shallow ulcer. The ulcerated border is elevated, sometimes pearly (Fig. 7-59B). Regional lymph nodes are involved late. It is more frequent in men and 95% are on the lower lip. Biopsy all the ulcers >2 weeks old.

Lip chancre. The initial lesion of syphilis occurs at the inoculation site. The lip is the most common extragenital site of primary syphilitic chancre; usually the upper lip is involved. The lesion is discoid, without sharply defined borders and can be moved over the underlying tissues. It soon ulcerates to exude a clear fluid teeming with *Treponema pallidum*. The regional lymph nodes are involved early and feel larger and softer than carcinomatous nodes. Serologic tests for syphilis are frequently negative while the chancre is present.

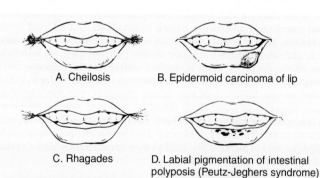

A. Cheilosis   B. Epidermoid carcinoma of lip

C. Rhagades   D. Labial pigmentation of intestinal
                     polyposis (Peutz-Jeghers syndrome)

FIG. 7-59 Some Lip Lesions. A. Cheilosis. B. Epidermoid carcinoma of lip: notice the sharply demarcated elevated edges with the ulcerating base, typically located at the mucocutaneous junction. **C. Rhagades. D. Signs of Peutz–Jeghers syndrome.**

Molluscum contagiosum. A nodular growth in the lip may ulcerate to discharge caseous material. The ulcer border may be elevated. The lesion is caused by Molluscipoxvirus. The resemblance to carcinoma may be striking, so biopsy may be required.

Rhagades. The white radial scars about the angles of the mouth are stigmata of previous syphilitic lesions (Fig. 7-59C).

Actinic keratosis. A dry, flat, light-colored precancerous growth occurs on the lip producing scaling; it bleeds easily.

Lip pigmentation—Peutz–Jeghers syndrome. Multiple pigmented brown to black spots on the lips resemble freckles (Fig. 7-59D), but freckles are uncommon on the mucosa. This autosomal dominant syndrome is associated with intestinal polyposis and increased risk for gastrointestinal cancer.

Lip telangiectasias—hereditary hemorrhagic telangiectasia. The most obvious lesions occur on the buccal mucosa, tongue, and lips. See page 153.

Oral Mucosa and Palate Signs

Xerostomia, Sjögren syndrome. See Sjögren Syndrome, page 241 and Xerostomia page 234.

Buccal pigmentation—Addison disease. Small patches of pigment in the buccal mucosa are common in blacks and other darkly pigmented races. In whites, however, dappled brown pigment in the cheek's lining strongly suggests Addison disease or Peutz–Jeghers syndrome.

Retention cyst. An obstructed mucous gland produces a blue-domed translucent cyst anywhere on the buccal surface.

Mucosal sebaceous cysts (Fordyce spots). The lip, cheek, and tongue mucosa show isolated white or yellow, sometimes slightly raised, spots <1 mm in diameter. Often a bit of white sebum may be expressed from the lesion. They are painless and harmless.

Koplik spots (measles). Koplik spots are the earliest diagnostic sign of measles and they are pathognomonic. One or two days before the exanthem appears, small white spots appear opposite the molars, and sometimes elsewhere, on the buccal mucosa (Fig. 7-60B). Each is surrounded by a narrow red areola.

Lichen planus. The lesions are thin, bluish-white, spiderweb lines resembling leukoplakia. Circumscribed areas of flattened papules on the flexor surfaces of the wrists and the mid shins support the diagnosis of lichen planus (Chapter 6, page 138).

Leukoplakia. These precancerous lesions occur at sites of chronic irritation from ill-fitting dentures or smokeless tobacco. Tobacco and alcohol are cocarcinogens. The first lesion is a whitened hyperkeratotic plaque. On the tongue, one or more areas on the dorsal surface show obliteration of the papillae with

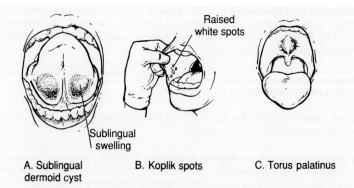

FIG. 7-60 Some Lesions of the Oral Cavity. A. Sublingual dermoid cyst. B. Koplik spots. C. Torus palatinus.

thin white lesions that are wrinkled and sometimes pearly. Persistent lesions coalesce and enlarge, becoming chalk white, thickening and becoming more firm than adjacent mucosa. Biopsy is indicated.

Thrush, candidiasis. Oral infection with *Candida* spp. occurs in patients who are diabetic, immunosuppressed (e.g., HIV, immunosuppressant drugs), inhaled corticosteroids or have received broad spectrum antibiotics. The lesions may be painless or cause mouth soreness, and the white plaques are easily removed with a tongue blade. Less commonly, the mucosa is erythematous and thin, without the white plaques. Pain with swallowing suggests concomitant *Candida* esophagitis.

Telangiectasias—hereditary hemorrhagic telangiectasia. Early and obvious lesions occur on the buccal mucosa, tongue, and lips. See Chapter 6, page 116.

Oral vesicles, blisters, and ulcers. Several diseases cause oral vesicles or bullae, often with multiple ulcerations. The major disease mechanisms are infection and immune-mediated processes. Larger ulcers are caused by tissue destruction from infection, neoplasm, or metabolic causes.

Herpes simplex. Primary herpes simplex infection causes severe stomatitis with painful vesicles that rupture forming shallow ulcers which heal slowly.

Herpangina. Coxsackievirus 16 infection results in fever and sore throat. Exam shows small vesicles or whitish papules on the soft palate.

Lichen planus. Painful chronic ulcers may be surrounded by characteristic lacy white mucosal lines.

Disseminated histoplasmosis. A persistent oral ulcer can be the presenting sign of disseminated histoplasmosis. Diagnosis is made by biopsy.

Cicatricial pemphigoid. Autoantibodies against hemidesmosomes in the basal layer of the mucosa and skin lead to separation of the epithelial layers with blister formation. Pain is mild to moderate. The incidence increases with age. Oral lesions may be accompanied by skin lesions (Chapter 6, page 147). The course is chronic and recurrent. It must be distinguished from pemphigus vulgaris (Chapter 6, page 146).

- *Stevens–Johnson syndrome.* This is a severe allergic reaction with generalized involvement of the skin and mucous membranes. The most common cause is medication exposure. Early recognition, withdrawal of the offending agent, and supportive therapy may be lifesaving.

Aphthous ulcer (canker sore). A few small vesicles appear in crops on the tip and sides of the tongue and on the labial and buccal mucosa. After the vesicle has ruptured, the lesion is a small, round, painful ulcer with a white floor, yellow margins, and narrow surrounding erythematous areola. The cause is unknown. Recurrent or persistent aphthous ulcers are seen in Crohn disease and Behçet syndrome.

Mucous patches (condyloma latum). This is the common lesion of secondary syphilis, occurring on the tongue and buccal and labial mucosae regardless of the site of the primary lesion. The patches are round or oval, 5–10 mm in diameter, slightly raised, and covered by gray membrane. They may ulcerate slightly. They feel indurated and are painless. Regional lymphadenopathy is common.

Osteonecrosis. Ionizing irradiation, especially of the mandible, suppresses normal bone turnover leading to acute or delayed bone necrosis with ulcerated overlying mucosa. Bisphosphonate therapy (especially intravenous bisphosphonates for malignant hypercalcemia and myeloma) also suppresses bone turnover and is associated with bone necrosis and mucosal ulceration. Patients present with one or more slowly progressive often painful ulcerations exposing underlying bone. A history of irradiation or bisphosphonate use is essential for making the diagnosis. Formerly, exposures to white phosphorus in the munitions industry caused a similar syndrome called *phossy jaw*.

Mucositis. The bone marrow and oral and intestinal mucosae are the body's most rapidly proliferating tissues. Cytotoxic chemotherapy transiently stops proliferation leading to impaired mucosal repair. Mouth ulcers occur 5–10 days after a cycle of cytotoxic chemotherapy. They may occur at any time during chronic oral alkylating or antimetabolite therapy.

Reddened parotid duct orifice—mumps. The parotid (Stensen) duct orifice, opposite the upper second molar, becomes reddened in mumps and other acute parotitis.

Bony palate protuberance—torus. This common anatomic variation is a bony knob or ridge in the midline of the hard palate. It is harmless.

Arched palate. There are many causes for high-arched palate. It is common in Marfan and Turner syndromes.

Cleft palate. A midline opening in the hard palate results from congenital failure of fusion of the maxillary processes. Usually associated with cleft lip, it also occurs in isolation. Its severity varies from a complete cleft of the entire soft and hard palate, including the alveolar ridge, to a partial cleft of the soft palate alone.

Bifid uvula. This results from incomplete fusion of the soft palate and may be accompanied by disoriented palatal muscles. Test elevation of the uvula. Deviation of the uvula and soft palate asymmetry suggest a muscular abnormality.

Teeth and Gum Signs
Wide interdental spaces. This occurs congenitally and is acquired in acromegaly as the jaw enlarges.

Caries. Tooth cavities can be subtle or obvious. Decreased saliva following irradiation or with sicca syndrome increases risk for caries.

Enamel loss. Enamel is destroyed by regurgitated stomach acid and acidic water in swimming pools with excessive chlorination. Enamel loss suggests bulimia nervosa.

Fluoride pits. Opaque chalk-white spots, 1–2 mm in diameter, are scattered on the surface of multiple teeth, indicating exposure to large amounts of fluoride during childhood.

Notched teeth—Hutchinson teeth. In congenital syphilis the permanent upper central incisors are misshapen, and the tips are notched (Fig. 7-61A). They are smaller than normal, and peg topped, resembling the frustum of a cone. Notching, interstitial keratitis, and labyrinthine deafness are the *Hutchinson triad*.

Periapical abscess. An abscess forming within bone at the root tip increases intraosseous pressure producing severe pain. Suspect an abscess when tapping the tooth accentuates toothache pain. Tender swelling in the adjacent gum and a draining sinus tract may form.

Bleeding gums. Gum bleeding signals local gum lesions or systemic blood vessel or hemostatic disorders. The patient complains of bleeding with brushing or notices blood in expectorated phlegm.

Gum recession. In older persons, the gingival margins may recede exposing the rough, lusterless cementum, below the enamel border.

Periodontitis. Adherent dental plaque inflames the gums leading to recession and erosion of the dental ligament. The receding gums are inflamed with deep pockets (>3 mm) between gum and tooth. The roots are exposed, and the teeth may be loose (Fig. 7-61B). The breath is often foul, and the gums bleed easily. A particularly virulent form is associated with methamphetamine abuse, *meth mouth*.

Necrotizing stomatitis (trench mouth, vincent stomatitis). Inflammation of the gums and adjoining mucosa is caused by a symbiotic infection with

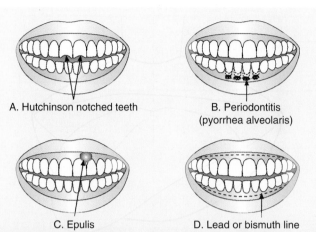

FIG. 7-61 Dental Abnormalities. A. Hutchinson notched teeth. B. Periodontitis: In the drawing, some of the lower teeth are involved: the gums are retracted, and pus is exuding from behind the gingival margins. **C. Epulis:** It is sessile, lighter in color than the gums. **D. Lead or bismuth line** in the gums.

Borrelia vincentii and *Fusobacterium plauti-vincenti.* Punched-out ulcers on the gums are covered with a gray–yellow membrane. The infection can remain localized to the gums or extend to pharyngeal structures, including bone.

Swollen gums—scurvy. The gums are deep red or purple and become swollen, tender, spongy and bleed easily. Other signs are subperiosteal hemorrhages and perifollicular purpura.

Gingival hyperplasia. Increasing gum volume occasionally covers the teeth. Phenytoin is the most common cause. In monocytic leukemia, gums infiltrated with monocytes have a similar appearance.

Epulis. This fibrous tumor of the gum arises from alveolar periosteum and emerges between the teeth. It is a nontender sessile mass (Fig. 7-61C), lighter in color than the gum, and rarely pedunculated. A similar tumor, but bright red, is a fibroangiomatous epulis.

Blue gums—lead and bismuth lines, quinacrine. With chronic exposure to lead (occupational) or bismuth (therapeutic), blue lines appear on the gums ~1 mm from the gingival margin where the heavy metals are deposited. The line, appearing solid to the unaided eye (Fig. 7-61D), is composed of small, discrete dots. Chronic quinacrine ingestion colors the gums diffusely blue or purple.

Tongue Signs

Dry tongue without longitudinal furrows. The surface dries from mouth breathing or lack of saliva. Tongue volume remains normal, so longitudinal furrows don't develop.

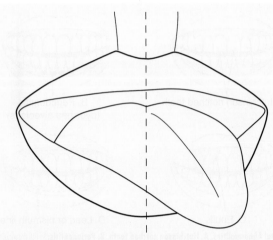

FIG. 7-62 Paralysis of the Left Side of the Tongue. Deviation is toward the paralyzed side.

Dry tongue with longitudinal furrows. Longitudinal furrows develop when tongue volume is reduced. This is a reliable sign of severe volume depletion.

Enlarged tongue. The tongue is enlarged in Down syndrome, cretinism, and adult myxedema. It increases in size during development of acromegaly and amyloidosis. Transient swelling occurs with glossitis, stomatitis, neck cellulitis, and angioedema. Lymphatic obstruction by carcinoma and superior vena cava obstruction often lead to enlargement.

Tremor. Tongue tremor is seen with increased sympathetic activity as in hyperthyroidism, alcohol and drug withdrawal, and anxiety.

Fasciculation. Denervation leads to spontaneous motor unit firing. Fasciculation is characteristic of bulbar poliomyelitis, West Nile virus encephalitis, and amyotrophic lateral sclerosis.

Shortened frenulum (tongue-tied). The frenulum is congenitally short limiting protrusion and preventing the tongue tip from reaching the roof of the mouth, thus impairing articulation of lingual consonants.

Limited tongue protrusion—carcinoma. See page 240.

Geographic tongue. This is a harmless condition of unknown cause. The tongues surface develops circular areas of smooth red epithelium, without papillae, surrounded by light-yellow rings of piled-up cells (Fig. 7-63B). The patches heal in a few days and are succeeded by new ones in other areas. *DDX:* Median rhomboid glossitis is lifelong and does not change over time.

Hairy tongue. Hyperplasia of filiform papillae entangled with an overgrowth of mycelial threads of *Aspergillus niger* or *Candida albicans* gives the tongue

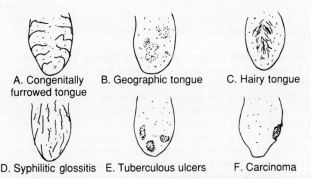

FIG. 7-63 Tongue Surface Patterns. A. Congenitally furrowed tongue. B. Geographic tongue. C. Black hairy tongue. D. Syphilitic glossitis. E. Tuberculous ulcers. F. Carcinoma: A typical location of carcinoma of the tongue is on the lateral edge.

a hairy appearance. Patients are asymptomatic. The distal two-thirds of the dorsum looks as if it were growing short hairs, usually black (Fig. 7-63C) but occasionally green from the fungus or because of chewing gum containing chlorophyll. It is seen in debilitated patients and after antibiotics.

Congenital furrows (scrotal tongue). This is a harmless condition, frequently inherited. The median sulcus is deep and the dorsal surface is interrupted by deep transverse furrows (Fig. 7-63A). It must be distinguished from the longitudinal furrowing in syphilitic glossitis.

Hairy leukoplakia. Epithelial hyperplasia results from Epstein–Barr virus (EBV) infection in patients with AIDS. The sides of the tongue have elongated "hairy" filiform papillae.

Atrophic glossitis. Nutritional deficiency results in impaired mucosal proliferation. The very high turnover rate of cells in the oral mucosa and tongue makes it susceptible to nutritional deficiencies. The tongue's extreme sensitivity explains the prominent symptoms. The patient complains of dry tongue, intermittent burning, and paresthesias of taste. The tongue becomes smaller, its surface slick and glistening, and the mucosa thins. In the advanced stages, there is considerable pain and swelling. The color is pink, red, or blue-red with atrophied hyperemic papillae appearing as small punctate red dots. **CLINICAL OCCURRENCE:** *Vitamin B₁₂ Deficiency:* Pernicious anemia, postgastrectomy, blind intestinal loop, extreme vegetarian diets, fish tapeworm (*Diphyllobothrium latum*) infestation; *Folic Acid Deficiency:* Megaloblastic anemia of pregnancy, chronic liver disease; *Other Causes:* Iron deficiency anemia, idiopathic gastritis, mixed B-complex vitamin deficiency, idiopathic.

Pellagra. Dietary deficiency of niacin (nicotinic acid and nicotinamide) is the cause. Initially, the patient complains of tongue burning with hot or spicy foods; the tongue appears normal. Later, the burning is constant. The tongue tip and borders become reddened; later the erythema spreads and the tongue swells. The denuded surface presents a fiery-red mucosa with ulcerations and indentations from teeth. After treatment, the tongue is pallid and atrophied. Other signs are Diarrhea, Delirium, and Dermatitis (*the three Ds*).

Magenta cobblestone tongue—riboflavin deficiency. Dietary riboflavin deficiency causes mild tongue burning. Swollen hyperemic fungiform and filiform papillae produce rows of reddened elevations suggesting cobblestones. Edema at the bases of the papillae produces the magenta color, contrasting with the fiery red pellagrous tongue, in which the epithelium is denuded. Cheilosis and angular stomatitis are common. A painless gray papule at one or both corners of the mouth enlarges and ulcerates producing indolent fissures with piled-up yellow crusts that leave permanent scars. Similar lesions can occur at the ocular canthi and nasolabial folds. Superficial keratitis and conjunctival injection are common.

Nonspecific glossitis. Pharyngeal infections may also involve the tongue, producing redness and swelling. The tongue may burn and feel tender.

Strawberry tongue (raspberry tongue). Streptococcal or staphylococcal infection release exotoxins (e.g., scarlet fever, toxic shock syndrome). The lingual papillae become swollen and reddened. According to Osler, the name *strawberry tongue* was given to the stage when the inflamed and hyperplastic papillae show through a white coat. Later, the epithelium desquamates, carrying away the coat and leaving a fiery-red, denuded surface surmounted by hyperplastic papillae; this has also been termed a strawberry tongue, others preferring the more accurately descriptive term *raspberry tongue*. During the desquamated period, taste is diminished.

Menopausal glossitis. Ascribed to estrogen deficiency, intense burning and slight mucosal atrophy occurs at menopause or in other estrogen deficiency states. The symptoms and signs improve with estrogen administration.

Syphilitic glossitis. The furrows of syphilitic glossitis are mainly longitudinal and deeper than the congenital type. The intervening epithelium is desquamated (Fig. 7-63D).

Herpetic glossitis. A painful inflamed tongue with longitudinal fissures has been described with herpes infection in HIV-infected patients.

Leukoplakia. Thin and white, often wrinkled or pearly areas obliterate the papillae. Later, the lesions coalesce, thicken, and become chalk white. In advanced stages, they look like dried, cracked white paint. Leukoplakia is a premalignant condition.

Dental ulcer. A projecting tooth or an ill-fitting denture causes ulceration on the sides or undersurface of the tongue. The ulcer margin may be elevated and surrounded by induration, suggesting carcinoma. Removal of the irritating surface should result in a trend toward healing in a few weeks. Lacking improvement, biopsy is indicated.

Sublingual mass—ranula. Cystic distention of sublingual or submandibular salivary ducts is caused by obstruction at the orifice. Because it looks like a frog's belly, Hippocrates used the Greek word for "little frog" to describe this lesion. A translucent mass is seen beside the frenulum and may extend to the other side. Bimanual palpation often tracks the mass to the submandibular gland. Transillumination reveals the submandibular duct traversing the upper part of the cyst.

Sublingual varices—caviar lesions. With aging, superficial sublingual veins develop varicosities resembling a mass of purple caviar (Chapter 6, Fig. 6-18A, page 131). They are of no clinical significance.

Posterior lingual mass—lingual thyroid. A lingual thyroid arises from a thyroglossal duct remnant. It presents as a round, smooth, red, nontender mass at the base of the tongue, near the foramen cecum. It may be the only functioning thyroid tissue.

Pharynx Signs

Oropharyngeal soft tissue hypertrophy. Enlargement of the tongue's base and narrowing of the pharynx by soft tissue hypertrophy combine to compromise the airway, especially when the tongue relaxes during sleep in the supine position. Normal oropharyngeal structures visualized with the patient sitting and the tongue relaxed in the floor of the mouth predict both the ease of tracheal intubation and the risk of upper airway obstruction during sleep. The *modified Mallampati score* is based upon visualization of the complete tonsillar bed, base of the uvula, and soft palate. Loss of visualization proceeds sequentially. A score of 1 means all structures are visualized; 2 means the full tonsillar bed is not seen; 3 means the base of the uvula is not seen; and 4 means the soft palate is not seen. Scores of 3 and 4 indicate high-risk.

Tonsil enlargement—hyperplasia. Children's tonsils are large, shrinking at puberty. Normal adult tonsils seldom protrude beyond the faucial pillars. Hyperplasia, usually bilateral, is usually attributed to chronic infection, but it may be associated with obesity, hyperthyroidism, or lymphoma.

Tonsillar exudates. Bacterial and viral infections produce a purulent tonsillar exudate which may spread to the lateral and posterior pharyngeal walls. The most common causes are viral infections, including acute mononucleosis (EB virus) and Group A streptococcal pharyngitis (see page 250 for a complete discussion).

Uvula edema. Allergic or nonallergic angioedema causes edema of the uvula and has occurred with thrombosis of an internal jugular vein containing a central venous line. Edema of the uvula together with bronchitis, asthma, and rhinopharyngitis suggests inhalational injury, often from recreational drug use (e.g., recent heavy smoking of marijuana, crack cocaine, hashish).

Larynx and Trachea Signs

Stridor. Extrathoracic airway narrowing worsens as transtracheal pressure increases during inspiration. A high-pitched sound is heard during inspiration,

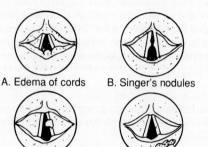

A. Edema of cords   B. Singer's nodules   C. Contact ulcers

D. Polyp of vocal cord   E. Carcinoma of   F. Squamous cell
                              piriform sinus   carcinoma

FIG. 7-64 Laryngeal Lesions in the Mirror. A. Laryngeal edema: The mucosa on the vocal cords, arytenoid prominences, and epiglottis is swollen and glistening. **B. Singer's nodules:** Apposing swellings on the free margins of the vocal cords at a distance one-third posteriorly in their extent. **C. Contact ulcers** opposed on the free margins of the cords at their junctions with the arytenoid cartilages. **D. Laryngeal polyp** on the free margin of the left cord. **E. Laryngeal carcinoma** in the left piriform sinus. **F. Squamous cell carcinoma** along the anterior half of the right cord.

having the same pitch and intensity throughout inspiration indicating a high degree of airway obstruction. Stridor is almost always accompanied by significant dyspnea. It is caused by mass lesions, such as carcinoma, which restrict vocal cord mobility or reduce the size of the glottic aperture, by bilateral vocal cord paralysis, which limits the effective glottic opening, or a swollen epiglottis in acute epiglottitis or inhalation injury.

Laryngeal edema. The signs of laryngeal obstruction range through hoarseness, dyspnea, and stridor. Inspection through the mirror is diagnostic. Glistening, swollen mucosa is seen on the vocal cords, arytenoid prominences, and epiglottis (Fig. 7-64A). Laryngeal edema may occur with acute laryngitis, lymphatic obstruction by neoplasm or abscess, radiation, anaphylaxis, angioedema, myxedema, and trauma to the larynx from instrumentation.

Hoarseness. Paralysis, edema or infiltration of a vocal cord, and vocal cord masses change the vibratory response to airflow. Hoarseness focuses attention on the larynx. A multitude of disorders cause hoarseness. **CLINICAL OCCURRENCE:** *Recent Onset—Overuse:* Shouting, cheering; *Infection:* Upper respiratory infections, chlamydia, diphtheria, measles; *Drugs:* Anticholinergic drugs, strychnine (laryngeal spasm), aspirin aspiration (chemical burn), potassium iodide, and uremia (cord edema); *Angioedema:* Insect bites, drug allergy, angiotensin-converting enzyme inhibitors, hereditary angioedema; *Foreign Body:* Food aspiration, after endotracheal intubation; *Laryngeal Spasm:* Croup, tetany, tetanus; *Burns:* Inhalation of irritant gases, swallowing of hot or caustic liquids. **Chronic Course—Occupational Overuse:** In the clergy, orators, singers, teachers; *Foreign Body:* Food aspiration, prolonged endotracheal intubation; *Lack of Mucus:* Sjögren syndrome; *Chronic Vocal Cord Inflammation:* Nonspecific chronic laryngitis, gastroesophageal reflux, alcoholism, gout, tobacco smoking; *Cord Edema:* Myxedema, chronic nephritis; *Surface Lesions:* Keratosis, pachyderma, herpes, leukoplakia, pemphigus; *Ulcers:* Tuberculosis, syphilis, leprosy, SLE, typhoid fever, trauma, contact ulcer; *Neoplasm:* Vocal nodules, sessile or pedunculated polyp, vocal process granuloma, vallecula cyst, leukoplakia, carcinoma in situ, epidermoid carcinoma, papilloma, angioma; *Innervation of cords:* Compression of recurrent laryngeal nerve by aortic aneurysm, large left atrium of the heart, mediastinal neoplasm, mediastinal lymphadenopathy, retrosternal goiter, injury during thyroidectomy; *Weak Cord Muscles:* Debilitating diseases, severe anemia, myasthenia gravis, myxedema, hyperthyroidism, normal aging process; *Laryngeal Bones and Cartilages:* Perichondritis of cricoid or arytenoids, ankylosis of cricoarytenoid joints (rheumatoid arthritis); *Larynx Compression:* Retropharyngeal abscess, tuberculosis of cervical vertebrae, neoplasm of pharynx, large goiters, actinomycosis; *Neck Irradiation*.

Vocal cord paralysis. The recurrent laryngeal nerves are susceptible to injury in the neck and chest inferior to the larynx. In unilateral cord paralysis, the affected cord may be immobilized near the midline or slightly more laterally in the paramedian position. In the latter case, vocal cord approximation is poor, and the voice is husky. During phonation, laryngoscopy shows the normal cord crossing the midline to meet the abducted immobile cord. In bilateral cord paralysis, the cords are usually fixed near the midline, so the voice is normal, but dyspnea is extreme and inspiratory stridor with strenuous exertion is pronounced. Cord paralysis is associated with thyroidectomy, aneurysm of the left aortic arch (left cord), mitral stenosis with enlarged left atrium (left cord), and mediastinal tumors.

Cricoarytenoid joint ankyloses. Inflammatory or traumatic arthritis limits motion at the cricoarytenoid joint. There is limited or absent motion of the true cords, resembling paralysis. Hoarseness and voice weakness are common. Passive mobility, tested by an otolaryngologist, is absent in ankylosing, but present with paralysis. If the joints are not completely immobilized, crepitus over the larynx may be heard with a stethoscope. It may be so insidious that dyspnea is not recognized. Causes are rheumatoid arthritis and prolonged contact with an esophageal feeding tube.

Polypoid corditis. The entire free margins of the true cords are loose and sagging, hoarseness resulting from imperfect approximation of the edematous cords. Causal factors include voice strain, irritation from alcohol and tobacco, and upper respiratory allergy or infection.

Vocal nodules (singer's nodules). With voice overuse, apposing 1–3 mm nodules form on the free margins of the true cords at the junction of the anterior one-third and the posterior two-thirds (Fig. 7-64B). Early lesions appear red, fibrosis later turns them white.

Laryngeal contact ulcer. Apposing ulcers occur on the free edges of both vocal cords at their junctions with the arytenoid cartilages. The irregular ulcer borders cause hoarseness (Fig. 7-64C). They usually are caused by overuse, trauma or instrumentation. Granulation tissue develops on one or both ulcers; enlargement can cause airway embarrassment.

Larynx neoplasm. See Syndromes page 240 below.

Salivary Gland Signs

Xerostomia. Dry mouth is caused by mouth breathing, obstructed salivary ducts, irradiation, and Sjögren syndrome. *DDX:* Dry eyes and salivary gland enlargement accompany Sjögren syndrome (page 202).

Sialorrhea (ptyalism). Sialorrhea is excessive saliva production, but it often refers to any condition of overabundant saliva, from rapid secretion, inability to swallow, production of viscid difficult to swallow saliva, or failure of the lips to contain the saliva.

CLINICAL OCCURRENCE: The common causes are poor neuromuscular control of the lips, tongue, and perioral soft tissues. Other causes are drugs, intoxicants, and local inflammation stimulating salivary secretion. *Drugs:* Mercury, copper, arsenic, antimony, iodide, bromide, potassium chlorate, pilocarpine, aconite, cantharides, carbidopa-levodopa; *Stomatitis:* Aphthous ulcers, septic ulcers, suppurative lesions, periodontal disease, chemical burns; *Specific Oral Infections:* Diphtheria, syphilis, tuberculosis; *Single Oral Lesions:* alveolar abscess, epulis, salivary calculus; *Reflex Salivation:* Gastric dilatation, gastric ulcer or carcinoma, acute gastritis, pancreatitis, hepatic disease.

Enlarged salivary glands. Salivary gland enlargement can indicate local or systemic disease. Painless enlargement of a single gland suggests tumor or an obstructed duct. A painful enlarged gland suggests acute viral or suppurative bacterial infection. Painless enlargement characterizes indolent mycobacterial and fungal infections. Generalized salivary gland enlargement suggests a systemic disease involving the salivary glands either primarily or secondarily, or excessive salivary stimulation (e.g., bulimia).

CLINICAL OCCURRENCE: *Degenerative/Idiopathic:* Sarcoidosis; *Infections:* Bacterial (staph, gonorrhea, syphilis, trachoma, actinomycosis); viral (mumps, EBV, hepatitis C, HIV); mycobacterial (tuberculosis); fungal (histoplasmosis); *Inflammatory/Immune:* Sjögren syndrome, amyloidosis; *Metabolic/Toxic:* Diabetes mellitus, metal sensitivity (lead, iodide, copper); *Neoplastic:* Primary salivary gland tumors, lymphoma, Warthin tumor; *Psychosocial:* Bulimia, chronic alcohol consumption.

Painless bilateral parotid enlargement. Parotids enlarge in a number of conditions: its mechanism is unknown.

CLINICAL OCCURRENCE: *Endocrine:* Diabetes mellitus, pregnancy, lactation, hyperthyroidism; *Degenerative/Idiopathic:* Fatty salivary gland atrophy; *Inflammatory/Immune:* Sjögren syndrome, sarcoidosis, amyloidosis; *Metabolic/ Toxic:* Malnutrition (cirrhosis, kwashiorkor, pellagra, vitamin A deficiency), poisoning (iodine, mercury, lead), drugs (e.g., thiouracil, isoproterenol, sulfisoxazole), obesity, starch ingestion; *Neoplastic:* Lymphocytic leukemia, lymphoma, salivary gland tumors; *Psychosocial:* Bulimia nervosa, stress.

Acute nonsuppurative parotitis. There is brawny induration of the parotid region, with swelling in front of the tragus, and behind the mandible and earlobe, pushing it outward. The skin is warm and there is pain, accentuated by mouth opening or chewing, and exquisite tenderness. Fever is common.

The duct orifice can be red, occasionally discharging pus. One or both sides may be involved. Mumps is the classic cause; occasionally bacterial infection is responsible. Iodine allergy can cause the same symptoms.

Acute suppurative parotitis. Acute bacterial parotid infection is seen in debilitated, immunosuppressed, and previously irradiated patients. The gland is swollen, tender, and painful; induration and pitting edema are often present, accompanied by high fever. The duct orifice discharges pus. Multiple abscesses may form, but fluctuance is difficult to detect.

Chronic suppurative parotitis. Repeated episodes of duct obstruction produces chronic inflammation without fever or pain.

Submandibular duct obstruction. When there is a history of a mass appearing after meals, but no mass on exam, give sips of lemon juice and watch for swelling. A new mass, or enlargement of a preexisting swelling, is diagnostic of duct obstruction. Compare duct orifices on each side. Using bimanual palpation, feel for a calculus or mass. Press the gland in the submandibular triangle and look for drainage.

Neck Signs

Stiff neck. Pain and limited neck motion direct attention to the neck's muscles, bones, and joints. Be sure the mental status is normal and there are no signs of meningeal inflammation (Chapter 14, page 670) before evaluating for other causes. **CLINICAL OCCURRENCE:** *Congenital:* Torticollis, syringomyelia, Chiari syndromes; *Degenerative/Idiopathic:* Fibromyalgia, myofascial pain syndrome, stiff-man syndrome, Parkinson disease; *Infectious:* Pharyngitis, laryngitis, prevertebral or retropharyngeal abscess, cervical lymphadenitis, meningitis; *Inflammatory/Immune:* Osteomyelitis, epidural abscess, tuberculosis, RA, ankylosing spondylitis, polymyalgia rheumatica; *Mechanical/Traumatic:* Acquired torticollis, trauma to cervical vertebrae (fracture, dislocation, subluxation, disk herniation), muscles and soft tissues (e.g., whiplash), cervical spondylitis, spinal stenosis; *Metabolic/Toxic:* Strychnine, hypercalcemia, tetanus; *Neoplastic:* Thyroid cancer, lymphoma, oropharyngeal carcinoma, metastatic carcinoma; *Psychosocial:* Malingering, pending injury litigation.

Torticollis (wryneck). Hematoma or partial rupture of the sternocleidomastoid during parturition results in unilateral muscle shortening and congenital torticollis. Dystonic drug reactions, e.g., to phenothiazines, frequently precipitates torticollis. The head may tip to one side, the dystonic sternocleidomastoid being prominent. If tipping is present but the muscles are not prominent, straighten the head causing the sternal head of one muscle to tense more than the other. In long-standing torticollis, the face, and even the skull, may be asymmetrical. *DDX:* Distinguish the head tilt of torticollis from head posture correcting for vertical squint or ocular muscle palsy, *ocular torticollis* (Chapter 14, page 662): slowly but firmly straighten the neck while watching the eyes for squint. Asymmetrical erosion of the occipital condyle from rheumatoid arthritis or neoplastic disease results in cranial settling in a tilted position.

Meningitis. The neck is held stiffly in slight or extreme dorsiflexion from pain and reflex muscle spasm. Forceful neck anteflexion results in involuntary flexion at the hips, knees, and ankles, *Brudzinski sign*, indicating meningeal irritation. See Chapter 14, page 671.

- *Septic thrombophlebitis of the internal jugular vein (Lemierre syndrome).* Local infection in the face or oropharynx leads to septic thrombophlebitis of the internal jugular vein. This is a medical and surgical emergency, mandating early recognition. The patient is systemically ill with fever, chills, and signs of septicemia. Septic emboli to the lungs cause multiple pulmonary abscesses [Bliss SJ, Flanders SA, Saint S. A pain in the neck. *N Engl J Med*. 2004;350:1037–1042].

Midline Cervical Mass

Thyroglossal cysts and fistulas. Cysts arise from midline thyroglossal duct remnants (Fig. 7-12, page 171). Thyroglossal cysts appear at any time in life. Some cysts are translucent. A fistula results from drainage of an inflamed cyst or incomplete excision of a thyroglossal remnant. The sinus tract opens in or near the midline. Cysts occur at various levels, presenting diagnostic challenges.

Suprahyoid level. A thyroglossal cyst immediately above the hyoid bone (Fig. 7-65A) must be distinguished from a sublingual dermoid cyst, visible under the tongue as a white, opaque body shining through the mucosa.

Subhyoid level. The midline cyst is between the hyoid bone and thyroid cartilage. Sometimes swallowing hides the mass temporarily under the hyoid. Dorsiflexing the neck and opening mouth, causes the cyst to reappear (Fig. 7-65B).

Thyroid cartilage level. At this level a thyroglossal cyst may deviate from the midline, usually to the left, the forward pressure of the thyroid cartilage pushing it aside. To distinguish the mass from an enlarged lymph node, have the patient protrude the tongue maximally. A thyroglossal duct cyst is tugged upward.

Cricoid cartilage level. In this region, a thyroglossal cyst must be distinguished from a pyramidal lobe mass. Tongue protrusion tugs the cyst upward.

Pyramidal thyroid lobe. See the preceding discussion on thyroglossal cyst at the cricoid level. The pyramidal lobe may extend from the thyroid isthmus to the hyoid bone (Fig. 7-66A). The base on the isthmus is usually wider than the projection's height. It may be palpable in Hashimoto thyroiditis.

Suprasternal notch mass—dermoid cyst. A nonpulsatile fluctuant mass in the suprasternal notch (*Burns space*) frequently is a dermoid cyst. The mass doesn't adhere to the trachea, or move upward with tongue protrusion.

Suprasternal mass—tuberculous abscess. Other than being slightly less fluctuant, this has the same characteristics as the dermoid cyst. It arises from an apical lung abscess or by drainage from deep cervical lymph nodes.

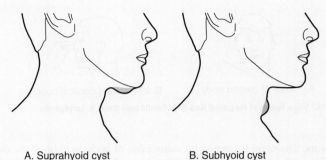

A. Suprahyoid cyst   B. Subhyoid cyst

FIG. 7-65 Thyroglossal Cysts and Sinuses. A. Suprahyoid cyst: This is above the hyoid bone. **B. Subhyoid cyst.**

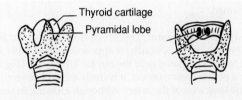

Thyroid cartilage
Pyramidal lobe

A. Pyramidal lobe of thyroid gland   B. Delphian nodes

FIG. 7-66 Thyroid-Associated Masses. A. Pyramidal lobe of thyroid gland. **B. Delphian nodes.**

Pulsatile suprasternal notch mass—aorta or innominate artery. Occasionally, the aortic arch or innominate artery elongates, bowing the vessel up into the suprasternal notch. This is not necessarily evidence of aneurysmal dilatation.

Lateral Cervical Masses: Intermittent or persistent cystic feeling masses in lateral neck compartments usually arise from normal structures that have become, or are intermittently, distended. The history, exact location, and characteristics of the mass usually identifies the probable etiology. Solid masses in these locations frequently arise in lymph nodes and suggest neoplasms, usually malignant. A fluctuant lymph node mass suggests infection, suppurative bacteria if acute and tuberculosis if chronic.

Branchial cyst. Embryonic branchial cleft remnants undergo cystic enlargement, usually in adults. Commonly, there is a single cystic mass just anterior but deep to the upper third of the sternocleidomastoid. The mass feels slightly soft and resilient; intercurrent inflammation makes it tender and firm. Aspirated fluid appears to be pus, but oil droplets may be seen floating on the surface.

Branchial fistula. Arising from a branchial cyst, the fistula may be either congenital or have developed from an inflamed cyst. Probing usually discloses a blind end in the lateral pharyngeal wall. Fistulas become intermittently infected.

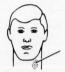 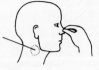

A. Tumor of carotid body   B. Intermittent cervical pouches

FIG. 7-67 Single Tumors of the Lateral Neck II. A. Carotid body tumor. B. Laryngocele.

Hygroma. The mass is formed by many cysts of occluded lymphatic channels. The soft, irregular, and partially compressible mass is usually present from childhood. It occupies the upper third of the anterior cervical triangle but may extend downward or under the jaw. Its brilliant translucence distinguishes it from all other cysts. Its size may vary from time to time and it may become inflamed.

Carotid body (glomus) tumor. This arises from the carotid body chromaffin tissue, can be familial or sporadic. It appears in middle life and grows very slowly. The mass is palpated near the carotid bifurcation (Fig. 7-67A). Usually shaped like a potato (*potato tumor*), it is freely movable laterally, but cannot be moved in the long axis of the artery. Although growing in the carotid sheath, it does not always transmit arterial pulsations. Early it may feel cystic, later becoming hard. Pressure on the tumor sometimes slows the heart rate producing lightheadedness. Some tumors produce vasoactive amines, and palpation can produce pupillary dilatation and hypertension, a useful diagnostic sign. Regional extension upward along the carotid sheath eventually occurs in 20%.

Zenker diverticulum (pharyngeal pouch). A pharyngeal diverticulum occurs cephalad to the cricopharyngeus muscle. The patient complains of gurgling in the neck, especially during swallowing. Regurgitation of food is common while eating or lying on the side. An intermittent swelling may be seen in the side of the neck, usually the left. If not apparent, the swelling may be induced by swallowing water. Pressure on the distended pouch causes regurgitation of old food.

Laryngocele. Herniation of a laryngeal diverticulum through the lateral thyrohyoid membrane causes intermittent neck swelling (Fig. 7-67B). Blowing the nose will often induce an air-filled swelling that is resonant to percussion. It is usually caused by chronic severe coughing or sustained blowing on a musical instrument.

Cavernous hemangioma. As in other parts of the body, the swelling is soft, compression partially empties the cavity of blood and refilling is slow. A faint blue color under the skin may be discerned.

Thyroid Signs
Tracheal displacement and compression by goiter. A large or strategically located goiter can cause tracheal compression and/or displacement (Fig. 7-68). Patients complain of tightness or pressure in the throat. Stridor is

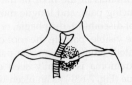

Tracheal displacement
by retrosternal goiter

FIG. 7-68 Tracheal Displacement: The retrosternal goiter on the patient's left compresses the trachea transversely pushing it to the right. The tracheal deviation can be demonstrated by palpation.

rarely the presenting complaint. The trachea is most vulnerable to compression at the thoracic inlet, especially in small patients with short necks. Usually the trachea is narrowed transversely. Small degrees of compression are not apparent from history or physical exam. With severe narrowing, slight pressure on the lateral thyroid lobes produces stridor (*Kocher test*). Lateral trachea deviation in the neck is present when the midpoints of the tracheal rings are not centered in the suprasternal notch (Fig. 7-68).

Tender thyroid—thyroiditis. See page 258.

Thyroid bruit. As the thyroid undergoes hyperplasia the increased blood flow produces a *thyroid bruit*, suggesting Graves disease. *DDX:* A thyroid bruit may be confused with a carotid bruit; the latter radiates to the angle of the jaw. An aortic murmur originates at the base of the heart and can be followed into the neck. A venous hum has a different pitch and is abolished by light compression of the jugular vein.

Thyroid enlargement—goiter. See page 256.

Thyroid nodules. See page 258.

Enlarged Delphian lymph nodes. A few lymph nodes are normally present in the thyrohyoid membrane. When enlarged, they are termed the Delphian because they may foretell thyroid cancer. Enlarged Delphian nodes indicate either subacute thyroiditis or thyroid cancer (Fig. 7-66B).

HEAD AND NECK SYNDROMES

Squamous Cell Cancers of the Head and Neck: Tobacco and alcohol are cocarcinogens for aerodigestive system squamous cell carcinoma. Muscle infiltration by neoplasm limits functions, e.g., tongue protrusion with deep cancers. Regional lymph node spread may be the first sign of disease. The enlarging nodes are stony hard. Lymph node biopsy is contraindicated since it violates tissue planes adversely affecting prognosis. Aspiration cytology is indicated for suspicious nodes. Complete panendoscopic evaluation of the upper aerodigestive tract is necessary in all cases to establish the primary site and disease extent, and for treatment planning.

Tongue carcinoma. Carcinomas in the floor of the mouth are often symptomatic, ulceration producing pain, and tongue motion causing discomfort. If the patient complains of discomfort, dysphagia, or inability to protrude the tongue, yet no lesions are visible, palpate the root of the tongue. Inspection usually reveals an ulcerated, whitish lesion. On palpation it is harder than surrounding muscle. Carcinoma is usually seen on the sides, base, and undersurface of the tongue (Fig. 7-63F) as an ulcerating mass with rolled and everted margins. It is not tender unless ulcerated. A unilateral neoplasm hindering muscle action, causes deviation toward the side of the lesion. Fixation to the mandible and metastases to submental or anterior jugular lymph nodes occur early.

Tonsil carcinoma. Human papilloma virus, especially type 16, causes more than half of tonsillar cancers. The patient complains of earache from referred pain. The breath is foul with a bleeding ulceration. Palpation discloses characteristic tonsil induration.

Larynx neoplasms. Larynx tumors are benign or malignant, pedunculated or sessile, localized or infiltrative. Infiltrative lesions are malignant. Localized masses must be biopsied for diagnosis (Figs. 7-64E and F)

Scalp, Face, Skull, and Jaw Syndromes
Headache. See Chapter 14, page 651, for a full discussion of headache. Discussed below are regional causes of headache related to extracranial disease.

Fever. Many febrile illnesses are associated with headache. The location varies, the pain may be slight or severe, throbbing or steady. Pain is thought to arise from distention of the cranial arteries.

Giant cell arteritis, temporal arteritis. See Chapter 8, page 361. Temporal headache resulting from ischemia in the temporal artery distribution are constant and relatively severe. Scalp tenderness is often present and exquisite scalp sensitivity is nearly diagnostic. Search for nodularity and decreased temporal artery pulsation.

Occipital neuritis. Pain over the ear and posterior scalp suggests occipital neuritis from occipital nerve entrapment.

Paranasal sinusitis. See page 248.

Ice cream headache. Applying cold to the palate triggers intense medial orbital pain. It is precipitated by eating very cold foods, classically ice cream, and lasts 2–120 seconds. It may be more common in migraineurs.

TMJ pain. Pain in front of the ear, episodic or constant, worsened with eating, and accompanied by clicking or grating sensations is typical of TMJ disease (Fig. 7-69). Common causes are trauma and being edentulous. Loss of correct maxilla-mandible spacing for chewing places abnormal forces on the TMJ. Other diseases affecting the TMJ are RA, rheumatic fever, SLE, gout, Sjögren syndrome, and familial Mediterranean fever. *DDX:* Pain in the side

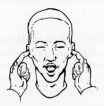

FIG. 7-69 Palpation of the TMJ. Place the tips of your index fingers in each external acoustic meatus and have the patient open and close his mouth. Clicking or crepitation is felt with TMJ arthritis; the joint will be tender if rheumatoid arthritis is the cause.

of the head with chewing suggests giant cell arteritis with claudication of the masticators. The mechanical symptoms identify TMJ pain. TMJ tenderness distinguishes RA from rheumatic fever.

Periorbital abscess. In suppurative ethmoid sinusitis, pus may extend through the lateral sinus wall forming an abscess between the ethmoid plate and periosteum lining the orbit. This is accompanied by fever, pain on eye movement, and edema between the inner canthus and the bridge of the nose. The edematous region is tender, and edema may extend to both lids. The pus may push the globe slightly downward and laterally. No chemosis is present. Surgical drainage is essential.

Orbital cellulitis. A periorbital abscess may extend producing diffuse orbital cellulitis. Invasion is heralded by a chill, high fever, and dull pain in the eye. The eyelids become edematous, particularly near the inner canthus, and chemosis develops. Ultimately, the eye becomes fixed. The patient appears very ill and requires immediate surgical care.

Eye Syndromes

Sjögren syndrome—keratoconjunctivitis sicca. Lymphocytes infiltrate the salivary and lacrimal glands with loss of exocrine function. This autoimmune disorder was first described as keratoconjunctivitis sicca and xerostomia in rheumatoid arthritis patients. Primary Sjögren syndrome is relatively common with symptoms of fatigue, dry mouth, eyes, and other mucosal surfaces, arthralgias and arthritis, and nephritis. Both central and peripheral neurologic symptoms may be present. In addition to rheumatoid arthritis other autoimmune diseases may accompany the syndrome. There is an increased risk of non-Hodgkin lymphomas.

Graves ophthalmopathy. Mucopolysaccharide deposition and fibrotic degeneration of the extraocular muscles and orbital fat displace the globe forward, impairing eye movement. Acquired bilateral exophthalmos is most commonly associated with Graves disease. The proptosis occurs independently of thyroid function, so the patient may be hyperthyroid, euthyroid, or hypothyroid. The proptosis is often permanent, although treating acute infiltration and edema may lead to resolution. Accompanying signs are lid edema, periorbital swelling, lid lag, lid retraction, and scleral show (page 175). Proptosis may initially be unilateral, raising concern for other intraorbital pathology. Patients may present with diplopia because of asymmetric muscle involvement.

Down syndrome (trisomy 21). The four ocular signs of Down syndrome are an epicanthic fold persisting after age 10 years; unilateral or bilateral slanting eyes in which the lateral canthus is elevated >2 mm above a line through both medial canthi; *Brushfield spots*, accumulations of light-colored tissues in a concentric band of the outer third of the iris; and hypoplastic iris seen as dark discoloration of the iris.

Uveal tract inflammation—uveitis (iritis, iridocyclitis, and choroiditis). The uveal tract, the vascular layer of the eye, is inflamed. It may involve only the iris (iritis), extend to the ciliary body (iridocyclitis), or involve the choroid (choroiditis) or retina (retinitis). Iritis is characterized by ciliary flush and miosis, accompanied by deep pain, photophobia, blurring, and lacrimation. The inflamed iris may adhere to the anterior lens forming *posterior synechiae*, manifest by pupil irregularity. Cells cast off into the anterior chamber form a sterile *hypopyon* (Fig. 7-34B). Yellow deposits or white dots of aggregated inflammatory and pigmented cells, *keratic precipitates*, appear on the cornea's posterior surface. Uveitis, most commonly idiopathic, also results from trauma, infection, allergy, sarcoidosis, collagen vascular diseases, and autoimmune conditions such as ankylosing spondylitis.

Red eye. A red eye may be caused by a benign self-limited condition or indicate serious sight-threatening eye disease. *DDX:* Generalized redness of the bulbar and tarsal conjunctivae, with minimal discharge and no visual loss, is usually viral conjunctivitis or blepharitis. Localized lid redness and swelling suggests hordeolum or chalazion. Severe photophobia, ciliary flush, visual loss, elevated intraocular pressure, corneal haze, acute proptosis, and acute scleritis require urgent evaluation by an ophthalmologist.
CLINICAL OCCURRENCE: *Benign Disorders:* Environmental irritant, allergic and viral conjunctivitis, external hordeolum (sty), internal hordeolum (chalazion), and blepharitis; *Serious Disorders Requiring Urgent Ophthalmology Referral:* Acute keratitis (herpes simplex, bacterial, trauma, foreign body), gonococcal and chlamydial conjunctivitis, acute glaucoma, acute iridocyclitis, uveitis, and acute scleritis.

Glaucoma. Increased intraocular pressure produces ischemic damage to the nerve fibers at the optic disk. A progressive increase in cup-to-disk ratio discovered by sequential observations suggests increasing intraocular pressure (Fig. 7-37). Early damage leads to nasal steps and arcuate defects. Later, there is general visual field constriction from optic nerve injury from increased intraocular pressure or vasculopathy of the nerve head (Fig. 7-39C). Detection of early visual field loss requires automated perimetry. Pupillary dilation is often present.

Narrow angle glaucoma. Drainage of aqueous from the anterior chamber is obstructed by narrowing the chamber angle and/or increasing aqueous production. Acute symptoms are extreme ocular pain with nausea and vomiting, and loss of vision. Chronic symptoms include halos around lights, tunnel vision, ocular pain, and headache. Chemosis, corneal edema, ciliary flush, and a fixed dilated pupil are seen on exam.

Open angle glaucoma. There is increased aqueous secretion and obstruction to outflow with normal chamber angles. The most common type of glaucoma, it occurs in older persons who may see colored halos around lights and experience insidious, painless blindness.

Sudden vision loss. *This always requires urgent attention by an ophthalmologist.* Visual loss is usually monocular resulting from detached retina, vitreous hemorrhage, retinal artery occlusion (embolus, thrombus, or vasculitis), optic nerve compression, or anterior ischemic optic neuritis (AION), arteritic and nonarteritic. Transient 5–15-minute unilateral visual loss (*amaurosis fugax*) is usually caused by embolic retinal artery occlusion. On fundoscopy, refractile cholesterol emboli may be seen at retinal artery bifurcations. Loss of vision in one visual field (right or left *hemianopsia*) indicates a lesion between the optic chiasm and visual cortex. Patients are often unaware of this visual field loss. Sudden bilateral visual loss with nystagmus and/or confusion suggests thiamine deficiency, from dietary deficiency or increased metabolic demand.

Monocular visual loss—amblyopia. Monocular visual loss in an otherwise normal eye occurs during visual development in the first few years of life from one of the three causes: misalignment of the optic axes (*strabismus*), large differences in refractive error between the two eyes (*anisometropia*), or deprivation of vision in one eye resulting from bilateral severe refractive errors. Amblyopia causes preventable visual loss in ~3% of the population. Early childhood screening, recognition, and treatment helps to prevent and, in some cases restore visual acuity.

Ear Syndromes

Acute external otitis. A variety of organisms can cause inflammation, but the usual offenders are *Pseudomonas aeruginosa*, or, less commonly, streptococci, staphylococci, or *Proteus vulgaris*. This may be the result of increased pH in the canal ("swimmer's ear"). Pain may be mild or severe and is accentuated by movement of the tragus or pinna. The epithelium appears either pale or red; it may swell closing the canal and impairing hearing. The tragus may also swell. A discharge is often present. Fever is not uncommon. Tender, palpable lymph nodes may appear in front of the tragus, behind the pinna, or in the anterior cervical triangle.

Chronic external otitis. Bacteria and fungi are the chief causes, although it can accompany a chronic dermatitis, e.g., seborrhea or psoriasis. Pruritus, not pain, is the chief symptom. Ear discharge may be present. The epithelium of the pinna and meatus is thickened and red; it is abnormally insensitive to the pain during instrumentation.

Malignant (necrotizing) external otitis. *Pseudomonas aeruginosa* invades the soft tissues, cartilage, and bone of patients with diabetes mellitus. Although some patients have minimal clinical findings, others experience pain, discharge, and fever with swelling and tenderness of the tissues around the ear. Auditory canal exam may reveal edema, redness, granulation tissue, and pus obscuring the TM. Complications are osteomyelitis of the mastoid, temporal bone, and skull base with involvement of CNs, especially CN-VII. Otolaryngology consult is mandatory.

Middle ear glomus tumor. Fibrovascular tumors arise from glomus bodies in the jugular bulb or middle ear mucosa. They present with pulsatile tinnitus in the involved ear. Sometimes the glomus jugular type is associated with paralysis of CN-IX and CN-XI which pass through the jugular foramen. Glomus tumors appear as red masses behind the TM. Identical tumors arise from the carotid artery bifurcation. Rarely, tumors are multiple, malignant, and/or secreting vasoactive amines. If biopsied, they bleed profusely. Familial forms occur.

Acute otitis media with effusion (serous otitis media). Eustachian tube obstruction prevents middle ear aeration. Resorption of trapped air produces negative middle ear pressure leading to an effusion, while atmospheric pressure displaces the TM inward. This usually follows an upper respiratory infection. Initially, the TM retracts around the malleus, becoming more distinct and curving the light reflex (Fig. 7-28B). Later, serous amber fluid is seen behind the TM (Fig. 7-28C). A fluid meniscus forms a fine black line, and sometimes air bubbles are visible (Fig. 7-28E).

Acute suppurative otitis media. Bacteria from the nasopharynx (*Streptococcus pneumonia, Haemophilus influenza, Moraxella catarrhalis*) enter the middle ear via the Eustachian tube; fluid in the chamber favors purulent infection. Throbbing earache, frequently with fever and hearing loss, is the chief complaint. The bright red and lusterless TM bulges obliterating normal landmarks (Fig. 7-28D). Perforation rapidly relieves pain and pus appears in the canal. If the infection extends into the mastoid air cells, pressure on the mastoid process may elicit pain. Fever and constitutional symptoms are more prominent in children than adults. *DDX:* Movement of the pinna and tragus does not cause pain, unlike acute external otitis.

Acute mastoiditis. The mastoid air cells communicate with the middle ear. Usually, mastoid infection results from inadequate treatment of acute suppurative otitis media. The symptoms of otitis gradually increase and there is low-grade fever. The eardrum is lusterless and edematous. Deep pain is elicited by percussing the mastoid process. Clouding of the mastoid air cells on imaging confirms the diagnosis. Bone destruction becomes evident after 2–3 weeks. Extension can cause a subperiosteal abscess of the mastoid process. Less commonly, erosion of bone damages the facial nerve (CN-VII) with facial paralysis. Extension through the inner table can cause meningitis, epidural abscess, or abscess of the temporal lobe or cerebellum. Infection of the internal ear can produce labyrinthitis.

Chronic suppurative otitis media. This is associated with a permanent TM perforation. A marginal annulus perforation is more common than a central defect. The chief symptom is painless aural discharge. Hearing is always impaired. Discharge volume may wax and wane, but recurrence is invariable.

Painless discharge accompanying a URI suggests an old perforation. Pain and vertigo indicate a complication, e.g., subdural irritation, brain abscess, or labyrinth involvement.

Cholesteatoma. In chronic suppurative otitis media with a deep retraction pocket in the attic or posterior superior quadrant of the TM, the squamous epithelium of the meatus may grow into the attic of the tympanic cavity. Desquamation produces a caseous mass of cells, keratin, and debris, which, becoming infected and slowly enlarging, extends into the mastoid antrum ultimately eroding bone. Patients have ear fullness, pain, headache, and hearing loss. Signs include chronic foul-smelling suppurative middle ear discharge, hearing loss, and a pearly gray mass visible with the otoscope.

Hearing loss. Sensorineural loss (nerve deafness) results from disorders of the cochlea or acoustic nerve (CN-VIII). Conductive loss means failure to conduct TM vibrations to the neurosensory apparatus. Causes of sensorineural loss include hereditary deafness, congenital deafness, trauma, infections, drug toxicity, and aging (*presbycusis*). Unilateral hearing loss and tinnitus may be the first symptoms of an acoustic neuroma. Conductive loss occurs with external acoustic meatus obstruction, TM and middle ear disorders, and fixation of the stapes by bone overgrowth (*otosclerosis*). Hearing loss screening involves questioning patient and family members about hearing difficulty. Follow affirmative or equivocal responses with the whispered voice test.

Dizziness. Symptoms described as dizziness may arise from problems in the inner ear, CN-VIII, or vestibular nucleus; from loss of proprioception due to peripheral neuropathy or visual impairment; from autonomic dysfunction or intravascular volume depletion; and from anxiety and other psychiatric disorders. This common complaint requires a careful history. *Never suggest descriptive terms (spinning, lightheaded, unsteady, etc.). The patient must describe the symptoms without using the word dizzy.* From the description, put the symptoms into one of four general categories: 1. true vertigo (an illusion or hallucination of motion); 2. near syncope (e.g., orthostatic lightheadedness, and hypotension); 3. postural unsteadiness caused by sensory abnormalities or weakness; and 4. the last group, for whom no clear physiologic explanation is suggested.

CLINICAL OCCURRENCE: *Endocrine:* Hypothyroidism, pregnancy, hypoparathyroidism, aldosteronoma; *Degenerative/Idiopathic:* Multisystem atrophy, migraine, absence seizures, peripheral neuropathy; *Infectious:* Meningitis, encephalitis, brain abscess, syphilis; *Inflammatory/Immune:* Vestibular neuritis; *Mechanical/Traumatic—Ears:* Utricular trauma from skull fracture, otosclerosis, leakage from tears in the oval or round windows, perilymph fistula; *Mechanical/Traumatic—Eyes:* Muscle imbalance, refractive errors, glaucoma; *Metabolic/Toxic:* Nutritional: Pellagra, alcoholism, vitamin B_{12} deficiency; cerebral hypoxia, fluid and electrolyte disturbances; *Neoplastic:* Brain tumors (primary, metastatic); *Psychosocial:* Panic attack, generalized anxiety disorder; *Vascular:* Hypotension, orthostatic hypotension.

Vertigo. When the head is at rest, persistent stimulation of the semicircular canals or vestibular nucleus produces a hallucination of motion. With the eyes open or closed the surroundings seem to be whirling or spinning about. Nausea and vomiting accompany severe vertigo. The first task is distinguishing between positional vertigo, which is common and usually benign, and spontaneous vertigo unrelated to position. Next, identify the cause as peripheral (labyrinth, CN-VIII) or central (brainstem). Nausea and vomiting are more common with peripheral lesions. Despite severe discomfort, the patient can stand and walk with peripheral lesions. With central lesions, they may be unable to stand without falling. Also, peripheral vertigo tends to improve with prolonged fixation of the eyes. *Signs Distinguishing Central from Peripheral Vertigo:* 1. *Bidirectional nystagmus:* The direction of the nystagmus changes with alteration of gaze without changing head position. It always has a central etiology. 2. *Head impulse test:* With the patient fixing his gaze on your nose, quickly turn the head about 45 degrees to the right and then left. If the eyes move to restore fixation, indicating an abnormal vestibuloocular reflex, the cause is peripheral. 3. *Vertical squint:* Perform the cover–uncover test (page 175) with the gaze directed first upward then downward. Movement of either eye to restore fixation on uncover indicates a central cause. 4. *The Dix–Hallpike Maneuver:* See page 173. A positive test indicates a labyrinthine disorder. 5. *The Fukuda Stepping Test:* Standing upright with the eyes closed and the arms outstretched, have the patient march in place, keeping the eyes closed. Rotation of >30 degrees is a positive test indicating asymmetric inner ear function [Froehling DA, Silverman MD, Mohr DN, Beatty CW. The rational clinical examination. Does this dizzy patient have a serious form of vertigo? *JAMA.* 1994;271:385–388].

CLINICAL OCCURRENCE: *Peripheral Labyrinthine System:* Serous labyrinthitis, perilymph fistula, labyrinth fistula, viral labyrinthitis, otosclerosis, otitis media with effusion, benign paroxysmal positional vertigo, Ménière disease, motion sickness, cholesteatoma, temporal bone fracture, postural vertigo; *Central Labyrinthine System:* Migraine, vertebrobasilar insufficiency, brainstem or cerebellar hemorrhage or infarction, posteroinferior cerebellar artery thrombosis, infarction of the lateral medulla (Wallenberg syndrome), cerebellopontine angle tumors, intra-axial tumors (pons, cerebellum, medulla), craniovertebral abnormalities causing cervicomedullary junctional compression, multiple sclerosis, encephalitis, meningitis, intracranial abscess (temporal lobe, cerebellum, epidural, subdural), trauma; CN-VIII infections (acute meningitis, tuberculous meningitis, basilar syphilitic meningitis), trauma, tumors.

Acute labyrinthitis (vestibular neuritis). This is the most frequent cause of vertigo. The patient gradually develops a sense of whirling that reaches a climax in 24–48 hours. Nausea and vomiting may occur. The patient seeks comfort in the horizontal position; raising the head may induce vertigo. The patient is incapacitated for several days. The symptoms gradually subside, and disappear in 3–6 weeks. There is no accompanying tinnitus or hearing loss.

Benign paroxysmal positional vertigo (BPPV). Dislodged calcium deposits (otoliths), usually in the posterior labyrinth, move in response to gravity eliciting a feeling of motion. This is most common in older individuals and may occur after head trauma or acute labyrinthitis. The onset is sudden, often when rolling over in bed or arising in the morning. There is no headache or fever. There is often intense nausea and inability to stand. Symptoms are minimized by avoiding any head motion. After a 1–2-second latent period the Dix–Hallpike maneuver (page 173) produces mixed vertical and rotational nystagmus, the fast components toward the dependent ear and upward toward the forehead. The nystagmus may be accompanied by profound vertigo and nausea. Canalith repositioning is curative, but recurrences are not uncommon.

Labyrinthine hydrops (Ménière disease). There is swelling of endolymphatic labyrinthine spaces and degeneration of the organ of Corti. There are sudden attacks of whirling vertigo, tinnitus, and neurosensory hearing loss with intervals of complete freedom from vertigo. Attacks last hours but not days. Hearing loss and tinnitus persist. Fluctuating slowly progressive hearing loss predominates on one side. Tinnitus also fluctuates, accentuating before an attack. The disease is self-limited. The cause is unknown. Labyrinthine tests are normal or hypoactive on the involved side.

Vascular disease. Transient vertigo may be caused by arterial spasm or obstruction producing low flow. Severe prolonged symptoms suggest thrombosis or dissection of a brainstem artery. There is sudden vertigo with nystagmus, loud tinnitus, and sudden deafness. Partial recovery is usual in 3–4 weeks.

Trauma. Skull fracture through the inner ear, concussion, or a loud noise induces symptoms like a stroke. Tinnitus and hearing loss are present. Labyrinthine tests show delay and hypoactivity on the affected side.

Trauma. *Damage to CN-VIII or brainstem nuclei.* Lesions, at either level, produce vertigo and nystagmus. Disorders of CN-VIII (e.g., acoustic neuroma) are accompanied by hearing loss, which is absent with brainstem lesions, except when other CNs are also damaged.

Nose and Sinus Syndromes

Rhinosinusitis. Infection, allergic inflammation, or irritation of the respiratory epithelium lining the nose and paranasal sinuses lead to hyperemia, edema, increased mucous production, and exudation of inflammatory cells. Patients experience congestion, nasal and postnasal discharge, sneezing, facial pressure, and sometimes fever. Diagnosis depends upon an accurate history noting time of year, exposures, and current infectious disease activity in the home and community. *DDX:* Rhinovirus infections do not cause sore throat or fever. Fever, purulent or bloody discharge, or pain in the upper teeth beginning several days after onset of a cold suggests suppurative sinusitis. Sneezing and itchy eyes suggest allergic rhinosinusitis with allergic conjunctivitis.

Acute rhinitis—the common cold. Rhinoviruses, and many others, infect the nasal and sinus mucous membranes causing inflammation and increasing nasal secretions. The sinuses are involved in 75% of patients. Most people have 4–6 episodes annually. The onset is abrupt with a watery discharge (*rhinorrhea*) and sneezing, often with malaise and mild myalgia, but without fever or sore throat. Nasal secretions may become purulent, possibly accompanied by fever and malaise. Mucosal edema obstructs nasal passages. Symptoms last 3–10 days. Severe local pain suggests bacterial sinusitis.

Chronic rhinitis. Chronic bilateral rhinorrhea suggests chronic environmental irritants (dust, smoke, perfume, dry or cold air), allergic rhinitis (seasonal or perennial), rhinitis medicamentosa, or vasomotor rhinitis.

Atrophic rhinitis. The patient complains of nasal discomfort or stuffiness. The membranes are dry, smooth, and shiny, and studded with crusts. A foul odor (*ozena*) may be present. The cause is unknown.

Allergic rhinosinusitis. IgE-mediated mast cell degranulation follows exposure to specific allergens to which the patient has been sensitized by previous exposure. Nasal and ocular itching, rhinorrhea, and lacrimation are accompanied by sneezing. Headache is common. The mucosa is usually pale, swollen, and edematous, but may be dull red or purplish. Allergic rhinitis is seasonal or perennial. Common allergens are pollens, molds, animal danders, house dust mite, and cockroach antigens. Seasonal symptoms are associated with exposure to pollens (trees in the spring; grasses in the summer; ragweed in the fall) or to antigens associated with a specific environment. Perennial allergic rhinitis suggests environmental antigens in the home, e.g., house dust mite and/or animal danders (usually cats).

Vasomotor rhinitis. Environmental, hormonal, and drug exposures cause nasal vasodilatation increasing mucous production by nonallergic mechanisms. Environmental irritants, e.g., smoke, perfumes, strong odors, and cold air, are a common cause. Pregnancy and therapeutic estrogens and progestins have been implicated. Chronic vasomotor rhinitis reflects persistent mucosal overreaction to environmental exposures.

Rhinitis medicamentosa. Using topical vasoconstrictors for more than a few days leads to rebound hyperemia on withdrawal, triggering more medication use. Looking like allergic rhinitis, the history of nasal vasoconstrictor use, and absence of eosinophils in nasal secretions suggest the diagnosis.

Suppurative paranasal sinusitis. Most viral upper respiratory infections are accompanied by sinus inflammation. Obstruction of the narrow sinus orifices leads to mucous accumulation which becomes infected by bacteria (*S. pneumoniae, H. influenzae, Moraxella* spp.) leading to suppurative sinusitis. The maxillary sinus with its dependent antrum and superiorly positioned orifice is at greatest risk. Severe face pain 7–14 days after onset of an acute upper respiratory infection suggests complicating acute suppurative bacterial sinusitis. Pain and pressure without fever earlier in the illness suggests sinus obstruction requiring decongestants [Williams JW, Simel DL. The rational clinical examination. Does this patient have sinusitis? Diagnosing acute sinusitis by history and physical exam. *JAMA*. 1993;270:1242–124]. Extension beyond the sinus into surrounding soft tissue and bone is a serious complication, the symptoms and signs being specific to the sinus involved. Transillumination may reveal an opaque maxillary or frontal sinus and plain films may show clouding of the sinus or a fluid level. CT imaging is definitive. Pain is not present with chronic inflammation or infection of the paranasal sinuses. *DDX:* Many patients with migraine are misdiagnosed with "sinus headaches." Nasal and sinus symptoms are common with migraine and cluster headache. Persistent or progressive symptoms raise concern for serious diseases, e.g., Wegener granulomatosis, nasopharyngeal carcinoma, and lethal midline granuloma.

Maxillary sinusitis. There is dull throbbing pain in the cheek and the ipsilateral upper teeth. Thumb pressure reveals localized maxillary tenderness. Examination discloses a reddened, edematous mucosa and swollen turbinates. A purulent blood-tinged discharge may be seen. Pus in the posterior middle meatus may be seen in the nasopharyngeal mirror. *DDX:* Painful teeth from maxillary sinusitis must be distinguished from dental apical abscess where only one tooth is painful and is tender when tapped.

Frontal sinusitis. There is pain above the supraorbital ridge and pressure there elicits tenderness. Ipsilateral eyelid edema is infrequent.

Ethmoid sinusitis. Pain is medial to the eye, seemingly deep in the head or orbit. Although lid edema is common, there is no localizing tenderness.

Sphenoid sinusitis. There is pain either behind the eyes, in the occiput, or in the vertex of the skull; no tenderness is elicited.

Chronic suppurative sinusitis. When a purulent nasal discharge persists >3 weeks, subacute or chronic sinusitis is suspected. Sinus pain is not prominent and tenderness is frequently absent. Exam after instilling a vasoconstrictor may reveal the source of the pus. *DDX:* Chronic suppurative sinusitis, especially with unusual organisms (e.g., fungi like *Aspergillus* spp. or *Mucor* spp.) or resistant to medical therapy, suggests common variable immunodeficiency.

- **Sinusitis and ocular palsies—cavernous sinus thrombosis.** Usually infection spreads from the nose through the angular vein to the cavernous sinus, where septic thrombosis occurs. This is the most feared complication of nasal infections because it can cause blindness and death. There are sudden chills, high fever, and pain deep in the eyes. The patient becomes prostrate and may rapidly become comatose. Early, there is ocular palsy involving the oculomotor (CN-III), trochlear nerve (CN-IV), or abducens nerve (CN-VI) within the cavernous sinus. Both eyes are involved early, with immobilization of the globes, periorbital edema, and chemosis. Death may occur within 2–3 days. *DDX:* Selective ocular palsy occurs early in cavernous sinus thrombosis, whereas orbital abscess produces complete immobilization of the globe gradually, without preliminary disorder of a single nerve. Bilaterality strongly suggests cavernous sinus thrombosis.

Midline granuloma. The cause is unknown, but some classify it as an angiocentric immunoproliferative lesion. Inflammation is attended by granuloma formation. It is most common in fifth and sixth decades, with a slight preference for women. Symptoms include sneezing, nasal stuffiness, obstruction, and pain. Signs are rhinorrhea, nasal congestion, and paranasal sinusitis progressing to inflammation and ulcerations of the nasal septum, palate, and nasal ali. Advanced disease is indicated by destruction of midfacial structures including pharynx, mouth, sinuses, and eyes with death from cachexia, pneumonia, meningitis, or hemorrhage. Indolent ulceration and mutilation suggest the diagnosis. *DDX:* Unlike granulomatosis with polyangiitis (Wegener), there is no systemic involvement or primary vasculitis.

Oral Syndromes (Lips, Mouth, Tongue, Teeth, and Pharynx)

Acute pharyngitis. The chief problem is distinguishing treatable bacterial pharyngitis from viral infection. Use antigen detection and throat culture to make a specific diagnosis when this is felt necessary.

Viral pharyngitis. Pharyngeal inflammation accompanies many viral infections, the most common are EBV, respiratory syncytial virus (RSV), parainfluenza, influenza, adenovirus, and coxsackievirus. The patient complains of sore throat, often with mild rhinorrhea and hoarseness. In influenza, the patient is febrile and usually complains of malaise, myalgia, and often a moderately sore throat and rhinorrhea. Oral inspection discloses swelling of mucosal lymphoid tissue on the posterior oropharyngeal wall, seen as elevated oval islands (Fig. 7-70). The mucosa may be dull red and the faucial pillars slightly edematous. Herpes simplex produces painful ulcers of the posterior pharynx, soft palate, buccal mucosa, and/or tongue, with punched-out edges surrounded by a rim of erythema.

Streptococcal and staphylococcal pharyngitis. Onset is often sudden, throat pain is severe, and the temperature rises to 39.5°C (103°F) or higher. The pharyngeal mucosa is bright red, swollen, and edematous, especially the fauces and uvula, and studded with white or yellow follicles. When the tonsils are present, they are swollen and stippled with prominent follicles. Tender, swollen cervical lymph nodes are common. Group A *Streptococcus* is much more common than *Staphylococcus*. *Scarlet fever* presents as an extremely painful throat with few follicles but brilliant red oropharyngeal mucosa extending forward to end abruptly near the back of the soft palate and fauces, as if red paint had been applied. Streptococcus is the presumptive cause unless proven

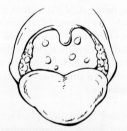

FIG. 7-70 Granular Pharyngitis in Viral Infections. Elevated islands of lymphoid tissue are seen in the oropharyngeal mucosa. The mucosa is only slightly reddened; seldom is there any edema or exudate.

otherwise. *DDX:* Hoarseness and cough are decidedly uncommon with bacterial pharyngitis, either arguing strongly against empiric antibiotic therapy.

- *Acute epiglottitis.* Bacterial infection of the epiglottis produces severe edema which can compromise the airway leading to asphyxiation. The condition is both more common and more dangerous in children. Patients present with sore throat and painful swallowing, decreased voice, and signs of pharyngitis. Stridor and the need to sit erect to breathe indicate impending airway compromise.
- *Pharyngeal diphtheria.* The fauces first become dull red and a patch of white membrane appears on the tonsil or oropharyngeal mucosa which is reddened, swollen, and edematous. The membrane becomes thick, gray or yellow, and tenaciously adherent to the mucosa, which bleeds when it is removed. The membrane spreads rapidly to other structures including the larynx. The cervical lymph nodes are enlarged and tender, and the patient is quite ill, with severe constitutional symptoms. A pharyngeal membrane requires culture on media appropriate for the diphtheria bacillus. *DDX:* The throat is not nearly as sore as in streptococcal pharyngitis. A membrane limited to a tonsil must be distinguished from Vincent angina (acute necrotizing ulcerative stomatitis) in which the membrane is limited to the tonsil and not tenacious and unaccompanied by severe constitutional symptoms.

Oropharyngeal candidiasis (thrush). Shiny, raised white patches, surrounded by an erythematous rim, appear on the posterior pharynx, buccal mucosa, and tongue. They may be painful. An atrophic erythematous mucosal lesion without white exudate also occurs. If there is pain on swallowing, Candida esophagitis is likely, especially in the immunosuppressed or diabetic patient.

Infectious mononucleosis. An acute acquired infection of lymphocytes with EBV leads to lymphadenopathy and atypical circulating lymphocytes. The identical clinical picture can be caused by acute HIV, CMV, HHV6 and toxoplasma infections. Sore throat is the most common symptom, accompanied by slight fever, malaise, cough, and headache. The pharynx is red and edematous, often with enlarged tonsils coated with exudate, making distinction from streptococcal infection difficult. The tonsils may reach the midline and impair speech and, rarely, respirations. There may be petechiae on the palate and uvula. The cervical lymph nodes are usually enlarged and tender. Disproportionate cervical lymph node enlargement suggests a generalized disease, so the physician should search for axillary and inguinal lymphadenopathy and splenomegaly. A morbilliform rash, conjunctivitis, splenomegaly, and occasionally jaundice with a tender, enlarged liver are seen.

Difficulty swallowing—dysphagia. Swallowing is a complex voluntary and reflex event requiring normal sensory and neuromuscular function of the tongue, mouth, and pharynx. Impairment of any of these structures can produce difficulty swallowing. Patients generally attach symptoms to the oral, pharyngeal, or esophageal phase of swallowing. Careful patient observation during attempts to swallow thin and thickened liquids, soft foods, and solid boluses helps identify the site and nature of the problem. Speech therapists should assist with the evaluation and videofluoroscopy. See also page 190, and Chapter 9, page 411.

CLINICAL OCCURRENCE: *Congenital:* Cerebral palsy, intellectual impairment; *Endocrine:* Hypothyroidism; *Degenerative/Idiopathic:* Parkinson disease, hypoglossal nerve palsy; *Infectious:* Tonsillitis, quinsy, mononucleosis, epiglottitis, mumps, retropharyngeal abscess, chancre, gumma, actinomycosis, rabies, oral and esophageal herpes simplex, *Candida*; *Inflammatory/Immune:* Myasthenia gravis, amyloidosis, Sjögren syndrome, scleroderma; *Mechanical/Traumatic:* Fractures, jaw dislocation, TMJ ankylosis, irradiation; *Metabolic/Toxic:* Botulism; *Neoplastic:* Sarcoma of the jaw, carcinoma; *Neurologic:* Stroke, bulbar paralysis, pseudobulbar paralysis, bilateral facial nerve palsy, myasthenia gravis, diphtheritic palsy, hypoglossal nerve palsy, Parkinson disease; *Psychosocial:* Hysteria; *Vascular:* Stroke.

Peritonsillar abscess (quinsy). Pyogenic infection of the tonsil spreads into the peritonsillar and pharyngeal spaces. The affected side is very painful and edematous. Mouth opening is always limited and may be difficult because of muscle spasm (*trismus*). An anterior abscess between the tonsil and anterior faucial pillar is easily seen, displacing the uvula to the opposite side (Fig. 7-71A). The adjacent soft palate is edematous and bulging. When the abscess is posterior to the tonsil, earache accompanies the sore throat and the tonsil is pushed forward, much of the swelling is hidden from direct vision. Surgical drainage is necessary.

Retropharyngeal abscess. Pus accumulates between the pharynx and the prevertebral fascia. This is most common in children <5 years old. With the tongue depressed, oropharyngeal swelling is seen on the posterior pharyngeal wall, and gentle palpation (Fig. 7-71B) discloses a unilateral soft swelling. In the nasopharynx, or opposite the larynx, the swelling is never directly visible. Suspect nasopharyngeal swelling when nose breathing is impaired (often attributed to adenoids), and laryngeal swelling with respiratory distress or difficulty swallowing. Urgent surgical drainage is necessary to avoid airway obstruction.

Aberrant right subclavian artery (dysphagia lusoria). The right subclavian artery, arising anomalously from the descending aorta distal to the left subclavian artery (Fig. 7-72), to reach the right axilla crosses left to right and upward, either behind the esophagus, between the esophagus and trachea, or rarely anterior to the trachea. In the first two positions, it puts pressure on the esophagus. Symptom starts in adolescence or early adulthood with difficulty swallowing solid food. An esophagram shows a pressure notch in the esophagus.

Larynx Syndromes

- **Acute laryngeal obstruction—aphonia, choking ("the cafe coronary").** An acutely obstructed larynx requires instant treatment. Even physicians may fail to recognize and treat laryngeal obstruction in time to save a life. Usually during a meal, the victim rises suddenly with a look of panic or anguish, often with a hand to the throat, unable to speak or breathe. Ask

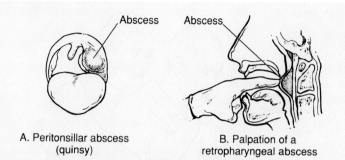

A. Peritonsillar abscess
(quinsy)

B. Palpation of a
retropharyngeal abscess

FIG. 7-71 Lesions of the Oral Cavity. A. Peritonsillar abscess (quinsy). B. Palpation of a retropharyngeal abscess: The sagittal section shows the relation of the abscess to the palpating finger. The gloved finger feels a boggy indentable mass as it presses gently against the anterior surfaces of the vertebral bodies.

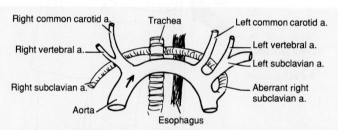

FIG. 7-72 Aberrant Right Subclavian Artery. The right subclavian artery arises in the descending aorta, distal to the origin of the left subclavian artery. It crosses the midline either behind the esophagus, between the esophagus and the trachea, or anterior to the trachea. In either of the first two patterns, the artery may compress the esophagus producing difficulty in swallowing, "dysphagia lusoria." A transverse compression band in the esophagram suggests the diagnosis.

the patient if he/she can speak. He/she may rush from the room, with face rapidly changing from pale to blue. This behavior is presumptive evidence of choking (in contrast, myocardial infarction permits speech and breathing), and there are fewer than 5 minutes in which to intervene before death.

The Heimlich maneuver (Fig. 7-73). Stand behind the victim wrapping your arms around their waist. Grasp your fist with the other hand, placing the thumb side of the fist against the victim's abdomen between the navel and xiphoid. With a quick upward thrust press your fist deep into the abdomen; repeat several times, if necessary. Heimlich calculated that his maneuver could forcefully expel approximately 940 mL of residual and tidal air at an average pressure of 31 mm Hg, enough to force the bolus out.

Acute laryngitis. The most common cause of hoarseness, acute viral laryngitis, is often accompanied by an unproductive cough, producing pain or a burning dryness in the throat. The true cords are reddened, their edges rounded by swelling. Erythema of other laryngeal membranes is present; edema of the larynx is common.

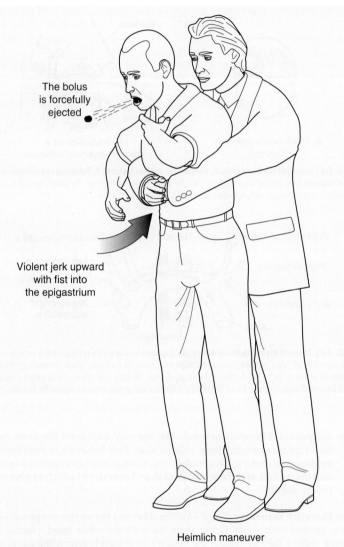

The bolus
is forcefully
ejected

Violent jerk upward
with fist into
the epigastrium

Heimlich maneuver

FIG. 7-73 Heimlich Maneuver. This is used to dislodge foreign bodies from the larynx. Standing at the subject's back, encircle the subject's waist with your arms. Grasp your fist with the other hand and give it a sudden forceful jerk that thrusts the fist upward into the subject's epigastrium. Repeat until the obstructing bolus is forcefully expelled from the throat.

Croup. Acute upper airway narrowing occurs with infection, allergy, foreign body, or neoplasm and is accompanied by a hoarse, brassy cough and dyspnea. Parainfluenza infection causing acute laryngotracheobronchitis is the most frequent cause in children redundant. *Inflammatory croup* is an acute laryngitis. The cords may appear normal and edema may be greatest in the sub-epiglottic region. Attacks increase danger of asphyxia.

In *spasmodic croup*, the child awakens with a barking cough, dyspnea, and stridor; cyanosis is frequent. The larynx looks normal. Recovery is sudden and complete. The cause is unknown.

Chronic laryngitis. Hoarseness and unproductive cough are usually present. Pain is negligible. The true cords are dull and thickened or edematous and polypoid. Frequently, the false cords are similarly affected. Chronic laryngitis is associated with chronic overuse of the cords, tobacco smoking, syphilis, and tuberculosis of the cords complicating cavitary pulmonary tuberculosis.

Hysterical aphonia. When viewed the cords are normal. The organic causes of aphonia are readily diagnosed by inspecting the larynx. Even before laryngeal examination, hysterical aphonia is demonstrated by the patient's ability to make a sharp normal cough.

Laryngeal dyspnea. Shortness of breath has many causes (Chapter 8, page 294). In laryngeal disease, dyspnea indicates advanced obstruction, milder obstruction producing hoarseness and stridor. In laryngeal dyspnea, the harder the attempt to inhale, the greater the obstruction. Exhalation is unopposed, so quiet breathing is more efficient.

Paradoxical vocal cord motion. During inspiration, the vocal cords paradoxically close narrowing the airway and producing wheezing. Patients often present with episodic wheezing and shortness of breath unresponsive to treatment appropriate for asthma. On auscultation, the wheeze is loudest over the larynx, not the lungs. Diagnosis requires direct visualization of the cords during an episode.

Dysphonia plicae ventricularis. Intermittent or chronic hoarseness occurs when the false vocal cords close over the true cords instead of remaining passive during phonation. A single cord examination may disclose no abnormality; with repeated examinations, one eventually coincides with the false cords closing partially or completely over the true cords. When this occurs, the voice breaks, as in a boy whose "voice is changing." The false cords may also be active when the true cords are separated by tumor, cricoarytenoid arthritis, voice abuse, or emotional instability.

Speech disorders. See Chapter 14, page 705.

Salivary Gland Syndromes

Dry mouth—xerostomia. Generalized abnormalities of salivary gland function result in inadequate wetting of the mucosa. The patient complains of a dry mouth and difficulty swallowing dry foods such as crackers. The patient is often consuming liquids attempting to wet the mouth. Extensive caries are frequent, often leading to loss of teeth. Common causes are anticholinergic drugs, head and neck irradiation, and immune salivary gland destruction in Sjögren syndrome (page 202). Ask about dry eyes and xerophthalmia.

Parotid tumors. Parotid neoplasia is benign or malignant. *Pleomorphic Adenoma (Mixed Parotid Tumor)* presents as a firm, painless, nontender nodule, slightly above and in front of the mandibular angle and, less commonly, just anterior to the tragus. It may remain benign for years, growing very slowly. Rarely, it suddenly becomes malignant, with rapid growth and metastases. The second most common benign neoplasm is the *Warthin tumor (papillary cystadenoma lymphomatosum)*, commonly occurring in the parotid tail in older men. It is bilateral more often than other salivary gland tumors. Malignancy is suggested by pain and tenderness, rapid tumor growth, facial nerve paralysis, and fixation to the skin or underlying tissues. Biopsy is necessary because the several tumor types require different management.

Salivary calculus—sialolithiasis. Calcium phosphate stones frequently form in the salivary ducts. The cause is unknown. The stone is in the submandibular gland or duct in ~85% of patients with salivary calculi. Submandibular swelling, with or without pain, occurs suddenly while the patient is eating, and subsiding within 2 hours. The sequence may be invariable for several years and is pathognomonic. Occasionally, the gland becomes infected or the duct obstructed. With a parotid duct stone, gland swelling may persist for several days. In all three glands, calculi are frequently identified by palpation. Approximately 80% of the calculi are calcified, so they can be seen by radiography without contrast. Intraoral dental radiographs are excellent for demonstrating the calculi. A noncalcified impalpable stone can be detected by sialography.

Submaxillary and sublingual gland diseases. These glands are subject to the same diseases as the parotid, with slight variations. Rarely, mumps involves the submandibular gland and not the parotid; it is more common to have the both involved. Ranula involving the sublingual or submaxillary gland is described on page 231.

Thyroid Syndromes
Hypothyroidism. See Chapter 5, page 97.

Hyperthyroidism. See Chapter 5, page 97.

Thyroid Goiters and Nodules
Goiter. Thyroid enlargement is caused by hyperplasia of thyroid tissue, infiltration with foreign substances (e.g., amyloid), infection, or neoplastic growth (primary thyroid cancers, lymphoma, or metastatic disease). Though often unaware of a problem, patients might complain of a neck mass or fullness. The goiter may be evident as a bilobed fullness in the neck above the suprasternal notch moving superiorly with swallowing. Tangential light helps visualization. Determine the size of each lobe and isthmus, its extent within the neck or retrosternal space, consistency (smooth, a single nodule, multinodular), fixation to surrounding structures, tenderness, and the presence or absence of regional lymph node enlargement, including Delphian nodes. Determine thyroid function as hypothyroid, euthyroid, or hyperthyroid. Clinical classification of goiters is based upon whether the goiter is focal or diffuse, nodular or non-nodular, toxic (hyperthyroid) or nontoxic (euthyroid or hypothyroid).

Diffuse nontoxic goiter. Defects in thyroid hormone synthesis limit effective hormone production so TSH stimulation leads to diffuse thyroid enlargement. All parts of the gland are smooth, enlarged, and firm. The surface can be slightly irregular (*bosselated*), but circumscribed nodules are absent. Frequently called *colloid goiter*, or *endemic goiter*, the terms are not always applicable, sporadic cases occurring in nongoitrous regions. The gland is often more than twice normal size.

CLINICAL OCCURRENCE: *Physiologic Euthyroid Hyperplasia:* **Before** menstrual periods, females from puberty to 20 years of age, pregnancy; *Hypothyroid:* Iodine deficiency, antithyroid drugs, thiocyanates, paraaminosalicylic acid, phenylbutazone, lithium, amiodarone, and rarely iodides, inherited defects of thyroid enzymes, chronic thyroiditis.

Nontoxic multinodular goiter. The nodules are polyclonal proliferations with less-efficient thyroid hormone production than normal thyroid tissue. This is usually found in women >30 years of age. The gland may be small or large. The significant feature is two or more distinct parenchymal nodules. The nodules may vary in consistency in the same goiter. Thyroid hormone secretion is low or normal.

Diffuse toxic goiter—Graves disease. See Chapter 5, page 98. The thyroid is smooth, diffusely enlarged and a bruit may be heard. The ophthalmopathy occurs independently of goiter and thyroid function.

Toxic multinodular goiter. Autonomous function of one or more nodules produces elevated hormone levels. This often arises from a long-standing nontoxic multinodular gland. The onset is usually gradual with signs of hyperthyroidism, e.g., atrial fibrillation, weight loss, diarrhea. The gland is bilaterally enlarged with multiple nodules apparent by palpation or ultrasound.

Retrosternal goiter. When a goiter's lower border cannot be palpated in the neck, especially when the neck is short, consider retrosternal extension. Rarely, the goiter is entirely retrosternal, rising into the neck only with increased intrathoracic pressure, e.g., a Valsalva. This is a *plunging goiter*. Increased retromanubrial dullness is uncommon. A goiter in the superior thoracic aperture may compress other structures, causing cough, dilated upper thoracic veins and rarely facial edema from pressure on the internal jugular vein (Fig. 7-74), dyspnea from airway compression during sleep, dyspnea when the head is tilted to the side or the arms are held up beside the head, and/or hoarseness from pressure on the recurrent laryngeal nerve. Tracheal compression is inferred by dyspnea or the *Kocher sign* in which pressure on the lateral lobe produces stridor. The trachea may be displaced laterally (Fig. 7-59). *Pemberton Sign:* Have the patient sit holding the arms up beside the head for a few minutes. Venous suffusion, facial cyanosis, and dyspnea imply thoracic inlet obstruction. *DDX:* The internal jugular vein is rarely compromised, so the facial cyanosis and neck edema associated with superior vena caval obstruction are absent. For unknown reasons, retrosternal goiter is associated with a high incidence of hyperthyroidism.

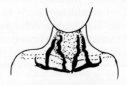

Venous engorgement
by retrosternal goiter

FIG. 7-74 Venous Engorgement: compression of the external jugular vein by a retrosternal goiter produces engorgement of the superficial branches in the skin of the neck and clavicular regions.

Solitary thyroid nodule. A solitary nodule is a benign or malignant neoplasm, cyst, or a dominant nodule in a multinodular gland. Many nodules solitary by palpation are found to be part of a multinodular process by ultrasound. Fine-needle aspiration of solitary nodules is the diagnostic procedure of choice. Thyroid irradiation in childhood increases the risk for carcinoma. Finding an isolated nodule in an atrophic thyroid gland suggests a *Plummer nodule* or toxic adenoma.

Toxic adenoma. Thyroid-stimulating hormone receptors are constitutively activated resulting in thyroid hormone overproduction. The symptoms and signs of hyperthyroidism accompany a single nodule in an otherwise atrophic gland.

Epithelial carcinoma. Malignant thyroid cancers are classified as papillary, follicular, and anaplastic. Thyroid cancer is more common in women and after radiation exposure, presenting in most cases as a painless nodule. Anaplastic cancer spreads widely and rapidly, whereas papillary and follicular cancers spread regionally before widely metastasizing.

Medullary carcinoma. Neoplasia of thyroid C-cells producing calcitonin is sporadic, inherited alone, or inherited as a multiple endocrine neoplasia (MEN) syndrome 2A or 2B. Screen all patients with a family history of MEN-2A or MEN-2B, and those with a family history of medullary carcinoma.

Thyroiditis. Thyroid gland inflammation, usually autoimmune, is common, especially in women after beginning childbearing. The thyroid is damaged by antibody- or cellular-cytotoxicity, or via induction of apoptosis. Disrupted follicles release preformed thyroid hormones directly into the circulation resulting in clinical hyperthyroidism and suppressing TSH and iodine uptake. Several distinct syndromes are identified by their clinical pictures. Graves disease, though not usually thought of as thyroiditis, is an immune-mediated disease often leading to thyroid failure. In addition to autoimmunity, viral and bacterial infections occur. *DDX:* The elevated T4 and T3, low TSH and low iodine uptake distinguish thyroiditis from Graves disease, toxic adenomas, and toxic multinodular goiter. Thyroid hormone ingestion might be identified by history but may be surreptitious. Graves disease produces a diffuse, smooth goiter.

Subacute thyroiditis—De Quervain thyroiditis, viral thyroiditis. Acute painful thyroid inflammation is caused by viral infection or postinfectious inflammation. Anterior neck pain is the presenting symptom, often aggravated by swallowing. The pain frequently refers to the ear, so the complaint can be earache. The gland is unusually firm and rather small, and it frequently contains one or more, often tender, nodules. The patient is euthyroid or hyperthyroid in the acute phase.

Hashimoto thyroiditis. Chronic lymphocytic infiltration leads to loss of functioning tissue and fibrosis. This is the most common cause of acquired hypothyroidism and is more common in women, the prevalence increasing with age. The symptoms are related to hypothyroidism; neck symptoms are rare. Most patients become hypothyroid with time. The gland is uniformly firm and nontender, may be diffusely enlarged, but is often normal or small. A rare encephalitis, *Hashimoto encephalitis*, is unrelated to thyroid function and responds to corticosteroids. *DDX:* Other autoimmune diseases more common in patients with Hashimoto thyroiditis include type-1 diabetes, Addison disease, vitiligo, rheumatoid arthritis, and systemic lupus.

Postpartum thyroiditis. Following delivery, the thyroid becomes inflamed in association with thyroperoxidase antibodies. Symptoms begin 2–6 months postpartum. Hyperthyroidism is most common, often followed by a period of hypothyroidism. It is more common in patients with thyroid autoimmunity before pregnancy. Self-limited, requiring only symptomatic therapy, it frequently recurs with subsequent pregnancies. *DDX:* Although a goiter may be present, the thyroid is nontender and may not appear a likely source of the problems. Mild symptoms of both hyper- and hypothyroidism are often misattributed to postpartum psychosocial stresses including inadequate sleep, mood changes, and family stress.

Reidel thyroiditis. The thyroid gland is densely fibrotic with fibrosis extending into the surrounding tissues. It is related to other IgG-4-related fibrosing conditions. Patients present with compressive symptoms of the esophagus, trachea, neck veins, or recurrent laryngeal nerves. Women in midlife are most often affected. Thyroid function is usually preserved. The gland is hard and fixed.

Acute suppurative thyroiditis. Infection of the thyroid gland by bacteria or fungi often extends from branchial cleft remnants. There is acute pain and fever. The gland is slightly enlarged, asymmetric, and fluctuance may be noted.

CLINICAL VIGNETTES AND QUESTIONS

CASE 7-1

A 25-year-old woman presents with pain in her left eye associated with decreased vision. She describes a blacked out spot in the middle of her visual field. These symptoms have progressed over the last 24 hours. The eye pain worsens with eye movement. She has never had symptoms like this previously and denies any significant past medical history.

QUESTIONS:
1. What is the differential diagnosis for this patient's presentation?
2. What is the most likely diagnosis?
3. What findings might you expect on physical examination?

CASE 7-2

A 26-year-old woman presents for evaluation of headache and double vision. She has had a sinus infection for 10 days. This morning she woke up with a sharp headache behind the eye and double vision. Her husband noted some swelling around the right eye this morning. Her temperature is 38.7°C.

QUESTIONS:
1. What is your differential diagnosis for this patient's presentation?
2. What is the most likely diagnosis?
3. What cranial nerve deficit would be most likely in this patient and why?
4. What are predisposing risk factors for this condition?

CASE 7-3

A 26-year-old ethnic Lebanese man complains of painful oral ulcers. He has had four episodes in the preceding 11 months. He has also had painful genital ulcers that have healed but left scars. When the genital ulcers occurred he was evaluated for STDs; that evaluation was unrevealing.

QUESTIONS:
1. What is the differential diagnosis for this patient?
2. What is the most likely diagnosis?
3. What other findings are needed to confirm this diagnosis?
4. What is pathergy?

CASE 7-4

An 8-year-old boy is brought to the emergency department by his parents due to fever, sore throat, and difficulty breathing. He seems to be more comfortable sitting slightly forward. He has not ingested or inhaled any foreign material. He has not received routine vaccinations due to religious objection by his parents. On examination he is in mild respiratory distress and he is drooling. There is audible stridor. His epiglottis appears cherry red.

QUESTIONS:
1. What is the differential diagnosis for this patient's presentation?
2. What is the most likely diagnosis?
3. What would be the likely pathogen?
4. What are the common causes of stridor in adults?

CASE 7-5

A 15-year-old girl presents with right sided neck pain. She has been ill for 6 days. She was diagnosed 4 days ago with strep pharyngitis and started amoxicillin. Two days ago she started to have fevers, rigors, and increasing right-sided neck pain. It is painful when she swallows. She has a cough and pleuritic pain with deep breaths. She appears ill, her temperature is 38.3°C, and her oropharynx has mild posterior erythema without exudates. Her neck has tender lymphadenopathy, fullness on the right side, and pain with flexion, extension, and rotation.

QUESTIONS:
1. What is your differential diagnosis?
2. What is the most likely diagnosis and why?
3. Which bacteria is likely to be isolated from this patient's blood cultures?

CASE 7-6

A 52-year-old man presents with dizziness associated with nausea and vomiting. Over the last 24 hours he has had a sense that the room is spinning. He is most comfortable lying in bed looking at the ceiling light fixture. He is able to walk though it increases his sense of spinning. His medical history is notable for hypertension and hypothyroidism. A recent TSH was normal. He denies tinnitus or hearing loss.

QUESTIONS:
1. What information from the history helps differentiate central versus peripheral vertigo?
2. What physical examination findings help differentiate central versus peripheral vertigo?
3. Based on the history what is the most likely diagnosis?

CASE 7-7

A 72-year-old woman presents to the emergency room with sudden onset of left eye pain and decreased vision. She and her husband were at a movie. She developed the pain as the lights went down. She describes blurred vision with halos around lights. She has pain around her eye and a diffuse headache. She is nauseated but has not vomited. Her physical examination reveals significantly reduced visual acuity, scleral injection, and a ciliary flush. The pupil is not reactive and the funduscopic examination is obscured by a cloudy cornea.

QUESTIONS:
1. What is the most likely diagnosis?
2. What precipitated this condition and why?
3. What factors predispose or cause this condition?
4. What medications can precipitate this condition?

CHAPTER 8

The Chest: Chest Wall, Pulmonary, and Cardiovascular Systems; The Breasts

SECTION 1
Chest Wall, Pulmonary, and Cardiovascular Systems

MAJOR SYSTEMS AND PHYSIOLOGY

The Thoracic Wall: The skeletal and muscular shell of the thorax encloses the heart and lungs, powers breathing, and is the mechanical platform for arm and neck motion. It is bounded anteriorly by the sternum and ribs, laterally and posteriorly by ribs, and supported posteriorly by the spine. The inferior boundary is the diaphragm and rib margins. Superiorly, it is bounded by the clavicles and soft tissues of the neck. The thoracic wall includes the bodies of 12 thoracic vertebrae, 12 pairs of ribs, and the sternum.

Bones. The thorax resembles a truncated cone, each pair of ribs having a greater diameter than that above, making the rib cage much smaller at the top than at the base. The ribs are separated by intercostal spaces numbered from the rib above. The first rib slopes slightly downward from back to front. Each succeeding rib has a greater slope, the intercostal spaces widening from top to bottom.

Sternum. The sternum (Fig. 8-1) consists of the *manubrium, body, (gladiolus),* and *xiphoid cartilage.* There is a fibrocartilage (rarely synovial) joint between the manubrium and body; mobility at this joint is slight. While it is cartilaginous at birth, the xiphoid begins calcifying in childhood and this continues throughout life. The xiphoid is commonly monofid, lance shaped and caudally oriented. Variations are very common and include bifid and trifid divisions, xiphoidal foramina as well as ventral and dorsal projections. When angulated forward, the xiphoid can be mistaken for an abdominal mass.

Ribs. Each rib is a flattened arch. All sternal rib ends continue as *costal cartilages.* The first to seventh ribs are usually termed *true ribs or vertebrosternal because* their costal cartilages join directly to the sternum. The costal cartilage of the first rib connects to the manubrium at a fibrous joint. The other six true ribs attach to the sternum by synovial joints. The second rib attaches to both the manubrium and body with two synovial joints. The eighth to twelfth ribs

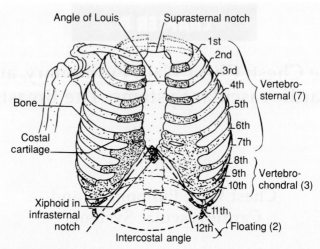

FIG. 8-1 The Bony Thorax. The left clavicle is removed exposing the underlying first rib. The xiphoid and rib cartilages are stippled. Note the surface landmarks: the suprasternal notch, the angle of Louis, and the infrasternal notch. The two lower rib margins form the intercostal angle.

are *false ribs* without anterior attachment to the sternum. The eighth, ninth, and tenth ribs are *vertebrochondral*, each costal cartilage usually joining the cartilage of the rib above. The 11th and 12th ribs are *vertebral or floating ribs* without anterior attachment. Important variations include supranumerary ribs such as the more common variation cervical rib articulated to the C7 vertebral body as well as the rare variant of lumbar ribs.

Thoracic wall muscles. The ribs are pulled together by contraction of the *internal and external intercostal muscles* attaching to adjacent rib margins and spanning the intercostal spaces. With the first rib fixed by scaleni contraction, contracting the intercostals, levatores costarum, and serratus posterior superior rotates the ribs upward. Fixing the last rib by quadratus lumborum contraction while contracting the subcostals and transversus thoracis rotates the ribs downward.

The Respiratory System: The thoracic respiratory system is composed of the trachea entering superiorly, the lungs with their branching airways, arterial, venous and lymphatic vascular channels, and the *pleura* lining both the lung (*visceral pleura*) and chest wall and mediastinum (*parietal pleura*).

Respiratory excursions of the thorax. At the end of passive expiration, thoracic volume is at its normal minimum or functional residual capacity. Inspiration increases thoracic dimensions anteroposteriorly, transversely, and vertically, expanding lung volume. Volume varies as the third power of changes in linear dimension, so relatively small changes in thoracic cavity height, width, and depth produce large volume changes. Normal *passive expiration* results from elastic recoil of the lungs and chest wall. Forced expiration

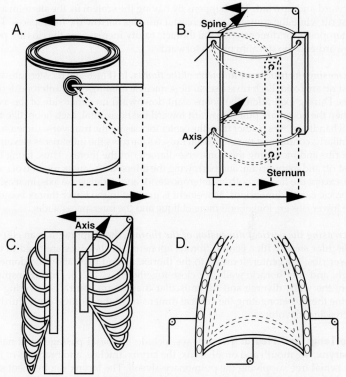

FIG. 8-2 Models Illustrating Thoracic Respiratory Movements. A. At rest, the handle of a cylindric paint can hangs obliquely, so its center and the side of the pail are equidistant from the central axis of the cylinder. When the handle is raised to the horizontal, the center of the handle diverges from the side increasing the distance from the central axis. **B.** In this model, two parallel rigid hoops pierce two vertical sticks. Elevation of the front stick (representing the sternum) increases the distance between it and the other stick (representing the spine). The differences in the points of the arrows show this change in the anteroposterior diameter. **C.** The semicircular ribs hang from the sternum and the spine, like the hoops in B and the bucket handle in A. Elevation of the sternum and the lateral bows of the ribs during inspiration increases both the transverse (as in A) and the anteroposterior (as in B) diameters of the thorax. **D.** Inspiratory volume is further augmented by depression of the diaphragm.

occurs with contraction of abdominal and chest wall muscles resulting in greatly accelerated airflow.

Increasing the anterior–posterior diameter of the thorax. The chest is like a cylindrical pail with its wire handle bowed in a semicircle of slightly greater diameter than the cylinder (Fig. 8-2A). When the handle hangs obliquely, the distance from its center to the cylindric axis is the radius of the pail. Raising the handle toward the horizontal moves it away from the side of the pail. In Figure 8-2B, a straight piece of wood represents the thoracic spine, a vertical stick is the sternum at end expiration (*dotted*), and the dotted hoop is a pair of ribs. Pulling the sternum and the first rib upward rotates the costal ring forward and upward. This happens by having the scaleni fix the sternum and first rib while the contracting intercostal muscles narrow the interspaces. The anteroposterior dimension of the thoracic cavity increases as the ribs are pull upward and the sternum moves forward.

Increasing the transverse diameter of the thorax. In (Fig. 8-2C) the sternum and first rib are fixed. Each rib is a separate semicircle rotating on an anteroposterior axis. During expiration, the hoops slant downward on either side of the axis. When the hoops are pulled upward toward the horizontal, each hoop, like the pail handle, moves further from the center increasing the transverse dimension. Similarly, contracting the intercostal muscles narrows the interspaces elevating the ribs and increasing the transverse diameter of the thorax. Thus, fixing the first rib and manubrium, and narrowing the interspaces causes rotation of each rib, except the first, on both an anteroposterior and a transverse axis, increasing thoracic cavity dimensions. Movement is greatest in the lower thorax because the lower ribs are longer and more oblique and the interspaces wider.

Increasing the vertical dimension of the thorax. The diaphragm is an elliptic muscular sheet with a central fibrous aponeurosis. Its edges are fixed to the lower ribs, the center domes into the thorax. At end expiration the dome is high, and the thoracic walls are close together (Fig. 8-2D). During inspiration, the walls diverge and the muscular diaphragm contracts lowering its dome thereby elongating the vertical dimension of the thoracic cavity further increasing its volume.

The Lungs and Pleura: The airways include the nasal passages and nasopharynx, the mouth and oropharynx, the larynx, trachea, and branches of the bronchial tree supplying the pulmonary alveoli. The larynx is a frequent site of obstruction, either from intrinsic swelling or by vocal cord paralysis.

The bronchial tree. The trachea bifurcates asymmetrically at the carina into *right and left mainstem bronchii.* The left bronchus diverges at a greater angle from the trachea than the right bronchus. Therefore, foreign bodies are most likely to lodge in the right main stem bronchus. The right bronchus sends a *lobar bronchus* to the three *pulmonary lobes,* the left bronchus branches into two lobar bronchi. Each lobar bronchus subsequently divides into bronchopulmonary segments. Although highly variable, the upper lobes typically have 3 segments while the lower lobes have five segments on the right but four on the left. The heart lies caudal to the tracheal bifurcation and the aorta arches from front to back over the left mainstem bronchus. Interposed between the aorta, trachea and left main bronchus is the *left recurrent laryngeal nerve,* which descends in front of the aortic arch, loops under it, and ascends on the lateral aspect of the trachea into the neck. A dilated, aneurysmal aortic arch can produce a tracheal tug by pulsating downward against the left bronchus. Similarly, a dilated aorta as well as mediastinal adenopathy can compress the left recurrent laryngeal nerve against the left bronchus, paralyzing the left vocal cord.

Lungs. Think of the lungs as clusters of pulmonary alveoli around subdivisions of the bronchial tree. The right lung has upper, middle, and lower lobes. The left lung has upper and lower lobes. The lobes are separated by

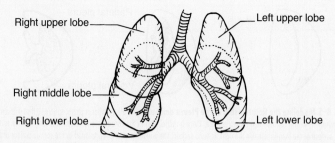

FIG. 8-3 The Lobes of the Lungs. The transparent diagram shows the anterior aspects of the pulmonary lobes and their main bronchi. Note the three divisions of the right main bronchus and the more direct line with the trachea on the right side. The dotted line shows the posterior extent of the lower lobes.

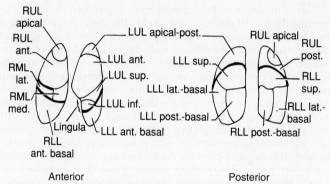

FIG. 8-4 Lung Segments. Each lobe is divided into segments. The thick lines are the anatomical fissures, readily identified on inspection of the lung and often in radiographs. The thinner lines are established only by careful dissections of injected preparations. In the abbreviations the first capital letter designates right or left; the second, upper, middle, or lower, and the third L is for lobe. Note that the lingula, composed of the superior and inferior segments of the left upper lobe, is near the heart corresponding in many respects to the right middle lobe.

infolded visceral pleura, the *lobar fissures* which limit air passage between lobes. However, fissure variations are common and many are incomplete or partial and permit air passage between adjacent lobes. The shape of the lungs is molded by the rib cage peripherally and the heart centrally. The molding indentation of medial edge of the left lung is termed the *cardiac notch*. Each lobe is divided into bronchopulmonary segments, consisting of the cluster of alveoli supplied by a single first branch of the lobar bronchus (Figs. 8-3 and 8-4). Segments are not demarcated by fissures. However, if present, extra fissures may follow these boundaries. The lingula of the left upper lobe is homologous with the right middle lobe.

The pleura. The relationship of each lung to its pleura is visualized by imagining a sphere of thin plastic material from which the air is being evacuated

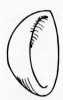
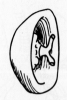
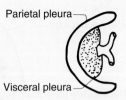

Parietal pleura

Visceral pleura

FIG. 8-5 Modeling the Relationship of the Pleura and Lung. Deflate a rubber or plastic sphere so that it assumes a hemisphere with a concave and convex surface. Place a model lung in the concavity and cement the lung surface to the inner surface of the hemisphere. On the right, in cross section, the parietal pleura is represented by the convex surface of the hemisphere; the cemented layers represent the visceral pleura. To complete the model, exhaust the hemisphere of air, replacing it with a little fluid to lubricate the inner surface. This geometry should be visualized while examining the chest and when looking at radiographs, remembering that the pleural surfaces are anterior, lateral, medial, and inferior.

(Fig. 8-5). As the sphere collapses, one-part invaginates forming a hollow hemisphere with convex and concave layers in apposition. The convex layer, representing the *parietal pleura*, is cemented to the inside of the thoracic cavity. The lung fills the concavity, which represents the *visceral pleura*. The parietal pleura is adherent to the thoracic wall; the visceral pleura is fixed to the lung surface and lines the interlobar fissures. The two apposing layers form the *pleural cavity*, containing only enough fluid for lubrication. The parietal pleura has the greater area, extending inferiorly on the ribs and diaphragm some distance below the lower tip of the lung forming the costophrenic sinus. This permits the lungs to move within the thoracic cavity, each descending part way into this sinus during deep inspiration. Between the two layers of pleura is a potential space, normally with a negative pressure relative to the atmosphere. This negative pressure maintains lung distention and transfers the inspiratory forces of diaphragm flattening and chest expansion to the lung. Air in this space, *pneumothorax*, destroys mechanical coupling of chest motion to lung expansion. The parietal pleura contains sensory nerve endings, but the visceral pleura is anesthetic.

Lung and pleura mechanics. When a normal lung is removed it partially collapses from its elastic recoil becoming much smaller than its hemithorax. Normal lung volume is maintained by adherence to the thoracic wall of the parietal and visceral pleurae. Atmospheric pressure resists any force tending to separate the pleural layers. During passive expiration, about negative –4 to –5 cm of water intrapleural pressure is maintained by elastic recoil of the lung and thorax. During inspiration, the pleural pressure decreases further to –8 to –10 cm of water because additional elastic recoil is produced by stretching the lung as the thorax expands.

The Cardiovascular System

The circulation. The circulatory system includes the heart, the blood and its conducting vessels, the lymph and its ducts, and the vessel walls. Since the heart and much of the aorta are intrathoracic, consideration of the circulatory system starts in the chest. Blood returning from the extremities enters the chest from the abdomen and lower extremities via the *inferior vena cava (IVC)*, and from the arms and head via the axillary and jugular veins, which merge into the *brachiocephalic veins* and *superior vena cava (SVC)* in the mediastinum. The heart is suspended from the great vessels (aorta, pulmonary artery, pulmonary veins, IVC, and SVC) within the pericardium, allowing the heart free motion during ventricular contraction.

The cardiac conduction system. The heart's normal pacemaker is the *sinoatrial (SA)* node located in the right atrial wall near the entrance of the SVC (Chapter 4, Fig. 4-1, page 54). It originates rhythmic waves of excitation that spread quickly through both atria until they reach the *atrioventricular (AV) node* near the posterior margin of the interatrial septum. The AV-node delays conduction during atrial systole. The impulse then passes down the *bundle of His*, which divides into *right and left bundle-branches* to the muscle of the right and left ventricles via the *Purkinje network*. Normal conduction is very rapid, arriving nearly simultaneously in both atria, and, after AV delay, in both ventricles. Deviations in the timing or pathways taken by these electrical waves cause changes in rate, rhythm, and electrical pattern of the P, QRS, and T waves of the electrocardiogram (ECG). The electrical signals trigger mechanical muscle contraction via the process of *electrical–mechanical coupling*.

Heart movement and function. Because myocardial muscle fibers form a complete spiral, contraction during systole decreases all cardiac dimensions. The apex rotates forward and to the right, approaching the chest wall and frequently causing a visible and palpable thrust, the *apical impulse*, in early systole marking the palpable onset of cardiac contraction. The heart has extremely high oxygen and energy requirements and the highest oxygen extraction of any organ. As a result, it is particularly sensitive to decreased blood flow. Blood flow within the heart and lungs is dependent upon complete functional separation of the cardiac chambers by intact interatrial and interventricular septa and functional valves. Valve closure, turbulent blood flow, and heart contraction can be felt and auscultated through the chest wall.

Peripheral arteries. Blood is distributed to the body through the major branches of the aorta, which are easily examined where they leave the chest (carotid and axillary arteries) or abdomen (femoral arteries). Blood pressure measurement and an estimate of blood flow are easily performed by physical examination.

Leg veins. Knowledge of normal leg vein functional anatomy has many clinical applications including differentiation of superficial from deep venous thrombosis and surgical planning. The *great saphenous vein* begins at the mediodorsal side of the foot, continuing upward along the medial edge of the tibia, and passing the knee behind the medial femoral condyle. In the thigh, it runs subcutaneously to the femoral canal, emptying into the *femoral vein*. The *small saphenous vein* begins at the lateral side of the foot, curving under and behind the lateral malleolus, continuing upward in the posterior midline, and finally diving into the *popliteal vein*. Valved *communicating veins* connect the saphenous veins to the *deep calf veins* and the great saphenous to the femoral vein. Superficial veins course through the cutaneous and subcutaneous tissues and are not surrounded by muscle. In contrast, deep veins by convention are completely surrounded by muscle. Normal flow is from superficial to deep veins and thence proximally driven by skeletal muscle contraction compressing the veins within the muscle compartments (*the muscle pump*).

Antegrade flow is assured by competent venous valves. Thrombosis in superficial veins is less likely to embolize because of the absence of muscular compression while deep venous thrombosis typically is associated with high potential to embolize into the vena cava and pulmonary arteries.

SUPERFICIAL THORACIC ANATOMY

The Chest Wall: The sternum's subcutaneous anterior surface has landmarks used in inspection and palpation. The heads of the clavicles are the sides of the *suprasternal notch*, its base is the superior edge of the manubrium (Figs. 8-1 and 8-6). The junction of the manubrium and body, (gladiolus), where the second rib articulates, forms the sternal angle (*angle of Louis*), a landmark for identifying ribs and interspaces. At the inferior end of the sternal body a slight depression, *the infrasternal notch*, is formed by the junction of the 7th rib costal cartilages. The xiphoid cartilage is palpable below this notch.

The bony thorax is a truncated cone narrowing superiorly. This narrowing is partially obscured by the overlying clavicles, shoulders, and upper chest and arm muscles giving the body a broad shouldered, squared-off contour. The clavicles, sternum, and lower ribs are palpable in most patients with normal body mass; portions of most other ribs can be seen or palpated. The first rib is overlaid by the clavicle. The pectoralis major and female breasts limit palpation of ribs anteriorly, and the latissimus dorsi covers some ribs behind the axilla. The scapulae, overlying the posterior chest wall lateral to the spine, cover parts of the second through seventh ribs. With the arms at the sides, the inferior scapular angle is at the seventh or eighth intercostal space, a landmark for counting ribs posteriorly (Fig. 8-7). Bilaterally, the inferior margins of the seventh, eighth, and ninth costal cartilages meet in the midline forming the *infrasternal angle* (intercostal angle). An oblique line drawn from the head of the clavicle to the anterior axillary line on the ninth rib approximately locates the *costochondral junctions* of the second to tenth ribs. The lower ribs with large radii, superficial location, and extensive anterior cartilage are vulnerable to injury. Upper ribs are less susceptible to mechanical injury because of their smaller radius of curvature and overlying muscles.

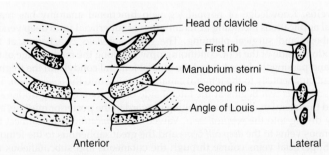

Head of clavicle

First rib

Manubrium sterni

Second rib

Angle of Louis

Anterior

Lateral

FIG. 8-6 The Angle of Louis. The adjacent edges of the manubrium and gladiolus form the angle of Louis. This is a landmark for counting ribs anteriorly because the second rib abuts the junction that forms the angle. The costicartilage of the second rib articulates with the fibrocartilage between the manubrium and the body and with the edges of both bones.

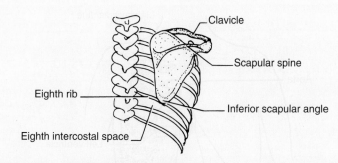

FIG. 8-7 Surface Landmarks of the Posterior Thorax. Note the relation of the scapulae to the ribs. The inferior angle of the scapula is usually at the eighth interspace allowing identification of the eighth rib posteriorly for counting posterior ribs.

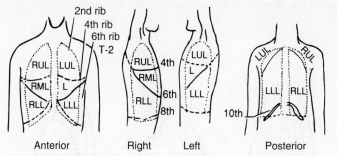

FIG. 8-8 Topography of the Five Lobes of the Lungs. The solid lines are the pulmonary fissures; the broken lines are projections. The boundary of the lingula (L) is hypothetical.

The *scapula* is overlaid with skeletal muscle and glides on the chest wall. Its medial border, inferior angle, lateral border, *spine, acromion*, and *coracoid process* are palpable in most patients with normal body mass. The lungs extend to the thoracic apex and may extend superiorly into the base of the neck where they are vulnerable to penetrating injury. The right and left pleural spaces coapt in the anterior superior mediastinum but are separated posteriorly by the spine and mediastinum and anteriorly and inferiorly by the pericardial sack and heart. The heart lies retrosternally and to the left with the right ventricle retrosternal and the left ventricle left lateral and posterior. The liver and spleen are below the diaphragm deep to the lower ribs. Deep inspiration flattens the diaphragm pushing them toward the costal margins where the liver and an enlarged spleen can be palpated. The *axillary folds* are formed by the pectoralis major anteriorly and the subscapularis and latissimus dorsi posteriorly.

The Lungs and Pleura: The topography of the five lung lobes has some clinical applications. In Figure 8-8, note that the anterior aspect of the right lung

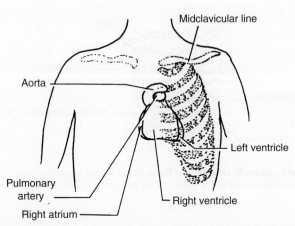

FIG. 8-9 Precordial Projections of the Anterior Surface of the Heart. The entire central area of the precordium is a projection of the right ventricle. The left border and apex are formed by the left ventricle; the right atrium is the right border.

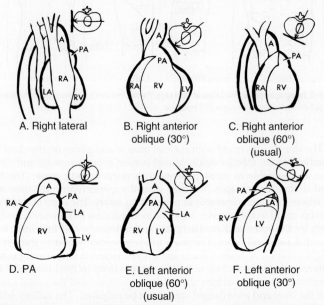

FIG. 8-10 X-ray Silhouettes of the Heart. The positions are named for the aspect of the patient's thorax that faces the cassette (except for the PA view). Angles are measured between the direction of the X-ray beam and the plane of the patient's back. The heavy lines on the silhouettes indicate distinctive segments used in diagnosis.

is formed almost entirely of the right upper and middle lobes, the posterior aspect containing only the upper and lower lobes. In the left lung, the upper and lower lobes present both back and front.

The Heart and Precordium: The anterior chest over the heart and aorta is the *precordium*, normally extending vertically from the second to the fifth intercostal space and transversely from the right sternal border to the left midclavicular line in the fifth and sixth interspaces. With an enlarged or displaced heart, the precordial boundaries shift. In *dextrocardia*, all signs described here are in the opposite hemithorax.

Figure 8-9 depicts the normal heart's projection on the precordium, and Figure 8-10 shows the basic projections on chest X-rays and fluoroscopic imaging used during coronary angiography. The aortic arch lies behind the manubrium. The sternum's right edge, from the third to fifth interspaces, is roughly the right heart border formed by the right atrium. The right ventricle lies anteriorly under the sternum and left lower ribs. The left ventricle, forming the cardiac apex and a slender area of the left heart border, sits posterior to the right ventricle. Thus, the right ventricle forms most of the heart's anterior surface but neither right or left heart border.

PHYSICAL EXAM OF THE CHEST AND MAJOR VESSELS

Inspection of the Rib Cage and Thoracic Musculature

Chest wall. With the patient upright or supine, inspect the chest wall from the foot of the bed looking for structural deformities that might restrict respiratory excursion. Observe several respiratory cycles noting the amplitude of chest movement, respiratory rate and rhythm. Look for signs of respiratory distress including labored inspiration with visible contraction of sternocleidomastoid muscles during inhalation and contraction of abdominal musculature during forced exhalation. Observe for other signs of respiratory compromise including sternal notch retractions, intercostal retraction, and paradoxical abdominal movements in which the abdomen moves upward and into the thorax during inhalation rather than downward and outward. Palpating with the palms can confirm asymmetric and dyskinetic chest wall motion.

Thoracic spine. With the patient standing or sitting, inspect the spine's cervical, thoracic and lumbar curves from the side. Observe for exaggerated, smooth forward curvature, (kyphosis), focal or angular, sharp forward curvature, (gibbus deformity), and exaggerated backward curvature of the lumbar spine, (lumbar hyperlordosis). From the back, assess the spine for straightness in the cranial to caudle dimension. Observe for lateral curvature of the spinous processes indicating scoliosis. To accurately detect and characterize the degree of scoliosis, palpate and mark each spinous process. The complete spine exam is described in Chapter 13 on page 539.

Palpating the Rib Cage and Thoracic Musculature

Trachea. Check for tracheal deviation by placing your index finger in the suprasternal notch and judging the space between the clavicles and each lateral tracheal border. Alternatively, feel for the tracheal rings in the middle of the suprasternal notch. If the apex of the rings touches the middle of the fingertip, the trachea is midline.

Thoracic wall. Palpate if there is chest tenderness, subcutaneous emphysema, (air crepitus), cysts or masses, breast lumps, or draining sinuses. Examine the soft tissues and large thoracic muscles for tenderness. If tender, characterize the movements that increase or diminish pain. Examine the costal cartilages and palpate the costochondral junctions and xiphisternal joint for tenderness. Palpate the ribs for point tenderness, swelling, bony crepitus, and pain on chest compression.

Testing upper chest excursion. Place a hand over the clavicle on each side of the patient's neck with palms against the upper anterior chest wall and curl the fingers firmly over the superior edges of the trapezii. Then extend your thumbs so their tips meet in the midline (Fig. 8-11A). Have the patient inspire deeply permitting your palms to move freely with the chest while your fingers are anchored on the trapezii. The upper four ribs move forward with inspiration, the thumbs diverging laterally an equal distance. Asymmetric excursion suggests a lesion on the lagging side in the chest wall, pleura, or upper lobe of the lung.

Testing midchest excursion anteriorly. With fingers high in each axilla and thumbs abducted, place the palms firmly on the anterior chest. Move the hands medially, dragging skin to provide slack until the thumb tips meet in the midline at the level of the sixth ribs (Fig. 8-11B). Have the patient inspire deeply letting your hands follow the chest movements. The thumbs should move apart. A unilateral lag indicates a lesion in the wall, pleura, middle lobe of the right lung, or lingula of the left lung.

Testing lower chest excursion posteriorly. The patient sits or stands with his back toward you. Place your fingers in each axilla, with the palms applied firmly to the patient's chest, so your index fingers are one or two ribs below the inferior scapular angles. Provide slack by pressing the soft tissues while pulling your hands medially until your thumbs meet over the vertebral spines (Fig. 8-11C). Have the patient inspire deeply, following the chest movements with your hands; your thumbs should move apart. A unilateral lag indicates a lesion in the wall, pleura, or lower lobes.

Testing costal margin excursions. With the patient supine, place your hands so the extended thumbs lie along the inferior edges of the costal margins, with their tips nearly touching (Fig. 8-11D). Have the patient inspire deeply, letting your thumbs follow the costal margins. Normally, the thumbs diverge. Diminished divergence or convergence indicates flattening of the diaphragm.

Examining the Lungs and Pleura: Examination of the lungs and pleura is necessary to screen for subclinical thoracic disease and in the initial evaluation of all patients with suspected cardiopulmonary disease. Accurate classification of breath sounds, cardiac sounds, chest percussion and assessment of tactile fremitus establish the likelihood of significant disease, permit initial

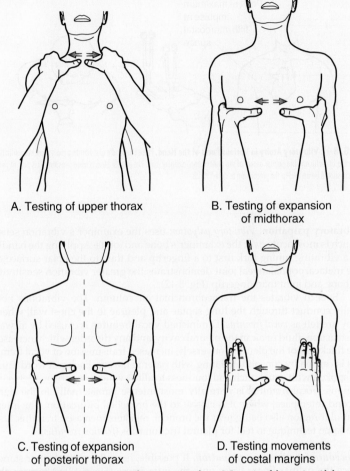

A. Testing of upper thorax

B. Testing of expansion of midthorax

C. Testing of expansion of posterior thorax

D. Testing movements of costal margins

FIG. 8-11 Testing Thoracic Movement. A. The upper anterior thorax. B. Expansion of the anterior mid-thorax. C. Expansion of the posterior thorax. D. Movement of costal margins.

characterization of disorders and provide essential context for accurate interpretation of imaging studies. Importantly, diagnostic imaging of the chest is static and cannot provide complete information on airflow, blood flow and musculoskeletal dynamics. Physical exam is rapid, can be performed in all clinical situations, and does not require additional equipment or remove caregivers from the patient. Some life-threatening conditions must be identified rapidly and primarily by physical exam such as central airway obstruction, tension pneumothorax, asthma, and pericardial tamponade. Other conditions require concurrent physical examination and imaging studies for accurate classification including musculoskeletal trauma and pleural effusions.

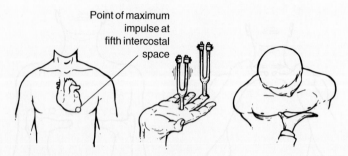

FIG. 8-12 Vibratory Acuity in Various Parts of the Hand. Place the handle of a vibrating tuning fork sequentially on the fingertip and the palmar aspect of the metacarpophalangeal joint: the palmar base is more sensitive. This part of the hand should be applied to the precordium to detect thrills.

Vibratory palpation. *Vibratory palpation* uses the examiner's vibration sense which is most acute over the examiner's bone and joints. Applying the handle of a vibrating tuning fork first to a fingertip and then to the volar surface of the metacarpophalangeal joint demonstrates the greater vibration sensitivity of bone and joint than fingertip (Fig. 8-12).

Speech vibrates the tracheobronchial air column. The vibrations normally conduct through the lung septae and pleurae to the chest wall where they are felt as *vocal fremitus*. Diminished vocal fremitus is caused by airway obstruction, fluid or air in the pleural cavity, and any disorder which increases the thickness of the pleura. Conversely, increased transmission of vocal fremitus is caused by consolidated lung with patent airways. Each test word must be spoken with equal pitch and loudness to allow valid comparisons between regions. Vocal fremitus is normally most intense parasternally in the right second interspace, where it is closest to the bronchial bifurcation. The interscapular region also being near the bronchi, registers increased fremitus. Use the same technique to feel for pleural friction rubs (*friction fremitus*).

Procedure for vibratory palpation. If possible, have the patient sit or stand. Place the palmar finger bases onto the interspaces (Fig. 8-13). Alternatively, use the ulnar side of the hand and fifth finger. Ask the patient to repeat the test words "ninety-nine" or "one–two–three," using the same pitch and intensity of voice each time. If vibrations are not felt, have the patient lower the pitch of their voice. Compare symmetrical parts of the chest sequentially with the same hand. It is better to compare two sensations sequentially with the same hand than to compare simultaneous sensations from two hands. When the lower thorax is reached, ascertain the point at which fremitus is lost. In the absence of a pleural lesion, this indicates the lung bases. Compare this with the position obtained by percussion and auscultation.

Chest percussion. Tissue density is evaluated by percussion. See Chapter 3, pages 30-32 for a discussion of percussion techniques. For best results, press the pleximeter finger into the intercostal spaces parallel to the ribs, then strike a series of blows with the plexor. Percuss the back with the patient sitting and

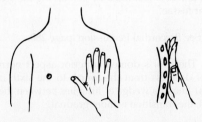

FIG. 8-13 Detection of Vocal Fremitus by Vibratory Palpation. Symmetrical points on the chest are palpated sequentially with the same hand and the strength of vocal fremitus is compared in different regions. The palpating hand is applied firmly to the chest wall with palm in contact with the wall, and vibrations are sensed with the bases of the fingers.

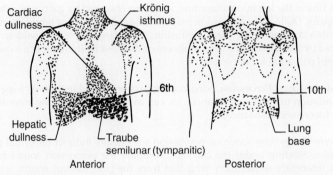

FIG. 8-14 Percussion Map of the Thorax. The entire lung surface is normally resonant. At the apices, a band of resonance, the Krönig isthmus, runs over the shoulders like shoulder straps. Hepatic dullness ranges downward from the right sixth rib merging into hepatic flatness. The Traube semilunar space of tympany extends downward from the left sixth rib; it is variable in extent, depending upon the amount of gas in the stomach. Posteriorly, the dullness below the lung bases begins at about the tenth rib.

the anterior chest with the patient sitting and supine. Both sonorous percussion and definitive percussion techniques are used to assess the density of the lungs (sonorous technique) as well as the symmetry and border of chest structures (definitive technique).

Definitive chest percussion. Definitive thoracic percussion outlines the borders between lung resonance and the dullness of the heart, spleen, upper liver border, and lumbar muscles below the lung bases. Definitive chest percussion is used to assess the position of the diaphragm, cardiac borders and to identify diaphragmatic asymmetry and pleural effusions (Fig. 8-14). When the patient is unable to sit, examine in the right and left lateral decubitus positions acknowledging that this introduces problems in interpretating percussion sounds (see pages 304-305 and Fig. 8-31). The boundary between resonant lung and tympanitic gastric bubble outlines the *Traube space.* The *Krönig isth-*

mus over the lung apices is identified by percussing the area of resonance in the supraclavicular fossae.

Cardiac dullness. See Precordial Percussion, page 280.

Hepatic dullness. The liver's domed superior aspect normally produces a transverse zone of dullness from the fourth to the sixth interspaces in the right midclavicular line. If a wedge of lung lies between the upper liver border and chest wall, the transition is more gradual.

Gastric tympany. The stomach usually contains an air bubble producing tympany in Traube space. Because the left diaphragm is lower, the upper tympanitic border is somewhat lower than the upper border of liver dullness on the right.

Splenic dullness. The spleen produces a dull oval between the ninth and eleventh ribs in the left midaxillary line; it is often obscured by gastric or colonic tympany. Dullness in this region may be enlarged by solid or liquid stomach or colon contents or by pleural effusion. An enlarged spleen is seldom obscured by gas. Enlarged splenic dullness or dullness in Traube space requires careful palpation for the spleen.

Sonorous Chest Percussion. Sonorous percussion is used to identify lung hyperinflation (increased resonance), as well as atelectasis and lung consolidation (decreased resonance).

Anterior lungs. Use sonorous percussion with heavy indirect bimanual percussion. Starting under the clavicles, compare the percussion sound from each interspace sequentially with that from the contralateral region, working downward to hepatic dullness on the right and Traube space on the left (Fig. 8-14). Also, percuss the lateral thorax. Except for cardiac dullness, the anterior chest should be resonant.

Lung apices. The lung apices extending slightly above the clavicles can produce a band of resonance over each shoulder, widening at its scapular and clavicular ends. The narrowest part, the *Krönig isthmus*, lies atop the shoulder. Reproducibility of this finding is low. With the patient sitting or standing, sound each supraclavicular fossa. On the right place the examiner's left thumb in the right supraclavicular fossa (Fig. 8-15A) where it is struck by the plexor finger of the right hand. For the pleximeter in the left fossa, the examiner's left arm is put around the patient's back the left long finger is curling anteriorly over the trapezius into the fossa (Fig. 8-15B). Apical lung fibrosis, dense pleural scarring or tumor infiltration diminishes the resonance.

Posterior lung and diaphragm excursion. Use sonorous percussion with the patient sitting or standing, the spine slightly flexed, and the shoulders pulled forward. Begin at the top and work downward comparing right to left sequentially and listening for asymmetry. The scapula and muscles impair resonance in proportion to their mass, but should produce symmetric changes. Switching from deep sonorous percussion to light definitive percussion technique, the inferior lung margins can normally be detected at about the ninth

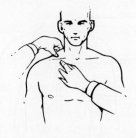
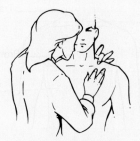

A. Percussion of right apex   B. Percussion of left apex

FIG. 8-15 Percussion of the Lung Apices. Bimanual indirect percussion is applied in the usual fashion, except for the use of the pleximeter. See the text for descriptions.

rib on the left and the eighth interspace on the right (Fig. 8-14). The transition between lung resonance and muscle dullness (or flatness) is gradual. Mark the lung bases during quiet respiration, then have the patient inspire deeply holding the breath while you percuss at full inspiratory capacity. The bases should move downward 5–6 cm reflecting flattening of the diaphragm.

Chest auscultation. Air moving in the tracheobronchial tree produces vibrations perceived as sounds. Lung and heart sounds have a frequency between 60 and 3000 cycles per second. Sounds are produced by turbulent air movement in normal, dilated, or narrowed airways, or during passage through the vocal cords. Diminished or absent breath sounds indicate airway obstruction or pleural disease. Additional sounds such as wheezes, stridor or crackles indicate airways disease, parenchymal disease or both.

Lung auscultation. If possible, have the patient sit. When recumbent, the back should be examined by turning the patient from side to side. With the patient breathing through the mouth, deeper and slightly more forcefully than usual, listen with the stethoscope's diaphragm anteriorly at the apices working downward comparing right to left sequentially. Then, listen to the back, again starting at the apices and working downward. Compare the lower lung margins as determined by auscultation, percussion, and fremitus.

Breath sounds are described as *vesicular, bronchovesicular, bronchial, asthmatic, cavernous,* or *absent.* Note also their quality and pitch and the relative duration of inspiration and expiration (Fig. 8-16). If *crackles* are heard, note whether they persist or disappear after a few deep breaths. If crackles are not heard, test for *posttussive crackles* by listening after a cough, particularly at the end of expiration. If an abnormality is found, test front and back for *whispered pectoriloquy* by having the patient whisper test words, such as "one–two–three." Test similarly with the spoken voice for *bronchophony* (Auscultation of Voice Sounds, page 307). Be alert for friction rubs, bone crepitus, and other unusual sounds.

Bedside sputum inspection. Collect sputum from a productive cough in a transparent plastic cup. Note the color, viscosity, presence of blood, or odor,

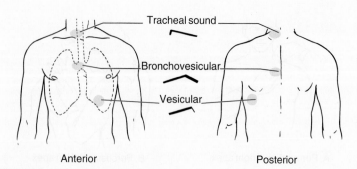

FIG. 8-16 Breath Sounds Map in the Normal Chest. The areas of the lungs that are unlabeled have normal vesicular breathing.

and estimate the daily volume. Attempt to identify any soft tissue elements, mucous plugs, blood, bronchial casts, or concretions.

Examining the Heart and Precordium: Despite advances in diagnostic technology, the cardiovascular physical exam remains an essential skill for the expert physician. Practice with mentoring by an expert is critical for learning the heart exam. Simulation technology also facilitates training. The physical exam is both sensitive and relatively specific for the diagnosis of valvular heart disease.

The cardiovascular exam is presented here in a convenient sequence emphasizing the precordium and careful neck and extremity exams. A complete cardiovascular evaluation also requires, if indicated, supplementary procedures such as electrocardiography, echocardiography, CT, MRI, scintigraphy, or cardiac catheterization.

Precordial inspection. Stand or sit at the patient's right-side shining a light across the anterior chest, preferably from the left-side. Look for the *apical impulse* which is visible in 20% of normal people. With your line of sight across the sternum look for precordial heaves.

Precordial palpation. Pulsations, lifts, heaves, and thrills can be felt in the precordium. Palpate with the palm, first examining areas of visible pulsation. Even when not visible try to identify the *apical impulse* in approximately the left fifth interspace 7–9 cm from the midline; it should be ≤2 cm in diameter. The impulse is synchronous with early ventricular systole. Palpate the entire precordium for the presence and strength of right and left ventricular thrusts. When present, a thrill or friction rub can be identified as systolic or diastolic by its relation to the apical impulse.

Precordial percussion. Percuss the precordium identifying the borders of cardiac dullness (*definitive percussion*). With the left arm abducted, locate the *left border of cardiac dullness* (LBCD): starting over resonant lung near the axilla, percuss the fifth, fourth, and third interspaces moving medially until cardiac dullness is encountered (Fig. 8-17). Measure the distance from the

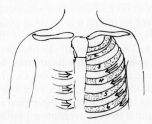

FIG. 8-17 Pattern of Precordial Percussion. The fifth, fourth, and third intercostal spaces on the left are percussed sequentially, as indicated by the arrows, starting near the axilla and moving medially until cardiac dullness is encountered.

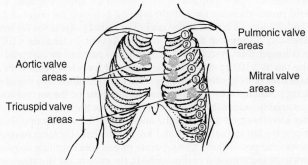

Pulmonic valve areas

Aortic valve areas

Mitral valve areas

Tricuspid valve areas

FIG. 8-18 Cardiac Valve Areas for Precordial Auscultation. These are the areas where the sounds originating from each valve are best heard; the areas are not necessarily closest to the anatomic location of the valves.

midline to the LBCD in the fifth interspace. The *right border of cardiac dullness* (*RBCD*) is normally behind the sternum so its position is not certain. When the heart border is displaced rightward, the RBCD can be identified. No conclusion about heart size can be drawn by percussing only the LBCD in isolation. With hydrothorax or thickened pleura, percussion of the heart border may be impossible. Assess the width of *retromanubrial dullness*; in the adult a width >6 cm suggests an anterior mediastinal mass or aortic aneurysm. All suspected abnormalities require correlation with the clinical presentation and confirmation by chest radiography, echocardiography or both.

Precordial auscultation. Proper stethoscope use is described in Chapter 3. The same principles apply to heart and lung auscultation. Listen in each primary valve area (Fig. 8-18). Timing of heart sounds is especially important. Use the apical impulse, or, if absent, the carotid upstroke to mark the onset of ventricular systole. Map the radiation of abnormal sounds on the precordium.

Auscultating heart rate and rhythm. Auscultate the apical ventricular rate comparing it with a peripheral arterial pulse. If the rate is regular and not bradycardic, counting for 15 seconds and multiplying by 4 is sufficiently accurate.

Any difference between the auscultated apical and palpated arterial rates is a *pulse deficit*. Pulse deficit occurs whenever ventricular systole generates a stroke volume insufficient to produce an arterial pulse wave; it is frequent with premature beats, bigeminal rhythm, and atrial fibrillation. **The ECG is the gold standard for heart rate, as not all electrical events produce an audible mechanical event, especially at high heart rates.** After counting the heart rate, listen carefully for an *irregularity of rhythm*. Dysrhythmias are harder to detect when the diastolic intervals are either very long or very short, that is, with particularly slow or fast heart rates. Determine if an irregularity has a relation to respirations and if there is a repeating pattern of beats.

Auscultating heart sounds: S1 and S2. Normally, auscultation reveals paired sounds, usually distinct in intensity and pitch, with each cardiac cycle (Fig. 8-19). Identification of the first (S1) and second heart (S2) sounds is essential because they mark the beginning and end of ventricular systole. The sound synchronous with an apical impulse is S1. Without an apical impulse, palpate the carotid pulse, allowing for a slight interval between the onset of cardiac systole and the wave's arrival in the neck. The radial pulse is too far from the heart to reliably distinguish the heart sounds. At ventricular rates <100 bpm, diastole is longer than systole, so the first of the pair can be accepted as S1. When the rate is >100 bpm try to slow the heart for a few beats with a Valsalva maneuver or by gently massaging either carotid sinus. The initial sound after a long pause must be the first heart sound. Finally, the second sound is almost invariably louder than the first at the base of the heart.

After identifying S1 and S2 at the apex, move the stethoscope short distances along the left sternal border and toward the base (*inching*) tracing each sound across the precordium. Use separate passes concentrating sequentially on the intensity (accentuated or diminished), the quality, the duration, and the presence of splitting of the sounds. Prolonged sounds can be differentiated from murmurs by their abrupt beginning and ending; murmurs have a gradual onset and end. A sound that begins abruptly but ends gradually is probably a heart sound followed by a murmur. Cardiac auscultation is difficult to master. It requires mentored practice listening to many normal and abnormal hearts to recognize the range of normal and correctly identify abnormal sounds.

Auscultating heart murmurs. Listen for heart murmurs only after S1 and S2 have been positively identified. Decide whether a sound of abnormal length is a split heart sound or a heart sound *and* murmur. Now turn your attention to the systolic interval between S1 and S2. Decide if there is any audible sound in this interval by assuming that a heart sound is the shortest perceptible sound and that anything appreciably longer may be heart sound and murmur. A prolonged sound starting abruptly and dwindling is probably a heart sound followed by murmur. One developing gradually and ending abruptly is likely a murmur and heart sound. Carefully examine each valve area using the diaphragm and listen at the apex and lower left sternal border with the bell. Cover the intervening spaces by inching the stethoscope short distances each time. Once a murmur is identified, ascertain its characteristics:

Timing. Determine in what part of the cardiac cycle the murmur occurs, (i.e. systolic or diastolic), and whether it is early, middle, or late in the interval, by reference to the first and second heart sounds.

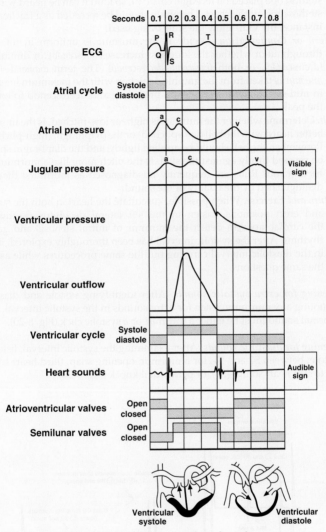

Seconds	0.1	0.2	0.3	0.4	0.5	0.6	0.7	0.8

FIG. 8-19 Relation of the Heart Sounds to Other Events in the Cardiac Cycle.

Location. Ascertain where on the precordium the murmur has maximum intensity.

Intensity. Grade intensity by the following scale: *Grade I,* barely audible with greatest difficulty; *Grade II,* faint but heard immediately upon listening. *Grades III, IV, V, and VI* are progressively louder: *Grade IV* requires the presence of a palpable thrill; *Grade V,* loud enough to be heard with the stethoscope placed on its edge; *Grade VI*, so loud it can be heard with the stethoscope off the chest. The grade should be recorded as a fraction, for instance, III/VI to show the scale being used.

Pattern or Configuration. Decide if the murmur is uniform in intensity throughout or whether the loudness increases (*crescendo*), or diminishes (*decrescendo*), or both (*crescendo-decrescendo*). The term *diamond-shaped murmur* is taken from the graphic depiction with the maximum intensity in mid-systole, with a crescendo preceding and decrescendo following the peak.

Pitch. Determine whether the murmur is high- or low-pitched. Is the murmur better heard with the bell (low-pitched) or the diaphragm (high-pitched)? Remember, the bell should be applied lightly, and the diaphragm should be pressed firmly against the skin. Is the pitch more like a murmur or a friction rub? Rubs are frequently misdiagnosed as murmurs; they are distinguished by the quality of the sound.

Posture and Exercise. When possible, auscultate the heart in both the supine and erect positions. Listen in the left lateral decubitus position at the cardiac apex to detect the murmur of mitral stenosis and gallop rhythms. After the systolic interval has been thoroughly explored, listen in the diastolic interval carrying out the same procedures while asking the same questions.

Listening for extra systolic sounds. After identifying systole and diastole, and noting any murmurs, listen for extra sounds in the systolic interval. Any abnormal sound must be either a murmur or a systolic click (Fig. 8-20).

Listening for diastolic sounds. After examining the systolic interval, listen in diastole, between S2 and S1, for a murmur, opening snap, third heart sound (S3), fourth heart sound (S4), or pericardial knock (Fig. 8-20).

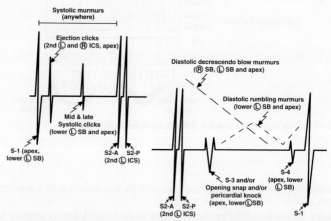

FIG. 8-20 Timing of Heart Sounds, Clicks, Opening Snap, and Murmurs Within the Cardiac Cycle. ICS, intercostal space; SB, sternal border; S2-A, S2-in aortic area; S2-P, S2 in pulmonic area.

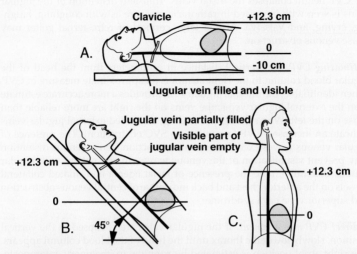

FIG. 8-21 Response of the Jugular Blood Column to Changes in Posture. The anteroposterior diameter of the thorax at the fourth interspace is ~20 cm; from this point, the vertical distance to the superior border of the clavicle is ~15 cm in the erect position. The right atrium is located at the midpoint of an anteroposterior line from the fourth interspace to the back. In any posture, a horizontal plane through this point is the zero-pressure level. In this figure, a slightly elevated venous pressure of 12.3 cm is assumed. **A.** With the patient supine, the horizontal plane 12.3 cm above the zero level is above the neck; at normal venous pressure the jugular vein is filled. **B.** With the thorax at 45 degrees, the blood column extends midway up the jugular, so the head of the column is visible. **C.** In the erect position, the head of the column is concealed within the thorax, 2.7 cm below the upper border of the clavicle.

Examining the Blood Vessels: Clinicians must be familiar with the accessible arteries and veins. These arteries are usually palpable: temporal, common and external carotid, axillary, brachial, radial, ulnar, common iliac, femoral, popliteal, dorsalis pedis, and posterior tibial (Chapter 4, Fig. 4-2). The abdominal aorta may be palpable. Visible veins are the external jugular, cephalic, basilic, median basilic, great saphenous, and veins on the hands and feet.

Measurement of arterial blood pressure. See Chapter 4, page 64.

Venous pressure. *Central venous pressure* (*CVP*) is measured at the level of the right atrium (RA). When erect, this is at the anterior fourth intercostal space. Proximal and superior to the RA are, in order, the SVC, the two subclavian veins, and the two subcutaneous *external jugular veins* in the neck above the clavicles. The vertical height of the blood column above the RA is the CVP, normally about 10 cm (Fig. 8-21A). Peripheral veins below CVP level are filled with blood; those above are collapsed. In adults, the upper clavicular border is ~13–18 cm above the RA, so the external jugular veins collapse when the patient is erect (Fig. 8-21C). As the thorax reclines blood rises into the neck veins becoming visible in the jugular veins (Fig. 8-21B). The arm and forearm veins distend to the same level as the SVC. In the horizontal position, all peripheral veins are filled (Fig. 8-21A). Raising the arm above the CVP height collapses the distal veins. Transient distention of the jugular veins is seen with increased intrathoracic pressure as with coughing, laughing, crying, and Valsalva. Also, a large cervical or retrosternal goiter may cause venous obstruction.

Estimating CVP. The vertical distance in centimeters from the head of the jugular blood column to the right atrium is an approximate measure of CVP. When identifiable, the internal jugular vein provides a more accurate estimate than the external jugular veins; the veins on the right are more reliable than those on the left. When sitting or standing, distended external jugular veins indicate an increased CVP (assuming no SVC obstruction). The presence of jugular venous waves excludes central obstruction. Tense venous distention may prevent visualization of the venous waves. In any patient with jugular venous distention, note the presence of facial edema and dilated collateral vessels on the anterior chest and back indicative of central venous obstruction and superior vena cava syndrome.

Indirect CVP measurement. If the jugular veins are collapsed in the vertical position, slowly lower the thorax until the head of the blood column appears. The right atrial position is estimated by running an imaginary anteroposterior line from the anterior fourth interspace halfway to the back; a horizontal plane through this point is the zero level for measuring venous pressure (Fig. 8-21B). The vertical distance in centimeters from this plane to the head of the blood column is the approximate CVP. The angle of Louis (sternal angle) is another reference point for estimating CVP. It is ~6 cm above the RA in most positions, though not always. Jugular venous pulsations >3 cm vertically above this landmark indicate elevated venous pressure.

Alternate indirect CVP measurement. Place the patient supine with an arm hanging over the bedside. Raise the arm slowly until the distended arm or hand veins collapse. The vertical distance from the zero level to the point of collapse estimates the CVP. Select a vein as close to the heart, for example, the cephalic, basilic, or median basilic veins (Fig. 8-22). There is great variation in the caliber and superficiality of the arm veins.

Venous pulsations. The venous pulse wave can be demonstrated in the external jugular veins if not obscured by overlying tissue. Venous pulsation is readily distinguished from an arterial pulse by being impalpable. There are three upward components to the venous pulse wave (Fig. 8-23) and two prominent descents. The *a-wave* results from right atrial systole; the *c-wave* is principally caused by expansion of the underlying carotid artery and is usually not visible. The a-wave peak is followed by an *x-descent*, initially because of atrial relaxation and later of downward movement of the tricuspid valve with right ventricular systole. The rising *v-wave* is produced by right atrial filling with the tricuspid valve closed. The peak of the v-wave is followed by the *y-descent* associated with tricuspid valve opening at onset of right ventricular diastole. Correctly identifying the waves and descents requires careful correlation with the cardiac cycle. The rapid descents are usually better appreciated than the slowly rising waves. The *x-descent* is normally the most readily observed portion of the jugular pulse, and its nadir is approximated by S2. The peak of the a-wave is normally the most prominent wave and occurs at about S1.

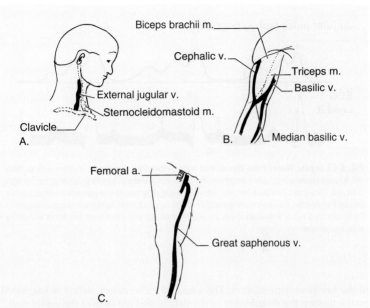

FIG. 8-22 Visible Veins and Venous Pressure Measurements. A. Veins of the neck. B. Veins of the arm. C. Veins of the thigh and leg.

Venous pulsations are also seen as lateral neck expansion and contraction occurring with filling and collapse of the internal jugular veins and their tributaries. This is best seen from the foot of the bed. In a few persons, pulsations occur in the superficial veins of the arms, forearms, and hands. A disproportion in the number of a-waves and ventricular systoles indicates a dysrhythmia, but the waves are difficult to see consistently. Failure to identify an expected venous pulse may indicate obstruction of veins proximal to the right atrium.

Capillary pulsation. Press down on the tip of a fingernail until the distal third of the nailbed blanches. With each heartbeat, the border of pink extends and recedes. This a prominent sign in aortic regurgitation known as *Quincke pulse*, but it can be seen to a lesser degree in many normal persons.

Examining the Arterial Circulation in the Extremities: Large named arteries normally have visible or palpable pulses. Their occlusion is recognized by regional ischemia. In the complete physical exam, assess the circulation by (1) bilateral palpation of the pulse volume in brachial, radial, femoral, dorsalis pedis, and posterior tibial arteries; (2) palpation for skin temperature changes; (3) inspection for varicose veins, edema, pallor, cyanosis, and ulceration of the arms and legs; and (4) inspection of the retinal vessels. Complaints of pain, coolness, or numbness in an extremity or signs of enlarged veins, masses, swellings, localized pallor, redness, or cyanosis lead to special examinations

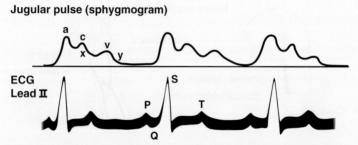

FIG. 8-23 Jugular Venous Pulse Waves. Heart action is reflected in the jugular vein. The waves should be timed with the apical impulse or heart sounds, remembering that a perceptible time elapses between cardiac events and their signs in the neck. The a-wave is the rebound from atrial systole. The bulging of the tricuspid valve cusps early in ventricular systole produces the c-deflection. The v-wave results from atrial filling while the valve is closed, together with an upward movement of the AV valve ring at the end of ventricular systole. The x-descent comes with atrial relaxation and the y-descent with opening of the tricuspid valve.

of the peripheral circulation. The cause of a circulatory deficit is suggested by the history, the distribution of the deficit, and the state of the vessel wall.

Skin exam for circulation. When a part is below heart level, pooled venous blood obscures evidence of arterial flow. Venous pressure is rarely >30 cm above that of the right atrium, whereas the systolic arterial pressure is >120 cm above the same reference point. Thus, lifting the hand or foot above the right atrium to a height exceeding the venous pressure, drains the masking venous blood pool permitting evaluation of tissue color produced by the arterial inflow. The most reliable signs of a regional perfusion abnormality are a temperature or perfusion discrepancy between symmetrical parts at the same external temperature.

Skin color. Color is imparted by blood in the venules of the skin's subpapillary layer and its melanin content. Examining for circulatory changes in dark-skinned individuals is difficult. Rather, focus attention on the mucous membranes, nail beds, and palms. When the arterial flow is nil and the veins empty, the skin is chalky white. Partial but inadequate arterial supply produces red or cyanotic skin, depending on the effect of external temperature and amount of pooled blood in the venules.

Skin temperature. Temperature reliably indicates skin perfusion. Normal flow is principally governed by arteriolar constriction or dilatation. Internal body temperature is maintained within narrow limits, partly by heat dissipation from the skin. In clothed persons, the skin of the head, neck, and trunk is warmer than that of the extremities, and the digits are cooler than the proximal hands and feet. Peculiarly, normal digits adjust their temperature to only one of the two levels. The fingers are somewhat cooler (32°C [90°F]) than blood temperature (37°C [98°F]) when the air temperature exceeds 20°C (68°F). If the air temperature is below 16°C (60°F), finger temperatures drop to approximately 22°C (72°F); no intermediate level is maintained.

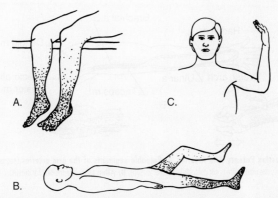

FIG. 8-24 Circulation of the Skin in Extremities. A. The legs are dependent to observe the color of the skin and nail beds. Arterial deficit produces a violaceous color from pooling of the blood in the venules because of loss of venomotor tone as a result of hypoxia. **B. While the patient is supine**, the foot is elevated above the level of venous pressure (15 cm [6 in.] above the right heart or 25 cm [10 in.] above the table when the patient is supine). Elevation drains the foot of venous blood, so the skin color reflects only the presence of arterial blood. The elevated leg is compared with the opposite extremity. **C. The hand is raised above the heart level,** so the skin color is produced exclusively by arterial blood.

Examining for arterial deficit. In a draft-free room at ~22°C (72°F) the extremities are normally exposed for 10 minutes while the complete physical exam is being performed. This duration of exposure can be used to assess the health of the skin and vasculature in the extremities. Coldness and pallor of the skin should not be routinely demonstrated with this exposure in normal patients. Have the patient sit, hanging the legs from the table or bed, comparing the skin color of both feet looking for pallor, deep redness, pale blueness, deep blueness, or a violaceous color (Fig. 8-24A). With the back of your hand or fingers feel the skin temperature from the feet up the legs. Compare comparable sites on each leg in sequence noting whether an increase in temperature is gradual or sharply demarcated. Have the patient lie supine. Grasp the patient's ankles and elevate the feet >30 cm (12 inch) above the right atrium. Note any change in skin color (Fig. 8-24C). If the color does not change, have the patient dorsiflex the feet five or six times, wait several minutes, then observe the feet for color changes induced by exercise. Allow the feet to hang down again and note the time for the color to return. Note how quickly color returns to an area blanched by finger pressure.

Inspect the feet carefully for evidence skin atrophy, loss of lanugo hair on the dorsa of the toes, thickening or transverse ridging of the nails, and ulceration or patches of gangrene. Examine the arms similarly by exposing them for 10 minutes and then observing the color in dependency and when elevated well above heart level (Fig. 8-24B). Repetitively opening and closing the fists discloses latent color changes. Note the time for color return in dependency.

Examining large arm and leg arteries. Palpate the walls of accessible arteries for increased thickness, tortuosity, and beading. A spastic artery feels like a

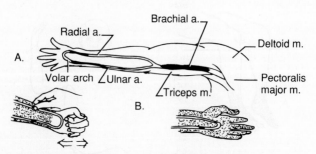

FIG. 8-25 Testing Patency Arm Arteries. A. Palpable segments of the arm arteries (segments in solid black). Frequently the ulnar pulse is not palpable in normal persons. **B. Allen test.** See the text for details.

small cord. Compare the pulse volume at symmetric arterial levels. Be careful not to mistake the pulse in your own finger for that of the patient.

Doppler ultrasound. Small portable instruments may be used at the bedside and these can more precisely evaluate the arterial circulation particularly for patients with significant peripheral vascular occlusive disease. When pulses are not palpable, Doppler ultrasound is required to distinguish nonpalpable flow from total arterial occlusion.

Arms. Listen for a bruit in the supraclavicular fossa over the *subclavian artery*. Only the brachial artery in the upper arm and the radial and ulnar arteries at the wrist are palpable. With the forearm flexed 90 degrees, palpate the *brachial artery* on the medial arm in the groove between the biceps and triceps muscles (Fig. 8-25A). Palpate the *radial artery* on the wrist's flexor surface just medial to the radial styloid. Palpate the *ulnar artery* on the wrist's flexor surface just medial to the distal ulna; it lies deeper than the radial artery and may not be palpable. Determine radial and ulnar artery patency with the *Allen test* (Fig. 8-25B). With the patient sitting and hands supinated on the knees, grasp the right wrist, with your thumbs on its flexor surface. Have the patient make a tight fist, then compress both the radial and ulnar arteries with your thumbs. Have the patient open the hand. The skin should be pale and remain so while both arteries are compressed. Take your thumb off the radial artery; the palm and fingers should quickly turn pink as flow returns. Delayed flush or no flush indicates partial or complete radial artery obstruction. Repeat the process, this time removing pressure from the ulnar artery. Return of flow is normally somewhat slower from the ulnar artery, but absence of flush is pathologic. Repeat this sequence on the other hand.

Legs. Palpate the *abdominal aorta* deeply between the xiphoid and the umbilicus. Palpate the *common femoral arteries* just below the inguinal ligaments, equidistant between the anterior superior iliac spines and the pubic tubercles (Fig. 8-26). Feel for *popliteal* artery pulsation with the patient supine and the legs extended. Place a hand on each side of the patient's knee with your thumbs anteriorly near the patella and the fingers curling around so the tips

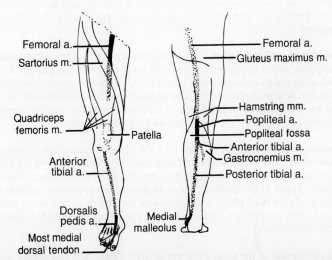

FIG. 8-26 Palpable Lower Limb Arteries. The palpable segments of the arteries are in solid black. The femoral artery is palpable only a short distance below the inguinal ligament at the midpoint between the anterior superior iliac spine and the pubic tubercle. The popliteal artery lies vertically in the popliteal fossa; it can be felt only by compressing the contents of the fossa from behind against the bone. The posterior tibial artery can be felt as it curls forward and under the medial malleolus. The palpable segment of the dorsalis pedis artery lies just lateral to the most medial of the dorsal tendons of the foot (the flexor of the great toe) over the arch of the foot.

rest in the popliteal fossa. Firmly press the fingers against the lower femur or upper tibia feeling for arterial pulsation. A normal popliteal artery may not be palpable. Palpate the *posterior tibial artery* in the groove between the medial malleolus and Achilles tendon. It may be more easily palpable with the foot passively dorsiflexed. Locate the *dorsalis pedis artery* on the dorsum of the foot just lateral to and parallel with the extensor hallucis longus tendon. In normal persons aged >45 years, either the dorsalis pedis or posterior tibial pulse frequently will not be palpable, but not both in the same foot.

Ankle brachial index. A quantified measure of arterial function is the *ankle-brachial index (ABI)*. The ABI is calculated from measurements of the systolic blood pressure in the brachial artery and the posterior tibial and/or the dorsalis pedis artery. The systolic pressure is taken as the inflation pressure of a standard blood pressure cuff that results in total arterial occlusion. The test is performed after the patient is at rest in the supine position for 10 minutes. Most commonly, the cessation of arterial pulses are assessed with a handled Doppler instrument. The ABI is the ratio of the ankle systolic pressure to the highest right or left brachial systolic pressure. A normal ABI is >0.9–1.4. An ABI greater than 1.4 indicates noncompliant, calcified arteries found in advanced atherosclerosis. Occlusive peripheral vascular disease in the lower extremity is indicated by the degree of abnormality with 0.75 to 0.9 mild, 0.6 to 0.75 moderate, and <0.6 severe ischemia. An ABI <0.5 suggests severe arterial disease and potential for limb threatening ischemia. Importantly, the

ABI should be interpreted within the context of clinical signs and symptoms such as claudication, paresthesias, weakness, and palpation of both the skin and pulses.

Examining Large Limb Veins: Adequate drainage of blood from the extremities requires patent veins, muscle contraction to pump blood proximally by compressing veins, and competent perforating and deep venous valves limiting retrograde flow. Failure of any one of these results in venous stasis which increases filtration pressure in the distal capillaries and post-capillary venules producing edema, stasis pigmentation, and/or skin ulceration.

Examining large arm and leg veins. With the patient supine, look for signs of venous stasis. Have the patient stand and check for dilated arm and leg veins. Elevate each extremity determining how rapidly the veins collapse; failure to promptly empty indicates obstruction. If obstruction is present, palpate the venous walls for hard plugs of thrombus or hard cords of fibrosis. If patent varicose veins are present, additional special tests may be used to assess for incompetent valves.

Laboratory exam of the large limb veins. Techniques such as Doppler ultrasound, impedance plethysmography, venography, and MRI can determine the patency and valve competence of the large limb veins.

CHEST, CARDIOVASCULAR, AND RESPIRATORY SYMPTOMS

General Symptoms

Chest pain. Chest pain often causes fear of ischemic heart disease, but has many noncardiac causes. Chest pain occurring without physical signs requires a careful history to categorize the attributes of pain. Focus on all the locations where pain is felt and solicit where it is most intense and if the pain radiates. Specific attention to the effect of exertion and rest on pain intensity is also important. Chest pain intensity should be quantified on a 10-point scale and changes over time and with treatment or intervention should be noted. Remember to evaluate chest pain and most other symptoms using a standard approach such as *PQRST: provocative-palliative factors, quality, region-referral, severity, and timing*. Interpret the characteristics of the chest pain within the contex of the patient's risk for major cardiovascular disease by simultaneously assessing the patient's ischemic cardiac disease risk factors.

Deep retrosternal or precordial pain and the six-dermatome band. See Six-Dermatome Pain Syndromes, page 350. Dermatomes T1–T6 cover the chest wall from the neck to beneath the xiphoid, and extend down the anteromedial aspect of the arms and forearms (Fig. 8-27). The first four dermatomes contain sensory afferents from dorsal roots of T1 to T4 and the lower cervical and upper thoracic sympathetic ganglia. In the ganglia and spinal cord, the fibers communicate with one another superiorly and inferiorly. The mediastinal, thoracic, and abdominal organs are also supplied by sensory afferents and parasympathetic efferents via the vagus nerve (CN X). The myocardium, pericardium, aorta, pulmonary artery, esophagus, and mediastinum have sensory fibers in these pathways. Disorders in any of these structures produce deep, visceral, and poorly localized pain. Spinal segments T5 and T6 receive

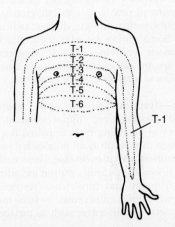

FIG. 8-27 The Six-Dermatome Band. Dermatomes T1–T6 form a band covering most of the thorax and extending down the anteromedial aspect of the arms and forearms. Sensory pathways from the viscera of this entire region are so interconnected that stimulation of any part can produce the same patterns of chest pain.

sensory fibers from the lower chest wall, the diaphragm and its peritoneal surface, the gallbladder, pancreas, duodenum, and stomach. Injury to these structures causes deep, visceral, poorly localized pain very similar in quality to that of the upper band. Deep visceral retrosternal pain in the precordial region or epigastrium is typical of pain from the structures supplied by spinal segments T1–T6, including the sympathetics. It is *not* specific for heart disorders. Neuroanatomy explains the structural basis for this clinical observation. Pain arising from T1–T4 usually has maximal intensity retrosternally or in the precordium, often extending with less intensity into the neck and/or down the anteromedial aspect of one or both arms and forearms. Pain arising in T5 and T6 is most often maximally intense around the xiphoid and/or in the back inferior to the right scapula, but pain can extend into the T1–T4 distribution through posterior sympathetic connections, making it indistinguishable from pain arising above the diaphragm. *The location of pain only indicates that its source is somewhere in the six-dermatome band (the myocardium, pericardium, aorta, pulmonary artery, mediastinum, esophagus, gallbladder, pancreas, duodenum, stomach, or subphrenic region).*

CLINICAL OCCURRENCE: *Congenital:* Hypertrophic cardiomyopathy; *Endocrine:* Retrosternal thyroid; *Degenerative/Idiopathic:* Esophageal spasm, gastroesophageal reflux; *Infectious:* Infectious pericarditis and pleuritis, granulomatous mediastinal lymphadenopathy, myocarditis, subphrenic abscess; *Inflammatory/Immune:* Esophagitis, pericarditis, sarcoidosis, pleuritis, myocarditis, postcardiotomy syndrome, pancreatitis, cholecystitis, gastritis; *Mechanical/Traumatic:* Pneumothorax, esophageal rupture, esophageal obstruction (extrinsic, foreign body, neoplasm, web, or ring), esophageal diverticulum, gastric perforation; *Metabolic/Toxic:* Acid or alkali ingestion;

Neoplastic: Carcinoma (primary or metastatic) of the esophagus, pericardium, lung, mediastinum, pleura; lymphoma; thymoma; teratoma; testicular cancer; *Neurologic:* Postherpetic neuralgia, diabetic radiculopathy, intercostal neuritis; *Psychosocial:* Somatization disorder, panic attack, hypochondriasis, malingering, Munchausen syndrome; *Vascular:* Myocardial ischemia (coronary atherosclerosis, spasm, embolism, thrombosis, vasculitis), central pulmonary embolism (PE) and infarction, aortic dissection.

Shortness of breath—dyspnea. Dyspnea is the result of abnormal gas exchange (decreased oxygenation, hypoventilation, hyperventilation) and/or increased work of breathing from impaired respiratory mechanics. Physiologically, dyspnea may result from pulmonary parenchymal disease, airways disease, pulmonary vascular disease, chest wall and neuromuscular disease as well as disorders of cardiac output including valvular disease, arrhythmias, cardiomyopathy and constrictive/restrictive pericardial disease. Dyspnea may result from anemia caused by bone marrow and bleeding disorders as well as metabolic disorders such as metabolic acidosis, sepsis and hyperthyroidism.

Dyspnea means difficult breathing, both a symptom and a sign. The complaint can be shortness of breath, running out of breath, being unable to take a deep breath, smothering, or chest tightness. Often accompanying dyspnea are tachypnea, increased respiratory excursions (*hyperpnea*), tense scaleni and sternocleidomastoid, flaring alae nasi, and a distressed expression. Identify associations of dyspnea, e.g., exertion versus dyspnea at rest and on standing or lying down. Rare patients seem unaware of dyspnea despite having to pause for breath in the middle of a sentence or even when they have cyanosis or resting tachycardia. These patients may be at risk for death from disorders such as asthma since they can present for clinical care late in the course of their disease and *in extremis*.

Significant comorbid psychiatric disease including depression and anxiety may be present in patients with ventilatory disorders. Psychiatric symptoms may be early and dominant features of cardiopulmonary disease. Acutely, hypoxemia and respiratory acidosis may cause delirium and abnormal behavior. For patients with chronic cardiopulmonary disease such as chronic obstructive pulmonary disease, pulmonary fibrosis or congestive heart failure, the rate of psychiatric comorbidity is high and these patients should be screened for this psychiatric co-morbidity. Conversely, because of direct effects on respiratory drive and symptom perception, primary psychiatric disorders such as anxiety as well as some pain syndromes may also result in profound sensations of dyspnea. Indicators of primary psychiatric disease include disproportionately severe symptoms compared to physical findings, normal lung auscultation, normal pulse oximetry, normal ECG and normal chest X-ray.

CLINICAL OCCURRENCE: *Decreased Fraction of Inspired Oxygen:* high altitude; *Airway Obstruction—Larynx and Trachea:* Infections (laryngeal diphtheria, acute laryngitis, epiglottitis, Ludwig angina), angioedema, trauma (hematoma or laryngeal edema), neuropathic (abductor paralysis of vocal cords), foreign body, tumors of the neck (goiter, thyroid and thymus carcinoma, primary tracheal tumors, lymphoma), extrinsic compression by aneurysm or esophageal tumor, ankylosis of the cricoarytenoid joints; vocal cord dysfunction syndrome; *Bronchi and Bronchioles:* Acute and chronic bronchitis, asthma, retrosternal goiter, aspirated foreign bodies, bronchiectasis, bronchial stenosis; *Abnormal Alveoli—Alveolar Filling:* Pulmonary edema, pulmonary infiltration (infectious and aspiration pneumonia, carcinoma, sarcoidosis, pneumoconioses), pulmonary hemorrhage, pulmonary alveolar proteinosis; *Alveolar Destruction:* Pulmonary emphysema, pulmonary fibrosis, cystic disease of the lungs; *Compression of Alveoli:* Atelectasis, pneumothorax, hydrothorax, abdominal distention; *Restrictive Chest and Lung Disease:* Paralysis of the respiratory muscles (especially the intercostals and the diaphragm), myasthenia gravis thoracic deformities (kyphoscoliosis, thoracoplasty), scleroderma or burns of the thoracic wall, pulmonary fibrosis; *Abnormal Pulmonary Circulation:* Pericardial tamponade, pulmonary artery stenosis, arteriovenous shunts in heart and lungs, pulmonary thromboembolism and infarction, other emboli (fat, air, amniotic fluid), arteriolar stenosis (primary pulmonary hypertension, irradiation); *Oxyhemoglobin Deficiency:* Anemia, carbon monoxide poisoning (carboxyhemoglobinemia), methemoglobinemia and sulfhemoglobinemia, cyanide and cobalt poisoning; *Abnormal Respiratory Stimuli:* Pain from respiratory movements, exaggerated consciousness of respiration (effort syndrome), hyperventilation syndrome, secondary respiratory alkalosis (increased intracranial pressure, metabolic acidosis).

Orthopnea–shortness of breath when lying down. This may occur as the result of redistribution of extracellular fluid from the periphery to the lungs, an elevated diaphragm from obesity or ascites, or muscular weakness exacerbated by upward pressure of the abdomen on the diaphragm and thorax when supine. Consciously or unconsciously, most patients with orthopnea sleep and rest with their head and chest elevated, often in a seated position. Estimate severity by the number of pillows required or if the patient sleeps in a chair to achieve a comfortable sleeping position. Many patients also have *paroxysmal nocturnal dyspnea*. Ask about orthopnea specifically and observe the patient for several minutes while supine.

Paroxysmal nocturnal dyspnea. With recumbency, fluid from edematous extremities is redistributed to the vasculature and lungs increasing pulmonary capillary pressure (PCWP) and, in extreme cases, causing pulmonary edema. Sudden paroxysms of breathlessness occur with recumbency, often accompanied by orthopnea and coughing. Sitting or walking for a few minutes relieves the dyspnea. Airway disorders such as asthma may also result in nocturnal dyspnea accompanied by sudden awakening, cough and wheezing. Unlike fluid-redistribution related paroxysmal nocturnal dyspnea, these patients do not typically have edema or preceding orthopnea and they may improve rapidly with inhaled bronchodilators.

Platypnea–shortness of breath on standing. With standing, pulmonary arteriovenous shunts may increase right-to-left shunting resulting in decreased oxygen saturation (*orthodeoxia*) and shortness of breath. Platypnea is characteristic of the *hepatopulmonary syndrome* (see page 346) seen with advanced liver disease. Patients complain of shortness of breath and weakness on standing, relieved by sitting or lying. They have stigmata of advanced liver disease including cutaneous spiders and ascites caused by portal hypertension.

Chest Wall Symptoms
Chest pain with tenderness. See Chest Wall Signs, pages 300-301.

Lung and Pleura Symptoms:
Shortness of breath—dyspnea. See page 294.

Cough. Cough is a sudden, forceful, noisy expulsion of air from the lungs. A cough has three stages: preliminary inspiration, glottis closure with respiratory muscle contraction, and sudden opening of the glottis producing an outward blast of air. The sensory nerve endings for the cough reflex are branches of the vagus (CN X) in the larynx, trachea, and bronchi. Exudates in the pharynx or bronchial tree, foreign body irritation, and tracheobronchial inflammation each trigger cough. Cough can also be induced by external acoustic meatus stimulation via the auricular branch of the vagus, and by esophageal stimulation from acid reflux. Coughing is characterized as voluntary or involuntary, single or paroxysmal. A *productive cough* raises sputum. Chronic unexplained coughs are most commonly caused by chronic post-nasal drip, gastroesophageal reflux, or asthma. *DDX:* A *brassy cough* is nonproductive with a strident quality occurring with narrowing of the trachea or glottal space, most commonly with laryngitis or epiglottitis, but also with laryngeal paralysis, vocal cord neoplasm, or aortic aneurysm. In pertussis a long strident inspiratory noise, a *whoop*, precedes the cough.
   CLINICAL OCCURRENCE: *Congenital:* Tracheoesophageal fistula, mediastinal teratoma; *Endocrine:* Substernal thyroid; *Degenerative/Idiopathic:* Emphysema, gastroesophageal reflux; *Infectious:* Sinusitis, pharyngitis, laryngitis, epiglottitis, tracheobronchitis, pneumonia, bronchiectasis, lung abscess, subphrenic abscess, typhoid; *Inflammatory/Immune:* Inhaled allergens, asthma, chronic bronchitis, interstitial lung disease, vasculitis, Goodpasture syndrome, relapsing polychondritis, endobronchial amyloidoma; *Metabolic/Toxic:* Tobacco smoking, inhaled irritants, angiotensin-converting enzyme inhibitors; *Mechanical/Traumatic:* Cervical osteophytes, inhaled foreign bodies, acute and chronic aspiration, tympanic membrane irritation, mediastinal mass and lymphadenopathy; *Neoplastic:* Cancer of the larynx and lung, endobronchial adenoma, thymoma, mediastinal lymphoma, metastases to the lung; *Psychosocial:* Cough tics and habits; *Vascular:* Congestive heart failure (CHF), vasculitis (Wegener, Churg–Straus), aortic aneurysm, pulmonary embolism , pulmonary hemorrhage.

Chest pain intensified by breathing. See Chest Wall Syndromes, page 339.

Respiratory pain—intercostal neuralgia. Irritation of an intercostal nerve produces sharp, lancinating, stabbing pain along the nerve's course. The pain is frequently intensified by respiratory motion, trunk movements, or exposure to cold. Tenderness along the nerve is diagnostic. Pain is greatest near the vertebral foramen, in the axilla, or at the parasternal line, corresponding to the nerve's major cutaneous branches.
   CLINICAL OCCURRENCE: Herpes zoster, diabetes mellitus, tabes dorsalis, mediastinal neoplasm, neurofibroma (an intercostal mass may be felt), perineural cysts (Tarlov cyst), vertebral tuberculosis, or obesity with nerve stretching.

Herpes zoster (shingles). See Chapter 6, page 144.

Cardiovascular Symptoms
Chest pain. See Chest Pain page 292 and Myocardial Ischemia Six-Dermatome Pain Syndromes page 350.

Palpitation. Palpitation, awareness of heart action, is described as pounding, fluttering, flip-flopping, skipping a beat, missing a beat, stopping, jumping, and/or turning over. The frequency, regularity, rate, and intensity vary with the cause. Ask whether the sensation is a single extra beat, a pause, or a series of beats. If the latter, ask whether it starts and ends abruptly or gradually, whether it is fast or slow, and whether it is regular or irregular. Have them tap out the rhythm with their finger. Identify precipitating circumstances and associated symptoms preceding, accompanying or following the palpitations. Next, perform a physical exam and obtain an ECG. Ambulatory or home-based electrocardiographic monitoring is recommended for patients who tolerate the palpitations poorly, have heart disease, syncope, falls or sustained palpitations.

Claudication—exertional limb pain. Exercising muscle has high oxygen and energy requirements. Energy is stored, but oxygen must be continuously delivered to meet the increased demand. Inability to increase blood flow during exertion produces ischemic muscle pain relieved by rest. Anemia increases symptoms by loss of oxygen-carrying capacity, whereas polycythemia increases blood viscosity slowing capillary flow. The patient usually complains of calf pain at a fixed walking distance requiring him/her to stop or sit for relief. It is consistently reproducible. Claudication can occur in any exercising muscle; be alert for reproducible exertional extremity or gluteal pain. Pulses are usually diminished or absent in the popliteal, dorsalis pedis, and/or posterior tibial arteries of the affected leg.
CLINICAL OCCURRENCE: Atherosclerotic, thrombotic or embolic obstruction of major leg arteries is most common. Exertional buttock and/or thigh pain may be true claudication or pseudoclaudication from spinal stenosis. Predisposing factors are tobacco use and diabetes.

Unilateral claudication in the young—popliteal artery entrapment syndrome. Entrapment of the popliteal artery by the medial head of the gastrocnemius muscle is a congenital anomaly. A young person develops unilateral claudication with absent or diminished pulses in the ipsilateral popliteal and dorsalis pedis arteries.

Cold hands and/or feet. This is caused by regional vasoconstriction to conserve heat. Examine carefully for decreased peripheral pulses or skin changes suggesting ischemia.

CHEST, TRACHEA, AND RESPIRATORY SIGNS
Chest Wall Signs
Thoracic spine abnormalities. See Musculoskeletal Signs, Chapter 13, page 559, for a complete discussion. Thoracic spine and chest wall deformities can decrease chest compliance, limit respiratory excursions and increase

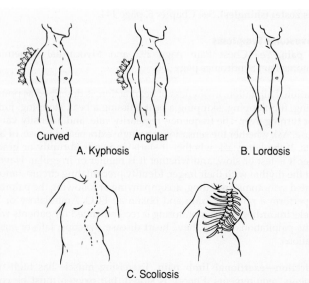

Curved   Angular

A. Kyphosis   B. Lordosis

C. Scoliosis

FIG. 8-28 Curvatures of the Spine Affecting the Thorax. A. Kyphotic thorax. B. Lordotic thorax. C. Scoliotic thorax. Note the narrowing of the rib interspaces on the right and the accentuation of the interspaces, posterior humping of the chest, and elevation of the shoulder on the left.

the work of breathing. In either *curved or angular kyphosis* (Fig. 8-28A), the spinal flexion can fix the thorax in the inspiratory position with increased anterior posterior diameter and horizontal ribs. Curved kyphosis appears identical to the barrel chest of pulmonary emphysema, but the auscultatory signs of emphysema are absent. Conversely, accentuating the lumbar lordosis throws the thoracic spine backward flattening the thoracic cage, creating an expiratory position (Fig. 8-28B). Lateral thoracic spine curvature is usually accompanied by some rotation of the vertebral bodies; only the lateral deviations of the spinous processes are visible (Fig. 8-28C). Minor functional scoliosis has a single lateral curve, usually with convexity to the right. Structural curves in the thorax are associated with an opposite compensatory curve inferiorly, the line of spinous processes forming an S-shape. The spinous processes always rotate toward the concave side. On the convex side, vertebral rotation flattens the ribs anteriorly and bulges the posterior chest, lifting the shoulder and lowering the hip. Viewed from the back, the posterior bulge becomes more prominent with spine anteflexion (Chapter 13, Fig. 13-13, page 540).

Rib cage abnormalities. Rib cage deformities are congenital, or acquired from surgery, poor nutrition, trauma, or adaptation to changes in the heart, lungs, and/or diaphragm.

Rib mass. Masses on ribs are caused by callus around an old fracture or fibrous dysplasia, neoplasm (e.g., chondrosarcoma), myeloma, desmoid tumor, metastasis of carcinoma, angioma, eosinophilic granuloma, and bone

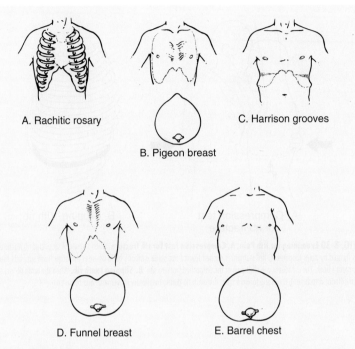

FIG. 8-29 Deformities of the Thorax. A. Rachitic rosary. B. Pigeon breast. C. Harrison grooves. D. Funnel breast. E. Barrel chest.

cysts, including osteitis fibrosa cystica. An intercostal nerve neurofibroma may cause visible or palpable swelling near the neck of the rib.

Pigeon breast (pectus carinatum). The sternum protrudes from the narrow thorax like the keel of a ship (Fig. 8-29B). It can be congenital or acquired. In *rickets*, a skeletal disorder caused by prolonged vitamin D deficiency in childhood, the softened upper ribs bend inward, forcing the sternum forward increasing the AP dimension at the expense of the width. Vertical grooves form in the line of the costochondral junctions persisting after the rickets heals. Pigeon breast also occurs in *Marfan syndrome*. A similar but asymmetric deformity occurs in severe *primary kyphoscoliosis*.

Harrison groove (Harrison sulcus). During active rickets, the protuberant rachitic abdomen pushes the plastic lower ribs outward on a fulcrum formed by the diaphragm's costal attachments. The line of bending forms a groove or sulcus in the rib cage extending laterally from the xiphoid process, with flaring of the cage below the groove (Fig. 8-29C). The deformity remains when the rickets heals.

Rachitic rosary. The sternal ends of rachitic ribs bulge at their costochondral junctions. In severe cases of rickets, the outward bulging produces knobs

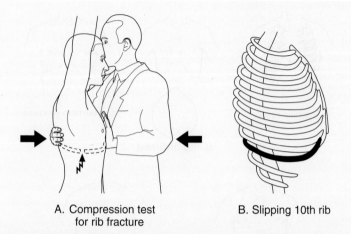

A. Compression test   B. Slipping 10th rib
for rib fracture

FIG. 8-30 Examining for Rib Pain. A. Compression test for rib fracture. When the site of suspected rib fracture is located by point tenderness, the sternum is pushed toward the spine with one hand whereas the other hand supports the patient's back. The maneuver will elicit pain at the untouched fracture site. **B. Slipping tenth rib.** When the tenth rib lacks an anterior attachment, it can slip forward upon the ninth rib during respiratory movements and cause pain.

at the costochondral junctions (Fig. 8-29A) that resolve completely with treatment.

Funnel breast (pectus excavatum). The reverse of the pigeon breast, the lower costal cartilages, inferior sternum, and xiphoid process are retracted toward the spine. Its most mild form is an oval pit near the infrasternal notch. A more severe deformity forms when the entire lower sternum sinks, significantly diminishing the thorax's AP dimension (Fig. 8-29D). Rickets and Marfan syndrome are causes, but many cases are unexplained.

Barrel chest. Emphysema with chronic airflow obstruction increases residual volume leading to increased AP chest diameter, horizontal ribs, and a depressed diaphragm. Since both the AP and the transverse chest dimensions enlarge, the ribs become nearly perfect circles (Fig. 8-29E).

Chest and respiratory pain with tenderness. The distinction between respiratory pain with tenderness and chest pain with tenderness is artificial, many conditions presenting in either manner, or with both pain at rest and with respirations. The patient may recognize the pain as superficial, sharp, and well localized. The skin and subcutaneous tissues, fat, skeleton, or breasts can be the site of pain. Careful chest exam localizes the pain to specific structures.

Skin and subcutaneous structures. Inflammation, trauma, and neoplasm in these tissues offer no diagnostic problem, provided they are considered and searched for. The presence of bruises, lacerations, ulcers, hematomas, masses, trigger points, or tenderness is usually diagnostic.

Chest wall pain. Have the patient point to the site of pain. Four maneuvers identify chest wall pain. (1) Palpate the chest wall for tenderness by applying firm, steady pressure to the sternum, costosternal junctions, intercostal spaces, ribs, and pectoralis major muscles and their insertions. (2) Adduct the arms horizontally by lifting one arm after the other by the elbow and pulling it across the chest toward the contralateral side, with the head rotated toward the ipsilateral side. (3) Extend the neck as the arms are pulled backward and slightly upward. (4) Put vertical pressure on the head. If any of these tests reproduces the patient's pain, the problem is in the chest wall.

Costochondritis and Tietze syndrome. This is a common cause of chest pain. The onset may be sudden or gradual. The pain is usually dull and may be intensified by respiratory motion and shoulder movements. The only physical sign is tenderness at the costochondral junction. There is no swelling and there are no X-ray findings. In *Tietze syndrome*, the pain is accompanied by tender, fusiform swelling of one or more costal cartilages, often that of the second rib. The overlying skin is reddened. Pain may radiate to the shoulder, neck, or arm. There is no lymphadenopathy. The pain may subside in a few weeks or persist for months, whereas the swelling can persist after the pain and tenderness subside. The cause is unknown, and the condition must be distinguished from osteitis, periostitis, rheumatic chondritis, and neoplasm of the ribs.

Rib fracture. Movement of rib fragments causes well-localized, sharp, lancinating pain. The patient complains of chest pain with breathing. Usually there is a history of chest trauma. Without a history of trauma, symptoms can suggest pleurisy. Ask about recent severe coughing. Inspiration is limited, and palpation discloses point tenderness on a rib. The fracture and/or crepitation may be felt. With one hand supporting the back, compressing the sternum with the other hand elicits pain at the untouched fracture site (Fig. 8-30A).

Cough fracture. The fracture is caused by a shearing force on the rib anterior to the serratus anterior attachment, that pulls the rib upward, and posterior to the abdominal external oblique attachment, that pulls the rib downward. Repeated coughing leads to structural fatigue and a *stress fracture*. Any rib from the second to the eleventh, most commonly the sixth, can break. After coughing for some time, pain develops with respiratory movements and coughing. The typical signs of fracture of a rib are present. If rib palpation is not performed, pleurisy may be misdiagnosed.

Xiphisternal arthritis. The pain is reproduced by palpating the xiphoid cartilage.

Slipping cartilage. The ligament between two ribs, commonly between the ninth and tenth costal cartilages, is weak or ruptured. When breathing or with movement, the tenth rib overrides the ninth producing an audible or palpable click (Fig. 8-30B). The pain may be falsely attributed to intraabdominal disease.

Palpable pleural friction rub. The inflamed pleural surfaces, having lost their lubricating fluid, rub together during breathing producing vibrations like two pieces of dry leather rubbing together (*dry pleurisy*). The rub is heard with the stethoscope or unaided ear as a creaking sound.

Inspiratory interspace retraction. Airway obstruction or decreased lung compliance leads to increased negative inspiratory intrapleural pressure collapsing the intercostal spaces. The inward movement is usually most evident in the lower chest. Sudden, violent retractions occur in tracheal obstruction and severe paroxysms of asthma.

Diminished chest excursion. This points to a lesion in the underlying chest wall, pleura, or lung; causes include pain, fibrosis, or consolidation. The restricted movement may be best observed from the foot of the bed.

Localized chest bulging during expiration—flail chest. Fracture of several contiguous ribs or the separation of several contiguous costal cartilages destroys chest wall integrity. Negative intrathoracic pressure during inspiration pulls the segment inward, while rising intrathoracic pressure during expiration bulges it outward. The paradoxical chest movements decrease minute ventilation and can contribute to respiratory failure in trauma victims. Concurrent lung contusion, hemothorax, pneumothorax and inspiratory splinting secondary to severe pain should be ruled out in patients with flail chest.

Inspiratory convergence of costal margins. When the dome of the diaphragm is flattened, contraction pulls the costal margins inward rather than upward. The normal outward flare of the lower costal margins decreases. Inspiration may move the lower ribs inward. A flattened diaphragm can be caused by pulmonary emphysema with air trapping, large pleural effusions or pneumothorax.

Fluctuant intercostal masses and sinuses. These findings usually indicate an abscess. An abscess lacking surrounding inflammation (*cold abscess*) is usually tuberculosis in a nearby rib. Actinomycosis frequently produces lung abscesses that invade through the chest wall. An abscess may form when an untreated pleural empyema points through the interspaces.

Subcutaneous and mediastinal emphysema. Air can enter the chest wall from the neck, from esophageal rupture, or directly from the lung. Rupture of alveoli permits air to travel beneath the visceral pleura to the hilum of the lung, then along the trachea into the neck. The thoracic wall is involved secondarily by migration from the neck. When a fractured rib or penetrating foreign-body punctures the pleura, air travels across the pleura to the thoracic wall causing emphysema in the deep muscle layers and later the subcutaneous tissues. Crepitus is the sensation imparted small globules of air moving in the tissues under the palpating fingers. Soft-tissue crepitus can be the first clue to rupture of the alveoli, pleura, or esophagus. The air invading the mediastinum may produce a distinctive systolic precordial sound described as a crunch, the *Hamman sign*. Soft tissue compression in the neck can produce massive neck and face swelling accompanied by cyanosis.

Pulsating sternoclavicular joint. There is an enlarged major vascular structure impinging posteriorly on the manubrium. It is seen with dissection of the aortic arch, ruptured saccular aortic aneurysm, persistent right aortic arch, or fusiform aneurysms of the innominate, carotid, or subclavian artery.

Trachea Signs

Lateral deviation of the trachea. At the level of the suprasternal notch lateral deviation is caused by a mass higher in the neck, such as cervical goiter or enlarged lymph nodes (Chapter 7, page 238, Fig. 7-68), or by a mediastinal shift within the chest. Below the suprasternal notch, an eccentric retrosternal goiter can push the trachea to one side. The trachea and mediastinum deviate to the opposite side with pleural effusion and tension pneumothorax. Atelectasis and reduced lung volume from fibrosis of the lung or pleura displace the trachea to the ipsilateral side.

Trachea fixation. Palpate the cricoid cartilage or tracheal rings with the thumb and index finger and ask the patient to swallow. Normally, the larynx and trachea rise cephalad. Grasp the trachea gently and move it side to side; usually, it is easily mobile. Fixation is normal when the neck is extended. Abnormal fixation occurs with pulmonary emphysema, adhesive mediastinitis, aortic aneurysm, and mediastinal neoplasm.

Lung, Pleura, and Respiratory Signs

Hiccup. Hiccup is a sudden involuntary diaphragm contraction producing an inspiration interrupted by glottis closure causing a characteristic sharp sound. It is thought to be mediated centrally through the phrenic nerve, by direct phrenic nerve stimulation, or by direct irritation of the diaphragm. The contractions occur two or three times each minute.

CLINICAL OCCURRENCE: *Hiccough Without Organic Disease:* Excessive laughter, tickling, aerophagia, tobacco smoking, alcohol ingestion; *Central Nervous System Diseases:* Encephalitis, meningitis, vertebrobasilar ischemia, intracranial hemorrhage, intracranial tumor, uremia, degenerative changes in brain and medulla, tabes dorsalis; *Mediastinal Disorders:* Phrenic nerve trauma, enlarged mediastinal lymph nodes (tuberculosis, malignant neoplasm, fibrosis), obstructed bronchus, adherent pericardium, enlarged heart, myocardial infarction (MI), obstructed esophagus; *Pleural Irritation:* Pneumonia with pleurisy; *Diaphragm and Abdominal Disorders:* Diaphragmatic hernia, subphrenic abscess, subphrenic peritonitis, hepatic neoplasm, gumma or abscess, stomach cancer, infarcted spleen, acutely obstructed intestine, acute hemorrhagic pancreatitis, after upper abdomen operations, diaphragm stimulation by cardiac pacemaker.

Hemoptysis. Cough productive of blood is hemoptysis. The bleeding lesion may be anywhere from the nose to the alveoli. Expectorated blood usually comes from the upper respiratory tract while blood in the bronchial tree induces coughing. Patients may not distinguish which is occurring, so both upper and lower respiratory tract disorders must be considered. Coagulopathy and thrombocytopenia may contribute to the severity and volume of hemoptysis, but rarely cause significant hemoptysis in the absence of other significant disease.

CLINICAL OCCURRENCE: *Upper Respiratory Tract:* Epistaxis, bleeding from the oropharynx, gum bleeding, laryngitis, laryngeal carcinoma, hereditary hemorrhagic telangiectasia; *Tracheobronchial Tree:* Acute and chronic bronchitis, trauma from coughing, bronchiectasis, bronchial carcinoma, broncholiths, foreign-body aspiration, erosion by aortic aneurysms; *Lungs:* Infections (pneumonia, especially caused by *Klebsiella*, lung abscess, tuberculosis, fungal infections, amebiasis, hydatid cyst), pulmonary embolism with infarction, trauma, pulmonary hemorrhage (vasculitis, especially granulomatosis with polyangiitis-Wegener, Goodpasture syndrome), idiopathic pulmonary hemosiderosis, lipoid pneumonia; *Cardiovascular:* Mitral stenosis, CHF, arteriovenous fistula, anomalous pulmonary artery, hypertension; *Hematologic:* Thrombocytopenia, leukemia, hemophilia, anticoagulant mediations.

Snoring. Snoring is produced by vibrations of the lax soft palate during sleep, often in association with obstructive sleep apnea. A similar sound results from uncleared secretions in the upper respiratory tract. When the latter occurs during severe illness, it is frequently a grave prognostic sign, the death-rattle.

Stridor. A high-pitched whistling or crowing sound is caused by inspiration through a narrow glottis. It occurs with vocal cord edema, neoplasm, diphtheritic membrane, pharyngeal abscess, and foreign body in the larynx or trachea. It may signal impending airway closure and asphyxiation.

Vibratory Palpation

Diminished or absent vocal fremitus. Thickened pleura, pleural effusion, pneumothorax, or loss of lung parenchyma (e.g., emphysema) reduce transmission of vibrations to the chest wall diminishing or eliminating vocal fremitus.

Increased vocal fremitus. Tense lung septae and fluid-filled alveoli increase transmission of vibrations. Consolidating pneumonia and inflammation around a lung abscess in contact with a bronchus or cavity in the lung, transmits bronchotracheal vibrations more efficiently than air-filled alveoli, increasing vocal fremitus.

Sonorous Percussion

Normal dullness in the lateral decubitus position. If a patient can't sit, percuss the back with the patient on one side then the other. This is not optimal since it is difficult to interpret the percussion sounds. The damping effect of the mattress causes a band of dullness nearest the bed. Directly above this band is an irregular area of dullness caused by lung compressed by the body's weight. If body weight causes a lengthwise sag, the spine flexes laterally compressing the chest wall and lung in the upward hemithorax. This produces another area of dullness (Fig. 8-31).

Abnormal sonorous percussion. Abnormally distributed normal sounds can be pathologic. The lung is normally resonant. As consolidation occurs its density increases producing, successively, impaired resonance, dullness, and flatness. Thickened pleura produces dullness. Pleural fluid gives dullness to flatness in a dependent distribution.

Dullness replacing resonance in the upper lung. This suggests neoplasm, atelectasis, or consolidation.

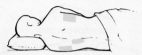

FIG. 8-31 Areas of Percussion Dullness Created by the Lateral Decubitus Position. The lowest green-shaded area is dull from compression of the thorax against the mattress. Immediately above, dullness is produced by compression of the lung from the body weight. In the opposite lung, dullness results by lateral deviation of the spine as it follows the sag in the mattress and compresses the lung.

Dullness replacing resonance in the lower lung. Pleural effusion, pleural thickening, and elevation of the diaphragm are specific to this area; neoplasm, atelectasis, and consolidation are other causes.

Flatness replacing resonance or dullness. Almost invariably, flatness results from massive pleural effusion.

Hyperresonance replacing resonance or dullness. When hyperresonance replaces resonance, or the area of hepatic and cardiac dullness is resonant or hyperresonant, consider emphysema. Asymmetric hyperresonance is suggestive of pneumothorax, or the interposition of gas-filled gut are suggested.

Tympany replacing resonance. This occurs almost exclusively with a large pneumothorax and tends to be unilateral. Tension pneumothorax is associated with tracheal deviation to the opposite side, elevated jugular venous pressure, tachycardia, and hypotension.

Auscultating Breath Sounds: Several breath sounds with distinctive qualities are recognized, all characterized by rising pitch during inspiration and falling pitch during expiration (Doppler effect). The duration and force of inspiration and expiration affect the breath sounds.

Normal breath sounds—vesicular breathing. While the ratio of inhalation to exhalation measured by air flow and chest movement in normal breathing is approximately 1:2, this is not consistently reflected by auscultation in normal subjects. Quiet tidal breathing produces vesicular breath sounds characterized by a longer inspiratory than expiratory phase (Fig. 8-32), the later portion of expiration being silent. Vesicular breath sounds are normal over the entire lung, except over the manubrium and in the upper interscapular region, where bronchovesicular sounds are heard. Breath sounds are faintest over the thinner portions of the lungs.

Cogwheel breathing. This is identical with vesicular breathing except that inspiration is broken by short pauses, giving the impression of jerkiness (Fig. 8-32). It has no pathologic significance.

Bronchovesicular breathing. Bronchovesicular bronchial breathing arise from more efficient sound transmission through compressed or consolidated lung.

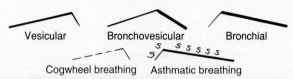

FIG. 8-32 Distinguishing Features of Breath Sounds. In the diagrams, the vertical component indicates rising and falling pitch, the thickness of the lines indicates loudness, and the horizontal distance represents duration. Inspiration is longer in **vesicular breathing,** expiration in **bronchial breathing. Bronchovesicular breathing** is a mixture of the two. Normally vesicular breathing is heard over most of the lungs, except that bronchovesicular breathing occurs over the thoracic portion of the trachea, anteriorly and posteriorly. Bronchial breathing does not occur in the normal lung. In **cogwheel breathing,** the inspiratory sound is interrupted with multiple breaks. **Asthmatic breathing** is characterized by a much prolonged and higher-pitched expiratory sound than is found in bronchial breathing. Asthmatic breathing is usually, but not always, accompanied by wheezes.

It is intermediate between vesicular and bronchial breathing. Inspiration and expiration are of roughly equal duration (Fig. 8-32), though expiration can be a bit longer. It is normal over the manubrium and the upper interscapular region. Compression or consolidation of the lung causes breath sounds to become bronchial.

Bronchial breathing (tubular breathing). In contrast to vesicular breathing, bronchial breath sounds have a shorter inspiratory than expiratory phase (Fig. 8-32) and are usually louder. Bronchial breathing does not occur in the normal lung.

Tracheal breathing. Tracheal breathing is normal in the suprasternal notch and over the sixth and seventh cervical spines. It is more harsh and hollow than bronchial breathing.

Wheezes. Wheezes arise from turbulent airflow and vibrating partially obstructed small airways. Wheezes are heard predominantly during expiration. They occur when airways are narrowed by bronchospasm, edema, collapse, or by intraluminal secretions, neoplasm, or foreign body. They are diffuse in asthma and bronchitis, usually accompanying prolonged expiration. An isolated wheeze may signal bronchial obstruction by a tumor or foreign body. Wheezing is neither sensitive nor specific for detecting airflow obstruction.

Asthmatic or obstructive breathing. In asthma, expiration is several times longer than in bronchial breathing, and the pitch is much higher. Expiration is active, not passive, and may require significant effort. Frequently, but not always, asthma is accompanied by wheezes audible without the stethoscope. (Fig. 8-32). Emphysema produces a similar breath sound profile, but wheezing is absent, and the sounds are less intense.

Crackles (rales). Crackles result from the opening and closing of alveoli and small airways during the respiratory cycle. In pulmonary edema fine crackles are produced by air bubbling through small fluid-filled distal airways.

Inspiratory crackles resemble the sound of hairs being rubbed together. They are heard in the bases with interstitial lung disease, fibrosing alveolitis, atelectasis, pneumonia, bronchiectasis, and pulmonary edema, and often in the apices with tuberculosis.

Rhonchus. Rhonchi are low-pitched gurgling sounds produced by liquid within the larger airways. They clear or change significantly after an effective cough.

Amphoric breath sounds. These are produced by an open pneumothorax or a large empty superficial cavity communicating with a bronchus. Amphoric breath sounds resemble blowing air over the mouth of a large bottle.

Auscultating Voice Sounds: In normal lungs whispered words are faint and the syllables indistinct, except over the main bronchi. Consolidation, atelectasis, and fibrosis improve sound transmission resulting in louder and more distinct words. Because of their pitch and loudness, whispered and spoken voice sounds are more useful than breath sounds in detecting pulmonary consolidation, infarction, and atelectasis. Spoken voice sounds are not as useful as whispered sounds since they are too loud for subtle discrimination.

Whispered pectoriloquy. Consolidated lung transmits whispered syllables distinctly, even when the pathologic process is too small to produce bronchial breathing. This is particularly valuable in detecting early pneumonia, infarction, and atelectasis.

Bronchophony. Spoken syllables are normally heard indistinctly. With lung consolidation syllables are distinct and sound close to the ear.

Egophony. This is a form of bronchophony in which the spoken "Eee" is changed to "Ay," with a peculiar nasal or bleating quality. This arises from compressed lung below a pleural effusion, and occasionally with lung consolidation.

Auscultating Abnormal Sounds
Rubs (pleural friction rub). See page 301.

Continuous murmur. The continuous murmur of a pulmonary arteriovenous fistula increases in intensity with inspiration. In patients with coarctation of the aorta, continuous murmurs may be heard below the left scapula and over the intercostal and internal mammary arteries from the collateral circulation.

Systolic crunching sounds. See Esophageal Rupture, page 355.

Interpreting Pulmonary and Pleural Signs: The findings of thoracic inspection, palpation, percussion, and auscultation must be synthesized to suggest a pathophysiologic process or diagnosis. The signs of altered lung density are the starting point for differential diagnosis. It is useful to draw a chest diagram like those in Figures 8-33 and 8-34 to depict your findings and generate hypotheses.

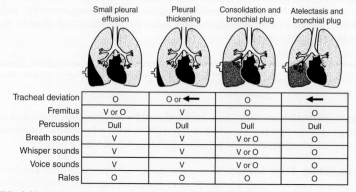

	Small pleural effusion	Pleural thickening	Consolidation and bronchial plug	Atelectasis and bronchial plug
Tracheal deviation	O	O or ←	O	←
Fremitus	V or O	V	O	O
Percussion	Dull	Dull	Dull	Dull
Breath sounds	V	V	V or O	O
Whisper sounds	V	V	V or O	O
Voice sounds	V	V	V or O	O
Rales	O	O	O	O

FIG. 8-33 Thoracic Disorders with Dullness and Diminished Vibration. ○, absent; V, diminished; ←, direction of deviation.

	Small consolidation	Thick-walled cavity	Massive consolidation	Large pleural effusion
Tracheal deviation	O	O	O	→
Fremitus	N or Λ	N or Λ	Λ	O
Percussion	Slight dullness	Slight dullness	Dull or flat	(a) Hyperresonant (b) Flat
Breath sounds	Bronchovesicular or bronchial	Bronchovesicular or amorphic	Bronchial	O or loud bronchial
Whisper sounds	N, O, or Λ	Pectoriloquy	Λ	O or Λ
Voice sounds	N, O, or Λ	Λ	Λ	O or Λ
Rales	+ or O	+	+	O

FIG. 8-34 Thoracic Disorders with Dullness and Accentuated Vibration. ○, absent; N, normal; +, present; Λ increased; →, direction of deviation.

Dullness and diminished vibrations

Pleural effusion and pleural thickening. Unless the fluid is trapped by loculations in the non-dependent regions of the chest, dullness occurs in the lowermost chest (Fig. 8-33, left). Because the costophrenic sulcus is higher in front, the dull region is a transverse band broadest posteriorly and laterally. The superior border of dullness can be difficult to percuss accurately because the fluid layer forms an upward-pointing wedge. Shifting dullness is not usually demonstrable. Since air is absent, there is no succussion splash. With a small amount of fluid respiratory excursions are normal. In pleurisy an antecedent friction rub disappears when an effusion forms. Pleural fluid dampens vibrations from the bronchotracheal air column, so vocal fremitus, breath sounds, and whispered and spoken voice transmit poorly. Small pleural effusions do not shift the mediastinum. Any longstanding pleural effusion may organize producing pleural fibrosis with the same distribution of dullness as the effusion. The thicker the pleura, the more it obstructs sound transmission and the denser the percussion note. Extensive fibrosis pulls the trachea to the affected side. Neoplasms, asbestosis, and mesothelioma also cause pleural thickening.

Pleural fluid. Fluid accumulates in the pleural space because of transudation from the pleural and pulmonary vessels (increased venous hydrostatic pressure, decreased oncotic pressure, capillary leak), increased pleural fluid production (inflamed pleura or pleural neoplasm), decreased pleural fluid absorption (lymphatic obstruction, systemic venous hypertension), or bleeding into the pleural space. Pleural fluid produces a dull or flat note to percussion. The lung field immediately above the the fluid can be hyperresonant (*skodaic resonance*) from distended air-filled alveolae above the compressed region. The distribution of dullness is dependent. With substantial amounts of fluid, the trachea is pushed to the unaffected side (Fig. 8-34). Vocal fremitus is absent. Occasionally, loud bronchial breathing is heard through the fluid from the compressed lung, the unwary mistaking it for consolidation. Fluid is distinguished from consolidation by diminished breath sounds and absent fremitus with fluid, and bronchial breath sounds with E-to-A change in consolidation. Massive pleural effusion obscures the lung fields on radiographs so that no appraisal of the parenchyma is possible. In contrast, when the patient with a hydropneumothorax stands, the fluid level falls below much of the lung, permitting lung visualization (Fig. 8-35) [Case with differential diagnosis: Quing DA, Mark EJ. Case 8-2002–A 56-year-old woman with a persistent left-sided pleural effusion. *N Engl J Med.* 2002;346:843–850].

CLINICAL OCCURRENCE: *Increased Transudation:* CHF, hypoalbuminemia (cirrhosis, nephrotic syndrome), PE, SVC syndrome; *Increased Production:* Mesothelioma, metastatic cancer, infections (bacteria, mycobacteria, viral, parasites, fungi), pulmonary infarction, pancreatitis, mediastinitis, collagen-vascular diseases (e.g., RA, systemic lupus erythematosus [SLE], drug-induced lupus, vasculitis), after heart or lung surgery, uremia, Meigs syndrome, pleuropericarditis peritoneal dialysis; *Decreased Absorption:* Lymphatic obstruction (lymphoma, lymphatic carcinomatosis, irradiation, surgical injury), CHF, SVC syndrome; *Bleeding:* Ruptured aortic aneurysm or dissection, trauma, postoperative.

Pulmonary consolidation with bronchial plugging. Consolidated lung produces dullness. Bronchial plugs block vibrations from the air column, so vocal fremitus, breath sounds, and whispered and spoken voice are absent (Fig. 8-33, middle right). The trachea is not displaced. Bronchial plugging, usually transitory in lobar pneumonia, is recognized by the sudden loss of air transmission. Imaging distinguishes between pleural effusion and pulmonary consolidation. Upper chest dullness on physical exam excludes effusion.

Atelectasis with bronchial plug. The volume of atelectatic lung is diminished. When a considerable amount of lung is atelectatic, the dense mass is pulled toward the chest wall by the negative intrapleural pressure shifting the

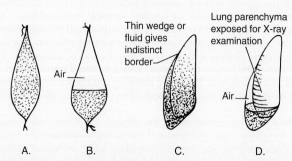

FIG. 8-35 **Models Illustrating Pleural Effusion and Pneumothorax. A. Suspend a plastic bag filled with water,** noting its contour. **B. Introduce air forming an air-fluid level,** the contour changes, and a succussion splash occurs with shaking. **C. An uncomplicated pleural effusion:** note the tapering upper wedge, or meniscus, of fluid. **D. Hydropneumothorax:** when air is introduced, a fluid level forms and the meniscus largely disappears.

trachea to the affected side. The collapsed lung is dull because its density is increased. The bronchial plug prevents transmission of air vibration, so vocal fremitus and breath and voice sounds are absent (Fig. 8-33, right). *DDX:* Tracheal deviation distinguishes atelectasis from consolidation with bronchial plug and from pleural effusion. Dullness and decreased breath sounds at the left scapular tip can be caused by a large pericardial effusion compressing the LLL (*Ewart sign*).

Pneumonia with small consolidation. A small, deeply placed consolidation may produce impaired resonance or dullness, depending on its size and distance from the chest wall. The dense lung efficiently transmits airway sounds, so vocal fremitus is increased and bronchovesicular or bronchial breathing and crackles may be heard (Fig. 8-34, left). Fever, chills, and productive cough are accompanied by tachypnea and tachycardia. The consolidation produces whispered pectoriloquy and bronchophony. Small regions of consolidation must be distinguished from a small cavity lying near a bronchus. A definitive diagnosis requires imaging. Pneumonia, granulomatous lung infiltrates, neoplasm involving bronchus, rheumatoid arthritis (RA), and sarcoidosis may all produce these findings.

Dullness with accentuated vibration
Pneumonia with lobar consolidation. The dense lung causes dullness or flatness on percussion. Consolidated lung in contact with a bronchus efficiently transmits vibrations so vocal fremitus is pronounced, there is bronchial breathing, and whispered and spoken voice produce pectoriloquy and bronchophony (Fig. 8-34, middle right). Crackles are frequently present. Lung volume is unchanged, so the trachea is midline. These finding are classically found in lobar pneumonia, but occasionally in lung neoplasms and pulmonary infarction. *DDX:* Consolidation can be confused with a thick-walled cavity, the distinction being made by imaging. Massive pleural effusion gives dullness and transmits loud bronchial breath sounds above the effusion, but the trachea is usually displaced to the unaffected side.

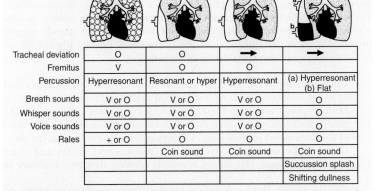

	Pulmonary emphysema	Closed pneumothorax	Tension pneumothorax	Hydropneumothorax
Tracheal deviation	O	O	→	→
Fremitus	V	O	O	
Percussion	Hyperresonant	Resonant or hyper	Hyperresonant	(a) Hyperresonant (b) Flat
Breath sounds	V or O	V or O	V or O	O
Whisper sounds	V or O	V or O	V or O	O
Voice sounds	V or O	V or O	V or O	O
Rales	+ or O	O	O	O
		Coin sound	Coin sound	Coin sound
				Succussion splash
				Shifting dullness

FIG. 8-36 Thoracic Disorders with Resonance Impaired Vibration. O, absent; V, diminished; +, present; →, direction of deviation.

Thick-walled cavity. Dullness, increased vocal fremitus, bronchovesicular breathing, and pectoriloquy indicate consolidation (Fig. 8-34, middle left). Amphoric breathing or cracked-pot resonance is rarely heard, but even these signs can occur in consolidation without cavity.

Resonance and hyperresonance
Pulmonary emphysema. Loss of interstitial elasticity and interalveolar septa leads to air trapping increasing lung volume. The air trapping holds the chest in the inspiratory position producing a barrel chest. The diaphragm is flattened, so the costal margins move out sluggishly or converge during inspiration (Fig. 8-36, left). The lungs are hyperresonant throughout because of their low density. Air pockets transmit vibrations poorly so vocal fremitus, breath sounds, heart sounds, and whispered and spoken voice are diminished or absent. When the breath sounds are audible, they are faint and harsh, distinctively lacking the rustling quality of vesicular breathing; this may antedate recognizable X-ray evidence of emphysema. The expiratory phase of respiration usually exceeds the inspiratory phase in proportion to the patient's degree of airflow obstruction. The elevated clavicles and flattened diaphragm in severe emphysema with air trapping cause the thyroid cartilage to be low in a shortened neck and it descends <4 cm toward the suprasternal notch with full inspiration. The thyroid is often in a retrosternal position and not palpable. Crackles are not consistently heard in homogenous emphysema and when present suggest concurrent bronchitis, pneumonia or interstitial lung disease. Similarly, concurrent wheezing suggests an acute exacerbation of chronic obstructive pulmonary disease or overlap syndrome with asthma and bronchial hyperactivity.

Closed pneumothorax. When the air leak between lung and parietal pleura is intermittent or self-limited, a closed pneumothorax forms. If the enclosed air volume is small, the lung remains partially inflated, and the mediastinum is not displaced (Fig. 8-36, middle left). An open pneumothorax with pleural adhesions preventing lung collapse and tracheal displacement presents similarly. Vocal fremitus, breath sounds, and whispered and spoken voice are usually diminished or inaudible. The chest is resonant or hyperresonant. Frequently, pneumothorax cannot be distinguished from a normal or emphysematous chest by percussion alone. Asymmetric breath sounds suggest pneumothorax on the quieter side. The trachea may deviate toward the affected side during inspiration (*pendular deviation*).

- *Open pneumothorax.* In open pneumothorax there is continuous and open air leak between lung and pleural cavity so the pneumothorax is at atmospheric pressure. The affected lung completely collapses and the mediastinum may be drawn toward the unaffected side by elastic recoil of the unaffected normal lung. Overlying the pneumothorax, the chest wall is hyperresonant or tympanitic. Fremitus and breath and voice sounds are absent. The patient is usually severely dyspneic and may be cyanotic.

- *Tension pneumothorax.* A one-way tissue valve permitting air entry into the pleural space during inspiration prevents its expulsion during expiration, the intrapleural pressure rapidly increasing. The affected lung is collapsed and the increasing intrapleural pressure causes extreme tracheal deviation, compression of the unaffected lung, and decreased venous return to the heart (Fig. 8-36, middle right). Decreased respiratory excursion, a distended tympanic hemithorax, and tracheal deviation away from the affected side are diagnostic of tension pneumothorax. There is deep cyanosis, severe dyspnea, and shock; release of air from the pleural cavity is lifesaving.

Hydropneumothorax. Upper thoracic hyperresonance or tympany with inferior dullness suggests hydropneumothorax or massive pleural effusion (Fig. 8-36, right). In either case, the trachea can be displaced to the unaffected side. In hydropneumothorax, the hyperresonant region does not transmit fremitus, breath sounds, or voice sounds. The lung above a simple hydrothorax transmits well. With hydropneumothorax, percussion easily identifies the fluid level; the level is vague in simple effusion. Shifting dullness is readily demonstrated by percussion with hydropneumothorax. The air-filled cavity carries bell tympany, and a succession splash may be demonstrated.

Sounds suggesting hydropneumothorax. Fluid moves silently in a cavity devoid of air. When the cavity contains both air and fluid, body movements cause a succussion splash, audible to patient and examiner. Grasp the patient's shoulders shaking the thorax while listening with and without a stethoscope. An abdominal *succussion splash* is present in the normal and dilated stomach. A thoracic succussion splash suggests hydropneumothorax, but a fluid-filled stomach herniating into the thorax through a diaphragmatic hernia can also produce the splash. Occasionally, a *falling-drop sound* is heard, resembling a drop of water hitting a fluid surface. A metallic tinkle may be heard when air bubbles emerge through a small bronchopleural fistula below the fluid level; when the fistula is larger, the air may gurgle, a *lung-fistula sound*.

Sputum Signs

Bloody sputum—hemoptysis. Priority is to identify the likely anatomic site of hemorrhage. *Blood-streaked sputum* is most commonly caused by inflammation in the nose, nasopharynx, gums, larynx, or bronchi. If occurring only after severe paroxysms of coughing, it is attributed minor airway trauma. Pink sputum, from blood mixing with respiratory secretions in the alveoli or bronchioles, is characteristic of pneumonia and pulmonary edema. *Massive bleeding* occurs with erosion of a bronchial artery by cavitary tuberculosis, aspergilloma, lung abscess, bronchiectasis, embolism with infarction, bronchogenic carcinoma, or a broncholith. *Alveolar hemorrhage*, from pulmonary vasculitis or blunt chest trauma, may not produce bloody sputum until the degree of hemorrhage and anemia is severe. Frankly bloody hemoptysis in the setting of trauma, recent cardiac or thoracic surgery, tracheostomy or aneurysm may be associated with life-threatening arterial-bronchial or arterial-tracheal fistula.

Bloody gelatinous (Currant-Jelly) sputum. Copious tenacious, bloody sputum is prominent in pneumonia caused by *Klebsiella pneumoniae* or *Streptococcus pneumoniae*.

Rusty sputum. In pneumococcal pneumonia, minor frank hemoptysis may precede purulent sputum containing degraded blood.

Frothy sputum—pulmonary edema. Alveoli flooded with transudated fluid, yield thin blood tinged sputum containing air bubbles suggesting pulmonary edema of any cause.

Purulent sputum. Inflammatory cells, predominately polymorphonuclear leukocytes, enter the airways and alveoli in response to lower airway infection. The exudate may be yellow, green, or dirty gray. Scant purulent sputum is typical of acute bronchitis, resolving pneumonia, and a small tuberculous cavity or lung abscess. Copious purulent sputum occurs with lung abscess, bronchiectasis, or bronchopleural fistula communicating with an empyema. Fetid sputum characterizes anaerobic infection and/or lung abscess. Lung abscesses with minimal connection to the airways do not produce much sputum.

Stringy mucoid sputum. In asthma there is increased mucous production and mucous plugging or small, and sometimes large, airways.

Broncholiths. Sputum broncholiths originate in calcified lymph nodes eroding a bronchus or from calcareous granulomas in silicosis, tuberculosis, or histoplasmosis. They may suggest the source of pulmonary hemorrhage [Harris NL, McNeely WF, et al. Case 14-2002. Case records of the Massachusetts General Hospital. *N Engl J Med*. 2002;346:1475–1482].

CARDIOVASCULAR SIGNS

Interpretation of physical signs from inspection, palpation, and precordial percussion assumes normal anatomic relations of the heart and chest wall. With thoracic deformity, e.g., kyphoscoliosis and pectus excavatum, caution is advised.

Inspection
Dyspnea (shortness of breath). See page 294.

Pallor. See Chapter 6, page 127.

Cyanosis. See Chapter 6, page 127.

Palpation
Edema. Extracellular fluid partitions between the vascular and interstitial compartments by a net equilibrium between hydrostatic and oncotic pressures. Normally, intravascular fluid flows into the extravascular interstitial space in the precapillary arterioles and capillaries since hydrostatic pressure (intravascular > interstitial) is only partially offset by the opposing oncotic pressure (intravascular > interstitial). In the postcapillary venules, lower intravascular hydrostatic pressure is more than compensated by intravascular oncotic pressure, resulting in interstitial saline flowing back into the intravascular space. Concomitantly, interstitial fluid, proteins, and cells are returned to the blood from the interstitial space and via lymphatics. Altering one or more of these forces upsets this equilibrium. Increasing venous pressure in CHF produces dependent edema; venous occlusion can result in localized edema. Obstructed lymphatics lead to lymphedema. Low plasma albumin (the plasma protein contributing most to oncotic pressure) lowers the plasma oncotic pressure, permitting edema to form that may first appear where tissue pressure is low, e.g., the periorbital tissue. Increased capillary permeability causes edema that is not dependent. Tissue inflammation, triggered by bacterial, chemical, thermal, or mechanical means, increases capillary permeability creating localized edema.

Excessive interstitial fluid accumulation, either localized or generalized, is *edema*. Extensive generalized edema is *anasarca*. In adults, ~4.5 kg (10 lb) of fluid must accumulate before pitting edema is detectable. Edema is demonstrated by gently pressing a thumb into the skin against a bony surface, e.g., the anterior tibia, dorsum of the foot, or sacrum. When the thumb is withdrawn, an indentation persists.

The *distribution of edema* is important diagnostically. Responding to gravity, dependent edema first appears in the feet and ankles, or over the posterior calves or sacrum in supine patients. As the dependent fluid volume increases, a fluid level may be detected, which seldom rises above heart level. Anasarca is recognized at a glance when it obliterates superficial landmarks. Chronic edema leads to fibrosis of the subcutaneous tissues and skin so they no longer pit on pressure, *brawny edema*. Symmetric edema affecting both legs suggests a problem in the pelvis or more proximally, whereas edema limited to the arms and head suggests SVC obstruction.

Edema limited to one extremity suggests a local problem with vascular channels or local inflammation. Edema formation is the same whether it is generalized or local. To evaluate local edema, the examiner must consider the local anatomy of the arteries, veins, lymphatics and soft tissues, the presence of any inflammatory or structural disease, and then form hypotheses as to the likely mechanism and anatomic site of the problem.

Exclusive dependence upon bedside exam can overlook cardiovascular causes of bilateral leg edema, so consider BNP measurement and/or echocardiography estimating right heart pressures, RV and LV size and function, and tricuspid valve function. The following approach, based upon the anatomic distribution of edema, is diagnostically useful.

CLINICAL OCCURRENCE: *Localized Edema—Inflammation:* Infection, angioedema, contact allergy; *Metabolic/Toxic:* Gout; *Insufficiency of Venous Valves:* With or without varicosities; *Venous Thrombosis:* Postoperative, immobilization, prolonged air or automobile travel; *Venous or Lymphatic Compression:* Malignancies, constricting garments; *Chemical or Physical Injuries:* Burns, irritants and corrosives, frostbite, chilblain, envenomation (insects, snakes, spiders); *Congenital:* Amniotic bands, arteriovenous fistulas, Milroy disease; *Bilateral Edema Above the Diaphragm:* SVC obstruction; *Bilateral Edema Below the Diaphragm:* CHF with elevated jugular venous pressure, including pulmonary hypertension from left heart abnormalities, intrinsic pulmonary disorders, right heart abnormalities, and constrictive pericarditis; *Portal Vein Hypertension or Obstruction:* Cirrhosis, portal vein thrombosis, schistosomiasis; *IVC obstruction:* Thrombosis, extrinsic compression, pregnancy; *Loss of venous tone:* Drugs (calcium channel blockers, angiotensin-converting enzyme inhibitors, other vasodilators), convalescence, lack of exercise; *Generalized Edema—Hypoalbuminemia:* Nephrotic syndrome, cirrhosis, chronic liver disease, protein losing conditions (e.g., enteropathy, burns, fistulas); *Renal Retention of Salt and Water:* Corticosteroids, NSAIDs; *Increased Capillary Permeability:* Sepsis, systemic inflammatory response syndrome, interleukin-2, idiopathic capillary leak syndrome.

Idiopathic edema. Recurrent and chronic edema occurs in women in the third to fifth decades without heart, liver, or kidney disease or venous or lymphatic obstruction. Affective disorders and obesity may coexist. Possible mechanisms include mild persistent precapillary arteriolar dilatation, exaggerated capillary leak on standing, and inappropriate chronic diuretic administration, often started for minor peripheral edema (*diuretic-induced edema*). Each mechanism inappropriately activates renin–aldosterone leading to salt and water retention.

Heat-related edema. Pitting ankle edema often occurs in normal adults within 48 h of arriving in the tropics from a temperate climate, or in temperate zones when weather changes from cool and dry to warm and humid. It spontaneously resolves with acclimatization.

Angioedema. Painless subcutaneous soft-tissue edema begins abruptly and spreads to involve several centimeters of tissue with diffuse borders. Erythema is not prominent. Angioedema often involves the face, lips, or tongue and laryngeal involvement is life threatening. Causes include hereditary absence of C1 esterase, allergen exposure, and angiotensin-converting enzyme inhibitors.

Apical impulse, point of maximal impulse (PMI). Careful examination of the apical impulse yields useful information about heart size, force of LV contraction, obstruction to LV ejection, and stroke volume.

Increased amplitude. Increased force of LV contraction increases the apical impulse amplitude. Common causes are LV hypertrophy (arterial hypertension, aortic stenosis, aortic regurgitation, mitral regurgitation) and/or increased contractility (exertion, emotion, hyperthyroidism).

Decreased amplitude. Reduced contractility, as in congestive heart failure, weakens the PMI, and, if accompanied by LV dilatation, it becomes more diffuse.

Enlarged, sustained apical impulse. Contraction against increased afterload prolongs left ventricular ejection time. Therefore, rather than the normal brief tap, aortic stenosis and systemic hypertension produce an enlarged sustained apical impulse.

Displaced to the left. Volume overload dilates the LV. If contractility is normal, the PMI is enlarged, brisk, and displaced laterally, but is not sustained. Causes of LV volume overload are aortic or mitral regurgitation and intracardiac shunts. Other causes of leftward displacement are right pneumothorax, left pleural adhesions, or left lung volume loss.

Displaced to the right. This is seen with left pneumothorax, right pleural adhesions, right lung volume loss, and dextrocardia.

Shifted downward. Severe emphysema flattens the diaphragm pulling the heart and mediastinum downward. The PMI may be felt just inferior to the xiphoid.

Right ventricular impulse. Normal right ventricular contraction does not produce a palpable impulse. A dilated, hypertrophied or forward displaced RV may produce a palpable impulse. A palpable precordial impulse near the left sternal edge in the third, fourth or fifth interspace and medial to the apex impulse almost always reflects right ventricular pressure or volume overload. With severe mitral insufficiency, the enlarged left atrium produces a sternal or parasternal impulse peaking with S2, whereas true right ventricular impulses peak during systole. Slight impulses move just the interspaces, while more advanced disease lifts the lower sternum with each beat.

CLINICAL OCCURRENCE: *Right Ventricular Hypertrophy (pressure overload):* Pulmonic stenosis, pulmonary hypertension, mitral stenosis; *Right Ventricular Dilation (volume overload):* Tricuspid or pulmonary valve insufficiency, left-to-right intracardiac shunts; *Forward Displacement of the Heart:* Tumors behind the heart, enlarged left atrium; *Right Ventricle Protuberance:* Right ventricular aneurysm; *Hyperdynamic Circulation:* Exertion, emotion, hyperthyroidism.

Other impulses
Epigastric pulsation. Normal in thin people after exertion, it is also seen with inferior displacement of the heart in emphysema. Most frequently, it reflects normal aortic pulsation. Abdominal aortic aneurysm (AAA) should be considered.

Pulsations at the Base. An impulse may be felt over the pulmonary conus, just to the left of the sternum in the second or third interspace, in pulmonary hypertension and/or with increased pulmonary blood flow from large left to right shunts. Ascending aortic aneurysm may produce pulsations in the right second interspace.

Thrills. Turbulent blood flow produces audible murmurs and palpable thrills when transmitted to peripheral structures. The vibrations feel like holding a purring cat. Since auscultation is more sensitive than palpation, thrills are associated with more intense murmurs (grade IV/VI). Thrills must be localized and timed to the cardiac cycle. *DDX:* In mitral stenosis, diastolic and presystolic thrills may be felt at the apex. Severe aortic stenosis causes a systolic thrill in the second right interspace and carotid arteries. The thrill from a ventricular septal defect (VSD) is felt in the fourth and fifth interspaces near the sternum.

Palpable friction rubs (friction fremitus). Occasionally a pleural or pericardial friction rub is palpable (see Acute Pericarditis, page 352).

Percussion
Shifted cardiac dullness. Estimating the distance of the cardiac apex from the midsternal line (MSL) by percussion only detects gross changes in heart size.

Left border shifted leftward. The LBCD is normally 7–9 cm left of the MSL. *DDX:* Leftward shift is caused by LV dilatation (RBCD normal or right-shifted), pericardial effusion (RBCD right-shifted, muffled heart sounds, paradoxical pulse), and displacement of a normal-sized heart to left by right pneumothorax, right hydrothorax, left pleural adhesions, or left lung atelectasis with left-shifted mediastinum.

Left border shifted rightward. Consider pulmonary emphysema with a normal midline heart, a prominent lingula anterior to the heart preventing accurate percussion of LBCD, and displacement rightward from right lung fibrosis or atelectasis, left pneumothorax, or left hydrothorax.

Right border shifted rightward. Causes include cardiac dilatation, pericardial effusion, left pneumothorax, left hydrothorax, right lung atelectasis, right pleural adhesions, and dextrocardia.

Right border shifted leftward. Causes include left lung atelectasis, left pleural adhesions, right pneumothorax, and right hydrothorax.

Enlarged cardiac dullness. The area of cardiac dullness expands when the right or left border is displaced laterally without the other moving, or both borders are displaced in opposite directions, e.g., by cardiac dilatation and pericardial effusion.

Wide manubrial dullness. Dullness >6 cm suggests aortic aneurysm, retrosternal goiter, thymus tumor, lymphoma, or metastatic carcinoma.

Auscultating Heart Sounds
First (S1) and second (S2) heart sounds. During ventricular systole intraventricular pressure rises rapidly closing the mitral and tricuspid valves and,

shortly thereafter, opening the aortic and pulmonic valves (Fig. 8-19). Tensing of the AV valves is associated with S1; tensing of the aortic and pulmonic valves is associated with S2. *The normal heart sounds are NOT caused by the leaflets slapping together.* Rather, the high-frequency components of these sounds are probably caused by the closed valves tensing producing abrupt deceleration of blood that vibrates the heart, vessels, and blood column. The contracting ventricles force blood silently into the aorta and pulmonary artery. When the ventricles relax, intraventricular pressure falls. Initial aortic and pulmonic valve leaflet apposition occurs prior to the high-frequency components of S2. The pressure gradient between each artery and the more rapidly declining intraventricular pressures abruptly stretches elastic leaflet tissue producing the second heart sound. S2 is heard when arterial flow is near zero but just before brief retrograde flow occurs. The heart sounds are usually loudest on the precordium nearest their origin: S1 from the AV valves at the apex and lower left sternal border; S2 from the semilunar valves at the base. S2 is louder than S1 at the base. Occasionally, S2 at the apex may be as loud or louder than S1. The intensity of S1 and S2 varies with the stress on the valve leaflets.

First heart sound, S1—onset of ventricular systole. S1 marks the beginning of ventricular systole, approximately synchronous with the apical impulse. S1 is usually louder than S2 at the cardiac apex and can be heard throughout the precordium. At the base, S1 is less loud than S2.

Splitting of S1. S1 splits with asynchronous tricuspid and mitral valves tensing. Slight splitting of S1 is a common normal finding. Wide splitting occurs with right bundle-branch block, which delays right ventricular contraction.

Accentuated S1. Thickened mitral valve leaflets with preserved mobility and increased force of LV contraction accentuate S1. This occurs in mitral stenosis, tachycardia from fever, hyperthyroidism, exercise, emotion, and hypertension.

Diminished S1. When the mitral and tricuspid valves are closely approximated at the onset of systole, their tensing is less forceful as seen with weak ventricular contraction, aortic insufficiency, prolonged PR interval, and heavily calcified mitral valve leaflets. Attenuation of heart sounds by obesity, emphysema, and pericardial and/or pleural effusion also diminishes S1.

Variable and intermittently very loud S1 (Bruit de Canon). Variable ventricular diastolic filling and asynchronous atrial and ventricular contraction change the intensity of S1 from beat to beat. Atrial fibrillation, atrial flutter with varying block, complete AV block, frequent premature beats, and ventricular tachycardia are each a cause.

Second heart sound, S2—onset of ventricular diastole. Tensing of the closed semilunar aortic (A2) and pulmonic (P2) valves produces S2, normally A2 slightly preceding P2. The more compliant and distensible an artery, the less closely the arterial pressure follows the pressure in the ventricle ejecting into that artery, a phenomenon known as *hangout*. Thus, the aorta's lower compliance compared to the PA causes the interval between completion of LV systole and A2 to be shorter than that between the completion of RV systole

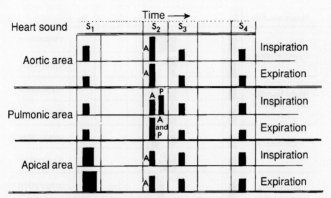

FIG. 8-37 Normal Physiologic Variations in the Heart Sounds. Duration is represented on the horizontal axis and intensity of the heart sounds on the vertical axis. The S1 is prolonged during inspiration. The aortic component of the second sound (A2) is audible over the entire precordium, but (P2) the weaker pulmonic component is heard only in the left second intercostal space. During expiration, the aortic and pulmonic components of S2 fuse. With inspiration the splitting of S2 widens. Splitting of S2 is normal only in the pulmonic area; it is pathologic elsewhere.

and P2, so A2 precedes P2 (Fig. 8-37). Aortic pressure is much higher than PA pressure making A2 louder than P2. Compare the intensity of A2 and P2 in the second left intercostal space. In adults, only A2 is heard at the apex; hearing both A2 and P2 suggests that P2 is abnormally loud.

Effect of respiration on S2. Inspiration delays PV closure resulting in inspiratory splitting of S2 by decreasing intrathoracic pressure leading to increased venous return and pulmonary compliance. In children and adolescents, the inspiratory split of S2 is wider than in older adults. In recumbent young persons, S2 may not fuse into a single sound with expiration. Fusion should occur during expiration when sitting, so failure to fuse suggests an unusually wide split. With advancing age, the normal split narrows and inspiratory splitting of S2 may not be detectable, even in recumbency. The variable splitting of S2 with the respiratory cycle distinguishes the triple S1-A2-P2 sounds from other sounds such as lower pitched noises including S3 and S4.

Accentuated A2. Increased pressure on the closed aortic valve increases A2. Arterial hypertension is most common, but it can occur with ascending aortic aneurysm.

Diminished A2. A2 is decreased when the valve is rigid and immobile or the pressure on the valve and aortic root at end systole is lower. Arterial hypotension and a heavily calcified AV in aortic stenosis diminish A2.

Accentuated P2. P2 is accentuated in primary or secondary pulmonary hypertension, atrial septal defect (ASD), truncus arteriosus, and in adolescence (Fig. 8-38).

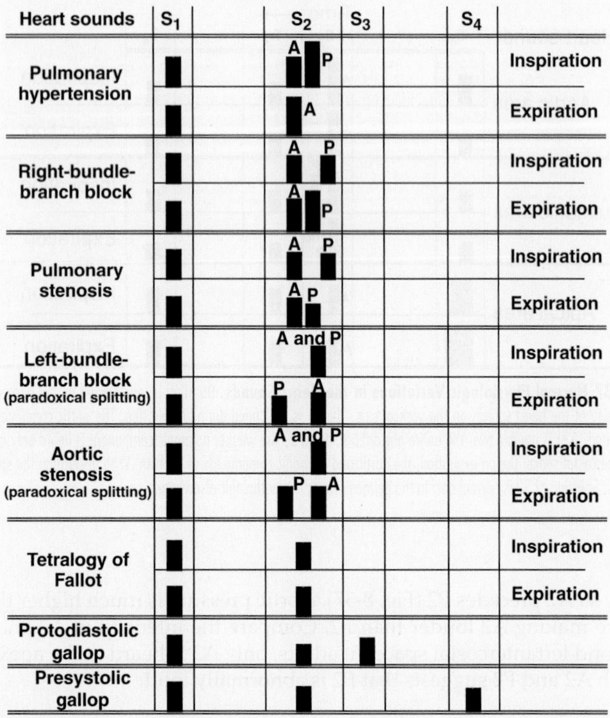

Heart sounds	S₁	S₂	S₃	S₄	
Pulmonary hypertension	■	A P			Inspiration
	■	A			Expiration
Right-bundle-branch block	■	A P			Inspiration
	■	A P			Expiration
Pulmonary stenosis	■	A P			Inspiration
	■	A P			Expiration
Left-bundle-branch block (paradoxical splitting)	■	A and P			Inspiration
	■	P A			Expiration
Aortic stenosis (paradoxical splitting)	■	A and P			Inspiration
	■	P A			Expiration
Tetralogy of Fallot	■	■			Inspiration
	■	■			Expiration
Protodiastolic gallop	■	■	■		
Presystolic gallop	■	■		■	

FIG. 8-38 **Pathologic Variations in the Heart Sounds. Pulmonary hypertension** causes an increased P2. **Right bundle-branch block** delays right ventricular emptying, increasing the normal split and accentuating P2. **Pulmonic stenosis** also delays P2 but decreases its intensity. In **left bundle-branch block** and **aortic stenosis**, LV ejection is delayed so A2 coincides with P2 and the normal expiratory movement of P2 causes paradoxic splitting during expiration.

Diminished P2. Diminished pulmonary artery pressure reduces tension on the pulmonic valve. Pulmonic stenosis is the most common cause (Fig. 8-38).

Widened inspiratory S2 split. This indicates either delayed PV tensing or early AV tensing. P2 delay occurs with right bundle-branch block, ASD, and pulmonic stenosis. Early AV closure valve occurs with severe MR (Fig. 8-38).

Reversed or paradoxic S2 split. Delays in LV ejection cause A2 to occur with or after P2. During inspiration there is a single sound, or closely approximated sounds; expiration increases the split. This is seen in hypertrophic cardiomyopathy with dynamic LV outflow obstruction, valvular aortic stenosis, left bundle-branch block, and RV pacing (Fig. 8-38).

Triple rhythms and gallops. These low-pitched sounds are best heard in a quiet room. Listen specifically for triple heart sounds (couplets alternating with single sounds) resembling a horse's gallop. The couplet may be either a normal S2 followed closely by an audible S3 or an audible S4 preceding a normal S1. Differentiating S3 from S4 requires correctly identifying S1 and S2. The galloping rhythm is most evident at rates >100 bpm. Some reserve "gallop" for an S3 and/or S4 *and* a rate >100 bpm. At very fast rates S3 and S4 fuse creating a mid-diastolic *summation gallop*.

S3, ventricular or protodiastolic gallop. Reverberation of ventricular muscle and blood, decelerating at the end of rapid early ventricular filling, produces the S3 (Figs. 8-20 and 8-38). S3 closely follows S2 in early diastole. It has the cadence of Kentucky: ken.... TUCK..eh. By whispering "ken .... TUCK..eh" to yourself as you listen, timing "ken" to S1 and "TUCK" to S2 you can train your ear to listen for the low-pitched S3 coincident with "eh." A left ventricular S3 is best heard at the apex with the patient lying 45 degrees to the left side; a right ventricular S3 is best heard near the lower left sternal border. S3 is best heard in expiration and is accentuated by increasing venous return by exercise, abdominal pressure, or flexing the knees on the abdomen. An S3 is normal in children, young adults, and in pregnancy. After the third decade it may indicate myocardial systolic dysfunction with increased LV end-diastolic pressure and elevated left atrial pressure. It is also seen, although of less concern, in hyperkinetic circulatory states (fever, anemia, and hyperthyroidism) or by very rapid ventricular filling from mitral regurgitation or a large left-to-right shunt with a VSD.

S4, presystolic or atrial gallop. S4 is caused by the vibrating LV muscle, mitral valve apparatus, and LV outflow tract produced by atrial contraction (Figs. 8-20 and 8-38). S4 occurs after atrial contraction but before S1. The cadence is Tennessee: "te..NUH … ..see." This is the most difficult to hear of all heart sounds; listen at apex with patient in left lateral decubitus position. As you listen, whisper to yourself "te..NUH … .see," timing "NUH" to S1 and "see" to S2; train your ear for the S4 coincident with "te." S4 is low pitched, identical to S3. The S4 always indicates a high pressure, powerful atrial contraction, most often associated with decreased ventricular compliance. S4 is heard with a thickened and/or noncompliant left ventricle, as with LVH, aortic stenosis, subaortic stenosis, hypertension, and acute ischemia or infarction from coronary artery disease (CAD).

Summation gallop, mid-diastolic gallop. High heart rates compress diastole moving S3 and S4 together giving the impression of a single sound or a rumbling murmur. Vagus stimulation may slow the rate enough to reveal the four sounds.

Early systolic ejection sound—ejection click, aortic ejection sound. The aortic root suddenly tensing at the onset of LV ejection and sudden doming of a stenotic yet flexible noncalcified aortic valve are causes (Fig. 8-20, page 284). At the onset of LV ejection in early systole, a click is heard at the base and apex. It is unaffected by inspiration and usually loudest at the base. Ejection clicks occur with a dilated aortic root from ascending aortic aneurysm, coarctation, hypertension, valvular aortic stenosis, a bicuspid aortic valve, or aortic regurgitation.

Early systolic ejection sound—ejection click, pulmonic ejection sound. See Aortic ejection sound above and Fig. 8-20. This is a click at the onset of right ventricular ejection, occurring with pulmonary valve stenosis or dilatation. It is best heard in the left second interspace during early systole. In some cases, a loud click fuses with S1 making S1 sound louder. The closer the sound is to S1, the more severe the stenosis. Pulmonic clicks may decrease or disappear with inspiration.

Mid or late systolic click—mitral valve prolapse. This click is heard at the apex in mid or late systole; it can be intermittent (Fig. 8-20). It is unchanged by respiration but can be delayed or abolished by squatting from standing or raising the legs, both of which increase LV end-diastolic volume. The click may first become apparent or, if already audible, will move toward S1 as the LV end-diastolic volume decreases with standing or Valsalva. It is sometimes associated with a late systolic murmur of mitral insufficiency. Most individuals are otherwise normal, although mitral prolapse occurs with increased frequency in Marfan syndrome and myxomatous mitral valve degeneration.

Diastolic snap—mitral opening snap. When LV pressure drops below LA pressure, stenotic but still flexible (noncalcified) mitral valve leaflets that are tethered at their commissures buckle or bow into the left ventricle producing a snap. The diastolic rumble begins a few hundredths of a second later (Fig. 8-20). The snap is best heard at the apex but may radiate to the base and left sternal border, simulating a widely split S2. This sign is characteristic of rheumatic mitral stenosis.

Diastolic snap—tricuspid opening snap. See mitral opening snap above. Usually associated with other rheumatic valvular abnormalities, this snap is difficult to identify.

Prosthetic heart valves. Prosthetic heart valves are common. It is advisable to be familiar with the various valve types and their auscultatory features.

Auscultating Extracardiac Sounds: These relatively uncommon precordial sounds are often mistaken for murmurs. Extracardiac sounds may move about within a specific part of the cardiac cycle, distinguishing them from the S1, S2, S3, and S4.

Diastolic sound—pericardial knock. With constrictive pericarditis ventricular filling stops abruptly in early diastole producing vibrations known as a pericardial knock. Knocks are higher pitched than S3 and are heard widely over the precordium. They can be earlier than S3 and increase with inspiration (Fig. 8-20).

Pericardial friction rub. Two inflamed pericardial surfaces rubbing together create a sound which seems closer to the ear than a murmur. Pericardial effusions often do not cover the entire pericardium, so rub and effusion can coexist. Listen during full expiration with the patient prone or sitting and leaning forward. Rubs are scratchy, grating, rasping, or squeaky. In ~50% of cases the rub is triphasic, in systole and early and late diastole. In one-third it is systolic and late diastolic. The rest are heard only in systole. Rubs are often intermittent.

Mediastinal crunch (Hamman sign). See Subcutaneous and mediastinal emphysema page 302 and Spontaneous esophageal rupture page 355.

Venous hum. High-velocity flow in the internal jugular veins, especially the right, produces a humming sound. Hums are usually heard in both supraclavicular fossae and often in the second and third interspaces near the sternum. They are low pitched, persist throughout the cardiac cycle, and frequently increase during diastole. Hums are intensified by sitting or standing; they do not vary with respirations. The hum is readily abolished by light pressure on the jugular veins beside the trachea. They are frequently mistaken for an intracardiac murmur. Venous hums can be normal. They are more common with hyperthyroidism and anemia.

Auscultating Heart Murmurs: In normal vessels and heart chambers, blood flow at rest is laminar and silent. Murmurs result from turbulence (vortices) developing near the vessel wall–bloodstream interface as the blood passes an obstruction or dilatation (vortex-shedding theory). Imagine 60 cm of pliable rubber tubing attached to a water faucet. When the faucet is turned on, a flow velocity can be attained that will not vibrate the tubing, because the flow is laminar and smooth. At this flow, slightly constricting the tubing causes vibrations distally. Similarly, increasing the flow without constriction induces turbulence. In a normal heart, murmurs are induced when the velocity of blood flow is increased by high output states such as exercise, anemia, pregnancy, or hyperthyroidism, that is, a flow murmur. Blood flowing over obstructions or through unusual openings in the circulation creates turbulence and collision currents resulting in murmurs.

Murmurs should be described by their location, pitch, and timing in the cardiac cycle. The quality of a murmur is of some diagnostic value. Ventricular filling murmurs involving diastolic flow across the AV valves are relatively low pitched because of the pressure gradients are low; blood flowing through narrow orifices with higher pressure gradients cause high-pitched murmurs. Accurate categorization of these features is necessary to establish the likely diagnosis. Figures 8-39 to 8-41 show the anatomy and murmur of each major condition.

Systolic Murmurs: Systolic murmurs may occur in early, mid, or late systole. Murmurs heard throughout systole are *pansystolic* or *holosystolic*. Blood moving across a rising then falling pressure gradient produces a *crescendo–decrescendo* murmur reflecting accelerating then slowing flow, e.g., aortic stenosis. The murmur, starting soon after S1, intensifies to a maximum at mid-systole, then tapers off disappearing before S2. Blood flowing continuously from a high-pressure region to one of low pressure produces a pansystolic murmur of almost uniform intensity typical of atrioventricular valve regurgitation. It is usually possible to distinguish the systolic murmurs of organic disease from those of little significance occurring only in early systole or mid-systole [Etchells E, Bell C, Robb K. The rational clinical examination. Does this patient have an abnormal systolic murmur? *JAMA.* 1997;277:564–571]. Echocardiography is an important adjunct for evaluating pathological systolic murmurs since some lesions are misdiagnosed even by experienced observers. Common errors are underestimating the severity of aortic stenosis because of decreased LV function, failing to identify combined mitral and

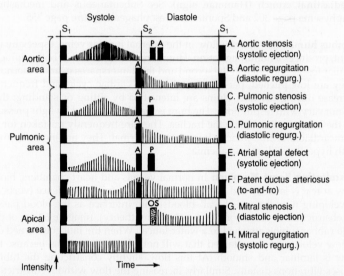

FIG. 8-39 Common Pathologic Heart Murmurs. The diagrams are drawn to represent intensity of the heart sounds and murmurs on the vertical axis and duration on the horizontal axis. Pitch is depicted by the spacing of the shading: wider spacing lower pitch. "A" and "P" refer to the aortic and pulmonic components of the S2. "OS" indicates the opening snap of the mitral valve in mitral stenosis. Note that the systolic ejection murmurs are inaudible at either end of systole and attain maximum intensity at mid-systole (in this diagram they form the upper halves of diamond-shaped figures of the phonocardiogram). Systolic regurgitant murmurs are pansystolic. The configuration of the diastolic ejection murmur of mitral stenosis terminates in a crescendo caused by superimposition of atrial contraction. Although the diastolic regurgitant murmurs are pandiastolic, in aortic and pulmonic regurgitation, the late diastolic part is seldom heard.

aortic murmurs, and missing aortic insufficiency in association with aortic systolic murmurs.

Benign, innocent, physiologic, functional, nonpathologic basal systolic murmurs. These murmurs can be produced by increased flow velocity and decreased blood viscosity. Most commonly heard in the second left interspace, they have medium pitch and a reusually grade I-II/VI. They are best heard when supine and tend to disappear with sitting or standing. They are infrequently transmitted to the neck. Functional murmurs occur in normal adults with anemia, fever, anxiety, exercise, hyperthyroidism, or pregnancy. Approximately 50% of normal children have functional systolic murmurs.

Aortic valve stenosis. Progressive commissural fusion and leaflet fibrosis result in a small valve orifice impeding LV ejection (Fig. 8-40C). **The Murmur:** Classically the murmur is heard in the second right interspace, but almost as often it is audible along the left sternal border in the third and fourth interspaces and at the apex. In ~15% of cases, it is loudest at the apex. Regardless of the site of maximal intensity, it transmits to the carotid arteries. Loud murmurs can be accompanied by systolic thrills at the base and in the carotids. Onset is very shortly after S1, when intraventricular pressure first exceeds

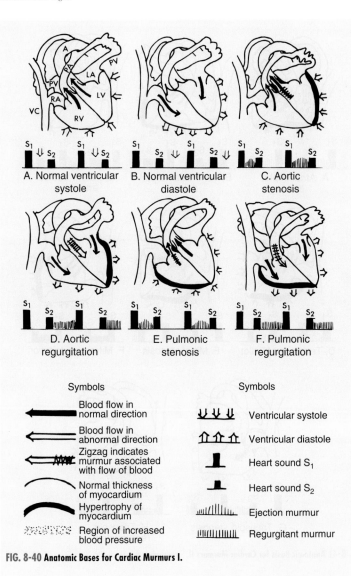

Symbols

← (solid arrow)	Blood flow in normal direction
← (outline arrow)	Blood flow in abnormal direction
◁〰〰	Zigzag indicates murmur associated with flow of blood
⌒	Normal thickness of myocardium
⏜ (thick)	Hypertrophy of myocardium
░░░	Region of increased blood pressure

Symbols

⇓ ⇓ ⇓	Ventricular systole
⇧ ⇧ ⇧	Ventricular diastole
▮	Heart sound S_1
▬	Heart sound S_2
⣿⢸⣿⣄	Ejection murmur
⎸⎹⎸⎹⎸⎹	Regurgitant murmur

FIG. 8-40 Anatomic Bases for Cardiac Murmurs I.

A. Normal ventricular systole

B. Normal ventricular diastole

C. Aortic stenosis

D. Aortic regurgitation

E. Pulmonic stenosis

F. Pulmonic regurgitation

aortic pressure. It ceases at or before S2. It is diamond shaped, initially rising (crescendo) then falling (decrescendo) in intensity (Fig. 8-39). As stenosis worsens the murmur's peak moves later in systole, i.e., *late peaking*. The murmur is usually harsh, medium pitched, and audible with the bell and diaphragm. Occasionally it sounds like gull's call or a dove cooing. With decreased LV contractility, it decreases in intensity and duration. **Heart Sounds:** In moderate and severe aortic stenosis accompanied by significant valve leaflet calcification,

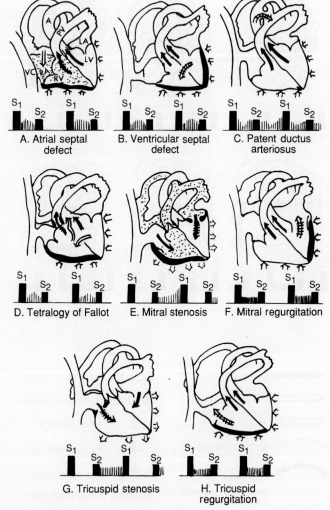

FIG. 8-41 Anatomic Basis for Cardiac Murmurs II. Same symbols as in Fig. 8-40.

A2 is soft or absent at the apex. If the valve is stenotic but not calcified (as in congenital aortic stenosis), S2 may split during expiration (paradoxically) reflecting delayed aortic valve closure (Fig. 8-38). Normal inspiratory splitting of S2 suggests mild stenosis. When a stenotic valve remains flexible, an ejection or early systolic click, caused by doming of the valve, precedes the murmur in early systole, but disappears when the valve calcifies. An apical S4 is common. **Precordial Thrust:** Left ventricular hypertrophy accentuates the precordial apical thrust. In the left lateral decubitus position, a double apical

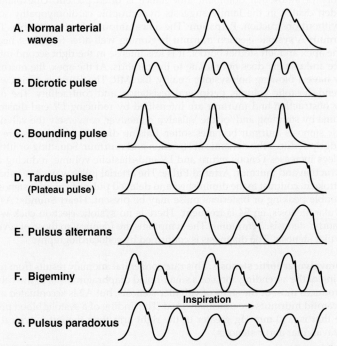

A. Normal arterial waves

B. Dicrotic pulse

C. Bounding pulse

D. Tardus pulse (Plateau pulse)

E. Pulsus alternans

F. Bigeminy

Inspiration

G. Pulsus paradoxus

FIG. 8-42 Arterial Pulse Contour. A. Normal pulse contour. B. Dicrotic pulse. C. Bounding or collapsing pulse. D. Tardus or Plateau pulse. E. Pulsus alternans. F. Bigeminal pulse. G. Pulsus paradoxus.

thrust is sometimes felt, the first impact reflects atrial contraction, the second reflects LV systole. **Arterial Pulse:** Severe aortic stenosis produces a slowly rising carotid pulse contour (*tardus or anacrotic pulse*, Fig. 8-42D) felt as a sustained push rather than the normal brief tap. Decreased pulse amplitude is often palpable, but it is best assessed by calculating pulse pressure. Physical findings do not reliably assess the severity of aortic stenosis. *Symptoms:* Aortic stenosis can be asymptomatic until severe, when exercise induces dyspnea, angina, or syncope. The most common etiologies are rheumatic valvulitis, valve sclerosis, and congenital bicuspid valve. **X-ray Findings:** Aortic valve calcification may be seen on plain chest radiographs. **DDX:** The systolic murmur of aortic sclerosis without stenosis is shorter and accompanied by normal heart sounds at the base. The apical systolic murmur of MR has a blowing quality and is often holosystolic. A systolic diamond-shaped murmur occurs with both valvular and subvalvular stenosis.

Hypertrophic obstructive cardiomyopathy (IHSS). Asymmetric LV hypertrophy with prominent hypertrophy of the basal interventricular septum is associated with dynamic outflow obstruction starting shortly after the onset of systole. Obstruction is caused by apposition of the anterior mitral leaflet to the hypertrophied septum. Mitral insufficiency may occur as well. A family history of autosomal dominant inheritance is often present. Unexplained sudden deaths in the family suggests hypertrophic cardiomyopathy with or without obstruction. **Palpation:** The apical impulse is often double. **The Murmur:** A systolic ejection murmur beginning well after S1 is best heard at the apex and left sternal border. It is less intense in the right second interspace and usually does not radiate to the carotids. At the apex, the murmur may have a blowing holosystolic quality, like MR. The murmur varies with LV end-diastolic volume, peripheral resistance, and contractility. The outflow obstruction and murmur are intensified by reducing LV end-diastolic volume by standing and/or the Valsalva maneuver, conversely the valvular aortic stenosis murmur becomes softer. Raising diastolic blood pressure by handgrip reduces the dynamic obstruction and murmur. Squatting or lifting the legs increases venous return and LV end-diastolic volume, reducing the obstruction and murmur. **Arterial Pulse:** The arterial pulse wave has a sharp upstroke in contrast to the diminished and delayed pulse of valvular stenosis. A double peaking or bisferiens pulse may be present. **Heart Sounds:** As in valvular stenosis, an S4 is frequent. There is no systolic ejection click with subaortic stenosis. **Symptoms:** The symptoms are identical to those of severe valvular stenosis. The diagnosis is confirmed by echocardiography.

Supravalvular aortic stenosis. This rare congenital anomaly results from narrowing of the ascending aorta or a small-holed diaphragm distal to the valve. It produces most of the signs of valvular stenosis, but A2 is accentuated and the carotid murmurs are unusually loud. The finding of a systolic blood pressure that is >10 mm Hg greater in the right arm than the left is typical of supravalvular aortic stenosis.

Aortic valve sclerosis. Aortic sclerosis is caused by leaflet thickening and calcification (sclerosis) without significant obstruction (stenosis). A medium-pitched murmur of moderate intensity is heard in the aortic region and may be heard at the apex. It is often brief, confined to early systole, and is usually softer than an aortic stenosis murmur. The murmur may be faintly heard in the carotids. A2 is usually present at the apex. *DDX:* Because the murmur is seldom loud or long or accompanied by an abnormal carotid pulse, it shouldn't be confused with aortic stenosis. Preservation of A2 at the apex speaks against severe calcific aortic valvular stenosis.

Valvular pulmonic stenosis. Pulmonary stenosis is usually congenital, alone or with the tetralogy of Fallot. It can be acquired with carcinoid tumors. A diamond shaped ejection murmur is loudest in the second left interspace (Figs. 8-39C and 8-40E). Its intensity, configuration, and pitch resemble an aortic stenosis murmur, but its intensity increases with inspiration. Carotid transmission may occur (left > right). Slow RV ejection delays P2 widely splitting S2. Lower pulmonary artery pressure reduces the intensity of P2 (Figs. 8-20 and 8-39C). An early ejection click indicates valvular rather than infundibular stenosis. An accentuated precordial thrust or sternal lift indicates RVH. *DDX:* The murmur resembles the pulmonary flow murmur of an ASD, but P2 is not diminished with ASD.

Infundibular pulmonic stenosis. The infundibulum is the funnel-shaped portion of the right ventricular chamber leading to the pulmonary artery.

Congenital narrowing produces a form of pulmonic stenosis. In contrast to valvular stenosis, the ejection murmur and the systolic thrill are usually in the third left interspace and there is no ejection click. Although this lesion may be isolated, it is usually accompanied by a VSD, as in the tetralogy of Fallot.

Ostium secundum ASD. Overfilling of the right ventricle, due to a congenital left-to-right interatrial shunt, causes the high-volume, high-velocity flow across the pulmonic valve (Fig. 8-41A). A medium-pitched murmur is heard in the second or third left interspace with maximum intensity a little before mid-systole (Fig. 8-39E). This murmur is sometimes accompanied by a low-pitched diastolic flow murmur along the lower left sternal border from increased flow through the tricuspid valve. S2 is widely split, and usually the split is fixed. P2 is not diminished. *DDX:* The murmur may be indistinguishable from pulmonic stenosis. Compared to pulmonic stenosis, it is usually lower pitched, peaks earlier in systole, and rarely becomes as loud.

Ostium primum ASD. The congenital opening in the interatrial septum is near the AV valves and often associated with a cleft mitral valve leaflet. There is a harsh systolic murmur at left sternal border and, if MR is present, an apical systolic murmur transmitted to the axilla. Sometimes a mid-diastolic murmur is heard at the lower left sternal border. S2 is accentuated with fixed splitting during inspiration and expiration. The right ventricular impulse is prominent. If MR is present, the LV apical impulse may be accentuated and laterally displaced.

Coarctation of the aorta. See also Coarctation of the aorta, page 368. The coarctation is in the descending aorta, so the murmur is heard best in the posterior interscapular area, and faintly heard, if at all, on the anterior chest. A continuous bruit can sometimes be heard over the sternum from the dilated internal mammary arteries.

Ventricular septal defect. Congenital VSDs occur alone and in Eisenmenger and Fallot syndromes. Blood flows from the high pressure left ventricle into the much lower pressure right ventricle through an opening in the interventricular septum (Fig. 8-41B). VSD is more common in the membranous than muscular septum. The high-pitched murmur is typically pansystolic with peak intensity in the fourth and fifth left interspace. It may be transmitted over the entire precordium and to the interscapular region. With muscular septal defects, the murmur may not persist throughout systole. The intensity and harshness diminish and the midsystolic accentuation is lost when pulmonary hypertension supervenes. Loud murmurs may be accompanied by a thrill. When the defect is large S2 may be accentuated. *DDX:* With pulmonary hypertension, imaging may be needed to distinguish VSD from persistent ductus arteriosus. Faint murmurs must be distinguished from benign systolic murmurs. VSD may complicate MI, typically at the cardiac apex; large acquired defects are rapidly fatal.

Tricuspid regurgitation (TR). Right ventricular contraction produces backflow of blood into the right atrium and major veins, with a pulsatile increase in CVP (Fig. 8-41H). Faint murmurs are in early systolic, loud murmurs are heard throughout systole, both augmenting with inspiration. They are high pitched and blowing, best heard with the diaphragm. Maximum intensity is along the lower left sternal border and may be sharply localized or transmitted to the apex. Right ventricular. hypertrophy may be present with a palpable right ventricular precordial thrust. When severe, tricuspid insufficiency produces engorged neck veins with prominent v-waves and hepatic pulsation. There are no characteristic heart sound changes. *DDX:* The location of maximum intensity, large jugular v-waves, and augmentation with inspiration is diagnostic. Congenital TR occurs with Ebstein anomaly. It is acquired in rheumatic heart disease, right ventricular failure, endocarditis, carcinoid tumor, and pulmonary embolism.

Mitral regurgitation. MR results from myxomatous degeneration of the valve, endocarditis, rheumatic valvulitis, ruptured chordae, papillary muscle ischemia or rupture, MI, and a dilated mitral valve ring due to LV dilatation. Blood flows back through the mitral orifice at almost constant velocity throughout systole (Fig. 8-41F). With severe MR, the left ventricle empties prematurely, so A2 is early, widely splitting S2. **The Murmur:** Classically, this loud high-pitched murmur with maximum intensity at the apex begins with S1, continues throughout systole, and ends at or near S2 (Fig. 8-39H). However, many variations occur. The murmur may mask S1, begin with S1 and decrescendo to end in early-to-mid systole, or begin in mid-to-late systole and crescendo to end with, or even after, S2. Faint murmurs are well localized; loud murmurs are transmitted to the axilla. Eccentric jets may produce murmurs with radiation to the base and carotids, or to the lung bases and spine. There is insignificant variation with phases of respiration or rhythm irregularities. A rumbling diastolic murmur from the increased flow volume across the mitral valve may be heard. **Heart Sounds:** S1 is often diminished or difficult to appreciate being embedded in the murmur. S2 is widely split with severe regurgitation. A2 may be difficult to appreciate at the apex being lost in the terminal portion of the murmur. An S3 is sometimes heard with moderate or severe MR. **Palpation:** Accentuation and lateral displacement of the apical thrust suggest LV hypertrophy and dilatation, respectively. An increased left parasternal thrust or lift may reflect the enlarged left atrial systolic rather than right ventricular disease. *DDX:* The murmur must be distinguished from aortic stenosis which is often loud at the apex as well as at the base. Comparison of the duration and quality at the apex and base differentiates the two.

Mitral valve prolapse—midsystolic click and apical late systolic murmur. The valve undergoes myxomatous degeneration, producing redundant leaflet tissue (especially the posterior leaflet), an enlarged valve annulus, and elongated chordae tendineae. As the ventricular volume decreases during systole, one or more valve leaflet scallops billow, prolapsing backward into the atrium and losing coaptation with resultant MR. This occurs in 2% to 5% of the population, more frequently in women. It can be inherited, probably as an autosomal dominant with reduced expression in males. **The Murmur:** The systolic crescendo murmur is heard best at the apex in mid to late systole. It is usually short, relatively high pitched, and blowing, persisting into S2. It may transmit to the back left of the spine. In unusual cases, it is described as cooing, honking, or whooping. It may be inaudible or so loud as to be heard without a stethoscope. It typically moves closer to S1 on standing (decreased venous return, smaller LV volume) and becomes shorter and later in systole when squatting or recumbent (increased venous return, larger LV volume). Auscultation during a Valsalva maneuver while erect may reveal a murmur inaudible at rest with the patient supine. **Heart Sounds:** A clicking sound is sometimes heard during mid-systole, coincident with the onset of the murmur; the click may occur without a murmur. **Associated Dysrhythmias:** Ventricular premature beats, paroxysmal atrial tachycardia, atrial fibrillation, sinus bradycardia, periods of sinus arrest, and positional atrial flutter may all occur in association. **Noncardiac Signs:** The incidence of chest wall abnormalities is increased, particularly pectus excavatum. Mitral valve prolapse is common in Marfan syndrome. **Symptoms:** Most persons are asymptomatic. A minority develop easy fatigue, shortness of breath, nonanginal chest pain, palpitation, or syncope. **Complications:** There is an increased relative risk for cerebral transient ischemic attacks, chordae tendineae rupture, congestive cardiac failure, endocarditis, and sudden death, though these are rare.

- **Ruptured interventricular septum, papillary muscle, or chordae tendineae.** Sudden appearance of a loud pansystolic murmur and hemodynamic shock suggests rupture of the interventricular septum, a chorda or papillary muscle, or severe papillary muscle dysfunction. There may be a precordial thrill; severe pulmonary edema occurs with chordae or papillary muscle injury. The murmur is usually grade II-IV/VI; however, severe mitral insufficiency can be associated with a surprisingly soft murmur. When the septum ruptures, there are signs of right-sided failure, low cardiac output, and poor peripheral perfusion. Prompt recognition and treatment can be lifesaving.

Diastolic Murmurs: Early, mid, and late diastolic murmurs are almost always pathologic and reflect valve leaflet dysfunction. Flow from the aorta or pulmonary artery back into a ventricle results in a diastolic regurgitant murmur beginning with S2 that may persist throughout diastole. The diastolic murmur of mitral stenosis does not start with S2 because ventricular pressure continues to fall after S2 until it becomes less than atrial pressure (the period of isovolumic relaxation).

Aortic regurgitation (aortic insufficiency). Flow driven by the decreasing transvalvular pressure gradient from early to late diastole produces the decrescendo murmur. The high pitch is caused by blood being forced through a relatively small orifice at high pressure (Fig. 8-40D). **The Murmur:** The high-pitched blowing decrescendo murmur immediately follows S2; it may not last throughout diastole (Fig. 8-39B). The murmur is best heard with the diaphragm held firmly against the chest while the patient is leaning forward in full expiration. The point of maximum intensity is in the right second or left third interspace. There is often an accompanying aortic systolic murmur. Transmission down the right rather than the left sternal border suggests aortic root aneurysm. **Heart Sounds:** S1 is usually normal; A2 may be accentuated. **Palpation:** Accentuation and lateral displacement of the apical thrust suggest LV hypertrophy and dilatation. Arterial Pulse: The pulse has a collapsing quality. Vasodilatation, high pulse pressure, and pistol-shot sounds may be found. Nailbed pulsation is easily seen. *DDX:* The quality and location do not distinguish aortic from pulmonic regurgitation, but maximal intensity in the aortic area, an accentuated and displaced apical thrust, increased pulse pressure, brisk carotid upstrokes, pulsus bisferiens, and Duroziez sign all favor AI. Common causes are rheumatic valvulitis, congenitally bicuspid aortic valve, and endocarditis. Marfan syndrome, aortic dissection, sinus of Valsalva aneurysm, and aortic valve annular ectasia are less common. Syphilitic aortitis is increasingly uncommon.

Pulmonic regurgitation. Most commonly the result of pulmonic valve ring dilation in pulmonary hypertension which leads to backflow of blood from the pulmonary artery into the right ventricle resulting in RV volume and pressure overload (Fig. 8-40F). **The Murmur (Graham Steell):** Indistinguishable in quality and timing from aortic regurgitation, it is usually softer and transmits less widely (Fig. 8-39D). The point of maximum intensity is in the second or third left interspace. In the absence of pulmonary hypertension, the murmur is medium to low pitched. **Heart Sounds:** P2 may be accentuated. **Palpation:** A right ventricular precordial thrust may be palpable. Pulmonary valve regurgitation occurs with pulmonary hypertension of any cause (mitral stenosis, left-sided heart failure, pulmonary emphysema, idiopathic pulmonary hypertension, congenital heart lesions, obstructive sleep apnea, chronic pulmonary emboli) and after pulmonary valvotomy.

Tricuspid stenosis. Tricuspid stenosis results from rheumatic valvulitis, congenital heart disease, and carcinoid tumors. Right atrial contraction against the stenotic valve orifice causes presystolic accentuation of the murmur and giant a-waves in neck veins. Impedance to right ventricular filling leads to elevated CVP (Fig. 8-41G). **The Murmur:** The diastolic murmur is low pitched and rumbling and has a presystolic crescendo when atrial fibrillation is absent. It is best heard with the bell lightly placed. When stenosis is mild, the murmur is late diastolic. With increasing severity, it is heard in mid and even early diastole. Increased venous return during inspiration accentuates the murmur. **Venous Pulse:** Giant a-waves are present. The CVP progressively increases as stenosis worsens. **Heart Sounds:** S1 is accentuated. Sometimes a tricuspid opening snap is identified. **Palpation:** The point of maximum intensity is sharply localized at the lower-left sternal border in the fourth or fifth interspace. In severe stenosis, signs of central venous congestion (elevated CVP, hepatomegaly, ascites, edema) are found, mimicking right ventricular failure. *DDX:* The murmur can usually be distinguished from that of mitral stenosis by its location and inspiratory accentuation. The diastolic rumble accompanying severe TR or a large ASD identical to the mid-diastolic rumble of tricuspid stenosis.

Mitral stenosis. In mild mitral stenosis ventricular filling is minimally delayed and the period of rapid filling shortens, resulting in a mid-diastolic murmur. With moderate or severe stenosis, ventricular filling is prolonged, so atrial systole increases the pressure gradient across the valve, producing a presystolic crescendo murmur. The accentuated S1 results from thickened but flexible leaflets. Pulmonary hypertension produces the accentuated P2. The opening snap is attributed to thickened but flexible leaflets, tethered at their commissures, bulging into the left ventricle when atrial pressure exceeds LV pressure; the snap is absent with immobile leaflets (Fig. 8-41E). **The Murmur:** This low-pitched rumbling murmur is heard best in the left lateral position near the apex. It is usually sharply localized, so the bell must be placed lightly directly on the apex. Sometimes, a loud murmur is discovered only by carefully inching the bell over the entire apex. In mild stenosis the murmur is middiastolic. As the orifice narrows, the murmur starts earlier and ends later, until it is almost pandiastolic. There is always a pause after S2 before the murmur begins. A long murmur often has a presystolic crescendo (Fig. 8-39G). **Heart Sounds:** S1 at the apex is accentuated if the thickened leaflets are mobile. If there is pulmonary hypertension, P2 is accentuated and occurs early but is still delayed by inspiration. When the murmur is loud, there is usually a mitral opening snap shortly after A2, heard best at the left sternal border between the second and fourth interspaces. This is commonly mistaken for a split S2. The opening snap disappears when the mitral cusps become calcified and rigid. **Palpation:** The murmur is often accompanied by a thrill at the apex in the left decubitus position. There is often a palpable right ventricular thrust indicating right ventricular hypertrophy. *DDX:* Tricuspid stenosis produces a similar murmur that is localized nearer the sternum. A similar diastolic apical rumble may be heard with increased mitral diastolic flow due to severe MR. The apical diastolic murmurs of aortic and pulmonic regurgitation have a blowing, not rumbling quality. Congenital stenosis is rare. Mitral stenosis nearly always results from rheumatic heart disease.

Aortic insufficiency. The Austin Flint or aortic insufficiency murmur is often associated with fluttering of the anterior mitral valve leaflet. However, neither this phenomenon nor others accompanying chronic aortic regurgitation seem consistently to correlate with this apical diastolic murmur. Authors vary on the criteria for diagnosis; the methods of Levine and Harvey are cited here. Some patients with severe AI and normal mitral valves have a murmur at the cardiac apex similar in pitch and timing to mitral stenosis. The examiner confronted with a combination of aortic and mitral murmurs must decide if the mitral valve is normal. AI is caused by rheumatic valvulitis, syphilis, or acute endocarditis. *DDX:* Accentuation of S1 or P2 favors organic mitral stenosis. The mitral valve opening snap is absent in the Flint murmur.

Continuous Murmurs: Murmurs heard throughout the cardiac cycle indicate turbulent flow occurs without interruption. Therefore, flow must be from a continuous high-pressure source to a low-pressure sump, e.g., from the aorta to the pulmonary artery or a vein, or across a fixed obstruction in the aorta.

Ductus arteriosus. A persistent ductus arteriosus is an arteriovenous fistula between the aorta and pulmonary artery (Fig. 8-41C) producing a continuous murmur throughout the heart cycle. The higher aortic pressure during ventricular systole increases the murmur's pitch. Uncorrected, the increased PA pressure leads to RVH and eventually right-to-left shunting with peripheral cyanosis confined to the lower extremities (*Eisenmenger physiology*). **The Murmur:** A murmur heard in the first and second left interspace throughout systole and diastole is usually caused by a persistent ductus. The murmur is medium pitched and rough, heard with the bell and diaphragm. Louder murmurs are harsh. There is typically a late systolic crescendo and a decrescendo after S2 producing a machinery murmur (Fig. 8-39F). Most frequently, transmission is to the interscapular region; occasionally it transmits down the left sternal border, sometimes to the apex. As pulmonary artery pressures approach aortic pressures, the murmur's diastolic portion may disappear. Pulmonary hypertension may lead to TR. Increased mitral flow can produce a diastolic rumble simulating mitral stenosis. **Heart Sounds:** S2 may be buried in the crescendo portion of the murmur. There is frequently a short pause between S1 and the murmur. **Palpation:** The precordial thrust of both ventricles can be accentuated. **Arterial Pulses:** With large shunts the peripheral pulse can have a collapsing quality like AI. *DDX:* Clubbing in the toes but sparing the fingers is seen with persistent right to left shunt in Eisenmenger physiology. The continuous murmur must be distinguished from a venous hum.

Coarctation of aorta. See Coarctation of the aorta, pages 329 and 368.

Coronary arteriovenous fistula and ruptured sinus of Valsalva aneurysm. These conditions present similarly with a continuous mid-precordial murmur; imaging is needed for differentiation. **The Murmur:** A continuous murmur with late systolic accentuation (machinery or to-and-fro) is audible on either or both sides of the lower sternum, often accompanied by a systolic or continuous thrill. *DDX:* Although the to-and-fro murmur has the same quality as that in ductus arteriosus, the location is sufficiently different to be distinctive. A mid-precordial to-and-fro murmur can occur with the combination of VSD and aortic regurgitation, but the quality of the systolic and diastolic components is distinct and there is no late systolic accentuation. Although a venous hum may be audible behind the upper sternum, its accentuation is diastolic, and it is abolished by pressure on the internal jugular vein.

Vascular Signs of Cardiac Activity: LV contraction maintains arterial blood pressure and produces palpable pulsations in all accessible arteries. Right atrial and ventricular contractions generate venous pulsations in the upper body. Because arterial pressure is normally ~16 times higher than CVP, arterial pulsations are palpable whereas venous pulsations are not. This is useful in determining the origin of visible pulsations.

Pulse contour and volume. The systolic arterial pressure contour is a function of aortic compliance, LV stroke volume, and the rate of flow from LV to aorta. These, in turn, are influenced by LV contractility and the size of the aortic valve orifice and LV outflow tract. The diastolic pressure contour reflects the run off during each cardiac cycle. The carotid pulse most accurately reflects the contour of the normal pulse contour and volume alterations are diagnostically significant.

Normal arterial pulse. The palpable primary wave is a swift upstroke to the peak systolic pressure, followed by a more gradual decline. A smaller upstroke caused by blood rebounding off the closed aortic valve, *the dicrotic wave*, occurs near the end of ventricular systole but is not usually palpable (Fig. 8-42A).

Twice peaking (dicrotic) pulses. There are two types of twice peaking arterial pulses (Fig. 8-42B). Most common is *pulsus bisferiens* with two palpable waves during systole. Less common is the *dicrotic pulse*, which has one wave palpable in systole and a second in diastole.

CLINICAL OCCURRENCE: Pulsus Bisferiens: Severe aortic regurgitation especially when associated with moderate aortic stenosis, hypertrophic subaortic stenosis, and hyperkinetic circulatory states, e.g., hyperthyroidism; Dicrotic Pulse: Very low cardiac output as with dilated cardiomyopathy or cardiac tamponade, especially in patients with normal aortic compliance.

Bounding or collapsing pulse (Corrigan pulse, water-hammer pulse). A large stroke volume and/or vigorous LV contraction generates a steep pulse upstroke followed by rapid decline as blood runs off from the aorta. With high pulse pressure the upstroke may be very sharp, whereas the down slope is precipitous (Fig. 8-42C). It may be accompanied by the pistol-shot sound. This is encountered in hyperthyroidism, anxiety, aortic regurgitation, persistent ductus arteriosus, and arteriovenous fistula.

Plateau pulse (pulsus tardus). Characteristic of severe aortic stenosis, the upstroke is gradual, and the peak delayed toward late systole (Fig. 8-42D). Carotid palpation reveals gentle, sustained lifting movements in contrast to the normal brief pulsatile tapping.

Absent pulses, pulseless disease. See Takayasu Aortitis, page 362.

Bigeminy (coupled rhythm). A normal beat is followed by a premature beat and a pause (Fig. 8-42F). If the premature beat occurs with a very short coupling interval so that ventricular filling is incomplete, it has a smaller stroke volume than the preceding normal beat and may not produce a palpable arterial pulsation and the radial pulse rate appears to be half the ventricular rate. This is detected by auscultating the rhythm over the precordium.

Pulsus alternans. Greater and lesser volume pulse waves alternate despite a normal rhythm and constant rate (Fig. 8-42E) signaling LV dysfunction. This may not be palpable but is detected while auscultating the blood pressure: as the cuff is slowly deflated every other beat becomes audible first, then, with further deflation, the rate appears to double as all beats are heard. *DDX:* This must be distinguished from bigeminal rhythm, in which a normal beat is followed by a premature beat.

Pulsus paradoxus. Normally, inspiration decreases intrathoracic pressure increasing venous blood flow into the chest and right ventricle, decreasing LV filling. The result is a small decrease in LV stroke volume and systolic blood pressure. In pericardial tamponade total heart volume (pericardial sac and chambers) is fixed. With inspiration the right heart volumes expand, bulging the septum leftward, resulting in further compromise of left heart volumes, exaggerating the fall in LV stroke volume and systolic arterial pressure. Labored breathing associated with exacerbations of obstructive airway disease also produces a paradoxical pulse. Under normal resting conditions the inspiratory fall in arterial systolic pressure is <10 mm Hg. A paradoxical pulse exists when inspiration creates a >10-mm-Hg drop in systolic arterial pressure. This is detected while auscultating blood pressure. Sometimes the exaggerated pulse volume swings can be palpated (Fig. 8-42G). Pericardial tamponade, pulmonary emphysema, and severe asthma are causes. *DDX:* In AV asynchrony pulse volume is variable so pulsus paradoxus cannot be accurately assessed.

Inequality of pulses. Disparity between right and left arterial pulse volumes is detected by simultaneous palpation and confirmed by taking the blood pressure at both sites. Arterial pressure differences between the arms must be interpreted cautiously: pressures not measured precisely simultaneously are >10 mm Hg different in up to 20% of normal individuals, whereas, when measured simultaneously by cuff, 5% or less show the same difference. Non-simultaneously measured systolic pressure differences of >10 mm Hg occur in almost 30% of hypertensive patients. Asymmetry suggests atherosclerosis, dissecting aneurysm or another arterial disease.

Dysrhythmias. See Chapter 4, page 57. Many dysrhythmias produce arterial beats of variable volume and disordered timing. Evaluate the disturbance from the precordial findings rather than the peripheral pulse. Ventricular contraction before the ventricle has had time to fill produces a peripheral pulse wave of diminished volume, or none at all. *The ECG, not palpation or auscultation, is the only way to accurately diagnose rhythm disturbances.*

Arterial Murmur or Bruit. Normal arteries are silent when auscultated. Turbulence is heard as a murmur and palpated as a thrill. Although murmur and bruit are literally synonymous, there is a tendency to reserve bruit for arterial sounds. The presence of a bruit does not necessarily indicate limited flow. Arteries become tortuous from arteriosclerosis or other circumstances and dilate with aneurysm. They may be constricted congenitally, by intimal proliferation, or by an atherosclerotic plaque. Dilated thyroid arteries with increased blood flow occur in Graves disease (here, the word bruit is often used). Blood flow through an arteriovenous fistula or large arterial collaterals, as in aortic coarctation, often produces bruits. A continuous murmur is produced by an arteriovenous fistula or a partially obstructed artery when the collateral circulation is poor, and the diastolic pressure is low distal to the obstruction.

Carotid bruit. Most of the blood flow to the brain and virtually all to the cerebral cortex comes through the internal carotid arteries. Despite collateral flow through the circle of Willis from the contralateral carotid and vertebrobasilar system, high-grade obstruction of one common and/or internal carotid artery is associated with high risk of disabling stroke. The neck should always be auscultated for bruits, and bruits should be evaluated by imaging. The degree of stenosis cannot be estimated by physical exam. Symptoms of cerebral ischemia in the distribution of the affected artery are associated with a substantial risk for stroke within hours to days.

Arterial sound—pistol-shot sound. This is produced by an arterial pulse wave front of higher than normal pulse pressure striking the arterial wall in the region being auscultated. When the stethoscope bell is placed lightly over an artery, particularly the femoral, a sharp sound like a gunshot is heard. Although commonly associated with aortic regurgitation, it also occurs in other conditions with high pulse pressure, e.g., hyperthyroidism and anemia.

Duroziez sign. Compressing the femoral artery with the stethoscope bell produces eddies and a systolic bruit. Continue listening while pressure on the bell is gradually increased. If, with further pressure a point is reached where a second murmur becomes audible, it is Duroziez sign. Most commonly encountered in severe aortic regurgitation, it occurs in other conditions with a high pulse pressure (Chapter 4, page 68). The second murmur is associated with an exaggerated forward acceleration of blood flow.

Venous signs of cardiac action. Cardiac action produces signs in the venous system by altering peripheral venous pressure and pulse contour and by producing venous congestion in the viscera.

Elevated CVP. Elevated CVP indicates overfilling of the intravascular space exceeding venous capacitance and/or impedance to filling of the right atrium or right ventricle. Impedance to right ventricular filling is often due to impaired outflow from the right ventricle causing elevated right ventricular end-diastolic pressure. When the venous pressure exceeds 10–12 cm of water under resting conditions, it is considered elevated. *DDX:* A generalized increase in venous pressure must be distinguished from SVC and/or IVC obstruction. Always assess whether the venous pressure appears uniformly elevated above and below the diaphragm; it must be if the *CVP* is elevated. Absence of signs below the diaphragm suggests SVC obstruction [Cook DJ, Simel DL. The rational clinical examination. Does this patient have abnormal central venous pressure? *JAMA.* 1996;275:630–634].

CLINICAL OCCURRENCE: Overfilling of the Vascular Space: Kidney failure, rapid infusion of fluids and blood products, chronic CHF with edema; Impedance to Right Heart Filling: Tricuspid stenosis or regurgitation, pericardial tamponade, constrictive pericarditis; Impaired Right Ventricular Outflow: Pulmonary hypertension, pulmonary embolus, pulmonic stenosis, right ventricular infarction.

Diminished venous pressure. This occurs in peripheral circulatory failure in the shock syndrome, usually associated with intravascular hypovolemia, diminished venous tone, and/or peripheral pooling. The peripheral veins are collapsed with the patient supine. See the discussion of Hypotension, Chapter 4, page 67.

Giant a-waves—tricuspid stenosis. See page 332.

Cannon a-waves. Right atrial contraction against a closed tricuspid valve produces retrograde ejection of blood into the central venous channels. Intermittent prominent venous pulsations are visible in the neck veins, *cannon a-waves.* They are identified as a-waves, since they are asynchronous with the apical impulse and carotid upstroke. They are easily obliterated by gentle pressure at the base of the neck insufficient to diminish the carotid pulse. *DDX:* Irregular cannon a-waves suggest that some atrial contractions are occurring simultaneously with ventricular contraction. A regular pattern of cannon a-waves suggests a fixed pattern of AV block, e.g., atrial flutter with 2:1 block. An irregular pattern with variable a-wave volume suggests AV dissociation, e.g., complete heart block. *An ECG is required to diagnose the rhythm.* Regular giant a-waves occurring consistently in synchrony with the heart sounds and arterial pulse suggests impedance to right atrial outflow, e.g., a noncompliant right ventricle or tricuspid stenosis.

Large v-waves in the venous pulse—TR. Tricuspid insufficiency allows the right ventricle to eject blood retrogradely into the central venous channels. Large v-waves are visible in the jugular veins and may be palpable as liver pulsation. The waves are v-waves since they are synchronous with the apical impulse and carotid upstroke.

Kussmaul sign and hepatojugular reflux. The right heart's inability to accommodate increased venous return gives rise to these signs. Position the patient so the jugular blood column is just visible above the clavicle. *Kussmaul sign* is present if the venous column doesn't collapse during inspiration. Next, with the patient breathing normally, place the right hand on the right upper abdominal quadrant pressing firmly upward under the costal margin for ≥10–15 seconds. *Hepatojugular reflux* is present if the jugular venous column rises and persists while abdominal pressure continues. Hepatojugular reflux is most commonly seen with early right heart failure. Both are seen with severe right heart failure, constrictive pericarditis, and right ventricular infarction.

Arterial Circulation Signs: Decreased arterial blood flow causes skin pallor, coldness, and tissue atrophy. Small-vessel pathology is often recognizable by cutaneous manifestations (page 288 and Chapter 6, page 127). Diseases affecting small arteries and arterioles, e.g., vasculitis, tend to be diffuse. Diseases of larger vessels cause regional hypoperfusion.

Warm skin. Normal skin temperature indicates adequate arterial flow. Normal nailbed color is red or pink.

Sharply demarcated warm and cool, pallid digits. Raynaud Syndrome. Raynaud syndrome occurs as the result of severe cutaneous arterial spasm most commonly in the fingers but may also occur in the ears, nose and toes. The primary manifestations are sharply demarcated cyanosis followed by pallor and numbness and painful parasthesias involving the affected area. As vasospasm resolves over minutes to hours, the skin may become erythematous and the pain intensifies before resolving. Raynaud's syndrome may occur idiopathically or secondarily in autoimmune disease and is often provoked by exposure to cold or emotional distress.

Atheroembolic disease. Embolization of cholesterol-rich atheroma to the small arteries produces hemorrhagic cutaneous infarcts and livedo.

Palpable purpura—vasculitis. See Leukocytoclastic Vasculitis, page 363.

Skin pallor and coldness—chronic arterial obstruction. Chronic progressive arterial obstruction induces collateral circulation and tissue accommodation to ischemia. Pallid cool skin strongly suggests regional hypoperfusion. It is normal in a cold environment but should rapidly resolve on exposure to warm air or water. Failure to do so suggests that the problem is not limited to the skin vessels but involves a major trunk artery. Pain may be present with exertion (*claudication*). The distribution of the arterial deficit depends upon the site of obstruction and the presence and extent of collateral circulation. Other useful signs are prolonged venous filling time, abnormal pedal pulses and a femoral bruit. Atherosclerosis is most common; less common causes are large vessel vasculitis (Takayasu aortitis, giant cell arteritis), Buerger disease, vasospastic disorders, and ergotism.

Dependent rubor and coldness—chronic arterial obstruction. See Examination of the Arterial Circulation in the Extremities, page 287, and Chronic extremity peripheral vascular disease, page 374.

Acute pain, skin pallor, and coolness—arterial embolus or thrombosis. Acute occlusion of a major peripheral artery resulting in cutaneous and muscular ischemia produces skin and nailbed pallor, cool skin, and ischemic pain. The pain is severe and not relieved by changing position. Embolic arterial occlusion is most common in native vessels, whereas thrombus is more common in prosthetic vascular channels. Urgent relief of obstruction is necessary to preserve the part. See acute extremity artery obstruction, page 374. The heart is the most common source of emboli (endocarditis, prosthetic valve, atrial fibrillation). Less commonly, an embolus arises from thrombus within an aortic aneurysm or paradoxical embolism via a patent foramen ovale.

Nodular vessels—polyarteritis nodosa. See page 362.

CHEST, CARDIOVASCULAR, AND RESPIRATORY SYNDROMES

Chest Wall Syndromes.

Chest pain intensified by respiratory motion. Pain accentuated by breathing, coughing, laughing, or sneezing usually indicates inflammation or injury to the ribs, cartilages, muscles, nerves, and pleurae of the chest wall. The specific area may also be tender. See Chest Wall Pain with Tenderness, page 301, as there is significant overlap between these categories.

Pleuritis and pleurisy. The parietal pleura has sensory fibers from the intercostal nerves that also give off twigs to the skin. The visceral pleura is anesthetic. Pleural pain is caused either by stretching of the inflamed parietal pleura or by separation of fibrous adhesions between two pleural surfaces. It is doubtful that pain is produced by the pleural surfaces rubbing together as pain often occurs without a friction rub and a rub is often present without pain. Pleural inflammation (*pleuritis*) produces knife-like shooting chest wall pain intensified by breathing, coughing, and laughing. Listen and palpate for a friction rub. Rubs are not constant, so frequently repeat the exam. Pleural effusion may develop. The diagnosis of *pleurisy* is made from the typical pain or the presence of a friction rub after excluding other causes of pleuritis, rib fractures, myositis, and neuritis. Pleurisy and a rub may precede radiographic evidence of pneumonia. Common causes of pleurisy include bacterial and viral pneumonia, tuberculosis, empyema, viral pleuritis, pulmonary infarction from embolus, mesothelioma, primary and metastatic lung neoplasm, and connective tissue diseases.

Diaphragmatic pleuritis and pleurisy. The peripheral diaphragmatic pleura is supplied by the fifth and sixth intercostal nerves so pain is felt near the costal margins. The central diaphragm (thoracic and peritoneal) is innervated by the phrenic nerve (C3–4), which also innervates the neck and supraclavicular

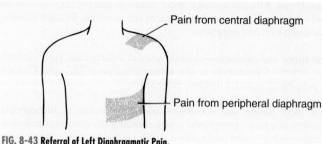

FIG. 8-43 Referral of Left Diaphragmatic Pain.

fossae. Thus, pain in the neck and supraclavicular region may result from irritation of the diaphragmatic pleura (Fig. 8-43). There is sharp shooting pain intensified by deep breathing, coughing, or laughing. Pain may be localized along the costal margins, epigastrium, lumbar region, or neck at the superior border of the trapezius or supraclavicular fossa, always on the same side. A pleural or pericardial friction rub may be present. *DDX:* The diagnosis of pleurisy is suggested when pain is accompanied by fever and a friction rub. Pleural effusion may appear later. A history of dysphagia, nausea or intraabdominal disease suggests disorders of the esophagus, pancreatitis, subphrenic abscess, peptic ulcer, splenic infarction or splenic rupture. Hiatal hernia can produce similar pain. Pericarditis with pleuritic pain (*pleuropericarditis*) should be considered.

Epidemic pleurodynia (Bornholm disease, devil's grip). Infection with group B coxsackievirus is a common cause. After a nonspecific prodrome, the patient is suddenly seized with sharp, knife-like thoracic or abdominal pain, intensified by breathing and movement, and accompanied by fever. The chest may be splinted, and the thighs flexed on the belly. Paroxysms of intense pain are separated by intervals of complete comfort. Cases are sporadic or epidemic. Mild pharyngitis and myalgias with tenderness of the neck, trunk, and limbs may be present. A friction rub is detected in 25% of cases. The sudden retrosternal pain suggests MI or dissecting aneurysm.

Chest wall twinge syndrome (precordial catch). The patient experiences brief episodes of nonexertional sharp pain or "catches" in the anterior chest, usually on the left side. Some patients report onset while bending over. The pains last from seconds to minutes and are aggravated by deep breathing and relieved by shallow respirations. The cause is unknown. The condition is common and harmless.

Rib fracture, periosteal hematoma, periostitis, intercostal myositis. See page 301.

Respiratory Syndromes.
Pneumothorax. Spontaneous rupture of a subpleural bleb, penetrating chest trauma and medical procedures may allow air to enter the pleural space

separating the lung and chest wall leading to failure of respiratory mechanics and lung collapse. Large sudden pneumothoraces may be accompanied by dyspnea and severe chest pain that is often unilateral but poorly localized. Vital sign changes are proportional to the degree of collapse and concurrent cardiopulmonary disease and include tachypnea, tachycardia and hypotension. With a large pneumothorax, the physical signs are distinctive: hyperresonant percussion, markedly diminished or absent fremitus, voice transmission, and breath sounds on the affected side, and tracheal deviation away from the affected side (page 311). Respiratory rib movements are decreased with persistent expiratory distention of the hemithorax. When tension pneumothorax develops, hemodynamic shock may occur within minutes and urgent diagnosis and treatment are necessary to prevent death. With a small pneumothorax, the only sign may be decreased breath sounds. On chest X-ray, lung markings are absent and often the visceral pleura is seen as a line. On thoracic ultrasound, pneumothorax is detected by noting the absence of sliding pleura and normal ultrasound reverberation through in the lung tissue. Tension pneumothorax is a hemodynamic diagnosis and when suspected must be managed prior to obtaining confirmatory X-rays.

CLINICAL OCCURRENCE: Pneumothorax results from rupture of a pleural bleb in pulmonary emphysema, and, occasionally, from inflammatory lung disease, such as sarcoidosis, fibrosis, or silicosis. Primary spontaneous pneumothorax is most often described in slender, healthy young persons with no discernible pulmonary lesion. Alveolar and pleural inflammation and necrosis secondary to septic embolism in bacterial endocarditis or *pneumocystis jiroveci* infection in HIV/AIDS may cause pneumothorax. Puncture of the lung by a fractured rib is the most common traumatic cause. In hospital-based settings, pneumothorax may be secondary to complications of mechanical ventilation (barotrauma), as well as procedural complications during central venous catheter placement, pacemaker insertion and lung biopsy procedures. The differential diagnosis of the sudden pain, dyspnea and hemodynamic changes must be distinguished from PE, MI, and acute pericarditis.

Acute bronchitis. Acute infection is usually viral, an atypical organism being less common. Airway inflammation produces persistent cough often with retrosternal burning pain. Fever is absent. Secretions in the bronchi and trachea produce rhonchi and, occasionally, wheezing. Secretions high in the trachea produce rhonchi that are heard throughout the thorax. The cough may be unproductive or tenacious, mucoid sputum may be raised. Usually, the airways are unimpaired so breath sounds are normal. *DDX:* Influenza, parainfluenza, and RSV are common. Chest X-ray is normal.

Pneumonia. Lung infection and inflammation are labelled pneumonitis or pneumonia. The process may be limited to the airways and alveolar airspaces or involve the pulmonary interstitium and vascular channels. The diagnostic challenges are to separate infectious from noninfectious pneumonia and then to identify the specific etiology. Key patient factors that determine risk for pneumonia as well as likely pathogens include immune status, age, tobacco use, inhalational exposures and preexisting lung disease. Onset is sudden or gradual, depending upon the etiology. Patients present with cough, dyspnea, fatigue, and, especially with infection, high fever, often with rigors. Physical findings range from minimal signs of airspace disease (bronchophony, whispered pectoriloquy) to respiratory failure with multilobar consolidation. Infectious pneumonia is separated into community-acquired and hospital-healthcare-associated categories. The approach to diagnosing specific etiologies of pneumonia is beyond the scope of this text.

CLINICAL OCCURRENCE: *Congenital:* Pulmonary sequestration (may be confused with pneumonia on chest X-ray); *Degenerative/Idiopathic:* Idiopathic interstitial pneumonia, eosinophilic pneumonia, alveolar proteinosis; *Infectious:* Bacterial, viral, tuberculosis, nontuberculous mycobacteria, rickettsia, fungi, Nocardia, pneumocystis, parasites; *Inflammatory/Immune:* Hypersensitivity pneumonitis, vasculitis, lymphomatoid granulomatosis, Goodpasture syndrome, lipoid pneumonia, collagen vascular diseases; *Mechanical/Traumatic:* Aspiration, lung contusion; *Metabolic/Toxic:* Inhalational injury, drug reactions, pneumoconioses; *Neoplastic:* Endobronchial neoplasm with post-obstructive infection, bronchioloalveolar cell carcinoma; *Vascular:* Vasculitis (Churg-Strauss, granulomatosis with polyangiitis).

- *Severe acute respiratory syndrome (SARS) and middle east respiratory syndrome (MARS).* Infection with coronaviruses cause severe lung inflammation leading to hypoxia and respiratory failure. The SARS outbreak in 2003 originated in China and spread rapidly but was controlled. In 2012 a different coronavirus causing the same syndrome was identified in Saudi Arabia and the Near East and entered the US in 2014. An initial flu-like illness is followed rapidly progressing pneumonia. The case fatality rate is high. Spread is by droplets. To make the diagnosis, a high index of suspicion is necessary with careful questioning about contact with infected or potentially infected people and travel to known areas of ongoing transmission. Current information is available at the Centers for Disease Control web site, www.cdc.gov.

Aspiration pneumonia. Aspiration of oral secretions, food, or regurgitated stomach contents causes mechanical airway obstruction with secondary inflammation (especially with low-pH gastric contents) and secondary infection often with anaerobic oral flora. The right middle and apical segment of the right lower lobe are commonly affected. Aspiration is common in association with impaired consciousness or swallowing. Coughing with meals and nocturnal regurgitation with cough and dyspnea suggest chronic aspiration. Necrotizing anaerobic infections lead to lung abscess with fetid sputum. Aspiration should be suspected when a patient presenting with pneumonia has a history of impaired consciousness or oropharyngeal neurologic dysfunction.

Lung abscess. Necrotizing organisms destroy lung tissue creating cavities with low oxygen tension, ideal for growth of microaerophilic or anaerobic organisms. A history compatible with aspiration is often present. The sputum is scant to intermittently copious, purulent, and foul smelling. Signs of consolidation may be present. If the cavity communicates with a bronchus and is only partially filled amphoric breath sounds may be heard (see Fig. 8-34, page 308). A fungus ball occurs when an old abscess cavity is colonized with *Aspergillus*.

Bronchopleural fistula with empyema. Bronchopleural communication is caused by an empyema draining through a bronchus or a lung abscess eroding into the pleural space. The presentation is chronic cough producing a large volume of purulent sputum. Sudden entry of pus into the pleural space produces severe prostration, chills, fever, and/or shock. Dullness with absent breath sounds in the lower hemithorax and a resonant region above—the whole devoid of breath sounds—suggests the diagnosis. A succussion splash may be heard.

- **Pulmonary embolism.** A dislodged deep vein thrombus (DVT) passes through the RA and RV into the pulmonary circulation. Large emboli obstruct the main pulmonary artery at its bifurcation or one of its branches producing acute pulmonary hypertension which in turn causes right ventricular pressure overload and RV failure with cardiogenic shock. Lung infarction initiates local inflammation. Ventilation–perfusion mismatching and intrapulmonary shunts cause hypoxia. DVT develops after surgery (particularly total hip and knee replacement), prolonged bed rest and air travel, immobilization, and venous stasis. Thrombophilia (factor-V Leiden, prothrombin gene mutations, antiphospholipid syndrome, protein C or S deficiency, mucinous adenocarcinomas, estrogens, pregnancy, etc.) increases DVT risk. Less-commonly embolized material are fat (from the marrow of fractured bones), air, amniotic fluid (when the fluid contains meconium, it is especially dangerous), and tumor tissue. Patients may be minimally symptomatic or present with sudden dyspnea, chest pain, and circulatory failure. *Symptoms:* Sudden dyspnea, with or without pain or tachypnea, is the key symptom. The pain is either pleuritic or a deep, crushing sensation in the six-dermatome band. Sometimes painless dyspnea resembles asthma because of the release of serotonin from platelets in the blood clot. Massive pulmonary embolus presents as syncope without other symptoms. *Signs:* Systemic effects (weakness, prostration, sweating, nausea, and vomiting) may predominate. Tachycardia is nearly always present. Fever occurs with infarction. Dyspnea, tachypnea, and cyanosis can be extreme. Hemoptysis, a pleural friction rub, and bloody pleural effusion strongly support PE with infarction. Massive infarction is indicated by shock, jaundice, and right-sided heart failure. A loud P2 and palpable precordial RV thrust indicate pulmonary hypertension. Sudden death is not uncommon. Occasionally, PE is accompanied by abdominal rigidity because the diaphragm is splinting adjacent to infarcted lung. A high index of suspicion is necessary to aggressively pursue the diagnosis as the next embolus may be fatal. Chronic recurrent pulmonary emboli lead to pulmonary arterial hypertension. *DDX:* Sudden onset of chest pain and/or dyspnea, tachypnea, or unexplained sinus tachycardia should raise the question of PE with or without infarction. The symptoms and signs may suggest asthma, bronchopneumonia, pleurisy, pericarditis, spontaneous pneumothorax, MI, acute pancreatitis, or perforated peptic ulcer.

Sleep-disordered breathing—obstructive and central sleep apnea. Sleep-disordered breathing results from either mechanical obstruction by redundant, lax oropharyngeal soft tissues (*obstructive sleep apnea*) or from decreased medullary respiratory drive (*central sleep apnea*). Hypoventilation and hypoxia at night produce frequent arousals, disrupting effective sleep. Patients are often, but not always, obese. They have daytime hypersomnolence and irritability and frequently have morning headaches and hypertension. Snoring is prominent but may not have been noted by the patient so history from the bed partner is critical. In prolonged disease, hypertension and fatigue or depression may be severe. Chronic nocturnal hypoxia leads to pulmonary hypertension and right heart failure. Physical risk factors for obstructive apnea are enlarged tongue, thickened oropharyngeal soft tissues (Mallampati score 3 or 4, Chapter 7, page 231) or neck circumference >43 cm (17 inches) in men or >40.5 cm (16 inches) in women.

Chronic cough. Patients present with chronic irritating cough and normal physical findings. Ninety percent of cases are caused by chronic postnasal drip, unsuspected asthma, and/or gastroesophageal reflux; evaluation for each is required. Angiotensin-converting enzyme inhibitors also cause chronic cough, which may begin months after starting the medication.

Pleural effusion. See page 308.

Lung cancer. Most primary lung cancers result from cigarette smoking or exposure to ionizing radiation. Patients present with symptoms and signs related to the chest (cough, hemoptysis, dyspnea, pneumonia, pleural effusion), regional symptoms (lymphadenopathy, SVC syndrome, brain mass), or systemic symptoms (weight loss, weakness, hypercalcemia, hyponatremia). Endobronchial lesions present as recurrent or slowly resolving pneumonia or atelectasis. *Bronchioloalveolar cell carcinoma* presents with cough, hypoxia, and diffuse infiltrates, often mistaken for infection. *Superior sulcus tumors* (neoplasms in the pulmonary apex, the upper mediastinum, or the superior thoracic aperture) produce *Pancoast syndrome* with severe neck, shoulder or arm pain.

Pulmonary edema. LV failure, mitral regurgitation, or acute lung injury result in interstitial pulmonary edema and alveolar flooding. An acute increase in LV end-diastolic pressure is transmitted across the mitral valve to the left atrium and pulmonary veins. Increased hydrostatic pressure in the pulmonary capillaries causes transudation of fluid into the pulmonary interstitium and subsequently the alveoli. Increased fluid in the lung decreases pulmonary compliance producing shortness of breath and cough. Alveolar flooding causes hypoxia and extreme respiratory distress. Severe dyspnea is accompanied by crackles, rhonchi, and gurgles throughout the lungs. Breathing is labored, with cyanosis and frothy sputum, often pink, occasionally bloody. Percussion is resonant, and auscultation reveals bubbling crackles and sometimes wheezes. *DDX:* In chronic heart failure pulmonary edema is often relapsing making the diagnosis obvious. It may occur suddenly with acute MI, especially with papillary muscle rupture and flail mitral valve leaflet. Occasionally, paroxysmal nocturnal dyspnea in cardiac patients closely resembles asthma with prolonged expiration and wheezing.

CLINICAL OCCURRENCE: *Degenerative/Idiopathic:* High altitude; *Infectious:* Hantavirus pulmonary syndrome; *Inflammatory/Immune:* Mismatched blood transfusion, hypertransfusion syndrome, SLE; *Mechanical/Traumatic:* LV failure-systolic and diastolic dysfunction (MI, cardiomyopathies, tachy- and bradyarrhythmias), mitral stenosis, mitral and aortic insufficiency (especially acute), PE, head trauma; *Metabolic/Toxic:* Acute lung injury (inhalation of noxious gases, aspiration, radiation, hemorrhagic pancreatitis, sepsis, drugs, fresh water drowning, etc.), intravascular heroin, snakebite; *Neoplastic:* Bronchioloalveolar cell carcinoma (not pulmonary edema, but may appear similar radiographically), lymphangitic carcinoma or lymphoma; *Neurologic:* Postictal, head trauma, subarachnoid hemorrhage; *Vascular:* Severe hypertension, intravascular volume overload (crystalloid, colloid, transfusions, kidney failure), subarachnoid hemorrhage.

Interstitial lung disease. Inflammation with cellular infiltration, interstitial edema, and/or collagen deposition thickens the alveolar walls and septa, decreases lung compliance, reduces lung volume, and impairs gas exchange. Inflammation may involve the entire alveolus. Granulomas, characteristic of some diseases, are diagnostically important. Patients present with chronic nonproductive cough and dyspnea. Thorough occupational and avocational exposure histories are critical to identifying respiratory irritants, toxins, and allergens. Physical exam shows resonant percussion, decreased breath sounds, and crackles of varying intensity, often at end-inspiration and usually most prominent at the bases. Chest X-ray shows increased interstitial markings, with or without alveolar signs. High-resolution CT may be diagnostic with characteristic patterns for specific entities.

  CLINICAL OCCURRENCE: *Congenital:* Tuberous sclerosis, neurofibromatosis, Niemann–Pick disease, Gaucher disease; *Degenerative/Idiopathic:* Idiopathic interstitial pneumonia (usual interstitial pneumonia), desquamative interstitial pneumonia, respiratory bronchiolitis-associated interstitial lung disease, acute interstitial pneumonia, cryptogenic organizing pneumonia, nonspecific interstitial pneumonia; after acute respiratory distress syndrome, radiation; lymphangioleiomyomatosis, amyloidosis, *Inflammatory/Immune:* Connective tissue diseases (SLE, RA, ankylosing spondylitis, systemic sclerosis, CREST syndrome [calcinosis cutis, Raynaud phenomenon, esophageal motility disorder, sclerodactyly, and telangiectasia], Sjögren syndrome, polymyositis–dermatomyositis) eosinophilic pneumonia, antibasement membrane disease (Goodpasture), idiopathic pulmonary hemosiderosis, graft-versus-host disease, with gastrointestinal or liver disease (Crohn disease, ulcerative colitis, primary biliary cirrhosis, chronic active hepatitis); *Metabolic/Toxic:* Inhaled substances (asbestosis, fumes and gases, aspiration pneumonia); with granulomas (hypersensitivity pneumonitis—organic dusts, e.g., farmer's lung, inorganic dusts—beryllium, silica); Drugs (antibiotics, amiodarone, gold, bleomycin, and other chemotherapy agents).

Hypersensitivity pneumonitis. Exposure to organic dusts at work or home elicits a chronic inflammatory response which can progress to irreversible fibrosis. Careful history is the key to diagnosis. Patients present with cough, shortness of breath, and increasing dyspnea, often with airflow obstruction on exposure to the agent. Exam may be normal or reveal crackles and wheezes.

Pulmonary-renal syndromes. There are antibodies to basement membrane in the glomerulus and pulmonary capillaries (Goodpasture), or vasculitis involving the lung and glomeruli (granulomatosis with polyangiitis) each causing pulmonary inflammation and/or hemorrhage and acute kidney injury. Goodpasture syndrome often presents acutely with dyspnea, hemoptysis, and cough. Granulomatosis with polyangiitis (Wegener) may be acute or subacute. Limited forms of both occur. Prompt diagnosis and treatment is required to preserve kidney function.

Sarcoidosis. Noncaseating granulomatous inflammation involves many organs singly or in combination. The cause is unknown. The lungs and hilar and mediastinal lymph nodes are most commonly affected. Patients may be asymptomatic or present with nonproductive cough and dyspnea accompanied by fever, malaise, weight loss, and night sweats. Lung exam is normal or shows crackles. Hepatosplenomegaly, lymphadenopathy, uveitis, cutaneous plaques, and salivary gland enlargement are other manifestations.

Hepatopulmonary syndrome. Pulmonary arteriovenous shunts enlarge with standing leading to decreased oxygen saturation (*orthodeoxia*) and shortness of breath. The cause appears to be circulating vasodilators usually metabolized in the liver. Patients have advanced liver disease with portal hypertension and portosystemic shunting, with or without cirrhosis. They complain of shortness of breath and weakness with standing and may become visibly cyanotic when upright. Symptoms are often relieved by sitting and always by lying down. Patients may become unable to sit or stand for any length of time. Physical exam shows stigmata of chronic liver disease including spider angiomata and ascites. Diagnosis is by bubble contrast echocardiography showing contrast in the left atrium in more than three but less than seven cardiac cycles.

Tracheal or bronchial obstruction. Complete obstruction of the trachea is incompatible with life. Partial obstruction by a foreign body, neoplasm, or other plug produces forceful prolonged inspiratory effort with retraction of the intercostal spaces, suprasternal notch, supraclavicular fossae, and epigastrium. A low-pitched rhonchus or stridor, may be heard over the chest and at the opened mouth during inspiration and expiration. In a ball-valve obstruction the rhonchus occurs only during inspiration or expiration. An isolated wheeze suggests a localized bronchial obstruction by bronchial adenoma, carcinoma, or foreign body. *Bagpipe sign*, another indication of partial bronchial obstruction, is an expiratory sound persisting after a short a forced expiration is abruptly stopped. If the obstructive rhonchus is heard on both sides of the chest, the affected side is the one with the palpable rhonchus. In obstruction of a large bronchus, trachea swings toward the affected side during inspiration and away from it with expiration. A moving foreign body can cause an audible slap with coughing or breathing. Slowly developing bronchial obstruction may be asymptomatic, but sudden obstruction causes severe dyspnea. Higher-pitched rhonchi arise from smaller bronchi. Causes of large airway obstruction include aspirated foreign bodies, intraluminal benign neoplasms (bronchial adenoma, amyloidoma), malignant neoplasm, relapsing polychondritis, extrinsic compression from mediastinal masses (retrosternal goiter, neoplasms, teratoma), laryngeal mass or paralysis, and tracheomalacia following prolonged endotracheal intubation.

Chronic obstructive pulmonary diseases. Expiratory airflow obstruction is the hallmark of asthma and chronic obstructive lung disease (COPD). In asthma the obstruction is initially fully reversible and may be either fixed or partially reversible in COPD. Air trapping increases residual volume sustaining an inspiratory chest position (flat diaphragm, horizontal ribs, increased anterior–posterior diameter, hyperresonance) which increases the work of breathing and decreases inspiratory capacity. The combination of history, physical signs, chest radiographic features, and pulmonary function testing allow differentiation.

Asthma. Asthma is an acquired syndrome of increased airway responsiveness to allergic and nonallergic stimuli resulting in airway inflammation, hyperplasia of mucous-producing goblet cells, and bronchial smooth muscle hypertrophy. All of these features decrease airway diameter and airflow resistance. Airflow obstruction affects exhalation more significantly secondary to the decrease in airway size during normal exhalation. Airway obstruction leads to air trapping and lung hyperinflation because of this differential effect on exhalation flows and exhaled lung volumes compared to inhalation. Active disease may be subclinical and asymptomatic patients may have significant airway inflammation. Between attacks, the patient is well, and the chest exam is normal. Asthma exacerbations begin with nonproductive cough and progressive dyspnea. Nocturnal awaking with coughing and chest tightness is common. Sitting and leaning over a table or chair back improves the dyspnea. The respiratory rate does not increase initially, but inspiration is short while expiration is prolonged and labored. The patient is often anxious. As air trapping flattens the diaphragm, the chest becomes hyperresonant maintaining an inspiratory position. During inspiration, the costal margins diverge only slightly or converge. In severe asthma attacks, the sternocleidomastoid and platysma muscles tense and the alae nasi flare with each inspiratory effort. Wheezing becomes less prominent as airway narrowing worsens. Auscultation discloses decreased air movement, wheezes, and coarse crackles. Localized absence of breath sounds suggests bronchial plugging. As the attack subsides, clear tenacious sputum is raised, and breathing gradually becomes less labored. Asthma can occur without wheezing. The only sign that consistently identifies severe asthma exacerbation is use of the accessory muscles of respiration. Severity is assessed by clinical history and bedside or home airflow measurements (Table 8-1). **DDX:** Wheezing occurs in acute bronchitis, without the labored respiration. When wheezing is limited to a single region, bronchial obstruction from foreign body or neoplasm must be considered. The sudden occurrence of LV failure or MR may closely simulate asthma with wheezes and crackles, and labored breathing may limit heart auscultation. Vocal cord dysfunction (i.e., paradoxical closure of the cords during inspiration) is suggested by wheezing that is loudest over the neck and is diagnosed by examining the glottis during an attack. The symptoms and signs of asthma are often relieved by inhaled bronchodilators. Spirometry confirms reversible airway obstruction.

Emphysema. Smoking, and rarely alpha-1 antitrypsin deficiency, lead to destruction of alveolar walls with loss of alveolar surface area. Decreased elastic recoil leads to expiratory collapse of terminal airways. Patients present with progressive dyspnea over months to years, often accompanied by gradual weight loss. At end-stage, patients often exhale against pursed lips, especially with exertion, the chest is hyperresonant, breath sounds are decreased and

TABLE 8-1 Asthma Clinical Severity Classification.

| Asthma Severity | Symptoms | | FEV_1; Peak Expiratory Flow Variability |
	Day	Night	
Mild intermittent	2 or less d/wk	2 or less nights/mo	$\geq$80; <20%
Mild persistent	>2 d/wk	>2 nights/mo	$\geq$80; 20%–30%
Moderate persistent	Daily	>1 night/wk	60%–79%; >30%
Severe persistent	Continual	Frequent	<60%; >30%

TABLE 8-2 Gold Criteria for COPD Severity.

Stage	Severity	FEV1 (% Predicted)	FEV_1/FVC
I	Mild	$\geq$80	<0.7
II	Moderate	<80	<0.7
III	Severe	<50	<0.7
IV	Very severe	<30 or <50 with respiratory failure or right heart failure	<0.7

exhalation is prolonged, (page 311). Wheezes and crackles are uncommon unless infection supervenes. Physical findings correlate poorly with the severity of airflow obstruction or abnormalities of gas exchange. Spirometry detects early obstructive airways disease. Severity is assigned using the Gold system (Table 8-2). Alpha-1 antitrypsin deficiency also produces liver disease that can dominate the presentation.

Chronic bronchitis. Chronic inflammation and secondary airway infection results from chronic exposure to tobacco smoke or indoor air pollution such as smoke from coal or wood-fired cooking stoves. Airways obstruction is prominent, and hypoxia is common. Patients with chronic bronchitis, with or without bronchiectasis, present with chronic cough productive of purulent sputum and progressive dyspnea. The clinical diagnosis is established when the cough is productive of sputum for over 3 months duration for two consecutive years. The lungs have diminished breath sounds and prolonged expiration and may have wheezing and inspiratory crackles. Physical findings correlate poorly with the severity of airflow obstruction or abnormalities of gas exchange and spirometry is required to confirm the diagnosis.

Bronchiectasis. Severe acute or chronic pulmonary infections damage the walls of small bronchi producing multiple chronically infected dilatations. Presentation is cough with purulent sputum and occasional hemoptysis or recurrent pneumonia. Sputum is copious and purulent. A resonant chest with coarse basilar crackles suggests bronchiectasis. Clubbing may be present. Chronic infection with nontuberculous mycobacteria is common. High-resolution CT imaging is diagnostic.

Churg–Strauss disease. See page 363.

Lymphomatoid granulomatosis. A variegated array of lymphatic cells, atypical lymphocytoid, plasmacytoid, and reticuloendothelial cells invade tissues and vessels. Nodules of varying size are found in the lungs, skin, kidneys, and central nervous system, usually sparing the spleen, lymph nodes, and bone marrow. In contrast to granulomatosis with polyangiitis (Wegener), the lung is always involved while the upper respiratory tract is usually spared. Transition to malignant lymphoma is common.

Cardiovascular Syndromes: Proper assessment of heart disease patients requires identifying the etiology, anatomic abnormalities, and physiologic disorders associated with the condition and the patient's functional capacity. For example, a formal diagnostic statement would be "rheumatic heart disease, inactive; mitral stenosis, right ventricular hypertrophy and dilatation, pulmonary congestion; atrial fibrillation; functional class II."

Etiology. Common etiologies are congenital (genetic and developmental), infectious, rheumatic, hypertensive, and ischemic.

Anatomy. List abnormalities of the aorta and pulmonary arteries, coronary arteries, endocardium and valves, myocardium, and pericardium. Congenital anatomic abnormalities are either cyanotic or noncyanotic (i.e., with or without significant right-to-left shunt).

Physiology. List disturbances in cardiac rhythm and conduction, myocardial, systolic or diastolic dysfunction, and clinical syndrome (e.g., anginal syndrome, CHF, cardiac tamponade).

Function. Two commonly used functional classification systems are:
  New York Heart Association classification of angina or dyspnea:
  Class I (No Incapacity). Although the patient has heart disease, the functional capacity is not sufficiently impaired to produce symptoms.
  Class II (Slight Limitation). The patient is comfortable at rest and with mild exertion. Symptoms occur only with more strenuous activity.
  Class III (Incapacity with Slight Exertion). The patient is comfortable at rest, but has dyspnea, fatigue, palpitation, or angina with slight exertion.
  Class IV (Incapacity with Rest). The slightest exertion invariably produces symptoms, and symptoms frequently occur at rest.
  Canadian Cardiovascular Society for angina:
  Class I. No angina with ordinary activity but angina occurs with strenuous or rapid or prolonged exertion.
  Class II. Slight limitation of ordinary activity (e.g., walking more than two level blocks or climbing more than one flight of stairs at a normal pace).
  Class III. Marked limitation of ordinary activity (walking one to two blocks on the level and climbing one flight of stairs).
  Class IV. Inability to carry on any physical activity without angina; angina may also be present at rest.

Six-dermatome pain syndromes. See Six-Dermatome Pain, page 350.

Myocardial Ischemia Six-Dermatome Pain Syndromes

Angina pectoris. Angina is caused by a temporary mismatch of myocardial oxygen demand and supply. Oxygen delivery abnormalities are simplified by rearranging the Fick equation: MVO_2 (myocardial oxygen consumption) = (coronary blood flow) × (myocardial arteriovenous oxygen difference). Because the arteriovenous oxygen difference is nearly maximal at rest, inadequate oxygen delivery is usually caused by inadequate coronary flow. Flow is directly proportional to the pressure gradient across the coronary bed (aortic diastolic minus coronary sinus pressure) and inversely proportional to resistance in the coronary arteries. Therefore, the most common cause of impaired oxygen delivery is atherosclerotic coronary artery obstruction. Vasospasm induced by cold or exertion may be superimposed. Increased myocardial oxygen demand is caused by increases in heart rate, myocardial contractility, ventricular systolic pressure, and/or ventricular cavity radius, regardless of a change in cardiac output or stroke volume.

Angina pectoris is a deep, steady pain or discomfort lasting 1–10 minutes in the six-dermatome region often accompanied by shortness of breath, anxiety, and/or diaphoresis. It is classically precipitated by exercise or anxiety and relieved by rest. Other precipitants are related to the cause of increased myocardial oxygen demand: examples of increased work are sinus tachycardia and atrial or ventricular tachycardias; digitalis, other inotropic agents, and anxiety increase contractility; hypertension and aortic stenosis increase systolic LV pressure; and, aortic regurgitation and systolic heart failure increase LV radius. Stable angina is reproducible, does not occur at rest without provocation, and does not awaken the patient at night. **PQRST**–Provocation: Stable angina has several classic provocations. (1) *Exertion*. An important characteristic of exertional angina is the lag period before the pain begins, and the time to subside with rest. Exertional pain without a lag period suggests another etiology. (2) *Postprandial*. Exertion after a heavy meal is common. (3) *Intense emotion*. Fear, anxiety, and sexual desire increase heart rate, blood pressure, and contractility. (4) *Cold*. Peripheral vasoconstriction and increased blood pressure and heart rate contributor. (5) *Positive inotropic or chronotropic drug effects*. Caffeine, amphetamines, and cocaine increase the heart rate and blood pressure. (6) *Anemia*. Oxygen delivery is reduced when the hemoglobin is <10 g/dL. Palliation: Rest, a warm environment, and nitroglycerin may each relieve an angina attack. *Complete relief of pain or other discomfort in the six-dermatome band after the administration of nitroglycerin is strongly suggestive of angina pectoris but is not diagnostic.* The pain of esophageal spasm also responds to nitroglycerin. If headache or flushing occurs without pain relief, stable angina is unlikely. Quality: Angina is usually described as crushing, aching, tightness, or pressure, frequently illustrated by clenching the fist over the sternum, the *Levine sign*. Region–Radiation: The pain occurs anywhere in the six-dermatome band. It is often most intense behind the sternum or in the precordium, radiating into the neck or throat, or down the medial aspect of either arm. Ischemia in the right coronary artery distribution can radiate to the interscapular region of the back. Less frequently, the pain is felt in the spine or right shoulder and arm. The rare patient complains of pain exclusively in the limbs or neck without chest pain. Severity: Pain may be mild, moderate, or severe, sometimes with a sense of impending death. Timing: The pain is continuous, not fleeting or lancinating, usually lasting from 1 to 10 minutes. **Physical Signs:** There may be no physical findings. S4 can occur during angina because the ischemic ventricle is less compliant. An S3 appears less often. An apical systolic mitral insufficiency murmur suggests papillary muscle ischemia. LV dyskinesia can cause a palpable precordial bulge or apical thrust. *DDX:* Anginal attacks are transient, (typically <10 minutes), which usually excludes MI, dissecting aneurysm, PE, and neoplasm. Atherosclerotic CAD is the most common cause, but less common causes of reduced coronary flow include vasculitis, aortic regurgitation, LV hypertrophy, anemia, and hypoxemia. Pain with swallowing and a sensation of food sticking suggest an esophageal source. The supine position often initiates gastroesophageal reflux pain. Pain from cholecystitis is often postprandial without concurrent exertion. Epigastric and/or right upper quadrant tenderness support gall-bladder disease. Walking induced pain in the shoulder girdle or spine and the chest without a lag period suggests musculoskeletal pain. Angina is clinically classified as follows:

Typical, or definite, angina. Substernal chest discomfort of characteristic quality and duration is provoked by exertion or emotional stress and relieved by rest or nitroglycerin.

Atypical, or probable, angina. This is defined as meeting two of the three characteristics of definite angina.

Noncardiac chest pain. This meets one or none of the typical angina characteristics.

Variant angina pectoris (Prinzmetal angina). Coronary artery spasm with ST-segment elevation occurs with or without angiographically detectable coronary narrowing. The pain quality and location resemble classic angina, but the pain occurs at rest and recurs in cycles, often at the same time each day. ST-segments on ECG are transiently elevated during pain suggesting myocardial injury. Pain is relieved promptly by nitroglycerin. Migraine and Raynaud phenomenon occur more commonly in patients with variant angina.

- *Unstable angina and MI.* The endothelium overlying an atherosclerotic coronary plaque may rupture exposing plaque contents to platelets and procoagulants initiating a platelet plug and fibrin clot. Vasoconstrictor substances are released resulting in intermittent or fixed arterial obstruction. Severe prolonged ischemia leads to myocardial necrosis. Lesser degrees of ischemia result in unstable angina syndromes and myocardial hibernation (decreased contractile function without pain or necrosis). Less common causes of acute coronary syndromes are coronary artery embolism and vasculitis. The transition from severe ischemia to infarction is gradual and depends upon the collateral coronary flow to the ischemic area, the contractile state of the myocardium, and the previous history of that myocardium. Myocardium subjected to repeated ischemic episodes, e.g., stable angina, is less susceptible to infarction.

Unstable angina. Patients present with new angina worsening in severity (more easily provoked and/or more difficult to relieve), lasting >15 minutes, occurring at rest and/or awakening the patient from sleep but *without myocardial necrosis.* Untreated patients have substantial risk of acute MI.

The **TIMI Risk Score** is used to estimate risk for rapid evolution to acute ST-elevation MI in patients with unstable angina and non-ST-elevation acute

MI. Give 1 point each for age ≥65 years, ≥3 traditional risk factors (CAD family history, hypertension, hypercholesterolemia, diabetes, current smoker), known ≥50% coronary stenosis, ST-segment changes, ≥2 anginal episodes in the preceding 24 hours, aspirin use in the last 7 days, and elevated CK or troponin. Scores of 0–2 are low risk, 3–4 intermediate risk, and ≥5 high risk.

Acute MI. MI occurs most commonly from the early morning hours to midday. The pain onset is usually not induced by exertion, nor does it remit with rest. The discomfort is identical to angina pectoris in quality, location, intensity, and constancy, but it lasts from 20 minutes to several hours. In some cases, the pain quickly increases to an intensity seldom experienced with angina; this may be sustained for hours, after which the pain subsides to a dull ache that can last days. The patient often complains of shortness of breath possibly related to increased LV end-diastolic pressure, depressed systolic function, or mitral insufficiency from papillary muscle dysfunction. Nausea and vomiting are common, particularly with inferior wall infarction. A sympathetic response is triggered with sweating, pallor, and cold moist skin. The heart rate may be slow, normal, or accelerated; similarly, blood pressure may be low, normal, or quite elevated. An S4 may be heard and the heart sounds are often muted. Crackles may appear at the lung bases. Life threatening cardiac rhythms can occur at any time. A pericardial friction rub appears in ~15% >24 hours after onset of the MI. Occasional MIs are painless, the diagnosis being suggested by the associated symptoms and signs. Large, uncompensated infarcts rapidly progress to cardiogenic shock and death characterized by hypotension, hypoxemia, decreased mental status and anuria.

MI terminology is based on EKG interpretation. Presentation with ST-elevations is an *ST-elevation infarction (STEMI).* Untreated, a STEMI develops Q-waves, becoming a *Q-wave MI.* If a Q does not form, it is a *non-Q-wave MI.* If no ST-elevation occurs, it is a *non-ST-elevation MI (NSTEMI).* An NSTEMI usually does not form a Q-wave, so is a non-Q-wave MI. If a Q-wave does appear, the NSTEMI is Q-wave infarction. *DDX:* Simple angina is excluded by the pain's long duration and lack of response to rest and nitroglycerin. Three potentially life-threatening disorders closely mimic the pain and presentation of MI: pulmonary embolism, (page 343), acute thoracic aorta dissection (page 354), and acute pericarditis (page 352). PE is suggested by clear lung fields and normal chest X-ray in the setting of marked dyspnea and hypotension. Dissection pain is more excruciating and reaches its peak more rapidly than MI pain. Prominent pain in the back makes dissection more likely, however, pain radiating to the back occurs with MI and may be absent with dissection. A new aortic diastolic murmur transmitting down the right sternal border, and/or asymmetrical pulses or blood pressures between extremities, suggests dissection, as does a widened superior mediastinum on chest X-ray. The pain of acute pericarditis may be severe and resemble MI though the pain may be intensified by reclining, breathing or swallowing. That pericarditis can be a sequela of MI adds potential confusion.

Inflammatory Six-Dermatome Pain Syndromes

Acute pericarditis. The visceral pericardium and inner surface of the parietal pericardium are anesthetic (Fig. 8-44), but the outer surface of the lower parietal pericardium is pain sensitive. The parietal pleura surrounds the anterior and lateral pericardium, accounting for pleural involvement from

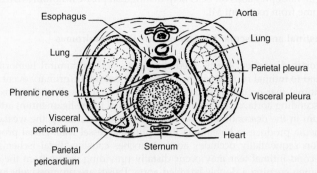

FIG. 8-44 Pleuropericardial Relationships. A transverse section of the lower thorax with anesthetic serosal surfaces represented by heavy beaded lines and pain-sensitive surfaces by lighter beaded lines. Note the proximity of the phrenic nerves and esophagus to the parietal pericardium, so pericarditis can produce pain in the phrenic nerve distribution or pain on swallowing.

pericarditis. Inflammation can involve the closely positioned esophagus and phrenic nerves causing dysphagia and phrenic pain. All these structures are innervated by fibers from the vagus and six-dermatome band. Phrenic nerve sensory fibers from the central diaphragm can be irritated in the lower pericardium causing neck pain at the superior border of the trapezius. **Symptoms:** Deep constant or pleuritic pain occurs in the six-dermatome band or the phrenic distribution. The location and quality of pain often resembles that of MI, but it is usually accentuated by breathing or coughing, worse in recumbency, and lessened while sitting and leaning forward. It may be intensified by swallowing. Pleuritic pain referred to the shoulder, particularly the left trapezius ridge, suggests pericarditis (Fig. 8-43, page 340). The pain may last for hours and is not relieved by nitroglycerin. Rarely, the pain is throbbing and synchronous with the heartbeat. **Signs:** Fever may follow the onset of pain. A transient pericardial friction rub is often heard. **ECG:** Widespread ST elevation followed by T wave inversion is diagnostic. The ST-T findings of pericarditis must be differentiated from the injury currents of infarction and normal early repolarization. *DDX:* Causes of pericarditis include infection, malignancy, rheumatic fever, collagen vascular diseases, trauma, uremia, or following MI or chest radiation. Until a pericardial friction rub appears or ECG signs develop, the steady pain suggests MI, dissecting aneurysm, pulmonary infarction, cholecystitis, or peptic ulcer. Pain on swallowing can suggest an esophageal lesion. The pleural pain must be distinguished from that of pleurisy, subphrenic abscess, and splenic infarction.

Post-cardiotomy syndrome. A hypersensitivity reaction to antigen derived from injured myocardium occurs several weeks after MI, cardiac surgery, or other heart injury. Findings are fever, pericarditis, pleuritis, pericardial and/or pleural effusions, and pneumonitis. Recurrences are common, usually with decreasing severity. The symptoms often respond dramatically to NSAIDs. Recurrent MI should be considered in patients with ischemic heart disease. The appearance of a pericardial friction rub, and absence of new Q-waves or

ST-segment depressions on ECG help distinguish post-cardiotomy (Dressler) syndrome from recurrent MI.

Mediastinal and Vascular Six-Dermatome Pain Syndromes

- **Aortic dissection.** Cystic medial necrosis and intramural hemorrhage lead to intimal rupture, or the intimal tear can be the primary event. The intimal tear occurs most commonly in the lateral wall of the proximal ascending aorta, or, less commonly, just distal to the ligamentum arteriosum in the descending aorta. Luminal blood penetrating the weakened media produces a hematoma that splits the vessel wall. Distal progression sequentially occludes aortic branches causing distal ischemia. A second intimal tear may occur distally providing egress from the false lumen creating a double-barreled aorta. Pulses are progressively lost in branches of the aorta, accompanied by loss of specific nerve functions. **Symptoms:** In 80% of cases, the onset is sudden, with excruciating pain in the precordium and/or the interscapular region that moves successively to the lower back, abdomen, hips, and thighs. The pain often suggests MI. Sometimes the onset is gradual without chest pain. **Signs:** Blood pressure is usually unaffected. Cardiogenic or hemorrhagic shock may occur with rupture into the pericardium or left pleural space respectively. *Proximal Progression:* A hematoma extending proximally from a tear in the aortic arch can distort the aortic valve ring separating the commissures to cause aortic regurgitation and a murmur transmitting down the right sternal border, occlude the coronary ostia causing an MI, produce hemopericardium with a pericardial rub and cardiac tamponade, and/or swell the base of the aorta pulsating the sternoclavicular joint. *Distal Progression:* When the hematoma extends away from the heart there is sequential asymmetrical decrease or loss of pulses in branches of the aorta and signs of nervous system injury. Carotid occlusion causes cerebral ischemia with localizing neurologic signs. Obstruction of the spinal arteries is indicated by paraplegia and anesthesia. Renal artery occlusion with infarction causes pain simulating renal colic. Aortic dissection may be rapidly fatal. **Chest X-ray:** Widening of the aorta, an enlarged aortic knob, or separation of calcified intimal plaques from the outer border of the aortic wall all suggest dissection. Imaging studies should be performed urgently when dissection is suspected. *DDX:* Most commonly, dissection occurs in association with cystic medial necrosis of the aorta, especially in patients with Marfan and Ehlers–Danlos syndromes. It occurs with less frequency in patients with hypertension, advancing age, during labor, and after penetrating or blunt trauma. Dissection may occur in a thoracic aortic aneurysm afflicted with aortitis from bacteria, syphilis, or giant cell arteritis.
- **Leakage and rupture of aortic aneurysm.** Expanding aneurysms are usually painless, but breach of the wall with leakage of blood into the surrounding tissue is accompanied by the sudden severe pain at the site of leakage or radiating into the body wall at that spinal segment. The pain is often accompanied by restlessness, diaphoresis, and tachycardia. The specific pain pattern reflects the site of leakage. Urgent evaluation and intervention required to prevent death. Complete rupture presents as

sudden severe pain followed shortly by death from rapidly progressive hemorrhagic shock.
- *Spontaneous esophageal rupture—Boerhaave syndrome.* Forceful vomiting precipitates chest or upper abdominal pain and severe dyspnea. Subcutaneous emphysema can dissect into the supraclavicular fossae accompanied by a precordial crunching sound from mediastinal emphysema (*Hamman sign*). *DDX:* The symptoms are common to MI, perforated peptic ulcer, cholecystitis, pancreatitis, esophagitis, hepatitis, nonperforating ulcer, and pneumonia. Radiographic demonstration of air in the mediastinum excludes all the foregoing in favor of ruptured esophagus.

Six-dermatome pain with dysphagia. See Chapter 9, page 432.

Subphrenic diseases. Lesions below the diaphragm usually present with abdominal pain, but there are frequent exceptions so consider subphrenic disorders with six-dermatome band pain. Subphrenic abscess, acute cholecystitis, peptic ulcer, acute pancreatitis, and splenic infarction are considerations.

Pulmonary artery embolism and pulmonary infarction. See page 343.

Pneumothorax. See page 340.

Other Cardiovascular Syndromes
Pulmonary edema. See page 344.

Cardiac dilatation. Dilatation of heart chambers is caused by poor systolic function or chronic volume overload. The dilated heart of trained athletes has a large stroke volume that maintains high cardiac output at relatively low heart rates, thereby minimizing myocardial oxygen demand. Heart enlargement, indicated by displaced apical impulse and borders of cardiac dullness or chest radiograph, implies dilatation of one or both ventricles. When the dilated heart also has depressed contractility, the elongated myocardial muscle fibers generate weak and often diffuse apical impulses. An apical impulse displaced leftward with a normal right heart border suggests LV dilation. *DDX:* Pericardial effusions will enlarge the heart silhouette and borders of dullness, but the apical impulse is usually undetectable, and the heart sounds are diminished.
CLINICAL OCCURRENCE: *Left Ventricular Dilation:* Aortic insufficiency, mitral insufficiency, ischemic cardiomyopathy, post-MI, dilated cardiomyopathy, viral myocarditis; *Right Ventricular Dilation:* Pulmonic insufficiency, tricuspid insufficiency, ASD with left-to-right shunt, right ventricular infarct, pulmonary hypertension with RV failure.

Myocardial hypertrophy. Hypertrophy, with or without dilation, is the result of pressure and/or volume overload or hypertrophic cardiomyopathy. Hypertrophied LV myocardium produces more powerful apical impulses than normal. The heart is not enlarged on physical exam without concomitant dilation (Fig. 8-45). Right ventricular hypertrophy can produce a palpable thrust over the right ventricle along the left sternal edge.
CLINICAL OCCURRENCE: *LV Hypertrophy:* Valvular aortic stenosis, mitral or aortic insufficiency, hypertension, hypertrophic cardiomyopathy; *Right*

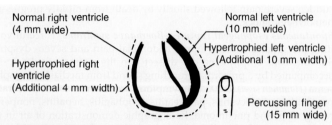

Normal right ventricle
(4 mm wide)

Normal left ventricle
(10 mm wide)

Hypertrophied left ventricle
(Additional 10 mm width)

Hypertrophied right
ventricle
(Additional 4 mm width)

Percussing finger
(15 mm wide)

FIG. 8-45 **Contribution of Myocardial Hypertrophy to the Area of Cardiac Dullness.** Without chamber dilatation, concentric cardiac muscle hypertrophy to twice its normal thickness and weight does not increase the area of cardiac dullness more than the width of the percussing finger. Therefore, after pericardial effusion is excluded, increased area of dullness must be attributed to dilatation.

Ventricular Hypertrophy: Pulmonic stenosis, ASD, pulmonary hypertension, hypertrophic cardiomyopathy.

Left ventricular congestive heart failure (CHF). CHF is the functional result of impaired LV contractility (*systolic dysfunction*) and/or decreased LV diastolic compliance (*diastolic dysfunction*). Decreased LV contractility leads to increased left ventricular end-diastolic pressure and volume, dilating the LV to maintain stroke volume at the expense of left atrial hypertension and pulmonary vein distention. The ventricular ejection fraction is preserved when congestion is principally caused by decreased diastolic compliance, i.e., diastolic dysfunction. Decreased cardiac output with renal hypoperfusion leads to salt and water retention, weight gain, and edema. Symptoms and signs are attributable to decreased cardiac output and volume expansion with pulmonary and peripheral vascular congestion. Early symptoms of LV failure are pulmonary congestion with dyspnea, orthopnea, nocturia, and cough. Crackles are heard in the lung bases. When venous capacitance is exceeded, congestion progresses to right ventricular failure with elevated CVP engorging the jugular veins. Even before the increase in CVP, a hepatojugular reflux sign can be demonstrated. Frequently an S3 develops. Arterial pressure response to the Valsalva maneuver correlates inversely with the left ventricular filling pressure: absence of the normal systolic pressure "overshoot" following release of the Valsalva, and failure of the BP to drop during the breath hold, suggest increased LV filling pressure. With biventricular failure, the liver can become large, tender, and painful. Chronic congestive hepatomegaly may produce capsular and parenchymal fibrosis without tenderness. Edema accumulates as right-sided or bilateral hydrothorax, ascites, and pitting edema of the ankles, legs, genitals, and abdomen. The lips, ears, and nail beds may be cyanotic. Impaired cerebral circulation may result in confusion and periodic breathing. The most common causes of CHF are chronic ischemic heart disease followed by dilated cardiomyopathy (pregnancy and postpartum, alcohol, hemochromatosis, idiopathic, secondary to viral infections), especially in younger patients. Diastolic heart failure is common in longstanding hypertension with LVH and hypertrophic cardiomyopathies. Restrictive cardiomyopathy results from amyloidosis, hemochromatosis, sarcoidosis, and other infiltrative diseases. *DDX:* Portal hypertension similarly, but without orthopnea or elevated jugular venous pressure. Metastatic carcinoma can produce ascites and chest effusions resembling cardiac failure.

CHF is staged according to the American College of Cardiology/American Heart Association staging system:

Stage A: Patients at substantial risk for heart failure but without structural heart disease or symptoms of heart failure.

Stage B: Patients with structural heart disease but without signs or symptoms of heart failure.

Stage C: Patients with structural heart disease with *prior or current* symptoms of heart disease.

Stage D: Patients with refractory heart failure (symptoms at rest despite maximal medical therapy) requiring specialized intervention.

Once a patient is assigned to a heart failure stage, he/she cannot be reclassified to a lower stage, e.g., reverting from Stage C to Stage B. This contrasts with the New York Heart Association and Canadian Cardiovascular Society classifications where patients move from class to class as symptoms change.

Right ventricular failure and cor pulmonale. Right ventricular failure results from myocardial damage and RV volume and/or pressure overload. Right and left ventricular function are interdependent, so primary LV failure is often accompanied by some degree of RV failure. When the CVP >22 cm, the liver enlarges, and above 25 cm ascites, edema, and orthopnea appear. Venous pressure is always high with RV failure, but it falls before other signs of failure resolve. The most frequent cause of right ventricular failure is advanced ischemic heart disease. *Cor pulmonale* is right ventricular failure due to pulmonary hypertension from primary pulmonary disease, either hypoxia induced vasoconstriction or obliteration of the pulmonary vascular bed.

CLINICAL OCCURRENCE: *Impaired Myocardial Function:* Ischemic heart disease (especially right ventricular infarction), hypertrophic and dilated cardiomyopathies, endomyocardial fibrosis (e.g., drugs, carcinoid syndrome), restrictive myocardial disease (e.g., amyloidosis); *Volume Overload:* TR, ASD with left-to-right shunt, pulmonic insufficiency; *Pressure Overload:* Primary pulmonary hypertension, secondary pulmonary hypertension—cor pulmonale (hypoxia caused by emphysema, cystic fibrosis, interstitial pulmonary diseases, pneumoconioses, hypersensitivity pneumonitis, pulmonary fibrosis, etc.), acute pulmonary embolus, chronic thromboembolic pulmonary hypertension, pulmonic stenosis, Eisenmenger complex, mitral stenosis, pulmonary venoocclusive disease.

Restrictive cardiomyopathy. Decreased diastolic compliance impedes ventricular filling leading to elevated ventricular end-diastolic pressure and reduced cardiac output. Systolic function is preserved. Patients present with dyspnea exacerbated by exertion and intermittent pulmonary congestion. Signs of right ventricular failure with edema, elevated CVP, and ascites may predominate. The heart is not enlarged. An S4 gallops is common. Causes are ventricular diastolic dysfunction, infiltrative heart disease (amyloid, sarcoid, hemochromatosis), and endomyocardial fibroelastosis. *DDX:* This must be distinguished from hypertrophic cardiomyopathy and constrictive pericarditis.

Hypertrophic cardiomyopathy. Inherited defects of myocardial contractile proteins lead to progressive hypertrophy, disorganized myocardial architecture, impaired diastolic relaxation, ventricular conduction abnormalities, and dysrhythmias. Asymmetric septal hypertrophy can produce dynamic obstruction to LV outflow during early systole. A family history of sudden death is common. Patients present with dyspnea, angina, and presyncope. Carotid upstrokes are brisk and may show a bisferiens pattern. An S4 is common. A characteristic murmur augmenting with Valsalva is heard with outflow obstruction (see Hypertrophic Obstructive Cardiomyopathy, page 327). Echocardiography is diagnostic.

Infective endocarditis. Heart valve infection leads to fibrin-platelet vegetations harboring the organism. Low virulence organisms, e.g., viridans streptococci, and HACEK organisms, have subacute presentations. High virulence organisms, e.g., *Staphylococcus aureus*, and fungi, rapidly destroy valves and so present acutely, with or without systemic emboli. *Subacute Bacterial Endocarditis (SBE):* Patients present with subacute or chronic fever, weight loss, arthralgia, myalgias, and signs of immune complex disease. *Acute Endocarditis:* Patients, often with a history of injection drug use, have fever and rigors. Peripheral emboli with organ infarction and metastatic infection are common. Systemic illness, especially with a new insufficiency murmur, should always trigger an endocarditis evaluation. The clinical diagnosis of infective endocarditis relies on the presence of positive blood cultures, echocardiographic findings consistent with endocarditis as well as associated findings such as peripheral embolic disease, vascular embolic disease, and immunologic phenomena such as glomerulonephritis, Osler's nodes and Roth's spots.

Nonbacterial thrombotic endocarditis (NBTE). Nonbacterial thrombotic endocarditis is the result of endocardial inflammation with sterile vegetations. Multiple large emboli suggest *marantic endocarditis* associated with occult neoplasms, most often a mucin-secreting adenocarcinoma. Libman–Sacks lesions (small vegetations composed of fibrin, lymphocytes, neutrophils and histiocytes) occur on the valves and endocardium of patients with SLE and antiphospholipid syndrome. Patients may be asymptomatic, have peripheral emboli, or present with progressive valve stenosis or regurgitation.

Valvular Heart Disease: These clinical conditions are discussed with their physical findings under the sections Cardiovascular Signs, page 313 and Auscultation of Heart Murmurs, page 282.

Congenital Heart Disease: Many patients with congenital heart disease survive into well into adult life. All clinicians should be familiar with the common syndromes. ASDs and small VSDs may be asymptomatic for decades, eluding diagnosis well into adult life.

Atrial septal defect. See page 329.

Ventricular septal defect. See page 329.

Persistent ductus arteriosus. See page 333.

Coarctation of the aorta. See pages 329 and 368.

Eisenmenger syndrome. An intra- or extra-cardiac left-to-right shunt connecting the pulmonary and arterial circul ations creates chronic volume and/ or pressure overload of the right ventricle and pulmonary arteries leading to severe pulmonary hypertension and, if left untreated, reversal of flow into a right-to-left shunt with peripheral hypoxemia and cyanosis. The RV and PA respond with hypertrophy and fibromuscular hyperplasia, respectively. Suspect Eisenmenger physiology when valve signs are coupled with cyanosis, decreased oxygen saturation not relieved with 100% oxygen, right-to-left shunt, clubbing of the fingers and/or toes, and polycythemia.

Tetralogy of fallot. The tetralogy is the combination of a VSD, obstruction to right ventricular outflow (usually infundibular pulmonic stenosis), an overriding aorta, and right ventricular hypertrophy (Fig. 8-41D, page 326).

Ebstein anomaly. The congenitally abnormal tricuspid valve, with small thin cusps and a portion originating below the AV ring, produces an atrialized portion of the right ventricle. Tricuspid insufficiency is not prominent; dysrhythmias are common.

- **Sudden cardiac death—cardiac arrest.** Cardiac arrest demands immediate treatment for any chance of survival. For 25% of patients, sudden cardiac death is the first symptom of severe CAD. Less common causes are hypertrophic cardiomyopathy (especially in young male athletes), coronary artery emboli, right ventricular dysplasia, Brugada syndrome, long-QT syndrome, and anomalous coronary artery anatomy. Public education seeks to teach all adults in basic cardiopulmonary resuscitation. Increasingly, automated defibrillators are present in public places to reverse fatal ventricular arrhythmias. All health care personnel should be trained in basic cardiopulmonary resuscitation (BCLS). Nurses and physicians should be trained in advanced cardiac life support (ACLS).

Mediastinal Tumors: Mediastinal masses rarely cause chest pain. Most attract attention by compressing normal structures or are found incidentally on chest X-ray. Signs suggesting a mediastinal tumor are dyspnea (retrosternal goiter), hoarseness and brassy cough (recurrent laryngeal nerve compression), *Horner syndrome* (superior cervical ganglion injury, Chapter 14, page 665), edema and cyanosis of the arms and neck (SVC obstruction), and chylous pleural effusion. Lymph nodes are enlarged in Hodgkin disease, non-Hodgkin lymphoma, carcinoma, germ cell tumors, or tuberculosis. Other masses are thymomas and teratomas (dermoid cyst). Dermoid cysts forming a tracheal fistula may produce the rare symptom of *trichoptysis*, coughing up of hair.

Pericardial Syndromes
Acute pericarditis. See page 352.

Postpericardiotomy syndrome. See page 353.

Pericardial effusion. Fluid accumulates within the pericardial sac because of infection, inflammation, malignancy, or transudation. Slowly accumulating fluid distends the pericardium compressing surrounding lung. Rapidly accumulating fluid is more likely to compress the heart chambers producing tamponade. Patients are asymptomatic or symptoms reflect the etiology (e.g., pain and fever with pericarditis; weakness, nausea and anorexia with uremia) or the hemodynamic consequences (e.g., shortness of breath and fatigue with tamponade). Signs include absent precordial impulse, decreased intensity and/or muffling of heart sounds, and low-voltage ECG. A rub may be present. Large effusions can cause dullness at the left scapular tip because of left lower lobe atelectasis (*Ewart sign*).

CLINICAL OCCURRENCE: *Congenital:* Familial Mediterranean fever, familial pericarditis; *Endocrine:* Hypothyroidism; *Degenerative/Idiopathic:* Sarcoidosis; *Infectious:* Bacterial, viral, tuberculosis, fungal, Whipple Disease; *Inflammatory/Immune:* Post-pericardiotomy, rheumatic fever, SLE, RA, ankylosing spondylitis, scleroderma, granulomatosis with polyangiitis, drug reactions; *Mechanical/Traumatic:* Trauma, post-irradiation; *Metabolic/Toxic:* Drug-induced, uremia; *Neoplastic:* Metastatic carcinoma, especially lung and breast, lymphoma; *Vascular:* MI, aortic dissection with rupture into the pericardium, chylopericardium, vasculitis.

Constrictive pericarditis. Progressive pericardial fibrosis restricts diastolic filling decreasing cardiac output. Symptoms are shortness of breath and fatigue. Signs are those of right heart failure: jugular venous distention, edema, ascites, and hepatic congestion. The initial pericardial injury is caused by pericarditis (viral, tuberculous, neoplasm), cardiac surgery, mediastinal irradiation, or uremia. *DDX:* It must be distinguished from restrictive cardiomyopathies and right ventricular failure.

Pericardial tamponade. Rapid or massive pericardial fluid accumulation compresses the heart impairing diastolic atrial and ventricular filling. Cardiac output falls and CVP rises. Patient are short of breath and fatigued and may rapidly progress to hypotension and circulatory collapse. The key physical signs are an elevated CVP with clear lung fields, no stigmata of chronic right ventricular failure, and a drop in systolic blood pressure during inspiration of >10 mm Hg (see pulsus paradoxus, page 335 and Fig. 8-42, page 327). Pulsus paradoxus may not be found in the presence of aortic insufficiency, left or right ventricular hypertrophy, or pulmonary hypertension. The heart size is usually normal by exam and chest X-ray. Suspected tamponade should be urgently evaluated by echocardiography. *DDX:* Easily confused with tamponade are acute PE, right ventricular infarction, constrictive pericarditis, and restrictive cardiomyopathy.

Disorders of the Arterial and Venous Circulations.

Vasculitis. Large vessel vasculitides are of unknown etiology. Vasculitis of medium-sized arteries may be associated with infection (polyarteritis nodosa with hepatitis B and C) or specific immunologic markers (granulomatosis with polyangiitis with c-ANCA). Small-vessel vasculitides are associated with immune complex deposition in the vessel walls. In some cases, the association with a specific infection is strong (e.g., mixed cryoglobulinemia and chronic hepatitis C infection); in others there is a strong association with serologic markers (e.g., microscopic polyangiitis and p-ANCA). Each involves vessel wall inflammation leading to vascular obstruction and end-organ damage. The current working classification for vasculitis syndromes

TABLE 8-3 Systemic Vasculitis Syndromes.

Size of the Vessel	Specific Diseases
Large arteries	GCA
	Takayasu arteritis
	Primary central nervous system vasculitis
Medium arteries[a]	Polyarteritis nodosa
	Kawasaki disease
	Eosinophilic granulomatosis with polyangiitis (Churg–Strauss syndrome)
	Granulomatosis with polyangiitis (Wegener granulomatosis)
Small vessels	Leukocytoclastic vasculitis (e.g., Henoch–Schonlein purpura, cryoglobulinemia, infections, drugs)
	Microscopic polyangiitis
	Urticarial vasculitis
	Systemic rheumatic syndromes
Pseudovasculitis[b]	Antiphospholipid syndrome
	Embolic phenomena (atrial myxomas, cholesterol, NBTE/Libman–Sacks endocarditis)
	Bacterial endocarditis
	Endovascular lymphoma

[a]May involve small vessels as well.
[b]May involve vessels of any size.
From Coblyn JS, McCluskey RT. Case 3-2003: case records of the Massachusetts General Hospital. A 36-year-old man with renal failure, hypertension, and neurologic abnormalities. *N Engl J Med.* 2003;348:333–342.

has proven helpful for selecting appropriate treatment. Vasculitides are classified by the size of the involved vessel, Table 8-3. The clinical manifestations depend upon the size and distribution of the vessels involved. Symptoms and signs are due to local ischemia and systemic inflammation. Skin involvement manifests as palpable purpura with or without skin infarction. Involvement of arteries to other organs gives signs specific to the organ affected, e.g., renal failure, transient ischemic attacks, stroke, and pneumonitis. The pattern of involvement suggests the size of the vessel and the specific vasculitis syndrome [Kathiresan S, Kelsey PB, Steere AC, et al. Case 14-2005: a 38-year-old man with fever and blurred vision. *N Engl J Med.* 2005;352:2003–2012].

- **Giant cell arteritis (GCA, temporal arteritis).** The cause is unknown. Histology shows segmental patchy medial necrosis in the temporal artery, with diffuse mononuclear infiltration and giant cells throughout the vessel wall. Thromboses are frequent. GCA affects major branches of the proximal aorta, especially the external carotid. Patients over age 50 present with fever and weight loss and may have headache, jaw claudication, and/or scalp tenderness. Visual symptoms forebode irreversible visual loss from retinal and ophthalmic artery occlusion. The headache is severe, persistent, and throbbing. *Polymyalgia rheumatica* (see Chapter 13, page 608) may antedate other manifestations or occur simultaneously. Systemic symptoms (fever, profound weakness, weight loss, malaise, and prostration) are common and may be the only manifestations of disease. Physical signs are few, but scalp tenderness and tortuous, tender, or nodular temporal arteries may be present. The overlying skin is often red and swollen. Vision is often impaired and ophthalmoplegia may be temporary or permanent. The retina may be normal or show evidence of retinal ischemia. Prompt diagnosis and treatment can prevent loss of vision. The typical ophthalmic finding is anterior ischemic optic neuropathy (AION, Chapter 7, page 207). The disk appears pale and swollen because the posterior ciliary arteries supplying the nerve head are obstructed. Aortic aneurysms (thoracic and abdominal) and dissection occur with increased frequency [Kelly NP, Gerhard-Herman M, Desai AS, et al. An unusual cause of leg pain. *N Engl J Med.* 2017;377;2267-72].

Takayasu aortitis. There is inflammation of the aorta and its major branches producing markedly reduced flow and thrombosis in the involved vessels. Patients are usually young women presenting with arterial ischemia symptoms. Absent pulses in arm or neck vessels (pulseless disease), carotid sinus sensitivity with head movement inducing syncope, and ocular disorders, such as cataract and retinal defects, form a characteristic triad.

Polyarteritis nodosa (PAN). Approximately a third of patients have chronic hepatitis B infection and HbSAg-HbSAb immune complexes have been found in the vessel walls. Causes of the other cases are not known. Transmural inflammation and necrosis of small and intermediate muscular arteries sometimes extends to adjacent veins and arterioles. Involvement is segmental with a predilection for arterial bifurcations and branch points. Vascular occlusion leads to tissue ischemia and necrosis. Aneurysms up to 1 cm in diameter are frequent. Symptoms include fever, weight loss, malaise, and pain in viscera and muscles. Skin lesions are common, especially on the legs, and subcutaneous nodules may be palpable along the course of vessels or nerves. Frequently involved organs are the kidneys (renal failure, hypertension), gastrointestinal tract (visceral infarction), heart (MI, pericarditis), liver (acute to chronic hepatitis), peripheral nerves (mononeuritis multiplex), skin (subcutaneous nodules over superficial vessels, palpable purpura, livedo reticularis), joints, and muscles (myalgias, arthralgias, arthritis). The lungs are rarely involved [Case records of the Massachusetts General Hospital. Case 3-2003. A 36-year-old man with renal failure, hypertension, and neurologic abnormalities. *N Engl J Med.* 2003;348:333–342].

Granulomatosis with polyangiitis (Wegener). The cause is unknown. Granulomatous inflammation of small arteries and veins is strongly associated with neutrophil anticytoplasmic antibodies to proteinase-3 (c-ANCA). Patients present with fever, malaise and signs of upper airway disease (sinusitis, obstructive, and/or destructive symptoms and signs), pulmonary involvement, and/or progressive renal failure. Other organ systems, including the skin, may be involved. Disease may be limited to the upper airway. It is most common in the fourth and fifth decades. Facial pain and epistaxis are caused by erosion of the nose (resulting in saddle deformity), sinuses, palate, or nasopharynx. The lungs may have infiltrates, nodules, and cavitations. The renal lesion is a rapidly progressive glomerulonephritis.

Eosinophilic granulomatosis with polyangiitis (Churg–Strauss syndrome). The cause is unknown. Eosinophilia is associated with nodular lung infiltrates and asthma. Patients present with signs and symptoms of asthma in association with eosinophilia and persistent slowly evolving abnormalities on the chest radiographs. Systemic symptoms and signs mimic polyarteritis nodosa. It may appear during tapering of corticosteroid treatment or introduction of leukotriene inhibitor treatment of asthma [Wolf M, Rose H, Smith RN. Case 28–2005: a 42-year-old man with weight loss, weakness, and a rash. *N Engl J Med.* 2005;353:1148–1157].

Microscopic polyangiitis. The cause is unknown and immune complexes and complement are not present in the vessel walls and granulomas do not form (*pauci-immune vasculitis*). There is a high prevalence of anticytoplasmic antibodies to myeloperoxidase (p-ANCA). Patients are systemically ill with fever, malaise, dyspnea, nonproductive cough, arthralgias, and myalgias. Acute rapidly progressive glomerulonephritis is common and pulmonary hemorrhage can be fatal. Except for the absence of airway involvement, it clinically is indistinguishable from granulomatosis with polyangiitis.

Leukocytoclastic vasculitis. Immune complexes lodge in the walls of terminal arterioles and venules inciting an inflammatory response that occludes vessels producing local tissue infarction. This common vasculitis most frequently affects the skin, particularly on the lower legs. The physical finding is purpura which is often palpable. The lesions come in crops that clear over days without scarring. Systemic symptoms (fever, malaise) and involvement of visceral organs including the kidneys (glomerulonephritis), lungs, gut, and rarely the heart and central nervous system, can occur. Precipitating events include infection, drugs, malignancies, and primary inflammatory disorders. Several distinct syndromes are identified, but overlap is frequent. *DDX:* This vasculitis must be distinguished from other causes of vasculopathy including disseminated fungal (e.g., histoplasmosis), viral (e.g., Rocky Mountain spotted fever) and bacterial infections (e.g., meningococcemia, gonococcemia), atheroembolism, scurvy, and thrombocytopenia.

Serum sickness. This hypersensitivity vasculitis is caused by antibodies against a widely disseminated exogenous antigen, most often penicillin. Deposition of antigen–antibody complexes in the subendothelial space elicits local inflammation. Headache and pruritus are accompanied by wheal formation at the site of subcutaneous or intramuscular injection. The urticaria spreads, and large areas of skin may become edematous. An erythematous rash is often present. Myalgias and arthralgias may be severe; nausea and vomiting may occur. Generalized lymphadenopathy is frequent.

Secondary vasculitis. This is a leukocytoclastic vasculitis occurring in association with another primary disease or condition inciting immune complex formation. Common causes are infections (endocarditis, HIV, EBV, etc.), primary inflammatory diseases (e.g., SLE, RA, Sjögren syndrome and polymyositis-dermatomyositis), serum sickness, and drugs (see below).

Idiopathic cutaneous vasculitis. This is an immune complex vasculitis limited to the skin and without an identifiable inciting event or exposure. It may be recurrent, and a burning sensation may precede the crops of purpura. Other skin signs that may accompany the purpura include urticaria, bullae, and erythematous macules. The lesions may itch.

Drug-induced vasculitis. Many drugs, especially the penicillins and sulfonamides, are associated with immune complex-mediated, typically cutaneous and/or urticarial, vasculitis. A p-ANCA positive small vessel vasculitis clinically identical to microscopic polyangiitis has been described with use of propylthiouracil, levamisole (adulterant in cocaine) and hydralazine. Drug-induced TTP-HUS (Chapter 6, page 152) may be confused with vasculitis.

Henoch–Schönlein purpura (anaphylactoid purpura). Onset often follows an infection. There is IgA deposition and inflammation in the small vessels of the skin, gastrointestinal tract, and kidneys. Patients, usually children or young adults, present with palpable purpura on the abdomen, buttocks and lower extremities, abdominal pain, fever, and heme-positive stools. Proteinuria and hematuria indicate glomerulitis. Nausea, vomiting, arthralgias, and myalgias are common. Urticaria may be present. The condition resolves spontaneously within a few days.

Behçet syndrome. This vasculitis of unknown cause is characterized by the triad of relapsing iridocyclitis, oral aphthous ulcerations, and genital ulcers. Most cases occur in Greece, Cyprus, Turkey, the Middle East, and Japan, but increasing numbers are reported in the United States. There is a high incidence of erythema nodosum and arthritis. A characteristic sign is the formation of sterile pustules at skin puncture sites, *pathergy*. Many patients have thrombophlebitis, neurologic disorders, or intestinal involvement. The disease is chronic with relapses and remissions.

Arteriovenous fistula: acquired. Communication between an artery and adjacent vein may be created surgically to facilitate venous access for hemodialysis or be caused by a stab or gunshot wound, diagnostic catheterization, or erosion from neoplasm or infectious arteritis. Hemorrhage after the inciting trauma is profuse but easily controlled. A thrill and bruit may develop some hours later. After the wound has healed, signs of chronic circulatory disturbance develop. Although fistulas may occur in any body part, signs are most evident when an extremity is involved (Fig. 8-46). Dilated veins and stasis dermatitis indicate venous congestion. Arterial hypoperfusion can produce distal gangrene. If extremity injury occurs before the epiphyses have closed, hypertrophy of the arm or leg can occur. A thrill and bruit are present throughout the cardiac cycle, with systolic accentuation. The skin temperature increases distal to the fistula. Paradoxically, these signs assure that an arteriovenous shunt established surgically to facilitate venous access remains patent. When the shunt is large, the dilated superficial veins become tense, venous pressure approaches arterial diastolic pressure, venous flow velocity increases, the RV dilates, arterial diastolic pressure falls, and cardiac failure may result. External compression, temporarily closing the fistula, produces a sharp slowing of the heart rate, called the *Branham bradycardiac sign*. Signs of abdominal or thoracic shunts are bruits and changes in venous and arterial pressure.

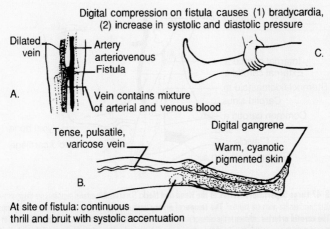

FIG. 8-46 Signs of Arteriovenous Fistula. A. A fistula between the popliteal artery and vein is shown behind the knee joint. **B. The superficial veins are greatly dilated** from blood under arterial pressure; they are tense to the touch and sometimes pulsatile. **Distal to the fistula,** the skin is warm from the arterial blood in the veins, cyanotic, and pigmented from hemostasis. Distal gangrene may occur. **At the site of the fistula** a thrill and bruit continuous throughout the cardiac cycle, with systolic accentuation, may be felt. With a large-flow fistula, the arterial pulse pressure is greater than normal. **C. Closure of the fistula by digital compression** slows the heart rate (*Branham bradycardiac sign*) and augments both systemic systolic and diastolic arterial pressures.

Congenital arteriovenous fistula. Cutaneous birthmarks are found in one-half of cases, so arteriovenous fistula should be considered when port-wine spots, blue-red cavernous hemangiomas, or diffuse hemangiomas are present. Frequently, congenital fistulas are quite small, so the signs associated with acquired lesions are not evident: thrills and bruits may be absent and the bradycardiac sign of Branham is less pronounced. The affected limb may be hypertrophied, and it may exhibit increased sweating and hypertrichosis. There is no history of trauma.

Circulatory Disorders in the Head, Neck, and Trunk: The large arteries and veins in the head, neck, and trunk are less accessible to inspection and palpation than those in the extremities (Figs. 8-47 and 8-48A). Vascular disorders in these regions frequently must be inferred from combinations of physical signs.

Carotid artery disease. The carotid arteries supply blood to the head and brain. Vascular symptoms and signs in the extracranial tissues supplied by the external carotid artery are unusual. The exception is frequent involvement by giant cell (temporal) arteritis producing jaw claudication and scalp tenderness. The internal carotid supplies the brain and eye and is frequently involved with atherosclerotic occlusive disease and atheroembolic events, e.g., amaurosis fugax and TIA. The most common sites for atherosclerotic obstruction are the carotid bifurcation, the carotid siphon, and the middle cerebral artery. Disease of the carotid bifurcation is frequently accompanied by a bruit audible in the neck. Carotid bruits with ipsilateral cerebral symptoms carry

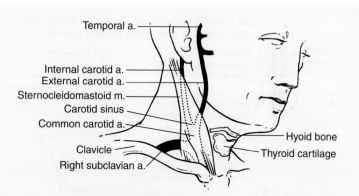

FIG. 8-47 Large Superficial Arteries of the Head and Neck. The accessible arterial segments are diagrammed in solid black; inaccessible parts are stippled. **The temporal artery** courses anterior to the ear and upward to the temporal bone. **The carotid arteries** are deep to the anterior margin of the sternocleidomastoid muscle. **The carotid sinus,** at the bifurcation of the common carotid, is level with the upper margin of the thyroid cartilage. A short segment of **the subclavian artery** is often palpable in the supraclavicular fossa.

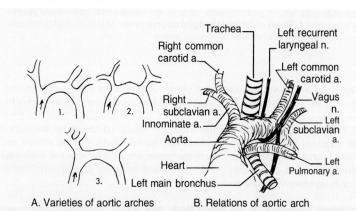

A. Varieties of aortic arches   B. Relations of aortic arch

FIG. 8-48 The Aortic Arch. A. Aortic arch variations. The normal pattern is only slightly more common than the other two. **1. The normal pattern** has a right innominate artery, branching into the subclavian and common carotid. There is no left innominate artery, the left subclavian and common carotid originating from the aorta itself. **2. There is both a right and left innominate. 3. The right innominate gives off the left common carotid** in addition to the right carotid and subclavian. **B. Anatomic relations of a dilated aortic arch.** Aneurysm of the aortic arch or dilatation of the left atrium may compress the left recurrent laryngeal nerve against the vertebrae or the left main bronchus producing paralysis of the left vocal cord, resulting in hoarseness or a brassy cough. Expanding downward, the arch impinges upon the left main bronchus depressing the trachea with each pulse wave, giving a physical sign called *the tracheal tug.*

a substantial risk for stroke within hours or days. Bruits without symptoms must be evaluated to assess the severity of obstruction.

Vertebral artery disease. The vertebral arteries are not accessible to direct examination. They join to form the basilar artery in the posterior fossa and collateralize the cerebral circulation via the posterior cerebral and posterior communicating arteries. Vertebral occlusive disease occurs because of atherosclerosis or dissection giving symptoms of brainstem ischemia (e.g., vertigo, dysarthria, dysequilibrium).

Arterial Aneurysms. Aneurysmal arterial dilatation may be congenital or result from cystic medial necrosis, atherosclerosis, hypertension, vasculitis, or infection. Aneurysms are *fusiform, saccular,* or *dissecting*. They may consume platelets and clotting factors. Similar physical signs are produced by fusiform and saccular dilatations, but the arterial dissection presents an entirely different clinical picture (aortic dissection, page 354). Pain accompanying an aneurysm suggests a penetrating aortic ulcer, leakage, or dissection of the arterial wall.

Thoracic aneurysms. The cause of thoracic aneurysms is multifactorial. Breakdown of structural proteins in the aortic media and adventitia leads to smooth muscle necrosis and development of cystic spaces filled with mucoid material (*cystic medial necrosis*). Predisposing factors include genetic abnormalities (e.g., Marfan syndrome), hypertension, pregnancy, inflammation (e.g., GCA, syphilis), and possibly atherosclerosis. Thoracic aneurysms are classified by their proximal extent, regardless of distal extension, into those involving the ascending aorta and those only involving the aorta distal to the left subclavian artery. The signs and symptoms are due to compression or distortion of adjacent structures and pain from medial dissection or sudden dilation without dissection. Dissection can occur prior to aneurysmal dilatation.

Ascending aortic aneurysms. These can produce aortic regurgitation from either dilation of the ascending aorta or proximal dissection extending to the valve ring and leaflets. The murmur characteristically transmits down the right sternal border rather than the left. A palpable thrust may develop in the right second or third intercostal spaces. The width of manubrial dullness is increased. Erosion of ribs and protrusion of a pulsatile mass can occur. Compression signs include hoarseness (recurrent laryngeal nerve traction), cough, wheezing, or hemoptysis (compression and/or erosion of bronchi). Acute six-dermatome chest pain may result from dissection or myocardial ischemia from dissection of coronary ostia (usually the right). Proximal dissection can rupture into the pericardium producing acute tamponade.

Aortic arch aneurysms. Retrosternal pain is frequent, radiating to the left scapula, left shoulder, or left neck. The dilated arch can compress the left recurrent laryngeal nerve against the trachea or the left main bronchus causing hoarseness and a brassy cough (Fig. 8-48B). Obstruction or dissection of the left subclavian artery causes delay and diminution of pulse volume and reduces left arm blood pressure by >20 mm. The dilated aortic arch can depress the left main bronchus producing a tracheal tug with each beat detected by grasping the cricoid cartilage lightly with the thumb and forefinger feeling the trachea dip with each pulse (Fig. 8-48B).

Descending aortic aneurysms. These are frequently silent and discovered incidentally. They may erode vertebral bodies causing back pain radiating around the chest via the intercostal nerves. Dissection can occlude spinal arteries producing paraplegia. Pain from dissection of descending thoracic aneurysms is like pain from acute MI or ascending aorta dissection, except that the most have pain in the back with or without anterior chest pain.

Abdominal aortic aneurysm (AAA). These are the most common aortic aneurysms. AAA involves all three layers of the aorta. The risk of rupture is directly related to its diameter. Aortic atherosclerosis is uniformly present and often widespread. AAA is uncommon in individuals younger than age 60, but prevalence increases with each decade. Major risk factors are atherosclerosis, cigarette smoking, and male sex. Family clustering has been noted. The width is estimated by placing the fingers on the lateral walls of the pulsatile mass just cephalad to the umbilicus. Pulsatile expansion is demonstrated by lateral as well as anteroposterior movement; this does not occur with a solid mass anterior to the aorta transmitting pulsations. Imaging is required for reliable measurement of size and changes over time. The presence or absence of abdominal or femoral bruits has no predictive value for the presence or absence of AAA. Pain in the mid to lower abdomen and the appearance of a pulsatile epigastric mass suggest recent expansion or leaking. Rapid enlargement in size may, however, be asymptomatic. Rupture is associated with severe pain in the abdomen, back, and/or inguinal areas, accompanied by hypotension. The sensitivity of abdominal palpation for the detection of AAA depends upon the size of the aneurysm and the patient's body habitus. Aneurysms >5 cm in diameter are at risk of rupturing and should be considered for elective surgery. Physical exam is only 75% sensitive for detecting aneurysms of this size. Diagnostic imaging is the preferred method of detection, and male smokers between 65 and 75 years of age are considered for screening. Iliac artery aneurysms, felt on deep palpation as pulsatile masses in the lower abdominal quadrants, are not rare and may rupture.

Dissecting aortic aneurysm. See page 354.

Mycotic aneurysms. These saccular aneurysms are the result of a weakened arterial wall resulting from infection, most frequently an embolic arteritis resulting from subacute bacterial endocarditis or septicemia. They can also develop as extensions of localized suppuration, actinomycosis, or tuberculosis. Mycotic aneurysms usually develop in vessels subject to bending and lightly protected by overlying muscles, e.g., the axillary, brachial, femoral, and popliteal arteries.

Coarctation of the aorta. A congenital stricture forms just proximal or distal to the aortic insertion of the ductus arteriosus (preductal or postductal). The most common constriction is distal to the left subclavian artery takeoff. The adult type almost invariably has a closed ductus. Tissue perfusion distal to the coarctation is maintained via high resistance chest wall collaterals perfusing at the expense of sustained central arterial hypertension. The collateral arterial circulation is via the left internal mammary artery and other left subclavian branches, to the left intercostal arteries (excepting the first two), the musculophrenic, and the superior epigastric arteries (Fig. 8-49). In most cases the collateral circulation allows the patient to remain asymptomatic into adulthood. There is hypertension in the arms with slight hypotension and a dampened pulse wave in the legs. A coincident bicuspid aortic valve

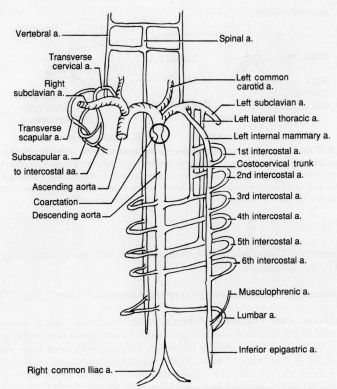

FIG. 8-49 Coarctation of the Aorta: Collateral Circulation. The diagram shows the collateral channels from the costocervical trunk and the internal mammary artery causing dilatation of the intercostal arteries. The circulation around the scapula is augmented by blood through the transverse cervical artery. The pulse volume in the arms is normal; in the femoral arteries it is diminished. The dilated scapular and intercostal arteries may be palpable in the back.

is common, so aortic systolic and/or diastolic murmurs may be heard. **The Murmur:** The murmur of the coarctation is heard best in the posterior inter-scapular area. The site of constriction is remote from the precordium, so the murmur is faint, if heard at all, on the anterior chest. When a murmur is audible anteriorly, it is usually a brief early systolic ejection murmur caused by an associated bicuspid aortic valve, often with an early systolic ejection sound. A continuous bruit from the dilated internal mammary arteries is sometimes heard over the sternum. **Arterial Pulses:** The dampened pulse wave in the distal aorta and its branches is most easily detected by palpating the femoral arteries. When the femoral pulses have good volume, a peak pulse lag between the radial and femoral arteries suggests coarctation. Palpable collateral circulation through the dilated intercostal arteries in the posterior intercostal spaces is diagnostic. Notching of the inferior rib margins posteriorly is visible on chest X-ray. Hypertension in young adults suggests the possibility

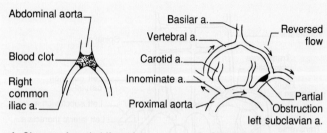

A. Closure of aortic bifurcation   B. Subclavian steal

FIG. 8-50 Two Syndromes of Large Artery Obstruction. **A. Obstruction at the aortic bifurcation (Leriche syndrome):** a short thrombus closes the lower part of the abdominal aorta and extends a variable distance down the common iliac arteries. The accessible segments of the femoral, popliteal, dorsalis pedis, and posterior tibial arteries are pulseless. Pain in the legs and intermittent claudication are the common symptoms. **B. Subclavian steal syndrome:** the most common site of narrowing is the left subclavian artery, although other sites have also been reported.

of coarctation. Coarctation is common in patients with the gonadal dysgenesis (Turner syndrome).

Aberrant right subclavian artery (dysphagia lusoria). Chapter 7, page 252.

Subclavian steal syndrome. Atherosclerotic subclavian artery stenosis proximal to the vertebral artery origin results in retrograde flow in the ipsilateral vertebral artery inducing brainstem ischemia with neurologic signs (Fig. 8-50). A bruit may be heard in the supraclavicular fossa, occasionally with a thrill. The arterial pulse volume and blood pressure are diminished in the affected arm. Symptoms and signs of cerebral ischemia are intermittent or continuous, ranging from vague dizziness to vertigo, slurring of speech, and hemiparesis. The neurologic signs and symptoms can be induced by exercising the affected arm.

Thoracic outlet syndromes—subclavian and brachial plexus compression. The roots of C5-T1 form the brachial plexus in the lateral neck between the scalenus medius and the scalenus anticus. The subclavian artery exits the rib cage over the first rib. Artery and nerves run together over the first and second ribs and under the clavicle and pectoralis minor into the upper arm. These syndromes are caused by compression of the nerves and vessels coursing between muscles and bones while making their exit from the neck (nerves) and chest (vessels) (Fig. 8-51). Symptoms, arising from brachial plexus compression, are largely sensory (paresthesias), and signs are those of positional arterial obstruction. Examine a patient presenting with subjective neurologic symptoms for signs of arterial compression.

Scalenus anticus syndrome. There is intermittent or constant pain and/or paresthesia in the ulnar aspect of the arm and hand, sometimes associated with weakness and wasting. *Adson Test,* Fig. 8-51a: Have the patient sit with the palms on the knees, chin high, and turned to the side being examined. Examine the radial pulse with breath holding in deep inspiration. A positive

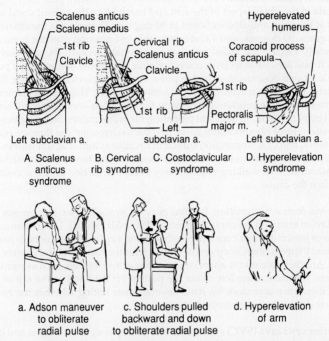

FIG. 8-51 Compression Syndromes of the Superior Thoracic Aperture. A. Scalenus anticus syndrome: the scalenus anticus muscle attaches to the transverse processes of the cervical vertebrae above and below to the first rib. Posteriorly and behind the subclavian artery, the scalenus medius attaches to the same bones. Hypertrophy of the bellies of the two muscles compresses the artery between them with motions such as turning the head to the ipsilateral side. This is tested by **the Adson maneuver (a),** where the patient sits with chin raised, head rotated to the left, and chest held in the inspiratory position. A positive test is marked by diminution or disappearance of the left radial pulse. The other side is tested similarly. **B. Cervical rib syndrome:** the diagram shows a cervical rib compressing the left scalenus anticus muscle and indirectly the subclavian artery. This may diminish the radial pulse and/or produce a partial brachial plexus peripheral neuritis. **C. Costoclavicular syndrome:** the geometry of the aperture may be such that rotating the clavicles downward and backward compresses the subclavian arteries against the first rib. This is tested (c) by having the patient seated in a chair and the examiner standing behind him pushing the shoulders downward and backward while an assistant feels for diminution of the radial pulses. **D. Hyperelevation of the arm:** in some persons thoracic geometry is such that hyperelevation of the arm causes the coracoid process to impinge on and compress the subclavian artery, diminishing the radial pulse (d).

test is dampening or obliteration of the radial pulse that resolves when the chin turns forward, still holding the breath. The syndrome is associated with muscular hypertrophy or edema after unusually vigorous arm use or with unusual occupations, such as weight lifters. Muscle spasm can result from poor posture, anomalous first rib, or cervical rib.

Cervical rib. In addition to producing scalenus anticus spasm (scalenus anticus syndrome, above), a cervical rib can directly compress the subclavian artery dampening the radial pulse in any position (Fig. 8-51B). Occasionally, the extra rib is palpable in the supraclavicular fossa. The rib may also compress the brachial plexus producing pain or paresthesias in the hand.

Costoclavicular syndrome. There is intermittent or constant pain and/or paresthesia in the ulnar aspect of the arm and hand. Have the patient stand with arms at the sides and elbows flexed at 90 degrees. Then elevate the elbows to 45 degrees, 90 degrees, and 135 degrees (this last position puts the hands on the head). Palpate the radial pulse and auscultate beneath the mid-clavicle at each position. Patients with costoclavicular syndrome obliterate the pulse in at least one position. A palpable pulse with a subclavicular systolic bruit indicates partial obstruction. *Costoclavicular Maneuver:* This test for clavicular compression of the subclavian artery on the first rib is specific but not sensitive. The patient sits, an assistant palpating his radial pulses. Standing behind the patient force his shoulders down and back narrowing the thoracic outlet (Fig. 8-51C and c). Compression sufficient to cause symptoms, diminishes the pulse volumes. Activities in which the shoulders are forced downward and backward, such as walking with a heavy backpack carried on the shoulders are often the cause.

Ischemia from arm elevation. In some persons, arm elevation compresses the subclavian artery on the coracoid process (Fig. 8-51D and d). The patient complains of intermittent or constant numbness and tingling in one or both hands or arms. Patients often sleep on their back with the hands behind or over the head. Another precipitant is working with the arms elevated, such as painting ceilings. *Hyperabduction Test:* Have the patient lift the hand to the top of the head then open and close his hand several times noting whether the radial pulse is diminished or abolished.

Superior vena cava (SVC) syndrome. The principal signs are edema and cyanosis of the head, neck, and both arms, edema of the face, both arms, and the upper third of the thoracic wall, and engorged venous without the pulsations normally transmitted from the right atrium (Fig. 8-52). The neck is enlarged by nonpitting edema (*Stokes collar*) and collateral veins may be visible on the chest and abdominal wall. Causes are mediastinal neoplasm, cervical or retrosternal goiter, thoracic aortic aneurysm, chronic mediastinitis (e.g., histoplasmosis), thrombosis from an indwelling intravenous catheter.

Inferior vena cava (IVC) obstruction. IVC occlusion impairs venous drainage from the legs and pelvis leading to development of collateral veins in the hemorrhoidal complex and abdominal wall. Renal vein thrombosis causes acute renal failure. **Acute IVC Obstruction:** It may be asymptomatic until lower extremity edema develops. Symmetrical rapidly progressive edema of both legs without evidence of heart or kidney disease suggests mechanical IVC obstruction. **Chronic IVC Obstruction:** Dilated superficial collateral veins with cephalad flow on the abdomen suggest chronic IVC obstruction. Visible collaterals can appear within a week of obstruction, the veins attaining maximal size in 3 months. To localize the obstruction, consider the vena cava in three segments (Fig. 8-52). Lower Segment (below the renal veins): The collaterals are distributed over thighs, groins, lower abdomen, and flanks. Leg edema, initially pitting, develops fibrosis with chronic venous stasis dermatitis. Pelvic congestion produces low back pain and genital edema. Middle Segment (above the renal veins and below the hepatic vein): The venous collaterals are large intra-abdominal veins without abdominal wall collaterals. Occlusion of the renal veins produces nephrotic syndrome. Gastrointestinal

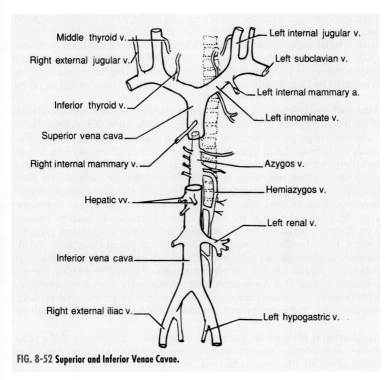

FIG. 8-52 **Superior and Inferior Venae Cavae.**

Labels on figure:
- Middle thyroid v.
- Right external jugular v.
- Inferior thyroid v.
- Superior vena cava
- Right internal mammary v.
- Hepatic vv.
- Inferior vena cava
- Right external iliac v.
- Left internal jugular v.
- Left subclavian v.
- Left internal mammary a.
- Left innominate v.
- Azygos v.
- Hemiazygos v.
- Left renal v.
- Left hypogastric v.

manifestations include nausea, vomiting, diarrhea, and abdominal pain. Malabsorption may develop. Upper Segment (above the hepatic veins): Venous collaterals form a prominent periumbilical plexus and large veins appear over the anterior abdomen. *Budd–Chiari syndrome* develops with hepatosplenomegaly, ascites, jaundice, and elevated transaminases.

CLINICAL OCCURRENCE: *Intraluminal:* Thrombosis, embolism, invading neoplasm, or extension from renal cell carcinoma; *Intramural:* Rare benign or malignant neoplasms; *External Pressure:* Hepatomegaly, lymphadenopathy, aortic aneurysm, surgical ligation, and pregnancy.

Disorders of Large Limb Arteries. Arterial disorders are occlusive or nonocclusive, and occlusion may be partial or complete. Four mechanisms cause arterial circulatory deficits: (1) extrinsic compression; (2) vasospasm; (3) luminal obstruction (intimal thickening, thrombus, embolus); or (4) arteriopathy (vasculitis, fibromuscular dysplasia). Temporary arterial compression is often related to extremity positioning. Vasospasm is recognized by the sharp border between ischemic and normal tissue. Intimal proliferation is inferred when the blood flow is diminished but still present. Complete occlusion is usually caused by embolism or thrombosis. Thrombosis is often the result of gradual, usually atherosclerotic, narrowing allowing development of collaterals with relatively mild symptoms coming on gradually. Sudden embolic or thrombotic occlusion causes severe pain and a cold white part. Arteriopathy such as vasculitis is usually inferred from the total clinical picture. When an acute arterial occlusion is suspected, determine the most distal site with adequate flow by noting the presence or absence of pulses along the vessel and palpate the vessel walls for signs of intrinsic disease. Urgent vascular imaging is required by Doppler ultrasound, and/or CT, MR, or contrast angiography.

Atherosclerosis. Atherosclerosis is characterized by degeneration and fibrosis of the media together with occlusive intimal proliferation. Arterial narrowing is the result of progressive intimal thickening, plaque formation with accumulation of cholesterol-rich lipid deposits, foam cells, and smooth muscle proliferation. Rupture of intimal plaques leads to thrombus formation. Arterial segments lengthen and, when the ends of a segment are anchored, the elongated vessel buckles producing visible and palpable tortuosity. Atherosclerosis may be diffuse or focal, often occurring at arterial bifurcations. In patients age >45, atherosclerosis is the major cause of arterial obstruction. Patients with diabetes mellitus have an increased risk inversely related to glycemic control. Hyperhomocysteinemia, congenital or acquired (folic acid and B_{12} deficiency), also increases risk for atherosclerosis and thromboembolic events. Atheromatous plaques may be felt in the walls of accessible arteries, the vessels feeling thick and noncompressible. Noninvasive vascular examination with Doppler ultrasonography and plethysmography are required for accurate diagnosis. Angiography with contrast or MRA is anatomically definitive.

Acute arterial obstruction. Occlusion of arteries to the organs of the head, thorax, and abdomen presents with symptoms referable to those organs, e.g., stroke, acute MI, PE, mesenteric, renal, and splenic infarction.

Acute extremity artery obstruction—embolism and arterial thrombosis. This is most common in the legs but does occur in the arms. The patient experiences sudden excruciating pain followed by numbness and weakness. Occasionally, anesthesia and weakness are presenting symptoms while the pain appears gradually. The distal extremity is pulseless and becomes pallid, the skin becoming cool. Venous pooling causes the skin distally to gradually become cyanotic while mottling occurs proximally; the cyanosis diminishes with limb elevation. Occasionally, the pain may be quite mild. Thrombosis is more likely when there are signs of diffuse vascular disease or a history of claudication. Embolism is likely with atrial fibrillation.

CLINICAL OCCURRENCE: *Thrombosis:* Atherosclerosis, thromboangiitis obliterans, vasculitis, infection, trauma, antiphospholipid syndrome, and sludging from polycythemia, hemoconcentration, cryoglobulinemia, or hyperglobulinemia; *Embolism:* Atrial fibrillation, mitral stenosis, endocarditis (infectious, NBTE), left atrial myxoma, LV mural thrombus post MI, and atheroembolism.

Chronic peripheral vascular disease (PVD). PVD is most common in the legs but can involve the arms. The patient complains of claudication and coldness progressing to continuous and/or night pain. Measure the ABI (page 291). Arterial insufficiency causes skin pigmentation, pallor, purplish discoloration fading with elevation, coldness, warm areas of collateral circulation, local hair loss, malnutrition of toenails, ulceration, and/or gangrene

(Figs. 8-24 and 8-53). Pulses are weak or absent and muscle wasting may be evident. Popliteal artery occlusion leads to collateral circulation via geniculate artery branches producing cold feet with especially warm knees or anteromedial lower thigh. ABI of <0.9 is associated with increased risk of cardiovascular morbidity and mortality. ABI <0.5 is more strongly associated with decreased physical activity than with claudication.

Pulseless femoral artery. When examining the abdomen, always palpate the femoral arteries. When a femoral pulse is diminished or absent, palpate the iliac pulses up to and including the aortic bifurcation located 2 cm below and slightly to the left of the umbilicus. The iliac arteries run in a line between the bifurcation and the midpoint of the inguinal ligament. The upper third is the common iliac, the lower two-thirds the external iliacs. Though these vessels may not be palpable in normal persons, finding asymmetry is significant. Bilateral decreased or absent femoral pulses suggest coarctation of the aorta, distal aortic thrombosis (*Leriche syndrome*, Fig. 8-50A, page 370), or dissecting aortic aneurysm. Unilateral absence suggests common iliac artery thrombosis. The significance of an absent or diminished femoral pulse is determined by the status of the distal pulses.

Thromboangiitis obliterans (Buerger disease). Beginning as an acute segmental panarteritis involving all three layers of medium-sized arteries, intimal granulation tissue ultimately causes arterial obstruction, producing tissue ischemia and necrosis. Thromboangiitis affects young male smokers and is often associated with superficial migrating thrombophlebitis. It usually presents between ages 20 and 40, a younger age than atherosclerosis. *DDX:* No physical signs distinguish Buerger disease from atherosclerosis. The distribution of affected vessels may differ from atherosclerosis, thromboangiitis having a predilection for the radial, ulnar, and digital arteries, in addition to affecting the lower extremities. Approximately 7% of Japanese patients are nonsmokers.

Raynaud disease and phenomenon. Intense spasm of the digital arteries and dermal vessels produces initial pallor, followed over minutes by filling of dilated cappillaries with deoxygenated venous blood producing cyanosis. Relaxation of arterial spasm flushes the capillaries with arterial blood producing the warm red phase of vasodilation. Approximately 80% of patients are young women. The sudden attacks are induced by cold exposure or emotional stress and last up to 60 minutes. Manifestations are unilateral or bilateral, most commonly in the fingers, though the toes are affected in 50% of cases. One to four fingers are involved, but rarely the thumbs. The terminal digits become chalk-white, numb and sweaty; intense cyanosis and pain succeeds the pallor. Sometimes either pallor or cyanosis is absent. During spontaneous recovery, or after warm water immersion, projections of hyperemia replace cyanosis until the digit becomes brilliant red. Hyperemia is accompanied by tingling, throbbing, and edema. After many attacks, trophic changes may appear in the nails and adjacent skin and small areas of gangrene may develop on the fingertips and toes. The term *Raynaud disease* is used when there is no associated condition and *Raynaud phenomenon* when it is associated with scleroderma, vibratory trauma, SLE, polyarteritis, peripheral neuropathy, thromboangiitis obliterans, or atherosclerosis.

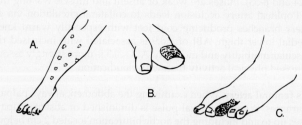

FIG. 8-53 Signs of Arterial Insufficiency. A. Poor wound healing. B. Nail dystrophy. C. Digital gangrene.

Raynaud phenomenon occurs more frequently in patients with migraine (26%) than in those without (6%). There is also an increased prevalence of chest pain and migraine in patients with Raynaud disease. *DDX:* Always inspect the nailbed capillaries (Chapter 6, page 107); abnormal capillaries are highly suggestive of scleroderma. The sequence of pallor, cyanosis, and redness is diagnostic when induced by cold exposure. Raynaud disease should not be confused with the vascular changes of complex regional pain syndromes (Chapter 4, page 75).

Acrocyanosis. Excessive arteriolar constriction is ascribed to increased sympathetic tone, although humoral factors may contribute. This is a benign painless condition in which the skin of the hands and feet is persistently cold, cyanotic, and moist. It is most common in young women. The skin is uniformly cyanotic, which worsens on cold exposure. Elevation and sleep abolish the cyanosis.

Digital gangrene. Gangrene of the finger and toe tips is caused by any disease or condition impairing peripheral perfusion. Causes include scleroderma, pneumatic hammer disease, atherosclerosis, thromboangiitis obliterans, cold agglutination disease, cryoglobulinemia, atheroemboli, sepsis, meningococcemia, vasopressor medications, antiphospholipid syndrome, warfarin skin necrosis (protein C deficiency), ergotism, and chronic renal failure.

Ergotism. Ergots induce intense constriction of peripheral blood vessels; some individuals are particularly sensitive. Ergot may be taken as a drug or eaten with dietary grain contaminated by a fungus. The first symptom is often burning extremity pain (*St. Anthony fire*) with loss of pulses in the hands and/or feet. Headache, weakness, nausea, vomiting, visual disturbances, and angina pectoris may occur. Cold skin and mottled cyanosis of the extremities follows. Finally, symmetrical gangrene involves the fingers and toes, sometimes extending proximally.

Cavernous hemangiomas. Congenital cavernous hemangiomas occur anywhere in the body. The limb is circumferentially enlarged and dilated, purplish, blood-filled, readily compressible sinuses raise the skin surface. This is distinguished from varicosities by a distribution not congruent with the large limb veins. With leg involvement standing may pool enough blood to cause orthostatic hypotension. Massive cavernous hemangiomas trap platelets producing thrombocytopenia, purpura, and bleeding (*Kasabach–Merritt syndrome*).

Aneurysms in the arms and neck. The subclavian, axillary, and brachial arteries are most commonly affected; the carotids are rarely involved. Trauma to the vessel wall is the most common cause; rarely, the vessels are involved by mycotic, necrotizing, or atherosclerotic aneurysms. The aneurysms are easily palpated.

Aneurysms in the legs. The most common sites are the femoral artery in the Scarpa triangle and the popliteal artery in its fossa. Atherosclerosis is the most common cause. The aneurysms are readily palpable.

Disorders of the Major Extremity Veins

Deep vein thrombosis. See Pulmonary Embolism, page 343. Intraluminal thrombus forms, usually in association with a lower extremity vein valve, with or without an inciting event. The thrombus can propagate proximally or distally and partially or completely occlude flow. Bland thrombus without inflammation appears more likely to dislodge. Leg veins are the most common identified source of PE. Hip and knee surgery have particularly a high incidence of associated DVT. Timely diagnosis facilitates initiation of appropriate therapy intended to prevent pulmonary embolus and diminish valve damage predisposing to future thrombosis and venous stasis. The history and physical exam separate patients into low-, intermediate-, and high-risk categories (Table 8-4). All patients in whom DVT is suspected should undergo further testing. Diagnostic algorithms constantly change, so consult current protocols. Early diagnosis can be lifesaving. Symptoms: Though often asymptomatic, tightness or a sense of fullness, aggravated by standing and walking, are noted. Signs: DVT may be accompanied by cutaneous *cyanosis* of the dependent foot and lower leg. Pitting edema of the foot, ankle, or leg that does not resolve overnight and venous engorgement on the feet persisting with the legs elevated to 45 degrees, suggest venous obstruction. Leg pain following the course of the thrombosed vein may be induced by sneezing or coughing, the pain disappearing when the vein is compressed proximal to the obstruction (*Louvel sign*). Palpation may detect tender vein segments. *Homan Sign:* With the knee in flexion, forcefully dorsiflex the ankle; calf or popliteal pain occurs in ~35% of DVT patients. Homan sign is neither sensitive nor specific for DVT.

Thrombophlebitis. As the name implies, thrombosis is accompanied by inflammation of the vein. Inflammation may either precede or follow clot formation. In addition to the signs and symptoms of thrombosis, pain and inflammation are prominent. When acute, the veins are painful and tender, and the overlying skin is red and hot. Adjacent muscles may cramp. Fever and leukocytosis are common. Acute femoral vein thrombophlebitis presents with excruciating pain, massive leg edema, and pallor from arterial spasm (*phlegmasia alba dolens*). The signs can suggest arterial embolism, but the pallor is less intense, there is more cyanosis, the femoral vein is tender, anesthesia is absent, and arterial pulses can usually be demonstrated by ultrasound. When the entire venous drainage of an extremity is obstructed, there is extreme

TABLE 8-4 Wells Criteria for Deep Venous Thrombosis Risk Stratification.

Clinical Feature	Score
Current cancer or within the last 6 mo	1
Paralysis, significant limb weakness or immobilization of one or both legs	1
Bedridden for >3 d or surgery within 4 wk	1
Localized tenderness along the deep veins	1
Entire leg swollen	1
Calf circumference >3 cm compared to the asymptomatic leg, 10 cm below the tibial tuberosity	1
Pitting edema greater in the symptomatic leg	1
Collateral (nonvaricose) superficial veins in the symptomatic leg	1
Alternative diagnosis as likely or more likely the DVT	2

Summary pretest risk estimation score observed prevalence of DVT:

Low	0 or less	3%
Moderate	1–2	17%
High	3 or more	75%

Adapted from Wells PS, Anderson DR, et al. Value of assessment of pretest probability of deep-vein thrombosis in clinical management. *Lancet.* 1997;350:1795–1798.

pain, massive edema, and deep cyanosis of the entire limb (*phlegmasia cerulea dolens*). Arterial and venous imaging are indicated.

CLINICAL OCCURRENCE: *Congenital:* DVT at an early age, at unusual sites (e.g. upper extremity, mesenteric vessels), a history of recurrent thromboses or emboli, a family history of DVT, or DVT with minimal trauma or minor surgery suggest congenital thrombophilia. Identified etiologies include activated protein C resistance, factor V Leiden mutation, proteins C and S deficiency, dysfibrinogenemia, homocystinuria, antithrombin III deficiency, and sickle cell disease. *Acquired:* Antiphospholipid syndrome (lupus-like anticoagulant, anticardiolipin antibodies), heparin-induced thrombocytopenia and thrombosis (HITT syndrome), leg fractures, limb surgery, trauma, prolonged inactivity (bed rest, international air travel, automobile travel), infection, cancer (especially mucin-producing adenocarcinomas), hyperhomocysteinemia, estrogen-containing medications, pregnancy, obesity, venous stasis and insufficiency, diabetes mellitus, polycythemia vera, idiopathic thrombocythemia, and paroxysmal nocturnal hemoglobinuria. Recurrent deep venous thrombosis may precede the diagnosis of cancer.

Post-phlebitic syndrome. Following proximal leg vein DVT, up to 50% of patients develop this syndrome. Pain and tenderness are slight, and the skin is normal or cool. The leg is swollen, initially with edema, but, if untreated, progresses to nonpitting fibrosis of the subcutaneous tissues and skin. Varicose veins may or may not be prominent. Venous stasis dermatitis is common. Severe cases can be disabling.

Superficial thrombophlebitis. Superficial vein thrombosis and inflammation occurs either alone or extends from the deep veins. Patients complain of tender red subcutaneous nodules or cords, often with a history of recent trauma. Superficial thrombophlebitis can mask coincident deep vein disease, so underlying DVT should be investigated. Superficial thrombophlebitis rarely causes life-threatening pulmonary embolus. *DDX:* Lymphangitis and other skin and soft-tissue infections can be confused with superficial thrombophlebitis, but the firm palpable venous cords are diagnostic.

Migratory superficial thrombophlebitis. Successive episodes of thrombophlebitis involve different veins in widely separated parts of the body. In a single episode, a segment of vein becomes tender, reddened, and indurated. Involution begins in a few days and the adjacent tissues become successively blue and yellow, often resolving with some skin pigmentation. Arm and leg veins are most commonly involved, but the subcutaneous veins of the abdomen and thorax may be affected. Although the lesions do not cause serious discomfort, this complex should prompt a search for an underlying disease. Migratory superficial thrombophlebitis is associated with antiphospholipid syndrome, thromboangiitis obliterans, Behçet syndrome, pancreatic carcinoma, and thrombophilic hematologic disorders, especially paroxysmal nocturnal hemoglobinuria.

Venous stasis. Vein occlusion and incompetent valves impair flow resulting in stasis changes. Occlusion is caused by external compression or luminal plugging by fibrosis, thrombus, or intravascular neoplasm. The pumping action of voluntary muscles is inhibited by bed rest and immobilization and dilated vessels exacerbate stasis. Dilated superficial veins drain poorly into smaller communicating veins. Deep vein dilatation causes their valves to become incompetent. Decreased capillary flow produces poor skin nutrition, chronic inflammation, and fibrosis. Signs of venous stasis are pitting edema, stasis pigmentation (hemosiderin), erythema, fibrosis, decreased skin elasticity, and ulceration (see Stasis Dermatitis, Chapter 6, page 135).

Varicose veins. Varicose veins are grossly dilated subcutaneous veins, often filling by retrograde flow from the deep veins because of incompetent valves in the perforating and deep veins. They are most common in legs (Fig. 8-54). Primary varicosities develop spontaneously; secondary varicosities result from proximal obstruction, e.g., pregnancy, trauma, and thrombophlebitis. When varicose veins are seen only in one extremity, extrinsic compression and an arteriovenous fistula should be considered. An AVM produces pulsation in the dilated veins.

Axillary vein thrombosis. This usually follows trauma or intensive arm use in hyperabduction, such as throwing. The entire arm swells and aches. The tissues are firm without pitting edema. The superficial veins at the superior thoracic aperture may be dilated. Poor collateral circulation results in cutaneous cyanosis. Axillary vein thrombosis is less likely to lead to lethal pulmonary emboli than deep venous thrombosis in the legs, but it does occur. *DDX:* When chronic, it must be distinguished from lymphedema. Both conditions produce solid, nonpitting swelling, but venous obstruction causes some cyanosis of the skin; the skin is pallid in lymphedema. Lymphedema of the arm was common after radical mastectomy.

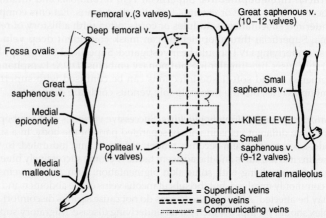

FIG. 8-54 Large Superficial Veins of the Legs. The great saphenous vein begins on the medial aspect of the foot, courses backward under the medial malleolus, up the medial aspect of the calf, behind the medial epicondyle, and then obliquely across the anterior thigh to the femoral vein as it enters the femoral canal beneath the inguinal ligament. **The small saphenous vein** begins on the lateral side of the foot, curves backward beneath the lateral malleolus, and then upward on the posterior surface of the calf to enter the popliteal fossa and join with the popliteal vein. The middle figure diagrams the **communications between the superficial veins (heavy solid lines) and the deep veins (broken lines) and the communicating vessels (dotted lines)**.

SECTION 2

The Breasts

BREAST PHYSIOLOGY

The Female Breast: The breast is a highly complex, specialized skin-related gland. The mammary glands are undeveloped in children and men. In women, ovarian estrogen production at puberty initiates development which reaches maturity in the childbearing years. Luteal progesterone secretion at onset of ovulation results in alveolar development. Other hormones, including prolactin, adrenocorticotropic hormone, corticosteroids, growth hormone, thyroxine, and androgens, play facultative roles in breast development and milk production. The mature breast is conical or hemispheric, containing 15–20 subdivided lobes, arranged radially, each with a separate excretory lactiferous tubule and nipple orifice. Considerable fat surrounds the glands, so discrete lobes are not ordinarily palpable. Vertical fibrous bands (Cooper ligaments) pass from the pectoralis fascia through the breast parenchyma to the skin, suspending the breast on the chest wall. A fascial cleft separates the deep surface of the breast from the thoracic wall, permitting some mobility.

The adult breast has four major components: stroma, ductal epithelium, glandular acini, and the myoepithelium, each influenced by a variety of hormones. The breast glands respond to pituitary and ovarian hormones. Follicular estrogens stimulate minimal mitotic activity, whereas luteal progesterone provokes significant cell division increasing breast size. If conception takes place, estrogens, progesterone, and prolactin stimulate extensive alveolar and ductal proliferation. With parturition progesterone suppression of prolactin ceases, allowing the epithelium to become actively secretory, releasing milk.

The Male Breast: The undeveloped male breast is easily examined. Unfortunately, exam is frequently neglected delaying recognition of serious disease. Men have residual breast anlage that will respond to hormones from adolescence to old age. Breast development is stimulated by abnormal hormone production, including hyperthyroidism, prolactin-secreting adenomas, acromegaly, testicular and adrenal tumors, and many drugs in addition to estrogens. Liver disease increases circulating estrogenic hormones so gynecotmastia is associated with advanced liver disease, particularly alcoholic cirrhosis.

SUPERFICIAL BREASTS ANATOMY

The breast's roughly circular contact with the pectoral fascia extends from the second to the sixth or seventh ribs with an axillary tail projecting laterally and superiorly along the axillary and serratus anterior fascia (Fig. 8-55).

The nipple lies slightly below and lateral to the center of the breast. It has papillae containing the lactiferous tubule orifices and pigmented skin extending onto the surface of the breast as the areola. Nipple and areola color vary from pink to brown, depending on the individual's complexion and parity. Both darken, and the areola enlarges after the second month of pregnancy. The sebaceous glands of Montgomery (areolar glands) form small elevations on the areolar surface. Their secretions protect the nipples during nursing. Areolar stimulation causes the subcutaneous radial and circular muscle fibers to contract producing nipple erection.

PHYSICAL EXAM OF THE BREASTS

The American Cancer Society and others provide guidelines for periodic breast cancer screening in women by breast exam and mammography. Also,

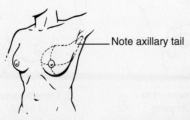

FIG. 8-55 Quadrants of the Breast. The hemisphere of the breast is divided into quadrants by imaginary vertical and horizontal lines intersecting at the nipple. The quadrants are named upper medial, upper lateral, lower medial, and lower lateral. Popularly, these quadrants are also named, respectively, upper inner, upper outer, lower inner, and lower outer. Note the protrusion of the upper lateral quadrant, called the axillary tail, in which breast tissue extends to the axilla.

regularly examine the male breast since breast cancer, and other conditions enlarging breast tissue in men, are easily identified on exam. The breasts are usually inspected and palpated with the patient sitting and supine. If the patient complains of a breast lump or a possible mass is detected, a more extensive exam is required. The breasts engorge before menses and during pregnancy, making the exam more painful and less accurate. The best time for breast exam is 5–7 days after onset of menses.

Breast Examination: The patient is examined sitting and supine, being certain to examine the creases under and between the breasts. If the patient has noted a lump, ask her to point it out. Always palpate the opposite breast first. Palpate both breasts in all four quadrants by compressing breast tissue between the three middle fingers pads and chest wall. Search for warmth, tenderness, and masses. When a mass is found, note its location, size, mobility, and consistency. Test for fixation to the underlying fascia by grasping the mass between thumb and forefinger attempting to move it back-and-forth transversely, then up-and-down. Repeat this procedure while the pectoralis muscle is tensed. Gently pinching the overlying skin reveals dimpling indicating that the mass is fixed to the skin (Fig. 8-56A). Transilluminate the mass to determine if it is opaque or translucent (Fig. 8-56B). Finish with regional lymph nodes palpation (Chapter 5, page 83 and Fig. 5-2).

Patient sitting with arms down. With the disrobed patient sitting, compare breast size and shape; the left may normally be slightly larger. Look for bulging or flattening of the contour, nipple displacement or retraction, skin dimpling, dilated superficial veins, or peau d'orange skin changes (Fig. 8-57A).

Patient sitting with arms raised. With the arms raised overhead, look for a shift in the relative position of the nipples, and for skin dimpling, or bulging (Fig. 8-57B).

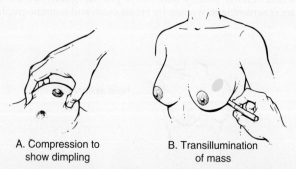

A. Compression to   B. Transillumination
show dimpling   of mass

FIG. 8-56 Further Breast Examination. A. Breast compression to accent dimpling: dimpling is a sign of shortening of the suspensory ligaments of the breast from neoplasm or inflammation. **B. Transillumination:** the density of a mass may, on occasion, be ascertained by transillumination of the breast; transparency probably means a cyst full of fluid; other masses are opaque.

Patient sitting with hands pressing hips. Pressing the hands downward on the hips puts tension on the breast ligaments arising from the pectoralis major fascia which can reveal dimpling. For a mass in the axillary tail, tense the serratus anterior muscle by having the patient press her hand downward on your shoulder (Fig. 8-57C).

Patient sitting with trunk bent forward. When the breasts are large and pendulous, having the patient lean forward so the breasts hang free from the chest wall facilitates inspection and palpation between the flats of both hands (Fig. 8-57D).

Patient supine. Most breast masses are detected in this position; proper technique is critically important (Fig. 8-57E). The entire breast from the second to sixth rib and from the sternal border to the midaxillary line is palpated against the chest wall. The lateral half of the breast is best palpated with the patient rolled onto the contralateral hip and the medial half with the patient supine, both with the ipsilateral hand behind the head. Palpate with the three middle finger pads rotating in small circular motions and moving in vertical overlapping passes from rostral to caudal and then caudal to rostral in the next pass. Vary finger pressure from light to medium to deep.

Nipple exam. Inspect the anterior trunk for supernumerary nipples. Look for fissures, scaling, excoriation, and nipple retraction or deformity.

BREAST SYMPTOMS

Breast Pain: The patient with pain or a lump in the breast often fears cancer. Many women will, at some time, experience breast discomfort significant enough to seek a physician's advice. Common causes of breast pain are engorgement during the luteal phase of the menstrual cycle, pregnancy, hematoma, cysts, mastitis and abscess, galactocele, and nipple disorders including fissures, inflammation, and epithelioma.

BREAST SIGNS

Breast Mass: Breast masses arise from cystic changes, benign proliferation of ductal or acinar tissue, infection, inflammation or fibrosis of the breast stroma, and neoplastic change in the ductal epithelium (ductal carcinoma) or the acinar tissues (lobular neoplasia). A breast mass must be accurately described noting its location (use the nipple as the center of a clock face: state the o'clock position and the radial distance from the nipple), size, shape, consistency (hard, firm, fluctuant, soft), texture (smooth, irregular), mobility (mobile, fixed to the breast tissue, pectoral fascia or skin), and tenderness. Thoroughly examine the regional lymph nodes (axillary, infraclavicular, and supraclavicular) for lymphadenopathy. Masses identified by the patient or clinician should never be ignored or be assumed to be benign. The patient's age and breast cancer risk factors should not deter evaluation of a breast mass. See page 386 for a discussion of common breast masses.

All masses persisting through one complete menstrual cycle and all masses in postmenopausal women require evaluation by a clinician experienced in the diagnosis and management of breast diseases and breast cancer. A normal mammogram or non-visualization of a palpable mass by ultrasonography does not exclude cancer.

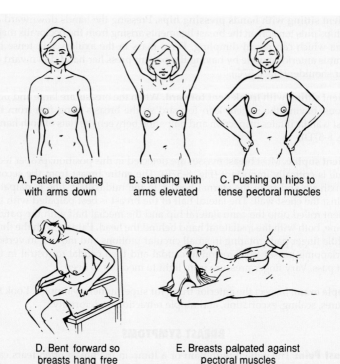

A. Patient standing with arms down

B. standing with arms elevated

C. Pushing on hips to tense pectoral muscles

D. Bent forward so breasts hang free

E. Breasts palpated against pectoral muscles

FIG. 8-57 Patient Positions for Breast Examination. The patient is stripped to the waist and sits facing the examiner. **A. The patient stands with arms at sides.** The examiner looks for elevation of the level of a nipple, dimpling, bulging, and peau d'orange. **B. The patient raises her arms.** Dimpling and elevation of the nipple are accentuated when there is a mass fixed to the pectoral fascia. **C. The patient pushes her hands down against her hips.** This flexes and tenses the pectoralis major muscles while the examiner attempts to move the mass to determine fixation to the underlying fascia. **D. Examining large and pendulous breasts.** The patient is asked to lean forward, so the breasts hang free from the chest wall, making; retraction and masses more evident. **E. In the supine position.** The examiner presses the breasts against the chest wall with the flat of his hand. The normal lobules are less prominent and significant masses are more distinctly felt.

Breast Tenderness (Mastodynia): During the luteal phase of the menstrual cycle and with pregnancy and lactation the breasts undergo glandular proliferation becoming larger, more engorged, and tender. Many women, in child-bearing years, have tenderness that varies through the menstrual cycle never resolving completely. The breasts can be firm and lobular but without distinct masses. Common causes of breast pain are engorgement during the luteal phase of the menstrual cycle, pregnancy, hematoma, cysts, mastitis and abscess, galactocele, and nipple disorders including fissures, inflammation, and epithelioma.

Breast Cysts: Cystic change in the breast creates single or multiple tender fluid-filled cysts. The patient has tenderness fluctuating through the menstrual cycle. Exam discloses one or more smooth, usually mobile, tender tense masses either fluctuant or firm. Ultrasonography or needle aspiration confirms the cyst.

Supernumerary Nipples (Polythelia) and Breasts (Polymastia): Extra nipples occur frequently in both sexes as minor developmental errors; rarely, they are associated with glandular tissue forming a complete breast. Supernumerary nipples are smaller than normal and often mistaken for moles. Close examination may disclose a miniature nipple and areola. Most occur in the mammary line (milk line) on the thorax and abdomen. They are found rarely in the axilla or on the shoulder, flank, groin, or thigh where they must be distinguished from moles.

Inverted Nipples: A common harmless developmental anomaly results in the nipple having a crater-like depression. Nipple retraction appearing after maturity suggests underlying neoplasm or inflammation.

Nipple Fissures: Breaks in the skin are usually caused by local infection, possibly in association with an unsuspected abscess.

Duct Fistula: A chronic draining wound close to the nipple and areola may be a fistula from an underlying duct.

Skin or Nipple Retraction: Acquired nipple retraction and skin dimpling are caused by shortened suspensory ligaments, and/or fixation to the underlying pectoral fascia by tumor or inflammation. Skin and nipple retraction and/or limited breast mobility on the chest wall suggest an underlying mass. Always examine for regional lymphadenopathy. Retraction can also be the result of previous mastitis, but that should not be assumed unless the evolution from acute mastitis to fixation and retraction has been personally observed.

Nipple Discharge: Abnormal breast secretions are concerning. Most causes are benign. Discharges are serous, bloody, or opalescent. Bilateral discharges usually result from hormonal influences. A pathologic condition is more likely if the discharge is unilateral. To detect nipple discharge, gently compress the nipple and areola between the thumb and forefinger. Cytology or breast biopsy may be necessary. Common causes of breast discharge are intraductal papilloma, fibrocystic disease, and sclerosing adenosis. Less common causes are chronic cystic mastitis, duct ectasia, galactocele, papillary cystadenoma, keratosis of nipple, fat necrosis, acute mastitis or abscess, tuberculosis, toxoplasmosis, and eczema of the nipple. Malignant lesions include ductal carcinoma, lobular carcinoma, sarcomas, and Paget disease of the nipple. Invasive breast cancers do not ordinarily cause a discharge.

Nipple Scaling and Excoriation—Paget Disease: An invasive malignancy extends along the ductal system, lactiferous tubules, and/or superficial lymphatics onto the nipple, areola, and skin, then further extends in the skin. Patients feel tingling, itching, and burning. The nipple, being reddened, scaling, and excoriated, appears eczematoid. Complete nipple destruction may occur.

Areolar Gland Abscess: The sebaceous glands of Montgomery become inflamed, forming tender, palpable abscesses in the periphery of the areola.

Unless drained, the abscess can become large and invade the breast. An underlying cancer with secondary infection should be considered.

BREAST SYNDROMES

The Female Breast

Breast masses. Breast masses arise from benign and malignant neoplastic change in the ductal or acinar epithelium, cystic changes, duct obstruction, infection, bleeding, infiltration by abnormal cells, or accumulation of intra- or extracellular substances, especially fibrosis. Some masses retain hormonal control; many do not. The important distinction is between benign and malignant lesions. Cysts are overwhelmingly benign and aspiration of nonbloody fluid with disappearance of the mass is diagnostic. Smooth regular borders and tenderness suggest an fibroadenoma. Tenderness is characteristic of inflammatory breast disease, with or without infection, but uncommon with cancer. Histology by aspiration cytology or biopsy is necessary to confirm benignity.

Premalignant and malignant masses. Most malignant neoplasms arise from the ductal epithelium, some having a strong genetic contribution (BRCA-1, BRCA-2). *Atypical ductal hyperplasia* is associated with an increased risk of subsequent in-situ or invasive ductal carcinoma. *Lobular neoplasia*, arising in the acinar lobules, is usually noninvasive but is associated with an increased risk for invasive ductal carcinoma. *Malignant lymphoma* may involve the lymph nodes and other breast tissues. The primary distinctions are between malignant and nonmalignant masses and invasive and noninvasive malignancies. The virtue in diagnosing a benign breast condition lies in excluding malignancy, which requires tissue. Discrete dominant lesions require biopsy for histologic diagnosis. Normal or nondiagnostic mammography must not prevent biopsy of a clinically suspicious mass. Neither surgeons nor radiologists have the certainty of pathologists. The evaluation of breast masses and their management is constantly evolving. Expert consultation is advised.

Breast cancer. There may be a dominant nontender breast mass in the breast. Suspensory ligament infiltration causes retraction revealed by dimpling, nipple deviation, and fixation to the pectoral muscles. Flattening of the nipple and a bloody or clear discharge indicate disease in the lactiferous tubules. Lymphatic obstruction produces cutaneous edema seen as *peau d'orange* (Fig. 8-58). Regional lymphadenopathy suggests lymphatic metastases. A solitary breast mass mandates a diagnostic biopsy. Occasionally, the presenting sign is a bloody discharge, enlarged lymph axillary nodes, or skin inflammation without a mass. **DDX:** The incidence of cancer in women <30 years of age is 1%, and there is a steady rise with increasing age; it is estimated that 1 in 9–10 women will eventually develop breast cancer. The median age at which the various pathologic breast abnormalities appear in women is known, and on that basis, probabilities are estimated. The data in Table 8-5 is from patients operated on at New York Medical College–Flower Fifth Avenue Hospitals during the period 1960–1975.

Inflammatory breast carcinoma. Breast cancer can present as an acute inflammatory disease, especially in the lactating breast. The appearance is like acute mastitis except that the entire breast is swollen and there is early involvement of the axillary lymph nodes. *DDX:* In acute mastitis, inflammation is usually limited to a single breast quadrant and lymphadenopathy is uncommon.

Fibrocystic breast disease. This includes a broad spectrum of benign pathologic conditions of the female breast. The specific pathologic diagnosis depends on the preponderance of one component over others. If the pathology is confined to stromal proliferation, fibroadenoma, virginal hypertrophy of the breast, and intracanalicular fibroadenoma may be diagnosed. When an abnormal ductal system predominates, micro or macrocystic disease, cystic mastitis, sclerosing adenosis, intraductal papilloma, and ductal ectasia involving the lactiferous sinus describe the changes. If the main change is in the terminal ductule and glandular elements, lobular hyperplasia is identified. Finally, myoepithelium hyperplasia leads to a diagnosis of myoepithelial hyperplasia of Reclus.

Fibroadenoma. Usually found in a young woman with large breasts, the ovoid or lobulated nodule has a firm, elastic, or rubbery consistency. It can be the size of a pinhead or quite large. The mass is nontender and freely movable, slipping easily in the breast tissue. It must be distinguished from dysplasia, carcinoma, and cystosarcoma phyllodes.

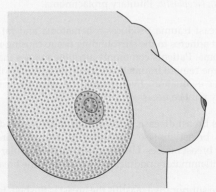

FIG. 8-58 Peau d'Orange. Cutaneous edema of the breast is indicated by skin that is indented deeply with holes, the accentuated orifices of the sweat glands, giving the appearance of an orange.

TABLE 8-5 Relationship of Breast Abnormalities and Age.

Diagnosis	Age Range (Median)
Fibrocystic disease	20–49 (30)
Fibroadenoma	15–39 (20)
Intraductal papilloma and ductal ectasia	35–55 (40)
Carcinoma	40–71 (54)

Fluctuant breast mass. Cysts are very common and must be distinguished from another fluctuant mass, e.g., lipoma or abscess. Fluctuance is demonstrated by holding the edges of the mass tightly to the chest wall with one hand while pressing its center with the fingers of the other hand. Abscess is often quite tender and has erythema. True lipomas are exceedingly rare, accounting for <1% of all breast lesions. Transillumination suggesting a cyst is confirmed by ultrasound or aspiration.

Galactorrhea. Prolactin from the anterior pituitary and progesterone and estrogen from the ovaries and placenta support lactation. Milk ejection is initiated by mechanical nipple stimulation sending afferent impulses to the hypothalamus, causing release of oxytocin from the posterior pituitary. Prolactin levels must be checked in patients with galactorrhea or amenorrhea. Pituitary prolactinomas elevate prolactin levels leading to galactorrhea and suppressing ovulation. Many physiologic states, clinical disorders, and drugs are associated with milk secretion.
CLINICAL OCCURRENCE: *Endocrine:* Pregnancy, adolescence, hypothyroidism, hyperthyroidism; *Degenerative/Idiopathic:* Uterine atrophy with amenorrhea and lactation (Frommel disease); *Infectious:* Herpes zoster, postencephalitis; *Inflammatory/Immune:* Mastitis; *Mechanical/Traumatic:* Mechanical nipple stimulation, suckling, chest wall trauma, thoracoplasty, pneumonectomy, mammoplasty, irradiation; *Metabolic/Toxic:* Drugs (phenothiazines, reserpine, methyldopa, oral contraceptive, tricyclic antidepressants, antihistamines, opiates); *Neoplastic:* Pituitary prolactinoma.

Fat necrosis. Breast trauma produces a hematoma and fat necrosis resulting in a scar that adheres to the surrounding tissue causing retraction which suggests carcinoma. Patients commonly attribute masses that turn out to be malignant to some remote traumatic incident, so a history of trauma should not deter further evaluation. Even though fat necrosis is inconsequential, excisional biopsy may be necessary.

Diabetic fibrous breast disease. Some women with type-1 diabetes develop diabetic fibrous breast disease presenting as one or more painless hard mobile irregular breast masses. Histology shows intralobular and perilobular B-lymphocyte inflammatory nodules with fibrosis in the breast fat.

Mastitis. In acute suppurative mastitis the breast is flushed, tender, hot, swollen, and indurated, frequently accompanied by chills, fever, and diaphoresis. Usually a single breast quadrant is involved. Inflammation often proceeds to abscess formation. Approximately two-thirds of cases occur during lactation. Inflammatory carcinoma must be considered, especially in the presence of nontender axillary lymphadenopathy.

Abscess. Usually a sequel of acute mastitis, there is a localized, hot, exquisitely tender and painful fluctuant mass frequently accompanied by chills and fever with leukocytosis.

Chronic breast abscess. Pus may become enclosed by a thick wall of fibrous tissue, presenting a nontender, irregular, firm mass requiring biopsy to exclude carcinoma.

Juvenile mastitis. A tender unilateral firm mass with signs of inflammation occurs beneath the nipple in young boys and in women 20–30 years of age. The condition is benign and resolves in a few weeks.

The Male Breast

Male breast cancer. Approximately 1% to 2% of breast carcinomas occur in men. The BRCA2 mutation increases the risk. The mass is apparent early because of the paucity of breast tissue. It begins as a painless induration with nipple retraction and fixation to the skin and deep tissues. The mass does not transilluminate. It must be distinguished from gynecomastia by fine-needle aspiration biopsy or excision. Mammography in the male is usually not helpful.

Gynecomastia. Circulating estrogens control breast development. Increased estrogen levels associated with puberty, liver disease, drugs, and endocrine abnormalities lead to proliferation of breast tissue in men. Gynecomastia is defined as a transient or permanent noninflammatory enlargement of the male breast. Physical exam reveals a finely lobulated often tender subareolar mass that is mobile on the chest wall. Increased nipple sensitivity is frequently noted by the patient. The mass may be small and unilateral. Gynecomastia developing bilaterally can reach the dimensions of the female breast. Hard masses or those with skin or chest wall fixation must be excised to exclude carcinoma.

CLINICAL OCCURRENCE: Idiopathic gynecomastia, appearing frequently at puberty, is usually unilateral. Hormonal stimulation with estrogens causes bilateral enlargement after castration, and in Cushing syndrome, hyperthyroidism, and testicular choriocarcinoma. Breast enlargement also occurs in liver cirrhosis. Refeeding gynecomastia occurs when patients with severe malnutrition are first fed. Gynecomastia may occur in association with leukemia, lymphoma, pulmonary carcinoma, familial lumbosacral syringomyelia, and Graves disease. Among the drugs occasionally causing gynecomastia are digitalis, isoniazid, spironolactone, phenothiazine, and diazepam.

CLINICAL VIGNETTES AND QUESTIONS

CASE 8-1

A 65-year-old man comes to the emergency room (ER) with acute short-ness of breath and hypotension. You are told by a medical student that the patient has pulsus paradoxus.

QUESTIONS:
1. What is pulsus paradoxus?
2. How do you assess for pulsus paradoxus?
3. What is the pathophysiology underlying this sign?

CASE 8-2

A 36-year-old Indian woman with a history of acute rheumatic fever presents with worsening shortness of breath especially with exertion. On auscultation she has an accentuated first heart sound, opening snap, and low-pitched diastolic murmur heard best with the bell.

QUESTIONS:
1. What is the most likely diagnosis?
2. Explain the physiology of the loud S1, the opening snap, and the diastolic murmur.
3. How would you estimate the severity of the valve lesion during physical examination?
4. What is Graham Steell murmur?

CASE 8-3

A 56-year-old man presents with dyspnea on exertion, orthopnea, and paroxysmal nocturnal dyspnea. Blood pressure is 140/50 and he has a bounding pulse. The apical impulse is displaced laterally and inferiorly and is diffuse and hyperdynamic. You hear a high-pitched, blowing decrescendo diastolic murmur.

QUESTIONS:
1. What is the diagnosis?
2. Describe physical examination findings which are associated with this diagnosis.
3. What is the common clinical presentation and some underlying causes of acute onset of this valve lesion?
4. What are some chronic conditions leading to this valve lesion?

CASE 8-4

A 55-year-old man comes for evaluation of worsening shortness of breath and ankle edema. He has an elevated JVD, bilateral crackles, and an S3 gallop.

QUESTIONS:

1. What causes S3 and S4 heart sounds?
2. Where and how are the S3 and S4 sounds best heard?
3. What is the significance of these heart sounds?

CASE 8-5

A 55-year-old man is referred to you by your nurse practitioner for evaluation of a heart murmur. You find a systolic crescendo-decrescendo murmur heard best at the right upper sternal border transmitted equally to both carotid arteries. An ejection click is heard just after S1. S2 is muffled.

QUESTIONS:

1. What is the most likely diagnosis?
2. What findings would you expect when examining his carotid arteries?
3. How do you differentiate this murmur from obstructive hypertrophic cardiomyopathy?

CASE 8-6

What is the differential diagnosis of:

QUESTIONS:

1. Elevated "a" waves?
2. Cannon "a" waves?
3. Absent "a" waves?
4. Elevated "v" waves?

CASE 8-7

A 54-year-old man is admitted after a few days of fever, chills, cough, and shortness of breath. He has had diarrhea and headaches as well. His temperature is 39.4°C and chest examination reveals crackles in the left lower lobe. Chest X-ray confirms left lower lobe consolidation. His laboratory workup reveals leucocytosis, mild AST and ALT elevation, hyponatremia, and hypophosphatemia.

QUESTIONS:

1. What are common pathogens responsible for community-acquired pneumonia?
2. What is the most likely pathogen in this patient?
3. What are some characteristic extrapulmonary features of *Myco-plasma pneumonia* infection?

CASE 8-8

A 25-year-old 2 ppd smoker presents to the emergency room with sudden onset of shortness of breath and right-sided pleuritic chest pain. On examination there is decreased chest excursion, hyperresonance to percussion, and diminished breath sounds on the right.

QUESTIONS:
1. What is the most likely diagnosis?
2. What are the characteristic signs and symptoms of this condition?
3. Describe the normal physiology and then the pathophysiology of this condition.
4. What are some causes of this condition?

CASE 8-9

A 30-year-old woman with asthma presents to the ER with significant respiratory distress and dramatic inspiratory stridor. She has had three previous episodes, each triggered by stress, and each lasting about 4 hours. She has dysphonia during these attacks. Albuterol nebulizers have had no beneficial effect. During these episodes stridor is heard, loudest in the neck, and less so in the chest.

QUESTIONS:
1. What is the pathophysiology of stridor?
2. What is the differential diagnosis of stridor?
3. What is the most likely diagnosis?

CASE 8-10

A 25-year-old male smoker comes to the ER with sudden shortness of breath and right-sided pleuritic chest pain. He is tachypneic, tachycardic, and the blood pressure is 90/50 mm Hg. Chest examination reveals decreased chest excursion on the right, hyperresonance to percussion, and absent breath sounds and fremitus. His trachea is deviated to the left.

QUESTIONS:
1. What causes hyperresonance to percussion, absent breath sounds and fremitus?
2. How can physical examination help in your differential diagnosis?
3. What is the most likely diagnosis?

CHAPTER 9

The Abdomen, Perineum, Anus, and Rectosigmoid

The history and physical exam are the foundation for differential diagnosis and efficient use of laboratory and imaging studies in evaluating abdominal symptoms. History delineates the character and sequence of symptoms. Knowing the anatomy and normal and abnormal physiology of the gut and its appended organs is essential to interpreting abdominal findings. As a condition evolves, frequent repetition of the exam yields valuable additional information.

The abdominal cavity is a shallow oval basin with a rigid W-shaped bottom made up of the vertebral column and back muscles. Heavy flank muscles form the sides and the diaphragm and pelvic floor muscles close either end. The brim is formed by the lower rib margins superiorly, and the pubic bones and ilia inferiorly. The anterior abdominal wall muscles and fascia, reinforced by two parallel rectus muscles attached to the ribs and pelvis, cover the abdominal cavity.

The abdominal viscera are solid or hollow. The solid viscera, the liver, spleen, kidneys, adrenals, pancreas, ovaries, and uterus, usually retain their shape and position as they enlarge. The liver, spleen, kidneys, and adrenals are shielded by the rib cage. The hollow viscera, the stomach, small intestines, colon, gallbladder, bile ducts, fallopian tubes, ureters, and urinary bladder, are not palpable unless distended by gas, fluid or solid masses.

Two systems are used to describe abdominal topography (Fig. 9-1). We use the division into quadrants by axial and transverse lines through the umbilicus.

MAJOR SYSTEMS AND THEIR PHYSIOLOGY

Alimentary System: The alimentary system converts ingested food into absorbable nutrients and fuels, and solid waste. This complex process includes ingestion, mastication, bulk transport, storage, mechanical disruption, mixing, and digestion of ingested food and absorption of nutrients coordinated with production, storage, transport, and carefully timed release of digestive enzymes and bile acids. It is a functional barrier to microorganisms, parasites, and toxic molecules.

The alimentary system starts at the mouth and ends at the anus. Its intraabdominal portion extends from the diaphragmatic hiatus to the anus. Normal motility and digestion require coordinated muscular and secretory activity mediated locally and systemically by neural and endocrine signals. The bowel is a muscular tube suspended by a mobile mesentery (stomach, small intestine, cecum, transverse and sigmoid colon) or anchored to the posterior abdominal wall (duodenum, ascending and descending colon) or pelvic floor (rectum). It is susceptible to intraluminal obstruction at narrow points (gastroesophageal junction, pylorus, ileocecal valve), to obstruction by extraluminal

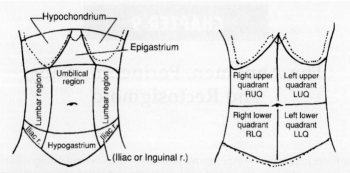

FIG. 9-1 Topographic Divisions of the Abdomen. On the left are the regions of the abdomen as defined in the Basle Nomina Anatomica terminology. Most of the nine regions are small, so that enlarged viscera and other structures occupy more than one. **On the right is a simpler plan with four regions**. This is preferred by most clinicians and is employed in this book. Many occasions arise when the quadrant scheme needs supplementing by reference to the epigastrium, the flanks, or the suprapubic region.

compression, and to twisting or kinking where suspended on a mesentery (especially the small bowel, cecum, and sigmoid). Symptoms referred to the abdomen include changes in appetite, pain, nausea, vomiting and altered stool character and frequency. Physical signs include changes in overall nutrition, abnormal abdominal contour, altered bowel sounds, solid-organ enlargement, increased peritoneal fluid, localized mass, and tenderness.

Hepatobiliary and Pancreatic System: The liver and pancreas parenchyma arise from condensation of mesenchymal cells around embryonic gut evaginations that become the biliary and pancreatic ducts. The pancreas releases bicarbonate, amylase, lipase, and proteinases in response to specific foods and duodenal contents. The pancreas also contains the islets of Langerhans, which release insulin, glucagon, and somatostatin in response to blood glucose changes. Portal venous blood from the gut, gallbladder, pancreas, and spleen percolates from the portal triads through a radial array of sinusoids to the central vein, hepatic vein and inferior vena cava (IVC). Hepatocytes process and remove toxic metabolic products and toxins absorbed by the gut eliminating them via the circulation or bile. They synthesize essential proteins including albumin, coagulation factors, lipoproteins, and transport molecules, and synthesize and secrete the bile salts necessary for fat digestion and absorption. Kupffer cells within the sinusoids are phagocytic antigen-presenting cells that clear bacteria from the portal circulation releasing cytokines into the systemic circulation.

Liver, biliary, and pancreatic symptoms include changes in food interest, nausea, vomiting, pain or discomfort associated with meals, and maldigestion altering stool consistency and frequency. Physical signs include changes in liver size, consistency, and shape, localized tenderness and masses, ascites, and systemic signs, e.g., jaundice, weight loss and bleeding.

Spleen and Lymphatics: See Chapter 5, page 82 for a discussion of the lymph nodes.

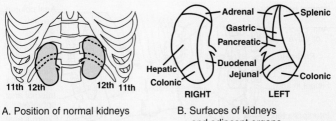

A. Position of normal kidneys

B. Surfaces of kidneys and adjacent organs

FIG. 9-2 Anatomic Relations of the Normal Kidneys. A. The position of the normal kidneys as viewed from the anterior surface of the abdomen. Note that the right kidney is lying in front of the twelfth rib, whereas the slightly higher left kidney is in front of the eleventh and twelfth ribs. **B. The anterior surfaces of both kidneys,** showing the regions touched by overlying viscera.

The spleen distributes arterial blood into complex sinusoids where senescent red blood cells, intracellular inclusions, and red cell membrane abnormalities are removed. The spleen also clears the blood of encapsulated bacteria and produces specific antibodies. The abdominal organs are rich in lymphatics, draining into lymph nodes in the mesentery and the hila of solid organs. These drain into the para-aortic nodes, mixing with lymph from the legs and pelvis, and ultimately into the thoracic duct. Few specific symptoms arise from alterations in these organs. A large spleen produces upper abdominal fullness; retroperitoneal lymph node enlargement or inflammation can present as flank and back pressure or pain. Fever, weight loss, and sweats may be the only symptoms of intraabdominal lymphoma. Moderate splenomegaly can be detected by physical exam, but intraabdominal lymph nodes are rarely palpable.

Kidneys, Ureters, and Bladder: See the discussion of urogenital function in Chapter 10.

The kidneys are in the retroperitoneum under the lower ribs (Fig. 9-2). The ureters run retroperitoneally along, then over, the psoas muscle, over the pelvic brim, and into the pelvis before entering the bladder. Obstruction of the renal pelvis or ureter, produces deep, poorly localized visceral pain in the abdomen, flank, pelvis, or testicles. Pain is referred to the flank and back from kidney enlargement or tissue invasion by inflammatory, infectious, or neoplastic processes. Physical signs are palpable kidney and bladder enlargement and pain on deep palpation.

SUPERFICIAL ANATOMY OF THE ABDOMEN AND PERINEUM

The Abdomen: Develop a complete mental image of the location and relationships of the abdominal organs, the mesentery and its attachments, and the arterial, venous, and lymphatic supply of each organ. Anchor this picture to superficial landmarks: the spine, ribs and costal margins, umbilicus, rectus muscle, inguinal ligament, ilia, and pubes. Associate this mental picture with the images presented by plain films, ultrasonography, CT, and MRI. This requires studying anatomy texts, reviewing imaging studies with your

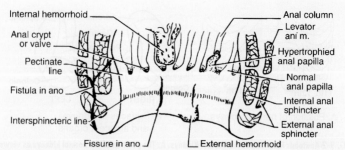

FIG. 9-3 Anatomy of the Anal Canal: Interior and Cross-Section. The anal columns (columns of Morgagni) descend vertically from the rectum and end in anal papillae that fuse to form the pectinate or dentate line; behind are the anal valves (crypts of Morgagni). The cut walls show the internal anal sphincter surrounded by the external sphincter that extends distally. The junction between the edges of the two sphincters forms the intersphincteric line. Internal hemorrhoids arise proximal to the pectinate line, external hemorrhoids distally. Two anal fissures are shown, one distal to a resulting hypertrophied papilla. A fistula (black and irregular) drains from an abscess in a rectal crypt (or valve) to the skin near the anus.

radiologist, and validating your picture by observing surgical procedures and postmortem dissections.

The Anus: Figure 9-3 depicts the anal canal. It is 2.5–4 cm long surrounded by two concentric layers of striated muscle: the involuntary internal sphincter and the voluntary external sphincter surrounding the internal sphincter. A band of the external sphincter extends beyond the distal end of the internal sphincter.

The Rectum: The rectum extends from rectosigmoid junction to the anal canal, ~12 cm. The distal end dilates to form the rectal ampulla. The rectum contains semilunar transverse folds, the valves of Houston; they are inconstant in number and position. The upper two-thirds of the rectum is covered by peritoneum. In men, the anterior peritoneal reflection extends to within 7.5 cm of the anal orifice as the rectovesical pouch; it is potentially accessible to the examining finger. In women, the rectouterine pouch extends downward anteriorly to within 5.5 cm of the anal orifice.

The Sigmoid and Descending Colon: The descending colon begins at the splenic flexure, descends retroperitoneally into left iliac fossa becoming the sigmoid colon at the iliac flexure. The sigmoid colon, suspended on its mesentery, extends from the iliac flexure to the rectum. The sigmoid forms a crude S by running transversely from the left ileum toward the right pelvis, doubling on itself passing leftward toward the midline and then downward becoming the rectum at about the third sacral vertebra.

PHYSICAL EXAM OF THE ABDOMEN

Examine the abdomen from the right side sequentially by inspection, auscultation, percussion, and palpation. Ensure a warm room, proper draping, and a pillow under the head. A pillow under the knees improves comfort while relaxing the abdominal muscles. Drape the legs and pelvis to the pubes

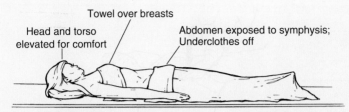

FIG. 9-4 Draping for Abdominal Examination. The patient lies supine on the examining table with a sheet or blanket covering the lower extremities up to the pubes. For women, the breasts are covered with a folded towel or gown. A small pillow supports the head. To further relax the abdominal muscles, a pillow can be placed to support the knees in slight flexion.

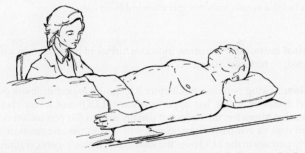

FIG. 9-5 Abdominal Inspection. The patient is supine with a single source of light shining across from feet to head, or across the abdomen toward the examiner. The examiner should sit in a chair at the right of the patient with her head only slightly higher than the abdomen so the physician can concentrate on the abdomen for several minutes, if needed.

(Fig. 9-4) with a gown covering a woman's breasts. If the patient presents with abdominal pain, initially avoid direct contact with the abdomen. Have the patient point to the painful area, and then, alternately, suck the abdomen in and push the stomach out while indicating areas of discomfort. Finally, have the patient cough. Pain with these maneuvers implies peritoneal inflammation.

Inspection: Do not rush inspection (Fig. 9-5). Low angle light from the side or the foot accentuates contours. Inspect for contour, distention, scars, engorged veins, visible peristalsis, and masses. Inspecting from the foot of the table reveals abdominal and thoracic asymmetry. Experience is necessary to learn normal abdominal contours and identify abnormal contours and distention.

Auscultation
Peristaltic sounds. Auscultate the abdomen before palpation. Learn to distinguish normal from the abnormal sounds associated with distinct types of abdominal pathology by auscultating during *every* abdominal examination. Listen with the bell in all four quadrants and the midline, listening for at least 5 minutes before concluding that bowel sounds are absent. Occasional weak sounds are not evidence of good peristalsis. High-pitched tinkles and rushes may denote partial obstruction.

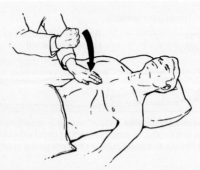

FIG. 9-6 Fist Percussion Over the Liver. The palm of the left hand is applied anteriorly to the lower ribs of the right hemithorax. The back of the applied hand is struck lightly with the fist of the right hand.

Abdominal murmurs. A murmur indicates turbulent blood flow in a dilated, constricted, or tortuous artery.

Percussion: During percussion (Chapter 3, page 30) expect dullness over the liver and tympany in the left upper quadrant (LUQ) and lower chest over the stomach. Otherwise, the abdomen usually gives a flat percussion note. An increased area of tympany is associated with gas in the abdomen or bowel. Routinely percuss in the LUQ over the lower ribs (*Traube's space*); dullness suggests an enlarged spleen. Dullness obliterating the gastric air bubble tympany can be caused by fluid in the stomach, feces in the colon, or an enlarged spleen. Bladder distention produces suprapubic dullness. Pain with percussion, especially pain remote to the site of percussion, suggests peritoneal inflammation (*rebound*). Gentle fist percussion performed with the heel of the hand on the ribs overlying the liver, spleen, and kidneys (Fig. 9-6) identifies pain caused by stretching or inflammation of the capsules surrounding these organs.

Percussion and palpation for costovertebral angle (CVA) tenderness. Press with one finger or thumb into the CVA between the spine and the twelfth rib (Fig. 9-2). Fist percussion at the same point can reveal deep tenderness.

Palpation: The anterior abdominal wall muscles resist palpation proportionally to their strength and tone. Minimize resistance by being gentle and explaining each step of the exam. If this is not effective, press firmly on the lower sternum with the left hand while palpating with the right. Inspiration attempted against this pressure relaxes the abdominal muscles. Examine symptomatic areas last, watching the patient's face for evidence of discomfort. Although usually performed supine, palpation while on either side or in the knee–elbow position can reveal masses not otherwise discernible. Standing is necessary to identify some hernias.

Light palpation. Start with light abdominal palpation searching for edges, tenderness, increased resistance, and masses. Some masses cannot be felt when pushing harder. With the palm and approximated fingers press gently to a depth of ~1 cm (Fig. 9-7A). Sweep gently over the surface beginning at the pubes and working up to the costal margins. A huge liver or spleen can be missed if the lower edge isn't located. Ticklishness tenses muscles impairing the exam. Patients are not ticklish to their own touch. Use this to advantage by putting the patient's fingers on yours as you examine (Fig. 9-7C). Use pressure on the stethoscope when auscultating to elicit tenderness. Tenderness to palpation but not the stethoscope pressure could suggest malingering.

Deep palpation. With the palm just touching the skin press the approximated fingers ever more deeply, feeling with the fingertip pads, while slowly

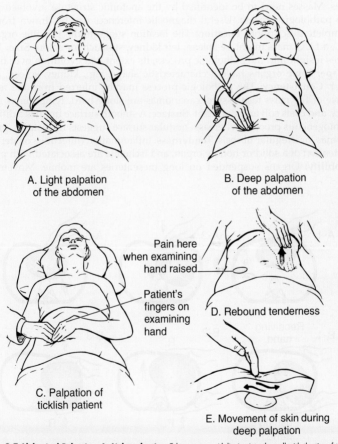

A. Light palpation
of the abdomen

B. Deep palpation
of the abdomen

Pain here
when examining
hand raised

Patient's
fingers on
examining
hand

D. Rebound tenderness

C. Palpation of
ticklish patient

E. Movement of skin during
deep palpation

FIG. 9-7 Abdominal Palpation. A. Light palpation. Take care to avoid digging into the wall with the tips of the fingers. **B. Deep palpation. C. Palpation of the ticklish abdomen. D. Rebound tenderness.** The hand is slowly pushed deep into the abdomen remote from the suspected tenderness, and then abruptly withdrawn. Pain in the affected region results from rebound of the tissue, usually a sign of peritoneal irritation. **E. Exploration during palpation.** When palpating the abdomen, especially deeply, the fingers remain relatively fixed to a place on the skin and the wall of the abdomen is carried with the fingers in a slow gentle to-and-fro motion to distinguish underlying masses and surfaces. The fingers do not glide over the skin but carry the skin with them.

moving them laterally and longitudinally 4 or 5 cm gliding the abdominal wall over the underlying structures (Fig. 9-7E). Examination can be *single handed*, but when resistance is strong use *reinforced palpation*, the fingers of one hand pressing on the distal phalangeal joints of the other, so the relaxed fingers can appreciate the tactile sensations (Fig. 9-7B). Measure small masses by grasping them between the thumb, middle, and index fingers. Bimanual palpation is used for large masses. When ascites is present, *ballottement* is useful. Where a mass is suspected thrust rapidly and sequentially more deeply into the abdomen; a tap on the fingertips indicates a mass (Fig. 9-8).

Characterizing a mass. Nearly all masses arise from previously normal tissues. Masses need to be identified by the anatomic structure involved and the pathologic process. Useful diagnostic inferences can be drawn from a complete description. **Location:** The location suggests the possible organs, e.g., a LUQ mass might be spleen, left kidney, stomach, or colon. **Size:** This gives insight into the pathologic process, its extent and evolution over time. **Shape:** Some organs have a characteristic shape, e.g., kidney, spleen, and liver. **Consistency:** The pathologic process may be inferred from the resistance of the mass to pressure: carcinomas are stony hard, lymphomas rubbery, and cysts soft and fluctuant. **Surface:** A smooth surface implies a diffuse homogeneous process, whereas a nodular surface suggests metastases, granulomas, or irregular fibrosis. **Tenderness:** Inflammation (infectious or sterile), distention of a solid or hollow organ, and ischemia are associated with pain. **Mobility:** Organs suspended on long mesenteries are mobile. Movement

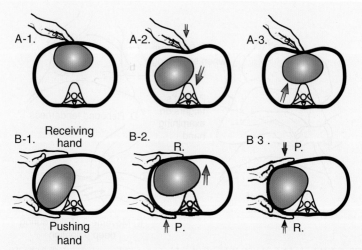

FIG. 9-8 Ballottement of Abdominal Masses. The term ballottement is applied to two somewhat different maneuvers. **A. One hand ballottement.** The approximated fingers abruptly plunge into the abdomen and are held there; a freely movable mass rebounds upward and is felt with the fingers. This is most commonly employed to feel a large liver obscured by free fluid in the abdominal cavity. **B. Bimanual ballottement. B1–2: determining the size of a large mass in the abdomen.** One hand (P) pushes the posterior abdominal wall, whereas the receiving hand (R) palpates the anterior abdomen. **B3: The receiving hand is now in the flank.** The pushing hand compresses the mass to get an estimate of its thickness.

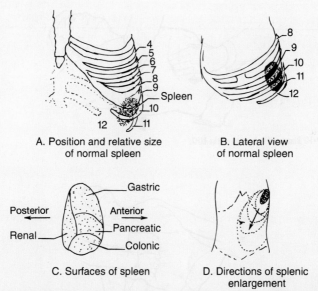

A. Position and relative size of normal spleen

B. Lateral view of normal spleen

C. Surfaces of spleen

D. Directions of splenic enlargement

FIG. 9-9 Anatomic Relations of the Normal and Enlarged Spleen. A. Position of the normal spleen, anterior view. The area of splenic dullness is in the left posterior axilla and usually <8–9 cm. **B. Normal spleen, left lateral view.** The spleen lies obliquely with its long axis along the tenth rib, its long borders coinciding with the ninth and eleventh ribs. **C. Anterior surface of the spleen.** The regions touching other viscera are indicated. **D. Enlarging spleen.** The directions in which the spleen enlarges are indicated by the dotted lines; the long axis of enlargement points downward and obliquely toward the symphysis pubis.

with respiration excludes a retroperitoneal location. **Pulsation:** This implies a location associated with a major artery. Aortic or major branch aneurysms must be assumed until excluded by imaging. Solid masses and tense cysts can simulate aneurysms by transmitting aortic pulsations.

LUQ palpation. Normal LUQ organs, including the spleen, are not palpable. The spleen is superficial while the left kidney is deep and closer to the midline. The spleen lies posterior-lateral under the left diaphragm, the lung separating it from the chest wall during deep inspiration. Its long axis parallels the tenth rib in the mid-axillary line (Fig. 9-9). The oblique orientation means that the vertical extent of mid-axillary splenic dullness describes its width. Feel for a moderately enlarged spleen or left kidney by standing on the patient's right side and using *bimanual palpation*. Lay the right hand on the abdominal wall in the LUQ with the fingertips 4–5 cm below the rib margin at the anterior axillary line. Place the left hand on the left mid-axillary chest wall at the eleventh and twelfth ribs with the fingers curling posteriorly. With the left hand lifting gently from the back the right hand palpates under the costal margin during deep inspiration (Fig. 9-10). The descending tip of an enlarged spleen touches the palpating fingertips. Repeat the procedure with the patient lying partially on his right side. In the *Middleton method*, the patient lies with his left fist beneath the left chest (Fig. 9-11). Standing on the patient's left side facing

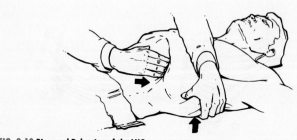

FIG. 9-10 **Bimanual Palpation of the LUQ.**

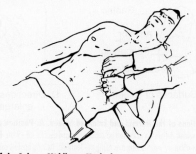

FIG. 9-11 **Palpation of the Spleen, Middleton Method.**

his feet, curl your fingers under the ribs feeling for the spleen tip during deep inspiration. Greatly enlarged spleens may be felt without bimanual palpation. Tympany over Traube's space, however, makes splenomegaly unlikely and obviates the need for extensive palpation maneuvers.

RUQ palpation. The RUQ contains the liver, gallbladder, hepatic flexure of the colon, and right kidney. *Bimanual palpation* is used for palpating the liver. The right hand is placed on the abdominal wall below the costal margin. The left hand is placed under the lower right chest lifting as the patient inspires deeply the right hand moving up and in (Fig. 9-12). As full inspiration is approached lift the fingertips toward the costal margin to catch the liver edge from below. Again, light fingertip pressure improves detection of the liver edge. To avoid missing an enlarged liver start well below the costa margin and move cephalad. An enlarged right kidney is felt as a fixed mass deep to the liver.

Palpation of the lower quadrants. RLQ and LLQ palpation are straightforward as there are normally no palpable organs, except for stool in the colon. The spine and sacral prominence are easily palpable in thin individuals and must not be confused with masses. *Psoas and obturator signs* should be performed in patients with abdominal pain (Fig. 9-13). With the patient flat or on their side, fully flex and extend both hips. Pain suggests inflammation of the psoas muscle or the overlying peritoneum. The *obturator sign* is elicited with the patient supine, and the hip and knee flexed to 90 degrees. Move the

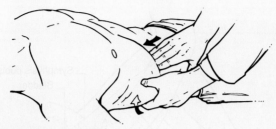

FIG. 9-12 Bimanual Palpation of the RUQ.

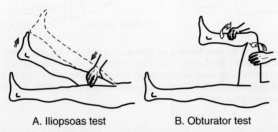

A. Iliopsoas test   B. Obturator test

FIG. 9-13 Testing for Irritated Iliopsoas and Obturator Muscles. Abscesses in the pelvis may be localized by demonstrating irritation of the more lateral iliopsoas or the medial obturator internus muscles. **A. Iliopsoas test.** The supine patient keeps his knee extended and is asked to flex the thigh against the resistance of the examiner's hand. Pain in the pelvis indicates irritation of the iliopsoas. **B. Obturator test.** The supine patient flexes the thigh to 90 degrees. The examiner moves the hip in internal and external rotation. Pelvic pain indicates an inflamed muscle.

hip fully through internal and external rotation; deep pelvic pain suggests inflammation of the obturator muscle or pelvic peritoneum.

Examining the abdomen and pelvis per rectum and vagina. (See the rectal examination below, the female pelvic examination in Chapter 11, page 486, and the male rectal examination in Chapter 12, page 511) A chaperone must be present during these examinations. Palpation via the rectum and vagina detects intrinsic disease of the rectum and vagina, allows examination of other structures of the male and female genitourinary tracts and the lower peritoneal cavity in the pelvis (Figs. 9-14 and 9-15). *Errors in the diagnosis of abdominal conditions are notoriously common when these examinations have been omitted.* Post-void vaginal exam is part of the abdominal exam of symptomatic women, even when speculum examination cannot be performed. Vaginal and rectal exams in the lithotomy position are preferred because masses will tend to fall on the examining finger. Wear lubricated gloves and use the index finger for rectal examination and the index and long fingers for the vaginal exam. Palpate the vagina first, then the rectum. For *bimanual palpation* bring the fingers of one hand pressing into the suprapubic abdominal wall toward the examining finger(s) in the rectum or vagina. When the exam is complete, provide tissues for the patient to clean themselves.

Examining for abdominal hernias. (See page 460.) Hernias are protrusions of abdominal contents through a weak point in the abdominal wall. Most

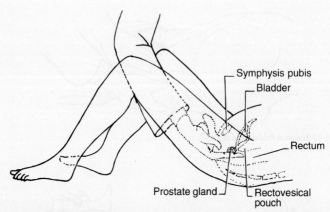

FIG. 9-14 Palpation of the Male Abdomen per Rectum. The examining hand is supinated. Anteriorly, the finger pad feels the prostate gland and seminal vesicles. Superiorly on the anterior rectal surface, the fingertip reaches the location of the rectovesical pouch of the peritoneum. Normally, this pouch is not palpable; in the presence of pus or a tender mass it may be perceived. Cancer cells may settle in this pouch from the abdominal cavity, producing a hard, nontender, transverse ridge, called a rectal shelf or Blumer shelf.

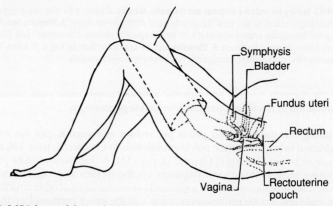

FIG. 9-15 Palpation of the Female Abdomen per Rectum. The finger pad feels the cervix uteri and the fundus uteri through the anterior rectal wall. Passing the finger inward, superior to the cervix, the fingertip reaches the location of the rectouterine pouch (Douglas pouch). Normally, this is not palpable; a tender mass is evidence of pus. See legend of Fig. 9-14 for Blumer shelf.

hernias have a peritoneal sac which may contain bowel, stomach, omentum, urinary bladder, colon, or even liver. Start with inspection. If the patient suspects a problem, have him demonstrate his observation. Many hernias are encountered unexpectedly, a bulge being seen at rest or appearing during maneuvers that increase intraabdominal pressure, e.g., cough or Valsalva. Palpate the abdominal wall defect and its contents. Omentum feels soft and nodular, whereas bowel is smooth and fluctuant. Gas in herniated bowel may cause peristaltic sounds or crepitation. If the hernia can be pushed back into the abdomen, it is *reducible*; if not, it is *irreducible* or *incarcerated*.

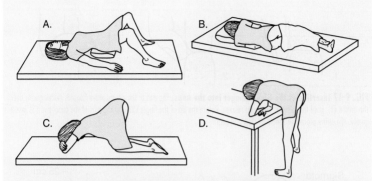

FIG. 9-16 Positions of the Patient for Rectal Examination. A. Modified lithotomy position. B. Left lateral prone position (Sims position). C. The knee–chest position. D. Bent over the table.

Zieman inguinal examination. See page 461.

Examining the Perineum, Anus, Rectum, and Distal Colon: The patient is examined in one of several positions (Fig. 9-16). The left lateral prone (Sims) and bent-over-table positions permit inspection of the perineum, palpation of the anal canal and rectum, and inspection of the anal canal and rectum with an anoscope. Raising the buttocks raised on a pillow facilitates exam in the lithotomy position. The anal canal cannot be examined in this position. The knee–chest and knee–elbow positions are uncomfortable for the patient and are reserved for special conditions such as evacuating colonic gas.

Inspecting the perineum. Whatever position is selected for the patient, the buttocks should be spread wide apart. Inspect the skin of the perineum and perianal region for signs of inflammation, sinuses, fistulas, excoriations, hemorrhoids, masses, and cutaneous lesions.

Examining the Anus.
Anal palpation. Ask the patient to breathe normally and explain the procedure as you go along. After gloving both hands, gently palpate for warmth, tenderness, and consistency around the orifices for sinuses and fistulas feeling for subcutaneous cords indicating tracks. Palpate between the anus and the ischial tuberosities, the site of ischiorectal abscesses. Inspect the mucocutaneous junction by everting the anal mucosa. Next, place the lubricated finger pad on the anal sphincter applying gentle pressure inward and somewhat anteriorly until the sphincter relaxes, admitting the fingertip (Fig. 9-17). The anal canal slants anteriorly, so the axis of entry is toward the umbilicus. Slowly advance while estimating sphincter tone, palpating the walls, and estimating the length of the anal canal. The exam is not painful unless a fissure in ano or thrombosed hemorrhoid is present. Palpation between the index finger in the canal and the thumb on the perineum can identify a soft tissue abscess or mass. *Without explicit indication do not perform a rectal exam on a neutropenic patient.*

Anoscopy. When anal pathology is suspected, view the anal canal using an anoscope. A good light must be available. The patient is placed in position

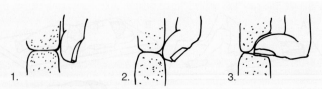

FIG. 9-17 Insertion of the Gloved Finger into the Anus. The pad of the gloved index finger is placed gently over the orifice (1), until the external sphincter relaxes. Rotate the tip of the finger (2) into the axis of the canal and (3) insert gently. The entire procedure should be slow and gentle.

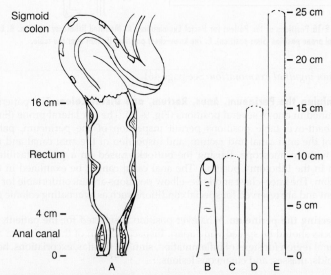

FIG. 9-18 Comparison of Lengths of Rectosigmoid Segments with Rigid Examining Instruments. All lengths are drawn to scale. **A. The rectosigmoid and anal canal. B. An average index finger (**10 cm long and 22 mm in diameter). **C. A typical anoscope. D. A proctoscope of 15 cm.**

(Fig. 9-16) and digital exam is done to exclude obstruction. Lubricate the ano-scope with the obturator in place, then gently insert the tip and tube aiming toward the umbilicus. Once fully inserted, remove the obturator to inspect the rectal mucosa and anal canal during slow withdrawal.

Examining the Rectum: The three parts to the rectal examination are palpa-tion of the lower peritoneal cavity (see above), palpation of adjacent internal urogenital organs (see Chapters 11 and 12), and exam of the rectum itself.

Rectal palpation. This is a continuation of anal canal palpation, the finger pushing beyond the anal canal to feel the walls of the ampulla. In the male, on the anterior wall, the finger sequentially palpates the anterior wall, pros-tate, seminal vesicles, and rectovesical pouch. Next, palpate the lateral walls, the hollow of the sacrum, and the coccyx. On the anterior wall of the female, the uterine cervix, uterine fundus (if retroverted), and rectouterine pouch are sequentially palpated. Palpate the rectal walls for masses and narrowing of the lumen.

Examining the Sigmoid Colon: The rectosigmoid and descending colon are inspected through a flexible sigmoidoscope (Fig. 9-18) which provides a wide field of view and can often be advanced to the splenic flexure without anesthesia. Indications for sigmoidoscopy are beyond the scope of this text.

ABDOMINAL, PERINEAL, AND ANORECTAL SYMPTOMS

Nonspecific Symptoms

Six-dermatome pain—esophageal discomfort. See Six Dermatome Pain, Chapter 8, page 350, and Chapter 9, page 432.

Acute abdominal pain. See also page 431. Knowing the innervation of each organ (somatic versus visceral, vagus, and/or sympathetic) helps interpretation of the patient's pain. Depending on the organ, some stimuli are painful, others are not, e.g., bowel distention is painful, laceration is not. Visceral pain is transmitted by vagal visceral afferent nerves and sympathetic afferent nerves. It is deep, boring, poorly localized pain frequently accompanied by autonomic features such as nausea, vomiting, and diaphoresis. Body wall and peritoneal pain, transmitted via the spinal somatic afferent nerves, is sharp and well localized. Acute severe abdominal pain, the *acute abdomen*, can herald benign or immanently life-threatening disorders. The specific diagnosis must be pursued with a sense of urgency since early surgical intervention will be lifesaving in some conditions (abdominal aortic aneurysm, bowel perforation) but is contraindicated in others (acute intermittent porphyria, sickle cell crisis). Accurate diagnosis relies on history, physical exam and imaging; laboratory tests are less helpful. Repeated exams by a single observer, be it day or night, are mandatory. Particularly important are the locations of pain and tenderness (Fig. 9-19), and change in location and variations in the quality of pain. Relatively few findings distinguish several conditions. For example, with intraabdominal visceral pain the patient may walk about, but if peritonitis supervenes, the patient holds very still to guard the abdomen. With acute pain patients usually seek care within a few hours of onset. Pain increased with walking, jumping, sneezing, or coughing is equivalent to the jar test (page 423) suggesting peritoneal inflammation. A pregnancy test must be obtained in all women of childbearing age with acute abdominal pain.

　　CLINICAL OCCURRENCE: *Congenital:* Meckel diverticulum, sickle cell crisis, pancreas divisum, angioedema; familial Mediterranean fever, AIP and variegate porphyria; *Endocrine:* Gastrinoma, adrenal insufficiency; *Degenerative/Idiopathic:* Diverticulitis, endometriosis, diabetic radiculopathy, transverse myelitis, mononeuritis multiplex; *Infectious:* Typhoid fever and enteritis; *Clostridium difficile* enterocolitis; viral gastroenteritis; visceral larval migrans; varicella-zoster virus; cytomegalovirus; viral hepatitis; tuberculous peritonitis and lymphadenitis; purulent peritonitis (spontaneous or secondary to perforation or penetration); *Inflammatory/Immune:* Pancreatitis, gastritis, esophagitis, autoimmune hepatitis, peritonitis, serositis, mesenteric

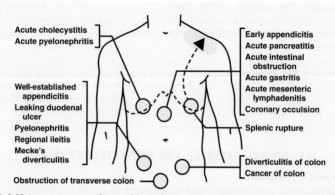

Acute cholecystitis
Acute pyelonephritis

Early appendicitis
Acute pancreatitis
Acute intestinal
obstruction
Acute gastritis
Acute mesenteric
lymphadenitis
Coronary occulsion

Well-established
appendicitis
Leaking duodenal
ulcer
Pyelonephritis
Regional ileitis
Mecke's
diverticulitis

Splenic rupture

Diverticulitis of colon
Cancer of colon

Obstruction of transverse colon

FIG. 9-19 Common Locations of Acute Abdominal Pain. In general, the painful spot is also tender, but not always. Note especially that the pain of acute appendicitis is in the epigastrium early and later in the RLQ. Pain in the spleen commonly radiates to the top of the left shoulder. These pains are ordinarily constant, in contrast to the intermittent pain of colic.

lymphadenitis, systemic lupus erythematosus (SLE), vasculitis, inflammatory bowel disease (Crohn disease, ulcerative colitis); *Metabolic/Toxic:* Familial Mediterranean fever, AIP and variegate porphyria, ingestions, heavy metal poisoning (lead, cadmium, arsenic, mercury), nonsteroidal anti-inflammatory drug (NSAID) gastroduodenitis, macrolide antibiotics; *Mechanical/Traumatic:* Deceleration injuries especially with improperly worn lap seat belts, may cause injury to the urinary bladder, bowel, mesentery, and intraabdominal vessels; fracture of a solid organ, perforation of bowel, bladder, or gallbladder, obstruction of the cystic, common bile, pancreatic ducts, ureter, ureteropelvic junction, or bowel by stones, masses, parasites, or bezoars; volvulus or strangulation of bowel in internal or abdominal wall hernias; penetrating and blunt trauma, abdominal cutaneous nerve entrapment; *Neoplastic:* Mass effect of tumors pressing on other structures or causing traction on bowel or mesentery, hemorrhage into tumor, ischemia and necrosis of tumor, erosion into or metastasis to blood vessels, nerves or adjacent organs; *Psychosocial:* History of physical, emotional or sexual abuse in childhood or as an adult; poisoning, substance abuse with drug seeking, drug withdrawal; *Vascular:* Abdominal aortic aneurysm or dissection, ischemic bowel, infarction of bowel or solid organs, vasculitis, mesenteric venous thrombosis or emboli (bland, septic, or atheroembolic), Henoch Schölein purpura, strangulation of hernias, rectus sheath hemorrhage, retroperitoneal hemorrhage.

Chronic and recurrent abdominal pain. Chronic pain is physiologically distinct from acute pain. The role of conditioning in the spinal cord and thalamus with chronic pain is under study, as is the decreased threshold to pain perception with visceral stimulation in some individuals with chronic abdominal pain. The pain pattern and associated symptoms help make inferences about pathophysiology, whereas location suggests the organs involved. Pain that is vague in onset but steadily worsens suggests progressive anatomic obstruction or mass effect. Intermittent symptoms suggest painful smooth-muscle contraction from visceral obstruction, relapsing infection, and recurring inflammation or ulceration. A careful history identifies precipitating factors (e.g., meals and type of food), timing (e.g., relation to menstrual cycle or starting new medications), and previous surgeries, symptoms, or illnesses that could help explain the current problem (e.g., adhesions from surgery or irradiation, trauma, infections, and travel). Nonspecific abdominal and pelvic pain is a common presentation of persons with a history of abuse. An empathetic, nonjudgmental history with specific questions relating to current safety, sexual practices, sexual abuse, and physical or emotional abuse is essential. Up to 30% of women presenting to a physician in the ambulatory setting have a history of abuse, and one-third of these have been abused within the last 12 months. The link between abuse and abdominal pain is not understood. Many thousands of dollars are wasted on fruitless laboratory and imaging investigations when a few minutes of directed history might have produced the diagnosis. If the history and physical exam do not suggest specific leads for further investigation, a barrage of laboratory and imaging tests are unlikely to be helpful. There is a tendency to project pain arising in the abdominal wall inward to intraabdominal structures. Identifying abdominal wall disorders avoids many unnecessary studies.

CLINICAL OCCURRENCE: *Congenital:* Malrotation, familial pancreatitis, polycystic kidney disease, porphyrias, familial Mediterranean fever, sickle cell anemia, Meckel diverticulum, cystic fibrosis, hereditary angioedema; *Endocrine:* Adrenal insufficiency, hypothyroidism; *Degenerative/Idiopathic:* Diverticulosis, diverticulitis, gastroesophageal reflux disease, gastritis, pancreatitis, ovarian cysts, arthritis of axial skeleton, AAA, gastric ulcer, endometriosis; *Infectious:* Whipple disease, viral hepatitis (B, C), tuberculosis, *Giardia*, duodenal and gastric ulcers, diverticulitis, chronic malaria, schistosomiasis, visceral larval migrans, leishmaniasis, hookworm, roundworms, bartonellosis (peliosis hepatitis), HIV, syphilis with tabes; *Inflammatory/Immune:* Ulcerative colitis, Crohn disease, gastritis, chronic pancreatitis, autoimmune hepatitis, chronic cholecystitis, sclerosing cholangitis, pancreatic pseudocyst, celiac disease, adhesions, peritonitis, SLE, sarcoidosis, retroperitoneal and mesenteric fibrosis; *Mechanical/Traumatic:* Partial bowel obstruction and strictures, cholelithiasis, nephrolithiasis, pancreatic duct stricture, sphincter of Oddi spasm and stricture, biliary stricture, dumping syndromes; adhesions; ureteral obstruction, ureteropelvic junction obstruction, chronic hydrosalpinx; *Metabolic/Toxic:* Heavy metal poisoning, porphyrias, ketoacidosis, uremia, NSAID gastropathy and gastric ulcer; *Neoplastic:* Splenic and retroperitoneal lymphoma, primary carcinomas of the esophagus, stomach, colon, pancreas, liver, bile ducts, gallbladder, ovary; metastatic cancer to the liver (especially from pancreas, colon, lung, breast, pancreatic islets, carcinoid), spleen (lymphoma), retroperitoneal lymph nodes (cervix, testis, lymphoma, melanoma, bladder), and peritoneal surface (especially ovary); *Neurologic:* Postspinal cord injury, postherpetic neuralgia, diabetic radiculopathy, diabetic autonomic neuropathy, abdominal cutaneous nerve entrapment; *Psychosocial:* History of domestic, sexual, or child abuse, substance abuse, opiate withdrawal; *Vascular:* Intestinal ischemia, vasculitis, atheroemboli, abdominal aortic or iliac aneurysm.

Nausea and vomiting. Nausea is an unpleasant sensation referred to the stomach often suggesting that vomiting is imminent. Vomiting is an involuntary integrated movement of pharyngeal and thoracoabdominal smooth and voluntary muscles to expel stomach contents. Nausea and vomiting are triggered by cortical (emotional), gastrointestinal (GI), vestibular, and chemical (via the central nervous system chemoreceptor trigger zone) stimuli; vomiting is coordinated by the brainstem. The violence and discomfort of nausea and vomiting often make them a presenting complaint. Vomiting is usually preceded by nausea. The history should include inciting events and exposures, the nature of the vomitus and its relationship to meals. *Variants of Vomiting: Projectile Vomiting* is a particularly forceful type associated with increased intracranial pressure and lacking antecedent nausea. *Retching* involves all movements of vomiting except that gastric contents are not expelled.

CLINICAL OCCURRENCE: *Congenital:* Pyloric stenosis; *Endocrine:* Adrenal insufficiency, pregnancy; *Degenerative/Idiopathic:* Pyloric stricture, gastroparesis, other GI motility disorders (e.g., scleroderma, pseudo-obstruction), Ménière disease, glaucoma; *Infectious:* Viral gastroenteritis, CNS infections, peptic ulcer (*Helicobacter pylori*); *Inflammatory/Immune:* Numerous disorders of the alimentary canal, biliary system, and pancreas, for example, hepatitis, pancreatitis, peritonitis; *Mechanical/Traumatic:* Upper GI obstruction; *Metabolic/Toxic:* Bacterial food poisoning; drugs—opiates, ipecac, chemotherapy agents, macrolide antibiotics, chemical toxins, many more; uremia, hepatic failure, ketoacidosis; cannabinoid hyperemesis; *Neoplastic:* Brain tumors, primary or metastatic; *Neurologic:* Autonomic reflexes associated with visceral stimulation, for example, myocardial infarction, ureteral stone, biliary colic, post-vagotomy, head injury with concussion, intracranial mass; *Psychosocial:* Offensive tastes, odors, and sights; severe pain; psychogenic; *Vascular:* Myocardial infarction, superior mesenteric ischemia (arterial or venous), migraine.

Abdominal bloating. See Distended Abdomen, page 416. A bloating sensation is caused by gaseous bowel distention, increased sensitivity to normal bowel gas, enlargement of abdominal or pelvic organs, ascites, and masses. Patients often try to induce burping, during which they swallow more gas. Smoking, carbonated beverages, and chewing gum also lead to swallowing gas. Patients with the irritable bowel syndrome have pain and complaints of distention at intestinal gas volumes not sensed by others.

Belching, flatus, and sensible peristalsis. See *Tympanites*, page 422, and Bloating Syndromes, page 444.

Site-Attributable Symptoms

Abdominal wall pain. Injury to the muscles, nerves, skin, and soft tissues of the abdominal wall, and pain referred from bones, nerve roots, and soft tissues of the spine may present as abdominal pain. Well-localized (fingertip precise) pain suggests somatic body wall pain. Band-like pain described as wrapping around the body suggests neuropathic pain, sclerotomal pain from bone lesions, or myotomal pain originating in the muscles, tendons, or ligaments at that segmental level. Pain exacerbated by specific motions and tenderness to palpation support this diagnosis.

CLINICAL OCCURRENCE: *Congenital:* Urachus abnormalities; *Degenerative/Idiopathic:* Xiphodynia; *Infectious:* Abscess, herpes zoster, pyomyositis; *Inflammatory/Immune:* Suture abscess, mononeuritis, polyneuritis, diabetic polyradiculopathy and amyotrophy, myositis; *Mechanical/Traumatic:* Abdominal cutaneous nerve entrapment (rectus abdominis nerve entrapment syndrome), abdominal wall hernia, abdominal wall muscle tear, rib cartilage injury, rib tip syndrome, spinal disc herniation, burns, retention sutures, foreign bodies; *Metabolic/Toxic:* Diabetic neuropathy; *Neoplastic:* Desmoid tumors, lipoma, sarcoma, metastases; *Neurologic:* Complex regional pain syndrome, postherpetic neuralgia, mononeuritis multiplex, diabetic amyotrophy; *Psychosocial:* Abuse, somatization, malingering; *Vascular:* Vasculitis with mononeuropathy or polyneuropathy.

Esophagus, Stomach, and Duodenum Symptoms

Regurgitation. See Heartburn below. Regurgitation is reflux of esophageal and stomach contents into the mouth or upper airway without active vomiting. It is passive, occurring under the influence of normal body positions and activities, suggesting poor esophageal sphincter function or increased intraabdominal pressure. Unlike vomiting, regurgitation may not be volunteered as a complaint. Ask about regurgitation while lying down, at night, or after meals. Regurgitation while fasting produces a sour bitter taste (water brash or pyrosis), whereas postprandial regurgitation returns food. Regurgitation of food more than 2 hours after eating suggests achalasia or delayed gastric emptying.

CLINICAL OCCURRENCE: *Congenital:* Abnormal lower esophageal sphincter (LES) and upper esophageal sphincter tone; *Degenerative/Idiopathic:* Decreased LES tone with or without hiatal hernia, achalasia; *Infectious:* Chagas disease; *Inflammatory/Immune:* Esophagitis, scleroderma, CREST syndrome; *Mechanical/Traumatic:* Achalasia, gastric outlet and upper intestinal obstruction, gastroparesis; *Metabolic/Toxic:* Alcohol, tobacco, caffeine, peppermint, uremia; *Neoplastic:* Esophageal or gastric cardia cancer.

Heartburn. Regurgitation of gastric acid or bile produces chemical irritation in the esophagus with or without esophagitis. Patients complain of burning retrosternal pain aggravated by alcohol, tobacco, caffeine, large fatty or acidic meals and obesity, frequently occurring after meals. Symptoms increase with recumbency and are decreased by antacids. Gastroesophageal reflux caused by decreased LES tone is the most common cause.

Difficulty swallowing—dysphagia. See also Chapter 7, pages 190 and 251. Swallowing is a complex neuromuscular activity involving both consciously controlled striated muscles and smooth muscle innervated by the autonomic system and the intestinal myenteric plexus. Abnormalities in voluntary motor function of the pharynx, smooth-muscle function, salivary function, or mechanical obstructions in the pharynx or esophagus lead to dysphagia. Have the patient indicate where the difficulty is felt. Ask if the problem is greater with liquids or solids. *DDX:* Ask whether they cough or choke with swallowing indicating a pharyngeal or laryngeal problem. Regurgitating food after meals may indicate esophageal obstruction by mass or achalasia. If swallowing is painful (*odynophagia*), infection, neoplasm, or erosions are likely.

Dysphagia lusoria (aberrant right subclavian artery). See Chapter 7, page 252. Pain is rarely present. The esophagram shows a transverse indentation produced by an anomalous right subclavian artery arising from the descending aorta.

Pain with swallowing—odynophagia. See Six-Dermatome Pain with Dysphagia in Syndromes, page 432.

Hematemesis. Bloody emesis indicates recent or active bleeding in the nose, mouth, pharynx, esophagus, stomach, duodenum, or, less frequently, the tracheobronchial tree. Bright red blood is arterial whereas dark blood is either venous or has been in the stomach for some time. Exposure to gastric acid and pepsin give blood a brown coffee grounds appearance. Ask the patient to estimate the volume of blood lost. Patients frequently overestimate the amount, especially if mixed with water, as in a sink or toilet bowl. Occasionally, the patient has difficulty distinguishing between hematemesis and hemoptysis, especially when coughing induces vomiting. Hematemesis following prolonged and violent retching or vomiting is characteristic of a mucosal tear at the gastroesophageal junction (*Mallory–Weiss tear*). If a bleeding site is not evident in the nose, mouth, or pharynx, upper endoscopy should be performed for diagnosis and possible therapy.
CLINICAL OCCURRENCE: *Congenital:* Hereditary hemorrhagic telangiectasia (HHT) (Osler–Weber–Rendu), Dieulafoy lesion; *Endocrine:* Gastrinoma (Zollinger–Ellison syndrome), hyperparathyroidism; peptic ulcer, *Degenerative/Idiopathic:* Duodenal diverticulum, gastritis; *Infectious: H. pylori* ulcers; *Inflammatory/Immune:* Gastritis, esophagitis; *Mechanical/ Traumatic:* Mallory–Weiss tear, portal hypertension (esophageal and gastric varices), foreign bodies, gallstone erosion; *Metabolic/Toxic:* NSAID gastropathy; *Neoplastic:* Cancer of the esophagus, stomach, and pancreas; *Psychosocial:* Factitious; *Vascular:* Arteriovenous malformations, gastric antral vascular ectasia, esophageal and gastric varices, portal gastropathy, thrombocytosis, coagulation defects.

Small Intestine and Colon Symptoms
Diarrhea. See Syndromes page 445.

Constipation. See Syndromes page 451.

Fecal incontinence. Loss of bowel control results from severe diarrhea of any cause, rectal inflammation, damage to the anal sphincters, or loss of normal sensory, autonomic, or voluntary muscle function. Vaginal delivery commonly injures the anal sphincter and pelvic nerves accounting for the large female predominance of fecal incontinence. Fecal and urinary incontinence are most common in women, especially those in institutions. Evaluation of mental status, and vaginal, neurologic, and rectal exams, including anal sensation and sphincter tone and strength, are necessary. Look for dementia, a flaccid anal sphincter, rectocele, rectal prolapse, impacted feces, mass, and sacral nerve deficit. Further evaluation requires specialty consultation.
CLINICAL OCCURRENCE: *Congenital:* Cerebral palsy, mental retardation, meningomyelocele; *Endocrine:* Hyperthyroidism; *Infectious:* Herpes simplex, gonorrhea or cytomegalovirus proctitis, dysentery syndrome caused by bacterial infection, infectious diarrhea, perirectal abscess; *Inflammatory/Immune:* Ulcerative colitis, Crohn disease, ulcerative proctitis, microscopic colitis, amyloidosis; *Metabolic/Toxic:* Drugs, especially cathartics, laxative abuse; *Mechanical/Traumatic:* Fissure, fistula, fecal impaction, pelvic floor relaxation,

rectal prolapse, rectocele; *Neoplastic:* Anal or rectal carcinoma, metastatic invasion of the sacral plexus or spinal cord; *Neurologic:* Dementia, cauda equina syndrome, transverse myelitis, sacral plexopathy, weakness or immobility, Parkinson's, peripheral neuropathy including diabetes, postherpetic neuralgia; *Psychosocial:* Malingering, psychosis; *Vascular:* Ischemic colon, stroke.

Pruritus ani. Pruritus is the symptom, and excoriation and perianal skin thickening (lichenification) are the signs. Patients may have a maddening, uncontrollable desire to scratch, but relief is very short-lived. Pinworms are common in children and in adults with young children. When the involved skin is moist, the etiology may be bacterial or fungal infection (*Candida*). Poor hygiene, contact allergies, irritation from bathroom tissue, and perianal dermatitis of unknown cause are also common.

Pain with bowel movements. See Anal Fissure, page 426.

Pelvic Symptoms

Pain in the perineum. Perineal pain accompanies many pelvic disorders and can involve somatic or sacral sympathetic afferents. Take a history and perform a physical exam looking for pathology involving the rectum, anus, scrotum and its contents, vagina, pelvic floor muscles, pelvic bones, and perineal skin.

CLINICAL OCCURRENCE: *Infectious:* Intertrigo, candidiasis, condyloma, vaginitis, cervicitis, urethritis, cystitis, prostatitis, epididymitis; *Inflammatory/ Immune:* Eczema, nonbacterial prostatitis, Bartholin gland inflammation; *Mechanical/Traumatic:* Thrombosed hemorrhoids, fissure in ano, fistula in ano, anal ulcer, cystocele, rectocele, testicular torsion or trauma, proctalgia fugax; *Neoplastic:* Anal, rectal, bladder, prostate, vaginal, cervical, and uterine cancer; intramedullary tumors.

Pelvic pain. See Abdominal Pain, pages 407 and 410 and Pelvic Pain, Chapter 11, page 489.

Blood in the feces. Blood in the bowel eventually passes in the feces, its appearance depending on the volume of blood, the bleeding site, and the transit time. Partially digested blood appears as bright blood, black loose stools or frank melena. Small volumes of blood, insufficient to change stool color or character, is occult bleeding. Immunochemical tests specific for human globin chains quantifies occult blood loss.

Black tarry stools—Melena. Fifty to sixty milliliters of blood in the stomach exposed to gastric acid and digestive enzymes produces a black, sticky (tarry) stool. Black, but not tarry, stools occur with ingestion of iron, bismuth and some fruits (e.g., black cherries and blueberries) or leafy green vegetables (e.g., spinach and collard greens). Difficulty cleaning the sticky stool from around the anus characterizes melena but not other causes of black stools. Melena can have a reddish hue and an acrid-sweet odor similar to creosote.

Bloody red stools—Hematochezia. Blood unchanged by passage through the gut usually has entered the bowel in the colon, or passed very quickly through the gut. Blood is cathartic so large bleeds stimulate rapid transit. Blood mixed with stool suggests bleeding onto partially formed stool in the colon. The source of blood on the surface of an otherwise normal stool is near the anus.

CLINICAL OCCURRENCE: *Congenital:* Congenital polyps and hamartomas; HHT; pseudoxanthoma elasticum; von Willebrand disease; hemophilia; Meckel diverticulum, Dieulafoy lesion; *Degenerative/Idiopathic:* Arteriovenous malformations, colonic diverticulosis, duodenal diverticulum; *Infectious:* See Acute Bloody Diarrhea, page 447, *C. difficile* colitis, typhoid enteritis, leptospirosis, herpes simplex esophagitis and proctitis, parasites; *Inflammatory/ Immune:* Immune thrombocytopenia, ulcerative colitis, Crohn disease, gastritis; *Mechanical/Traumatic:* Mallory–Weiss tear, ulcers, intussusception, anal fissure, anal fistula, fecal impaction, epistaxis, swallowed blood; *Metabolic/ Toxic:* Vitamin K deficiency, scurvy, heavy metal poisoning, NSAIDs; *Neoplastic:* Polyps or cancer anywhere in the GI tract, cancer invading the bowel wall, for example, pancreatic cancer, gastrinoma (Zollinger–Ellison syndrome); *Psychosocial:* Factitious; *Vascular:* Thrombocytopenia, arteriovenous malformations, ischemic bowel, erosion of AAA into the gut, gastric antral vascular ectasia, esophageal varices, gastric varices, portal gastropathy, hemorrhoids.

ABDOMINAL SIGNS

Inspection

Jaundice. Technically, jaundice means yellow. Medically, jaundice means bilirubin staining of tissues and fluids. Bilirubin stains all tissues, but jaundice is most intense in the face, trunk, and sclerae. Jaundice is usually visible when the serum concentration of conjugated bilirubin exceeds 3 mg/dL. Jaundice is less visible in artificial light than daylight. Long standing jaundice may acquire a green hue. Yellow skin is also caused by carotene and rare chemical toxins, conditions that must be distinguished from jaundice.

Normal Bile Pigment Cycle. When senescent erythrocytes are destroyed in the spleen and other reticuloendothelial tissues, hemoglobin is metabolized to unconjugated bilirubin, iron, and globin. Unconjugated bilirubin is insoluble in water and circulates bound to albumin, so it is not filtered by the kidneys. The liver takes up unconjugated bilirubin, combining it with glucuronic acid to form water-soluble conjugated bilirubin. Conjugated bilirubin is excreted into the bile and gut where bacterial enzymes convert it to urobilinogen. Most urobilinogen is lost in the feces, but some is reabsorbed and re-excreted in the bile (enterohepatic circulation) and urine. Excess water-soluble conjugated bilirubin in the blood is filtered by the kidneys and excreted in the urine. Jaundice occurs with markedly increased production or impaired hepatocellular uptake or conjugation of unconjugated bilirubin, excretion of conjugated bilirubin, or obstruction of the intra- or extrahepatic bile ducts.

Scleral Color. Bilirubin is distributed uniformly throughout the sclera, in contrast to the yellow subscleral fat that collects in the periphery, farthest from the limbus. Carotene does not stain the sclerae.

Pruritus. Itching often accompanies obstructive jaundice and biliary cirrhosis. The intensity of the itching is usually proportional to the bilirubin concentration and the duration of jaundice.

Urine Color. Conjugated, but not unconjugated, bilirubin is excreted in the urine. High urine concentrations impart a dark-yellow to brown color and a shaken specimen produces yellow foam, the bile salts lowering the surface tension of water. Jaundice without urine darkening suggests unconjugated bilirubinemia. *Acholic Feces:* In complete biliary obstruction or with severe hepatocellular loss, the stools are malodorous and appear white or gray like clay.

Unconjugated hyperbilirubinemia. Hemolysis produces unconjugated bilirubin faster than maximal liver uptake, conjugation and excretion. Impaired hepatic uptake or conjugation are less common causes. Stool color is normal. Increased bilirubin in the gut leads to elevated urinary urobilinogen. The urine contains no bilirubin because only water-soluble conjugated bilirubin is excreted in the urine. Tests for intrinsic liver disorders are negative.

CLINICAL OCCURRENCE: *Increased Production—Hemolysis of Normal Red Cells.* Autoimmune hemolytic anemia, transfusion hemolysis, hemolysis from chemicals, drugs, or infections. *Red Cell Defects.* Sickle cell disease, thalassemia, glucose-6-phosphate dehydrogenase (G-6-PD) deficiency, pyruvate kinase deficiency, paroxysmal nocturnal hemoglobinuria. *Ineffective Erythropoiesis.* Thalassemia major, folate, and vitamin B12 deficiency. *Miscellaneous.* Absorption of hematoma, pulmonary infarction. *Deficient Hepatic Uptake.* Sepsis, fasting, hypotension, and drugs. *Deficient Hepatic Conjugation—Congenital:* Gilbert syndrome, Crigler–Najjar syndromes; *Acquired:* Advanced hepatocellular disease, sepsis, competitive inhibition by drugs metabolized to glucuronides.

Conjugated hyperbilirubinemia. This results from impaired excretion of conjugated bilirubin into the bile canaliculi or obstruction of biliary flow through the canaliculi, intrahepatic, and extrahepatic bile ducts to the duodenum. The feces may be acholic in which case the urine lacks urobilinogen but contains bilirubin. The serum alkaline phosphatase is elevated out of proportion to the transaminases. Clinically, it is important to distinguish mechanical extrahepatic obstruction from intrahepatic obstruction resulting from mechanical obstruction or altered hepatocyte and canalicular function (*cholestasis*). In extrahepatic obstructive jaundice dilated bile ducts are seen by ultrasonography.

CLINICAL OCCURRENCE: *Intrahepatic Cholestasis—Congenital:* Dubin–Johnson syndrome, Rotor syndrome; *Acquired:* Hepatocellular disease, drugs (especially sex steroids), sepsis, hypotension, primary biliary cirrhosis. *Extrahepatic Obstruction—Intrinsic:* Gallstones, biliary sludge, biliary carcinoma, sclerosing cholangitis, stricture, parasites; *Extrinsic:* Pancreatic carcinoma, porta hepatis lymphadenopathy, pancreatitis, pancreatic pseudocyst.

Mixed hyperbilirubinemia. This results from combined hepatocellular and biliary tract injury which is common in advanced hepatobiliary disease of almost any etiology. The plasma contains both conjugated and unconjugated bilirubin. The serum transaminase level depend upon the amount of active hepatocellular injury and the remaining hepatocyte mass. The alkaline phosphatase is variably elevated. The primary etiology of hepatobiliary injury needs to be distinguished from the secondary consequences (e.g., cirrhosis or pigment stones). More than one process may be present. The stools may be acholic. Accurate diagnosis requires careful history, serologic testing and liver biopsy.

Distended abdomen. The abdomen is distended by the accumulation of fluids or tissue (Fig. 9-20). Examples are obesity, gas, ascites, solid organs enlargement (e.g., hepatomegaly, splenomegaly, polycystic kidneys, ovarian cysts, fibroids), obstruction of hollow organs (stomach, small and large intestine, bladder, gallbladder), neoplasms (benign or malignant), and pregnancy. See Abdominal Distention, page 444 Tympanites, page 422 and Ascites see below.

Ascites. Peritoneal fluid accumulates by one or more of several mechanisms: transudation of fluid from the liver surface because of portal hypertension; obstruction of peritoneal lymphatic drainage; decreased plasma oncotic pressure; and increased peritoneal fluid production with peritoneal carcinomatosis or inflammation, usually infectious. Each mechanism presents with a

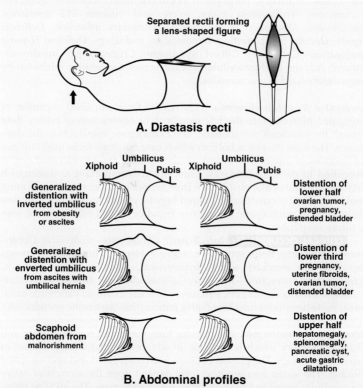

A. Diastasis recti

B. Abdominal profiles

FIG. 9-20 Visible Abdominal Signs. A. Diastasis Recti. This is abnormal separation of the abdominal rectus muscles. It is frequently not detected when the patient is supine unless the patient's head is raised from the pillow so that the abdominal muscles are tensed. **B. Abdominal profiles.** Careful inspection from the side may give the first clue to abnormality, directing attention to a specific region and prompting search for more signs.

recognizable clinical pattern. The profile of a fluid-filled abdomen is a single curve from xiphoid to pubes (Fig. 9-20B). The umbilicus is sometimes everted. Four signs characterize free fluid, but ultrasonography is definitive:

1. *Bulging flanks* produced by fluid pressure on the sidewalls (Fig. 9-21B);
2. *Tympany* atop the abdominal curve, regardless of the patient's position, caused by mobile gas-filled bowel afloat on the ascitic fluid (Fig. 9-21A);
3. *Shifting dullness.* With the patient supine, percuss the level of dullness in the flanks marking it on the skin. Then turn the patient on one side for a minute and percuss the new level of dullness. Considerable shift indicates the presence of fluid (Fig. 9-21C).
4. *A fluid wave* is demonstrated by tapping a flank sharply with one hand the other receiving the impulse on the opposite flank after a perceptible time lag (Fig. 9-21D). Mesenteric fat produces a similar wave, so the fat is blocked by having the patient or an assistant press the ulnar surface of their hand into the midline of the abdomen. A wave passing this block is usually caused by free fluid. These signs will not detect less than 500 mL of peritoneal fluid.

Ascites—an approach to differential diagnosis. A useful physiologic approach to the differential diagnosis of ascites is based upon assessing the likely mechanism of fluid accumulation. *Increased Central Venous Pressure:* Right ventricular failure, pulmonary hypertension, constrictive pericarditis,

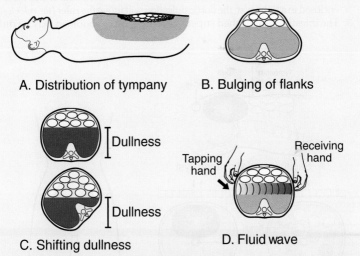

A. Distribution of tympany   B. Bulging of flanks

C. Shifting dullness   D. Fluid wave

FIG. 9-21 Signs of Ascites. A. Distribution of tympany. In the supine position, free fluid causes the gas-filled gut to float, so an area of tympany forms at the top of the bulging wall. **B. Bulging flanks.** The free fluid pushes the flanks outward, so they bulge toward the table or the bed. Fat in the mesentery also will cause this when the abdominal muscles are weak. **C. Shifting dullness.** The dependent fluid causes an area of dullness in the lowest part which shifts to remain lowest with changes in position of the body. **D. Fluid wave.** A fluid wave, elicited by tapping one side of the abdomen, is transmitted to the receiving hand on the opposite side. The waves take perceptible time to cross the abdomen.

tricuspid valve stenosis or obstruction. *Hepatic Vein Obstruction:* Budd–Chiari syndrome, thrombosis, proximal IVC obstruction or thrombosis. *Obstruction of the Hepatic Sinusoids and Intrahepatic Portal Veins:* Cirrhosis from any cause, primary biliary cirrhosis, amyloidosis, schistosomiasis, neoplastic infiltration. *Portal Vein Obstruction:* Portal vein thrombosis, pylephlebitis, extrinsic compression by lymph nodes or masses in the porta hepatis. *Peritoneal Irritation:* Acute or chronic peritonitis, neoplastic implants (especially ovarian cancer), tuberculosis. *Decreased Oncotic Pressure:* Nephrotic syndrome, hepatocellular dysfunction, repeated large volume paracentesis, protein-losing enteropathy, malnutrition. *Thoracic Duct or Lymphatic Obstruction (Chylous Ascites):* lymphoma, metastatic neoplasm, trauma, surgical injury, trauma to thorax or abdomen, tuberculosis, filariasis, intestinal lymphangiectasia. *Miscellaneous:* Myxedema, benign ovarian adenoma with ascites and hydrothorax (Meigs syndrome), starvation edema, and wet beriberi (thiamine deficiency and hypoproteinemia are only contributing factors).

Ovarian cyst. See Female Reproductive Tract Syndromes, Chapter 11, page 502. Large ovarian cysts filling the abdomen must be distinguished from ascites. Because they are thin walled and filled with fluid they can evert the umbilicus and produce a fluid wave and shifting dullness. The pelvic examination is not diagnostic. Three signs help identify these cysts (Fig. 9-22):

1. Careful inspection of the abdominal profile reveals two curves instead of one.
2. When a ruler is pressed transversely across the abdomen, the pulsations of the abdominal aorta are not transmitted with free fluid. If the fluid is enclosed in a tight cyst, the aortic pulsation will move the ruler (*the ruler test*).
3. The intestines are pushed superiorly, so the lower abdomen may be dull.

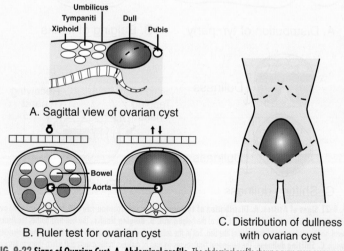

FIG. 9-22 Signs of Ovarian Cyst. A. Abdominal profile. The abdominal profile shows a curve more pronounced in the lower half. The gas-filled intestines, producing tympany, fill the superior half of the cavity, instead of floating to the top. **B. The ruler test. C. Distribution of dullness.**

Obesity. Abdominal obesity results from excessive caloric intake and/or re-distribution of adipose tissue caused by hormonal factors, especially gluco-corticoids. Fat is deposited in the retroperitoneum, mesentery, organs, and abdominal wall. Obesity causes a uniformly rounded abdomen and increased girth (Fig. 9-20). The umbilicus, adhering to the peritoneum, is deeply buried. Adiposity is usually evident in other parts of the body. Men accumulate more visceral and mesenteric fat than women. Because generalized obesity is obvi-ous, the challenge is to determine if other causes of abdominal distention are also present.

Pregnancy. The breasts are engorged, fetal movements and parts may be felt, the cervix is softened, and the fetal heart should be audible. With a molar pregnancy, there will be no signs of a fetus. A gravid uterus can resemble a large ovarian cyst (Fig. 9-20).

Feces. A large accumulation of feces, as in megacolon, may cause disten-tion. A history of chronic constipation and chronic laxative use are common. Disorders of the myenteric plexus, advanced age, and use of anticholinergic drugs are other causes. Soft deformable intraabdominal masses may be pal-pated; rectal examination may show stool in the vault. Tympanites is usually absent.

Depressed abdomen—scaphoid abdomen. In extreme malnutrition the abdominal wall sinks inward toward the vertebral column, forming a depres-sion, bounded superiorly by the costal angle and inferiorly by the wings of the ilia, making the shape of an ancient Greek boat, a *skaphe* (Fig. 9-20B). The abdominal contents are more visible and more readily felt than normal mak-ing it easy to overestimate the size and significance of structures that are nor-mally not palpable.

Scars and striae. See Chapter 6, page 118.

Engorged veins. The abdominal wall veins are scarcely seen unless the skin and subcutaneous fat are thin. Engorged veins are seen through a normal abdominal wall. The veins distend when normal venous drainage is obstructed increasing collateral flow. The low pressure (<30 cm H_2O) normal venous system is easily obstructed by extrinsic compression. Slow venous flow also increases the risk for thrombosis. Obstruction of portal venous drainage from the abdominal viscera is most common (see Portal Hypertension, page 430). Chest and abdominal wall collaterals also follow obstruction of the IVC distal to the hepatic vein, iliac veins, femoral veins, superior vena cava, brachioce-phalic, and subclavian veins. The pattern of distended veins on the abdomen, chest, and extremities, together with the direction of flow, accurately predicts the site of obstruction. Abdominal wall veins do not have valves, so flow can be in either direction, but it is always away from the site obstruction. Above the umbilicus flow is normally cephalad; below the navel it is caudad. The direction of flow is the direction of most rapid refilling of an empty venous segment (Fig. 9-23). IVC obstruction causes cephalad flow in the lower abdo-men (*flow reversal*). Portal obstruction increases normal cephalad flow in the upper abdomen and caudad flow in the lower abdomen. SVC obstruction

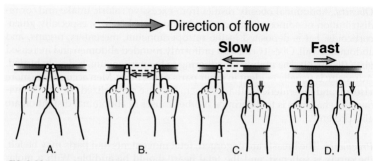

FIG. 9-23 Testing Direction of Blood Flow in Superficial Veins. A. The examiner presses the blood from the veins with his index fingers in apposition. **B. The index fingers slide apart,** milking the blood from the intervening segment of vein. **C. Pressure upon one end of the segment is released,** observing the time of refilling from that direction. **D. Repeat the procedure,** releasing the other end first. The flow of blood is in the direction of the faster flow.

causes reversed caudad flow in the upper abdomen. Very rarely, engorged veins form a knot around the umbilicus called *caput medusae*.

CLINICAL OCCURRENCE: *Mechanical/Traumatic:* Extrinsic compression from mass lesions (superior vena cava, IVC, and their major tributaries), obliteration of hepatic sinusoids (portal hypertension), strictures caused by traumatic or iatrogenic injury (surgery, instrumentation, or irradiation); *Vascular:* Thrombosis caused by intravenous catheters or pacemakers (subclavian, jugular, brachiocephalic, femoral), spontaneous thrombosis from congenital or acquired thrombophilia (any vein, superficial or deep).

Visible peristalsis. Normal contractions of the stomach and intestines may be visible, under a thin abdominal wall, as slow undulations. Visible peristaltic waves through a wall of normal thickness usually reflect increased amplitude and strength of peristalsis. They appear as oblique ridges beginning near the LUQ and gradually moving downward and rightward. Parallel ridges may form a ladder pattern. The waves are slow requiring several minutes of bedside observation with the eyes near the abdominal level. Abnormally powerful waves indicate obstruction. *Borborygmus,* intestinal rumblings heard without a stethoscope, in conjunction with visible peristalsis and pain suggest partial or complete bowel obstruction.

Visible pulsations. The aorta can cause visible epigastric pulsation, the amplitude increasing with wide pulse pressure, tortuous aorta, or aneurysm. A pulsatile mass can be an aneurysm or a solid mass overlying the aorta. An aneurysm expands laterally as well as anteroposteriorly. Ultrasonography or CT is diagnostic.

Diastasis recti. If the two abdominal rectus muscles lack their normal midline attachment, raising the feet reveals the separation as a midline bulge. This may be visible or evident only on palpation (Fig. 9-20A). With the abdomen relaxed no abnormality is seen.

Everted umbilicus. Increased intraabdominal pressure, usually from ascites, everts the umbilicus without a true hernia.

Umbilical fistula. This may discharge urine through a patent urachus, pus from a urachal cyst or tract or an intraabdominal abscess, or feces from a connection with the colon.

Umbilical calculus. Poor hygiene leads to accumulation of dirt and desquamated epithelium in the umbilical cavity producing a hard mass often with inflammation.

Bluish umbilicus (Cullen sign). A blue coloration around the umbilicus indicates retroperitoneal bleeding.

Ecchymoses on abdomen and flanks (Grey Turner sign). First associated with hemorrhagic pancreatitis, it is seen with retroperitoneal hemorrhage of any cause. The blood dissects along the deep tissue planes to the skin of the lower abdomen, groin, and flanks. The stage of hemoglobin degradation determines the color from blue-red, to blue-purple, to green-brown.

Auscultation

Decreased or absent bowel sounds, ileus. Listen for at least 5 minutes *by the clock* before accepting absent bowel sounds. Occasional weak tinkles are not evidence of good peristalsis. High-pitched tinkling sounds and rushes may be heard in partial obstruction. Ileus is never a primary problem, except in intestinal pseudo-obstruction, but indicates a metabolic/toxic, inflammatory, or infectious process.

CLINICAL OCCURRENCE: *Endocrine:* Myxedema; *Degenerative/Idiopathic:* Intestinal pseudo-obstruction; *Infectious:* Peritonitis; *Metabolic/Toxic:* Electrolyte abnormalities: hypokalemia, hypomagnesemia, hypocalcemia; uremia; drugs: opiates, anticholinergics; *Mechanical/Traumatic:* Advanced intestinal obstruction; *Neurologic:* Spinal cord injury; *Vascular:* Mesenteric ischemia.

Increased bowel sounds. Increased peristalsis indicates bowel irritation usually resulting from luminal toxins, irritants, or early obstruction. History and other exam findings usually distinguishes diarrheal illness from obstruction.

Succussion splash. Air and fluid in the stomach can produce audible splashes with movement or palpation. A loud splash and distention suggests gastric dilatation often caused by gastroparesis or outlet obstruction.

Peritoneal friction rub. A friction rub with breathing, movement, peristalsis, or palpation indicates peritoneal inflammation (Fig. 9-24). Like a pleural rub, it sounds like two pieces of leather rubbing together.

CLINICAL OCCURRENCE: *Infectious:* Liver or splenic abscess, perihepatitis (Fitz–Hugh–Curtis syndrome); *Mechanical/Traumatic:* After liver biopsy; *Neoplastic:* Hepatocellular carcinoma, liver metastases, peritoneal mesothelioma; *Vascular:* Splenic infarction.

Abdominal bruits. Bruits imply arterial flow through a narrowed or tortuous artery (generally systolic only), or large volume high to low pressure flow, e.g. an arteriovenous malformation (both systolic and diastolic). Hepatic arteriovenous malformations are common in HHT. Hepatocellular carcinoma

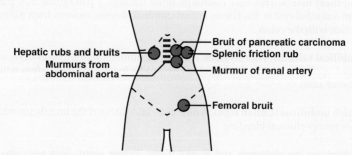

FIG. 9-24 Abdominal Bruits and Rubs. Green shading indicates the optimum areas for the auscultation of each sound.

frequently produces a harsh arterial bruit that is either systolic or continuous with systolic accentuation. Rarely, a venous hum is audible over a hepatic hemangioma or in the dilated periumbilical flow associated with a patent umbilical vein (Cruveilhier–Baumgarten syndrome). A continuous systolic-diastolic bruit can occur with a renal arteriovenous fistula. Renal artery stenosis is found in approximately two-thirds of patients with systolic renal artery bruits. These murmurs are soft, medium- or low-pitched, and most commonly heard just above and to the left of the umbilicus (Fig. 9-24).

Percussion

Tympanitic percussion—tympanites. Tympanites indicates the presence of free air in the abdomen from perforation or excessive gas within the bowel from obstruction, abnormal motility, or swallowed gases. Signs of tympanites are abdominal distention, a large area of tympany, and an abdominal profile describing a single curve (Fig. 9-20B). Mechanical obstruction from intraluminal mass, extrinsic compression, intussusception, or volvulus commonly produces noisy tympanites, vomiting, and colicky pain. Tympanites may not be present with obstruction proximal to the ligament of Treitz, the gut being too short to contain much gas and fixed in the retroperitoneum. Rather, proximal obstruction causes gastric distention with localized LUQ tympany. With prolonged obstruction the distended stomach can drop to the pelvic brim. Nonmechanical obstruction from decreased bowel motility, which can be diffuse or segmental, produces silent tympanites, anorexia, and nausea, without colic or vomiting. Both types of obstruction can occur sequentially or together. Tympanites can occur with normal bowel sounds and no vomiting (see Obstruction Syndromes, page 453. A small amount of intraperitoneal gas cannot be identified by physical exam. Without peritonitis, bowel sounds can be normal and pain absent. The amount of pain, tenderness, and guarding is proportional to the severity of chemical peritonitis (e.g., bile or gastric acid) or infection from perforated bowel.

 CLINICAL OCCURRENCE: *Intraluminal Gas—Congenital:* Lactase deficiency, fructose malabsorption; *Degenerative/Idiopathic:* Intestinal pseudoobstruction, lactase deficiency; *Infectious:* Small bowel bacterial overgrowth; *Inflammatory/Immune:* Megacolon from ulcerative colitis or Crohn disease; *Mechanical/Traumatic:* Volvulus, ileus, endoscopic procedures, air contrast barium enema, aerophagia, carbonated beverage ingestion, bowel obstruction;

Metabolic/Toxic: Toxic megacolon, lactase deficiency, artificial sweeteners; *Neurologic:* Ileus following spinal cord injury; *Psychosocial:* Factitious disorders; *Vascular:* Ileus from ischemia. **Pneumoperitoneum**—*Degenerative/Idiopathic:* Ruptured diverticulum, perforated ulcer, pneumocystoides; *Infectious:* Typhoid fever with perforation; ruptured diverticular abscess; *Inflammatory/ Immune:* Perforated megacolon; *Mechanical/Traumatic:* Perforating abdominal wounds, perforating ingested foreign bodies, volvulus with perforation, post-paracentesis, post-laparoscopy, post-hysterosalpingogram, peritoneal dialysis; *Neoplastic:* Perforated colon cancer; *Vascular:* ischemic bowel with perforation.

Abdominal pain with percussion. See Rebound tenderness below.

CVA tenderness. Percussion pain and tenderness to palpation indicate inflammation of the kidney or surrounding soft tissues, e.g., pyelonephritis.

Palpation

Tenderness. Tenderness is caused by inflammation of the abdominal wall, peritoneum, or a viscus. Solid organs are tender when their capsule is stretched. When a tender area is found during abdominal exam, repeat palpation of the spot while the patient raises their head off the pillow or feet off the table. If the tenderness is unchanged or worsens, an abdominal wall disorder is likely. If the tenderness diminishes, an intraabdominal process is more likely.

Rebound tenderness. The inflamed peritoneum is painful with direct pressure or movement, especially when two inflamed surfaces slide over one another. Because the peritoneum has somatic sensory afferents, the site of pain is well localized. Press the fingertips gently into the abdomen, then suddenly withdraw them watching the patient's face (Fig. 9-7D). Pain worsened after withdrawal is rebound tenderness. The pain can occur at the site of pressure or remote from it. If a site of inflammation is suspected, do your first maneuvers in the other quadrants. An alternate and less-painful method is the use of light percussion. Rebound tenderness is a reliable sign of peritoneal inflammation. Another test for peritoneal irritation is vigorously moving the patient's pelvis from side to side. Jar Tenderness (Markle Sign). The patient stands on the floor, knees straight, rises on the toes, then drops onto the heels. Note the location and severity of pain. This is useful when tense abdominal muscles prevent testing rebound tenderness. A false-positive is uncommon. Finding of jar tenderness by the heel-drop test localizes peritoneal irritation, especially in the pelvis. Abdominal pain on running or walking is equivalent. **CLINICAL OCCURRENCE:** *Congenital:* Familial Mediterranean fever, acute intermittent and variegate porphyria; *Endocrine:* Ectopic or tubal pregnancy; *Infectious:* Pelvic inflammatory disease, intraabdominal abscess; diverticulitis; *Inflammatory/Immune:* Peritonitis, appendicitis; cholecystitis, regional enteritis (Crohn disease), familial Mediterranean fever, acute intermittent and variegate porphyria; *Mechanical-Traumatic:* Intraabdominal bleeding; *Vascular:* Infarction of abdominal organs.

Cutaneous hyperesthesia and allodynia. See Chapter 14, page 675. In acute appendicitis, an area of hyperesthesia is frequently found in the RLQ preceding perforation.

Subcutaneous crepitus. See Chapter 6, page 118.

Voluntary muscular rigidity. Increased abdominal wall muscle tone results from failure to relax, a cold room or examining hands, and anxiety. The rigidity interferes with effective deep palpation. It is distinguished from involuntary rigidity by being abolished with suitable maneuvers (pages 398–399).

Involuntary muscular rigidity. Peritoneal irritation causes reflex abdominal wall muscle spasm. Involuntary rigidity persists despite relaxing maneuvers. Attempting a sit-up without using the arms is painful. Involuntarily rigid muscles are not necessarily tender and must be distinguished from abdominal wall masses. Reflex rigidity may be unilateral, whereas voluntary rigidity is bilaterally symmetrical. Assess symmetry by comparing muscle tension right to left in upper and lower quadrants.

Subphrenic abscess. Pus collects under either diaphragm secondary to suppurative lesions in the liver or spleen, or elsewhere in the abdomen, e.g., a perforated appendix. Suspect subphrenic abscess in patients with unexplained fever or anorexia. There may be nothing directing attention to the region. An elevated hemidiaphragm suggested by percussion is confirmed by X-ray. Pleural effusion, evidenced by percussion dullness, decreased breath sounds, and decreased fremitus, can occur on the affected side. Suspect gas under the right diaphragm when tympany is found over the normal area of hepatic dullness. Tenderness and edema in specific locations suggests the involved subphrenic space (Fig. 9-25): *Right Anterior Superior Space*, under the right costal margin in front of the liver, between the sixth and tenth right intercostal spaces anteriorly; *Right Anterior Inferior Space*, below the right anterior costal margin behind the liver; *Left Anterior Superior Space*, under the left costal margin anteriorly, between the sixth and tenth left interspaces in the midclavicular line; *Left Anterior Inferior Space*, under the left costal margin in the mid axillary line; and *Left Posterior Inferior Space*, over the left twelfth rib.

Abdominal masses. See Abdominal Masses, page 455. If sufficiently large or close to the abdominal wall, masses produce resistance to light palpation. Light palpation determines only the presence of a mass and its location. Note whether the shape and location correspond to abdominal muscles or resembles a viscus. Describe the mass by location, size, shape, consistency, surface, tenderness, and mobility. Not all masses are intraabdominal. Intramural masses remain palpable when the abdominal muscles are tensed; intraabdominal masses become less distinct (Fig. 9-26). *DDX:* Rectus hematoma is frequently mistaken for an intraabdominal mass.

Shallow abdominal cavity. Enlarged paraaortic and/or mesenteric lymph nodes (retroperitoneal lymphadenopathy) can fill the retroperitoneal space. The nodes are covered with fascia and abdominal viscera, making the floor of the abdominal cavity seem more accessible than normal. The abdominal cavity seems shallower than normal, but without definite masses, discrete nodes not being felt. (Fig. 9-27). Retroperitoneal nodes are best visualized by CT or MRI. Lymphoma, metastatic germ cell tumors, and granulomatous diseases

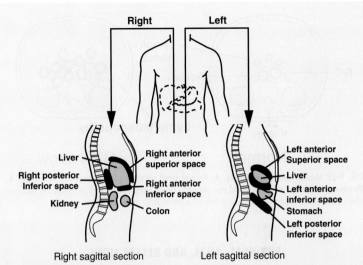

FIG. 9-25 Locations of Subphrenic Abscesses. The loci are in the right midclavicular line, behind the costal margin, and the LUQ. Posteriorly, the region of the right kidney should be examined.

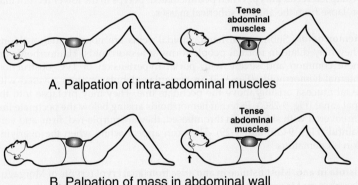

FIG. 9-26 Distinguishing Between Intramural and Intraabdominal Masses. Palpate the mass while the patient raises his head from the pillow. When the abdominal muscles tense, the intraabdominal mass moves away from the palpating hand, whereas the intramural mass remains accessible.

are most common. The massively enlarged kidneys of polycystic kidney disease also produce this finding.

Nodular umbilicus (Sister Mary Joseph nodule). Intraabdominal carcinoma, especially gastric cancer, can metastasize to the navel.

Pulseless femoral artery (Leriche syndrome). Always palpate the femoral arteries during abdominal exam. See Chapter 8, page 375 for further discussion.

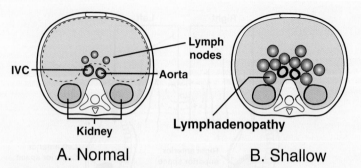

FIG. 9-27 Shallow Abdominal Cavity. A. Normal small paraaortic lymph nodes are not palpable. **B. Massive enlargement of prevertebral and preaortic lymph nodes.** These cannot be distinguished from other retroperitoneal masses by palpation; they give the impression that the abdomen is shallower than normal.

PERINEAL, ANAL, AND RECTAL SIGNS

Inspection

Pruritus ani. See symptoms page 413.

Prolapsed rectal polyp. When pedunculated, polyps in the lower rectum may prolapse from the anus as spherical masses.

Hemorrhoids. Submucosal hemorrhoidal veins are normal anal cushions. They may dilate in normal people forming hemorrhoids. Hemorrhoids are more common and severe with portal hypertension or IVC obstruction. Internal hemorrhoids (Fig. 9-3) are irregular globular masses covered with rectal mucosa arising above the pectinate line. They may prolapse into the anal canal (Fig. 9-28C). External hemorrhoids arising below the pectinate line are covered with skin. When thrombosed, they are purple-red, firm, and very painful (Figs. 9-28B and 9-29). They can appear white when the overlying skin is edematous.

Fistula in ano. Most fistulae in ano arise from anal crypt (crypts of Morgagni) abscesses and track to the perianal skin. Look for a small sinus track opening in the perianal skin (Fig. 9-28D). The internal orifices of the tracks are just above the pectinate line (Fig. 9-3 page, 396). Do not probe fistulas from the skin. Gentle palpation around the external orifice may reveal the track as a subcutaneous cord. The origin is inferred from the location of the fistula on the perineum (Fig. 9-30A). *DDX:* Chronic lesions stimulate a hypertrophied anal papilla (*sentinel pile*). Multiple fistulas suggest Crohn disease or tuberculous proctitis.

Fissure in ano. Anal sphincter spasm causes the extreme pain associated with fissures. If the patient presents with pain, do not attempt a digital rectal exam before inspecting the mucosa by retracting the skin on both sides looking for the fissure posteriorly (Fig. 9-30B). It is an extreme unkindness to the patient to attempt further examination without giving either local anesthetics or

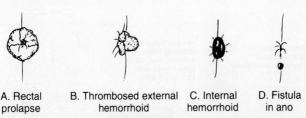

A. Rectal   B. Thrombosed external   C. Internal   D. Fistula
prolapse   hemorrhoid   hemorrhoid   in ano

FIG. 9-28 Some External Anal Findings. A. Rectal prolapse appears as a red doughnut of most rectal mucosa protruding through the anus. **B. Thrombosed external hemorrhoids** are semispheric masses of erythematous skin at the mucocutaneous junction with the anus. **C. Internal hemorrhoids** are mucosal masses sometimes seen through the retracted anus. **D.** Fistulas opening on the skin are accompanied by a papule of hypertrophied skin on the margin of the orifice.

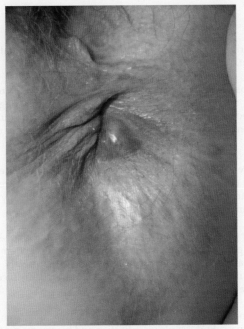

FIG. 9-29 Hemorrhoid. External Hemorrhoid with a small skin break that resulted in bleeding.

analgesics. The fissure is a slit-like separation of the superficial anal mucosa, suggesting a longitudinal tear. It rarely becomes an ulcerating crater.

Sentinel pile. This term is applied to two structures. More commonly, it refers to a hyperplastic skin tag found external to a fissure in ano. Resembling an external hemorrhoidal tag, it is also called a *fibrous anal polyp.* The name also is applied to a hypertrophied anal papilla internal to a fissure in ano (Fig. 9-3).

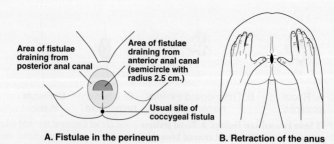

A. Fistulae in the perineum   **B. Retraction of the anus**

FIG. 9-30 Examination of the Perineum. A. Fistulae in the perineum. The dark blue semicircular area anterior to the anus, with a radius of 2.5 cm, indicates the location of fistulae draining from the anterior surface of the anal canal (Salmon law). Anal fistulae draining to the skin in the light blue area arise in abscesses from the posterior surface of the canal. A coccygeal (pilonidal) fistula is usually in the midline, near coccyx or sacrum. **B. Retracting the anus.** This is a method of stretching the anal orifice to inspect for fissure in ano, external hemorrhoids, or prolapsing internal hemorrhoids or polyps.

This lesion arises from the pectinate line, whereas an internal hemorrhoid arises above it.

Rectal prolapse. When the patient strains as if to defecate, the rectal mucosa everts below the sphincter (Fig. 9-28). When symptoms suggest prolapse but the procedure fails to demonstrate it, have the patient squat and strain in the position for defecation. The prolapse can be mucosal or complete.

Palpation

Anal stricture. Congenital strictures present as narrow crescentic folds at the rectal end of the anal canal. Fibrous strictures in the same region usually result from surgery for internal hemorrhoids. Radiation therapy can produce a sharply delimited stricture.

Carcinoma of the anus. Squamous cell carcinoma of the anal skin is caused by human papillomavirus infection. It is most common in homosexual men practicing anal-receptive intercourse. Its incidence is greatly increased in HIV-infected men. The tumor presents as an exophytic or ulcerating mass narrowing the anal canal.

Rectal carcinoma. Cancer may cause plateau-like, nodular, annular, or cauliflower rectal mass. Endoscopic visualization and biopsy are essential.

Fibrosis of anal sphincter muscles. The entire canal is narrowed so the finger feels encased in a rigid tube. This frequently produces fecal impaction.

Tight sphincter—apprehension. The most common cause of a tight anal sphincter is apprehension. Preliminary reassurance should be combined with a gentle and slow examination. When the sphincter tightens, stop advancing until the sphincter relaxes. Though the procedure may be uncomfortable, it should not be painful. When the sphincter is in spasm that cannot be relaxed by gentleness, suspect a fissure.

Relaxed sphincter—lacerated anal muscles. Childbirth, injury during surgery, and sexual abuse each damage the anal sphincter. Partial sphincter lacerations are more common than lacerations completely disrupting the sphincter. If the laceration extends through the anal canal the edges of the anus are either separated or form an irregular line. When the anus is retracted by pulling the skin from each side, a dimple may be visible in the posterior anal ring. The sphincter feels weak when the finger is inserted. Ultrasonography confirms the defect. See Fecal Incontinence, page 412.

Atonic muscles. Damage anywhere in the peripheral or central sensory and motor systems controlling the sphincters produces decreased tone. The finding should prompt a careful neurologic examination.

Rectal Blumer shelf. Debris accumulating in the pelvis from neoplasms or inflammation elsewhere in the abdomen or pelvis is felt through the anterior rectal wall as a hard shelf in the rectovesical or rectouterine pouch. Peritoneal metastases from a primary carcinoma higher in the abdomen are most common. It also occurs from pelvic inflammatory disease in women and prostatic abscess in men.

Mistaken normal structures. The cervix, a vaginal tampon, and a pessary felt through the anterior rectal wall can be misinterpreted as a neoplasm. When the uterus is retroverted, the normal fundus may similarly mislead. Occasionally, a loop of normal colon in the pelvic pouches is felt as a soft and freely movable mass not easily confused with cancer.

Rectal polyps. Some polyps are difficult to palpate , especially if sessile. They are easily missed since they are soft and may be mobile.

Coccygeal tenderness. When pain in the region of the coccyx is exacerbated by sitting or defecation test for tenderness in the sacrococcygeal joint during digital rectal exam. With the index finger in the rectum on the anterior surface of the coccyx press the posterior surface of the bone with the thumb on the skin outside. Moving the bone anteriorly and posteriorly elicits pain in the joint. The coccyx may be displaced from previous injury.

Fecal impaction. Symptoms may be vague. The patient may complain of constipation or obstipation, but sometimes there is diarrhea, the fecal stream passing around the impaction producing incontinence. The debilitated or postoperative patient may only be restless or have fever or anorexia. Barium suspensions administered for X-ray examination commonly cause impaction. The rectum is filled with hard, dry masses of feces. These are removed by breaking up and extracting the pieces with the examining finger.

Coccygeal sinus (pilonidal sinus). A congenital track extending from the coccyx or sacrum to the perineum drains to the exterior, usually in the midline posterior to the anus (Fig. 9-30). The sinus is lined with epithelium and hairs, hence the alternate name pilonidal. When blocked, it can form a tender dimple or bulge just below the coccyx or on one side, usually the left.

Ischiorectal abscess. An abscess forms within the pelvic floor muscles and tissue spaces between the rectum and the ischium. This is often associated with neutropenia. Because it is deep-seated there may be no signs on inspection. Tenderness on deep palpation between the anus and ischial tuberosity identifies the site.

Anal intermuscular abscess. Abscesses between the muscles of the anus cause agonizing pain during defecation and discomfort during sitting. In high abscesses, a tender mass is felt just above the anorectal junction. Low abscesses are most frequently found by palpating the distal end of the anal canal between two fingers.

ABDOMINAL, PERINEAL, AND ANORECTAL SYNDROMES

Hepatobiliary and Pancreatic Syndromes

Portal vein thrombosis. When occlusion occurs rapidly, symptoms of hepatic and/or mesenteric vascular congestion (anorexia, pain and tenderness, ileus, distention, diarrhea, and vomiting) occur before signs of portal hypertension. Ascites and splenomegaly follow rapidly. Infarctions of the upper GI tract may occur. Slowly developing obstruction presents as ascites or signs from vessels forming the portosystemic shunts. Occlusion occurs after surgical manipulation of the portal vein, septic thrombophlebitis of the portal vein (*pylephlebitis*), trauma, polycythemia vera, neoplastic invasion of the vein lumen, or prolonged debilitating illness. Clinical suspicion should lead to imaging.

Portal hypertension. Any obstruction to the blood flow in the portal vein, liver (presinusoidal, sinusoidal, post-sinusoidal), or hepatic veins produces portal hypertension. Increased portal pressure causes splenic congestion with splenomegaly, development of venous collaterals about the esophagus, the rectum, and the abdominal wall, and production of ascites because of increased hydrostatic pressure in the liver capsule and mesenteric veins (Fig. 9-31). Search for splenomegaly, visible collateral veins, and ascites. Collaterals veins can be seen in the anus, abdominal wall, esophagus, and proximal stomach. Hemorrhoids may be portal collaterals, but their occurrence from local causes is so common that their presence is rarely diagnostic. Dilatation of the periumbilical veins can produce a venous rosette around the navel, a *caput medusae*, but it is rare. The common demonstrable collaterals are dilated superficial veins in the abdominal wall between the umbilicus and the lower thorax containing blood flowing upward, in the normal direction. When the veins are greatly dilated, a venous hum with systolic accentuation may be heard below the xiphoid process, over the epigastric surface of the liver, or around the navel. The hum comes from varices in the falciform ligament. Dilated veins in the lower esophagus and gastric cardia produce esophageal varices and portal gastropathy visible during endoscopy. Ascites is painless and may be mild, moderate, or severe. *DDX:* Portal obstruction with ascites and ankle edema may be mistaken for right heart failure. Both conditions can produce pleural effusions, hepatomegaly, ascites, and ankle edema. Engorged neck veins and orthopnea are frequent with heart failure but absent with portal hypertension. Causes of portal hypertension are hepatic vein thrombosis,

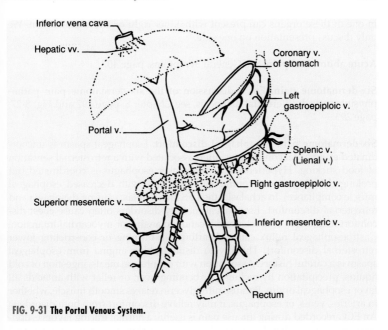

FIG. 9-31 The Portal Venous System.

liver cirrhosis, intrahepatic tumors and cysts, granulomatous liver diseases, portal vein thrombosis, and septic thrombosis of the portal vein.

Hepatic vein thrombosis—Budd-Chiari syndrome. Hepatic vein thrombosis causes hepatic sinusoidal congestion obstructing portal flow through the liver producing portal hypertension. The acutely distended liver capsule is painful. The onset may be abrupt, with abdominal pain and vomiting. The liver is tender and enlarges rapidly. Mild jaundice can be present. Ascites rapidly accumulates. Shock may ensue, with death in a few days. IVC obstruction at or above the hepatic vein produces similar symptoms and additional signs related to the legs. If the initial stage is survived, the chronic findings appear [Chung RT, Iafrate AJ, Amrein PC, et al. Case 15–2006: A 46-year-old woman with sudden onset of abdominal distention. *N Engl J Med.* 2006;354:2166-2175]. Budd-Chiari syndrome is associated with cirrhosis, acute or subacute liver disease caused by abscess, malignancy or trauma, polycythemia vera, paroxysmal nocturnal hemoglobinuria, myeloproliferative disorders, and thrombophilic states including oral contraceptive use.

Chronic hepatic vein occlusion. This late phase of the Budd–Chiari syndrome is marked by portal hypertension, ascites, hepatomegaly, and secondary hepatocellular failure. Sudden onset and lack of alcohol intake or hepatitis suggests the correct diagnosis.

Acute Abdominal Pain Syndromes. The abdomen contains the following paired organs: kidneys, ureters, adrenals, renal and iliac arteries and veins, and ovaries. A disease or syndrome associated with abdominal pain arising in one of these organs can present with either right or left lateralization. We only discuss presentation on one side.

Acute abdominal pain. See General Symptoms, page 407.

Six-dermatome pain. For a discussion of the six-dermatome pain pathophysiology and differential diagnosis, see Chapter 8, page 292 and Fig. 8-27, page 293.

Six-dermatome pain—esophageal discomfort. Esophageal spasm is uncoordinated esophageal contractions often associated with a retrosternal sensation of food sticking. Hypertensive or nutcracker esophagus is coordinated but prolonged high-pressure contractions (probably with decreased esophageal muscle compliance). In achalasia, the LES fails to relax, causing dysphagia and retrosternal discomfort. Esophageal motility disorders often cause chest discomfort identical in character and location to angina or myocardial infarction. Gastroesophageal reflux causes heartburn, a burning or constricting lower retrosternal discomfort. The key to distinguishing angina from esophageal spasm is a careful history. Association with dysphagia, meals, ingestion of cold liquids, precipitation by reclining or bending over, or relief with antacids all favor esophageal origin. Because nitroglycerin relaxes smooth muscle, whether in arteries, veins, or esophagus, it may relieve discomfort from both disorders. An ECG recorded during intense pain is useful; a normal tracing favors esophageal pain, although it does not exclude cardiac ischemia. *The presence of a hiatal hernia has no diagnostic significance in the differential diagnosis of chest pain.*

Esophageal pain and dysphagia. Mechanical disruption of normal swallowing and activation of esophageal nociceptors produces these findings. Some of the more frequent causes are discussed below.

Esophageal laceration—Mallory–Weiss tear. Esophageal laceration near the esophagogastric junction follows severe retching and vomiting. Hematemesis follows the retching and vomiting. Bleeding is usually self-limited.

Acute esophagitis. Retrosternal pain intensified by swallowing is caused by prolonged vomiting, nasogastric tubes, pill esophagitis, corrosive esophageal burns, acute infections (herpes simplex, *Candida spp.*, cytomegalovirus), and reflux of gastric acid or bile.

Chronic esophagitis. Inflammation causing pain and dysphagia persists for weeks or months and may be complicated by ulceration and/or intestinal metaplasia (Barrett esophagus), a premalignant lesion. Progressive fibrosis produces esophageal stricture. Acid reflux is the most common cause. Irradiation, infections (HIV, *Candida*, herpes, and cytomegalovirus) are less common.

Esophageal achalasia. Unremitting forceful LES contraction causes functional obstruction at the gastroesophageal junction dilating the proximal esophagus. Symptoms include weight loss, dysphagia and regurgitation of food, saliva, and esophageal secretions. Chest pain may be present. Cough, especially after meals or with recumbency, suggests aspiration.

Zenker diverticulum. This is a pulsion diverticulum in the posterior hypopharynx protruding downward between spine and esophagus. It fills with food, causing dysphagia and regurgitation of putrefied food. Occasionally, there is retrosternal pain. An esophagram visualizes the pouch.

Plummer–Vinson syndrome. Severe iron deficiency is associated with a postcricoid esophageal web demonstrated by esophagram that explains the dysphagia in some, but no anatomic basis for the dysphagia is found in many patients.

Esophageal cancer. Adenocarcinomas at or just above the gastroesophageal junction are increasing in frequency; squamous cell carcinomas predominate more proximally. Dysphagia usually precedes pain by weeks or months. The pain sometimes radiates to the neck or back. Chronic esophagitis with metaplasia (Barrett esophagus) substantially increases the risk for developing adenocarcinoma.

Foreign body. Swallowed rigid objects lodge at the level of the aortic arch or diaphragm, causing pain and dysphagia.

Acute abdominal pain

- **Acute peritonitis.** Acute infection and/or sterile chemical irritation of the peritoneum produce an intense inflammatory response with transudation of intravascular fluid into the peritoneal space. This can be complicated by bleeding and/or bacterial infection (sepsis) related to the inciting event. Common causes are penetrating trauma, rupture of the bowel, and bowel infarction. There are three symptom stages. (1) *Stage of Prostration (Primary Shock).* The patient experiences a sudden, excruciating epigastric pain, frequently collapsing. The pain soon spreads over the entire abdomen. The patient is anxious, pale, and diaphoretic. Respirations are shallow because moving the diaphragm is painful. Retching or vomiting occurs. Hypothermia and hypotension are common. The initial stage may last from a few minutes to several hours. (2) *Stage of Reaction (Masked Peritonitis).* This brief respite for the patient may deceive the inexperienced physician. The blood pressure rises, the skin becomes warmer, and the generalized abdominal pain and tenderness become less intense. The thighs are flexed for comfort and the patient moves cautiously because of pain. Involuntary boardlike rigidity results from abdominal muscle contraction and shallow respiration. The pelvic peritoneum is tender on rectal exam. Intraperitoneal free fluid is rarely demonstrated. Gas under the diaphragm is suggested by a diminished area of RUQ liver dullness. (3) *Stage of Frank Peritonitis.* The classic signs of advanced peritonitis appear. Ileus distends the abdomen, vomiting resumes and persists with increasing violence, and the temperature declines to subnormal levels. The entire abdomen is tender, but rigidity may lessen in the late stage. Dehydration and pain produce the classic *facies hippocratica*, with hollow features and anxious expression. An expedited team approach to the evaluation and management of suspected peritonitis minimizes morbidity and mortality through rapid diagnosis and combined medical and surgical treatments.

- *Spontaneous bacterial peritonitis.* Portal hypertension produces transudative ascites with a low **serum-albumin-ascites-gradient (SAAG)** and low in immunoglobulins. Bacteria seeded from the gut lead to infection with minimal localizing symptoms. Patients have advanced liver disease. They may present with fever or confusion without abdominal pain or tenderness. If the serum albumin ascites gradient is <2.1 and there are >250 PMNs/mm³ in the ascites fluid, treatment should be started pending culture results.
- *Solid organ rupture.* Blunt trauma to the lower thorax, back, and/or abdomen can fracture kidneys, liver, or spleen. The fracture and hemorrhage may be contained by the surrounding capsule, but rupture of the capsule acutely or delayed by hours or days results in severe hemorrhage. Upper quadrant and flank pain are present, and tenderness may be present anteriorly or posteriorly. Renal fracture results in gross hematuria unless the ureter is obstructed. Fracture of solid organs must be sought emergently by CT.
- *Volvulus.* Volvulus most commonly occurs in the sigmoid colon (90%) or the cecum (10%) where the gut is suspended on a long mesentery. Twisting compromises blood flow, forms a closed loop of distended bowel, and leads to ischemic perforation. A vague, tender mass may be felt. Frequently the only findings are distended bowel, tympany, pain, violent peristalsis, and vomiting. Early diagnosis and treatment are imperative. A bird beak cutoff of colonic gas may be seen on noncontrast X-rays. Colonoscopy can be both diagnostic and therapeutic.
- **Abdominal pain and pallor.** Abdominal pain accompanied by pallor is an ominous presentation requiring expeditious evaluation. Of greatest concern is hemorrhage from rupture of a major vessel or organ. Intense sympathetic activation, even without hemorrhage, may cause pallor and diaphoresis.
- *Ruptured ectopic pregnancy.* See Chapter 11, page 501.
- *Corpus luteum hemorrhage.* See Chapter 11, page 502.
- *Ruptured aortic or iliac aneurysm.* See page 436.
- *Bleeding peptic ulcer.* An ulcer eroding into a major vessel leads to life-threatening hemorrhage. Although bleeding may be preceeded by ulcer disease symptoms, it is not uncommon, especially for NSAID-induced ulcers, to present with painless hemorrhage and/or perforation. Blood should be sought in the stools and a nasogastric aspirate.
- *Hemorrhagic pancreatitis.* Pancreatic inflammation erodes blood vessels in the retroperitoneum, leading to hemorrhage into the necrotic pancreas and dissection of hemorrhage into the retroperitoneal spaces. See page 435 for complete discussion.

Acute Epigastric Pain: Visceral pain arising in the intestine from the stomach to the transverse colon is carried by the vagus nerve and projects to the epigastrium. In addition, somatic pain from the upper abdominal peritoneum and retroperitoneal structures is localized to the epigastrium.

- **Early acute appendicitis.** See Acute RLQ Pain—Appendicitis, page 440.

- **Perforated peptic ulcer.** Perforation causes leakage of acid, digestive enzymes, blood, bacteria, and bowel contents into the peritoneal cavity, lesser sac, or retroperitoneum. With free perforation, sterile peritonitis is followed by purulent peritonitis, septicemia, shock, and death. There may be a history of epigastric pain occurring 3 or 4 hours after meals and relieved by food or antacids. Occasionally, there are no antecedent symptoms, particularly in elderly patients taking NSAIDs. The patient describes sudden, excruciating pain in the epigastrium that spreads over the entire abdomen. Sometimes it intensifies in the suprapubic region because of the downward flow of gastric contents (Fig. 9-32). RLQ pain, tenderness, and rigidity may be pronounced, suggesting acute appendicitis. Without prompt diagnosis and treatment, generalized peritonitis will supervene.

Limited perforation of peptic ulcer. When the perforation is into a closed space, the released gastric contents are walled off producing a local abscess. The stage of prostration is mild, with the pain limited to the epigastrium or flank. The abscess forms in the subphrenic space or lesser peritoneal sac.

Acute gastritis. Inflammation of the gastric mucosa is caused by infection, chemical irritation, autoimmune injury, or drug-induced injury. Frequently, the cause is unknown. Symptoms are anorexia, nausea, and vomiting, sometimes with hematemesis, and epigastric pain with or without tenderness. Upper endoscopy is diagnostic revealing mucosal inflammation, erosions, and submucosal hemorrhage. Common causes are ingestion of aspirin, NSAIDs, alcohol, or contaminated food, uremia, infection with *H. pylori*, cytomegalovirus, herpes simplex, or enteroviruses, and autoimmune gastritis.

Acute pancreatitis. Auto-digestion of the pancreas, initiated by release of pancreatic enzymes into the parenchyma as a consequence of ductal obstruction, inflammation, ischemia or trauma, incites an intense sterile inflammatory response. The expanding inflammatory mass dissects within the retroperitoneum and occasionally ruptures into the peritoneum producing hypotension and shock. Secondary infection of necrotic tissue

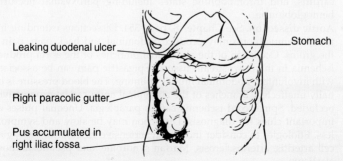

FIG. 9-32 Iliac Abscess from a Leaking Duodenal Ulcer. A perforated duodenal ulcer drains down the right paracolic gutter into the right iliac fossa, as indicated by stippling.

is common after the first few days. Without warning, the patient develops excruciating epigastric pain often with radiation to the back or flank. Irritation of the left hemidiaphragm causes pain radiating to the left shoulder via the phrenic nerve afferents. Occasionally, the pain spreads over the entire abdomen (generalized peritonitis) or primarily to the RLQ. The pain is knife-like with a boring quality, going directly through to the back. Because pain is aggravated when supine, the patient may sit leaning forward or curl up in the fetal position. Retching and vomiting are severe. The symptoms are more intense and prolonged than with a perforated stomach. Shock can occur. Since the process is confined to the retroperitoneum, there is often a disparity between the severity of symptoms and the paucity of abdominal findings. Epigastric tenderness is always present, but muscle rigidity is usually absent; when present, it is confined to the epigastrium. Occasionally a tender transverse mass is felt deep in the epigastrium. Two or three days after onset, blue or green ecchymoses can appear in the flank (*Turner sign*) or the umbilicus (*Cullen sign*) from extravasation of hemolyzed blood. Pseudocysts (an accumulation of blood, necrotic debris, and fluid in the retroperitoneum) are a late complication; they are rarely palpable. Acute pancreatitis may be an acute exacerbation of chronic, relapsing pancreatitis. Common causes of acute pancreatitis are alcohol and gallstones. Other causes include hypertriglyceridemia, pancreatic ductal obstruction and stricture, pancreas divisum, perforated peptic ulcer, ampulla of Vater dysfunction, mumps, and drugs.

- **Mesenteric ischemia.** The superior mesenteric artery and vein are most commonly affected, by either embolism or thrombosis. Half of patients with arterial thrombosis have a history of postprandial abdominal pain. Arterial occlusion produces the typical clinical picture. There is sudden onset of severe epigastric pain minimally relieved by narcotics followed by distention, ileus, and vomiting. Blood may pass per rectum. There are few localizing signs though a tender mass may be palpated in the epigastrium. Venous thrombosis often presents atypically. There is a severe metabolic acidosis as endotoxemia and shock supervene. Common causes are atherosclerosis, atheroembolism, fibromuscular dysplasia, acute bacterial or fungal endocarditis, embolism of mural cardiac thrombus, nonbacterial thrombotic (marantic) endocarditis, and thrombophilic states including paroxysmal nocturnal hemoglobinuria.

- **Aortic dissection.** See Chapter 8, page 354. Dissections extending into the abdominal aorta may produce abdominal and back pain, pain in the groins. Occlusion of the abdominal branches of the aorta produces ischemia in the downstream tissues. Epigastric pain can be associated with involuntary abdominal muscle splinting. The blood pressure is initially unaffected. Branches of the abdominal aorta can be progressively occluded. Spinal cord ischemia causes paraplegia. Unequal pulses are important clues for diagnosis. Dissection may be slow and symptomless. Etiologies to consider include hypertensive vascular disease, giant cell arteritis, arteriosclerosis, Marfan syndrome, and pseudoxanthoma elasticum.

- **Abdominal aortic aneurysm leak and rupture.** AAA is often painless until it leaks blood into the adventitia and retroperitoneal space. Pain is moderate to severe, usually well localized, and often accompanied by nausea. Pain may radiate to one or both groins. Pain in the back and flank can dominate the presentation. Gentle palpation and urgent diagnosis are necessary.

Acute RUQ Pain: The liver, gallbladder, duodenum, head of the pancreas, right kidney, and pleural reflections of the right lung are the leading causes of RUQ pain. Failure to consider pneumonia with pleural involvement and myocardial infarction in the differential diagnosis can lead to inappropriate abdominal surgery.

Cholelithiasis with biliary colic. Gallstones, composed of cholesterol and/or bile pigments, rarely cause symptoms unless a stone obstructs the cystic duct, common bile duct, or pancreatic duct, or perforates the gallbladder wall. Forceful peristaltic contractions against a stone impacted in an obstructed duct produces colic. An attack of biliary colic may be uncomplicated or associated with acute cholecystitis, obstructive jaundice, and/or gallstone pancreatitis. Onset of pain in the epigastrium or RUQ is sudden with radiation to the inferior border of the right scapula (Fig. 9-33). The pain is severe, recurring in cyclic paroxysms, and associated with nausea and vomiting. During the attack, the RUQ is rigid. Ultrasonography is diagnostic. Calcified gallstones are seen on plain X-ray films. Gallstones are common in patients with hemolytic anemias and in certain racial groups, e.g., Native Americans. Stones are more prevalent with obesity, female sex, multiparity, diabetes, and some drugs.

Acute cholecystitis. Cystic duct obstruction, usually by gallstone impaction, results in distention and sterile inflammation of the gallbladder wall. *Acalculous cholecystitis* complicates surgical or medical illness with progressive gallbladder enlargement, ischemia, and rupture with high mortality. The

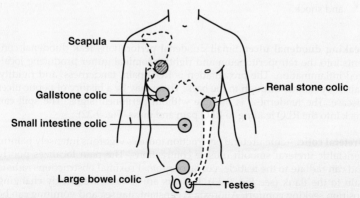

FIG. 9-33 Locations of Abdominal Colic. Colic is notable for its paroxysmal occurrence, severity, and crescendo–decrescendo cycling. It occurs when a hollow viscus is obstructed. Pain results from smooth-muscle contractions trying to overcome the obstruction. Note the radiation of gallstone colic from the RUQ to the angle of the right scapula posteriorly. The colic of renal calculus frequently radiates to the testis on the same side.

onset is acute or subacute, the pain is poorly localized, and may radiate to the top of the right shoulder. Episodes of mild postprandial RUQ pain may precede an acute attack. Nausea and anorexia are usual; vomiting, although less common, may be severe. The gallbladder, felt at the inferior margin of the liver, is tender. Pressing under the right costal margin as the patient inspires produces inspiratory arrest (*Murphy sign*). Fist percussion over the liver produces pain with acute cholecystitis and acute hepatitis. The abdomen is not rigid unless peritonitis is present. Sometimes the gallbladder is palpable as an exquisitely tender globular mass below liver edge. Fever is usual, but high fever or chills suggests ascending cholangitis or suppurative cholecystitis. Ultrasonography demonstrates the thickened, edematous gallbladder wall with luminal sludge or stones. Gallstones are the most common cause, including microlithiasis with sludge. Uncommonly, parasites, bacterial infection, and primary biliary cancer precipitate attacks. The diagnosis is confirmed with a radionuclide scan confirming cystic duct obstruction. Hospitalized patients who have been fasting for many days, can have false-positive radionuclide studies because the fluid-filled gallbladder does not easily contract.

- *Acalculous cholecystitis—gallbladder hydrops.* A dilated gallbladder with poor muscular contractions results in a thin tense edematous wall predisposed to rupture. This is an infrequent but serious complication of other serious medical and surgical illnesses. It is asymptomatic or accompanied by epigastric pain, nausea, and vomiting. There is fever and RUQ tenderness and a tender RUQ mass may be appreciated.
- *Acute RUQ pain—gallbladder rupture, bile peritonitis.* Gallbladder perforation is a consequence of an eroding stone, infection, ischemic necrosis, or postoperative leak. Bile is extremely irritating to the peritoneum, producing a chemical peritonitis. The initial picture suggests cholecystitis or gallstone colic, but the pain gradually spreads throughout the abdomen with signs of generalized peritonitis progressing to prostration and shock.

Leaking duodenal ulcer. Small duodenal perforations leak duodenal contents into the retroperitoneum and right abdominal gutter producing localized inflammation. The presentation is RUQ pain, tenderness, and rigidity. Pain may radiate through to the back. There may be a history of peptic ulcer disease. The tenderness is midline without peritoneal signs. The spill can track into the RLQ leading to RLQ pain and mass (Fig. 9-32).

Ureteral colic. Acute ureteral obstruction induces vigorous intensely painful peristaltic ureteral smooth muscle contractions. The pain localizes poorly and can radiate to the testicle, vulva, or groin. Proximal obstructions radiate pain to the flank (see Fig. 9-33). Patients are restless, frequently changing position seeking comfort. Anorexia is constant, nausea and vomiting can be severe. Microscopic hematuria is expected and sometimes gross hematuria occurs. A calcium-containing stone may be seen on plain X-ray films. *DDX:* Patients with peritonitis, pancreatitis and leaking aneurysms prefer to hold still, not move.

Acute pyelonephritis. Infection, usually ascending from the bladder, produces inflammation and swelling in the kidney, distending the capsule and producing pain. Upper quadrant and flank pain is poorly localized and exacerbated by fist percussion at the CVA. The pain may be severe and accompanied by nausea. RUQ tenderness is deeper and less severe than with acute cholecystitis. Urinalysis and culture are usually diagnostic. In women with recurrent infections or men with a first infection, suspect congenital or acquired anatomic abnormalities in the urinary tract (stones, tumor, diverticulum, etc.).

Renal or pararenal abscess. Often complicating urinary tract obstruction, progressive necrotizing pyelonephritis spreads into the perinephritic space and can track along tissue planes into the pelvis. The patient has abdominal pain radiating into the groin with CVA tenderness and fever. If the cortex, but not the medulla, has been seeded by bacteremia, pyuria may be absent.

Acute hepatitis. Acute hepatic inflammation resulting from hepatocyte injury and secondary inflammation is a consequence of infections, alcohol, or drugs. Acute parenchymal swelling distends Glisson capsule causing pain. Fever, malaise, and anorexia are usually present. Smokers may lose their taste for cigarettes. The entire liver edge is tender, blunt, and smooth. Fist percussion over the liver produces a dull aching pain. Jaundice appears after several days.

Pleurisy. Right lower lobe pneumonia can present with RUQ pain and no findings on abdominal exam. When breathing accentuates pain, breaths become shallow. A pleural rub and signs of pneumonia should be sought. Chest X-ray is mandatory when evaluating upper abdominal pain.

Acute LUQ Pain: The spleen, stomach, left kidney, splenic flexure of the colon, and pleural reflections of the left lung base are the most likely sources of LUQ pain.

Splenic infarction. The spleen is highly vascular, and the sinusoidal structure creates a low redox environment susceptible to ischemic injury. Severe, sharp pain develops in the LUQ with splinting of the abdominal muscles. Pain frequently radiates to the top of the left shoulder. Fever and leukocytosis may be present. A splenic friction rub may be heard. CT identifies splenic infarction resulting from emboli (e.g., endocarditis), vasculitis, or in situ vascular occlusion (as with sickle cell disease). Splenomegaly from polycythemia vera, chronic myelocytic leukemia, and myelofibrosis can also lead to infarction.

Ruptured spleen. A spleen enlarged by infectious mononucleosis, sepsis, or infarction can rupture either spontaneously or with minimal trauma. Large, soft spleens have been ruptured by palpation. Intense pain occurs in the LUQ, radiating to the top of the left shoulder (*Kehr sign*). The pain may be accentuated by elevating the foot of the bed, increasing contact between peritoneal blood and the diaphragm. Abdominal CT scan is diagnostic.

Pyelonephritis, ureteral colic, and pararenal abscess. See RUQ pain above.

Pleurisy. See RUQ pain above.

Acute RLQ Pain: The cecum, appendix, and terminal ilium are usually located in the RLQ, each with unique inflammatory disorders.

- **Acute appendicitis.** Obstruction of the appendix leads sequentially to inflammation, transmural inflammation involving the peritoneum, ischemia, perforation, and localized or generalized peritonitis. Appendicitis usually results from impaction of fecal material or foreign matter in the appendicular lumen. Less commonly, carcinoid tumors, vasculitis, or lymphoma are implicated. Initial pain, mediated by vagal afferents, is poorly localized, accompanied by nausea and vomiting, and referred to the epigastrium. Local peritonitis, sensed by peritoneal somatic afferent nerves, is sharper locating to the appendix, commonly the RLQ. Generalized peritonitis pain is diffuse sharp and accompanied by generalized abdominal and systemic signs. Poorly localized epigastric pain without epigastric tenderness is usually the first in a predictable sequence of symptoms and signs. Nausea or vomiting may occur. As the pain worsens, it shifts to the RLQ accompanied by fever and leukocytosis. Until localization occurs appendicitis is often not considered. With a different sequence of events, the diagnosis of appendicitis should be questioned. Deep tenderness often starts a little more than halfway between the umbilicus and the anterior superior iliac spine. When the appendix is retrocecal there is less RLQ tenderness. With pelvic appendicitis the RLQ is not tender, but the peritoneal pouches may be tender on rectal examination.

- *Acute appendicitis with perforation.* Cecal edema and inflammation, felt as a tender mass (*phlegmon*), is indistinguishable from contained perforation with abscess. Perforation without containment transiently reduces the pain, only to increase over a couple of hours as generalized peritonitis with intense involuntary abdominal muscle rigidity supervenes. Variant presentations occur depending on the location of the appendix. *Extrapelvic appendix.* With retrocecal perforation the back muscles are inflamed with tenderness below the twelfth rib on the right. Psoas irritation causes the right hip to be held in flexion or rigid extension. Flexing and extending the thigh against resistance aggravates the pain (*iliopsoas test*, Fig. 9-13A, page 403). An appendiceal abscess lying medially behind the ileum can involve the right ureter causing painful urination and pyuria. *Intrapelvic appendix.* When the appendix is in the true pelvis there is diffuse suprapubic pain and the abdominal muscles are not rigid. Bladder and rectal irritation causes painful urination and tenesmus. Rectal exam discloses a tender mass in the peritoneal pouch. If the abscess contacts the obturator muscle, flexing the thigh and rotating the femur internally and externally produces suprapubic pain (*obturator test*, Fig. 9-13B). Typhlitis, Crohn disease, pelvic inflammatory disease, ovarian disease, and ectopic pregnancy are frequently in the differential.

- **Neutropenic enterocolitis (typhlitis, cecitis).** Neutropenia, particularly following chemotherapy for acute leukemia, is associated with acute inflammation of the cecum, progressing rapidly to ischemia with bloody diarrhea and perforation. Aerobic gram-negative bacteria play a role and bacteremia is common. Symptoms and signs are like acute appendicitis, although the patient may be more toxic early on. CT reveals the thick cecal wall.

Terminal ileitis (Crohn disease, regional enteritis). See page 448.

Perforated peptic ulcer. See page 435.

Acute LLQ Pain: The left lower quadrant is filled with colon which is the source of most LLQ pain.

Diverticulitis. Diverticulosis is common and usually asymptomatic. Obstruction of a diverticulum can lead to inflammation, abscess, and perforation (diverticulitis). LLQ pain and tenderness may be accompanied by muscular guarding. Pelvic diverticulitis cannot be distinguished clinically from pelvic appendicitis, though prior diverticulitis and appendectomy favor diverticulitis. CT is required to distinguish between perforations of a right-sided diverticulum, a colon cancer, or a ruptured appendix.

Acute Suprapubic Pain: Acute suprapubic pain most often results from pelvic pathology. Visceral pain from the pelvic organs localizes poorly until the peritoneum is involved.

- **Urinary bladder rupture.** Blunt abdominal trauma can burst a full bladder. Pelvic fractures can directly lacerate the bladder. Perforation is into the peritoneal cavity or retroperitoneum. Urine leaking into the peritoneal cavity produces mild peritonitis with suprapubic pain and tenderness. The usual bladder is not felt above the prostate on rectal or vaginal exam. Urine leaking into the retroperitoneum dissects to the perineum producing palpable bogginess about the rectum and vagina on rectal exam. Scrotal swelling can occur, but it is not as pronounced as after a severed ureter.

Acute salpingitis (pelvic inflammatory disease). See Chapter 11, page 498.

Ovarian torsion. An ovarian cyst or mass increases the likelihood of the ovary twisting on its mesentery producing strangulation. Sudden pelvic pain is accompanied by vomiting and tenderness over the ovarian mass.

Ectopic pregnancy. See Chapter 11, page 498.

Diabetic radiculopathy (diabetic amyotrophy). Acute abdominal and/or thoracic pain follows ischemic or inflammatory radiculopathy of one or more thoracic and/or lumbar spinal nerves. This is unrelated to the duration or control of the diabetes. Dermatomal pain and allodynia and weakness of the muscles supplied by affected nerves are demonstrable by careful physical exam. This is often mistaken for an acute intraabdominal event because of the acuity and severity of the pain. The pain persists for 6 to 24 months or longer. EMG is diagnostic.

Subacute Abdominal Pain Syndromes
Diabetic radiculopathy (diabetic amyotrophy). See above.

Abdominal angina (visceral ischemia, intestinal ischemia). The increased intestinal oxygen demand required for digestion and absorption of food following a meal exceeds the supply because of mesenteric artery obstruction. Because of limited collaterals, the bowel perfused by the inferior mesenteric artery is most vulnerable. Visceral ischemia is characterized by the triad of postprandial pain, anorexia from fear of eating, and weight loss. The pain is usually in the upper abdomen or periumbilical and sometimes radiates to the back. It is typically intermittent, coming on 30 minutes after eating and persisting from 20 minutes to 3 hours. Sometimes there is no relationship between meals and pain. Diarrhea, occasionally bloody, is frequent. Sometimes a short systolic bruit is heard in the epigastrium or umbilical region. *DDX:* Similar symptoms are seen with mesenteric vein occlusion though these patients develop gastric and esophageal varices.

Pancreas carcinoma. Pain results from acute or chronic pancreatitis or invasion of retroperitoneal structures and celiac plexus. Retroperitoneal invasion causes constant, dull, poorly localized pain in the mid epigastrium, flank, or back. When the head of the pancreas is involved painless persistent jaundice is the rule. As the tumor enlarges, the triad of pain, weight loss, and jaundice is nearly universal. The first sign of pancreatic carcinoma may be migrating superficial thrombophlebitis (Chapter 8, page 379), recurrent deep vein thromboses (*Trousseau syndrome*), or nonbacterial thrombotic endocarditis (*marantic endocarditis*, Chapter 8, page 358).

Rectus hematoma. The epigastric artery and vein run vertically within the rectus sheath. Hemorrhage within the sheath above the arcuate line is confined within the sheath, but hemorrhage below the arcuate line dissects into the lateral abdominal wall. Inciting events are direct trauma, coughing, paracentesis, and operative injury. Debilitated and anticoagulated patients are especially susceptible. The mass may be tender and painful. Though often mistaken for an intraabdominal mass, the hematoma remains palpable when the abdominal wall is tensed, while an intraabdominal mass is obscured (Fig. 9-26, page 425). Ultrasonography or CT is diagnostic.

Chronic and Recurrent Abdominal Pain

Chronic abdominal pain. See page 408. Pain is the presenting symptom for many chronic abdominal disorders. Chronic disease usually produces less severe pain in the same location as an acute process (Fig. 9-19, page 408).

Recurrent abdominal pain. Recurrent pain suggests an intermittent mechanical problem, a partially treated inflammatory disorder, or an episodic metabolic/toxic syndrome.
CLINICAL OCCURRENCE: *Congenital:* Porphyria, sickle cell disease, familial Mediterranean fever, other familial fever syndromes; *Degenerative/Idiopathic:* Chronic pancreatitis, sphincter of Oddi dysfunction; endometriosis; *Infectious:* Chronic hepatitis, schistosomiasis, *H. pylori* ulcers and gastritis; *Inflammatory/Immune:* SLE, autoimmune gastritis; *Mechanical/Traumatic:* Biliary colic, ureteral colic, adhesions, and partial bowel obstruction; *Metabolic/Toxic:* Lead poisoning; cannabinoid hyperemesis; *Neoplastic:* Partial bowel obstruction from luminal masses; *Psychosocial:* Domestic, sexual, and child abuse; *Vascular:* Mesenteric ischemia.

Cannabinoid hyperemesis. Long-term use of cannabis leads to cyclic episodes of nausea, epigastric or periumbilical abdominal pain, and hyperemesis. Most commonly patients are under age 50 and use cannabis daily. Hot showers relieve the symptoms temporarily leading to compulsive showering. Symptoms resolve with cessation of use.

Abdominal wall pain syndromes. Look for point tenderness (*trigger points*) not abolished by contracting the abdominal muscles, sensitivity to light touch by clothing (*hyperesthesia* or *allodynia*), abdominal wall defects (with or without hernia), masses, surgical and varicella-zoster scars, and abdominal wall weakness or asymmetry. Injecting local anesthetic into trigger points frequently answers the diagnostic question. *DDX:* Fully examine the spine for disorders referring pain to the abdomen.

Abdominal cutaneous nerve entrapment. Anterior cutaneous nerve branches from T7 to L1 become entrapped as they pass through the rectus sheath. Entrapment can occur from overuse of the rectus muscles or weight gain increasing traction on the nerve. The pain usually occurs lateral to the entrapment site and is increased by tensing the rectus muscles. Pain is reproduced by pressure over the small fascia defect marking the exit site and is relieved by trigger point injection.

Chronic epigastric pain. See the discussion of Acute Epigastric Pain, page 434.

Xiphoid-sternal arthritis. Epigastric or retrosternal pain radiates around to the back and is reproduced by palpating the xiphoid-sternal joint. Injecting local anesthetic gives complete relief. *DDX:* This may be mistaken for angina pectoris, peptic ulcer, hiatal hernia, biliary colic, or chronic pancreatitis if the xiphoid cartilage is not specifically palpated.

Peptic ulcer. Peptic ulcer is caused by *H. pylori* infection, NSAIDs, or gastrin-secreting islet cell tumor (Zollinger–Ellison syndrome). Ulcer pain is caused by gastric acid irritating exposed nerves. Epigastric pain occurs predictably 1–4 hours after meals and is relieved by food, H2 blockers, and antacids. The symptoms are similar whether the ulcer is gastric, pyloric, duodenal, anastomotic, or marginal. Ulcer pain is aggravated by fasting, drinking alcohol, or coffee. The pain is described as gnawing, aching, burning, or hunger and is felt in the epigastrium near the xiphoid, sometimes radiating to the back. The pain varies from mild discomfort to severe and may awaken the patient from sleep. Untreated, ulcer symptoms may recur with periods of pain lasting from a few days to several months. Frequently there is moderate tenderness localized to the epigastrium. Endoscopy is diagnostic.

Pyloric obstruction. Usually obstruction results from scarring of the pylorus from peptic ulceration. Pain is not invariable but, if present, it ranges from vague discomfort to colicky epigastric pain, usually soon after eating. Emesis of undigested food eaten many hours or days before can occur. Abdominal palpation may elicit a succussion splash. Anatomic outlet obstruction must be distinguished from pylorospasm caused by peptic ulcer and gastroparesis.

Postgastrectomy syndrome. Losing gastric storage capacity and pyloric sphincter function after subtotal gastrectomy often causes uncontrolled dumping of hypertonic stomach contents into the small intestine. The large amount of fluid in the small bowel and increased intestinal motility contribute to the symptoms. Gastric stapling procedures create a defunctionalized pouch which can develop inflammation (pouchitis) and the small remnant stomach can be a source of postprandial discomfort. *Early Dumping Syndrome* occurs shortly after eating, the patient experiences epigastric discomfort without pain, weakness, sweating, nausea but not vomiting, tachycardia, palpitation, and epigastric fullness. Reclining may relieve the symptoms. Foods with high osmotic loads exacerbate the symptoms. *Late Dumping Syndrome* occurs more than 2 hours after eating with symptoms of sweating, trembling, weakness, hunger, nausea, vomiting, and, rarely, syncope.

Chronic pancreatitis. See page 450.

Gastric carcinoma. Pain is usually preceded by anorexia, weight loss, and weakness. The pain is a steady, unremitting ache in the epigastrium, sometimes radiating to the back, or resembles peptic ulcer pain.

Chronic RUQ pain. See the discussion of RUQ Pain, page 437.

Chronic cholecystitis with or without cholelithiasis. See page 437.

Hepatocellular carcinoma. Hepatocellular carcinoma arises in a cirrhotic liver, particularly following chronic hepatitis from hepatitis B and/or C viruses. Abdominal pain is the most common symptom. A hard, nodular, localized liver mass with centrifugal extension may be palpable, sometimes with an overlying peritoneal friction rub. A bruit may be heard.

Metastatic carcinoma. Pancreatic and colon cancers frequently metastasize to the liver via the portal vein. Metastases from lung and breast cancer are also common. Poorly localized upper abdominal pain or discomfort, usually without abdominal distention or mass, is a common presentation. Most often the liver is diffusely stony hard. When a single discrete liver mass is felt, also suspect hepatocellular carcinoma or abscess. Peritoneal friction rubs and bruits are rare.

Bloating and Distention Syndromes: Bloating and distention are common complaints associated with mechanical or functional bowel obstruction and abnormal digestion. These symptoms are often unaccompanied by abdominal distention or obstruction on exam. Visceral hyperalgesia may explain this discrepancy.

Stomach distention. Gastroparesis is a consequence of reflex loss of gastric tone following abdominal surgery or upper intestinal inflammation, autonomic neuropathy as in diabetes, vagotomy, or decreased bowel motility associated with chronic illness and bed rest. In acute distention, the patient, often bedridden from another disorder, becomes acutely more ill with vomiting, upper abdominal distention, and hypotension. The greatly dilated stomach fills the epigastrium, rarely reaching to the pelvis. There is tympany on LUQ percussion and often a succussion splash. Visible peristalsis can be present initially. Later, weak or absent peristaltic sounds indicate ileus. Nasogastric suction yielding a large volume of fluid resolves the distention. The major provocative factors are pain, abdominal trauma, and immobilization. Postoperative cases are common. Chronic gastroparesis is more frequent, less dramatic, and more difficult to diagnose. Glucose control in diabetics is difficult because of the irregular gastric emptying. Nausea and emesis of undigested food several hours after eating suggests gastroparesis. Diabetes mellitus is the most frequent cause, but other causes of visceral autonomic neuropathy should be considered.

Ascites. See page 416.

Irritable bowel syndrome. See page 452.

Lactose and fructose intolerance. See page 448.

Diarrhea Syndromes
Diarrhea. Diarrhea is >200 g of stool per day on a Western low-residue diet. "Diarrhea" is also used to describe watery or loose stools, or increased stool frequency. Several general pathophysiologic mechanisms underlie increased fecal volume and stool water loss. *Osmotic diarrhea* results from ingestion of nonabsorbable osmotically active solutes that draw water into the bowel. *Secretory diarrhea* results from increased normal secretions (e.g., Zollinger–Ellison syndrome) or secretion of abnormal fluid into the lumen (e.g., cholera). *Inflammatory/immune diarrhea* results from inflammation of the bowel wall with exudation of fluid, proteins and cells, usually combined with increased motility and decreased absorption. Increased bowel motility decreases the time available for absorption of solutes (small intestine) and water (colon). *Malabsorption and maldigestion* cause diarrhea, the former from loss of effective absorptive surface (e.g., celiac disease), and the latter from inadequate digestion of food (e.g., pancreatic insufficiency). *Short bowel syndrome* results in loss of absorptive surface (surgical resection or fistulas) and bile acid malabsorption producing colonic irritation. First, determine exactly what is meant by diarrhea, and if it is acute, chronic, or recurrent. Second, obtain a detailed description of the stools, their frequency, and pattern. Ask specifically about nocturnal diarrhea, which is always pathologic. Third, focus on exposures (travel, drugs, previous surgery, dietary habits, contact with others with a similar illness), and associated symptoms (anorexia, nausea, vomiting, fever, weight loss, or abdominal pain). On completion of the history formulate a hypothesis for the diarrhea's pathophysiologic mechanism(s). During physical exam look for signs of weight loss, volume depletion, increased bowel motility (borborygmi), and abdominal distention and/or tenderness. Laboratory evaluation is usually not required for suspected viral diarrhea. If you suspect a bacterial or protozoal etiology, stool culture and tests for bacterial and protozoal antigens are necessary. Always inspect atypical stool. Diarrhea in

HIV infected patients is a complex clinical problem with multiple infectious and noninfectious causes. Consultation with a specialist in HIV-related diseases is recommended. *Patterns:* Recognizing several relatively distinct diarrheal syndromes helps form a concise differential diagnosis: acute diarrhea, dysentery syndrome, diarrhea with maldigestion/malabsorption, steatorrhea, diarrhea with weight loss, or diarrhea with bloody stools.

Acute nonbloody diarrhea. Diarrhea lasting <2 weeks, and not preceded by recurrent or relapsing episodes, is acute diarrhea. Infectious and toxic causes are most common.

CLINICAL OCCURRENCE: *Infectious:* Enteroviruses, Rotavirus, noroviruses (e.g., Norwalk agent), enterotoxigenic *Escherichia coli, Salmonella, Shigella, Campylobacter* spp., *Giardia, Cryptosporidium,* cyclospora, amebiasis, *C. difficile, Vibrio cholerae; Metabolic/Toxic:* Food poisoning (*Bacillus cereus,* staphylococcal, *Clostridium perfringens*), antibiotic-associated diarrhea, alcohol, osmotic laxatives, sugar-free candy and foods, drug withdrawal; *Vascular:* Ischemic colitis.

Traveler's diarrhea. Travelers ingest contaminated food and water containing the colonic flora of their host country. Often within a week of arrival travelers experience 1–5 days of self-limited watery diarrhea, abdominal cramping, and anorexia. The most common organism is enterotoxigenic *E. coli. Shigella, Salmonella, Campylobacter, V. cholerae, Giardia, Cryptosporidium,* and viruses can have the same presentation.

Viral gastroenteritis. Infection of the bowel epithelium causes loss of absorptive function. Systemic signs may be absent, mild (Norwalk), or severe (rotavirus, norovirus). Commonly epidemic, there is sudden onset of nausea, vomiting, and explosive diarrhea, with or without abdominal cramps. Myalgia, malaise, and anorexia, usually without fever, are common. Diarrhea and vomiting subside within 48 hours though lassitude may persist for several days. The stools consist of water and fecal remnants; blood, pus, and mucus are absent. Common causes are rotavirus, noroviruses, adenovirus, caliciviruses, enterovirus, and coronavirus. Specific diagnosis is not required.

- *Cholera.* Cholera toxin inhibits gut Na+ absorption and activates Cl– excretion, producing severe secretory diarrhea. Waterborne *V. cholerae* infection is locally endemic in some countries, sometimes triggering epidemic and pandemic disease. There is sudden abdominal cramping, vomiting, and voluminous watery stools containing flecks of mucus (rice-water stools) progressing to dehydration, electrolyte imbalances, prostration, shock, and death.

Food intolerance. Ingestion of specific foods causes local and systemic allergic reactions. Symptoms are nausea, vomiting, abdominal cramping, and diarrhea. Angioedema can occur. Identification of the allergen can be difficult. Shellfish, peanuts, cow's milk, and cereals are common culprits.

Food poisoning. Usually, preformed bacterial exotoxins are ingested in contaminated food. *B. cereus* also causes a longer incubation diarrhea probably from exotoxin production in the gut. Severe cramping abdominal pain, nausea, vomiting, diarrhea, and prostration begin 1–6 hours after a meal, resolving within hours. Large groups of diners are frequently affected. Specific foods are clues to the etiology: potato salad, mayonnaise, and cream pastries—*Staphylococcus aureus*; meat, poultry, legumes—*C. perfringens*; fried rice—*B. cereus*.

Chinese restaurant syndrome. This is attributed to monosodium glutamate, a seasoning used in Asian cooking. It is characterized by severe headache, burning sensations, and feelings of pressure about the face starting 10–20 minutes after eating. Occasionally, chest pain, prostration, gastric distress, and pain in the axillae, neck, and shoulders develop.

Acute bloody diarrhea. Acute bloody diarrhea indicates compromise of the bowel mucosa, usually in the colon. Infections that either invade the mucosa or produce toxic epithelial necrosis are most likely. Chronic inflammatory bowel diseases can present with diarrhea both initially and with relapse. Patients present without pain or with abdominal pain and tenesmus (*dysentery syndrome*). Fever and leukocytosis suggest an enteroinvasive organism with risks of local complications and systemic spread. Painless bleeding in otherwise healthy individuals suggests bleeding from a structural abnormality (Meckel diverticulum, diverticulosis, polyp, or cancer).

CLINICAL OCCURRENCE: *Congenital:* Meckel diverticulum; *Inflammatory/ Immune:* Ulcerative colitis, Crohn disease; *Infectious:* Bacteria (*Campylobacter jejuni, Salmonella* spp., *Shigella* spp., enterohemorrhagic *E. coli* 0157:H7), protozoa (*Entamoeba histolytica, Balantidium coli*), cytomegalovirus; *Mechanical/ Traumatic:* Rectal foreign body; *Metabolic/Toxic:* Heavy-metal poisoning (arsenic, mercury, cadmium, copper, iron); *Neoplastic:* Villous adenoma with malignant change; *Vascular:* Ischemic colitis.

Dysentery. Dysentery is a syndrome of abdominal cramping and painful defecation with stools containing pus and blood, indicative of colon and rectal inflammation. Dysentery is an infectious diarrhea often with mucosal invasion and ulceration. Dysentery is distinct from simple gastroenteritis. Stool culture and testing for ova and parasites are required; sigmoidoscopy may be useful. Common etiologies are bacterial (*C. jejuni, Salmonella* spp., *Shigella* spp., enterohemorrhagic *E. coli* including 0157:H7) and protozoa (*E. histolytica, B. coli*, strongyloidiasis).

Amebiasis. Ingestion of water contaminated with *E. histolytica* leads to ulcerations in the colon and terminal ilium, and liver abscess. Acute infection may be fulminant with cramping abdominal pain, bloody diarrhea, and tenesmus. Exam reveals fever, diffuse abdominal tenderness, dehydration, and weight loss. Subacute infection has milder abdominal cramps, diarrheal stools containing mucus or blood, often alternating with intervals of normal function and exam may find fever and RLQ tenderness. Liver abscess is suggested by spiking fevers, prostration, and RUQ pain with mildly abnormal liver tests.

Ulcerative colitis. See Chronic Constant Diarrhea—Ulcerative Colitis, page 449. Although a chronic disease, its onset may be sudden, resembling acute dysentery.

Poisoning with heavy metals or drugs. The heavy metals (such as arsenic, cadmium, copper, or mercury) may be ingested accidentally or with suicidal or homicidal intent. Nausea, vomiting, cramping abdominal pains, and bloody diarrhea begin soon after ingestion.

Chronic intermittent diarrhea. Diarrhea lasting more than 2 weeks is chronic and less likely to be infectious. Intermittent diarrhea implies a disease with a relapsing-remittent course (e.g., Crohn disease) or an interaction of the host and the environment, particularly the diet (e.g., lactase deficiency). Most causes of chronic persistent diarrhea can also present as chronic intermittent diarrhea.

Irritable bowel syndrome. See page 452.

Lactase deficiency (lactose intolerance). Deficiency of small bowel mucosal lactase leads to incomplete digestion of lactose, the disaccharide in cow's milk. The lactose is fermented by colonic bacteria producing gas and diarrhea. This is more common in Blacks and Asians than in Caucasians. Eating milk products produces watery diarrhea and gas, often with abdominal cramps. Patients often do not make the association because of the ubiquitous presence of milk products in the diet. Milk product avoidance leads to prompt resolution and is the treatment of choice. Malabsorption of sorbitol in sugarless candies causes a similar picture.

Fructose intolerance. Some individuals are unable to absorb fructose in the quantities ingested, especially those who consume substantial amounts of soft drinks sweetened with high fructose corn syrup. The unabsorbed fructose creates an osmotic diarrhea and increased intestinal gas when fermented by colonic bacteria. Symptoms and signs are identical to lactose intolerance.

Regional enteritis (Crohn disease, terminal ileitis). Transmural granulomatous inflammation of the small and large intestine results in blood loss and interferes with gut motility and absorption. Presenting symptoms are attacks of RLQ colic commonly accompanied by diarrhea. Weight loss may be severe. Perforations, strictures, and fistulas are common complications including perianal fistulas and anal stricture. Colon involvement is segmental with skip areas. Extraintestinal manifestations (oligoarthritis, spondylitis, pyoderma gangrenosum) may be the presenting complaint. Barium in the small bowel may show strictures, fistulas, loss of mucosal detail, and tubular thickening of the submucosa. Diagnosis is by endoscopic biopsy with gross and microscopic examination of resected tissue. *DDX:* The first attack of ileitis may be clinically indistinguishable from acute appendicitis, although diarrhea usually precedes the attack and a RLQ mass may be appreciated early in the course. If similar prior episodes have occurred, the probability is strong for chronic ileitis with an exacerbation. Consider infection with Yersinia, Salmonella, Shigella, tuberculosis, amebiasis, and cytomegalovirus.

Ulcerative colitis. See page 449.

Chronic constant diarrhea. Chronic constant diarrhea suggests an unremitting underlying structural or functional process involving digestion, absorption, bowel motility, or metabolism. The history (age of onset, exacerbating or palliative maneuvers), comorbid conditions, and characteristics of the stools are critical to a parsimonious differential diagnosis.

CLINICAL OCCURRENCE: *Congenital:* Cystic fibrosis, lactase deficiency, celiac disease; *Endocrine:* Hyperthyroidism, adrenal insufficiency, carcinoid syndrome, pheochromocytoma; *Degenerative/Idiopathic:* Irritable bowel syndrome, chronic pancreatitis, diverticulitis; *Infectious:* Giardia, HIV/AIDS and opportunistic infections, microsporidiosis, cyclosporiasis, Whipple disease, small bowel bacterial overgrowth, intestinal parasites; *Inflammatory/ Immune:* Ulcerative colitis, Crohn disease, microscopic colitis, mastocytosis, chronic pancreatitis, celiac disease, amyloidosis; *Mechanical/Traumatic:* Short-bowel syndrome, enterocolic fistulas, radiation enteritis; *Metabolic/ Toxic:* hyperthyroidism, lactase deficiency, drugs (metformin, proton pump inhibitors, misoprostol, colchicine, digitalis, antacids), bile salt-induced, laxative abuse, nonsteroidal anti-inflammatory drugs, alcohol; *Neoplastic:* Mastocytosis, villous adenoma, pancreatic islet cell tumors (producing vasoactive intestinal peptide, gastrin, glucagon, etc.), small-bowel lymphoma; *Neurologic:* Autonomic neuropathies; *Psychosocial:* Laxative abuse; *Vascular:* Vasculitis.

Ulcerative colitis. There is intense confluent chronic mucosal inflammation and ulceration with crypt abscesses beginning at the rectum and extending proximally. The mucosa is red, edematous, and friable, the slightest touch causing bleeding. Often the entire rectosigmoid is covered by purulent exudate obscuring the multiple ulcers. The clinical picture varies from acute dysentery with fever, abdominal pain, tenesmus, bloody diarrhea, and weight loss to mild abdominal discomfort with mostly formed stools and little blood. The rectum is always involved, and inflammation extends proximally in continuity. The extent of the disease varies from only rectal involvement to pancolitis. In long-standing disease, the lumen is contracted and irregular with pseudopolyps. The terminal ileum may be inflamed and dilated, in contrast to the constriction found in regional enteritis. Diagnosis is made by endoscopic inspection and biopsy. Disease duration greater than 10 years and pancolitis, but not the severity of symptoms, are associated with an increased risk for colon cancer. Ulcerative colitis must be distinguished from Crohn colitis, ischemic colitis, amebiasis, and bacillary infections.

Amyloidosis. See Chapter 5, page 87. Amyloidosis gives rise to chronic diarrhea, hypomotility, obstructive symptoms, ulceration, hemorrhage, and protein-losing enteropathy.

Zollinger–Ellison syndrome. A gastrinoma, usually in the pancreas or duodenum, produces large amounts of gastrin stimulating excessive gastric HCl secretion leading to diarrhea and producing ulcers in esophagus, duodenum, and jejunum. Recurrent attacks of epigastric pain, nausea, vomiting, and diarrhea can be accompanied by malabsorption and weight loss. Suspect excess gastric secretion when severe ulcer disease and diarrhea occur in the absence of *H. pylori* infection.

Carcinoid syndrome. Liver metastases from a carcinoid tumor in the GI tract produce large amounts of serotonin. See Carcinoid Syndrome, Chapter 6, page 147. Symptoms include recurrent diarrhea, nausea, vomiting, and abdominal pain. Intermittent migratory flushing of face and neck occur with rapid color changes between red, white, and violet. Right-sided heart failure may develop from endomyocardial fibrosis with tricuspid insufficiency.

Chronic diarrhea and malabsorption (maldigestion–malabsorption syndrome). *Maldigestion* results from failure to deliver sufficient pancreatic enzymes and bile salts into the duodenum, inadequate mixing of luminal contents, or insufficient time in the small bowel for digestion to occur. *Malabsorption* results from damage to the small-bowel epithelium or bypass or loss of absorptive surface area. *Steatorrhea* occurs when triglycerides are not digested or absorbed because of poor micelle formation or insufficient pancreatic lipase secretion. Fat appears in the stool as triglycerides. Frothy, greasy, and foul-smelling stools suggest steatorrhea. Weight loss is common despite a good appetite. Fat-soluble vitamins (A, D, E, and K) are malabsorbed and deficiency syndromes may be the presenting complaint. Microscopic exam of stool stained with Sudan III shows fat globules.

Small bowel bacterial overgrowth (Blind Loop syndrome). Decreased small intestinal motility leading to stasis, loss of protective gastric acid, and decreased ileocecal valve function increase the risk for bacterial overgrowth and the blind- or stagnant-loop syndrome. Bacteria consume nutrients, including vitamins, leading to malnutrition and vitamin deficiency, particularly vitamin B12. The patient presents with diarrhea, abdominal bloating, flatus, steatorrhea, weight loss, macrocytic anemia, and sometimes feculent belching. Because the bacterial overgrowth is responsible for the malabsorption, a short course of antibiotics should lead to demonstrable improvement. Common antecedent conditions include surgically created blind pouches, enteroenterostomies, long afferent loops, strictures, fistulous communications, and small bowel diverticula. Tapeworms can produce a similar picture.

Chronic pancreatitis and pancreatic insufficiency. Chronic pancreatitis results from alcohol, drugs, or ductal strictures. Extensive loss of pancreatic tissue leads to inadequate endocrine and exocrine function producing diabetes and steatorrhea. Chronic pancreatitis is characterized by episodes of abdominal pain and stools that are soft, loose, frothy, and malodorous, frequently floating on water. The repeated attacks of pain are identical to acute pancreatitis. Alcohol abuse and mild forms of cystic fibrosis are common causes. A palpable pancreatic pseudocyst may develop. Pancreatic calcification is diagnostic.

Celiac disease (gluten-sensitive enteropathy, nontropical sprue). In persons with specific HLA-DQ2 alleles, ingestion of gluten (gliadin) from wheat flour induces chronic mucosal and submucosal inflammation producing characteristic flattening of the villi and chronic malabsorption. Patients present with fatigue, cramping, diarrhea, steatorrhea, and weight loss without anorexia. A family history may be present, and patients frequently have made dietary modifications. The stools are soft, frothy, and malodorous from unabsorbed fat. Unexplained iron deficiency, hypocalcemia, neuropathy, dermatitis herpetiformis, and weight loss without complaints of diarrhea are common presentations.

Whipple disease. Invasion of the intestinal mucosa and lamina propria with *Tropheryma whippelii* produces foamy macrophages filled with glycoprotein leading to lymphatic obstruction and malabsorption. Dissemination produces arthritis, lymphadenopathy, and anindolent meningitis. Presentation can be at any age, most commonly in white men in their fourth and fifth decades. Migratory polyarthralgias and polyarthritis may precede intestinal symptoms and weight loss. Abdominal symptoms are cramping and episodic diarrhea with fatty, foul-smelling stools. There is generalized malaise and weakness; cough and dyspnea can occur. Fever is intermittent and may be accompanied by hypotension, edema, lymphadenopathy, and emaciation. CNS infection causes slowly progressive chronic meningitis.

Giardiasis. *Giardia* organisms adhere to the brush-border of enterocytes in the duodenum and upper small bowel impairing absorption of nutrients leading to diarrhea and weight loss. A travel history and exposure to surface water potentially contaminated by livestock and wildlife is useful. Stool antigen testing is available.

Cystic fibrosis. An autosomal recessive disease usually diagnosed in childhood. Patients with mild disease may present in adult life with pancreatic insufficiency, rhinosinusitis, and recurrent pulmonary symptoms.

Enteroenteric fistula. A fistula between the proximal and distal bowel produces diarrhea with undigested food in the feces and/or fecal emesis. The diarrhea may be intermittent and results, in part, from bacteria overgrowth in the proximal gut. Malabsorption of nutrients, fluids, and electrolytes causes weight loss, hypoproteinemia, and dehydration. Fecal belching and vomiting suggests gastrocolic fistula.

Constipation Syndromes
Constipation. Bowel motility is under autonomic control and requires an intact myenteric plexus. Multiple factors, including luminal contents, drugs, emotional state, physical activity, and acquired habits (bowel training) affect stool frequency and character. Defecation requires a coordinated sequence of involuntary and voluntary muscular contractions and relaxations. Failure to properly sequence these events prevents effective defecation. Patients and physician use "constipation" to mean any combination of infrequent stools, hard desiccated stools, or stools that are difficult to pass. In the evaluating constipation, each factor must be investigated as several may be operative at one time. First, determine the patient's baseline bowel movement pattern, the onset of the current difficulty, and any therapeutic interventions undertaken. Many people do very well with two or three evacuations a week. Patients often describe the gradual development of abdominal fullness. Acute or subacute constipation developing on a lifelong history of normal bowel movements requires investigation. Chronic constipation of years' duration may indicate an underlying disorder of the bowel wall, a gut motility problem, or poorly coordinated defecation. *Dyssynergy* results from failure to relax the voluntary sphincter during rectal contraction.

CLINICAL OCCURRENCE: *Congenital:* Hirschsprung disease; *Endocrine:* Hypothyroidism, hyperparathyroidism, pregnancy; *Degenerative/Idiopathic:* Intestinal pseudoobstruction; diverticulosis, diverticulitis; *Infectious:* Chagas disease, toxic megacolon; *Inflammatory/Immune:* Scleroderma (progressive systemic sclerosis), amyloidosis; *Mechanical/Traumatic:* Excessive fiber intake, mechanical obstruction by stricture or mass, irradiation, anal fissure; *Metabolic/Toxic:* Drugs, including opiates, anticholinergics, tricyclic antidepressants, and many others; hypokalemia, hypomagnesemia, hypercalcemia; *Neoplastic:* Colon polyps, colon and anal cancers; *Neurologic:* Spinal cord injury, sacral plexus lesions, multiple sclerosis, Parkinson disease, irritable bowel syndrome; *Psychosocial:* Eating disorders, substance abuse (opiates), depression, dyssynergistic defecation; *Vascular:* Stroke.

Intestinal obstruction. See Obstructive Syndromes below.

Fecal impaction. There may be no discomfort, or the patient may complain of constipation, tenesmus, or inability to defecate. Diarrhea is a frequent complaint because liquid stool passes around the impaction. Digital rectal exam reveals hard fecal masses that must be removed manually. Common inciting factors are immobilization, bed rest, dehydration, anticholinergic medications, dementia, and barium for GI contrast X-rays.

Irritable bowel syndrome. This common cause of constipation is characterized by periods of constipation alternating with bouts of diarrhea. Either symptom may be the main complaint. The triad of symptoms is long-standing intermittent constipation, scybalous stools, and abdominal pain relieved by defecation. The cause is uncertain, although many patients have increased sensitivity to visceral discomfort (*visceral hyperalgesia*).

Laxative abuse, atonic colon. Chronic stimulant laxative use leads to loss of colonic sensation and reflexes producing an adynamic, dilated colon dependent upon laxatives for defecation. The patient has a long history of constipation, fancied or real. The stools may be alternately voluminous and scanty. Abdominal palpation often reveals large fecal masses.

Dyssynergistic defecation. Normal defecation requires contraction of colonic and rectal smooth muscle and simultaneous relaxation of the internal (involuntary) and external (voluntary) sphincters. Failure of this coordinated process leads to attempts to defecate against a closed anal sphincter producing constipation. Patients complain of difficulty defecating and having to strain excessively even with soft stools. On examination, they may be unable to voluntarily relax the external sphincter.

Megacolon. Lifelong constipation with occasional passage of an enormous formed stool suggests megacolon. Causes are congenital (Hirschsprung disease) or acquired defects in the intrinsic myenteric innervation of the colon such as idiopathic intestinal pseudoobstruction and Chagas disease.

Drug effects. Many drugs slow bowel motility, including opiates, anticholinergic drugs, antihistamines, chronic laxative use, and overuse of bulk laxatives. Pill bezoars have been described. Medication history is key with attention to laxative and enema use. Ophthalmologic medications are systemically absorbed and can affect gut function.

Bowel Obstruction Syndromes.
Noisy tympanites with colic and vomiting—mechanical obstruction. These findings suggest localized bowel obstruction with the increased force of peristaltic contraction proximal to the obstruction producing colic and proximal bowel distension. Decompression occurs by vomiting retained luminal contents. Mechanical obstruction is probable. Tympanites is present when the obstruction is distal to the mid jejunum. Increased peristalsis proximal to an obstruction produces frequent, loud peristaltic sounds (*borborygmi*) accompanied by cramping and colic. With partial obstructions high-pitched high-pressure-to-low-pressure sounds ("rushes") may accompany the pain. Vomiting appears earlier and is more intense the more proximal the obstruction. Distal obstruction may result in feculent emesis which classically indicates colonic obstruction in a person with an incompetent ileocecal valve or a cologastric or coloenteric fistula. Colic is almost invariably present from the onset. In general, the more proximal the obstruction, the more severe the symptoms. **Proximal Small Intestine:** Epigastric pain is intense, and vomiting is early and severe. If the vomitus contains bile, the obstruction is beyond the second portion of the duodenum. Abdominal distention limited to the epigastrium appears late. **Distal Small Intestine:** Symptoms are less severe, vomiting is delayed, but the vomitus may have become feculent. Diffuse abdominal distention gradually develops. **Colon:** The colon narrows beyond the splenic flexure making the descending and sigmoid regions most susceptible to obstruction. Pain is less than in small bowel obstruction. Vomiting is late and may be fecal. Constipation is invariable but only after empting stool below the obstruction which delays recognition. An empty rectal ampulla devoid of gas is strong presumptive evidence of colon obstruction. **CLINICAL OCCURRENCE:** *Infectious:* Parasites, diverticular abscess; *Inflammatory/Immune:* Crohn disease, diverticulitis with stricture; *Mechanical/Traumatic:* Adhesions (most common), gallstone impaction, bezoars, foreign body, pyloric stenosis, volvulus, hernias (internal and abdominal wall), intussusception, external compression from intraabdominal cysts and neoplasms; *Neoplastic:* Benign and malignant tumors.

Bezoars. Bezoars are concretions of hair (trichobezoar), plant fibers (phytobezoar), or medicines (aluminum hydroxide gel or polystyrene sodium sulfonate) formed in the GI tract. They present with obstructive symptoms when they lodge at the pylorus (gastric outlet obstruction) or ileocecal valve (small-bowel obstruction). They can cause mechanical erosion of the bowel wall leading to ulceration, bleeding, and pain.

Strangulated hernias. See page 460.

Intussusception. Intussusception is the invagination of bowel into the lumen of adjacent bowel. The enfolded portion always points down the fecal stream. There are four types: ileum into ileum, ileum into ileocecal valve, ileocecal valve into colon, and colon into colon (Fig. 9-34). This is the most common cause of intestinal obstruction in infants. In children it is frequently preceded by a viral infection; in adults, neoplasm in the intestinal wall is usually the cause. In addition to obstructive symptoms, mucus, and sometimes blood, is passed. The pathognomonic sign is an oblong mass in the right or upper mid-abdomen and absence of bowel in the RLQ (*Dance sign*) [Berger DL, Mohammadkhani M. Case 26-2002 — An 87-year-old woman with abdominal pain, vomiting, bloody diarrhea, and an abdominal mass. *N Engl J Med.* 2002;347:601–606].

Colon cancer. After adhesions this is the most common cause of intestinal obstruction in persons over age 50. Gradually increasing constipation culminates in low intestinal obstruction. Obstruction near the hepatic flexure distends the cecum forming a painful, rounded RLQ mass. Distal cancers cause gradual distention of the sigmoid and/or descending colon which is readily palpated in the LLQ.

Volvulus. See page 434.

Silent tympanites without colic or vomiting—ileus. A silent abdomen and distended bowel suggests diffuse ileus without mechanical obstruction resulting from decreased bowel motility and muscular tone. Abdominal tympany is always present and peristaltic sounds are diminished or absent. When

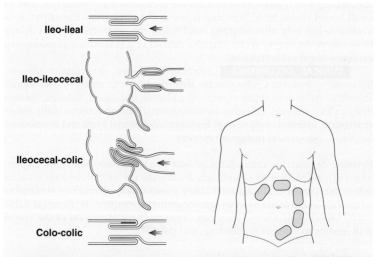

A. Types of intussusception   **B. Location of intussusception**

FIG. 9-34 Intussusception. This is the prolapse of one segment of intestine into an adjoining segment. **A. The four types of intussusception.** The lumen enfolds in the direction of fecal flow, as shown by the arrows. In the colocolic type the stippling indicates a neoplasm which usually causes the telescoping. **B. Locations.** The usual sites of palpable masses are shown as sausage-shaped outlines; these are usually in the colon.

present, abdominal pain is mild, and colic is absent. Vomiting is uncommon, but anorexia and nausea are expected.

CLINICAL OCCURRENCE: *Infectious:* Peritonitis (spontaneous bacterial peritonitis in cirrhosis, perforated bowel, perforating neoplasm, ruptured colonic diverticulum or diverticular abscess, tuberculosis, penetrating abdominal trauma, surgical wound dehiscence), *C. difficile* colitis, amebic colitis, typhoid fever, *Giardia*, Whipple disease; *Inflammatory/Immune:* Sterile peritonitis from perforated stomach or duodenum, bile, ruptured bladder, enzymes released by acute pancreatitis, ruptured ovarian cyst, blood (e.g., bleeding from follicular cyst), recurrent serositis syndromes (e.g., SLE, familial Mediterranean fever, familial Hibernian fever), inflammatory bowel disease (ulcerative colitis, Crohn disease), toxic megacolon; *Mechanical/Traumatic:* Manipulation of the gut (abdominal surgical procedures, abdominal trauma), adhesions, tumors, volvulus, intussusception, parasites; *Metabolic/Toxic:* Hypokalemia, hypothyroidism, acidemia or alkalemia, diabetic ketoacidosis, uremia, heavy metal poisoning, porphyria, toxic megacolon or any major metabolic disorder, drugs (opiates, anticholinergics, vinca alkaloids, ganglionic blocking agents); *Neurologic:* Trauma to the axial skeleton, spinal cord injury, compression fracture, herpes zoster, urinary retention, fecal impaction, aerophagia; *Vascular:* Mesenteric arterial embolism or thrombosis, mesenteric venous thrombosis, hypotension, ischemic bowel.

Abdominal Masses
Rectus sheath hematoma. See page 442.

Parenchymal organ enlargement. The liver, spleen, adrenals, and kidneys enlarge in several ways: an expanded cell mass (normal or abnormal, e.g., neoplastic infiltration, inflammatory cells, infection), intra or extracellular deposition of material (fat, amyloid, mucopolysaccharides, etc.), vascular congestion, or cystic change. History and physical exam suggest a mechanism directing a judicious selection of laboratory and imaging studies to determine the mechanism.

CLINICAL OCCURRENCE: *Congenital:* Horseshoe kidney, infiltration by cells of the reticuloendothelial system (e.g., lipopolysaccharidases); *Degenerative/Idiopathic:* Single or multiple cysts; *Infectious:* Granulomatous diseases (fungal infections, tuberculosis), chronic infection and parasitosis (amebiasis, hydatid disease); *Inflammatory/Immune:* Infiltration by cells of the reticuloendothelial system (e.g., histiocytosis syndromes), granulomatous diseases (sarcoid), extracellular protein deposition (amyloidosis); *Mechanical/Traumatic:* Obstruction of normal effluent systems (hydronephrosis, hepatic vein obstruction), enlargement of fluid-containing hollow organs as a consequence of outflow obstruction (e.g., urinary retention and gallbladder hydrops); *Metabolic/Toxic:* hypertrophy of normal tissue as a consequence of increased functional demands (e.g., splenomegaly in hemolytic anemias), accumulation of intracellular inclusions (steatosis, glycogen storage diseases and lipopolysaccharidases); *Neoplastic:* Primary neoplasms, infiltration by metastatic neoplasm either diffusely or focally, extramedullary hematopoiesis; *Vascular:* Renal and hepatic vein obstruction.

RUQ Mass. The liver, gallbladder, and right kidney are most likely to present as RUQ masses. Less common are pancreatic pseudocysts and colon masses.

Enlarged liver, hepatomegaly. The liver fills the anterior RUQ behind the ribs. The left lobe extends leftward to the midclavicular line, though it is rarely palpable. The liver has convex and concave surfaces; the concave inferior surface tips backward and downward. The relatively heavy liver is suspended from the diaphragm by the coronal ligaments (Fig. 9-35). The diaphragm's support is augmented by the hilar vessels and the combination of negative intrathoracic pressure and positive intraabdominal pressure produced by the abdominal wall muscles. There are two axes of liver rotation, a transverse axis near the attachment of the coronary ligaments and an anteroposterior axis near the hilum, to the left of the center of mass. Downward rotation through the transverse axis presents more of the anterior surface below the costal margin (Fig. 9-35B). Downward rotation about the anteroposterior axis results in a tongue of liver appearing in the right flank (Fig. 9-35A). Rotation is expected with any condition that lowers the dome of the diaphragm, decreases the normal amount of abdominal fat, or decreases abdominal muscle tone. Many normal livers are readily palpable just below the costal margin. The edge roughly parallels the costal margin (Fig. 9-35A). Liver size is estimated by measuring from the upper border of hepatic dullness to a lower border determined by palpation or percussion, but estimates of liver size based on percussion are notoriously inaccurate. Many clinical impressions of hepatomegaly are not confirmed with imaging or autopsy because the rotations of the normal liver are not appreciated. The surface should be examined for consistency and nodularity. Tenderness can be elicited by direct palpation or by fist percussion. Percussion tenderness occurs in acute cholecystitis and

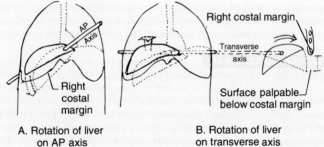

A. Rotation of liver on AP axis   **B. Rotation of liver on transverse axis**

FIG. 9-35 Rotations of the Normal-Sized Liver Making it Palpable Beneath the Costal Margin. The liver is suspended by its coronary ligaments and is fixed to the prevertebral fascia by its hilar blood vessels behind the right costal margin. The diaphragm could not hold a 1500-g liver if not assisted by the negative intrapleural pressure above it, and the positive pressure of abdominal contents, below. Depression of the diaphragm or relaxation of the intraabdominal pressure permits the normal liver to fall beneath the costal margin and become palpable (ptosis). With the diaphragm fixed, the liver may rotate on one or two axes to become palpable. Depression of the diaphragm increases the amount of palpable surface permitted by rotation. **A. The** normal-sized **liver can rotate on an anteroposterior axis near its left side.** With this counterclockwise rotation the lower border appears below the costal margin, forming an angle with the costal margin. **B. The** normal-sized **liver can rotate on a transverse axis.** The liver edge presents below and approximately parallel to the costal margin. This is distinguished from liver enlargement only by the inward curve of the anterior surface.

hepatitis. Palpate over the liver for friction rubs and auscultate for bruits. The coincidence of these two signs indicates a high probability of hepatic carcinoma.

CLINICAL OCCURRENCE: *Congenital:* Polycystic kidney disease, glycogen storage disease, lipopolysaccharidases, hemochromatosis; *Infectious:* Liver abscess (bacterial or amebiasis), echinococcal cyst, viral hepatitis, schistosomiasis, leishmaniasis; *Inflammatory/Immune:* Amyloidosis; *Mechanical/Traumatic:* Hematoma, CHF, tricuspid insufficiency, pulmonary hypertension, cor pulmonale, constrictive pericarditis, hepatic vein thrombosis; *Metabolic/Toxic:* Steatosis, rickets; *Neoplastic:* Hepatocellular carcinoma, metastatic carcinoma (especially colon, pancreas, lung, breast), islet cell carcinoma and carcinoid, biliary carcinoma, histiocytosis syndromes, leukemic infiltration, lymphoma, myelofibrosis/extramedullary hematopoiesis; *Vascular:* Hemangioma, infarction, hematoma.

Pulsatile liver. The liver may directly transmit the aortic pulse wave. Alternatively, retrograde flow from the central veins during ventricular systole can expand the liver volume. Expansile pulsation is demonstrated by placing the hands on opposite sides of the liver and observing that the surfaces move apart in systole. Tricuspid insufficiency is the usual cause.

Nonalcoholic fatty liver disease (NAFLD); nonalcoholic steatohepatitis (NASH). Fat accumulates in hepatocytes in type 2 diabetes, obesity, hypertriglyceridemia, and with older age, initially without inflammation. Inflammation (NASH) leads to fibrosis and cirrhosis in some patients. Both conditions are asymptomatic until cirrhosis, portal hypertension, and hepatic insufficiency appear. Transaminases may be elevated during this asymptomatic period.

Hemochromatosis. Homozygous or compound heterozygous recessive mutations prevent suppression of hepatic hepcidin release resulting in excessive enterocyte absorption of iron. Parenchymal iron accumulation causing tissue injury results in multiple organ's dysfunction, including liver cirrhosis, heart failure, diabetes mellitus from islet cell damage, arthritis, pituitary insufficiency, and melanism. Phenotypic expression is much higher in men. Women are protected during childbearing years by regular menstrual blood loss. Iron accumulation is asymptomatic. Skin color may be bronze, blue-gray, brown, or black, accentuated in the flexor folds, the nipples, recent scars, and in parts exposed to the sun. The pigment is melanin, although hemosiderin is also increased. Skin color change may antedate hepatic cirrhosis and diabetes by several years. When major organ damage occurs, lassitude, weight loss, joint pain, abdominal pain, and loss of libido may be seen. Signs are diffuse bronze skin pigmentation (melanin), hepatomegaly, splenomegaly, spider angiomas, loss of body hair, edema, ascites, peripheral neuropathy, arthropathy, and testicular atrophy. Early diagnosis and therapeutic phlebotomy avoids organ damage. Iron overload resulting from hypertransfusion in refractory anemias produces a similar syndrome.

Enlarged tender gallbladder. See Cholecystitis, page 437.

Enlarged nontender gallbladder. Common bile duct obstruction leads to progressive gallbladder distention. A palpable nontender gallbladder is caused by distention with stones, acalculous cholecystitis, and gallbladder hydrops in which mucous cells continue to secrete despite cystic duct obstruction. Chronic cystic duct obstruction usually produces a contracted gallbladder. A palpable nontender gallbladder (*Courvoisier sign*) implies gallbladder dilatation due to carcinoma in the head of the pancreas rather than a common duct stone since stones cause chronic cholecystitis and a scarred contracted gallbladder wall. There are many exceptions. Carcinoma of the gallbladder produces a hard, irregular, moderately tender mass.

Enlarged kidney. The right kidney lies lower than the left. The kidneys are contained posteriorly by the psoas and the twelfth rib while the liver (right) or spleen (left) prevent extension superiorly (see Fig. 9-2, page 395 for the anatomic relationships of the kidneys). Therefore, enlarging kidney push forward and downward into a position similar to an enlarged spleen or liver, only deeper. The kidney contour is always rounded in contrast to the relatively sharp liver and spleen edges. The left kidney is differentiated from the spleen by its deep location and lobulated surface which must not be mistaken for the splenic notch. Since the kidneys are in the retroperitoneum they do not move with deep inspiration like the spleen and liver. In thin persons, the lower pole of the right kidney may be palpable whereas the left is not. Because their shapes are so dissimilar, there is usually no difficulty distinguishing kidney from liver. Rarely, a protruding renal mass may be confused with hydrops of the gallbladder or pancreatic pseudocyst.

CLINICAL OCCURRENCE: *Congenital:* Polycystic kidney disease, horseshoe kidney, compensatory hypertrophy opposite absent kidney; *Degenerative/Idiopathic:* Cysts; *Inflammatory/Immune:* Amyloidosis; *Mechanical/Traumatic:* Hydronephrosis, hematoma; *Neoplastic:* Renal cell carcinoma and renal sarcoma, transitional cell carcinoma of renal pelvis and ureter.

Ptotic and transplanted kidney. The surrounding fascia holds the kidneys loosely within the superior retroperitoneal space; inferior displacement is not rare, even into the pelvis. Size and shape allow identification, but only if a displaced kidney is considered. Transplanted kidneys are placed in the pelvis where they are easily palpable above the inguinal ligament.

Epigastric masses. Smooth nontender epigastric masses suggest enlargement or distention of normal organs; tenderness implies infection, hemorrhage, or inflammation. Irregular masses suggest neoplasm or a polycystic organ. The abdominal profile offers a clue to diagnosis (see Fig. 9-20, page 416). Acute gastric dilatation produces visible distention in the epigastrium and LUQ. A pulsatile mass is an aortic aneurysm until proven otherwise. In the absence of acute illness, a smooth epigastric mass suggests a pancreatic cyst or pseudocyst. Enlargement of the left lobe of the liver also presents in the epigastrium. Liver and retroperitoneal masses are immobile on palpation, but the liver moves with respirations. Infections and neoplasms produce masses in the omentum, stomach, pancreas, left lobe of the liver, and transverse colon. A polycystic or horseshoe kidney sometimes presents as a midline epigastric mass. Massive periaortic lymph node enlargement may be palpable. Ultrasonography or CT is usually necessary to delineate the involved structure(s).

LUQ mass. A LUQ mass most likely arises from the spleen, kidney, left lobe of the liver, or colon.

Splenomegaly. The enlarged spleen retains its characteristic shape with the splenic notch on the medial edge near the lower pole. Enlargement displaces the lower pole downward from behind the thoracic cage and along its oblique axis toward the left iliac fossa. The lower pole may reach the pelvis and rarely crosses the midline. Many acute infections produce a moderately enlarged soft spleen with blunted edges while chronic disorders cause a firm or hard spleen with sharp edges. Tenderness indicates peritoneal inflammation from infection or infarction. Although uncommon, the spleen can rupture from over-vigorous palpation, most often in infectious mononucleosis. *DDX:* The enlarged spleen and left kidney may have the same general shape, but the kidney is deeper, rounded posteriorly, and never has a distinct edge. Kidney lobulations must not be mistaken for the splenic notch. Ultrasonography or CT is definitive.

CLINICAL OCCURRENCE: *Congenital:* Thalassemia minor and major, lipopolysaccharidases (Gaucher disease, Niemann–Pick disease); *Infectious:* Acute and chronic malaria, typhoid fever, SBE, abscess, schistosomiasis, congenital syphilis, leishmaniasis; *Inflammatory/Immune:* Hemolytic anemia, SLE, RA, pernicious anemia, amyloidosis; *Mechanical/Traumatic:* Chronic CHF, portal hypertension, hematoma; *Metabolic/Toxic:* Pernicious anemia; *Neoplastic:* ALL, lymphoma, CML, CLL; *Vascular:* Infarcts, vasculitis, hematoma.

Enlarged kidney. See page 458.

RLQ masses. The normal cecum is felt as an indistinct doughy slightly tender mass. Sometimes it is fluctuant. Tuberculosis, pericecal or appendiceal abscess, Crohn disease, and carcinoma produce firm masses in the cecum and terminal ileum.

LLQ masses. Irregular plastic fecal masses in the sigmoid are occasionally mistaken for neoplasm. Fecal masses move or disappear in a couple of days. A spastic sigmoid colon is felt as a cord about the diameter of the little finger, lying vertically about 5 cm medial to the left anterior superior iliac spine; the cord can be rolled under the fingers and is slightly or moderately tender. A tender LLQ mass suggests diverticular phlegmon or abscess.

Suprapubic and pelvic masses. Suprapubic masses most often arise within the pelvis. Pelvic and rectal exam is required for a complete description. Pelvic masses arise from the colon, the female or male pelvic organs, and rarely from accumulation of neoplastic or inflammatory debris on the pelvic floor.

Pregnancy. All pubescent and post-pubescent women prior to menopause who present with a pelvic or suprapubic mass are assumed to be pregnant until proven otherwise.

Distended urinary bladder. A chronically obstructed urinary bladder may reach the umbilicus, usually in the midline. The patient may have minimal urinary symptoms or complain of incontinence (because of overflow). The mass is dull to percussion, fluctuant, painless, and disappears with catheterization. It can be mistaken for a neoplasm when a diverticulum disrupts its symmetry. It must be distinguished from ovarian cyst and pregnancy in the female.

Ovarian cyst. See 418.

Pelvic abscess. Pelvic abscesses result from suppurative disease of pelvic organs, perforation of pelvic or abdominal organs, dissection of abdominal wall infections, and lymphatic extension of regional infections. Knowledge of the specific anatomy of the male and female pelvis is necessary for interpreting the exam. In the male, a tender, rounded mass, felt through the anterior rectal wall, superior to the prostate gland, is likely to be a pelvic abscess in the rectovesical pouch. Similarly, in the female, a mass felt through the anterior rectal wall superior to the cervix uteri is probably an abscess in the rectouterine pouch. These abscesses result from perforation of the appendix or a colonic diverticulum, salpingitis, or prostatitis.

Other abdominal masses. The masses previously described involve tissues generally localized to a specific region. However, a mass can form anywhere in the gut. Volvulus (page 434) is usually in the sigmoid colon or the cecum but may occur elsewhere. Intussusception (page 453) occurs primarily in children. An abscess can present as a mass in any part of the abdomen. Abscess should be suspected when a mass is palpated in a region normally devoid of solid organs. Colon cancer and inflammatory masses associated with Crohn disease may be found virtually anywhere in the abdomen or pelvis. Except for intussusception, these conditions so not have distinctive physical findings.

Abdominal, Inguinal, and Other Hernias
Strangulated hernia. Occlusion of venous return from herniating gut or omentum produces swelling and edema preventing reduction. The gradual increase in pressure ultimately prevents capillary and arterial flow; gangrene and perforation may quickly ensue. Pinching and strangulation of only a partial circumference of the gut wall produces a *Richter hernia*. Most commonly a previously recognized hernia presents as a painful mass producing intestinal obstruction. Strangulated bowel is painful, feels firm, but is usually not tender. Forceful attempts at reduction may result in rupture of strangulated gut or reduction en masse, where the hernia sac accompanies the loop of bowel without relieving the strangulation.

Incisional hernia. Palpate for a defect in the abdominal wall underlying an operative scar. Have the patient perform a Valsalva maneuver or raise their head off the pillow. Herniation occurs adjacent to the scar (Fig. 9-36).

Epigastric hernia (fatty hernia of the linea alba). Preperitoneal fat protrudes between the fibers of the linea alba, usually without a peritoneal sac. The

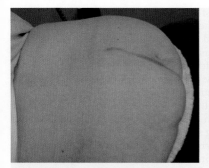
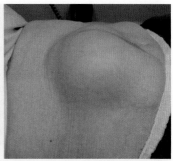

FIG. 9-36 Abdominal Wall Hernia. This hernia is not evident when the patient is at rest on the exam table. Straining forces the abdominal contents into the hernia as the abdominal wall muscles contract.

patient can have midline pain in the epigastrium. To identify the hernia, have the patient stand while running a finger down the midline looking for a small nodule which is occasionally reducible.

Umbilical hernia. There is a defect in the abdominal fascia where the umbilical vessels and urachus exit the abdomen into the umbilical cord. A congenital hernia protrudes through the umbilical scar and has a complete fibrous collar continuous with the linea alba. The adult hernia is periumbilical, the collar is absent, and the upper part of the hernia is covered only by skin. The navel may protrude when intraabdominal pressure is increased by standing or Valsalva. These hernias are soft except when chronic inflammation has caused fibrosis. Umbilical hernias are very common in infants and tend to resolve spontaneously by 4 years of age. The adult type frequently develops during pregnancy, in long-standing ascites, or when intrathoracic pressure is repeatedly increased as in asthma, chronic bronchitis, and bronchiectasis.

Inguinal hernias
Zieman inguinal examination. This examination detects direct and indirect inguinal hernias and hernias into the femoral triangle, so it is effective in women and men. The patient stands to the examiners left side. Placing the palm of the right hand against the right lower abdomen spread the fingers slightly so the long finger lies along the inguinal ligament with the fingertip in the external inguinal ring (Chapter 12, Fig. 12-5B, page 512). The index finger is over the internal inguinal ring, and the ring finger lies over the femoral canal and the fascial opening for the saphenous vein. The patient takes a deep breath, holds it, and bears down as if to have a bowel movement. A hernia in any of the three sites is felt as either a gliding motion of the walls of the empty sac or as a protrusion into the sac. When the internal ring is closed by the index finger, any herniating mass cannot be an indirect inguinal hernia. The examination on the left is the mirror image of the right using the left hand.

Indirect inguinal hernia. The internal inguinal ring lies just above the midpoint of the inguinal ligament. In men, the spermatic cord emerges from the abdominal cavity through this ring, runs medially in the canal, exiting the subcutaneous external ring just lateral to the pubis, then drops over the brim of the bony pelvis into the scrotum. Inguinal hernias follow the course of the cord; they may extend only a small distance into the canal or descend into the scrotum. In the female, the round ligament corresponds to the spermatic cord and the hernia follows a similar course. In either sex, a small, indirect inguinal hernia may produce a bulge over the midpoint of the inguinal ligament at the abdominal (internal) inguinal ring (Fig. 9-37). To palpate the male inguinal canal, place the index fingertip at the most dependent part of the scrotum then gently lift it into the subcutaneous external inguinal ring by invaginating scrotum (Fig. 12-5A). When the patient coughs or strains a tap from the hernia sac may be felt on the fingertip. A larger hernia may feel like a mass in the canal. In the female, palpation of the inguinal canal is usually unsatisfactory.

Direct inguinal hernia. A hernia through the posterior wall of the inguinal canal is termed direct. The site of the weakness is *Hesselbach triangle*, bounded by the inferior epigastric artery, the lateral border of the rectus muscle and the inguinal ligament, Thus, it lies nearly directly behind the subcutaneous (external) inguinal ring. A bulge is produced close to the pubic tubercle, just above the inguinal ligament, medial to the site of an indirect hernia (Fig. 9-37). When examining the inguinal canal, coughing or straining produces an impulse on the pad not the tip of the finger. Direct hernias usually occur in men, are always acquired, and seldom cause pain.

Femoral hernia. The femoral nerve, artery, and vein lie lateral and just inferior to the midpoint of the inguinal ligament. Immediately medial to the vein is the femoral canal, a continuation of the femoral sheath, through which a hernia may bulge with increased intraabdominal pressure (Fig. 9-37). Large femoral hernias become irreducible and may push upward in front of the inguinal ligament where they can be confused with inguinal hernias. Palpating the hernia sac neck just lateral to and below the pubic tubercle confirms a femoral hernia. The neck of an inguinal hernia sac is above the inguinal ligament.

Obturator hernia. A peritoneal sac protrudes through the obturator foramen in the pelvis producing a fullness or mass in the femoral triangle. The fullness is not sharply defined because the sac is covered by the pectineus muscle. This rare lesion occurs almost always in older emaciated women with a history of weight loss. The hernia is rarely diagnosed before it has caused intestinal obstruction. The thigh on the affected side is usually held in semiflexion. Any hip motion produces pain. When the genicular branch of the obturator nerve is compressed, the pain extends down the medial thigh to the knee (*Romberg–Howship sign*). Palpation through the rectum or vagina may reveal a soft tender mass in the region of the obturator foramen. Obturator hernia must be distinguished from the far more common femoral hernia. When only a portion of the bowel circumference is strangulated (*Richter hernia*) obstruction does not occur. Pain may occur late, only after perforation or sepsis has occurred.

Spigelian hernia. A peritoneal sac with considerable extraperitoneal fat penetrates the linea semilunaris to lie within the abdominal wall covered only by

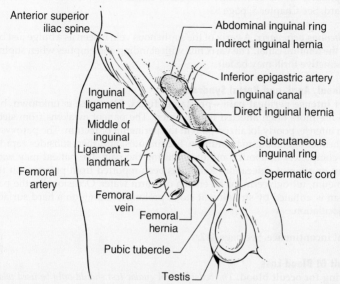

FIG. 9-37 Hernias in the Inguinal Region. Inguinal hernias. The inguinal ligament stretches from the anterior superior spine of the ilium to the pubic tubercle. The flattened tube of the inguinal canal lies just above and parallel to it, between the superficial and deep layers of abdominal muscles. The lateral end of the canal opens posteriorly into the abdominal cavity through the abdominal inguinal ring (internal ring). The internal ring is not palpable, but it is just above the midpoint of the inguinal ligament. The medial end of the canal opens anteriorly into the subcutaneous tissue through the subcutaneous inguinal ring (external ring). In the male, this is where the spermatic cord emerges from the abdominal muscles. A hernia is indirect when it enters the canal from the abdominal cavity through the abdominal inguinal ring; a hernia entering medial to this ring is direct. In small hernias, the relation of the bulge to the midpoint of the inguinal ligament is diagnostic of direct or indirect. If the hernia is large, palpating the inguinal canal through the scrotum may determine the entrance site into the canal. The direct hernia is as an anterior bulging of the posterior wall of the inguinal canal. **Femoral hernia.** The femoral artery and vein emerge from the abdomen beneath the midpoint of the inguinal ligament, where the artery is palpable. The impalpable femoral vein is immediately medial to the artery and the femoral canal lies medial to the vein ~2 cm medial to the pulsating artery. A bulge in the region of the femoral canal on coughing or straining indicates a femoral hernia. A femoral hernia protruding upward in front of the inguinal ligament may be confused with an inguinal hernia. Careful palpation demonstrates that the inguinal canal is empty.

skin, subcutaneous fat, and aponeurosis of the abdominal external oblique muscle. It is usually asymptomatic until it strangulates. There is a tender abdominal wall mass 3–5 cm above the inguinal ligament. Examination is by inspection and palpation while the patient stands.

Other inguinal masses. Additional causes of a groin masses are lymph nodes, varix, aneurysms, lipoma, ectopic testis, ectopic spleen, and inguinal endometriosis.

Lymphadenopathy. Inflammation, infection, or neoplastic involvement of lymph nodes causes enlargement with or without tenderness. Inflammation and fluctuant lymph node swelling near the femoral vessels below the inguinal ligament is a so-called *bubo* occurring in chancroid, syphilis, and lymphogranuloma venereum. Neoplastic nodes are nontender and rubbery or hard. See Chapter 5, page 83.

Saphenous vein varix. A varix of the saphenous vein is seen as a bulge just below the femoral canal. The varix fills with standing and empties when supine; a distinctive thrill may be felt.

Perineal, Anal, and Rectal Syndromes

Brief intense perineal pain—proctalgia fugax. The cause is unknown, but men are more often affected than women. The patient awakens from sleep with intense, poorly localized pain in the perineum or rectum. The paroxysm reaches an agonizing maximum in 1–2 minutes, and then subsides rapidly and completely in about 5 minutes. During the pain, the patient may walk about or attempt defecation. Relief has been reported from pressure on the perineum, nitroglycerin, or an enema of warm water. Occasionally, the paroxysm is initiated by straining at stool, prolonged sitting on a hard surface, or ejaculation.

Fecal incontinence. See page 412.

Occult GI Blood Loss

Testing for occult blood. *The bedside stool guaiac test should only be used when recent GI bleeding is suspected by history or examining a stool.* False-positive guaiac results lead to misdirected evaluations. Occult blood screening for colorectal neoplasms is best done with immunochemical methods which are quantitative and far superior to guaiac testing. Bleeding from any site in the alimentary or the upper respiratory tracts can give a positive test for blood without discoloring the stool. But only guaiac testing (not immunochemical) detects upper GI bleeding (digested blood). The source of occult blood loss is sought by endoscopy.

GI bleeding associated with skin lesions. In some patients, GI blood loss is associated with skin lesions having their counterparts in the GI tract.

Peutz–Jeghers syndrome. See Chapter 7, page 223 and Fig. 7-59 page 222.

HHT (Rendu–Osler–Weber disease). Telangiectases on the face, nasal or buccal mucosa, and extremities suggest similar lesions in the GI tract.

Blue rubber–Bleb Nevus syndrome. Cutaneous cavernous hemangiomas, especially on the trunk or extremities, suggest similar lesions in the small intestine.

Ehlers–Danlos syndrome. Common signs are hyper elastic skin, hyper flexible joints, petechiae, and fragile skin.

Pseudoxanthoma elastic. See Chapter 6, page 151.

Neurofibromatosis (von Recklinghausen disease). See Chapter 6, page 151.

Amyloidosis (primary or secondary). See Chapter 5, page 87.

Malignant atrophic papulosis (Degos disease). This is a vasculitis of the skin and mucosa. Small, red papules on the skin become umbilicated, with porcelain-white depressed centers and dry scale. The border disappears, leaving a white patch. Patients may have acute abdominal pain with vomiting and bleeding which can progress to gangrene and peritonitis.

Schölein–Henoch purpura. See Chapter 8, Vasculitis, page 360.

Drugs. Aspirin and other NSAIDs produce erosive lesions which can bleed anywhere in the GI tract. Warfarin is associated with large bruises and bleeding in the GI tract.

Scurvy. See Chapter 6, page 152.

Kaposi sarcoma. Endemic Kaposi sarcoma presents as dark-blue nodules and plaques usually on the feet. HIV-associated Kaposi sarcoma frequently involves the mucous membranes of the mouth and GI and genitourinary tracts.

Mastocytosis. See Chapter 6, page 117.

ADDITIONAL READING

William Silen. *Cope's Early Diagnosis of the Acute Abdomen.* 22nd ed. New York, NY: Oxford University Press; 2010.

CLINICAL VIGNETTES AND QUESTIONS

CASE 9-1

A 25-year-old woman complains of feeling ill for a week with fevers, abdominal pain, nausea, vomiting, and anorexia. Her skin and eyes have become yellow over the last day. Her urine has become dark without dysuria. She has not had diarrhea or constipation. Her stool has become light colored.

QUESTIONS:
1. What is your differential diagnosis for this patient?
2. What additional history do you need?
3. What physical examination findings are you going to look for and why?

CASE 9-2

A 61-year-old man presents with left lower quadrant pain that has been increasing in intensity for 3 days. He has some relief after a bowel movement. He has had low-grade fevers and decreased appetite, but no nausea or vomiting. His chronic constipation has been worse over the week but he denies a change in stool caliber, or blood in the stool. He has not had any weight loss.

QUESTIONS:
1. What is the most likely diagnosis?
2. What physical examination findings might you expect?
3. What would be the significance of a psoas sign or obturator sign?

CASE 9-3

A 64-year-old man presents because of vomiting blood. He awoke, felt ill, and immediately vomited a large volume of bright red blood which he estimates as "at least a quart." He feels lightheaded, like he might pass out when he first stands up. His past medical history is unremarkable and he never sees doctors because he is never sick. He has smoked 1 pack of cigarettes per day for 50 years and drinks a fifth of whiskey and a 12 pack of beer every couple of days since his mid-twenties.

QUESTIONS:
1. What is your differential diagnosis?
2. What physical examination findings will be important to evaluate?
3. What history is typical of a Mallory–Weiss tear?

CASE 9-4

A 35-year-old woman complains of abdominal pain and increasing abdominal girth for several weeks accompanied by increasing dyspnea on exertion. Her only medication is an oral contraceptive. On examination she has mild icterus, a mildly protuberant abdomen, and dilated veins on her abdomen. Bowel sounds are normal and the abdomen is soft with right upper quadrant tenderness and hepatomegaly measuring 5 cm below the costal margin. She has 1+ pitting edema bilaterally.

QUESTIONS:
1. How can the direction of flow in the abdominal veins help with the diagnosis?
2. What is the most likely diagnosis?
3. What are predisposing risk factors for this condition?

CASE 9-5

A 35-year-old male construction worker presents with a lump in his left inguinal region that appeared last week as he was recovering from community-acquired pneumonia. It aches but is not red or painful. He has not had fever, chills, nausea or vomiting. The bulging seems worse at the end of the work day. He is obese with a BMI of 33.

QUESTIONS:
1. What are the anatomical relationships of direct and indirect inguinal hernias?
2. Describe the physical examination findings of both direct and indirect inguinal hernias.
3. Describe a femoral hernia and how to identify it.

CASE 9-6

A 60-year-old man complains of being told by his family that his skin has been turning yellow over the last 6 weeks. He has had progressive loss of appetite and has lost about 10 lb. He has not had fever, chills, night sweats, or known sick contacts. He denies abdominal pain, diarrhea, constipation, or change in stool. His urine has turned dark and he has increasing skin itching without a rash. On examination he is icteric and the abdomen is soft, nontender, and without masses or organomegaly.

QUESTIONS:
1. What is the differential diagnosis for this presentation?
2. What is the most likely diagnosis?
3. Describe other presentations of this condition.

CASE 9-7

A 45-year-old Caucasian man complains of diarrhea. He has had foul-smelling foamy stools that often leave an oily layer in the toilet bowl. He has lost 15 lb since the diarrhea began. He has subjective fevers but no night sweats or chills. He has joint pain primarily his knees and ankles for the last 18 months, without swelling or erythema. He feels fatigued but denies chest pain or tightness, or shortness of breath. His wife thinks that his skin is becoming grey in color, especially in the sun-exposed areas. You confirm the skin findings and identify scattered lymphadenopathy.

QUESTIONS:
1. What is your differential diagnosis for this presentation?
2. What is the most likely diagnosis?
3. What causes this condition?

CHAPTER 10

The Urinary System

OVERVIEW AND PHYSIOLOGY OF THE URINARY SYSTEM

The urinary system includes the kidneys, renal pelvis, ureters, urinary bladder, and urethra. The kidney filters the blood at the glomerulus, reabsorbs and secretes solutes and fluid in the renal tubules, and concentrates the urine in the medullary collecting ducts. Urine passes down the ureters to the bladder by gravity and peristalsis filling the urinary bladder. At the ureterovesical junction the ureters are compressed by detrusor muscle tone as they pass obliquely through the bladder wall. This compression increases during detrusor contraction preventing urine from refluxing into the ureters. The detrusor actively relaxes as the bladder fills maintaining a low pressure within the bladder until it reaches capacity. Further filling stretches the bladder wall rapidly increasing intravesical pressure. The urethra exits the bladder through the urethral sphincter and the urogenital septum. This sphincter has involuntary smooth muscle under parasympathetic and sympathetic control, and voluntary striated muscle innervated via the lumbosacral plexus. Continence requires tonic urethral sphincter smooth muscle contraction and active inhibition of detrusor contraction. Voiding requires detrusor contraction and simultaneous relaxation of the urethral sphincter muscles.

URINARY SYSTEM ANATOMY

The kidneys lie posteriorly partially under the 11th and 12th ribs lateral to L1–4 (Chapter 9, Fig. 9-2, page 395). They lie retroperitoneally enclosed in a tight capsule and surrounded by Gerota fascia. The ureters descend in the retroperitoneum over the psoas muscle and into the pelvis running laterally and then anteriorly to enter the bladder inferiorly on either side of the midline. The bladder lies behind and below the symphysis pubis in the anterior pelvis. The urethra exits the bladder through the urogenital diaphragm formed by pelvic floor muscles, entering the male prostate and penis or the female perineum. The male's proximal urethra is surrounded by the prostate gland and receives secretions from the prostate and seminal vesicles. The perineal portion of the female urethra is quite short. The urethral meatus is visible on inspection and the prostate is palpable during rectal exam. The other normal structures cannot be identified by physical exam.

EXAMINING THE URINARY SYSTEM

See also The Abdomen, Chapter 9; The Female Genitalia and Reproductive System, Chapter 11; and The Male Genitalia and Reproductive System, Chapter 12.

URINARY SYSTEM SYMPTOMS

Discolored Urine. See page 472.

Urethral Discharge. See page 474 and Urethritis page 479 and Chapter 12, page 523.

Ureteral Colic. See Abdominal Pain Chapter 9, pages 407 and 433 and ureteral colic Chapter 9, page 438. Vigorous contraction of ureteral smooth muscle against an obstruction is intensely painful. Obstructing stones in the renal pelvis, ureter, or bladder produce waves of severe acute pain, *ureteral colic*. The pain's location varies with the site of obstruction. Obstruction at the renal pelvis gives flank and upper abdominal pain. Ureteral obstruction produces pain in the upper abdomen, lower abdomen, pelvis, testicles, and perineum. Bladder outlet obstruction produces pain in the pelvis. The diagnosis is supported by an acute onset, absence of systemic symptoms other than nausea and anorexia, a personal or family history of urolithiasis, and microscopic hematuria without pyuria.

Frequent Urination without Polyuria. The average adult urinates about five or six times daily, the frequency depending upon fluid balance, renal function, individual habits, and the presence or absence of genitourinary tract irritation. Frequent urination is caused by increased urine volume (*polyuria*), decreased bladder capacity, or increased stimulation of the micturition reflexes by irritation of the genitourinary tract. The history, physical exam, measurement of 24-hour fluid intake and urine volume, volume of each voiding, and postvoid residual bladder volume usually identifies the correct cause(s).
   CLINICAL OCCURRENCE: *Congenital:* Small bladder capacity, ureterovesical reflux, urethral and meatal stricture; *Endocrine:* Atrophic vaginitis; *Degenerative/Idiopathic:* Benign prostatic hyperplasia, pelvic floor relaxation, cystocele, urethrocele; *Infectious:* Bacterial and viral pyelitis, cystitis, urethritis, vaginitis, salpingitis; *Inflammatory/Immune:* Interstitial and chemical cystitis, prostatitis, appendicitis; *Metabolic/Toxic:* Chemical cystitis, highly acidic urine; *Mechanical/Traumatic:* Pelvic floor relaxation, cystocele, urethrocele, bladder stone, extrinsic compression of the bladder or urethra, bladder wall fibrosis, urethral stricture, bladder neck obstruction; *Neoplastic:* Bladder cancer, prostate cancer, locally invasive cervical and rectal cancer; *Neurologic:* Spinal cord, cauda equina and sacral plexus lesions, autonomic neuropathy, detrusor instability; *Psychosocial:* Untrained bladder, voiding habits.

Frequent Urination with Polyuria. The adult male bladder holds ~500 mL; the adult female bladder holds somewhat less. The average urine output in 24 hours is 1200–1500 mL but is dependent upon the type and volume of fluid intake, sensible (vomiting, diarrhea) and insensible (sweating, respiratory) fluid losses, and the renal concentrating ability. Increased urinary volume (*polyuria*) is caused by increased osmotic load (e.g., diabetes mellitus), increased fluid intake, medications, dietary exposures, and/or decreased renal concentrating ability. The history, physical exam, and urinalysis establish the cause in most cases.
   CLINICAL OCCURRENCE: *Congenital:* Renal tubular defects (e.g., renal tubular acidosis type 1); *Endocrine:* Diabetes mellitus, central or renal

diabetes insipidus; *Degenerative/Idiopathic:* Chronic renal failure of any cause; *Inflammatory/Immune:* Interstitial nephritis; *Metabolic/Toxic:* Diuretic use, hypercalcemia, hypokalemia; *Mechanical/Traumatic:* Post-obstructive diuresis; *Psychosocial:* Excessive fluid intake, psychogenic polydipsia, alcohol and caffeine ingestion.

Nocturia. Urine production declines during sleep which is usually not interrupted by a need to urinate. Some people have habitual nocturia aggravated by high fluid intakes, especially of caffeinated or alcoholic beverages taken in the evening. Nocturia is common with disorders causing urinary frequency or polyuria. Edematous states (congestive heart failure, hepatic insufficiency, nephrotic syndrome, and chronic renal failure) are associated with nocturia caused by mobilization of dependent fluid from the lower extremities and abdomen during recumbency. Sleep disorders may cause nocturia as well. Reclining decreases bladder support contributing to nocturia in women with pelvic floor relaxation and after hysterectomy.

Urinary Incontinence. Involuntary loss of urine by children at night is *enuresis*. Urinary incontinence in adults should initiate an evaluation for the specific cause; most are treatable. See Urinary Syndromes—Incontinence, page 474.

Difficult Urination. Normal urination occurs with effortless bladder sphincter relaxation coordinated with detrusor muscle contraction. Difficulty initiating or maintaining a urine stream indicates obstruction to flow or decreased detrusor strength. The patient may complain of hesitation in starting the urinary stream, decreased force of urination, and/or dribbling at termination of urination. Occasionally, straining is required to maintain the stream.

CLINICAL OCCURRENCE: *Degenerative/Idiopathic:* Prostatic hyperplasia; *Infectious:* Tabes dorsalis, prostatitis; *Inflammatory/Immune:* Chronic sterile prostatitis; *Mechanical/Traumatic:* Urethral stricture or valve, bladder neck obstruction, bladder stone or clot, pregnancy, hematoma; *Neoplastic:* Urethral carcinoma, prostate cancer, uterine fibroid, vaginal cancer, cervical cancer; *Neurologic:* Detrusor weakness, multiple sclerosis, spinal cord injury or epidural compression, myelitis, syringomyelia.

Painful Urination (Dysuria). Inflammation of or breaks in the urethral epithelium, usually the result of infection or trauma, exposes the submucosa to acidic urine during urination resulting in pain in the penis or female urethra. Ask if the pain is greater at initiation, during, or at the end of voiding. Pain during urination occurs with urethral obstruction, urethritis, cystitis, vulvitis, and meatal ulcers. Pain after urination is more typical of bladder calculus, cystitis, prostatitis, and seminal vesiculitis.

URINARY SYSTEM SIGNS

See also Abdominal Signs, Chapter 9; Female Genital and Reproductive Signs, Chapter 11; Male Genital and Reproductive Signs, Chapter 12.

Urinary Retention. See Urinary Syndromes—Urinary Retention, page 475.

Determining Post-Void Residual Urine Volume. The *residual volume,* the volume of urine remaining in the bladder after a full voluntary voiding, is used to assess the adequacy of bladder emptying. The post-void residual volume is estimated by ultrasonography and measured directly by catheterizing the bladder. The risk for bladder infection increases sharply with residual volumes >100 mL.

Anuria and Oliguria. Bladder outlet obstruction is the most common cause of anuria and oliguria. Decreased urine production measured in the bladder results from a profound decline in glomerular filtration because of decreased renal blood flow and/or intrarenal or ureteral obstruction. The process must involve both kidneys or obstruct both ureters. Even with hypovolemia, normal kidneys continue to excrete >500 mL daily. In *oliguria*, the 24-hour urine output is 50–400 mL (4–25 mL/h). The output is 0–50 mL in *anuria*. Oliguria and anuria indicate advanced kidney dysfunction requiring immediate treatment. Acute kidney injury may occur unexpectedly and usually patients do not complain, which can delay recognition. Postrenal obstruction with hydronephrosis must always be excluded, even when another cause seems likely. For clinical occurrences see Urinary Syndromes—Acute Kidney Injury, page 475.

Discolored Urine. Normal urine is clear and yellow due to urea. Urine dilution or concentration changes the color's intensity but not the color itself. A true color change results from colored substances in the urine, either filtered from the blood or arising in the urinary tract itself. Increased urine opacity is caused by precipitation of solutes or addition of cellular material or mucous. For a complaint of abnormal urine color determine if the change is in the intensity of the normal yellow color or a true color change. Ask if the change is persistent or episodic and whether it is associated with activities, certain foods, medications, or other symptoms. Inspection and analysis of a freshly voided urine specimen should precede any further investigation. Patients describe any red discoloration as blood, a conclusion to avoid until proven. Often discolored urine is first identified by someone handling specimens, e.g., the porphyrias.

CLINICAL OCCURRENCE: *Colorless:* Urine of low concentration from excessive fluid intake, chronic glomerulonephritis, diabetes mellitus, diabetes insipidus; *Cloudy White:* Phosphates in an alkaline urine (the cloud disappears with the addition of acid), epithelial cells from the lower genitourinary tract, bacteria, pus, chyle (when the urine is centrifuged, chyle remains homogeneously distributed; milk fat added for malingering floats to the top); *Yellow:* Highly concentrated normal urine, tetracycline, pyridine; *Orange:* Urobilinogen, pyridium (antispasmodic that is orange in acidic urine and red in alkaline urine), rhubarb (food and purgative), cathartics (senna aloes), anthracyclines; *Red:* Beets, blackberries, aniline dyes from candy, freshly voided hemoglobin or myoglobin, pyridine, porphyrin, phenolphthalein (a cathartic, red in alkaline urine, colorless in acidic urine), cascara (cathartic), rifampin, doxorubicin; *Blue-Green:* Bilirubin (urine with yellow froth), methylene blue, *Pseudomonas* infection; *Black-Brown:* Highly concentrated normal urine, bilirubin (with yellow froth), acid hematin (hemoglobin standing in acidic urine), methemoglobin, porphyrin, phenol (black in large quantities), cresol, homogentisic acid, tyrosine; *Brown-Black After Standing:* Porphyrin (changed from exposure to sunlight), melanin (changed from exposure to sunlight), homogentisic acid (changed from bacterial alkalinization of the urine).

Hematuria. Asymptomatic microscopic hematuria is ≥3 red blood cells (RBCs) per high-powered field (HPF) on a properly collected urine specimen in the absence of an obvious cause. Dipstick identification of urinary heme is not specific for hematuria. Hematuria is distinguished from hemoglobinuria and myoglobinuria by finding erythrocytes in freshly voided urine collected within 1 hour after completely emptying the bladder. In all three cases urine testing for heme is positive. Gross hematuria is frequently noticed by men during urination. The pattern of gross hematuria may indicate the source of blood: *initial hematuria*—the urethra; *terminal hematuria*—a small hemorrhage from the bladder trigone; *total hematuria*—hemorrhage from the kidney or profuse bleeding from the bladder. Red cell casts prove a renal source. In most instances, hematuria demands a complete genitourinary tract investigation, including upper tract imaging, urine cytology, and cystoscopy.

CLINICAL OCCURRENCE: *Congenital:* Hemophilia, sickle cell disease, polycystic kidney disease; *Endocrine:* Menstruation; *Degenerative/Idiopathic:* Bladder diverticulum, polyps, prostatic hyperplasia, endometriosis, uremia, thrombocytopenia; *Infectious:* Urethritis, bacterial and viral (adenovirus 11) cystitis, prostatitis, pyelitis, schistosomiasis, malaria, yellow fever; *Inflammatory/Immune:* Interstitial cystitis, fever, glomerulonephritis, polyarteritis, microscopic polyangiitis, Goodpasture syndrome, Wegener syndrome; *Metabolic/Toxic:* Chemical cystitis (e.g., cyclophosphamide or ifosfamide), analgesic nephropathy, anticoagulants, scurvy, vitamin K deficiency; *Mechanical/Traumatic:* Blunt or penetrating trauma, urethral stricture, instrumentation, postsurgical, decompression of a distended bladder, heavy exercise (e.g., marathon runners), foreign body, stones, rupture, radiation, medullary necrosis; *Neoplastic:* Kidney, ureter, bladder, prostate cancers; *Psychosocial:* Factitious; *Vascular:* Bladder and prostatic varices, renal infarction, vasculitis, arteriovenous malformation.

- *Hemoglobinuria.* Urinary extracellular hemoglobin results from filtering plasma free hemoglobin or red blood cells lysing in the urine. It may produce red urine identical to myoglobinuria and hematuria. With intravascular hemolysis, hemoglobin binds to plasma haptoglobin; the hemoglobin–haptoglobin complex is not filtered by the normal glomerulus. When the binding capacity of haptoglobin is exceeded, free hemoglobin passes through the glomerular basement membrane and a freshly voided urine specimen usually contains hemoglobin casts, excluding hemolysis in the bladder. Hemoglobin gives positive chemical tests whether it is intracellular or extracellular; therefore hemoglobinuria is distinguished from hematuria by the absence of erythrocytes in freshly voided urine. Smaller myoglobin molecules are rapidly cleared from the blood and thus red tinged plasma would suggests hemoglobinuria rather than myoglobinuria. Spectroscopy is required to distinguish myoglobin from hemoglobin. At specific gravity < 1.006 the dilute urine causes hemolysis of RBCs in the bladder producing hemoglobinuria.

CLINICAL OCCURRENCE: *Congenital:* Glucose-6-phosphate dehydrogenase (G-6-PD) deficiency; *Endocrine:* Pregnancy and the puerperium; *Degenerative/Idiopathic:* Paroxysmal nocturnal hemoglobinuria; *Infectious:* Malaria, blackwater fever, typhus, gas gangrene, generalized anthrax, yellow fever; *Inflammatory/Immune:* Major transfusion reaction, autoimmune hemolytic anemia, hapten-associated hemolysis (quinine, sulfonamides), high-titer cold-agglutinin disease; *Mechanical/Traumatic:* March hemoglobinuria, mechanical heart valves, severe aortic and paraprosthetic mitral regurgitation, extracorporeal circulation, major burns, intravascular devices; *Metabolic/Toxic:* Oxidant drugs or fava beans in persons with G-6-PD deficiency (sulfonamides, sulfones, primaquine), envenomation by snake or spider bites, infusion of outdated, frozen, or improperly stored blood; *Psychosocial:* Injection of distilled water; *Vascular:* Microangiopathic hemolytic anemia–thrombotic thrombocytopenic purpura, hemolytic uremic syndrome, and malignant hypertension; renal infarction.

- *Myoglobinuria.* Myoglobin from damaged muscle colors the urine red and tests positive for heme (see Hemoglobinuria above). Muscle pain, crush injury, or prolonged muscle ischemia are usual; loss of consciousness associated with severe injury may obscure the history.

CLINICAL OCCURRENCE: *Congenital:* McArdle disease; *Inflammatory/ Immune:* Autoimmune hemolytic anemia, incompatible blood transfusion; *Mechanical/Traumatic:* Crush injuries, compression injuries caused by prolonged immobilization or impaired consciousness, electrical shock, compartment syndromes, intravascular hemolysis; *Metabolic/Toxic:* Severe hypokalemia, ingestion of quail (idiosyncratic), opiate and sedative abuse.

URETHRAL SIGNS

Urethral Discharge. Inflammation of the urethra and/or its exocrine glands distal to the urogenital septum creates purulent secretions which leak from the urethra between times of urination. Men complain of a penile discharge accompanied by staining of the underwear with pus or blood. Determine whether the discharge is clear or purulent, accompanied by painful and/or frequent urination and whether the patient has had any new sexual partners. Ask specifically about same-sex contacts and the use of condoms. In women, urethral discharge is confounded with vulvovaginitis.

CLINICAL OCCURRENCE: *Infectious:* Chlamydia trachomatis, Neisseria gonorrhoeae, Ureaplasma urealyticum, Trichomonas vaginalis, other sexually transmitted infections; *Inflammatory/Immune:* Reiter syndrome, Behçet syndrome; *Mechanical/Traumatic:* Urethral catheter and foreign bodies.

URINARY SYSTEM SYNDROMES

Hematuria: See Urinary Signs—Hematuria, page 473.

Loin Pain–Hematuria Syndrome—IgA Nephropathy. IgA accumulating in the glomerular mesangium disrupts the glomerulus. Patients present with painless hematuria or hematuria and loin pain, often following a mild viral infection. Progression is unpredictable, but only a minority develops end-stage renal disease.

Urinary Incontinence. Loss of bladder control results from abnormal genitourinary sensation, smooth muscle dysfunction (detrusor instability, overactive bladder, urge incontinence), an inadequate sphincter (stress incontinence), urinary retention leading to overflow, combinations of these (mixed incontinence), cognitive impairment, and inability to respond in time to reach a toilet. Most causes of urinary incontinence in adults are treatable so a specific physiologic and anatomic diagnosis is required. Determine the onset, pattern, precipitating factors, fluid intake, and measures taken by the patient to reduce the incontinence. Review all prescription and nonprescription medications and dietary supplements. Determine whether the patient feels an urge to void prior to the episode, whether coughing, sneezing, or laughing precede the episode, and the volume of urine lost. Having the patient complete a bladder journal for at least 2 weeks, recording fluid intake (type and amount), urine volume, and incontinent episodes greatly facilitates the evaluation.

CLINICAL OCCURRENCE: *Degenerative/Idiopathic:* Benign prostatic hyperplasia, cystocele urethrocele; *Infectious:* Cystitis, urethritis; *Mechanical/Traumatic:* Pelvic floor relaxation, sphincter injury from childbirth; *Neoplastic:* Prostate, bladder, cervix, and rectal cancers, especially with sacral plexus involvement; *Neurologic:* Spinal cord injury, epidural cord compression, cauda equina syndrome, stoke, dementia, autonomic and peripheral neuropathies, normal pressure hydrocephalus, multiple sclerosis, paralysis, muscular weakness and limited mobility.

Urinary Retention. Urine is retained in the bladder when mechanical outflow obstruction and/or loss of detrusor strength prevent complete emptying. Rapid increases in bladder volume lead to high wall tension, whereas slow increases increase bladder compliance and flaccidity. Retention is more common in men than in women. Acute urinary retention is usually painful, distinguishing it from painless anuria or oliguria. Seriously ill patients may be unable to communicate discomfort. Chronic retention develops gradually and is painless. The only symptoms may be frequent small volume urination or overflow incontinence. The patient may sense bladder fullness, but this is often absent. Suprapubic dullness and a rounded midline mass are found on exam. Measure the post-void residual volume by catheterization or ultrasonography.

CLINICAL OCCURRENCE: *Congenital:* Urethral valves; *Infectious:* Bacterial prostatitis, prostate abscess; *Inflammatory/Immune:* Nonbacterial prostatitis; *Mechanical/Traumatic:* Prostate hyperplasia, bladder stone, occluded catheter, urethral stricture or calculus, ruptured urethral; *Neoplastic:* Prostate and bladder cancer, locally invasive cervical or rectal cancer; *Neurologic:* Spinal cord injury, autonomic neuropathy, tabes dorsalis.

Acute Kidney Injury. Acute loss of renal function is *prerenal* (decreased effective renal blood flow), *renal* (glomerulonephritis, mesangial proliferation, tubular dysfunction, or interstitial inflammation), or *postrenal* (obstruction of the ureters or bladder). The physical exam assessing intravascular volume, cardiac output, and the presence of severe liver disease, identifies prerenal causes. Post-renal causes (obstruction) must be excluded. Urinalysis helps to distinguish between glomerular causes (microscopic hematuria, red blood cell casts, proteinuria) and tubulointerstitial disease (white blood cells in the urine, cellular and granular casts, decreased concentrating ability, salt wasting). Medications commonly cause or contribute to acute kidney injury. Congenital solitary kidney or a prior nonfunctioning kidney can be associated with acute kidney injury from unilateral events not normally associated with a sudden and dramatic loss of renal function. The following clinical classification is diagnostically more useful than pathologic categorizations.

CLINICAL OCCURRENCE: *Congenital:* Sickle cell crisis; *Endocrine:* Hyperparathyroidism (severe hypercalcemia), thyroid storm; *Degenerative/Idiopathic:* Advanced chronic renal failure of any cause; *Infectious:* Pyelonephritis, septicemia, hemorrhagic fevers, blackwater fever (malaria), bacterial endocarditis; *Inflammatory/Immune:* Vasculitis (see below), antiglomerular basement membrane disease (Goodpasture syndrome), systemic lupus erythematosus, progressive systemic sclerosis (scleroderma), serum sickness, retroperitoneal fibrosis; *Mechanical/Traumatic: Major Trauma.* Hypovolemic shock, crush syndrome, burns, heat prostration, hematoma, ruptured kidneys, myoglobinemia; *Instrumentation.* Retrograde pyelography and catheterization of ureters; *Postrenal Obstruction* (especially if one kidney is absent or poorly functioning). Renal calculi, cysts, tumor or mass obstructing the ureters, obstruction by crystals of uric acid, oxalic acid, cystine, or calcium; *Metabolic/Toxic: Medications.* Antibiotics (aminoglycosides, amphotericin-B, sulfonamides), nonsteroidal anti-inflammatory drugs, and hypersensitivity to any medication; *Toxins.* Myoglobin, radiologic contrast material, heavy metals (mercury, bismuth, copper, uranium, arsenic), organic solvents (carbon tetrachloride), inorganic phosphorus, carbon monoxide, paraldehyde, ethylene glycol, heroin, biologics (mushrooms, rattlesnake venom), methemoglobinemia; *Blood Transfusion.* Hemolysis from mishandled or incompatible blood; *Neoplastic:* Lymphoma, extensive cervical cancer causing bilateral ureteral obstruction, tumor lysis syndrome; *Vascular:* Hypotension of any cause (sepsis, hemorrhage, obstetrical complications), postoperative (especially with major vascular procedures—aortic resection, cardiotomy, repair of injuries to blood vessels, etc.—or hemorrhage), vasculitis (polyarteritis nodosa, microscopic polyangiitis, Goodpasture syndrome, granulomatosis with polyangiitis (Wegener), hypersensitivity angiitis, or vasculopathy (hemolytic uremic syndrome, thrombotic thrombocytopenic purpura, malignant and accelerated hypertension, abdominal aortic dissection, atheroemboli).

Interstitial Nephritis. Inflammation of the renal cortical and medullary interstitium (as distinct from the glomerular and vascular injury of glomerulonephritis) results in scarring, decreased tubular function, and progressive renal insufficiency. Injury may be acute (infection, drug induced) or chronic (toxins, drugs, infection, obstruction). Interstitial nephritis is often asymptomatic with abnormalities on urinalysis (pyuria, cellular casts, and proteinuria) and declining renal function the only findings.

CLINICAL OCCURRENCE: *Congenital:* Polycystic kidney disease, medullary cystic and sponge kidney, sickle cell disease, vesicoureteral reflux; *Infectious:* Acute and chronic pyelonephritis, viral infection (Epstein–Barr virus, cytomegalovirus, HIV, hantavirus), brucellosis, Yersinia, tuberculosis, leptospirosis, rickettsia, mycoplasma; *Inflammatory/Immune:* Drug allergy (penicillins, sulfonamides, etc.), Sjögren syndrome, Goodpasture syndrome, transplant rejection; *Mechanical/Traumatic:* Chronic obstruction, ureterovesical reflux, radiation; *Metabolic/Toxic:* Drugs (nonsteroidal anti-inflammatory drugs, diuretics, anticonvulsants, cyclosporin, and others), toxins (heavy metals, lithium, herbals, and others), hypercalcemia, hyperuricemia, prolonged hypokalemia; *Neoplastic:* Multiple myeloma, lymphoma, leukemia; *Vascular:* Accompanying glomerulonephritis and vasculitis.

Chronic Kidney Disease and Chronic Renal Failure. Causes of chronic loss of renal function are prerenal, renal, or postrenal. When the functioning nephron mass falls below a critical level the increased filtration by each remaining nephron required to maintain adequate solute clearance leads to progressive failure of these remaining nephrons, the vicious cycle leading to end-stage kidney disease. Weakness, anorexia, fatigue, and nausea are common symptoms. Pruritus and dyspnea are late occurrences. Slow progression leads to adaptive metabolic and hemodynamic changes which may be apparent on physical exam. Hypertension, extracellular fluid volume expansion causing edema, muscle wasting, and anemia are common. Less frequently, pericarditis, or soft-tissue calcifications may be found. The staging categories are listed in Table 10-1.

CLINICAL OCCURRENCE: *Note: The causes of acute renal failure are not repeated here. Congenital:* Polycystic kidney disease, Alport syndrome; *Endocrine:* Diabetes mellitus, the metabolic syndrome; *Infectious:* Chronic pyelonephritis, renal tuberculosis; *Inflammatory/Immune:* Glomerulonephritis, systemic lupus erythematosus; *Mechanical/Traumatic:* Bladder neck obstruction; *Metabolic/ Toxic:* Nonsteroidal anti-inflammatory drugs, acetaminophen; *Vascular:* Hypertension, atherosclerotic renal artery stenosis, atheroemboli, vasculitis.

Polycystic kidney disease. An autosomal dominant defect of renal tubular development produces massive enlargement of the kidneys and progressive renal failure. Presenting symptoms are flank pain, nausea, malaise, renal colic, and hematuria. Hypertension is common and the enlarged kidneys are often palpable.

TABLE 10-1 Staging of Chronic Kidney Disease

Stage	Description	Glomerular Filtration Rate (mL/min per 1.73 m^2)
0	Increased risk	$\geq$90, but with risk factors for chronic kidney disease (e.g., hypertension, diabetes, etc.)
1	Kidney damage with normal or increased GFR	$\geq$90
2	Kidney damage with mildly decreased GFR	60–89
3	Moderately decreased GFR	30–59
4	Severely decreased GFR	15–29
5	Renal failure	<15 or dialysis

National Kidney Foundation. K/DOQI clinical practice guidelines for chronic kidney disease: evaluation, classification, and stratification. Am J Kidney Dis. 2002;39(2 Suppl 1):S1-266.

Uremia. Uremia is a clinical syndrome associated with advanced renal failure. Though it includes azotemia, the symptoms do not necessarily parallel the degree of azotemia. Symptoms include increased fatigability, headache, anorexia, dyspnea, nausea, vomiting, diarrhea, hiccup, restlessness, and depression. Signs on physical exam include Cheyne–Stokes breathing, fetid breath, dehydration, pericardial friction rub, muscle twitching, delirium, and coma.

Glomerulonephritis (nephritic syndrome). Inflammation damages the glomerular capillary endothelium, basement membrane, mesangium, and/or epithelial podocytes destroying glomerular microstructure. Proteinuria and hematuria with red blood cell casts are diagnostic. Glomerulonephritis accompanies many systemic diseases, the signs and symptoms of that disease often predominating. Primary renal diseases often present with oliguria, edema, severe hypertension, and electrolyte disorders accompanying end-stage renal disease.

Nephrotic syndrome. Damage to the glomerular basement membrane increases filtration of low molecular weight proteins, particularly albumin, resulting in proteinuria when the tubular capacity to reabsorb the protein is exceeded. Albuminuria of >3.5 g in 24-hours or a urine protein/creatinine ratio of >3.5 is diagnostic. Hypertension, edema, hypoalbuminemia, and elevated serum cholesterol are frequently present. Complications include protein malnutrition and increased risk of thrombosis, particularly in the renal vein. Creatinine and blood urea nitrogen may remain normal. Nephrotic syndrome may complicate many forms of glomerular injury and is particularly common in diabetic nephropathy.

Urolithiasis. Stones form either from solutes accreting upon a nidus (usually calcium oxalate, but also uric acid) or because of chronic urinary tract infections with urea-splitting organisms (struvite stones). Microscopic or gross hematuria may occur intermittently, but most stones are asymptomatic until they obstruct a ureter or the bladder outlet. Pain is the presenting symptom, the site depending upon the location of the impacted stone (see Ureteral Colic, Chapter 9, page 438).

Uroepithelial Cancer (Bladder, Ureter, Renal Pelvis). Transitional epithelium undergoes neoplastic transformation under the influence of substances excreted in the urine. Risk factors include tobacco, industrial chemicals, and certain chemotherapy agents (cyclophosphamide, ifosfamide). Gross or microscopic hematuria is the only early sign. Advanced disease extends into pelvic and retroperitoneal organs causing pain, fistulas, and obstructions.

Kidney Cancer. Most renal cancers arise from the epithelium, some having inherited (von Hippel–Lindau syndrome) or acquired mutations of the von Hippel–Lindau gene. Tobacco smoke is a major risk factor for renal cell carcinoma. Renal cancers may invade the renal vein and inferior vena cava. They metastasize to the lungs and invade retroperitoneal structures, including bone, causing pain. Microscopic hematuria may be present. Flank fullness or pressure may be present prior to the onset of pain.

Urinary Tract Infection. Infection is usually by enteric organisms ascending the urethra. Metastatic infection most often affects the kidney. Sexually transmitted organisms predominate in the lower tract (urethra, urethral glands, and prostate). The presence of foreign bodies (catheters, stents, stones) or obstruction leads to persistent and complicated infections. Symptoms and signs depend upon the specific site of infection.

Urethritis and urethral syndrome. Infection is by sexually transmitted organisms (*N. gonorrhea*, *C. trachomatis*, genital mycoplasmas, or herpes simplex) or complicates prolonged catheterization. Burning dysuria and purulent discharge demonstrated by urethral stripping are nearly uniform. Untreated, progression to upper tract infection is possible. Dysuria, urgency, and frequency with negative cultures for bacteria and lack of response to antibiotics define the *urethral syndrome*. The etiology is poorly understood and may result from viral infection or sterile inflammation.

Cystitis. Ascending bladder infection is common in normal women because of urethral colonization with enteric (e.g., *Escherichia coli*) and vaginal flora and the short urethra. Cystitis in men suggests an anatomic, usually obstructing, abnormality. Residual urine volume >100 mL is associated with increased risk of infection. Inflammation of the bladder wall and trigone causes urinary frequency, urgency, dysuria, and a sensation of incomplete voiding. Untreated, infection can ascend to the kidneys.

Acute pyelonephritis. Bacteria ascend from the bladder or, less commonly, reach the kidney via the bloodstream. Infection involves primarily the renal medulla and collecting system but may extend to the cortex or perinephritic tissue forming an abscess. Symptoms are fever, chills, and flank pain. Physical exam reveals costovertebral angle percussion tenderness. Prompt diagnosis and treatment prevents bacteremia, urosepsis, and local suppurative complications.

Chronic pyelonephritis. Chronic kidney infection is caused by nonpyogenic bacteria, including slowly growing, often intracellular organisms, such as tuberculosis and brucellosis. Chronic pyelonephritis is often asymptomatic until systemic symptoms (fever of unknown origin, anorexia, weight loss) occur. Sterile pyuria is the only sign. See Interstitial Nephritis below.

Vesicoureteral reflux. Ureterovesical valve incompetence leads to urine refluxing from the bladder into the ureters, increasing ureteral and renal pelvis pressures, creating a functional obstruction. This is common in young children, especially girls, and during pregnancy. It is associated with recurrent infections in addition to producing pressure-induced kidney injury. It may be asymptomatic with only abnormalities on urinalysis (pyuria, cellular casts, and proteinuria) and declining renal function.

Interstitial Cystitis. A condition of unknown cause results in often painful bladder wall inflammation leading to fibrosis and decreased bladder capacity. Interstitial cystitis is most common in women presenting with urinary frequency and bladder pain but with negative cultures. Diagnosis is by excluding other causes of bladder pain and frequency through a complete urologic evaluation.

CLINICAL VIGNETTES AND QUESTIONS

CASE 10-1

A 45-year-old man with a recent history of severe diarrhea and fatigue is found to have acute kidney injury based on his elevated blood urea nitrogen (BUN) and creatinine (baseline kidney function is normal). Blood pressure is 140/80 mm Hg while lying down and after standing it drops to 100/60 mm Hg. His laboratory work-up is significant for BUN of 100 mg/dL and serum creatinine of 4 mg/dL. His urine sodium is <20 mEq/L, urine osmolarity is high, and urine microscopy reveals bland sediment.

QUESTIONS:
1. How do you approach the differential diagnosis of acute kidney injury in this patient?
2. What are the most important physical examination findings to assess?
3. What finding on urine microscopy will assist you?
4. What is the most likely diagnosis and why?

CASE 10-2

A 75-year-old man is evaluated for hypoalbuminemia, hyperlipidemia, and slowly progressive proteinuria developing since his squamous cell lung cancer resection a year ago. BP is 140/86 mm Hg. Physical findings are decreased breath sounds in the right lower lobe consistent with his previous surgery and 3+ lower extremity edema. Chest film reveals a new 2-cm nodule in the left upper lobe. Labs: BUN 17 mg/dL; creatinine 1.0 mg/dL; urinalysis 4+ protein, and few oval fat bodies/high power field; 24 hour urine collection reveals 15 g of protein.

QUESTIONS:
1. What is the name for this syndrome and what are its clinical features?
2. What is the differential diagnosis for this presentation in adults and children?
3. What is the most likely diagnosis?

CASE 10-3

A 42-year-old man with recently diagnosed Budd–Chiari syndrome comes in for evaluation of new anemia. His urine dipstick is positive for blood (3+) but his urine microscopy does not show any erythrocytes.

QUESTIONS:
1. What causes hemoglobinuria?
2. How is it differentiated from hematuria?
3. What is the differential diagnosis of hemoglobinuria?
4. What is the most likely diagnosis?

CASE 10-4

A 23-year-old woman with a URI develops gross hematuria. Urinalysis shows 1+ protein, 1+ blood, 20 to 30 dysmorphic RBCs, and urine protein-to-creatinine ratio is 1.4 (~1.4 g of protein in 24 hours). Complement tests are normal.

QUESTIONS:
1. How would you differentiate glomerular from nonglomerular hematuria?
2. What are the three causes of isolated glomerular hematuria?
3. What is the most likely diagnosis?
4. How is this patient's presentation different from postinfectious glomerulonephritis?

CASE 10-5

A 55-year-old man with a 40 pack-year smoking history comes for evaluation of red urine. The urine dipstick shows heme and the urine microscopy confirms hematuria.

QUESTIONS:
1. What is the initial laboratory test to evaluate red urine?
2. In which situations do false positive dipsticks for heme occur?
3. What are some risk factors for malignancy in a patient presenting with hematuria?

CASE 10-6

A 50-year-old man on lithium for bipolar disorder complains of frequent urination. His 24-hour urine output has been close to 5 L and his serum sodium is between 142 and 144 mEq/L most of the time.

QUESTIONS:
1. Define polyuria.
2. What are three causes of excessive water diuresis?
3. What are the main clinical features of each?
4. What is the most likely diagnosis?

CHAPTER 11

The Female Genitalia and Reproductive System

OVERVIEW OF FEMALE REPRODUCTIVE PHYSIOLOGY

Male and female external genitalia arise from identical embryologic anlage. Phenotype development depends on the presence or absence of testosterone. Lack of the SRY gene (typically found on the Y chromosome) leads to development of ovaries and female sex organs. The female reproductive organs include the ovaries, ovarian ligaments, Fallopian tubes, uterus, vagina, vaginal and introital glands of Bartholin, labia minora and majora, and the clitoris with its covering prepuce. The labia majora and clitoris are cognates of the scrotum and penis respectively. Ambiguous genitalia reflect development and maturation from a mixed genetic substrate or hormone environment.

Pituitary follicle-stimulating hormone (FSH) cyclically stimulates the ovaries to mature one ovum within a follicle. The follicle produces estrogen causing endometrial proliferation. When the serum estrogen level reaches a threshold, a luteinizing hormone (LH) surge from the pituitary causes egg release and then the corpus luteum forms at the site of ovulation. The latter secretes progesterone which transforms the proliferating endometrium to its secretory phase. The released ovum, captured by the fimbriated end of the Fallopian tube, travels down the tube to the uterus. If fertilized, the ovum may implant into the receptive endometrium establishing a pregnancy. If implantation does not occur, the corpus luteum involutes after approximately 14 days and progesterone levels decline steeply. When an ovulation cycle is complete and the withdrawal of progesterone occurs, the endometrium sloughs as menstrual bleeding. FSH again rises stimulating development of another follicle. Implantation of a fertilized ovum leads to development of the trophoblastic cells which secretes human chorionic gonadotropin (HCG), which maintain the corpus luteum and suppresses pituitary FSH and LH and stopping ovulation and menstruation. Ultimately when the trophoblastic cells become a functional placenta, the corpus luteum will involute.

ANATOMY OF THE FEMALE GENITALIA AND REPRODUCTIVE SYSTEM

At puberty, the *mons pubis* overlying the symphysis pubis (Fig. 11-1) becomes covered with hair, the *female escutcheon*. The hair forms an inverted triangle with a horizontal upper border.

The Vulva: The female external genitalia is the vulva or pudendum (Fig. 11-2B). The *labia majora* are elevated ridges extending inferiorly from the mons pubis nearly to the anus. They contain fat, blood vessels, nerves,

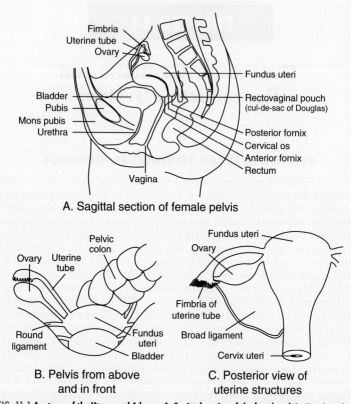

A. Sagittal section of female pelvis

B. Pelvis from above and in front

C. Posterior view of uterine structures

FIG. 11-1 Anatomy of the Uterus and Adnexa. A. Sagittal section of the female pelvis. Note the angle of the vagina with the vertical axis of the body, and the axis of the uterus perpendicular to the vaginal axis. The lips of the cervix are shown in the same plane as the anterior vaginal wall, which is shorter than the posterior wall. The rectovaginal pouch (cul-de-sac of Douglas) lies anterior to the rectal wall where it can be palpated during the rectal exam. The uterine fundus in the usual position is inaccessible to the rectal examining finger, but very close to palpation from the lower abdomen. **B. View of the pelvis from above and in front.** Note how the round ligament curves anteriorly and the uterine tubes curve posteriorly. **C. Posterior view of the uterus and broad ligaments (spread out).** Note the suspension of the ovary near the fimbriated end of the uterine tube. The uterine tube forms the upper border of the broad ligament.

and tissue resembling the dartos tunic in the scrotum. Medial to the labia majora are two smaller skin folds, the *labia minora*, running from the clitoris and uniting in a transverse fold, the *fourchette*, lying in front of the anus. The *clitoris*, the female erectile organ, is composed of two small corpora cavernosa surrounded superiorly by the prepuce and inferiorly by folds of the labia minora, the *frenulum*. Posterior to the clitoris is a cleft between the two labia minora, the *vestibule*, pierced by the *urethral meatus* and the *vaginal orifice*, posterior to the meatus. The vaginal opening is a median slit varying inversely with the size of the hymen. The *hymen* is a thin membrane covering part of the vaginal orifice. Commonly a perforate ring, widest posteriorly, the hymen may be cribriform, annular, fringed, or even imperforate. After

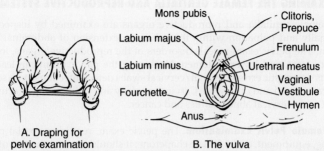

FIG. 11-2 Examination of the Vulva. A. Draping for pelvic examination. The patient assumes the lithotomy position with feet in stirrups projecting from the end of the examining table. A sheet is spread over the patient; the two lower corners are wrapped about the thighs and legs. The middle of the lower edge of the sheet is slackly draped over the lower abdomen. **B. Topographic anatomy of the vulva.** The recessed vestibule contains a relatively small vaginal orifice, surrounded by one of the usual patterns of unruptured hymen. Bordering the vestibule are the two projecting folds of often deeply pigmented skin, the labia minora. Anteriorly, accessory folds of the labia form the prepuce enclosing the clitoris. Lateral to the labia minora are two parallel ridges of skin and fat forming the labium majus.

rupture, the hymenal remnants heal as irregular folds of mucosa. Two pairs of glands open onto the vestibule: the *paraurethral (Skene) glands* open just inferior to the urethra and the *greater vestibular (Bartholin) glands* open on the posterior edge of the vaginal orifice.

The Vagina, Uterus, and Adnexa: From its orifice, the *vagina* extends posteriorly into the pelvis (Fig. 11-1). It is an elongated tubular collapsed space with a posterior wall ~ 9 cm long and a shorter 6–7.5 cm anterior wall. The walls reflect onto the *uterine cervix* located most commonly at the vagina's anterior apex. The vaginal recess behind the cervix is the *posterior fornix* and recesses on either side are *lateral fornices*. The vaginal mucosa is thrown into transverse rugae, separated by furrows of variable depths. The nulliparous cervix is a smooth button with a rounded face pierced by the *cervical os*. The parous cervix may be somewhat irregular and large with an oval-shaped cervical os. The anterior and posterior lips of the cervix usually contact the posterior vaginal wall. The *urethra* and *bladder* lie ventral to the anterior vaginal wall and the *rectum* lies behind the posterior wall. The peritoneal cavity extends behind the posterior fornix, interposed between the rectum and the cervix, forming the *rectovaginal pouch* (cul-de-sac of Douglas). The muscular uterus is shaped like an inverted pear, is mobile and can flex anteriorly or posteriorly from the fulcrum of the cervicovaginal junction. From each side of the uterine fundus a *Fallopian tube* curves laterally and posteriorly ~10 cm into the pelvis. The tubes, suspended by the *mesosalpinges*, are the upper borders of the *broad ligaments* spreading from the lateral edges of the uterus to the pelvic wall. The *uterus* and broad ligaments form a transverse septum dividing the pelvis into anterior and posterior fossae. The *ovaries* are on the posterior surface of the broad ligaments, medial to and below the fimbriated ends of the Fallopian tubes. They are suspended by the *ovarian ligaments* attached to the uterus and the *suspensory ligaments* attached to the pelvic wall.

EXAMING THE FEMALE GENITALIA AND REPRODUCTIVE SYSTEM

The female genitalia and reproductive organs are examined by inspection externally and palpation within the pelvis, an extension of abdominal palpation. The pelvic exam reveals disorders of the reproductive organs, lower urinary tract, and lower abdomen. Neglecting the pelvic exam can lead to serious diagnostic errors. Vaginal/cervical swabs detect infections, both sexually transmitted and otherwise. Cervical cytology and HPV testing effectively detect early cervical abnormalities and cancer.

The Female Pelvic Examination: The pelvic exam, requiring special positioning, equipment, and a female chaperone; it should come at the end of the physical exam. Always talk the patient through each phase of the exam. After emptying her bladder, the patient is positioned supine on the exam table with a sheet covering the abdomen, pelvis and legs. Sit on a low stool within reach of a side table holding specula, forceps, gauze, gloves, lubricating jelly, and the materials for cytology and cultures. Placing her feet in the foot-holders, expose the perineum keeping the lower corners of the sheet around her legs (Fig. 11-2A). Put on gloves and shine a bright light onto the perineum. The following sequence is suggested: (1) inspect the vulva; (2) insert the vaginal speculum; (3) collect specimens for cytology and microbiologic tests; (4) inspect the vaginal walls and cervix; (5) perform bimanual examination of the uterus and adnexa; and (6) finish with a rectovaginal exam if indicated.

Inspection and palpation of the vulva. Inspect the perineum for swelling, ulcers, lesions, and color changes (Fig. 11-2B). Separating the labia with thumb and forefinger inspect the clitoris, vestibule, urethral meatus, and vaginal orifice. Palpate for vestibular tenderness, then for Bartholin gland enlargement posterior-lateral to the hymen. Have the patient strain as if to defecate looking for bulging of the anterior or posterior vaginal wall or urine leakage.

Vaginal speculum exam. Speculum exam with lubrication options including jelly or mineral oil precedes digital exam (Fig. 11-3). Use a bivalve speculum of suitable size to separate the vaginal walls for inspection of the vagina and cervix and collection of samples for cytology and microbiology. A Pedersen speculum is typically adequate for women who have not had a vaginal delivery. Graves's speculums are best for parous or obese. Separate the labia minora at the level of the posterior fourchette, then, with the other hand holding the speculum blades closed, insert the speculum into the vagina with slight downward pressure to avoid pinching the urethra against the symphysis pubis. When the speculum tips reach the upper vagina, separate the blades while illuminating the vaginal cavity with a suitable light. Move the speculum handle so the blade tips expose the cervix then lock the blades open. If a discharge is present, determine whether it is from the cervical os or the vagina. Obtain a sample of the discharge for microscopic examination. If the cervical os is obscured by discharge, gently sponge it with a large, sterile cotton swab. Obtain specimens from the cervix for cytology and from the cervix and vagina for appropriate cultures. Collection of cytology from the cervix often causes some slight bleeding from the cervical ectropion and will stop without intervention in almost all cases. Inspect the cervix for color, lacerations, ulcers, and new growths. Inspect the cervical os for size, shape,

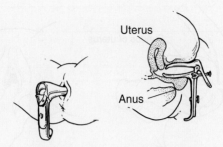

A. Insert speculum   B. Spread blades
                         of speculum

FIG. 11-3 Using the Vaginal Speculum. The labia minora are retracted laterally with the gloved index and middle fingers. The closed blades of the vaginal speculum are inserted in the vagina with the widths of the blades almost horizontal. **A. Speculum in position.** The closed speculum blades are well inserted at a 30-degree to 45-degree angle posteriorly. Then the blades separated and locked open. **B. A sagittal section shows the open speculum in proper position.** The upper shorter blade lifts the vault of the vagina exposing the cervix on the anterior vaginal wall.

color, discharge, and polyps. Unlock the blades and *inspect the vaginal walls* by rotating the speculum to expose the entire cavity. Finally, carefully withdraw the speculum while inspecting the mucosa, while at the same time allowing the speculum to close during this withdrawal.

Bimanual pelvic exam. Always use the same hand for vaginal exam, most commonly the examiners dominant hand. In these directions, the right hand is arbitrarily assigned to the vagina as the left hand palpates the abdomen. When possible, use two fingers for vaginal examination. Place the gloved right hand in this position: index and middle fingers straight and close together, thumb widely abducted, fourth and fifth fingers folded into the palm. Lubricate the straight fingers. Spread the labia with the left thumb and forefinger to avoid the discomfort of pulling pubic hair into the vagina. Put gentle downward pressure on the fourchette while inserting the two lubricated fingers into the vagina with the finger pads facing the anterior vaginal wall (Fig. 11-4A). Examine each structure systematically forming a mental picture of your observations. The *greater vestibular glands* (vulvovaginal glands or Bartholin glands) are examined with the forefinger inside the vagina and the thumb opposite and outside on the posterior part of the labium majus feeling the inner wall for abscess or tenderness (Fig. 11-4B). Evert that part of the vaginal mucosa looking for a red spot or pus at the opening of an inflamed duct. The normal glands and ducts cannot be seen or felt. The *urethra* is palpated for mobility, tenderness or induration in the midline of the anterior vaginal wall near the introitus. The *base of bladder* is similarly palpated halfway between the introitus and the cervix. Palpate the *vaginal wall* for tenderness, induration (from scars, granulomas, or neoplasm), strictures, septa, and adhesions (not to be confused with the normal transverse rugae). Next, examine the *cervix*. It normally feels like a button, with a convex face and a central depression, the consistency of the tip of the nose. Feel for nodules and ulcers and note any abnormality of shape, size, or consistency. Determine the axis

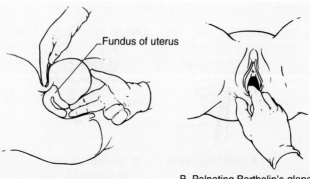

A. Bimanual pelvic examination

B. Palpating Bartholin's gland
(vulvovaginal gland)

FIG. 11-4 Bimanual Pelvic Examination. A. Palpation of the uterus. The index and middle fingers of the gloved right hand are inserted in the vagina with the tips of the fingers facing anteriorly and touching the cervix. The fingers of the left hand are pressed deep into the abdomen above the mons pubis, pushing the uterine fundus downward and forward toward the two vaginal fingers. The adnexa are examined similarly, except the vaginal fingers are placed to the side of the uterus and the abdominal fingers are pushed into the belly at a point 2–3 cm medial to the anterior superior iliac spine. Attempt to approximate the fingertips of the two examining hands. The abdominal fingers are pulled inferiorly to push the tube and ovary onto the tips of the vaginal fingers. **B. Palpation of the greater vestibular gland (Bartholin gland).** The index finger is inserted in the vagina near the posterior introitus. With the thumb pressing on the labium majus outside, the finger and thumb are approximated.

of the cervix; most commonly it faces posteriorly. Examine the *uterine corpus and fundus* bimanually by pushing the cervix anteriorly while the fingers of the left-hand press into the abdomen just above the symphysis. Estimate the size of the uterus, its axis, tenderness, mobility, and characterize any nodules. To examine the *adnexa*, place the vaginal fingers on one side of the cervix and push their tips superiorly and posteriorly as far as possible. With the fingers of the left hand, locate a point on the same side of the abdomen 2–3 cm medial to the anterior superior iliac spine. Push the abdominal fingers deep, their tips approaching the vaginal fingers while feeling for the uterine tubes and ovaries between the two hands. If the structures are not felt, move the fingertips of both hands inferiorly toward the pubis passing the adnexa between the two hands. Abdominal pressure should be deep but gentle. Pressing the two hands a little closer each time the patient expires avoids abdominal guarding. The abdominal hand displaces the structures while the vaginal hand feels them. The ovary and tube are usually not palpable. The normal *Fallopian tube* is ~4 mm in diameter, half the size of a pencil, with the consistency of rubber tubing. The normal *ovary* is ~3 cm × 2 cm × 2 cm. The ovary is soft and naturally tender to palpation. Look for enlargement or asymmetry of the adnexa, unusual tenderness, decreased mobility, and masses or induration. Examine the *pelvic floor*, noting the size of the introitus. With the fingers turned posteriorly, press the pelvic floor inferiorly and posteriorly to assess for loss of support.

Rectovaginal exam. Women with any rectal complaints, history of cancer, radiation etc or those over 50 years of age should have a rectovaginal exam.

After changing gloves, insert the gloved middle finger into the anal canal with the forefinger in the vagina, palpating the ***rectovaginal wall*** between the two fingers. A thickened rectovaginal septum or parametrium suggests spread of cervical carcinoma, puerperal infection, or pelvic inflammatory disease. Note distortion or defects in the circular ***anal sphincter muscle***, a common consequence of vaginal delivery. Next, palpate the ***anal canal*** for intrinsic lesions (see Chapter 9, page 428). Palpate the ***anterior rectal wall*** (posterior vaginal wall) for tenderness and masses then systematically examine the ***lateral and posterior rectum and ampulla***.

Pelvic examination via the rectum. The pelvis is best examined through the vagina; however, for virgins exam can be done via the rectum. While using the left hand to press on the lower abdomen as in the bimanual vaginal examination, palpate the pelvis. Through the anterior rectal wall, locate the cervix; attempt to feel the body and fundus of the uterus. This may be the only way to palpate a retroverted uterus. Insert your finger fully and palpate the anterior rectal wall in the region of the peritoneal rectovaginal pouch (cul-de-sac of Douglas; Fig. 11-1).

FEMALE GENITAL AND REPRODUCTIVE SYMPTOMS

General Symptoms

Pelvic pain. Pain arises from inflammation, usually from infection, distention of tubular structures or cysts, traction on serosal surfaces by masses or adhesions, hemorrhage, and invasion of sensitive structures by neoplasms or implantation of endometrial tissue. Visceral pain is poorly localized by the patient whereas serosal pain is usually well localized. Pelvic pain is common. Obtain a complete history of the pain pattern, its relationship to menses, ovulation, bowel movements, urination, and physical and sexual activity. Assess for the possibility of pregnancy. Chronic pelvic pain is typically multifactorial, thus it is vital to discuss history of trauma, (sexual, physical and emotional). Describe the pain quality using the patient's words. The patient must be relaxed and the pelvic exam gentle to localize the pain to a specific area or structure.

CLINICAL OCCURRENCE: *Congenital:* Imperforate hymen, porphyria; *Endocrine:* Ectopic pregnancy, functional ovarian cyst; *Degenerative/ Idiopathic:* Ovarian cyst (especially with hemorrhage or rupture), endometriosis, ovulation (mittelschmerz), diverticulosis; *Infectious:* Cervicitis, endometritis, salpingitis, pelvic inflammatory disease, tubo-ovarian abscess, cystitis, diverticulitis and diverticular abscess, appendicitis; *Inflammatory/ Immune:* Inflammatory bowel disease, appendicitis; *Mechanical/Traumatic:* Ovarian torsion, tubal pregnancy; *Neoplastic:* Any locally invasive cancer (e.g., cervical, endometrial, rectal, bladder), metastases, degenerating leiomyoma; *Psychosocial:* Physical, emotional, and sexual abuse; *Vascular:* Ovarian infarction (torsion).

Painful menstruation (dysmenorrhea). Primary dysmenorrhea results from uterine ischemia caused by myometrial contraction under the influence of prostaglandins released during menstruation. The most frequent complaint is severe suprapubic cramping. Backache and headache are less severe. Dysmenorrhea may disappear after a pregnancy. Prostaglandin inhibitors can be quite helpful and may be used prophylactically. Pain that accompanies menses arising from a pelvic source (e.g., endometriosis, pelvic neoplasms, and pelvic inflammations disease) is *secondary dysmenorrhea*.

Painful intercourse (dyspareunia). Mechanical stimulation of pelvic structures during vaginal intercourse can lead to pain preventing sexual enjoyment. Apprehension increases pain perception. Ask if the pain is felt during or after intercourse, and if felt superficially or deeply after penetration. Ask specifically whether the patient has sufficient stimulation to become sexually aroused, about the sufficiency of vaginal lubrication, whether the partner is so aggressive as to cause trauma, and about bleeding after intercourse. Inquire about sexual practices, including the use of foreign bodies as stimulants, rectal intercourse, and whether previous experiences have produced fear of intercourse (e.g., rape, incest, molestation, and physical and emotional abuse). Common causes are insufficient foreplay, inadequate lubrication, postmenopausal estrogen deficiency with atrophy of vaginal mucosa, vaginismus (reflex spasm of muscles around the lower vaginal opening), vulvar vestibulitis, lichen planus, perineal trauma and lacerations, pelvic and perineal infections, pelvic tumors, endometriosis, contact dermatitis.

Menstrual disorders. See Female Reproductive Syndromes. Menstrual Disorders, page 499.

Vulvar and Vaginal Symptoms
Vulvar pain. The vulva is somatically innervated, so pain is well localized. Infection, inflammation, and local trauma are the most common identifiable causes. *Dysesthetic vulvodynia* may be neuropathic and *vulvar vestibulitis* may have an inflammatory basis.

Vaginal pain—vaginismus. Painful contraction of the pubococcygeus muscle around the lower third of the vagina results in severe persistent or intermittent pain. The cause is unknown, and treatment is difficult. Intercourse is painful or impossible.

Vulvar pruritus. Vulvar itching is usually the result of obvious disease or chemical irritation of the vulvar skin. *Candida* (and other yeast) infection and lichen sclerosis are common etiologies. This symptom is also often associated with diabetes and obesity.

Vaginal bleeding. See Female Reproductive Tract Syndromes—Menstrual Disorders, page 499.

FEMALE GENITAL AND REPRODUCTIVE SIGNS
Vulvar Signs
Ambiguous genitalia—intersexuality. Refer to special works on this subject.

Genital ulcer. Trauma and sexually transmitted diseases are the most common causes. Painless ulcers are most typical of syphilis. Painful ulcers are most likely Herpes Simplex Virus (HSV). Ulcers increase the risk of acquiring and transmitting sexually transmitted infections (STIs) including HIV. Because of persistent warmth and moisture, ulcers tend to be both more painful and slower healing in women than men. See also Chapter 12, page 514.

CLINICAL OCCURRENCE: *Degenerative/Idiopathic:* Lichen sclerosis; *Inflammatory/Immune:* Behçet syndrome, vulvar vestibulitis, fixed drug reaction, lichen planus; *Infectious:* Herpes simplex types 1 and 2, chlamydia, syphilis, chancroid, lymphogranuloma venereum, HIV, cytomegalovirus, Epstein–Barr virus, granuloma inguinale; *Mechanical/Traumatic:* Inadequate lubrication during intercourse; *Neoplastic:* Squamous cell cancer.

Vulvar rash. Determine if the rash is acute or chronic, pruritic, weeping or scaling, associated with bleeding or pain, or with the use of topical and systemic medications, creams, and lotions.

CLINICAL OCCURRENCE: See also Vulvar Inflammation—Vulvitis, below. *Endocrine:* Atrophic vulvovaginitis; *Degenerative/Idiopathic:* Lichen sclerosis; *Infectious:* Candidiasis, dermatophytes, cellulitis, abscess of skin and mucosal glands; *Inflammatory/Immune:* Contact dermatitis; *Mechanical/Traumatic:* Abrasions and lacerations, tight-fitting clothing with poor ventilation; *Metabolic/Toxic:* Diabetes mellitus; *Neoplastic:* Bowen disease, vulvar carcinoma; *Psychosocial:* Pruritus vulvae, pruritus ani.

Vulvar inflammation—vulvitis. It occurs alone or is associated with vaginitis and discharge. The skin is often red, warm, and variably edematous and tender. Alternatively, the skin is thinned, atrophic or opaque, and white. The latter changes are common in lichen sclerosis and lichen planus.

CLINICAL OCCURRENCE: *Infectious:* cellulitis, candida, dermatophyte, *Inflammatory/Immune:* Contact dermatitis, vulvar vestibulitis, lichen planus, lichen sclerosis; *Mechanical/Traumatic:* topical irritants, tight-fitting clothing; *Neoplastic:* diffuse Bowen disease.

Atrophic vulvovaginitis. Estrogen withdrawal leads to skin which is thin, delicate, inelastic, and easily irritated and inflamed. A careful history focusing on menstrual pattern and symptoms of estrogen insufficiency, especially hot flashes and urinary urgency, point to the diagnosis. Examination shows absent rugae and a thin dry mucosa (page 493).

Vulvar swelling, masses, and growths. All normal vulvar structures are susceptible to neoplastic change. Infection with human papilloma virus or syphilis can produce condylomas. Evaluation is identical to other skin growths with special respect for the sensitivity of the tissues and the need to maintain cosmesis.

CLINICAL OCCURRENCE: *Infectious:* Syphilis (condyloma latum), human papilloma virus (condyloma acuminatum), histoplasmosis; *Inflammatory/Immune:* Granulomatous disease; *Mechanical/Traumatic:* Obstructed mucosal glands and Bartholin and Skene glands, epidermal inclusion cyst; *Neoplastic:* Bowen disease, melanoma, invasive squamous cell cancer.

Diffuse swelling of the vulva. Lymphatic obstruction produces lymphedema of the labia and surrounding tissues. Likewise, the labia will be edematous when systemic venous pressure is very high and dependent edema reaches above the inguinal ligaments, for example, advanced right ventricular failure or constrictive pericarditis. Irritation may produce hypertrophy of the labia. Look for local irritation and history and physical findings of systemic disease affecting the lymphatics or venous system.

Hematoma. A large, painful, bluish labial swelling may occur within a few hours after local trauma. Without a history of trauma, hematoma may be confused with cellulitis.

Labioinguinal hernia. Failure of the peritoneal pouch to obliterate in the fetus permits a hernia to descend from the abdomen into the labium majus. It presents with visible swelling and is analogous to a scrotal hernia in males.

Abscess of the greater vestibular gland (Bartholin gland abscess). The normal glands are not palpable, and their ducts are not visible. Bartholin gland cysts are common and typically asymptomatic. Infection of the cyst leads to an abscess which may track to the skin or toward the ischiorectal fossa. Cysts and smaller abscesses are found only by vaginal examination (Fig. 11-4B). Inflammation causes a red spot at the duct orifice, and pus may be expressed. If the abscess is large, the posterior labium is swollen and fluctuant, and the skin is tender, hot, and red.

Urethral Meatus Abnormalities
Urethritis. See also Urinary Syndromes, Urinary Tract Infections—Urethritis, Chapter 10, page 479. A purulent discharge from the meatus is usually caused by *Neisseria gonorrhoea*, *Chlamydia trachomatis*, genital mycoplasmas, or herpes simplex. Palpating the anterior vaginal wall beginning at the cervix and stroking toward the meatus reveals urethral tenderness and induration, and pus may be squeezed from the meatus. A urethral diverticulum may also produce pus.

Urethral caruncle. This papilloma appears as a small red mass in the meatus or the visible portion of the urethra. It usually occurs as a complication of urethritis. It may be tender and painful with urination.

Periurethral (skene) gland and duct inflammation. The periurethral gland (Skene gland) lies on either side of, and posterior to, the female urethra, just inside the meatus. It may become the site of chronic infection. If inflamed, the mouth of the duct is visible and red, when viewed by spreading the meatus.

Urethral prolapse. Slight gaping of the meatus is common in the multipara. When more severe, the urethral mucosa protrudes from the meatus becoming tender and inflamed.

Vagina Signs
Vaginal ulcers. The causes are the same as for ulcers of the vulva (page 490).

Vaginal discharge. A clear to slightly white vaginal discharge containing mucous, epithelial cells, and commensal bacteria (particularly lactobacilli) at a pH of 4.0 is normal. Infection and/or inflammation leads to increased mucous production and exudation of white blood cells from the mucosa, producing vaginal discharges. Depending upon etiology, discharges vary from thick white to thin, frothy, and bloody with variable odor, pH, and accompanying pruritus. Common causes are atrophic vaginitis, contact dermatitis, bacterial vaginosis, *Candida*, *Trichomonas*, cytolytic vaginosis, retained tampons, pessary, foreign body, vaginal and cervical cancers (often bloody).

Vaginitis. Inflammation of the vaginal mucosa from infection, allergy, or irritants leads to erythema. History and examination of the vaginal secretions usually yields a diagnosis.

CLINICAL OCCURRENCE: *Degenerative/idiopathic:* Vaginal atrophy; *Infectious:* *Candida*, *Trichomonas*, bacterial vaginosis, viral enanthems, cytolytic vaginosis; *Inflammatory/Immune:* Contact dermatitis, Behçet disease; *Mechanical/Traumatic:* Retained foreign body, inadequate lubrication during intercourse; *Neoplastic:* Diffuse Bowen disease.

Bacterial vaginosis. This is one of the most common causes of vaginitis in women of childbearing age. They present with a thick, off-white, malodorous discharge with a "fishy smell" and a pH >4.5. Diagnosis is confirmed by finding clue cells (exfoliated vaginal epithelial cells to which *Gardnerella vaginalis* adhere) in vaginal secretions. Cultures are of no value because *G. vaginalis* is present in 50%–60% of healthy women.

Vulvovaginal candidiasis. Itching, irritation, pain, dyspareunia, with erythema and edema characterize infection with *Candida* spp. The discharge has a normal vaginal pH (<4.6); pseudohyphae and neutrophils are seen in a 10% KOH preparation. Culture may be needed to confirm the diagnosis and distinguish it from less-common atypical yeast such as *glabrata*, which do not respond to usual treatments as well as potential noninfectious causes.

Trichomonas vaginitis. *Trichomonas vaginalis* produces a tender, reddened mucosa, studded with small hemorrhagic spots. The resulting malodorous discharge is yellow-green to gray and frequently frothy with a pH of 5.0–6.0. In a more chronic stage, the vaginal mucosa contains scattered red papules, giving a granular appearance. Rapid diagnosis may be made by suspending a bit of discharge in isotonic saline solution and finding many neutrophils and mobile trichomonads by microscopic examination. Urine sample can be sent for polymerase chain reaction testing for trichomonas.

Atrophic vaginitis. The vaginal mucosa is estrogen dependent and following menopause becomes thin, dry, and smooth without rugae. The thin and tender mucosa contains abraded patches and adhesions that bleed easily. Frequently, a serosanguineous discharge with a pH >6.0 results due to the lack of lactobacilli.

Cytolytic vaginosis. Overgrowth of *Lactobacillus* spp. produces a low vaginal pH leading to breakdown of epithelial cells and inflammation. The vaginal pH is 3.5–4.5, and microscopic examination shows few polymorphonuclear cells, cytolytic changes in the epithelial cells, and no evidence of *Candida*, *Trichomonas*, or bacterial vaginosis.

Blue vagina—cyanosis. The mucosa becomes cyanotic from local venous engorgement in pregnancy, a pelvic tumor, or congestive cardiac failure.

Vaginal neoplasm. Neoplasms in the vaginal mucosa may be primary or secondary to carcinoma of the uterus, rectum, bladder, or external genitalia.

Vaginal polyp. Polyps arise from the vaginal wall or extend from the cervix. Polypoid deformities of the vaginal apex following hysterectomy are common.

Rectovaginal pouch mass. Being the most dependent portion of the abdominal cavity, the rectovaginal pouch collects fluid, exfoliated cells, and mobile masses from within the abdomen. Masses include prolapsed ovary, bowel loops, carcinoma of the colon, implants of endometriosis or ovarian carcinoma, a rectal shelf formed by other intraabdominal cancer, or an accumulation of pus, fluid, or blood from abdominal lesions.

Rectovaginal fistula. The rectovaginal wall breaks down after extensive radiation, obstetrical trauma, surgery, Crohn disease, and malignancy. Fecal contamination of the vagina suggests a fistula from rectum to vagina. The mouth of the fistula may be palpable as a small indurated area in the posterior vaginal wall; the orifice may be visible on speculum exam. The rectal wall may also be indurated from scar tissue.

Pelvic floor relaxation. The muscular pelvic floor is pierced by the rectum, vagina, and urethra. Vaginal delivery stretches and may tear the muscles. These are repaired at the time of delivery, however many women note relaxation of the muscles. Tearing of the urethral and anal sphincters can also occur. Inadequate support of the pelvic organs leads to loss of sphincter functions and prolapse of tissues. Patients complain of incontinence, feelings of pressure and fullness, and visible or palpable prolapse of tissues. Pelvic floor physical therapy can greatly improve these symptoms once healed after delivery.

Enlarged introitus. When the hymen is ruptured, the vaginal orifice normally admits two fingers. When three fingers are accommodated, the introitus is enlarged, usually indicating pelvic relaxation from childbirth. This is typically asymptomatic and not pathologic.

Cystocele (bladder prolapse). When the patient stands or strains, the anterior vaginal wall containing a portion of the bladder bulges into the vagina and may emerge from the introitus as a soft, spherical tumor (Fig. 11-5B). This usually indicates pelvic floor injury during childbirth.

Rectocele (rectal prolapse). When the patient stands or strains, the posterior vaginal wall, containing a portion of the rectum, protrudes into the vagina and may emerge from the introitus (Fig. 11-5B). Exam in the left decubitus position may detect larger rectoceles as compared to exam of the supine patient.

Uterine prolapse. Loss of the normal ligamentous support for the uterus causes the cervix to protrude from the introitus on standing or straining.

Cervix Signs

Discharge—endocervicitis. The columnar epithelium of the endocervix is particularly susceptible to infection with gonococci, chlamydia, herpes, and genital mycoplasmas. A mucopurulent or purulent discharge emerges from the os (Fig. 11-5A). The cervical lips are usually inflamed and eroded. If tenderness is absent when palpating the uterine fundus, infection limited to the cervical canal is likely. Acute cervicitis is usually caused by gonococcal or chlamydia infection. Infection extending into the uterine cavity and tubes produces endometritis and pelvic inflammatory disease, which can lead to tubo-ovarian abscess, permanent hydrosalpinges and sterility.

Endometritis. See Uterine Signs—Endometritis, page 497.

Cervical ulcer. There is a loss of epithelium and sloughing of underlying tissue. Specific causes are herpes simplex, chancroid, syphilis, tuberculosis, and carcinoma. Biopsy is indicated when tests for infection are negative. This can result from the abrasion of a pessary or other chronic foreign body.

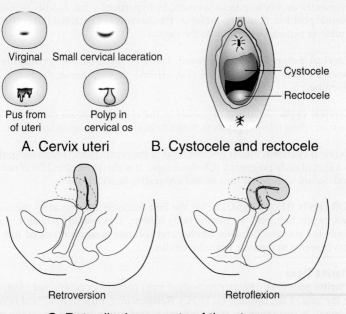

Virginal   Small cervical laceration

Cystocele

Rectocele

Pus from of uteri   Polyp in cervical os

A. Cervix uteri   B. Cystocele and rectocele

Retroversion   Retroflexion

C. Retrodisplacements of the uterus

FIG. 11-5 Some Pelvic Signs. A. Lesions of the cervix. The lacerations of childbirth leave various scars. Pus or a polyp may be seen coming out from the os. **B. Cystocele and rectocele.** When the patient is asked to strain as if to defecate, the introitus widens and bulging may develop anteriorly (cystocele) or posteriorly (rectocele). **C. Uterine displacements.** If the axis of the uterus remains straight and the whole organ is tilted, it is *retroversion*. If the axis of the uterus is bent, the condition is *retroflexion*.

Cervical carcinoma. A bloody discharge frequently follows straining or coitus. Whereas a cervical polyp is small and soft, a hard mass in the cervix suggests a neoplasm and should prompt cytology and biopsy. Chronic ulceration with induration is a late sign of carcinoma. Extensive ulceration, induration, and nodularity make the diagnosis obvious.

Lacerations. During vaginal delivery, the cervix frequently sustains laceration (Fig. 11-5A). Commonly, the tears are transverse and bilateral; occasionally, laceration is unilateral. Multiple tears produce a stellate appearance. Recently torn edges appear raw. Healing leaves scarred fissures or notches that can be felt on bimanual exam. The cleft lips may be everted. Overall, healing after repaired vaginal lacerations results in a visibly normal appearing vaginal introitus and patients are asymptomatic after adequate healing time.

Eversion or ectropion. Velvety red mucosa, without ulceration, extending outward from the cervical os usually results from migration of endocervical tissue onto the visible portions of the cervix.

Hypertrophic cervix. The hypertrophic cervix enlarges and elongates but retains its normal shape, whereas neoplasm distorts the shape. This most frequently occurs in parous women. In hypertrophy the fundus retains its normal position; in uterine prolapse, the cervix is not enlarged but only more visible as fundus descends into the vagina.

Cervical polyp. A soft, bright-red, benign tumor, usually pedunculated, emerges from the cervical os (Fig. 11-5A). It may cause discharge and bleeding.

Cervical cysts. Occlusion of glands in the cervical mucosa causes 1–3 mm clear or white retention cysts (*nabothian cysts*) visible on speculum exam.

Cervical cyanosis. Bluish discoloration of the cervix from venous congestion is a sign of early pregnancy (*Chadwick sign*). It is also present in 25% of normal and occurs with pelvic tumors and congestive heart failure.

Soft cervix (Hegar sign). During the first trimester of pregnancy the cervix and its junction with the uterine body softens. This is easily palpable; sometimes the contrast between fundus and isthmus is so pronounced that the cervix seems to separate from the fundus.

Uterine Signs
Uterine positions. The uterine body is most commonly positioned anteriorly in the axis of the cervix (Fig. 11-5C). *Retroversion*, present in 25% of normal women, is displacement of both fundus and cervix toward the spine with the cervix facing the anterior vaginal wall. The fundus may be felt through the anterior rectal wall. When freely movable it is asymptomatic; fixation suggests endometriosis or other scarring process. *Retroflexion* is posterior displacement of the fundus only, with the cervix in the normal position. The fundus is palpable through the posterior fornix and rectum. *Lateral displacement* of the uterus is caused by adhesions, adnexal or pelvic masses.

Tenderness—endometritis. Tenderness of the uterine body or fundus indicates endometrial infection. Endometritis is caused by sexually transmitted diseases (gonorrhea, chlamydia, and mycoplasmas) or by infection following childbirth or abortion or other instrumentation of the uterus.

Uterine enlargement. An enlarged uterus requires a specific explanation.

Pregnancy. Generalized uterine enlargement in a woman of childbearing age is considered a pregnancy until proven otherwise. Initially, the gravid uterus becomes more rounded. Other symptoms and signs of pregnancy are nausea with or without vomiting (morning sickness), fatigue, tenderness of the breasts, pelvic cramping, amenorrhea, cyanosis of the vaginal and cervical mucosa (*Chadwick sign*), softening of the cervix, and softening of the uterine isthmus (*Hegar sign*). Pregnancy testing is mandatory (via urine point of care or serum beta HCG testing). Ultrasonography can identify an intrauterine pregnancy as early as 5–6 weeks gestation and fetal heart tones should be heard around 6–7 weeks gestation. Ultrasound will likely also identify a corpus luteum or other simple ovarian cysts in early pregnancy. The height of the uterus reflects the stage of pregnancy: 12 weeks, at the pubis; 20 weeks, at the umbilicus; 36–40 weeks, at the xiphoid.

Leiomyoma (fibroid). A firm, often painless growth, firmly attached to the uterus, moves with the fundus. Fibroids are the most common benign tumor of the female genital tract. They are frequently multiple and can arise from multiple different uterine sites. Pedunculated fibroids hang off the surface of the uterus on a stalk, and subserosal or intramural are within the muscle of the uterus. Finally, submucosal or intracavitary fibroids impinge or are located within the uterine cavity. Intracavitary fibroids notoriously cause the most significant abnormal bleeding. An asymmetric gravid uterus is sometimes mistaken for a uterine fibroid in a woman of childbearing age. A markedly enlarged fibroid uterus may be felt above the symphysis pubis as a hard, multinodular mass. Vaginal exam demonstrates that the masses move with the cervix indicating attachment to the uterus. Transvaginal ultrasound, with or without intrauterine saline infusion, is the imaging test of choice for fibroid diagnosis.

Uterine neoplasm. With carcinoma and sarcoma, the uterus can be symmetrically or asymmetrically enlarged. There may be a bloody discharge. Leiomyosarcoma, cancer arising from a leiomyoma, is very rare and occurs in 0.4 to 0.64 per 100,000 women when benign fibroids occur in as many as 60% of women.

Endometrial neoplasm. With adenocarcinoma vaginal bleeding is the most common presentation. Clear cell and other more rare subtypes can present with watery discharge, pelvic pain, or endometrial thickening on ultrasound.

Adnexal Signs
Endometriosis. See Female Genital and Reproductive Syndromes, Endometriosis, page 503.

Adnexal tenderness. Pain arises from inflammation, usually infection, and from distention of tubular structures or cysts, traction on serosal surfaces by masses or adhesions, hemorrhage, and invasion of sensitive structures by neoplasms or implantation of endometrial tissue. Obtain a history of the pain pattern, its relationship to menses, ovulation, bowel movements, urination, and physical and sexual activities. The patient must be relaxed and the exam gentle to localize the pain to a specific area or structure.

CLINICAL OCCURRENCE: *Congenital:* Imperforate hymen, porphyria; *Degenerative/Idiopathic:* Ovarian cysts (especially with hemorrhage or rupture), ovulation (mittelschmerz), endometriosis, diverticulosis; *Infectious:* Cervicitis, endometritis, salpingitis, pelvic inflammatory disease, tubo-ovarian abscess, cystitis, diverticulitis and diverticular abscess, appendicitis; *Inflammatory/Immune:* Inflammatory bowel disease, appendicitis; *Mechanical/Traumatic:* Ovarian torsion, ectopic/tubal pregnancy; *Neoplastic:* Locally invasive cancer (e.g., ovarian, cervical, endometrial, rectal, bladder, metastatic); *Vascular:* Ovarian infarction (torsion), septic pelvic thrombophlebitis, ovarian vein thrombosis.

Adnexal mass—pelvic inflammatory disease (salpingitis, hydrosalpinx, pyosalpinx, tubo-ovarian abscess). Infection ascends from the cervix via the endometrium. Sexually transmitted organisms (gonorrhea, chlamydia, myco-plasmas) often initiate infection, but aerobic and anaerobic enteric florae are frequent components in advanced infection. Negative testing for STIs does not eliminate the possibility of pelvic inflammatory disease or a tubo-ovarian abscess. With acute infections, the Fallopian tubes are tender and swollen, frequently obscuring the separate adnexal structures. Moving the uterus and cervix is extremely painful, a sign called *cervical motion tenderness*. In chronic disease, the exudate and fibrosis around the tubes feels like an unyielding mass, *a frozen pelvis*. When adhesions or inflammation seal a tube at both ends it may fill with fluid or pus, respectively a *hydrosalpinx* or *pyosalpinx*, felt as a sausage-shaped mass and appears on ultrasound as a tubular fluid filled structure separate from the ovary. When the ovary and broad ligament are involved a tubo-ovarian *abscess* is formed. See also page 503, Sexually Transmitted Infections.

Pelvic abscess. See Abdominal Masses—Pelvic Abscess, Chapter 9, page 460.

Tubal mass—ectopic pregnancy. See page 501. Irregular vaginal bleeding and pelvic pain during childbearing years is an ectopic pregnancy until proven otherwise. Adnexal thickening or a mass may not be felt. Softening of the cervix and fundus occurs with tubal pregnancy, as with intrauterine pregnancy. Movement of the uterus and cervix is painful. A high index of suspicion is essential to ensure diagnosis and treatment for this life-threatening condition.

Ovarian mass—oophoritis. Inflammation enlarges an ovary, which is difficult to detect by palpation because inflammation also involves the tubes making component structure identification difficult.

Ovarian mass. Enlargement of an ovary requires a specific explanation.

Neoplasm. Both benign and malignant neoplasms affect the ovaries, diagnosis being made by surgical pathology. Physical exam, even in experienced hands, is not an effective screen for adnexal masses.

Endometriosis. Enlarged ovaries are common in endometriosis (Chapter 9, page 503).

Cyst. See Female Genital and Reproductive Syndromes—Ovarian Cysts, Chapter 9, page 418.

Rectal Signs: See Perineal, Anal, and Rectal Signs, Chapter 9, page 426.

FEMALE GENITAL AND REPRODUCTIVE SYNDROMES

Menstrual Disorders: Menstruation usually begins (*menarche*) between the ages of 12 and 15 years in temperate climates and at 9–10 years in the tropics. The anterior pituitary produces FSH and LH in response to pulsatile hypothalamic secretion of gonadotropin-releasing hormone (GnRH). FSH induces maturation of an ovarian graafian follicle by granulosa cell growth and follicular fluid formation. In combination with FSH, LH causes the theca interna to secrete estrogen. The mature follicle ruptures through the ovarian surface, releasing the ovum which enters the fimbriated end of a Fallopian tube. A fertilized ovum may implant in the endometrium. The ruptured ovarian follicle becomes the corpus luteum, whose cells secrete both estrogen but a preponderance of progesterone under the influence of LH and FSH. If the ovum is not fertilized, the corpus luteum gradually degenerates and scarifies turning into the corpus albicans. Ovulation occurs ~2 weeks before menstruation. When estrogen is the primary secretion (*follicular phase*), the endometrium undergoes proliferation. Later, when progesterone secretion predominates via the corpus luteum (*luteal phase*), the endometrium differentiates into secretory endometrium. Involution of the corpus luteum and steep decline in progesterone leads to sloughing of the endometrium as menstrual bleeding. The menstrual cycle usually recurs in periods of 21–35 days, although there is great variability. Menstrual flow lasts ~5 days. The usual blood loss during one cycle is 30-40mL, mostly during the first and second days, and chronic loss of more than 80mL is associated with iron deficiency anemia. Most women are unable to measure blood loss quantitatively, thus the number or frequency of saturated sanitary napkins or tampons is a surrogate measure. A menstrual pad is saturated when it contains 30–50 mL of blood. The menopausal transition usually begins between the ages of 40 and 55 years with an average age of completing menopause of 52 Menstrual disturbances may be caused by disorders of the anterior pituitary gland, hypothalamus, thyroid, ovary, or uterus. Another common cause is iatrogenic, such as abnormal bleeding while on an oral contraceptive pill or other hormonal supplement provided by a health care professional.

First it is necessary to establish the woman's normal menstrual pattern starting at menarche, including the menstrual cycle length, the amount and duration of normal flow, and her history of conception, live births, abortions, stillbirths, and contraception. Determine the time of the last normal cycle and then seek specific information about the current problem. It is important to differentiate problems of cycle length (early or delayed menses), duration of flow (protracted or short), quantity of flow (too much or too little), and associated symptoms (e.g., pain-dysmenorrhea). Terminology can be confusing so use clear descriptions, avoiding Greek and Latin obscurations. Evaluation of menstrual abnormalities requires a thorough history, complete pelvic exam, and evaluation of the woman's hormonal status, frequently combined with imaging (ultrasound) of the pelvis and/or endometrial sampling. Remember, pregnancy and menopause are the most common causes of a menstrual disorder.

Abnormal Uterine Bleeding—Heavy menstrual bleeding (AUB/HMB)—. AUB/HMB, previously referred to as menorrhagia, is menstruation persisting longer or a daily volume of flow greater than normal, often defined as >80 mL, however in practice it is based primarily on the individual patient's perception. Persistent blood loss with menorrhagia commonly causes iron deficiency with or without anemia.

CLINICAL OCCURRENCE: *Congenital:* Coagulation defects (thrombocytopenia, von Willebrand disease, hemophilia); *Endocrine:* Ovulatory dysfunction (anovulation, oligoovulation), perimenopause, hypothyroidism; *Degenerative/Idiopathic:* Endocervical and endometrial/cervical polyps, endometriosis, endometrial hyperplasia, adenomyosis; *Infectious:* Endometritis, salpingitis; *Inflammatory/Immune:* SLE; *Metabolic/Toxic:* Scurvy; *Neoplastic:* Uterine leiomyoma, carcinoma, leukemia. Other: Iatrogenic (i.e. medications, hormonal therapy, etc.).

Abnormal Uterine Bleeding—Inetermenstrual bleeding (AUB-IMB), previously referred to as metrorrhagia. AUB-IMB also refers to irregular bleeding that occurs outside of a patient's typical menstrual timing. Irregular and intermenstrual bleeding suggest an endometrial abnormality. There is significant overlap in etiologies between AUB-HMB and IMB. The most common causes are endometritis, uterine leiomyoma, ovulatory dysfunction, endometrial polyp, cervical polyps, cervical and endometrial cancer, pregnancy, ectopic pregnancy, threatened abortion, and retained products of conception.

Primary amenorrhea. Primary amenorrhea is failure to initiate regular menstrual cycles (*menarche*) at a chronologically appropriate age or at the latest by age 16. It results from genetic, hormonal, or anatomic abnormalities of sex chromatin, sexual differentiation, and/or sexual maturation. Severe psychological stress can result in amenorrhea in otherwise normal individuals. Correlate sexual and somatic maturation with chronological age and, if necessary, bone age. Obtain growth records to identify longstanding growth problems. Estimate the Tanner stage of secondary sexual development and confirm normal external genitalia by physical exam. Imaging studies may be needed to confirm the presence of normal vagina, uterus, and ovaries.

CLINICAL OCCURRENCE: *Congenital:* Delayed puberty, uterine agenesis, imperforate hymen (cryptomenorrhea), ovarian agenesis or dysgenesis (Turner syndrome), and other disorders of sex chromosomes; *Endocrine:* Hypo- and hyperthyroidism, hypopituitarism, androgens; *Mechanical/Traumatic:* Hysterectomy, oophorectomy, pelvic irradiation; *Metabolic/Toxic:* Lead, mercury, morphine, alcohol, malnutrition, chemotherapy, excessive exercise, obesity, debilitating diseases; *Neoplastic:* Androgen-producing tumors, prolactinoma, craniopharyngioma; *Psychosocial:* Anorexia nervosa, depression.

Gonadal dysgenesis—Turner syndrome (Monosomy X), ovarian agenesis. There is a congenital absence of one X chromosome and fibrotic ovarian remnants. The karyotype is XO with no Y and a diploid number of 45 in 80% of cases. Monosomy X is associated with negative (male pattern) sex chromatin of buccal mucosal cells and neutrophils. These patients may also show short stature, webbed neck, a shield-like chest, cubitus valgus, short metacarpals, lymphedema, and infantile female genitalia and breasts. Sexual maturation is delayed with primary amenorrhea and delayed growth of axillary and pubic hair. If menarche does occur, premature ovarian failure is common.

Secondary amenorrhea. Secondary amenorrhea is the cessation of menstrual cycles after previously normal cycles. Severe psychological stress, such as significant weight loss, eating disorder, or other significant stressors, can result in amenorrhea in otherwise normal individuals. Evaluation of secondary amenorrhea requires a detailed personal medical, psychologic and menstrual history, a family history, and physical exam with attention to signs of endocrine disease. Secondary amenorrhea is expected in midlife associated with the menopause transition as ovarian function begins to wane. Pregnancy is the most common cause of secondary amenorrhea in women of childbearing age.

CLINICAL OCCURRENCE: *Congenital:* Polycystic ovary syndrome, adrenal hyperplasia; *Endocrine:* Pregnancy, menopause, hyper- and hypothyroidism, hypopituitarism, primary ovarian failure, hormonal contraceptives, elevated prolactin, diabetes; *Infectious:* HIV, tuberculosis; *Inflammatory/Immune:* SLE, vasculitis; *Mechanical/Traumatic:* Hysterectomy, oophorectomy, pelvic irradiation, after uterine curettage; *Metabolic/Toxic:* Lead, mercury, morphine, alcohol, malnutrition, chemotherapy, excessive exercise, significant weight changes, obesity, debilitating diseases; *Neoplastic:* Androgen-producing tumors, prolactinoma; *Psychosocial:* Eating disorder, depression.

Polycystic ovary syndrome. Increased production of androgenic steroids by the ovary or, less commonly, the adrenal is associated with insulin resistance and impaired fertility because of anovulation. Genetic factors are important, although the genes and mode of inheritance are unknown. Patients may present in adolescence or, more commonly, the third or fourth decade of life with oligomenorrhea, amenorrhea, infertility, obesity, and excessive hair growth. Only about half the women with the metabolic abnormalities have polycystic ovaries. There is an increased risk for diabetes. Lab values may demonstrate insulin resistance, elevated testosterone, or DHEA.

Ectopic pregnancy. A fertilized ovum normally implants in the endometrium, but implantation can occur in the Fallopian tubes, ovary, cesarean scar, uterine interstitium, or peritoneum. Presentation varies with the implantation site. Pain and bleeding are frequent. Early transvaginal ultrasound is essential to the timely diagnosis of ectopic pregnancies. These pregnancies can never become viable and must be aborted surgically or pharmacologically to protect the woman from life-threatening hemorrhage.

Abdominal Pain and Pallor—Rupture and Hemorrhage from Tubal Pregnancy. Tubal pregnancy occurs when a fertilized ovum implants in a tube, most commonly scarred by pelvic inflammatory disease or previous surgery. Fetal growth stretches and finally ruptures the tube, which has become very vascular, resulting in sudden, large-volume intraperitoneal hemorrhage. Rupture of a tubal pregnancy usually occurs in the first 8 weeks of gestation, often change in menses has been noticed. Uterine bleeding or spotting is common. Typically, a previously healthy young woman suddenly develops agonizing poorly localized abdominal and pelvic pain. The abdomen is quiet on auscultation and increasingly tender, progressing to rigidity. Referred pain to one or both shoulders is common as hemoperitoneum irritates the diaphragm. The abdomen becomes distended and hemorrhagic shock can develop quickly. Serosal inflammation and premonitory minor bleeding, prior to frank rupture, may present as suprapubic or pelvic discomfort. Blood in the pelvis produces fullness in the fornices. A clot or liquid blood may be felt in the rectouterine pouch. One must suspect ectopic pregnancy in any fertile woman with acute abdominal pain. A pregnancy test must be obtained in all women of childbearing age with abdominal pain. Transvaginal ultrasonography is diagnostic. Ectopic pregnancy in other locations (ovary, broad ligament, cesarean scar or abdomen) can also present with pain and abdominal bleeding. Due to the life-threatening nature of this condition and the absolute necessity of timely diagnosis/treatment, ectopic pregnancy must be excluded before pursuing other causes of acute abdominal pain.

Ovary Disorders

Ovarian cysts. Cystic change in the ovary can arise from the follicles, corpus luteum, stroma, and ovarian epithelium. Cysts can be physiologic, degenerative, neoplastic (benign or malignant), or teratomas. Specific diagnosis is made by pathology. A firm or slightly fluctuant, nontender spheroidal mass is felt in the region of the ovary. Cysts extending just above the pelvic brim in the midline resemble a distended bladder and cannot be palpated vaginally. Persistence of the fluctuant mass after bladder catheterization suggests ovarian cyst, gravid uterus, or rectal sheath hematoma. Transvaginal ultrasonography is diagnostic. Large ovarian cysts can fill much of the abdomen and must be distinguished from ascites (see Abdominal Signs—Ovarian Cyst, Chapter 9 page 418).

Abdominal pain and pallor—Follicular and corpus luteum hemorrhage. The ovarian surface ruptures when the ovum is released from the follicle to enter the Fallopian tube. Pain is common (*mittelschmerz*), and persistent bleeding can occur, especially in women on chronic anticoagulation. The corpus luteum matures over 7–10 days so rupture of a corpus luteum cyst usually occurs around the onset of menses. Minor bleeding may be asymptomatic, but heavy bleeding produces the classic signs of intraabdominal hemorrhage. Ultrasonography shows free fluid in the peritoneal cavity and may detect the follicular or corpus luteum cyst. A negative pregnancy test will allow differentiation between this pain and pallor versus ectopic pregnancy.

Ovarian cancer. Malignant tumors arise predominantly from the epithelium, although germ cell and stromal tumors are not rare. BRCA-1 and BRCA-2 genotypes increase the risk for ovarian cancer. Screening for ovarian cancer is not currently recommended as there is no method proved to be effective in average risk populations. Ovarian cancer often presents as ascites after generalized peritoneal spread with the most common stage at presentation being advanced at IIIC.

Uterine Disorders

Endometrial cancer (adenocarcinoma). Risk is increased in women with increased estrogen levels in the absence of progesterone-induced cycling. Post-menopausal women who no longer have progesterone cycling from their ovaries are at increased risk given that they can have estrogen made in adipose tissues or given it iatrogenically. Endometrial carcinoma typically presents with abnormal uterine bleeding or postmenopausal bleeding. Obesity, unopposed estrogen therapy, a positive family history, and atypical endometrial hyperplasia are risk factors. Diagnosis is by endometrial biopsy. Given early signs of bleeding, quickly diagnosed endometrial adenocarcinoma typically is confined to the uterus and is treated surgically.

Vaginal cancer. This is a rare disease. Squamous cell carcinoma of the vagina is typically secondary to human papilloma virus infection. Clear-cell vaginal cancer was associated with the exposure of female fetuses to maternal diethylstilbestrol (DES), given to prevent spontaneous abortion (between the years 1938 and 1971).

Sexually transmitted infections. STIs can be asymptomatic, present locally as ulcers (genital ulcer page 490) inflammation (endocervicitis page 495 and endometritis page 497) and cervical discharge, or present as systemic disease. All sexually active women under the age of 26, or those with new or multiple partners, should be screened for STIs, per the CDC guidelines. The presence of one STI increases the risk of acquiring or transmitting others. Barrier contraceptives (condoms) are effective at decreasing the risk of acquiring an STI. All persons with an STI should be offered screening for HIV and syphilis which are often acquired without symptoms. Extension of infection to the tubes, ovaries, and broad ligament causes pelvic inflammatory disease (see page 498); female infertility is a frequent outcome due to tubal scaring after infection. In addition, several infectious diseases not usually defined as STIs can be acquired sexually, e.g., hepatitis B.

Infertility. The capacity to become pregnant with a viable fetus requires the coordinated functioning of complex physiologic systems in an anatomically normal woman. Failure of any component of this system can result in infertility. Initial evaluation focuses on assessing general health and nutrition, the menstrual history, and a physical examination to confirm normal sexual development and anatomy. Evaluation of the sexual partner is also required with a general health and nutrition history as well as a complete seminal fluid analysis. The etiology and evaluation of infertility is a complex subject. See specialized texts for further information.

Endometriosis. Normal-appearing endometrial tissue forms implants in ectopic sites including the ovaries, posterior surface of uterus, sigmoid colon, uterosacral ligaments, and, less often, distant sites such as pleura. Cyclical bleeding is associated with pain and development of adhesions. The exact cause is unknown. Patients present with dysmenorrhea and abdominal or pelvic pain that is often cyclical. Tender nodular masses surrounded with fibrosis may be felt. The ovaries are frequently enlarged with implants called *endometriomas*. The uterus may be fixed or painful with movement. Infertility is common, and diagnosis usually requires laparoscopy.

CLINICAL VIGNETTES AND QUESTIONS

CASE 11-1

A 28-year-old woman has sudden onset right lower quadrant pain radiating into her right groin. The pain started while she was jogging. She has developed nausea and vomiting, but has not had fever, chills, dysuria, hematuria, urgency, or hesitancy. Her medical history is notable for infertility and she is currently undergoing ovulation induction therapy. She has a blood pressure 112/60 mm Hg, heart rate 72 bpm, respiratory rate 14, and temperature 37°C. Her abdomen is not distended, bowel tones are normal, and there is tenderness and some guarding in the right lower quadrant without masses, organomegaly, or rebound tenderness.

QUESTIONS:
1. What is your differential diagnosis for this patient's presentation?
2. What findings on pelvic examination do you expect if this is an ovarian torsion?
3. What are some risk factors for ovarian torsion?

CASE 11-2

A 25-year-old woman complains of a painless genital ulcer on her labia. It started as a small red papule which then ulcerated. She denies fever, chills, sweats, dysuria, hematuria, urgency, or vaginal discharge. She has no medical problems and her only medication is an oral contraceptive. She has had six lifetime sexual partners and was once treated for chlamydia. Three weeks ago she had unprotected intercourse while on a Caribbean cruise. Her examination reveals a 2-cm nondraining ulcer with a raised edge on the labia majora. There is no urethral or vaginal discharge. There is painless inguinal lymphadenopathy.

QUESTIONS:
1. What is your differential diagnosis for this presentation?
2. What is the most likely diagnosis?
3. What are some long-term sequel of this disease?

CASE 11-3

A 27-year-old woman complains of vaginal discharge that started 2 days ago. She denies pain, discomfort, or urinary symptoms. She has never had this before. She is sexually active in a monogamous relationship with her husband of 5 years using an oral contraceptive for birth control. Her last menstrual cycle was 10 days ago and was normal. She denies systemic symptoms. Examination reveals a malodorous grayish white discharge; no erythema or inflammation is noted.

QUESTIONS:
1. What is the most likely diagnosis?
2. What are the predisposing risk factors for this condition?
3. Describe two other common infectious causes of vaginal discharge and how would they present.

CASE 11-4

A 13-year-old female is brought in by her mother for evaluation of primary amenorrhea. She is shorter than all of her school classmates and she has not had significant pubertal hair growth or development of breast buds.

QUESTIONS:
1. Name some causes of primary amenorrhea and their pathophysiology.
2. You suspect this patient has Turner's syndrome. What physical findings might you expect to see?

CHAPTER 12

The Male Genitalia and Reproductive System

OVERVIEW OF MALE REPRODUCTIVE PHYSIOLOGY

The same embryologic anlage produces female or male external genitalia depending on the level of testosterone. The SRY gene (typically found on the Y chromosome) leads to testicular development, with masculinization of the reproductive tract. When this gene is absent, ovaries develop with subsequent maturation of female sex organs. The scrotum and penis are cognates of the labia majora and clitoris, respectively. Ambiguous genitalia are the result of development and maturation with a mixed genetic substrate or hormonal environment.

The male reproductive organs are the testes, epididymis, vas deferens, seminal vesicles, prostate, and penis. The testes arise intra-abdominally and descend through the inguinal canal into the scrotum, usually by birth. Being slightly cooler than body temperature, scrotal location is more conducive to spermatogenesis. Luteinizing hormone causes testicular Leydig cells to produce testosterone. Spermatogenesis in the seminiferous tubules requires follicle-stimulating hormone (FSH) and paracrine Sertoli cell. Sperm collected in the epididymis travels up the vas deferens within the spermatic cord to the prostate and seminal vesicles. The spermatic cord also contains the testicular artery and vein and the lymphatics. Ejaculate contains sperm suspended in prostatic and seminal vesicle secretions.

MALE REPRODUCTIVE SYSTEM ANATOMY

At puberty, the mons pubes develops hair that extends onto the abdomen forming the triangular *male escutcheon*, with its superior apex near the umbilicus.

The Penis: The male reproductive system is designed to produce and store sperm cells that are to be deposited on the female cervix by forceful ejaculation of the sperm and spermatic fluids via the erect penetrating penis. The shaft of the penis contains three columns of erectile tissue, the two dorsolateral *corpora cavernosa* and the smaller ventral *corpus spongiosum* containing the urethra (Fig. 12-1). The three columns form a cylinder bound by fibrous tissue. Surrounding the urethral meatus at the tip of the penis is an obtuse cone of erectile tissue, the *glans penis*. The glans has a corona at its junction with the shaft. A flap of skin, the *prepuce* or foreskin, covers the glans. The *frenulum* is a fold of the prepuce extending into the ventral notch of the glans. Penile erection and ejaculation are complex physiologic processes which can

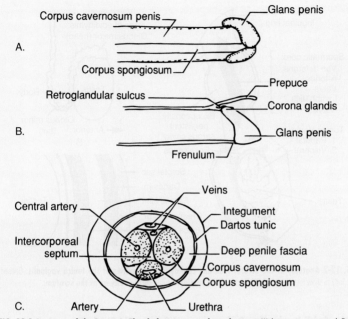

FIG. 12-1 **Structure of the Penis. A. The shaft in its ventrolateral aspect.** With integument removed. **B. A sagittal section of the shaft.** With integument included. **C. A cross-section of the shaft.**

be disrupted by vascular disease, drugs, nerve injury, endocrine abnormalities, and anxiety. Successful reproduction is dependent upon the coordinated functioning of this system.

The Scrotum: The scrotum is a sac of thin, rugous skin overlying the tightly adherent dartos muscle and fascia that form the *dartos tunic* (Fig. 12-2C). The sac, bisected by a median raphe, hangs from the root of the penis. Internally, it is divided into two halves by a septum formed by a fold of the dartos tunic. Each half contains a testis with its epididymis and spermatic cord. The scrotal contents slide easily in a fascial cleft between the scrotal wall and the covering of the testes and cords. The skin of the scrotum is deeply pigmented and contains large sebaceous follicles which often form cysts. The *dartos muscle* regulates testicular temperature by adjusting the size of the scrotum. Exposure to cold shrinks the sac conserving heat; warm temperatures enlarge the sac dissipating heat. In advanced age, the dartos muscle becomes relatively atonic. The dartos muscle functions independently of the *cremasteric muscles* that elevate the testes. The testicular artery, arising in the abdomen, reaches the testes via the inguinal canal and spermatic cord. The pampiniform venous plexus surrounds the artery from the testes through the inguinal canal. Venous blood flowing away from the testes cools the arterial blood by counter current heat exchange. Lymphatics from the scrotal contents drain via the spermatic cord to the pelvic lymph nodes. The scrotal vascular and lymphatic supply is in continuity with the perineum and its lymphatics drain into the inguinal lymph nodes.

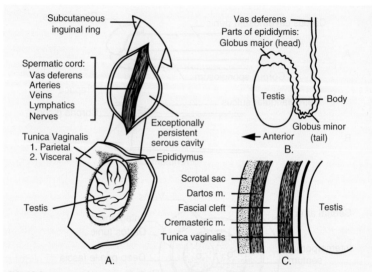

FIG. 12-2 Anatomy of the Scrotal Wall and Epididymis. A. Cavities of the tunica vaginalis. Opened anteriorly to show testis and cord. **B. Parts of the epididymis** and **cord. C. Layers of the scrotum.**

Testis, Epididymis, Vas Deferens, and Spermatic Cord: Toward the end of fetal development, the testes descend from the abdomen into the scrotum. The scrotal ligament, or *gubernaculum*, leads the testis into its scrotal position. The peritoneum covering the testes becomes the *processus vaginalis* extending with the testes through the inguinal canal into the scrotum. This peritoneal extension is normally obliterated within the spermatic cord. In the scrotum this serous membrane invaginates to surround each testis except for their posterior aspect forming the *tunica vaginalis* (Fig. 12-2A). Persistence of the *processus vaginalis* leads to congenital hernias and funicular hydroceles. The spermatic cord suspends the testis in the scrotum. The *testis* is a roughly $4.5 \times 2.5 \times 3$ cm smooth, solid ovoid with a nearly vertical long axis. The head of the *epididymis* caps the upper pole of the testis. The body of the epididymis forms an elongated inverted cone attached vertically to the posterior surface of the testis. The apex of the cone, or tail of the epididymis, approaches the lower pole of the testis (Fig. 12-2B). The epididymis is continuous with the *vas deferens*, which joins other vessels to form the spermatic cord. The *spermatic cord* consists of the vas deferens, arteries, veins, nerves, and lymphatic vessels, all held together by the *spermatic fascia*. From the testis, the cord extends upward, enters the external inguinal ring, passes through the inguinal canal, and exits at the internal inguinal ring where its components diverge. In the abdomen the vas deferens continues retroperitoneally until it lies behind the bladder and anterior to the rectum. It joins the seminal vesicle duct to become the *ejaculatory duct*.

The Prostate and Seminal Vesicles: The prostate contains glands dispersed in a stroma of smooth muscle and fibrous tissue. It is prone to hyperplasia with age. Its position is approximately 2 cm posterior to the symphysis pubis. It is

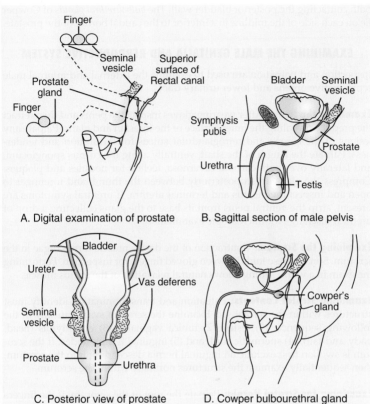

A. Digital examination of prostate

B. Sagittal section of male pelvis

C. Posterior view of prostate

D. Cowper bulbourethral gland

FIG. 12-3 Rectal Exam of the Male Genitalia. A. Relationship of the examining finger to the prostate and seminal vesicles. The lower section shows the finger at the prostate gland; the higher section shows the finger between the two seminal vesicles. **B. A sagittal section of the male penis and pelvic organs. C. A posterior view of the prostate, seminal vesicles, and vasa deferentia. D. Palpation of the Cowper bulbourethral gland.** There is one gland on each side of the urethra. The diagram shows a sagittal section of the male pelvis. The tip of the index finger is in the rectum with the pad facing the anterior rectal wall, between the inferior border of the prostate and the inner edge of the anal canal. The thumb is outside the rectum, pressing the perineum on the medial raphe toward the fingertip. A normal gland is not palpable; an inflamed gland is tender. If it contains pus, it forms a palpable mass from pea to hazelnut size (the round black spot).

walnut sized and shaped like an inverted, truncated cone with the base superior overlaid by the bladder. The apical surface faces inferiorly and rests on the *urogenital diaphragm* (Fig. 12-3B and C). The anterior and posterior surfaces are flattened. The *prostatic urethra* pierces superior surface, slightly anterior to the center, and runs inferiorly emerging through the inferior surface. The slightly convex posterior prostate surface is palpable through the rectal wall. A shallow *median furrow* divides the distal posterior surface into a right and a left lobe below the *transverse depression* made by the ejaculatory ducts which enter the prostate and converge to enter the urethra. The paired *ampullae* of the vas deferens are superior to the prostate and medial to the seminal vesicles, both contacting the posterior bladder wall. The *bulbourethral glands* of Cowper lie on each side of the midline just inferior to the caudal border of the prostate.

EXAMINING THE MALE GENITALIA AND REPRODUCTIVE SYSTEM

Inspection and palpation are used to examine the external and internal male reproductive organs and lower urinary tract.

Examining the Penis: After wearing gloves inspect the penis and then retract the prepuce revealing the inner surface of the foreskin and glans. Palpate any lesions of the corona and retroglandular sulcus for induration and tenderness. Palpate the length of the shaft, ventrally along the corpus spongiosum, and laterally over both corpora cavernosa, feeling for nodules and plaques. Compress the glans anteroposteriorly between the thumb and forefinger to open and inspect the meatus and terminal urethra. If urethral symptoms are present, strip the ventral penis from its base to the glans collecting a drop of urethral discharge for microscopic examination.

Examining the Scrotum: Contraction of the dartos muscle forms rugae in the scrotum. Spread these folds between gloved fingers for inspection. Performing the exam in a warm setting allows natural relaxation of the dartos muscle.

Examining Scrotal Contents: Palpation and transillumination identify most structures within the scrotal sac. Examine the scrotum systematically in the following sequence: (1) testes, (2) tunica vaginalis, (3) epididymis (head, body, and tail), (4) spermatic cord, and (5) inguinal lymph nodes. If the scrotum is swollen first exclude an inguinal hernia descending into the scrotum, then sequentially examine the structures normally within the scrotum.

Examining for Scrotal Hernia: Palpate the root of the scrotum; if the fingers can get above the mass, a hernia is excluded. With a finger in the external inguinal ring have the patient cough feeling for an impulse from a hernia. Inguinal hernias always descend in front of the spermatic cord and testes, so identify their positions relative to the mass. A swollen scrotum should be transilluminated using a cool light source in a darkened room. With the thumb and forefinger, pull the scrotal wall tightly over the mass. Place the light on the posterior scrotum shining light anteriorly through the mass. Determine whether the structure is translucent or opaque. Most hernias are opaque, although gas-filled of gut will transmit light. Listen with a stethoscope for peristaltic sounds.

Examining the Testes: Grasping each testis with a gloved hand examine each independently. Determine their size, shape, consistency, and sensitivity to light pressure. Transilluminate each, even if they feel normal; with a hydrocele an atrophied testicle may feel normal. Use ultrasonography to distinguish between intra-testicular and extra-testicular masses.

Examining the Epididymis: Locate the epididymis on the posterior surface of each testis. It is felt as a vertical ridge of soft nodular tissue extending from the upper to the lower pole. In ~7% of males the epididymis develops anteriorly, *anteversion of the epididymis*, in which case the tunica vaginalis will be posterior to the testis. Compare their component segments of head, body, and tail from right to left.

Examining the Spermatic Cord: It is easiest to examine the scrotal contents with the patient supine though palpation of varicoceles is best performed with the patient standing. Compare the spermatic cords at the neck of the scrotum by compressing each cord between the thumb and forefinger (Fig. 12-4). The normal vas deferens is a distinct hard cord that can be separated from the other cord structures. Trace the cords down to the testes. A varicocele looks and feels like a bag of worms. Other palpable structures are spermatoceles, which are separate from and superior to the testis, and epididymal cysts. The poorly delineated strands are nerves, arteries, and cremasteric muscle fibers. The vas may be congenitally absent, which may be due to a cystic fibrosis gene mutation or be associated with absence of the ipsilateral kidney.

Examining the Male Inguinal Region for Hernia: The index fingertip is placed at the most dependent part of the scrotum then is gently directed into the subcutaneous external inguinal ring by invaginating scrotum (Fig. 12-5A). When the patient coughs or strains, a hernia sac will be felt as a tap on the fingertip. A larger hernia may feel like a mass in the canal.

Zieman inguinal examination. See Inguinal Hernias, Chapter 9, page 461.

Male Rectal Exam

Palpating the prostate and seminal vesicles. Place the patient in the lithotomy position, the knee–chest position, the left-lateral-prone position (Sims),or bent-over-the-table position. Three of these have been considered elsewhere (Chapter 9, Fig. 9-16, page 405). In the bent-over-the-table position, the patient stands with legs apart, the trunk flexed on the thighs, and the elbows resting on the knees or the examination table. The procedural details are the same, whatever the position. Generously lubricate the gloved forefinger. Place the pad of the forefinger on the anal orifice. Applying light pressure while the patient gently

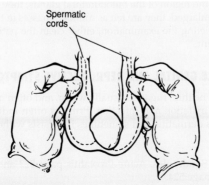

Spermatic cords

FIG. 12-4 Palpation of the Spermatic Cords. Each gloved hand simultaneously grasps a cord between thumb and index finger, comparing the two structures. Normally, the vasa deferentia are distinct cords. The other cord contents (arteries, veins, vessels, and nerves) are not distinguishable.

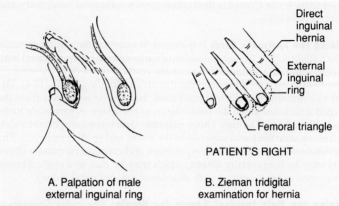

A. Palpation of male external inguinal ring

B. Zieman tridigital examination for hernia

FIG. 12-5 Examination of the Inguinal Regions for Hernia. A. Palpating the inguinal ring in the male. B. Zieman tridigital examination for hernia. The left side of the patient is examined from his left and with the examiner's left hand.

bears down relaxes the sphincter to admit the fingertip. Gradually ease the tip past the anal canal and into the rectal ampulla. Keeping the finger pad facing the anterior rectal wall, move the finger cephalad feeling the elastic bulging surface of the *prostate* (Fig. 12-3A). Identify the *median furrow* separating the lateral lobes and the *transverse furrow* forming the lower border of the *middle lobe*. Determine whether the prostate's surface is smooth or nodular; whether the consistency is elastic, hard, boggy, soft, or fluctuant; whether the shape is rounded or flat; whether the size is normal, enlarged, or atrophied; whether sensitivity to pressure is abnormal; and, whether there is normal mobility or fixation. The *seminal vesicles* are superior to the prostate on either side of the midline. They are ~7.5 cm long, so only their lower portions can be reached. They are usually not palpable being too soft; feeling them suggests disease. If felt, examine each for distention, sensitivity, size, consistency, induration, and nodules. Palpate the region of the bulbourethral glands; they are normally not palpable. When enlarged, they are felt as rounded masses in the anterior rectal wall. After completing the examination, either clean the patient or provide a tissue to the patient.

MALE GENITAL AND REPRODUCTIVE SYMPTOMS

Scrotal itching. The thin, rugated, usually warm, and often moist scrotal skin is susceptible to irritation and infection. Pruritus often indicates inflammatory or infectious dermatitis, but sometimes it persists without skin changes or evident cause.

Pelvic Pain. See Syndromes, Acute Prostatitis page 522 and Chronic Pelvic Pain Syndrome, page 524.

Pain in the Testis and Epididymis. The testis and epididymis are innervated by somatic and sympathetic nerves from lower thoracic roots. Pain from these structures frequently radiates to the epigastrium and/or hypogastrium. If the scrotal wall or tunica vaginalis is involved, the pain is well localized. Pain arising in the testis can be mild or excruciating and is frequently accompanied by nausea. Identify a relationship to activities, sexual activities, and signs of systemic or sexually transmitted disease. A complete sexual history is essential.

CLINICAL OCCURRENCE: *Congenital:* Very large hydrocele; *Degenerative/ Idiopathic:* Inguinal hernia, large varicocele; *Infectious:* Acute orchitis (mumps, echovirus, lymphocytic choriomeningitis virus, arbovirus group B), chronic orchitis (leprosy, tuberculosis), acute epididymitis (*Gonorrhea, Chlamydia, Escherichia coli, Mycoplasma*), and chronic epididymitis (leprosy, tuberculosis, syphilis, brucellosis); *Mechanical/Traumatic:* Blunt and penetrating trauma, testicular rupture, torsion, ureteral stone; *Neoplastic:* Testicular carcinoma, leukemia; *Neurologic:* Neuropathy; *Vascular:* Testicular infarction and hemorrhage.

Penile Curvature. See Male Genitourinary Signs—Plastic Induration of the Penis, page 517.

Erectile Dysfunction and Impotence. See Syndromes—Erectile Dysfunction and Impotence, page 523.

MALE GENITAL AND REPRODUCTIVE SIGNS

Penis Signs
Ambiguous genitalia—intersexuality. Consult texts on developmental anomalies.

Venereal wart or papilloma (condyloma acuminatum). Infection by human papillomavirus (HPV) causes formation of pointed villous projections that may be single or conglomerate (Fig. 12-6E). Warts can occur on the corona, in the retroglandular sulcus, and on the shaft. Warts are frequently found about the anus and occasionally in the urethra. Especially when moist, secondary infection produces ulceration. The verrucous appearance is distinctive. An exuberant growth with much ulceration must be distinguished from carcinoma by biopsy.

Condyloma latum. This is a cutaneous manifestation of secondary syphilis following infection with *Treponema pallidum*. A flat and warty growth (a *secondary syphilid*) occurs on the genitalia or anus (Fig. 12-6D). The flat appearance is diagnostic. When the lesion has an exuberant growth, it must be distinguished from the condyloma acuminatum and carcinoma.

Urethral discharge. See Urinary System Signs—Urethral Discharge, Chapter 10, page 474, and Male Genital and Reproductive Syndromes— Urethritis, Chapter 10, page 479 and 523.

Penis—hypoplasia and hyperplasia. Normal penis size varies widely. Striking discrepancies between penile size and the patient's age lead to the inference of hypoplasia or hyperplasia. Penile hypoplasia is either a feature of intersexuality or eunuchoidism occurring before puberty. In intersexuality,

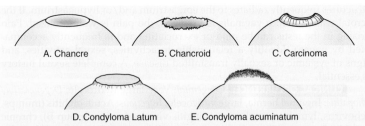

A. Chancre   B. Chancroid   C. Carcinoma

D. Condyloma Latum   E. Condyloma acuminatum

FIG. 12-6 Penile Lesions. A. Chancre. The border is smooth; there is no necrosis or suppuration. Induration surrounds the lesion, so it can be picked up like a disk. **B. Chancroid.** The border is irregular without induration and the center is necrotic. There is profuse suppuration. **C. Ulcerating carcinoma.** The necrotic ulcer may resemble chancroid but, with progression, is surrounded by induration and nodulation. **D. Condyloma latum.** This is the flat non-suppurating nodule of secondary syphilis. **E. Condyloma acuminatum.** The lesions are moist villous growths protruding above the skin. It may ulcerate.

distinction between a hypoplastic penis with hypospadias and a hyperplastic clitoris may be difficult or impossible without histologic examination of the gonads. Hyperplasia is caused by tumors of the pineal gland, hypothalamus, Leydig cells, or adrenal gland. An inaccurate impression of hypoplasia often occurs as men gain weight and abdominal girth.

Generalized penile swelling—edema. Fluid accumulates in the loose tissue of the penis in generalized edematous states of any cause and with obstruction of the penile veins or lymphatics. The penis, and usually the scrotum, is diffusely swollen without erythema, warmth, or tenderness. See also Scrotal Edema page 518.

Generalized penile swelling—contusion. Trauma to the penis, especially during erection, causes extravasation of blood, usually without pain. In a few days the penis and scrotum may be stained from degraded hemoglobin.

Generalized penile swelling—fracture of the shaft. Trauma during erection may rupture one or both corpora cavernosa. Severe pain occurs at the time of injury, with immediate subsidence of the erection and temporary relief of pain. Subsequent engorgement from extravasation of blood produces recurrence of pain. This is a urologic emergency. Rupture may not be distinguishable from contusion unless an operation is performed.

Genital ulcer. Ulceration of the penile shaft, glans, or foreskin occurs at the site of trauma or inoculation of sexually transmitted organisms. The character of the ulcer is diagnostically useful (Fig. 12-6). Inspect the base and edges and look for vesicles that ulcerate, noting especially the presence of pain. Palpate the ulcer base and surrounding tissue for induration. Carefully feel for regional lymphadenopathy. Because these are usually sexually transmitted infections (STIs), serologic evaluation for syphilis and HIV are indicated, as are counseling on safe sexual practices and condom use. **CLINICAL OCCURRENCE:** *Infectious:* Behçet syndrome, herpes simplex, syphilis, chancroid, lymphogranuloma venereum (LGV), molluscum contagiosum; *Mechanical/Traumatic:* Traumatic sex, tight-fitting clothing; *Neoplastic:* Penile cancer.

Syphilitic chancre (hard chancre). *Treponema pallidum* from sexual contact invades intact skin producing a silvery papule that erodes to form a superficial ulcer with serous discharge teeming with organisms. This is the primary lesion of syphilis (Fig. 12-6A). It commonly occurs on the glans or inner leaves of the foreskin but is occasionally on the shaft or scrotum. Rarely, it is extragenital, usually on the lips. The chancre is painless, usually single, round or oval, with a smooth, slightly raised border. The underlying induration permits the superficial lesion to be lifted as a small disk between the thumb and the forefinger. Inguinal lymph nodes painlessly enlarge without suppuration. The chancre appears before serologic tests for syphilis become positive. Dark field microscopic examination of the serous exudate demonstrates the organism confirming the diagnosis.

Chancroid (soft chancre). Suppurative infection caused by the bacillus *Haemophilus ducreyi* usually involves the genitalia, although it can be extragenital. The lesion begins as a small red papule that quickly becomes pustular enlarging to form a punched-out ulcer with undetermined edges (Fig. 12-6B). The base is covered with a gray slough, discharging pus profusely. Extensive necrosis ensues and multiple ulcers form. The lesions are quite painful. In one-third of the cases, the regional lymph nodes become swollen and tender (the *bubo*). These frequently suppurate. While the clinical appearance is quite typical, mixed infections must be excluded.

Lymphogranuloma venereum (LGV). LGV, caused by a rickettsia-like organism *Chlamydia trachomatis*, primarily involves the lymphatic system. The painless and evanescent initial lesion, an erosion <1 mm in diameter, is frequently overlooked. Occasionally, the penile lesion becomes vesicular, papular, or nodular. One or two weeks after infection, the inguinal lymph nodes become swollen and tender, matting together with areas of softening, and reddening of the overlying skin. Syphilis, chancroid, and herpes simplex need to be excluded. Multiple small fistulas form, discharging creamy pus or serosanguineous exudate. Healing occurs over many months with extensive fibrosis. A cicatrizing proctitis may be a late complication. The late clinical appearance is distinctive.

Herpes simplex. Local discomfort on the glans, prepuce, or shaft precedes characteristic grouped vesicles surrounded by erythema. The vesicles rupture, producing painful superficial ulcers that heal in 5–7 days. Recurrent relapsing painful vesiculation and ulceration is characteristic.

Behçet syndrome. Painful aphthous ulcers with yellowish necrotic bases, resembling those seen on the oral mucosa, occur singly or in crops that last 1–2 weeks.

Prepuce—phimosis. The orifice is too small for the foreskin to be retracted over the glans (Fig. 12-7A). The lips of the prepuce are pallid, striated, and thickened. The narrow orifice may obstruct urination. Retained smegma

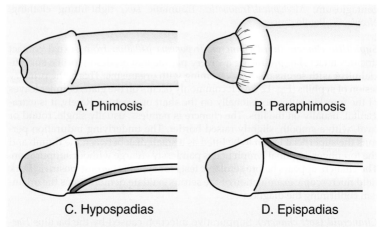

A. Phimosis   B. Paraphimosis

C. Hypospadias   D. Epispadias

FIG. 12-7 Structural Foreskin (Prepuce) Abnormalities. A. Phimosis. The tight orifice inhibits retraction of the foreskin over the glans. **B. Paraphimosis.** A foreskin with a small orifice has been retracted over the glans. The lips impinging on the retroglandular sulcus prevent return to the normal position. Edema develops in the foreskin, the skin of the shaft, and the glans. **C. Hypospadias.** A developmental anomaly in which the urethral meatus opens on the underside of the shaft. **D. Epispadias.** A developmental anomaly in which the urethral meatus is on the dorsum of the penis.

leads to inflammation and even calculus formation. The acquired type may be caused by adhesions to the glans from infection. Circumcision is curative.

Paraphimosis. A tight foreskin, once retracted, becomes edematous and cannot be returned over the glans (Fig. 12-7B). The edema impedes venous drainage from the glans causing swelling increasing the risk for necrosis of the glans. Manual replacement of the prepuce may be attempted. Surgical incision or circumcision may be necessary.

Glans—balanitis. Acute or chronic irritation, infection, or inflammation of the glans produces epithelial erosions or thickening with papules or plaques. In *erosive balanitis* the skin of the glans desquamates forming erosions and small ulcers which may become confluent and involve the entire glans. *Zoon's balanitis* is due to a plasma cell infiltration of unknown cause; it occurs mostly in uncircumcised middle-aged men. *Circinate balanitis* is characteristic of reactive arthritis (Reiter syndrome). Primary cutaneous diseases such as psoriasis, lichen planus, and lichen sclerosis et atrophicus affect the glans. Left unchecked, lichen sclerosis may extend to the distal urethra contributing to a urethral meatal stricture. Infections include *Candida*, HPV (condylomata), and syphilis (primary, secondary, and tertiary). Intraepithelial and invasive squamous cell cancers can mimic other causes of balanitis.

Carcinoma of the penis. Squamous cell carcinoma occurs in areas of irritation or inflammation on the foreskin, glans, or shaft. HPV infection and being uncircumcised increase risk. The primary lesion commonly involves the dorsal corona or the inner lip of the foreskin. A warty growth develops, ulcerates, and discharges watery pus. Parts of the tumor undergo necrosis and slough (Fig. 12-6C). Metastasis occurs, most often to the inguinal lymph nodes. Often, the clinical appearance is not sufficiently typical to distinguish this from condyloma, so biopsy is necessary.

Dorsal shaft—thrombosis of the dorsal vein. A thrombus in the dorsal vein of the penis causes a palpable cord in the midline dorsally ~1 mm in diameter. It is usually secondary to inflammation of the glans.

Dorsal shaft—varicose veins. Varicosities of the dorsal veins of the penis may be visible and palpable. They may be sufficiently large to require surgery.

Shaft—cavernositis. Inflammation causes an irregular hard mass in the lateral or ventral cavernous corpora usually accompanied by priapism and edema. Suppuration may occur, with drainage through the skin or urethra.

Priapism. Erection is sustained by reflex or central nerve stimulation, or by local mechanical causes, such as thrombosis, hemorrhage, neoplasm, injection of vasoactive agents, and inflammation in the penis. Prolonged, persistent, usually painful penile erection occurs without sexual desire. It may complicate leukemia, sickle cell anemia, and use of drugs for psychiatric disorders or erectile dysfunction. Urgent treatment is required.

Plastic induration of the penis (Peyronie disease). This chronic condition of unknown cause is characterized by irregular fibrosis of the septum or sheath of the corpus cavernosum extending into the tunica albuginea. It never affects the corpus spongiosum. It is considered a component of Dupuytren diathesis along with palmar and solar fibrosis. The patient may complain about the curvature during erection. Firm, nontender plaques (single or multiple) are felt in the lateral corpora cavernosa or dorsally over the intercorporeal septum. The plaques are not necessarily symmetrical.

Urethral Signs
Meatus stricture. Narrowing of the urethral meatus is detected by antero-posterior pressure on the glans. Strictures in other portions of the urethra are suggested by difficulty passing a urethral catheter.

Hypospadias. The urethral meatus appears on the ventral surface of the glans, the shaft, or at the penoscrotal junction (Fig. 12-7C).

Epispadias. Maldevelopment results in the meatus opening dorsally on the glans, shaft, or at the penoscrotal junction (Fig. 12-7D). It is often associated with exstrophy of the bladder.

Morgagni folliculitis. The follicles of Morgagni open into the urethra laterally, immediately behind the meatal lips. When the urethral mucosa is inflamed, the mouths of these ducts become prominent and pus can exude when the follicles are involved.

Papilloma. A benign tumor in the meatus may be visible when the orifice opens with bilateral pressure on the glans.

Acute urethritis. See also, Male Genital and Reproductive Syndromes—Urethritis, page 523. An acute indurating urethritis, especially resulting from infection from an indwelling catheter, may produce a palpable cord extending the entire length of the penis.

Periurethral abscess. Pus accumulating in the midportion of the penile urethra in the *Littre follicle* produces visible swelling.

Urethral stricture. A urethral tunnel stricture at the penoscrotal junction may be felt as a palpable, cord-like mass in the corpus cavernosum urethrae. Strictures in other parts of the penile urethra are usually not palpable.

Urethral diverticulum. When located at the penoscrotal junction, a diverticulum frequently produces a visible swelling felt as a soft midline mass.

Urethral carcinoma. A urethral neoplasm may occasionally be felt as an indurated mass in the corpus spongiosum.

Scrotum Signs

Edematous scrotum. Extracellular fluid collects in the dependent scrotum when venous or lymphatic outflow is obstructed or when urine extravasates from a ruptured urethra below the urogenital diaphragm. Acute lymphatic obstruction produces lymphedema that pits with pressure; when longstanding, it will be nonpitting. Pitting edema occurs when systemic venous pressure is very high and dependent edema reaches above the inguinal ligaments (e.g., advanced right ventricular failure, constrictive pericarditis, thrombosis of the pelvic veins or inferior vena cava, nephrotic syndrome), often in association with tense ascites.

- **Gangrenous scrotum.** A necrotizing polymicrobial mixed aerobic and anaerobic perineal infection (*Fournier gangrene*) is caused by gram-positive and gram-negative organisms, often with gas production. The rapid progression results from subcutaneous vascular thrombosis leading to gangrene of the overlying dermis. It is most common in diabetic patients beyond the sixth decade. Fever and signs of sepsis are accompanied by necrotic, foul-smelling, rapidly advancing gangrene of scrotum; crepitation may be present. Emergent wide surgical debridement and antibiotics can be lifesaving.

Sebaceous cysts. These common nodular lesions on the scrotal skin are benign. The white cyst content may be visible.

Blue papules—scrotal venous angioma (Fordyce lesion). Venous angiomas develop in the superficial scrotal veins in men older than 50. The papules are usually multiple, 3–4 mm in diameter and filled with venous blood coloring them dark red, blue, or almost black. They are of no significance.

Carcinoma of the scrotum. The neoplasm is like those in other skin areas. It is particularly common in workers with occupational exposure to tar or oil.

Testis, Epididymis, and Other Intrascrotal Signs

Undescended testis—cryptorchidism. During fetal development, the testicular descent is arrested in the abdomen, inguinal canal, or at the pubo-scrotal junction; other locations are possible. An undescended testis is frequently associated with a congenital inguinal hernia on the same side resulting from persistence of the saccus vaginalis. Either or both testes may be affected. An abdominal testis cannot be palpated. In the other locations, the testis is palpable, but smaller and softer due to atrophy. Undescended testis carries an increased risk of testicular cancer and decreased fertility.

Small testes—atrophy. The testis may be smaller than normal from Klinefelter syndrome or Prader–Willi syndromes. Atrophy may occur after infarction, trauma, mumps orchitis, cirrhosis, syphilis, filariasis, large varicocele, or surgical repair of an inguinal hernia.

Nontender testicular swelling—neoplasm. See Testicular Cancer, page 522.

Tender testicular swelling—testicular torsion. The testicle is suspended by the spermatic cord. If the testicle twists within the scrotum, the venous and lymphatic vessels, because of their thin walls and lower pressure, become obstructed before arterial inflow. The resulting engorgement progressively worsens arterial circulation leading to ischemia. Pain is acute and severe, and pain may be referred to the lower abdomen, mimicking an acute abdomen, like appendicitis. The testicle is abnormally high in the scrotum and lies horizontally with the epididymis located anteriorly. It is tender to palpation and feels irregular and edematous. Occasionally, the twist in the cord can be felt. Urgent surgical intervention is required to prevent decreased function or atrophy of the testicle and should not await confirmation by ultrasound or other maneuvers. Manual detorsion may be attempted while awaiting transport to the Operating Room (OR). *DDX:* Torsion is frequently confused with acute epididymoorchitis and strangulated scrotal hernia. Five distinguishing features are: (1) the affected testis is higher than normal due to the twisted cord and cremasteric muscle spasm; (2) palpation cannot distinguish between the testis and the epididymis—in acute epididymoorchitis the epididymis can usually be felt separately from the testis; (3) elevating and supporting the scrotum usually relieves epididymoorchitis pain—it does not decrease the pain of torsion (*Prehn sign*); (4) in torsion, the ipsilateral leg is often held in flexion; and (5) a secondary hydrocele, if present, contains serosanguineous fluid rather than the serous fluid of epididymoorchitis. Sometimes a strangulated hernia cannot be distinguished from torsion without operation.

Tender testicular swelling—acute orchitis. Inflammation of one or both testes occurs frequently in mumps, and occasionally with other infections. The testis is swollen, tender, and extremely painful. The inflammation may cause an acute hydrocele, but the edema and pain prevent accurate assessment. Primary or secondary epididymitis is often associated. Acute orchitis can be confused with testicular torsion.

Nontender intra-scrotal swelling. Normal and persistent fetal structures enlarge due to fluid accumulation or neoplasms. The differential diagnosis of painless intrascrotal lesions requires a complete knowledge of the normal and developmental anatomy including arterial, venous, and lymphatic circulations.

Hydrocele. Serous fluid accumulates in the cavity of the tunica vaginalis. Palpation reveals a smooth, resilient pear-shaped mass that tapers upward and disappears before reaching the root of the scrotum. The testis and the epididymis are usually behind the mass (Fig. 12-8B); with testicular anteversion these structures will be anterior (Fig. 12-8O). Transillumination reveals the testicle's shadow within the translucent mass. *DDX:* Hematoceles are opaque, spermatoceles arise from the epididymis behind the testis, and spermatic cord hydrocele occurs above the testis.

Hydrocele of the spermatic cord. When the saccus vaginalis around the spermatic cord fails to obliterate, a serous cavity persists forming a hydrocele. The sausage-shaped hydrocele is located above the testis and feels smooth and resilient. Like scrotal hydoceles, cord hydroceles readily transilluminate (Fig. 12-8K). If no other abnormalities are present, these findings are diagnostic. *DDX:* When associated with a hernia, spermatocele, or testicular hydrocele, the distinction may be impossible without ultrasound or operation. Occasionally, the hydrocele communicates with the peritoneal cavity, a *communicating hydrocele*, which is recognized by the fluctuation in size.

Hematocele. The tunica vaginalis is filled with blood, usually from trauma. The swelling resembles a hydrocele but is opaque to transillumination (Fig. 12-8C).

Hematoma of the cord. Trauma causes bleeding around the spermatic cord producing a boggy mass that is opaque to transillumination (Fig. 12-8L).

Chylocele. In filariasis, lymph accumulates in the cavity of the tunica vaginalis. The mass is translucent; distinction from hydrocele is made by aspirating the fluid.

Varicocele. Varicosities of the pampiniform plexus of veins form a soft, irregular mass in the scrotum. It occurs predominantly on the left side, occasionally it is bilateral, and almost never is exclusively on the right. Palpation discloses a soft "bag of worms" sensation that is rarely mistaken for anything else (Fig. 12-8N). *DDX:* A varicocele empties when the patient is supine. An indirect inguinal hernia containing omentum also may recede when the patient is supine. Place a finger over external inguinal ring, have the patient stand with your finger in place; the veins refill but the hernia will be held back.

Spermatocele. These are retention cysts of the epididymis. They are usually located in the head of the epididymis or behind the testis (see Hydrocele). They are usually small and translucent but can reach 10 cm (Fig. 12-8G). They are opaque on transillumination.

Syphilis. Nontender swelling and nodularity start in the globus major then extend to the body of the epididymis (Fig. 12-8J). The cause is inferred from positive serologic tests for syphilis.

Tuberculosis. Hard, nontender nodularity begins in the body of the epididymis. The epididymis becomes adherent to the scrotum, and sinuses may form (Fig. 12-8I). The cause is usually inferred from the presence of tuberculosis elsewhere.

Tender epididymal swelling—acute epididymitis. Infection of the epididymis ascends from the urethra, prostate, or seminal vesicles. Indwelling urethral catheters increase the risk of epididymitis. The painful, tender swelling of the epididymis may be accompanied by fever, leukocytosis, and pyuria. In young, sexually active men with multiple or new sexual partners, sexually transmitted organisms are expected; in men >40 years of age and in those with catheters, enteric organisms are common.

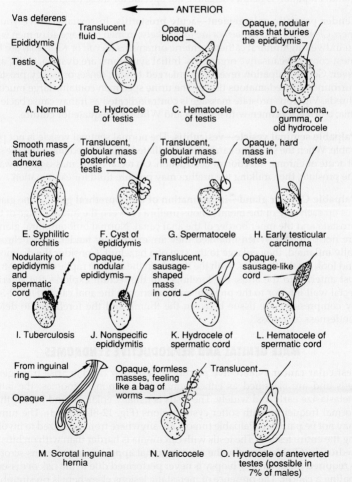

FIG. 12-8 Swellings of the Scrotal Contents. (See text for descriptions of Figure 12-8A to 12-8O.)

Thickening of the vas deferens—deferentitis. Inflammation and infection of the vas deferens usually ascends from other structures. If acute, the vas is tender and swollen. With chronic inflammation the vas may be thickened, indurated, and nodular (Fig. 12-8I), suggesting tuberculous or syphilis.

Prostate and Seminal Vesicle Signs

Nontender prostate enlargement. The prostate enlarges due to hyperplasia of the normal tissues, infiltration by chronic inflammatory or neoplastic cells, or a combination of these. Diffuse enlargement of normal consistency is expected as men age, most often representing benign prostate hyperplasia (page 524). Asymmetrical enlargement, stony hard nodules, diffuse hardness, and obliteration of the normal sulcii suggest prostate cancer (page 524). Chronic prostatitis, either infectious or primarily inflammatory, presents with a boggy or firm gland. Palpation is neither sensitive nor specific for these diagnoses.

Tender prostatic enlargement—acute prostatitis. In sexually active young men, *Chlamydia* and *Gonorrhea* are most likely; in men over age 40 or men with an indwelling urethral catheter, enteric organisms (*E. coli* or *Klebsiella*) are the most common causative organisms. Initial symptoms are dysuria, chills, and fever. Gentle palpation reveals an enlarged tender, tense, or boggy prostate surrounded by edematous tissue. The urine specimen contains large mucous shreds. Vigorous prostate massage is contraindicated as it may cause bacteremia; a urine specimen with bacteria and WBCs is adequate for culture.

Palpable seminal vesicle—vesiculitis. The normal seminal vesicle is not palpable. When the structure can be felt as a dilated or indurated mass, it is the site of acute or chronic infection or obstruction. On rectal exam, massaging toward the prostate, then milking the urethra may procure fluid for examination

Palpable Cowper gland—inflammation of bulbourethral gland. One gland lies on each side of the membranous urethra between the inferior edge of the prostate and the inner border of the anal canal. Normal bulbourethral glands are not palpable. When inflamed they are exquisitely tender. When chronically inflamed, they enlarge to the size of a hazelnut. Consider the diagnosis and look for the findings. With the thumb on the median raphe of the scrotum just anterior to the anus, the forefinger in the rectum explores the anterior rectal wall inferior to the prostate and superior to the anal canal (Fig. 12-3D) by compressing the tissue between the thumb and the forefinger to detect tenderness or a mass.

MALE GENITAL AND REPRODUCTIVE SYNDROMES

Testicular cancer. Ninety-five percent of testicular cancers arise from germ cells and are classified as either seminomas or nonseminomas; the latter metastasize early and widely. The testis is usually enlarged and harder than normal frequently with softer cystic regions (Fig. 12-8D and H). The tumor may not be palpable. Palpable tumors are anywhere from pea-sized to involving the entire testicle. The testis with carcinoma is harder than with orchitis or hydrocele. Orchiectomy by the trans-inguinal approach (never trans-scrotal) is required for diagnosis; biopsy is never performed due to the risk of disseminating a cancer. The presence of metastatic lesions elsewhere is presumptive evidence that a testicular nodule is neoplastic.

Inguinal hernia. See Chapter 9, Hernias, page 460.

Sexually transmitted infections. STIs can be asymptomatic, present locally as ulcers or inflammation, or present systemically. All sexually active men and women should be asked about a history of STIs. All persons with an STI must be screened for other STIs that could have been acquired asymptomatically, including HIV and syphilis. Hepatitis B and C, not usually considered STIs, can be acquired sexually. Barrier contraceptives (condoms) decrease transmission of STIs.

Syphilis. *Treponema pallidum* enters the body across an epithelial barrier disseminating to regional lymph nodes, then throughout the body. Primary syphilis presents as single, firm, painless, punched-out ulcer on or near the genitalia, lips, mouth, or a woman's breast, the *chancre*. Secondary syphilis occurs 6 weeks after the chancre with headache, sort throat, myalgia, malaise, itching, and a maculopapular rash on the soles, palms, and extremities. There may be lymphadenopathy, fever, and alopecia. Tertiary syphilis presents with various clinicopathologic pictures depending on tissues involved. Findings may include aortic insufficiency, tabes dorsalis, general paresis, and/or gumma formation.

Urethritis. Infection causes urethral inflammation with purulent urethral discharge. Sexually transmitted organisms, e.g., *Chlamydia*, *Gonorrhea*, and the genital *Mycoplasmas*, are the most common pathogens in young men. In men over age 40, enteric bacteria predominate. Urination causes burning pain; erection may be painful. The edges of the meatus may be reddened, edematous, and everted. A variable amount of pus or clear fluid discharges from the urethra. The dorsal lymphatic channels of the penis may be tender and palpable. Tender inguinal lymphadenopathy may develop. The diagnosis is made by inspection and finding mucous shreds and pus in the first few drops of a urine specimen. Prostatitis may complicate urethritis by extension of infection into the prostatic ducts. Urethritis, conjunctivitis, and arthritis are the triad of reactive arthritis (Reiter disease); urethritis frequently is the presenting sign.

Erectile dysfunction—impotence. Sexual arousal, rigid distention of the corpora cavernosum, orgasm, and effective ejaculation require intact endocrine, neurologic, and vascular function. Dysfunction anywhere in this complex and coordinated process can produce erectile dysfunction, the inability to sustain a penile erection of sufficient rigidity or duration for satisfactory coitus. Many patients do not volunteer their inability to sustain an erection or acknowledge the problem on a questionnaire. Ask specifically about sexual performance. Awakening with early morning erections argues against an organic cause (neurologic, vascular, or endocrine). A thorough history of the onset and progression of symptoms, libido, medications, surgery, and psychosocial issues is essential. Screening for depression, hypothyroidism, hypogonadism, and diabetes is useful. Full evaluation requires urology referral.

   CLINICAL OCCURRENCE: *Congenital:* Genetic disorders impairing sexual maturation (e.g., Prader Willi syndrome) or leading to hypogonadism (e.g., hemochromatosis); *Endocrine:* Primary hypogonadism, hypothyroidism, hypopituitarism, diabetes mellitus; *Degenerative/Idiopathic:* Hypertension, atherosclerosis; *Mechanical/Traumatic:* Postradical prostatectomy, radiation, long-distance bicycling; *Metabolic/Toxic:* Medications (antihypertensives, anxiolytics, antidepressants), alcohol, opiates, marijuana, chronic renal failure; *Neurologic:* Peripheral neuropathy, myelitis, spinal cord compression, multiple sclerosis, dementia; *Psychosocial:* Depression, anxiety; *Vascular:* Atherosclerosis, vasculitis.

Benign prostatic hyperplasia. Hyperplasia, particularly of the median lobe, places pressure on the bladder trigone narrowing the prostatic urethra. Benign prostatic hyperplasia affects older men. They present with urethral obstructive and/or irritative symptoms such as hesitancy, weak urinary stream, nocturia, and dribbling. The enlarged prostate often feels rubbery or firm. Size on exam does not predict obstruction since median lobe enlargement protrudes anteriorly away from the examining finger.

Prostate cancer. Local disease is usually asymptomatic; dysuria and obstructive symptoms can occur in advanced disease. One or more discrete nodules may be identified, or the entire gland may be stony hard obliterating the median furrow. Description should include size, presence or absence of normal landmarks, and extension beyond a single lobe or outside the prostate. Extension is palpable or inferred from fixation of the rectal mucosa to the posterior prostate surface.

Chronic prostatitis. Chronic prostatitis may be infective or sterile; often one is unsure. Patients present with pelvic discomfort and/or dysuria without discharge or systemic symptoms. A history of STI or acute prostatitis is often absent. The prostate may be normal, enlarged, diffusely softened (boggy) or firm; it is not tender. Routine urine cultures are negative. Prostate massage may identify an infection or evidence of inflammation, though it is often painful.

Chronic pelvic pain syndrome (prostadynia). Chronic deep, boring pelvic, and/or perineal pain is/are not rare in otherwise healthy men. The onset may be acute or insidious. Pain can wax and wane but rarely remits completely. There may be mildly decreased stream or hesitancy, but dysuria, urethral discharge, hematuria, and fever are absent. The cause is unknown but is likely due to pelvic floor dysfunction with muscle tightness that can be improved with biofeedback and pelvic floor physical therapy.

Reactive arthritis (Reiter syndrome). Reactive arthritis follows an STI or diarrheal illness. There is chronic recurrent inflammation of the urethra, conjunctivae, skin, periarticular tissue, and large joints. Patients present with urethritis, conjunctivitis, arthritis, back pain, and/or characteristic skin disease on the feet and glans penis. There is no diagnostic test, so diagnosis is clinically based on multisystem findings, compatible history, and absence of alternative diagnosis.

Behçet syndrome. Patients present with oral and/or genital aphthous ulcers. See Chapter 8, page 364.

Klinefelter syndrome. An abnormal complement of 47 chromosomes (XXY and variants) produces variable masculinization. Affected individuals are tall with long legs, atrophic testes, and gynecomastia. They have low fertility.

CLINICAL VIGNETTES AND QUESTIONS

CASE 12-1

A 22-year-old man complains of painful urination. He has burning during urination and some purulent urethral discharge. He has had multiple sexual partners in the last year.

QUESTIONS:
1. What is the differential diagnosis for his presentation?
2. How does his history and each of his symptoms influence your differential diagnosis?
3. What is the most likely diagnosis?
4. What is the triad of reactive arthritis (Reiter's syndrome)?
5. What infections frequently precede reactive arthritis?

CASE 12-2

A 25-year-old man presents with a painful lesion on the shaft of his penis. You observe grouped vesicles on an erythematous base.

QUESTIONS:
1. Which characteristics of the lesions help differentiate the causes of infectious genital ulcers?
2. What are the characteristics of inguinal lymphadenopathy in each disease?
3. What is the most likely diagnosis?

CASE 12-3

A 25-year-old man presents with genital ulcers.

QUESTIONS:
1. What are infectious causes of genital ulcers?
2. What are some of the noninfectious causes of genital ulcers?
3. What is the differential diagnosis for recurrent genital ulcers?

CASE 12-4

A 24-year-old man complains of dull, aching left scrotal pain most noticeable when standing and relieved by recumbency. Palpation discloses a soft "bag of worms" sensation.

QUESTIONS:
1. What is the most likely diagnosis?
2. What is the underlying pathophysiology?
3. It is more common on one side. Which side and why?
4. How do you differentiate this from an indirect inguinal hernia?

CASE 12-5

A 32-year-old man comes to your clinic with 2 days of left scrotal pain. Palpation reveals exquisite tenderness and a swollen indurated 1.5 cm nodular lesion on the posterior aspect of the testicle.

QUESTIONS:
1. What is the most likely diagnosis?
2. What reflex response helps differentiate this diagnosis from testicular torsion?
3. How is this reflex elicited?
4. How does the patient's age help in your differential diagnosis?

CHAPTER 13

The Spine, Pelvis, and Extremities

Patients with problems referable to the spine and extremities are classified by the type of symptom(s), its acuity, and its location(s). Symptoms are pain, tenderness, swelling, deformity, limited function (restricted motion, weakness), or unusual sensations like clicking and snapping. The symptoms are either localized to a single body part, affect two to four parts either simultaneously or sequentially, or are diffuse and either symmetrical or asymmetrical. Symptoms are acute, subacute, or chronic; when chronic, they may be slowly progressive. Describing the problem by symptom, site, acuity, aggravating or alleviating factors, and progression rapidly narrows the diagnostic possibilities. The exam then focuses on those specific body parts and signs.

When the problem is a single symptom in one location, the symptom, signs, and condition are inseparable and should not be thought of as separable descriptors. These will be addressed in the Symptom, Sign, or Syndrome section depending, somewhat arbitrarily, on which is the key to diagnosis, the symptom, the sign, or the whole picture.

Traumatic injuries will be discussed at the end of the Syndrome section, organized by site of injury.

MAJOR SYSTEMS AND THEIR PHYSIOLOGY

The musculoskeletal system has four major functional components: bones and ligaments, synovial and fibrocartilaginous joints, muscles and tendons, and nerves innervating the muscles. Tendons anchor muscle to bone, whereas ligaments anchor bone to bone. The shape and body contour are attributable to its bony structure and overlying muscles.

Bones: The ossified skeleton provides mechanical support for the body and protection for viscera within the body cavities, vertebral column, and skull. Mature bone forms by mineralizing osteoid laid down by osteoblasts on a cartilaginous matrix in the epiphyses of the long bones, endplates of the vertebrae, and cartilaginous structures (endochondral bones of the skull and face). *Cortical bone* forms a thick cortex surrounding a central hollow, the marrow space. *Trabecular bone* forms an intricate lattice laid down along the lines of stress within the marrow cavity. Bone reapbsorption by osteoclasts and formation by osteoblasts is continuous. Bone must maintain enough strength to resist the compression and tension applied by mechanical loading and muscle traction. Bone strength depends upon normal architecture, collagen, and mineralization; abnormality of any component results in susceptibility to fracture. The shape of mature bones is affected during skeletal matuaration by the muscles pulling at their anatomic origins and insertions. Muscles that insert on a small portion of bone and exert large forces deform the bone into prominences. Adjacent bones are connected by *ligaments*, collagenous bands continuous with the collagen of the bone itself. Ligaments stabilize the bones relative to one another and the intervening joints.

Joints: Joints separate articulated bones. *Fibrocartilage* separates bones at joints where motion is minimal, e.g., the intervertebral discs. *Synovial (diarthrodial) joints* separate bones where motion is extensive. The bone surfaces of diarthrodial joints are covered with *hyaline cartilage* built to resist repeated axial loading with minimal deformation while providing a smooth, virtually friction-free surface for motion. The avascular cartilage derives its nutrition by diffusion from the synovial fluid. The diarthrodial joints are enclosed within a synovial envelope of collagen lined with a single synovial cell layer that secretes the proteoglycans necessary for joint lubrication. Joint integrity is maintained by ligaments anchoring bone to bone and the muscles whose tendons cross the joint.

Muscles, Tendons, and Bursae: *Striated skeletal muscles* exert contractile force proximally on one bone at its origin and distally, via a variably elongated *tendon*, onto its insertion on another bone. Therefore, muscular contraction serves to change the relative position of the bones. Most muscles originate diffusely directly from the periosteum, whereas some attach by tendons at both their origin and insertion, e.g., the long head of the biceps. Tendons are elongated, relatively avascular collagen structures that are continuous at their origin with the interstitial collagen of the muscle and at their insertion with that of the bone. Tendons may lie free in the tissue but are often surrounded by synovial sheaths or bursae where they cross mobile joints or pass around bony prominences. *Bursae* are synovial-lined sacs serving to reduce friction between tendons or muscles and underlying bone. Muscles are highly vascular since they require maximal oxygen delivery to efficiently convert stored glycogen and fatty acids into effective mechanical power. Muscle is enclosed in an inelastic collagenous *fascia*. Muscle is susceptible to tearing from the force of its own contraction. Ischemic necrosis may occur when contracting with a compromised blood supply. Body contours result from muscles and subcutaneous fat overlying the skeleton. Asymmetry or abnormalities of body contour suggest changes in the underlying muscles, or less commonly, fat distribution.

SUPERFICIAL ANATOMY OF THE SPINE AND EXTREMITIES

See the descriptions of each anatomic location given under the sections on Physical Exam and texts on anatomy for artist's renditions.

The Axial Skeleton—Spine and Pelvis

Cervical spine. There are seven cervical vertebrae (Fig. 13-1A), three of which are specialized: C1 is the *atlas* (bearing a globe, like the Greek god after whom it is named); C2 is the *axis* about which the atlas rotates; and C7 is the vertebra prominens. Head nodding occurs chiefly at the *atlantooccipital joint*. Flexion and extension involve the occiput—C1 and C3–C7. All vertebrae permit lateral bending. Half of rotation occurs at the *atlantoaxial joint*, with the remainder distributed through the cervical spine. See Figure 13-1B for measurements of cervical motion.

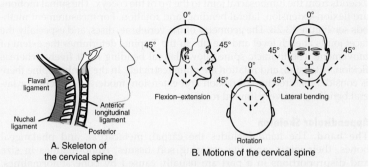

FIG. 13-1 **Anatomy and Motions of the Cervical Spine. A. The cervical spine. B. Motions of the cervical spine.** Normal range of motion exceeds the angles shown as points of reference.

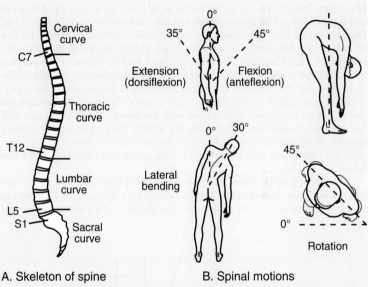

FIG. 13-2 **Bones and Motions of the Spine. A. Lateral view of the four spine curves. B. Spinal motions.** Flexion–extension, lateral bending, rotation.

Thoracolumbar spine and pelvis. There are 12 thoracic and five lumbar vertebrae, a fused mass of five sacral vertebrae articulating with the pelvic bones at the *sacroiliac (SI) joint*, and four coccygeal vertebrae. Viewed laterally, the vertebral column has four curves (Fig. 13-2A). Least pronounced is the *cervical curve*, concave backward beginning at C2 and ending at T2. The *thoracic curve* is convex backward, beginning at T2 and ending at T12. The *lumbar curve*, more pronounced in females, is concave backward from T12 to the lumbosacral joint. The *pelvic curve*, convex backward and downward, extends from the lumbosacral joint to the tip of the coccyx. The spinal motions are flexion–extension, lateral bending, and rotation. For measurement methods see Figure 13-2B. The geometry of the vertebrae, discs, and especially the facet joints at each level and the ribs in the T-spine, determines the extent of movement. The thoracic spine allows lateral bending most freely, whereas flexion, extension, and rotation are quite restricted. In the lumbar spine there is considerable freedom of flexion and extension, moderate capacity for lateral bending, and very limited rotation.

Appendicular Skeleton

The hand. The hand includes the carpal, metacarpal, and phalangeal bones, their joints, and the covering soft tissues. Abnormalities in size and disproportions in a part are usually caused by bone abnormalities. *Hand posture* reflects the relative tone of the finger and wrist flexors and extensors, the intrinsic hand muscles, and the presence or absence of joint disorders.

The wrist. The wrist includes the radiocarpal joint, the eight carpal bones in two parallel rows, and the overlying tendons and tendon sheaths (Fig. 13-3). The *radiocarpal joint* articulates a concave with a convex surface. The distal radius and the triangular *articular disk* capping the distal ulna form the proximal concave surface. The distal convex surface contains the curving sides of three proximal-row carpal bones: the *navicular*, *lunate*, and *triquetrum*. The *pisiform* does not participate because it lies on the volar aspect of the triquetrum. The navicular is most commonly fractured because the radius has wider contact with it than with the lunate, and the articular disk cushions the forces transmitted from the ulna to the triquetrum. The major *synovial cavity* lies between radius and the navicular. A minor cavity separates the distal ulna and the articular disk, extending proximally between the radius and ulna.

The topography must be known to properly examine the wrist (Fig. 13-4). ***Volar Aspect of the Wrist:*** The *pisiform* bone can be palpated as a bony prominence on the ulnar side, just distal to the palmar crease and

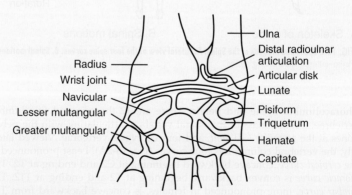

FIG. 13-3 Bones of the Wrist.

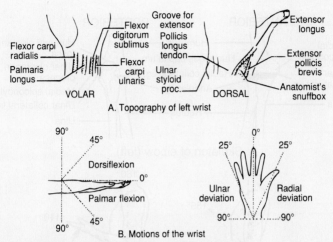

FIG. 13-4 **The Wrist. A. Topography of the wrist. B. Motion at the wrist.**

proximal to the base of the *hypothenar eminence*. Four tendons can be palpated and often seen. With the digits slightly flexed and muscles tensed, three tendons are apparent in most persons. From the ulnar to the radial side, they are the *flexor carpi ulnaris, palmaris longus,* and *flexor carpi radialis*. The palmaris longus is absent in ~10% of persons. With the fist clenched hard, the tendon of the *flexor digitorum sublimis* also appears between the flexor carpi ulnaris and the palmaris longus. **Dorsal Aspect of the Wrist:** The most conspicuous prominence is the *ulnar styloid process*. Extension of the thumb accentuates the borders of the *anatomist's snuffbox*, a recess formed between the *extensor pollicis longus and brevis*.

The forearm. The forearm extends from the elbow to the wrist. *Inspection* and *palpation* are used for examination. The radius and ulna articulate with the humerus proximally. They are connected by an *interosseous membrane* throughout most of their length. The radius and ulna are practically subcutaneous, so their entire length can be palpated. The *dorsal muscle mass* is formed by the wrist and finger extensor muscles which insert on the lateral humeral epicondyle. The *volar muscle mass* is the finger and wrist flexors inserting on the medial epicondyle.

The elbow. There are two articulations in the elbow. The hinged *humeroulnar joint* is formed by the semilunar notch of the ulnar olecranon process embracing and moving around the transverse drum of the spool-shaped *trochlea* of the distal humerus (Fig. 13-5A). When the elbow is in full extension, the *olecranon process* fits into the *olecranon fossa* of the humerus just above the trochlea. The *trochlea* forms the medial two-thirds of the lower humeral articulation. The lateral third is the rounded *capitulum* on which a cup-shaped depression in the radial head pivots and glides to form the *humeroradial joint*. The radial

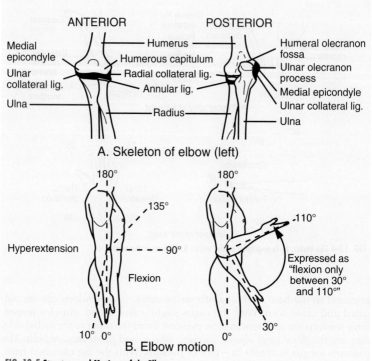

FIG. 13-5 **Structure and Motions of the Elbow.**

head is a squat cylinder rotating in the *annular ligament* during forearm prona-tion and supination.

Viewed from the back (Fig. 13-6), three bony prominences of the flexed elbow make an inverted equilateral triangle: the two basal points are the medial and lateral epicondyles of the humerus; the tip of the olecranon pro-cess is the apex. During full extension, the three points form a straight trans-verse line.

The shoulder. The shoulder girdle includes bones (humerus, scapula, clavi-cle, and sternum), joints (glenohumeral, acromioclavicular, sternoclavicular, and scapulothoracic), their ligamentous connections, and the overlying mus-cles, tendons, and bursae. The glenohumeral joint is a ball-and-socket articu-lation. The hemispheric *humeral head* fits into the shallow cavity formed by the scapular *glenoid* and its surrounding fibrous *labrum* (Fig. 13-7). The articulat-ing surfaces are enclosed by a short tube of *joint capsule*. The scapular *coracoid process* projects anterior and medial to the joint and the *acromion* forms a rigid fender above the joint. They are connected by the *coracoacromial ligament*. The clavicle connects to the acromion by the superior *acromioclavicular ligament*

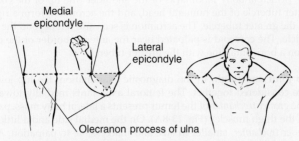

FIG. 13-6 Topographic Relations of the Elbow. A. Posterior View. In extension, the ulnar olecranon process lies on a straight line between the medial and the lateral epicondyles of the elbow. In flexion, the olecranon process moves downward to produce an inverted equilateral triangle between the three bony prominences. Any distortion of this triangle after trauma points to a fracture involving one or more of its points. **B. Anterior View.**

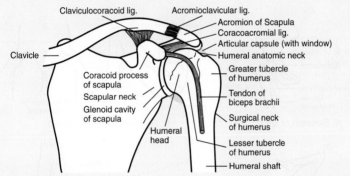

FIG. 13-7 Anatomy of the Shoulder Joint. An anterior window in the joint capsule exposes the inner attachment of the biceps brachii muscle.

and to the underlying coracoid process by the *coracoclavicular ligament*. From its origin within the joint capsule, the *tendon of the long head of the biceps* emerges anteriorly between the greater and lesser tubercles of the humeral head. A *synovial membrane* lines the joint capsule and forms a tubular sheath, extending distally to the surgical neck of the humerus, for the biceps tendon.

Great freedom of motion results from the shallow glenoid cavity, large articular surface of the humeral head, and absence of restraining ligaments; this also makes it vulnerable to dislocation. The *joint capsule* is loose, exerting little tension except in extreme positions. Muscle tension maintains shoulder stability. The *scapula* is held to the thoracic wall by its muscular attachments, its wing gliding freely over the thoracic muscles. Scapular movements add greatly to upper limb mobility; scapular motion must be distinguished from motion at the glenohumeral joint. The shoulder girdle is connected to the axial skeleton via the *acromioclavicular joint*, *clavicle*, and *sternoclavicular joint*.

The principal bony landmarks of the shoulder (the tip of the coracoid, the greater tubercle of the humeral head, and the acromion) form a right triangle at the greater tubercle. The acromion is seen and felt beyond the end of the clavicle. The coracoid is palpated near the anterior border of the deltoid muscle on a horizontal line with the greater tubercle.

The hip joint and thigh. In the diagnostic examination, the hip joint and thigh are considered together. The femoral axis slants medially toward the knee. The *greater trochanter* of the femur presents a lateral bony mass, palpable through the thigh muscles (Fig. 13-8A). On the medial side and a little distal is the *lesser trochanter*, smaller in size and inaccessible to palpation. Arising between the trochanters, the *femoral neck* slants proximally and medially, forming an angle with the femoral axis of 120–160 degrees. An increase in the angle produces lateral deviation of the femoral shaft, *coxa valga*, a decrease in the angle deviates the shaft medially, *coxa vara*. The neck is surmounted by the globular *femoral head*, which fits into the cupped *acetabulum* of the pelvis, forming a ball-and-socket joint. The hip permits flexion–extension, abduction–adduction, and internal–external rotation (Fig. 13-8C). An important

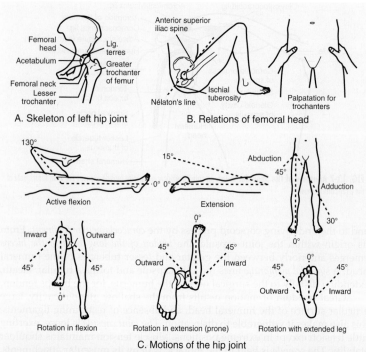

FIG. 13-8 Anatomy and Motions of the Hip Joint. A. Skeleton of the left hip joint. B. Relations of the femoral head. The greater trochanter lies on the Nélaton line between the anterior superior iliac spine and the ischial tuberosity. The relative positions of the femoral heads with respect to the trochanters can be compared on the two sides as illustrated. The thumbs are placed on the anterior superior iliac spines, while the fingers rest on the greater trochanters of the femora. Small disparities in distance are readily detected. **C. Motion at the hip joint.**

topographic relationship is defined by the *Nélaton line* extending from the *anterosuperior iliac spine* to the *ischial tuberosity*. With the thigh flexed, the line passes through the tip of the greater trochanter; an upward deviation of 1 cm is considered normal (Fig. 13-8B).

The knee. The knee region includes the *tibiofemoral* and *tibiofibular joints*, the *patella*, the adjacent segments of the femur, tibia, and fibula, their ligaments, menisci, and muscles. Viewed from below (Fig. 13-9), the articular surface of the femur has a horseshoe shape, with its open-end posterior. The horseshoe's two anteroposterior legs are formed by nearly parallel *lateral and medial femoral condyles*, separated by the *intercondylar fossa*. The surface of the anterior bow is indented by a shallow median groove curving upward onto the anterior femur, *the patellar articular surface*. Superior to the articular surfaces of the condyles are the *medial and lateral epicondyles*. Viewed from above, the articular surface of the tibia presents two lateral, almost flat, oval facets, the *medial and lateral tibial condyles*, separated by an *intercondylar fossa* with anterior and posterior segments. The lateral borders of the intercondylar fossa are

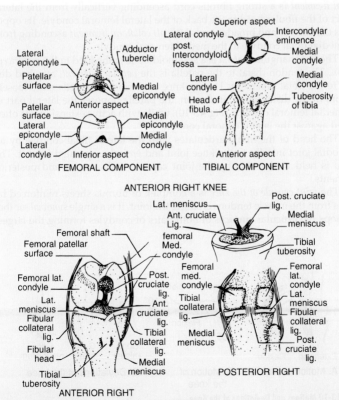

FIG. 13-9 Articular Surfaces and Ligaments of the Right Knee.

the *intercondylar eminences.* On the central anterior tibia, slightly below the joint, is the *tibial tuberosity.*

The *knee joint has three articulations:* a medial and a lateral condylar articulation and an anterior joint where the patella glides over the femur (Fig. 13-9). The femoral condyles may be likened to two thick disks with their edges resting on the almost flat tibial condyles. The small radius of curvature of the femoral condyles presents little apposing surface with the tibia in any position. The *lateral and medial menisci* are flattened crescents of fibrocartilage rimming the peripheral borders of the tibial condyles. Their radial cross-sections are wedge-shaped, with the thickest part outward. This arrangement deepens the articular surfaces of the tibial condyles and fills the space between the curved femoral condyles and the flatter tibial surface. The ends of their crescents attach medially to the intercondylar fossa.

The principal internal ligaments are the *anterior cruciate ligament (ACL)* and *posterior cruciate ligament (PCL),* named for the positions of their tibial attachments and their crossing arrangement (Fig. 13-9). The ACL begins in front of the anterior tibial intercondyloid eminence and passes upward, backward, and lateralward to the back of the lateral femoral condyle. The PCL attaches to the posterior intercondyloid fossa, passes upward, forward, and medially, to the front of the medial femoral condyle. The *lateral (fibular) collateral ligament* is a strong fibrous cord ascending vertically from the lateral aspect of the fibular head to the back of the lateral femoral condyle. Its opposite is the thinner and broader *medial (tibial) collateral ligament* ascending from the medial tibial condyle to the medial femoral condyle.

The flat triangular *patella* is a sesamoid bone embedded in the *quadriceps tendon.* The tendon distal to the patella is the *patellar ligament,* attached distally to the tibial tuberosity. During knee extension the patella rides loosely in front of the distal femur. In flexion, the patella opposes the lateral part of the medial femoral condyle (Fig. 13-10), while with active extension it is often pulled against the lateral femoral condyle.

The head of the fibula articulates with the lateral tibial condyle by an arthrodial joint inferior to the knee joint and entirely separated from it. The fibula is held to the tibia by the joint capsule and anterior and posterior ligaments.

The *joint capsule of the knee* is a complex of fibrous sheets reinforced by bands from the muscle tendons crossing the joint. It is a single *synovial sac* that envelops the articular surfaces of both pairs of condyles forming the largest

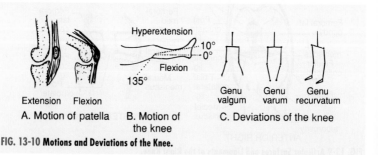

| Extension | Flexion |
| A. Motion of patella |

Hyperextension
10°
0°
Flexion
135°
B. Motion of the knee

| Genu valgum | Genu varum | Genu recurvatum |
| C. Deviations of the knee |

FIG. 13-10 Motions and Deviations of the Knee.

joint cavity in the body. A large *suprapatellar pouch* ascends anteriorly, first between the patella and the anterior aspect of the femur, then between the quadriceps tendon and a fat pad in front of the femur. Understanding the extent of this sac is diagnostically important.

The principal bursae of the knee are: (1) a bursa lying between the skin and the patella, the *prepatellar bursa*; (2) a smaller bursa between the skin and the patellar ligament, the *superficial infrapatellar bursa*; (3) a bursa between the skin and the tibial tuberosity; and (4) the *anserine bursa* medial and inferior to the knee joint between the tibia and the tendons of the *semitendinosus, gracilis,* and *sartorius* muscles. The suprapatellar pouch of the knee joint between the quadriceps tendon and femur is not a true bursa, though it functions as such. It may be erroneously called the suprapatellar bursa.

Full motion at the knee is flexion to >140 degrees and extension to 180 degrees or slightly beyond.

The ankle. The ankle joint is a hinged articulation between the proximal tibia and the distal talus. The superior talar articular surface is rounded superiorly, tips slightly medially, and is continuous with the flattened, nearly vertical, medial and lateral faces (Fig. 13-11). The upper curvature articulates with the flat surface of the lower tibia. At the sides of the joint the tibia's *medial malleolus* and the fibula's *lateral malleolus*, form the sides of a mortise articulating with the flat lateral talar surfaces to stabilize the joint medially and laterally. During ankle flexion and extension, the tibial surface glides over the curved surface of the talus changing the angle between leg and foot and rotating the leg medially on the foot with increasing dorsiflexion helping to transfer weight toward the medial foot and great toe during the stance and push-off phases of gait. The lower ends of the tibia and fibula are bound together by

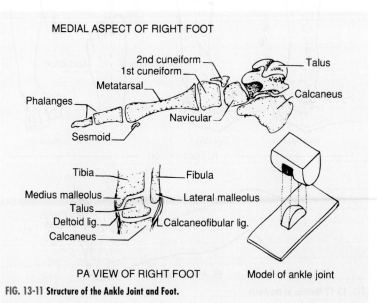

MEDIAL ASPECT OF RIGHT FOOT

2nd cuneiform
1st cuneiform
Metatarsal
Phalanges
Sesmoid
Navicular
Talus
Calcaneus

Tibia
Medius malleolus
Talus
Deltoid lig.
Calcaneus
Fibula
Lateral malleolus
Calcaneofibular lig.

PA VIEW OF RIGHT FOOT   Model of ankle joint

FIG. 13-11 Structure of the Ankle Joint and Foot.

the *anterior and posterior tibiofibular ligaments*. The medial malleolus is attached to the talus and calcaneus by a triangular band, the *deltoid ligament*. The lateral malleolus is attached below to the talus and calcaneus by the *calcaneofibular ligament* and the anterior and posterior *talofibular ligaments*. The joint capsule, lined with synovium, surrounds the articulation.

Ankle motions are dorsiflexion (extension) and plantar flexion (flexion) (Fig. 13-12). The only bony landmarks are the medial and somewhat lower lateral malleoli.

The foot. The foot is a complex structure designed to withstand the enormous forces transmitted bidirectionally between the body and the ground during walking, running, and jumping. It is both flexible and strong, and able to adapt to virtually any ground surface. It is divided into the *hindfoot* (talus and calcaneus), *midfoot* (navicular, cuboid and medial, intermediate, and lateral cuneiforms), and the *forefoot* (metatarsals, phalanges, and sesamoids). The hindfoot and midfoot are separated by the *transverse tarsal joint* separating the talus and calcaneus from the navicular and cuboid, respectively. The transverse tarsal joint is responsible for inversion and eversion. The midfoot is separated from the forefoot at the *tarsometatarsal joint*. The foot has two prominent arches: the *longitudinal arch* forms the instep medially from the tubercles of the calcaneus to the heads of the metatarsals; and, the mediolateral *metatarsal arch* from the first to the fifth metatarsal heads. The calcaneus is palpable on all but its superior and distal surfaces. The bones of the midfoot and forefoot are best palpated dorsally where they are not covered by

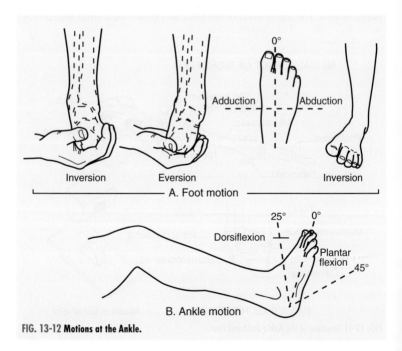

FIG. 13-12 Motions at the Ankle.

muscle. There is a bony prominence on the midlateral margin just above the sole formed by the tuberosity of the fifth metatarsal.

The foot can be visualized anatomically as a tripod constructed of a series of triangles, each with an apex and a base. The tripod has its apex at the tibiotalar joint and a triangular base made up of the calcaneus and the first and fifth metatarsal heads. This tripod allows stable weight bearing on uneven ground. One of the triangles is the longitudinal arch with its apex at the transverse tarsal joint and its base the calcaneus and first metatarsal head. Another is the metatarsal arch, with its base the first and fifth metatarsal heads and its apex the third metatarsal head. The tip of the great toe with the first and fifth metatarsal heads forms the stable triangular base for the pushoff phase of gait. Last, each toe forms a triangle with the apex at the proximal interphalangeal (PIP) joint and the base at the pad of the toe and the metatarsal head. These functionally interlocking structures give the foot extraordinary strength and dynamic stability. Any disruption of this complex architecture results in significant loss of function.

EXAMINING THE SPINE AND EXTREMITIES

The exam must integrate the observations of bones, joints, and muscles. Most clinicians examine anatomic regions in a sequence dictated by convenience, rather than examining each component sequentially. The exam also requires constant cross-referencing to the nervous and peripheral vascular systems.

Examining the Spine

Examining the cervical spine. STOP: *Following trauma or suspected neck injury, the cervical spine must ALWAYS be immediately IMMOBILIZED in a rigid collar PRIOR TO ANY MOVEMENT or examination of the patient.* In the absence of acute trauma, examine the patient in the seated position viewing the neck from the front, sides, and back for deformities and unusual posture. Have the patient point to the site of pain. Test active motions of the neck with the instructions: "chin to chest," "chin to right and left shoulder," "ear to right and left shoulder," and "head back." With the flat of the hand, palpate the paravertebral muscles for spasm, tender points or trigger points. Palpate and percuss the spinous processes for tenderness.

Examining the thoracolumbar spine and pelvis. STOP: *Following trauma or suspected spinal injury, the spine must ALWAYS be immediately immobilized on a back board PRIOR TO ANY MOVEMENT or examination of the patient.* In the absence of acute trauma, the patient should be gowned to allow easy observation of the spine while maintaining patient comfort. ***With the Patient Standing:*** **Inspect** from the back and side for deformity, muscle wasting, local swelling, abnormal curvature, or lateral deviations of the spine. If the spinal processes are not visible, palpate and mark each to disclose a scoliosis. When lateral curvature is present, have the patient bend forward observing the spine and the chest wall on either side of the spine. Note whether the spine straightens and any asymmetry of the chest wall. In structural scoliosis, one side is higher than the other (Fig. 13-13); with muscle spasm or ligament and joint disease, the chest is symmetrical. Tensing the glutei reveals wasting. **Percuss** each spinous process to elicit tenderness. Have the patient

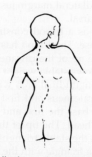

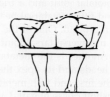

Scoliosis as demonstrated
by marking spinous processes

Scoliosis as viewed
with spine hyperflexed

FIG. 13-13 Structural Scoliosis. Inspection of the flexed spine from behind shows the unequal elevation of the two erector spinae muscle masses.

walk observing the gait. Hopping on each foot identifies muscle weakness and pain. Direct the patient to flex, extend, and laterally bend the spine without assistance. Test rotation by grasping the hips while the patient turns first one shoulder, then the other. **Palpate** for tenderness, muscles spasm, and tender or trigger points. ***With the Patient Supine:*** For comfort, have the head pillowed and the knees slightly flexed. Do the *straight-leg-raising test* (Fig. 13-14A) by grasping the ankle, with the knee held in extension, and lifting the lower leg to its limit. Note the location of pain, especially con-tralateral radiation indicating nerve root compression (*Lasèque sign*). With the straight leg elevated at a little-less-than-complete hip flexion, dorsiflex the foot looking for aggravation of pain. An alternative test is to gradually extend the flexed knee, with the finger pressing on the tibial nerve in the popliteal fossa; this produces pain if there is irritation of the lower lumbar nerve roots. ***With the Patient Prone:*** Have the patient turn from the supine to the prone position noting guarding, an indication of pain severity. For comfort, place a pillow between the table and the patient's pelvis. See if the muscle spasm and spinal deformity observed while erect persists in the prone position. Reexamine for areas of tenderness and deformity. A step deformity between L5 and S1 indicates *spondylolisthesis*. With the heel of the hand, press along the spinous processes. Pain from light pressure sug-gests approximating vertebrae with an intervening bursa; pain from deep pressure arises in intervertebral facets or disks. ***With the Patient Sitting:*** Examine for muscle wasting and check the knee and ankle reflexes.

Schober test for lumbar flexion. With patient standing erect, heels together, mark the spine at the lumbosacral junction (the L5 spinous process or the point where a horizontal line between the posterior superior iliac spines in-tersects the spine) and a second mark 10 cm above the first. Have the patient bend forward maximally, trying to touch the fingers to the toes. Normally, the distance between the marks increases by $\geq$5 cm. If the distance increases <4 cm, mobility is restricted.

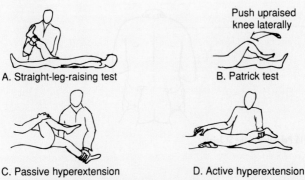

FIG. 13-14 Tests at the Hip and SI Joint. A. Straight-leg-raising **test.** The examiner lifts the supine patient's lower limb when the knee is held in extension. **B. Patrick test.** Lateral rotation of the hip is assessed by having the knee flexed and the foot of that leg placed on the opposite patella. The examiner then pushes the flexed knee down and out rotating the femoral head. **C. Passive hyperextension of the thigh (Gaenslen test).** While supine, the patient flexes the knee and femur on the affected side and holds the knee with the hands to eliminate lumbar lordosis. The examiner then hyperextends the unaffected thigh by letting it sink over the side of the table. In SI joint disease this maneuver evokes pain. **D. Active hyperextension.** With the patient prone and the abdomen resting on a pillow, the patient lifts the spine against the resistance of the examiner's hand; SI disease causes pain.

Additional exams for herniated disk. Test neurosensory function by assessing knee and ankle reflexes, flexion and extension strength at the knee and ankle, great toe extension strength, and sensation to touch. *Crossed-Straight-Leg-Raising Test:* With the patient supine, lift the unaffected leg holding the knee straight. With a herniated disk, this maneuver exacerbates the pain in the affected limb and may cause sciatic pain in the hitherto unaffected limb. This is considered by some to be pathognomonic for a herniated disk. *Reverse Straight-Leg-Raising Test:* With the patient lying prone and the knee flexed maximally on the thigh, quadriceps tightness in the anterior thigh is normally felt. With true disk disease, as the root tightens over the involved disk and abdominal compression increases subarachnoid pressure, pain is felt in the back or in a sciatic distribution on the affected side.

Testing the sacroiliac (SI) joint. Examine the patient while sitting facing away from you. Locate the posterior superior iliac spines by the dimples in the overlying skin or by placing your thumbs on the iliac crests (Fig. 13-15); follow the crests medially to the iliac spines. The portion of the SI joint most accessible to palpation is one fingerbreadth medial to the spines. As the patient bends forward slowly, press your thumbs deeply along the joint testing for tenderness. In the *Gaenslen test of the SI joint* (Fig. 13-14C), the supine patient holds the knee of the affected side with both hands, flexing the knee and the hip fixing the lumbar spine against the table; then the other thigh is hyperextended by pushing it downward over the side of the table. An affected SI joint will be painful. Active prone hyperextension of the spine (Fig. 13-14D) may aggravate SI pain when the patient attempts to lift the spine against the resistance of the examiner's hand held in the lumbar region.

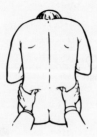

FIG. 13-15 Palpation of the SI Joints.

Low back pain—Magnuson pointing test for malingering. Low back pain is a favorite complaint of malingerers. Identify the painful spot by palpation marking it with a skin pencil. After completing the rest of the exam, palpate again for the painful spot. The patient with organic disease identifies the same point each time; the malingerer identifies a somewhat different spot.

Examining the Appendicular Skeleton: Examine all joints systematically from head to foot or in reverse sequence, comparing right and left. To minimize pain and guarding, support the joint to be examined. *Inspect* the bony landmarks, the joint's size and contour (visualizing the joint capsule's location), the overlying skin color, and any deformity (swelling, angulation, rotation, subluxation, contracture, or ankylosis). *Palpate* gently for skin temperature and tenderness in the skin, muscles, bursae, ligaments, tendons, fat pads, and joint capsule. The normal synovium is not palpable, whereas a thickened synovium feels "doughy" or "boggy." *Test the joint for effusion* by placing the finger(s) of each hand on opposite sides of the joint, then compress with one hand; an effusion will displace the receiving fingers. *Test active range of motion* by having the patient move the joint through its full range. *Test passive range of motion* by anchoring the joint proximally with one hand while the other gently moves the distal member to its full limits. Feel how the motion terminates: muscle spasm, gelling that improves with repeated movement, joint effusion, locking from loose bodies in the joint, and fibrosis cause *soft arrests*, whereas bony ankylosis causes a *hard arrest*. Palpate over the joint for crepitus with motion. *Test ligament integrity* by anchoring the bone proximal to the joint while gently displacing the distal bone in the plane to be tested. The muscles must be relaxed when testing ligament stability. Always compare right and left since normal ligament tightness is quite variable, from tight to loose ("double jointed").

The upper limb. This anatomic region includes the structures of the neck, shoulder girdles, upper arms, forearms, wrists, and hands. Its principle function is the placement and manipulation of the hands. The exam usually begins with the hands and works proximally, the sequence used here.

The hand. Hand structures are relatively superficial and easily examined. *Inspection:* The *fingertips* in extension form an arc with the apex at the middle finger. With flexion the finger tips align at the base of the thenar eminence with the nails in the same plane; if there is shortening or crossing of the fingertips then prior injury with shortening and/or rotation of the affected phalanges or metacarpal is present. Have the patient gently make a fist observing the *knuckles*, the distal metacarpal heads. There should be a smooth arc between the index and little fingers. A depressed knuckle indicates a shortened metacarpal. Observe the intrinsic hand *muscle bulk* on the dorsum of the hand and the web space between the thumb and index finger. Prominent tendons and bones occur with loss of muscle mass, usually resulting from ulnar nerve damage. Inspect the hand's palmar aspect for normal skin creases, thenar and hypothenar muscle mass, callosities, and palmar fascia thickening. Inspect the nails and finger tips for deformities, ulcers, and signs of previous trauma. *Palpation:* Examine each joint for bony prominences, synovial thickening, or effusion. Palpate the thenar, hypothenar, and first web space muscles both relaxed and with contraction. If bone injury is suspected, palpate the entire length of the bone. To detect tenderness, squeeze the palm front to back and laterally across the knuckles. *Functional tests of fingers:* Complete functional exam of the hands requires an in-depth understanding of the anatomy of the bones, muscles, tendons, ligaments, and nerves of the hand and forearm. Here, we present a screening examination. The fingers are named thumb, index, long or middle, ring, and little, or they are numbered one through five. The phalangeal joints are termed *distal interphalangeal (DIP), proximal interphalangeal (PIP),* and *metacarpophalangeal (MCP).* The aspects of the fingers are dorsal (extensor surface) and volar (flexor or palmar surface). Figure 13-16 illustrates the functional assessment of the joints. Muscle testing is described in Chapter 14, page 632. Test active flexion and extension against resistance at the DIP and PIP joints. The *superficial flexors* attach on the middle phalanx assisting flexion at the MCP and PIP. Flexion at the DIP is performed solely by the *deep flexors.* Next, test finger abduction and adduction; these movements are powered by the *interosseus* and *lumbrical muscles* innervated by the *ulnar nerve.* Test the thumb flexion and extension power at the MCP and IP, as well as abduction and adduction performed by the *thenar muscles* innervated by the *median nerve.*

The wrist. *Inspect* and *palpate* the wrists for asymmetry, swelling, tenderness, deformities, and crepitus. *Testing wrist motion:* Primary wrist motions are extension–flexion (dorsiflexion and palmar flexion) and radial–ulnar deviation; Figure 13-4 depicts the methods of measurement.

The forearm. Inspect the muscle masses for symmetry; often the dominant arm is better muscled. Assess for weakness and/or wasting. **Palpate** the radial and ulnar arterial pulses. Forearm motions are pronation and supination (Fig. 13-17). Test for active and passive range of motion and power against resistance. Pain with resisted motion is especially important and the sites of pain should be palpated.

The elbow. *Inspect* and *palpate* the region for deformity, tenderness, and swelling. Swellings are more common on the extensor surface. Subcutaneous nodules are often found in the *olecranon bursa* and distally in the ulnar region. *Testing Elbow Motion:* The movements of the humeroulnar joint are extension-flexion. Pronation–supination principally involves the humero-radial and the distal radioulnar joints. Measurements of these motions are

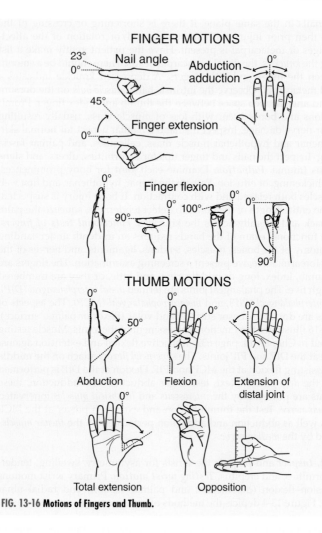

FIG. 13-16 **Motions of Fingers and Thumb.**

shown in Figure 13-5B. Test passive and active motion and strength by resisting active motion.

The shoulder. Examine the disrobed patient from front and back while sitting with the arms relaxed (Fig. 13-18). *Inspect* the shoulder anteriorly and the *scapula* posteriorly for deformities and muscle wasting; nearly everyone carries one shoulder higher than the other. *Palpate* the scapular spine, following it to the *acromion* and the *acromioclavicular joint*. Palpate the *sternoclavicular joint* for deformity or tenderness. Next, palpate the *subacromial space* and the *deltoid muscle* and its subdeltoid bursa. Palpate the tendons of *the rotator cuff*

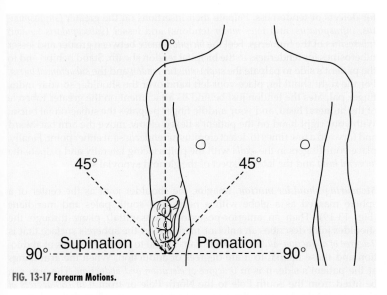

FIG. 13-17 Forearm Motions.

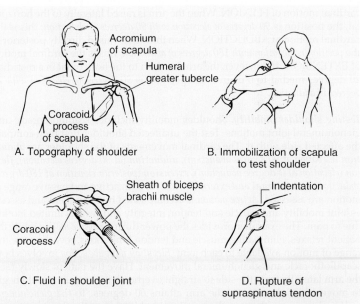

FIG. 13-18 Examination of the Shoulder Joint. A. Topography of the shoulder. The bony prominences of the humeral greater tubercle and the coracoid and acromial processes of the scapula form a right-angled triangle. **B. Immobilizing the scapula to test shoulder motion. C. Fluid in the shoulder joint.** The joint capsule distends around the biceps tendon. **D.** Supraspinatus tendon rupture.

for defects or tenderness. Palpate their insertions on the greater (*supraspina-tus*, *infraspinatus*, and *teres minor* tendons) and lesser (*subscapularis tendon*) *tuberosities* of the humerus. Feel the *bicipital groove* between greater and lesser tuberosities for tenderness in the bicipital tendon sheath. Stand behind and to the patient's side to palpate the *supraspinatus tendon* and the *subacromial bursa*. For the right shoulder, place your left hand over the shoulder so your index finger palpates the tendon just behind its attachment on the greater tubercle of the humeral head, and your middle finger palpates the subacromial bursa. With your right hand on the patient's flexed elbow, move the arm backward and forward a few times to detect crepitus or tenderness at either point. Finally, place your fingers in the *axilla* with the pulps facing laterally and palpate the *humeral head* and the lateral aspect of the glenoid synovial sac.

Measuring shoulder motion. Imagine the shoulder joint as the center of a sphere marked as a globe with a north and south poles and meridians (Fig. 13-19). Then an anterior-posterior (parasagittal) plane through the shoulder joint describes an anterior meridian on the sphere's surface that is *0 degree of abduction–adduction*. Meridians lateral to it mark degrees of abduc-tion and those medial to it are degrees of adduction. When the arm hangs at the patient's side, it is in *0 degree of elevation and abduction*. The arm can be lifted from the South Pole to the North Pole or from *0 to 180 degrees of elevation*. While elevating, the arm must follow in a meridian that designates abduction or adduction. If the arm is raised directly forward to the horizon-tal, the position is *90 degrees of elevation with 0 degree of abduction*; this is the cardinal motion of FLEXION. When the arm is raised laterally to the horizon-tal, the position is *90 degrees of elevation with 90 degrees of abduction*; this is the cardinal motion of ABDUCTION. When the arm is raised directly posteriorly, the *position is elevation with 180 degrees of abduction*; this is the cardinal motion of EXTENSION. If, however, the arm is raised to the horizontal in a meridian 20 degrees medial to 0 degree, the position is *90 degrees of elevation with 20 degrees of adduction*.

Testing shoulder mobility. Shoulder mobility includes scapulothoracic and glenohumeral joint motions. Test the unaffected shoulder first then compare the affected side with it. The cardinal movements of the shoulder are **abduc-tion** (*elevation at 90 degrees abduction*), **adduction** (*at 90 degrees elevation*), **flex-ion** (*elevation at 0-degree abduction*), **extension** (*posterior elevation at 180 degrees abduction*) and **internal and external rotation**. Both active and passive range of motion are assessed. *Active motion* is accomplished by the patient and assess-es joint mobility and muscle and tendon integrity and reveals limited motion due to pain. The examiner provides the power during *passive motion* while the patient relaxes, eliminating muscle and tendon limitations, revealing the full range of motion available to each joint. *Elevation with abduction* involves both scapulothoracic and glenohumeral movement. Have the patient slowly raise the arm laterally from the side to straight overhead; the scapula should begin to move when elevation of the arm attains 60 degrees. To *test glenohumeral motion alone*, grasp the scapular wing and hold it fast to the thorax with one hand while the patient's arm is resting at his side (Fig. 13-18B). Alternatively, place one hand on top of the acromion to stabilize the scapula. Have the patient elevate the arm laterally (90 degrees of abduction) as far as possible, with the scapula fixed. To *test adduction (at 90 degrees elevation)* rest the fingers of one

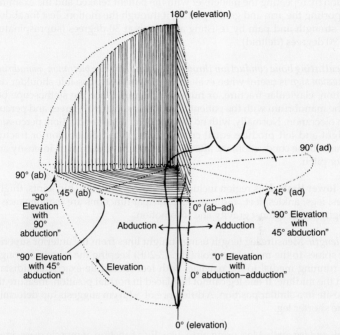

FIG. 13-19 Motions at the Shoulder. This terminology of shoulder motion can be confusing. The system presented here leaves no room for misinterpretation. **Elevation** is a movement of the arm along any meridian, measured from position at the south pole. Elevations along the meridian in the parasagittal plane passing through the shoulder joint are **flexion (forward) and extension (backward)**. Movement medial to this is **adduction**; movement lateral to the plane is **abduction**. When the arm is elevated in any meridian other than the parasagittal one, the motion is expressed as "elevation in abduction" or "elevation in abduction." The amount of deviation from the parasagittal plane is noted in degrees, for example, "elevation in 70 degrees of abduction."

hand on top of the patient's shoulder with your thumb behind, fixing the patient's scapula. Have the patient move the arm across the front of the chest as far as possible trying to place the wrist over the opposite shoulder. *Flexion* (*elevation at 0-degree abduction*) is tested by having the patient elevate the arm forward from rest to straight overhead in the anterior–posterior plane. For *extension* (*posterior elevation at 180 degrees abduction*), have the patient push the arm straight backward in the same plane to the limit of motion. *Test internal and external rotation* with the arm at 90 degrees of abduction and 90 degrees of elevation, starting with the elbow flexed at 90 degrees and the palm facing the floor. For *internal rotation*, ask the patient to lower the hand, palm down, as far as possible without moving the elbow. For *external rotation*, start from the neutral position and have the patient raise the hand, palm forward, as far as possible without moving the elbow. Repeat internal and external rotation with the elbow flexed 90 degrees and held at the side (0 degree of elevation and abduction). When there is a deficit in active motion, test passive range of motion by repeating the maneuver with the patient relaxed and the examiner supporting the arm and gently putting it through the motion. Test for abduction strength and pain by resisting abduction at 30 degrees (supraspinatus) and 90 degrees (deltoid).

Auscultating bone conduction through the shoulder. The *olecranon–manubrium percussion sign* is useful when evaluating patients with possible shoulder dislocation, clavicular fracture, or humeral fracture. Place the stethoscope bell on the manubrium with the patient's elbows flexed at 90 degrees and percuss each olecranon. Normally, with no disruption of bone conduction, percussion of right and left produce equal crisp sounds. When dislocation or fracture disrupts bone conduction, the affected side will have decreased intensity and duller pitch.

The lower limb. This region includes the pelvis, buttocks, hip joints, thighs, knees, legs, ankles, feet, and toes. Its principal functions are maintenance of upright stance against gravity and locomotion.

Leg length. Measure leg length using straight lines from the anterior superior iliac spines to the medial malleoli (Fig. 13-20E) keeping the tape in a straight line running medial to the patellae. Both feet should lie exactly equidistant from the midline. If one leg cannot be placed in normal position, measure the opposite in a similar position. A difference of >1.5 cm suggests hip deformity in the shorter leg.

Thigh and leg girth. Measuring girth, usually a function of muscle mass, identifies wasting not detected by inspection. Measure thigh circumference with a tape at symmetrical levels from the anterior superior iliac spines (Fig. 13-20D). Leg girth is measured at symmetrical distances below the tibial tuberosities.

The hip. The patient is disrobed from the waist down, covering the genitalia but not the buttocks. Have the patient point to the site of pain. An affected hip joint commonly causes pain in the inguinal region or in the buttock posterior to the greater trochanter. *Pain from the hip joint may be felt only in the knee; this has led to many diagnostic errors.* Begin with the patient standing. *Inspect* for a list to one side, asymmetry of the buttocks or other muscle masses, and scars or sinuses. Have the patient walk looking for gait abnormalities: swinging the leg from the lumbar spine suggests ankylosis; a waddling gait is typical of bilateral hip dislocation; the gluteal gait (*Trendelenburg gait*), the trunk listing to the affected side with each step, suggests gluteus medius weakness, or, rarely, unilateral hip dislocation. *Lateral tilting of the pelvis:* To determine if the pelvis is level, sit in front of the standing patient, with your thumbs on the anterior superior iliac spines; the interspinous line should be horizontal. Lateral tilting results either from adduction of one thigh or from shortening of the limb. Next, measure the distance between each greater trochanter and the anterior superior iliac spine. If the pelvis is not horizontal, place books or blocks under the foot of the shorter limb until the pelvis is horizontal, thus accurately measuring shortening.

Next, have the patient lie on the examining table. The following tests, except for extension, are done in the supine position.

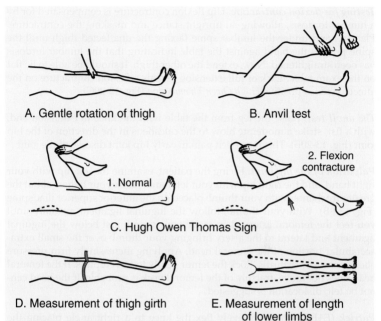

A. Gentle rotation of thigh

B. Anvil test

1. Normal

2. Flexion contracture

C. Hugh Owen Thomas Sign

D. Measurement of thigh girth

E. Measurement of length of lower limbs

FIG. 13-20 Tests of the Hip Joint and Thigh. A. Gentle rotation of thigh. B. Anvil test. C. Hugh Owen Thomas sign for flexion contracture: Flex the unaffected hip pressing the lumbar spine against the table. If opposite hip extension is impaired after eliminating the lumbar lordosis, it is a positive Hugh Owen Thomas sign. **D. Measuring thigh girth.** Mark a spot on both thighs measuring down from the anterior superior iliac spines. Measure the girth at each level. **E. Measuring leg length.** Approximate the legs or have them in the same relative position from the midline. Measure from the anterior superior iliac spine to the medial malleolus, with the tape running medial to the patella.

Testing rotation in extension. Because it is most gentle, this motion is tested first; if it is painful, all other maneuvers are done cautiously. With the patient supine, place a hand on each side of the lower thigh. Rotating it side-to-side watching the patella and/or the foot for the range of rotation (Fig. 13-20A).

Testing rotation in flexion. Flex the knee and hip to 90 degrees, then move the foot maximally both medially (*external rotation*) and laterally (*internal rotation*) (Fig. 13-8C).

Testing abduction. The patient lies supine with the legs together. Place a hand on the iliac crest grasping the ankle with the other hand. Gradually abduct the thigh until the pelvis moves, noting the angle attained (Fig. 13-8C).

Testing adduction. With each hand grasping an ankle, hold one leg down in extension while moving the other thigh across it (Fig. 13-8C). Note the angle attained from the neutral position. The thigh should cross the other at midthigh.

Testing for flexion contracture. Hip flexion contracture is compensated for by a lumbar lordosis, allowing an upright stance and masking the contracture. Place a hand under the lumbar spine flexing the unaffected thigh until the spine presses the hand against the table indicating that the lumbar lordosis has been straightened. Now, extend the other thigh. It should be able to lie flat on the exam table. Lack of full extension reveals a flexion contracture on the affected side, a positive *Hugh Owen Thomas sign* (Fig. 13-20C).

The anvil test. Raise the leg from the table with the knee in extension and, with a fist, strike a moderate blow to the calcaneus in the direction of the hip joint (Fig. 13-20B). This may elicit pain in early hip joint disease of the joint.

Palpation of the hip joint. Facing the patient, examine the left hip with your right hand, and the right hip with your left hand. Hook your fingers about the greater trochanter with your thumb placed on the anterior superior iliac spine (Fig. 13-8B). With your thumb, follow the inguinal ligament medially until you feel the femoral artery, then move your thumb just below the inguinal ligament and lateral to the artery bringing your thumb over the small extra-acetabular portion of the femoral head. Applying increasingly firm pressure elicits pain with arthritis. Rock the femur gently to feel crepitus. If the femoral head does not move, fracture of the femoral neck is probable. If the head cannot be felt, dislocation is suggested.

Patrick (FABER) test. Passively flex the knee to a right angle placing the foot on the opposite patella. Push the flexed knee toward the table as far as possible (Fig. 13-14B). This maneuver is also known by its acronym FABER (Flexion, ABduction, and External Rotation). Painless full external rotation (negative Patrick sign) excludes symptomatic hip and SI joint disease.

Test extension. With the patient prone, steady the pelvis with one hand while raising the limb posteriorly (Fig. 13-8C). Normal extension is ~15 degrees.

The knee. The normal movements of the knee are flexion and extension. For measurements, see Figure 13-10B.

Screening knee exam. Inspection: Have the legs and thighs uncovered; observe the patient standing and supine. Inspect the knee region for deformities, swelling, redness, and muscle wasting. Note the position of the patella. *Palpation:* With the patient supine, test swellings for fluctuance, joint effusion, crepitation with motion, and points of localized tenderness in the ligaments, bones, and along the joint line. Palpate for doughy synovial thickening obscuring bony landmarks. Test the range of flexion and extension, anterior and posterior mobility of the tibia on the femur, and the medial and collateral ligaments for laxity or pain. With a history of pain or locking, test for internal disorders as described on page 552.

Examining for knee effusion. Inspection may reveal bulging that obliterates the natural hollows on both sides of the patellar tendon and in the suprapatellar pouch. When extensive, it forms a horseshoe shape around the patella (Fig. 13-21A). *Palpate* with the patient supine and the knees extended. Gently press the thumb and fingers of the right hand against the anterior femoral condyles at the medial and lateral sides of the distal patella slightly proximal to the joint line. Slide the left hand down the distal thigh with constant pressure until the patella rests in the space between the thumb and the first finger. Apply pressure compressing the suprapatellar pouch. If effusion is present, a palpable and often visible fluid bulge appears under the palpating thumb and/or fingers. Lesser amounts of fluid is detected visually by compressing the swelling in one of the obliterated hollows beside the patella while watching for the hollow to slowly refill spontaneously or with compression of the suprapatellar pouch. Test for *patellar ballottement* (patellar tap or floating patella) by compressing the suprapatellar pouch, as described above, while the fingers of the other hand push the patella sharply against the femur (Fig. 13-21B). If enough fluid is present to elevate the patella from the femur, the brisk pressure on the patella forces it down against the femoral condyles with a palpable tap, the *patellar ballottement sign*.

Examining knee ligaments. This is part of the routine knee exam. Determine the degree of tightness or laxity of the anterior and posterior cruciates and both collateral ligaments. Always compare right to left since considerable individual variation exists for joint stability.

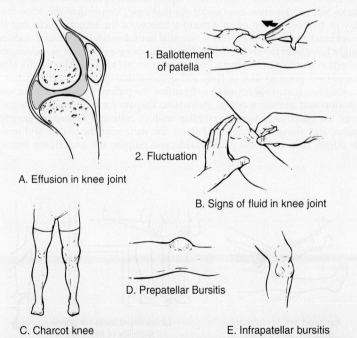

FIG. 13-21 Swellings of the Knee and Their Diagnosis. A. Knee effusion. B. Signs of knee effusions. C. Charcot knee. D. Prepatellar bursitis. E. Infrapatellar bursitis.

Collateral ligaments. With the patient supine, flex the knee to 10 degrees. Palpate the proximal and distal insertions and each ligament at the joint line. The rope-like *lateral ligament* is easily identified at the joint line posterolaterally. The broader *medial ligament* is more difficult to identify. Grasp the calf with one hand while the other hand supports and stabilizes the femur from behind with the thumb and fingertips on opposite joint margins overlying the collateral ligaments (Fig. 13-22). Stress the lateral then the medial collateral ligaments by exerting a varus then a valgus force on the calf while palpating over joint margin. Feel for separation of the tibia from the femur and look for medial or lateral displacement of the tibia.

Cruciate ligaments. Test the *anterior cruciate* with the *Lachman test* (Fig. 13-23A). Have the supine patient flex the affected knee to an angle of 30 degrees. Sit on the patient's foot to fix it. Grasp the upper part of the leg with your fingers in the popliteal fossa and your thumbs on the anterior joint line. Pull the head of the tibia toward you so it glides on the femoral condyles. Forward movement of >1 cm is a positive Lachman test, indicating ACL rupture. To test the *posterior cruciate*, start as in the Lachman test and observe for posterior sagging of the tibia. Then push the head of the tibia posteriorly. Displacement should be <5 mm. Always compare the two knees because considerable individual variability in ligament tightness is normal; asymmetry indicates previous injury.

The injured knee. Immediately after injury, muscle spasm and swelling may make full examination impossible. In that case, immobilize the knee for a day or two before the exam. Obtain a history of the trauma, including the exact mechanism of injury. This is essential to understanding which structures might have been injured. Ask which motions cause discomfort or locking and ascertain whether unlocking is sudden or gradual (as in muscle spasm). Have the patient point to sites of pain and demonstrate the position of fixation if locking has occurred. *Inspection:* Examine the patient supine; look for joint effusion and muscle wasting. *Palpation:* Palpate for tenderness, especially over the quadriceps tendon, patellar tendon, collateral ligaments, anserine bursa, and along the joint line. Palpate the surface of the patella and under its edges, then push the patella aside and palpate the underlying femoral

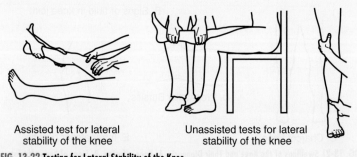

Assisted test for lateral   Unassisted tests for lateral
    stability of the knee   stability of the knee

FIG. 13-22 Testing for Lateral Stability of the Knee.

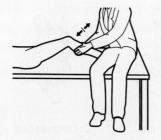 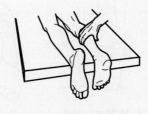

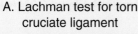

A. Lachman test for torn   B. Examination for ruptured
cruciate ligament   Achilles tendon

FIG. 13-23 Testing the Cruciate Ligaments and Achilles Tendon. A. Lachman test for a torn cruciate ligament. The patient is supine with the knee flexed at 30 degrees and the foot flat on the table. The examiner sits on the foot anchoring it, then pulls the head of the tibia toward himself testing the ACL. Forward motion of >1 cm is positive. Pushing the knee backward with the knee flexed at 90 degrees tests the PCL. **B. Examination for ruptured Achilles tendon.** The prone patient hangs the feet over the end of the table. Inspection shows less natural plantar flexion on the side of rupture. **Simmonds Test.** Squeeze the calf muscles transversely; a normal or partially ruptured tendon produces plantar flexion; complete rupture will not respond.

condyles. Put the knee through a full passive range of motion feeling a click with pain. A painless click is relatively unimportant as it may be normal, caused by tendons moving over a bony prominence. Observe the active range of motion and compare to the passive range of motion. Remember that joint effusion limits flexion and full extension.

McMurray test for meniscus injury. With the patient supine, grasp the injured knee with one hand with the fingers pressing the medial and lateral joint line (Fig. 13-24A). Grasp the heel with the other hand with the foot's plantar surface resting along the wrist and forearm. First, flex the knee until the heel nearly touches the buttock. To test the posterior half of the medial meniscus, rotate the foot laterally, and then slowly fully extend the knee. If a click is felt or heard during extension reproducing the sensation preceding pain or locking, the medial meniscus is torn. For the lateral meniscus, repeat the examination with the foot rotated medially.

Apley grinding test for meniscus injury. Have the patient lie prone on a couch (~2 feet (60 cm) high) (Fig. 13-24B). Grasp the foot with both hands, flex the knee to 90 degrees, and rotate the foot laterally. This should cause little discomfort. Now, resting your knee on the patient's hamstrings to fix the femur, pull the leg to further flexion holding the foot in lateral rotation; pain indicates a lesion of the MCL. Next, compress the tibial condyles onto the femoral condyles by placing your body weight onto the plantar surface of the foot, still in lateral rotation. Pain from this maneuver indicates tear of the medial meniscus.

Childress duck-waddle test for meniscus injury. This test is strenuous, reserve it for athletes (Fig. 13-24C). Have the patient squat and waddle on

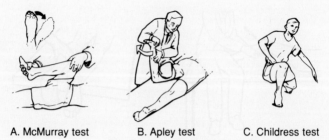

A. McMurray test   B. Apley test   C. Childress test

FIG. 13-24 Tests for Tear of the Medial Meniscus. A. McMurray test. B. Apley test. C. Childress test.

the toes, swinging from side to side. With rupture of the posterior horn of the meniscus complete flexion cannot be attained and pain or clicking occurs in the posteromedial joint.

The ankle. *Inspect* and *palpate* the ankle for edema, effusion, and tenderness. Test dorsiflexion and plantarflexion by grasping the heel firmly with the left hand to immobilize the subtalar joints while the right hand grasps the midfoot moving the ankle through the full range of flexion and extension. Test anterior stability by stabilizing the distal tibia with one hand while grasping the heel and pulling it directly forward with the other (*drawer test*). Test *inversion* and *eversion* stability by stabilizing the tibia as above while alternately firmly inverting and everting the heel. Increased mobility with each test indicates injury to the ankle ligaments stabilizing that motion. Always compare sides.

The foot. Inspect the shoes for uneven wear. Normal wear is on the heel's lateral edge. Wear on the medial heel and tilting of the vertical heel seam indicates abnormal foot mechanics. With the patient standing barefoot, inspect the heels from behind, the sides, and the front. Always compare right to left. Look for the normal slight outward angulation of the heel which should rotate medially when standing on the toes. Note any deformities (e.g., hammertoes or bunion), the height of the pedal arches, and alignment (a plumb line hanging from the mid-patella should point between the first and second metatarsals). Have the patient point to sites of pain and palpate each for tenderness and crepitus. With the patient supine, inspect the sole for calluses and palpate the fat pads under the calcaneus and metatarsal heads. Test motion by supporting the heel with one hand while moving the foot in dorsiflexion, plantarflexion, eversion, and inversion with the other hand (Fig. 13-12A).

Examining for flatfoot. The patient stands with the feet parallel, separated by ~10 cm. Note the height of the medial longitudinal arch. If it is flattened, see if it resumes a normal height when weight is removed. Test strength of the anterior leg muscles by having the patient stand on the heels. With the patient supine, test for shortening of the Achilles and peroneal tendons by dorsiflexion and inversion, respectively. Test eversion, which is limited in rigid flatfoot.

Muscle examination. See Chapter 14, The Neurologic Examination, page 632.

Brief Examination for Skeletal Injuries: STOP: If pain or other symptoms or signs lead you to suspect injury to the spine, IMMEDIATELY IMMOBILIZE the patient and obtain radiographic confirmation of stability before moving the neck or spine or proceeding with the exam. Trauma with enough force to injure major skeletal structures is frequently accompanied by internal visceral injuries, which ALWAYS take precedence over the skeletal injuries.

The following procedure rapidly evaluates an injured but conscious person to identify skeletal injury in the absence of specific complaints.

Head. Have the patient open and close his mouth and bite down while palpating the masseter muscles; if no pain is elicited, the facial bones are not affected. Palpate the zygomatic arch and nose for tenderness. Palpate the scalp for bruises and lumps. Press from opposite sides of the patient's head for pain suggesting a skull fracture.

Neck. Palpate the cervical vertebral spines before moving the neck. Have the patient roll his head gently from side to side while your fingers palpate the neck muscles for tenderness or spasm. Ask the patient to lift his head and place your hand under it. Ask the patient to push down with his head to assess his strength and discomfort.

STOP: If PAIN is elicited with any of these maneuvers, IMMEDIATELY IMMOBILIZE the neck and cease further movement or exam until the neck is cleared by adequate radiologic evaluation.

Chest. Ask the patient to take a deep breath; if this is painful, place your hands on opposite sides of the chest and squeeze. This will locate the point of tenderness of a rib fracture. Palpate the full length of each clavicle.

Spine. With the patient supine, slip your hand under his back, lifting the chest slightly and running your fingers down the spinous processes for tenderness and angulation. Determine if spine motion is limited.

STOP: If PAIN is elicited with any of these maneuvers, IMMEDIATELY IMMOBILIZE the spine and cease further movement or examination until the spine is cleared by adequate radiologic evaluation.

Arms and hands. Have the patient move, in succession, his fingers, hands, and arms through a full range of motion. Palpate each finger for phalangeal and metacarpal injuries. Shake both right and left hands asking the patient to twist his arm, with elbow both straight and flexed. If these maneuvers are painless with normal strength, injuries of hand, wrist, forearm, elbow, arm, shoulder, clavicle, and scapula are excluded.

Pelvis. With a hand on each anterior ilium press down, then put pressure on the symphysis pubis. Have the patient squeeze your clenched fist placed between his knees; lack of pain excludes fractures of pelvis and femora.

Legs and feet. Have the patient move first one leg, then the other, through a full range of motion. Palpate each toe. Have the patient stretch his legs flat on the table. Press his feet together and have him rotate them laterally against your resistance. Normal strength without pain on these maneuvers excludes major injuries of legs and pelvis.

MUSCULOSKELETAL AND SOFT TISSUE SYMPTOMS

Pain: Pain arising in bones, ligaments, and joints is well localized. Ask the patient to point with, a single finger, to where the pain is felt. Remember, pain from deep structures radiates to superficial sites having the same segmental innervation, e.g., femoral neck fracture may be felt as pain at the knee medially. Increased pressure within a closed medullary cavity is felt as severe, less well localized, boring aching pain. Acute injuries are described as sharp or stabbing pain. Pain elicited by movement and significantly relieved at rest indicates mechanical aggravation of a moving or supporting structure. By isolating the movement, the affected structures can be identified. Throbbing or pulsating pain suggests increased pressure in a closed or tightly encapsulated compartment being aggravated by arterial pulsation. Except for the intramedullary space, the compartment can be localized by squeezing or putting deep pressure on the tissues in the area of the pain.

Joint pain—arthralgia. Joint pain, with or without objective signs of inflammation, may precede arthritis by weeks or months. The onset, location, severity, and temporal pain pattern are important. Inquire for morning stiffness and whether activity makes the pain better or worse, and how quickly it remits with rest. Morning stiffness lasting >60 minutes suggests inflammation.

Bone pain. Mechanical injury, inflammation, infarction, increased intraosseous pressure, and stretching of the periosteum cause bone pain. Somatic afferent nerves carry the pain fibers and the pain is well localized, especially when the periosteum or endosteum is involved. Pain is often the only symptom of bone disease, although it may be accompanied by localized tenderness and swelling. Characteristically, bone pain is constant, well localized, worse at night and often intensified by movement or weight bearing. Bone pain refers to the nearest joint, but careful exam can usually distinguish articular from bone pain. Squeezing the overlying muscles excludes tender muscles as the pain source. Bone pain should prompt imaging.

CLINICAL OCCURRENCE: *Congenital:* Hemoglobin S and C (bone infarction), aseptic necrosis of the femoral head (Legg–Calvé–Perthes disease); *Endocrine:* Hyperparathyroidism (osteitis fibrosa cystica); *Degenerative/Idiopathic:* Paget disease, hypertrophic osteoarthropathy (HOA); *Infectious:* Osteomyelitis, syphilis, tuberculosis; *Inflammatory/Immune:* Eosinophilic granuloma; *Mechanical/Traumatic:* Fracture, tendon avulsion and rupture, ligament avulsion, epiphyseal plate injury; *Metabolic/Toxic:* Osteoporosis, osteomalacia, drugs (GCSF), erythropoietin; *Neoplastic:* Osteosarcoma, multiple myeloma, giant cell tumor, large cell lymphoma, Ewing tumor, metastases to bone, fibrosarcoma, chondrosarcoma; *Vascular:* Avascular necrosis (with glucocorticoids, hemoglobin S and C diseases).

Muscle pain—myalgia. Muscle pain is transmitted by somatic sensory neurons and is generally well localized. Pain results from trauma, repetitive or sustained contraction, inflammation, ischemia, and metabolic disturbances. Chronic myofascial pain is of unknown etiology, but probably represents alterations in the peripheral and/or central pain circuits. Pain is frequently referred to and from muscles and regional structures. History is the key to diagnosis: note the onset, duration, and character of the pain, its relationship to activity, rest, and symptomatic therapy. Myalgias accompanying systemic inflammatory illnesses are often more severe at night or with prolonged inactivity. The neuromuscular exam looks for wasting, hypertrophy, spasm, tenderness, trigger points, tender points, weakness, and fasciculations.

CLINICAL OCCURRENCE: *These are examples, only. Congenital:* McArdle disease (paroxysmal myoglobinuria); *Endocrine:* Hyper-/hypoparathyroidism, hypothyroidism; *Infectious:* Any acute infection, e.g., influenza, (less common but important: malaria, rubella, dengue, rat-bite fever, trichinosis, leptospirosis, typhus, rickettsiosis, Bartonella), epidemic pleurodynia, pyomyositis; *Inflammatory/Immune:* Rheumatic fever (RF), dermatomyositis, polymyositis, systemic lupus erythematosus (SLE), vasculitis, polymyalgia rheumatica (PMR); *Mechanical/Traumatic:* Trauma, strain, hematoma, march myoglobinuria, hypertonia, spinal stenosis; *Metabolic/Toxic:* Fever, acute hyponatremia, hypocalcemia, hypophosphatemia, hypomagnesemia, dehydration, diuresis, osteomalacia, drugs (statins and others); *Neoplastic:* Paraneoplastic myopathy and dermatomyositis; *Neurologic:* Fibromyalgia, neurogenic claudication; *Psychosocial:* Abuse; *Vascular:* Compartment syndromes, ischemia, atheroemboli, vasculitis.

Back pain. The pain is acute and/or chronic; the quality is sharp or aching. Think of back pain in terms of the anatomic structures that cause pain in, or radiate pain to, the back. Remember that pain from internal organs can refer to the back. Acute pain resulting from mechanical forces applied to the back is usually sharp and severe. Chronic pain, usually of an aching quality, follows acute injury or repetitive use injury.

CLINICAL OCCURRENCE: *Acute: Bones and Ligaments:* Fracture, dislocation, torn or avulsed ligament; *Cartilage:* Herniated intervertebral disk, diskitis; *Joints:* Reactive arthritis; *Muscles:* Strain, myositis, hematoma; *Nerves:* radiculopathy (disk compression, diabetes), epidural mass or abscess, subarachnoid hemorrhage, polio, tetanus; *Acute Referred Pain:* Dissecting aortic aneurysm, angina, retrocecal appendicitis, pancreatitis, cholecystitis, biliary colic, pneumothorax, pleurisy, nephrolithiasis, pyelonephritis. *Chronic: Bones and Ligaments:* Osteoporosis, osteomalacia, osteomyelitis, diffuse idiopathic skeletal hyperostosis (DISH), spondylolysis and spondylolysthesis, spondyloarthritides, tuberculosis, syphilis, Paget disease, primary or secondary bone neoplasm, spina bifida; *Cartilage:* Herniated intervertebral disk; *Joints:* Osteoarthritis (OA); *Muscles:* Chronic muscle strain, fibromyalgia, myositis; *Nerves:* Syringomyelia, Chiari malformation, arachnoiditis; *Chronic Referred Pain:* Esophageal carcinoma, peptic ulcer, chronic pancreatitis, pancreatic carcinoma, renal cell carcinoma, retroperitoneal lymphoma, hepatomegaly from any cause, spinal cord tumor, aortic aneurysm.

Upper arm, forearm, and hand pain. When pain is well localized to one part of an extremity, the diagnosis is relatively straightforward. However, pain is often diffuse throughout the upper limb, making an anatomic classification of causes useful. Limb pain can arise in non-musculoskeletal sites, e.g., pain referred to the upper arm by myocardial ischemia.

CLINICAL OCCURRENCE: Well-Localized *Pain:* Arthritis, bursitis, bone fracture, tendon rupture, tenosynovitis, cellulitis, muscle strain, neoplasm, ischemia and claudication; *Diffuse Pain:* Herniated cervical intervertebral disk, PMR, spondylitis, spinal tuberculosis, neoplasm of bone, Pancoast tumor, syringomyelia, radiculitis, carpal tunnel syndrome, ulnar tunnel syndrome, complex regional pain syndrome (reflex sympathetic dystrophy).

Pain in ulnar side of hand—ulnar tunnel syndrome. The ulnar nerve passes posterior to the medial humeral epicondyle in the ulnar groove, and then deep to the superficial flexors and above the deep flexors in the forearm, where it is stretched and compressed during vigorous muscular activity. Injury to the ulnar nerve at the elbow causes pain or numbness in the little finger, the ulnar half of the ring finger, and the ulnar side of the palm. Wasting of the hypothenar eminence and interosseus muscles results from prolonged compression. The ulnar nerve may be stretched or injured by a cubitus valgus deformity or an old elbow fracture. Other risk factors for ulnar entrapment include alcoholism and diabetes. Press on the ulnar nerve in its groove behind the median epicondyle; tingling in the ulnar distribution of the hand suggests ulnar tunnel syndrome.

Numbness, tingling, and pain—carpal tunnel syndrome. See Chapter 14, page 702.

Shoulder pain. Pain around the shoulder is common and may be poorly localized. Diagnosis requires identifying the anatomic region of pain, its quality, severity, and timing, and provocative and palliative movements. It is helpful to consider the conditions arranged by anatomic location. Focus attention on identifying the structures involved and shoulder stability. Several maneuvers are helpful in examining the shoulder but none definitively identifies instability.

CLINICAL OCCURRENCE: *Shoulder Joints:* Arthritis of sternoclavicular, acromioclavicular, and glenohumeral joints; subluxations of humeral head, acromioclavicular joint, sternoclavicular joint; *Bursae:* Subacromial and subdeltoid bursitis; *Tendons:* Supraspinatus tendonitis, tear of supraspinatus tendon (partial or complete), other rotator cuff tears, rupture of long tendon of the biceps, bicipital tenosynovitis; *Muscles:* Strain, fibromyalgia (tender points), myositis, hematoma, muscle rupture (complete or incomplete), PMR; *Bones:* Fractures of humeral neck, scapular neck, clavicle; snapping scapula; *Nerves:* Nerve compression by the scalenus anticus muscle (*scalenus anticus syndrome*), first rib and clavicle (*costoclavicular syndrome*); complex regional pain syndrome (*shoulder–hand syndrome*); *Vascular:* Aneurysm or thrombosis of the subclavian artery.

Pain referred to the shoulder. Pain is referred to the shoulder from many sites in the chest, especially those innervated by branches of the vagus nerve or cervical sympathetic chain. When the diaphragm is involved (phrenic nerve) patients present with aching or sharp pain usually felt over the top of the shoulder or in the trapezius at the base of the neck (see Pleuritis, and Chapter 8, Fig. 8-43, page 340). Myocardial ischemia pain is most often referred to the inner arms, jaw, and shoulder. Pain from nerve injury is often burning in quality and follows a dermatome. The following anatomic sites and conditions must be considered.

CLINICAL OCCURRENCE: *Cardiovascular:* Acute coronary syndrome and angina pectoris (to either or both shoulders), aortic aneurysm or dissection; *Pleura:* Pleuritis of the central part of diaphragm, pneumonia, tuberculosis, pneumothorax, or carcinoma of the superior sulcus (*Pancoast syndrome*); *Spleen:* (left shoulder only) Infarction, rupture; *Diaphragm:* Subphrenic abscess, leaking peptic ulcer; *Stomach and Duodenum:* Gastritis, peptic ulcer, gastric carcinoma; *Liver and Gallbladder:* Cholelithiasis, cholecystitis, hepatitis, hepatic cirrhosis or carcinoma, hepatic abscess; *Pancreas:* Chronic pancreatitis, carcinoma, calculus, or pseudocyst; *Nerves:* Herpes zoster, brachial plexitis, neoplasm of cervicothoracic vertebrae, myelitis, spinal cord tumor.

Hip, thigh, knee, and leg pain. In evaluating lower extremity pain, keep in mind that pain often results from unconscious redistribution of weight bearing secondary to an antecedent disorder. For example, limping on a chronically painful foot causes muscle strain in the back, pelvic girdle, and both lower limbs. Identify painful structures by palpable tenderness and pain accentuation with specific movements. Pain arising in somatic tissues (muscle, bone, tendon, and ligament) is usually well localized. Pain is referred to regional structures innervated by the same spinal segment, e.g., lesions of the femoral neck frequently produce pain in the medial aspect of the knee. For diagnostic purposes an anatomic approach is useful. Patients will often describe pain in the general region of a joint as arising from the joint, so maintain a broad view of "hip," "knee," and "ankle" pain.

CLINICAL OCCURRENCE: *Muscle:* Medication (statins), strains and tears, hematoma, PMR, fibromyalgia, ischemia and infarction, infection, tumors; *Soft Tissues:* Herniation of fat through muscle fascia, bursitis; *Tendons:* Tenosynovitis, strain and rupture; *Joints:* Arthritis (inflammatory, septic, crystal-induced, OA), dislocations, sprains; *Bones:* Fractures, neoplasms, osteomyelitis, osteoporosis, osteomalacia, aseptic necrosis, spondylolisthesis; *Arteries:* Thrombosis, embolism (thrombus, atheroma, fat, septic vegetations), vasculitis, aneurysm; *Veins:* Thrombosis, thrombophlebitis, venulitis, venous insufficiency; *Nerves:* Herniated intervertebral disk, epidural mass, contusion, vasculitis (mononeuritis multiplex), tabes dorsalis, neoplasms (especially neurofibromas), postherpetic neuralgia, peripheral neuropathies (e.g., diabetes and others).

MUSCULOSKELETAL AND SOFT TISSUE SIGNS

General Signs
Painless nodules near joints or tendons. Several diseases produce painless nodules in joint capsules, tendons, ligaments, or the surrounding connective tissue. *Rheumatoid nodules* in rheumatoid arthritis (RA) or acute RF are subcutaneous usually in the periosteum or the deeper layers of the skin over bony prominences. *Gouty tophi*, although usually in bursae, also form in the

Achilles tendon and pinna of the ear. The diagnostic *tendon xanthomas* of hypercholesterolemia occur in the hands and the Achilles and patellar tendons. *Juxtaarticular nodes* (*Jeanselme nodules*) occur near joints in syphilis, yaws, and other *treponemal diseases*. Periarticular *calcium deposits* occur in the CREST syndrome and tumoral calcinosis.

Synovial cyst—mucoid cyst. These are either bursae or tendon sheaths distended by fluid or protrusion cysts herniated by hydrostatic pressure from joint capsules. They are usually nontender and fluctuant. Protrusion cysts may collapse under pressure. Synovial cysts occur in RA, usually on the dorsal aspects of the PIP joints. In OA, they commonly occur over the DIP joints of the hands and feet. Cysts arising from the extensor sheaths of the wrists cause oval swellings on the dorsa of the hands called *ganglions*. The protrusion cyst of the knee is known as a *Baker* or *popliteal cyst*.

Noisy joints. Normal joint surfaces produce a smooth, gliding motion without palpable or audible friction or noise. Inflammation, cartilage injury, and loose bodies are often associated with clicks or crepitation on movement. Moving joints may emit several sounds. The knees or hips produce creaking. Crepitus, a grating sound that may be palpable, is produced by roughened cartilage surfaces rubbing together indicating significant joint surface damage.

Muscle tenderness. Pain reproduced by gently squeezing the muscles identifies pain arising in muscles distinguishing it from referred pain. Tonic muscle contraction is identified as palpable persistent muscle firmness. Both muscle and joint pain are intensified by movement. Neuritic pain is associated with tenderness over the nerve trunk radiating in the distribution of its branches. Chronic neuritic pain may trigger secondary tonic muscle contractions.

Increased joint mobility. Passive joint motion is restrained by ligaments attached to the bones across the joint. Muscle contraction also restrains active motion. Excessive motion implies a congenital or acquired ligament disorder. Acquired laxity from acute or chronic ligament injury is limited to the affected joint and the motion normally restrained by the affected ligament resulting in asymmetry between the affected and the unaffected side. Diffuse joint laxity results from congenital connective tissue disorders of the *Ehlers–Danlos syndromes*. Increased laxity of the skin, easy bruising, and poor scar formation are common manifestations of these syndromes. *Benign hypermobility syndrome* is more common and can be associated with loose joints, daytime pain and nighttime awakening with discomfort, especially after exercise. It is more common in females and is a cause of musculoskeletal pain in children and young adults.

Bone swelling. Swelling is detected by inspection and palpation, but the signs are rarely diagnostic. The location of the swelling in a long bone may be distinctive. Hamilton Bailey formulated the following diagnostic aids: (1) swelling in all diameters of the bulbous end of a long bone is most likely caused by *giant cell tumor*; (2) swelling on one aspect of a bone near the epiphyseal line is most likely an *epiphyseal exostosis*; (3) swelling in all diameters, beginning at the metaphysis and extending toward the center of gravity, may be *Brodie abscess, osteoid osteoma*, or *osteosarcoma*; (4) swelling in all diameters, at the center of gravity, may be *Ewing tumor, eosinophilic granuloma*, or *bone cyst*; and (5) consider that any localized bone tumor may be *metastatic from a distant primary*, so complete examination is indicated. X-ray findings may be distinctive, but biopsy is often indicated.

Bone nodule—occupational nodule. Repeated trauma during work or sport to a limited region of soft tissue and underlying bone may cause bosses of the bones with overlying calluses. Examples are *surfer's nodules* on the dorsa of the feet (from pressure on the surfboard as the surfer sits cross-legged) and *painter's bosses* on the subcutaneous surface of the tibia at the junction of the upper and middle thirds from standing on a ladder and resting the tibias against the next higher rung.

Trigger points—myofascial pain. Painful firm nodules or bands occur in muscles under frequent tonic contraction. The patient complains of pain, often with projection of pain in a nondermatomal pattern around the area and distally, e.g., into the arm from trigger points in the upper back and neck, or into the leg from trigger points in the pelvic girdle. The pain often has a burning quality. Motor strength and sensation are normal. Trigger points are characteristic of myofascial pain syndromes. They occur most commonly in large muscles of the back and proximal extremities. Injection of local anesthetic, heat, massage, and stretching, combined with avoidance or changes in precipitating postural activities, is effective therapy. Left untreated, changes may occur in central and peripheral pain pathways leading to chronic persistent pain syndromes.

Tender points—fibromyalgia. Persistent reproducible pain is elicited by palpating specific muscles. The patient does not complain of pain in these sites, unlike trigger points. Eighteen symmetrically located sites in the neck, back, and extremities have been standardized for the diagnosis of fibromyalgia (page 607).

Thoracolumbar Spine and Pelvis Signs
Dorsal protrusion from the spine—spina bifida cystica. Failure to fuse the neural arch of a vertebra is *spina bifida*. When the meninges form a sac protruding through the defective arch, it is a *meningocele* (Fig. 13-25A). When the sac contains spinal cord or cauda equina, it is a *myelomeningocele*. In *spina bifida occulta*, there is no protrusion of the meninges; the only external manifestation may be a skin dimple, a patch of hair, or a lipomatous nevus. The sac is covered by healthy skin and the local swelling is filled with spinal fluid making it fluctuant and translucent. With *myelomeningocele*, the overlying skin is frequently defective and transillumination may show cord or nerve fibers. Transmission of pressure from the open fontanelle to the meningocele suggests that the communication is wide. Sometimes, a sinus leads from a spina bifida occulta to the sacral skin, a congenital *sacrococcygeal sinus*, often mistaken for a pilonidal sinus.

Scoliosis. Scoliosis is most often idiopathic, occurring most commonly in adolescent girls. *Compensatory scoliosis* occurs with torticollis, thoracoplasty, congenital hip dislocation, and shortened lower limb. *Structural scoliosis*

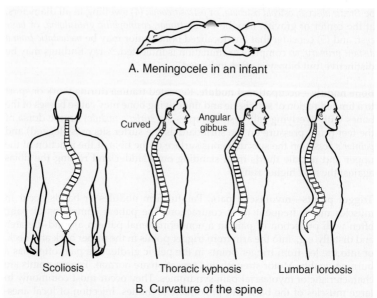

A. Meningocele in an infant

Curved

Angular gibbus

Scoliosis   Thoracic kyphosis   Lumbar lordosis

B. Curvature of the spine

FIG. 13-25 Spinal Disorders. A. Meningocele. B. Spine Curvatures.

occurs in congenital deformities and paralysis of back or abdominal muscles. Lateral thoracic spine curvature is usually accompanied by some vertebral body rotation but only the lateral deviation of the spinous processes is visible. Minor *functional scoliosis* forms a single lateral curve, usually with convexity to the right. With structural changes, the lateral thoracic curve produces an opposite compensatory curve inferiorly, the line of spinous processes forming an S-shaped curve. The spinous processes always rotate toward the concave side. On the convex side, the vertebral body rotation causes flattening of the ribs anteriorly and bulging of the chest posteriorly, elevation of the shoulder, and lowering of the hip. Viewed from the patient's back, the posterior bulge is augmented with anteflexion of the spine (Figs. 13-13 and 13-25). Lateral deviation with a single curve is usually postural disappearing with extreme spine flexion. An S-shaped or other complex curve may be compensatory or structural (Fig. 13-25B).

Kyphosis. The normal forward concavity of the thoracic spine is accentuated, producing a hunchback (Fig. 13-25B). A smooth curve results from faulty posture, rigid kyphosis of adolescence (*Scheuermann disease*), ankylosing spondylitis, Paget disease, osteoporosis (*Dowager hump*), acromegaly, and senile kyphosis. Of these, only the curve of faulty posture disappears with spine extension. An abrupt angular curve, a *gibbus deformity*, is caused by the collapse of one or more contiguous vertebrae (Fig. 13-25B), resulting from osteoporosis, osteomyelitis, tuberculosis, neoplasm (e.g., multiple myeloma), or trauma. In either *curved or angular kyphosis*, the spinal flexion may force the thorax permanently into the inspiratory position, with increased anteroposterior diameter and horizontal ribs. The distortion is identical with the barrel chest of pulmonary emphysema, but the auscultatory signs of emphysema are absent.

Kyphoscoliosis. The thoracic deformity of scoliosis is accentuated and compounded when kyphosis is also present. The thoracic cavity may be so reduced as to compromise cardiopulmonary function.

Backward spinal curvature—lordosis. The normal posterior concavity of the lumbar curve is accentuated (Fig. 13-25B). Weakness of the anterior abdominal muscles is a common cause. This occurs to counterbalance the protuberant abdomen in pregnancy and obesity. It compensates for other spinal deformities in spondylolisthesis, thoracic kyphosis, flexion contracture of the hip joint, congenital hip dislocation, coxa vara, and shortening of the Achilles tendons. Copper deficiency myopathy is associated with sway-back. Accentuating the lumbar curve throws the thoracic spine backward, the thoracic cage becoming flattened from the pull of the abdomen, resulting in an expiratory position of the ribs.

Low back pain with spinal indentation—spondylolisthesis. Most commonly L5 slips forward on S1 (Fig. 13-26A) because of an inherited defect of the lamina or fracture or degeneration of the articular processes of the neural arch. If symptoms occur, there is low back pain often referred to the coccyx or the lateral aspect of the leg (L5 dermatome). Inspection frequently discloses a

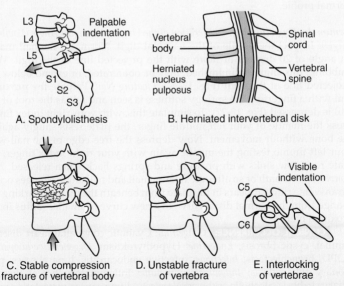

A. Spondylolisthesis

B. Herniated intervertebral disk

C. Stable compression fracture of vertebral body

D. Unstable fracture of vertebra

E. Interlocking of vertebrae

FIG. 13-26 Lesions of a Single Vertebra. A. Spondylolisthesis. B. Herniated intervertebral disk. C. Stable compression vertebral fracture. D. Unstable compression vertebral fracture. E. Interlocking or subluxation of vertebra.

transverse loin crease. Palpation of the lumbar spine reveals a deep recession of the spinous process of L5. There is restricted flexion of the lower spine.

Appendicular Skeleton, Joint, Ligament, Tendon, and Soft-Tissue Signs
Fingernail signs. See Chapter 6, pages 121.

Clubbing. Clubbing has intrigued physicians since Hippocrates. Recent evidence suggests that vascular endothelial growth factor (VEGF), reaching the systemic circulation either from the lung or via extra-pulmonary shunts, may be the cause of clubbing. Clubbing is reversible when the cause is removed. The three key observations are the floating nail base, loss of the unguophalangeal angle, and increased longitudinal convexity of the nail plate. Clubbing is painless and usually bilateral. With long-standing clubbing, the soft tissue and terminal phalanx become thickened, the convexity of the nail plate is extreme, and the fingers are bulbous. In the literal sense, the term "clubbing" should be reserved for this late stage, but it is now applied to the general process in all stages, from the first sign of floating nail. Convexity alone is seen in other conditions or as a normal variant. The floating nails and alteration of the unguophalangeal angle distinguish clubbing from all other conditions. The floating nail and flattened angle occur rapidly, e.g., within 10 days after a tonsillectomy complicated by lung abscess. With chronic illness of >6 months, the entire nail has abnormal convexity. The sequence of changes can occasionally be observed in a patient with subacute bacterial endocarditis. When first seen with a 3-month history of illness, a transition ridge is visible (Fig. 13-27). After treatment of the infection a second ridge appears, this one marking the transition between distal abnormal curvature and proximal normal profile.

Demonstrating clubbing. Obliteration of the Unguophalangeal Angle (Lovibond Angle): Inspect the profile of the terminal digit. Normally, the nail makes an angle of 20 degrees or more with the projected line of the digit. With clubbing, this angle is diminished, may be obliterated, or extend below the projected line of the digit (Fig. 13-27). *Floating Nail:* Palpate the proximal nail with a fingertip. The springy softness is seen and felt as the root of the nail is depressed (Fig. 13-27). To simulate this, with your right index finger press the mantle of your left middle finger; the plate rests snugly against the bone without movement. Now depress the free edge of the nail with your left thumb testing the mantle again with your right index finger; the plate root now sinks with pressure and springs back when released. *Nail Convexity:* A month or so after the floating nail and nail angle changes occur, a transverse ridge appears in the plate from beneath the mantle marking the change from the normal distal curve to a new curve of smaller radius in the proximal nail.

CLINICAL OCCURRENCE: *Congenital:* Cyanotic congenital heart disease, familial, cystic fibrosis; *Endocrine:* Hypothyroidism; *Degenerative/Idiopathic:* COPD, bronchiectasis; *Infectious:* Infective endocarditis, lung abscess, pulmonary tuberculosis; *Inflammatory/Immune:* Inflammatory bowel disease, biliary cirrhosis, alcoholic cirrhosis; *Neoplastic:* Lung cancer, metastatic cancer to lung, mesothelioma; *Vascular:* Hypertrophic osteoarthropathy, pulmonary arteriovenous malformations (including dialysis shunts).

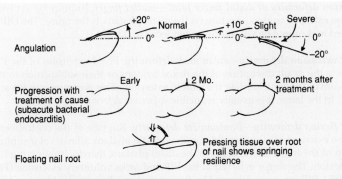

Angulation

+20° Normal +10° Slight Severe

0° 0° 0°

−20°

Progression with treatment of cause (subacute bacterial endocarditis)

Early 2 Mo. 2 months after treatment

Floating nail root

Pressing tissue over root of nail shows springing resilience

FIG. 13-27 Characteristics of Clubbed Fingers. There are three principal signs of clubbing of the fingers: 1. Angulation; 2. Curvature of the nail; and 3. Floating nail root.

Finger signs. Some finger abnormalities are considered with the hand; the more localized disorders are discussed here.

Thumb ulnar collateral ligament sprain. There is a history of a fall onto the palm, often while grasping an object with the thumb. The patient complains of pain in the MCP joint of the thumb and an inability to exert significant pressure on the pad of the thumb tip without pain or giving way. Exam shows tenderness and laxity of the ulnar collateral ligament.

Painless interphalangeal joint nodules—Heberden and Bouchard nodes. These are hard marginal osteophytes on the DIP and PIP joints, a form of OA. *Heberden nodes* of the DIP joints are nodules, 2–3 mm in diameter, one on either side of the dorsal midline (Fig. 13-30K). They are usually painless, motion is slightly limited, and deformity is progressive, but function is preserved. They are more pronounced on the dominant hand. Involvement begins in several joints most commonly in peri- or postmenopausal women. In women the condition is usually hereditary. A single Heberden node may result from trauma. Nodules on the PIP joints are *Bouchard nodes*. They occur with Heberden nodes, but somewhat less frequently than the latter.

Dactylitis—sausage digits. Enthesitis of one or more fingers produces diffuse "sausage-like" swelling with or without joint effusion. Dactylitis is seen in reactive and psoriatic arthritis and hand–foot syndrome of sickle cell or sickle–thalassemia disease. *Monarticular swelling—interphalangeal joint sprain.* A painful fusiform joint swelling may persist for several months. In most cases, there is a history of trauma.

Localized swelling—synovial or mucous cyst. A synovial cyst results from myxomatous degeneration of a joint capsule. A small, tense nodule, frequently mistaken for a sesamoid bone, appears over an interphalangeal joint. It may be so tense that it feels bony hard; usually, it is not fluctuant. Pressure may elicit slight tenderness. Often there is slight transverse mobility.

Flexion deformity of distal finger joint—mallet finger. Rupture or avulsion of the extensor tendon inserting on the distal phalanx is the cause. The DIP is flexed and cannot be voluntarily extended (Fig. 13-28A).

PIP extension deformity—swan neck deformity. Fixed extension of the PIP joint is the result disruption of the flexor tendons or their subluxation to the dorsum of the joint, holding the joint in extension. This is common in RA and SLE. In the latter, it is usually reducible, *a Jaccoud deformity.*

PIP flexion deformity—Boutonnière deformity. Rupture of the central band of the extensor tendon inserting on the middle phalanx allows volar subluxation of the intact lateral band to the distal phalanx thereby holding the PIP in flexion. The finger is flexed at the PIP and lacks voluntary extension (Fig. 13-28B). PIP extension followed by flexion may produce a palpable or audible click, as the lateral slips of the distal extensor tendons diverge and slip laterally over the head of the proximal phalanx, hence, buttonhole rupture.

Thumb flexion deformity—saluting hand. Thumb extension at the MCP and interphalangeal joint is performed by the extensor pollicis longus tendon; rupture leads to loss of function. The hand position approximates the hand position of an American military salute (Fig. 13-28C). The thumb is limply flexed and cannot be voluntarily extended. The tendon is often worn through by moving over the fragments of a Colles fracture.

Flexor tendon contracture. Tenosynovitis causes adhesions between a tendon and its sheath. Fibrotic shortening of tendons without synovial adhesions occurs in Volkmann ischemic contracture (page 600). The two mechanisms are distinguished with the wrist flexed by grasping the tip of the flexed finger

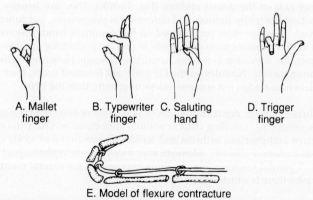

A. Mallet finger   **B. Typewriter finger**   **C. Saluting hand**   **D. Trigger finger**

E. Model of flexure contracture

FIG. 13-28 Acquired Flexion Deformities of the Fingers. A. Mallet finger. B. Boutonnière deformity.
There is permanent flexion of the PIP joint from rupture of the extensor tendon inserting on the middle phalanx. The position is like that employed when using a keyboard. **C. Saluting hand.** The thumb is limply flexed in the palm and cannot be voluntarily extended. **D. Trigger finger.** The fourth or ring finger moves painlessly into flexion. Extension is temporarily impeded, then occurs with a palpable snap. **E. Finger flexure contractures.** With sheath adhesions, passive motion is nil, even with wrist flexion.

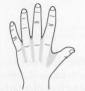

A. Interosseous atrophy   B. Thenar atrophy   C. Hypothenar atrophy

FIG. 13-29 Wasting of the Intrinsic Muscles of the Hand. Regions of atrophy are indicated by stippling.

pulling it into extension. With the slack provided by wrist flexion, the shortened tendon permits partial extension; adhesions to the sheath or palmar fascia prevent any extension (Fig. 13-28E).

Tight skin—sclerodactyly. See Scleroderma, Chapter 6, page 148. All digits are usually involved, Raynaud phenomenon is nearly always present, and cutaneous calcinosis may occur. Abnormal nail bed capillaries are common and should be sought.

Finger pad nodules
Osler nodes. Septic emboli from infective endocarditis lodge in cutaneous vessels producing microscopic abscesses. These pea-sized, tender bluish or pink nodules, sometimes with a blanched center, occur on the finger pads, palms, and soles of the feet in some patients with infective endocarditis.

Janeway spots. Janeway spots are only a few millimeters in diameter. They appear over hours to days as crops of erythematous or hemorrhagic, macular or nodular lesions. They occur in the palms, soles, and/or distal finger pads. Although painless and nontender, they may ulcerate. Most writers consider them hallmarks of bacterial endocarditis or mycotic aneurysm. Bacteria have been isolated from the lesions.

Circulatory disorders of the fingers. See Chapter 8, pages 287, 338 and 375.

Palm signs
Yellow palms—carotenemia. See Chapter 6, page 120.

Thenar wasting. The thenar eminence is formed by the bellies of *opponens pollicis, abductor pollicis brevis, and flexor pollicis brevis* innervated by the median nerve. Wasting suggests a lesion of the median nerve, most commonly carpal tunnel syndrome or severe OA at the base of the thumb. It accompanies wasting of all intrinsic hand muscles with axonal neuropathies (Fig. 13-29B).

Hypothenar wasting. The hypothenar eminence is formed by the bellies of *palmaris brevis, abductor digiti quinti, flexor digiti quinti, and opponens digiti quinti* innervated by the ulnar nerve. Wasting suggests damage to the ulnar nerve

(Fig. 13-29C). If both thenar and hypothenar wastings are present, consider cervical myelopathy.

Palmar fascia thickening—Dupuytren contracture. See page 598.

Granular palms—hyperkeratosis. Fingertip palpation discloses rough granular excrescences in the horny layer. The most common cause is chronic arsenic poisoning. A rare cause is *hyperkeratosis (tylosis) palmaris* et plantaris, an autosomal dominant disease associated with esophageal carcinoma.

Normal and abnormal hand posture
Position of repose. The relaxed posture of the hand is with the wrist slightly extended and the fingers and thumb flexed, the index finger less bent than the others (Fig. 13-30C). The hand assumes this posture to reduce painful tension on injured or inflamed soft tissues, tendons, muscles and/or bone.

Ulnar deviation or drift of fingers. The fingers deviate at the MCP joints toward the ulna and the MCPs may be subluxed (Fig. 13-30B). This results from MCP joint capsule hyperplasia stretching the capsules until the extensor tendons sublux to the ulnar sides of the joints.

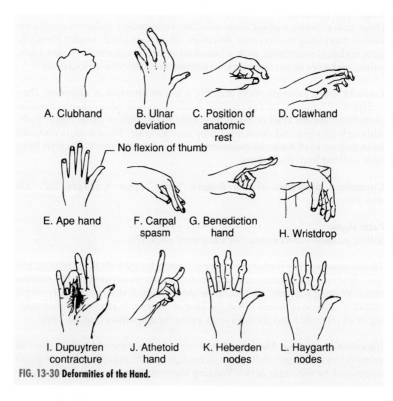

A. Clubhand   B. Ulnar deviation   C. Position of anatomic rest   D. Clawhand

No flexion of thumb

E. Ape hand   F. Carpal spasm   G. Benediction hand   H. Wristdrop

I. Dupuytren contracture   J. Athetoid hand   K. Heberden nodes   L. Haygarth nodes

FIG. 13-30 Deformities of the Hand.

Diabetic hand—diabetic cheiroarthropathy. In long-standing diabetes the soft tissues of the hand become thick and contracted bending the fingers into a slightly flexed position. Have the patient attempt to place the palms together; a space will remain between the opposing palms and fingers, the *prayer sign.*

Carpal spasm. The thumb is flexed on the palm, the wrist and MCP joints are flexed, the interphalangeal joints are hyperextended, and the fingers are adducted in the shape of a cone (Fig. 13-30F). All the hand muscles are rigid. The spasm is involuntary, usually painless, and cannot be relaxed by the patient. This posture occurs in tetany and *hand dystonia* associated with repetitive hand activities.

Clawhand. This results from the stronger pull of the *extensor communis digitorum* and the *flexor digitorum* against weak or paralyzed interosseus and lumbrical muscles. The claw reflects hyperextension at the MCP joints and flexion at the interphalangeal joints (Fig. 13-30D). Paralysis results from injury to the brachial plexus, ulnar and median nerve injuries, and syringomyelia, the muscular atrophies, or acute poliomyelitis.

Ape hand. Unable to flex, the thumb is held in extension (Fig. 13-30E). This occurs in syringomyelia, progressive muscular atrophy, and amyotrophic lateral sclerosis.

Benediction hand—preacher's hand. The ring and little fingers cannot be extended while the other digits move normally and, in extension, produce this posture (Fig. 13-30G). This occurs in ulnar nerve palsy, syringomyelia, and extensor tendon rupture in RA. It is named from the ecclesiastical gesture of pronouncing benediction. Do not confuse it with Dupuytren contracture.

Wrist-drop. Weak wrist extensors are unable to overcome gravity, so the hand drops from the wrist when the forearm pronates (Fig. 13-30H). The cause is radial nerve injury.

Athetoid hand. With athetosis, involuntary muscle contractions simultaneously flex some digits while hyperextending others, giving a resemblance to a writhing snake (Fig. 13-30J).

Large hands
Acromegaly and gigantism. See page 581. Soft-tissue overgrowth increases finger girth and thickens the palm forming a paw or spade hand. Arthritis is frequently present.

Hypertrophic osteoarthropathy (HOA). See page 580. All dimensions of the hands are increased, as in acromegaly, but HOA is invariably accompanied by finger clubbing.

Enlargement of one hand—hemihypertrophy and local gigantism. An entire side of the body may be enlarged in a congenital deformity known as hemihypertrophy. Local gigantism often results from a congenital arteriovenous fistula in the upper limb. In either case, the hand is normally proportioned.

Long, slender hands—arachnodactyly, Marfan syndrome. All the long bones of the hands are slender and elongated, often with hyperextensible joints. The *wrist sign* distinguishes elongated fingers from long, normal fingers. The patient encircles his own wrist, with his thumb and little finger proximal to the ulnar styloid process. Normally, the encircling digits scarcely touch, but in arachnodactyly they may overlap by 1–2 cm because of the long digits and narrow wrist. The *thumb sign* (*Steinberg sign*) may also be positive: when the fingers are clenched over the thumb, the end of the thumb protrudes beyond the ulnar margin of the hand (Fig. 13-31). Neither sign is specific for Marfan syndrome.

Interosseous wasting. The extensor tendons and metacarpals stand out on the dorsum of the hand due to loss of intrinsic muscle mass, most easily detected in the first dorsal interosseous between the thumb and index finger. Finger adduction and abduction are weak. Wasting suggests ulnar nerve injury (ulnar nerve entrapment at the elbow, diabetic neuropathy) or severe disuse (RA).

Dorsal hand swelling
Painless swelling. Edema arising from the deep spaces of the hand accumulates in the loose subcutaneous tissue dorsally, rather than the palmar surface, because of the restricting palmar fascia. Causes include infection, superior vena cava obstruction, anasarca, and *relapsing symmetrical seronegative synovitis with pitting edema* (RS3PE). Unilateral edema may also occur after occlusion of venous or lymphatic drainage in the upper arm.

Painful dorsal swelling. Infection and extensor tenosynovitis cause edema, erythema, and localized tenderness. Fluctuance may not be present even with

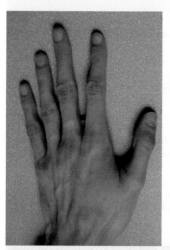
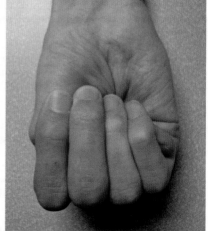

FIG. 13-31 Marfan Syndrome: Arachnodactyly and Positive Thumb Sign. These are signs of Marfan syndrome. The long thin fingers are notable and the tip of the thumb extends beyond the fifth finger when bent into the palm of the hand.

an abscess. A rare cause is *thyroid acropachy* associated with Graves disease and treatment of hyperthyroidism.

Wrist signs
Hypertrophic osteoarthropathy. See page 580.

Swollen wrist. Physical exam identifies the swollen structure. Periarticular edema in the subcutaneous tissues around the joint, but outside the synovium, pits with pressure. With thickening of the joint capsule and synovium the tissues feel boggy. When the synovial envelope is bulging and fluctuant, fluid is present. Effusion, pus, and blood are distinguished by aspiration.

Painful swelling or limited wrist motion—arthritis. With active inflammation, there is swelling accompanied by variable degrees of pain, warmth, and tenderness. The overlying skin may be warm and reddened. In RA there is swelling and limited motion, but no redness or excessive warmth. In contrast, with gout, pseudogout, and septic arthritis the joint is swollen, red, hot, and tender. Some presentation of Gout and Calcium pyrophosphate dihydrate deposition disease (CPPD) can look very similar to RA without any associated redness or warmth. Primary OA does not affect the wrist.

Localized swelling and tenderness—tenosynovitis. See page 600.

Localized painless dorsal wrist swelling—ganglion. This is a protrusion cyst of the joint capsule usually seen on the dorsum of the naviculolunate joint (Fig. 13-42D). It is painless, round, sessile, tense, translucent, and more prominent in flexion.

Dorsal angulation of the wrist—Madelung deformity. The wrist is deformed by a sharp protrusion upward (dorsally) of the lower ulna (Fig. 13-46C), best seen in pronation. This is caused by nontraumatic dorsal subluxation of the distal end of the ulna, usually in young women.

Forearm and elbow signs
Elbow deformity—cubitus valgus and varus. The normal elbow carrying angle is ~170 degrees on the lateral side of the arm and forearm, an angle <165 degrees is a valgus deformity, and one >175 degrees is a varus deformity (Fig. 13-32A). A difference of >10 degrees between right and left is also abnormal.

Elbow swelling—effusion. The elbow's synovial sac is loose and easily distended with fluid, giving a characteristic outline with fluctuant bulging posteriorly and on both sides of the olecranon process and triceps tendon (Fig. 13-32B). It is easily palpable between the lateral epicondyle, radial head, and olecranon. The elbow held in semiflexion accommodates maximal fluid volume. The joint may be distended by synovial fluid, pus, or blood.

Elbow arthritis. Any type of arthritis can involve the elbow joint. *Suppurative arthritis* produces painful swelling, with pus in the joint. *RF* and *RA* cause painful swelling; chronic RA often limits extension. *A loose body* is suggested

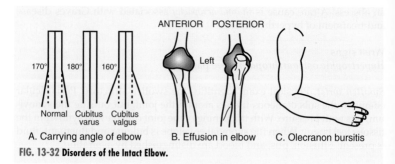

FIG. 13-32 Disorders of the Intact Elbow.

by locking. A unilateral enlarged, painless elbow may be *neurogenic arthropathy* (Charcot joint) and suggests syringomyelia.

Olecranon bursitis. Trauma, inflammation, infection, and gout cause effusion in the bursa overlying the olecranon process (Fig. 13-32C). The swelling is fluctuant. The location distinguishes it from fluid in the joint.

Elbow pain—lateral and medial epicondylitis. See page 601.

Upper arm signs. This region includes the humeral shaft and its covering muscles, principally the biceps and triceps.

Upper arm pain—bicipital tenosynovitis. See page 602.

Shoulder pain—coracoiditis. See page 602.

Bicipital humps—biceps rupture. The profile of the contracting biceps has one or two humps. One hump results from tendon or muscle sheath rupture (Fig. 13-47F). Rupture of the belly causes two humps. Rupture of the muscle may not greatly impair strength. Rupture occurs during lifting and is usually painful. Absence of this history suggests degeneration of the long-head of the biceps tendon in the shoulder joint, often associated with chronic impingement or shoulder synovitis. Rupture of the long-head tendon results in mild weakness.

Shoulder signs. See Figure 13-43. Full painless abduction excludes serious shoulder injury. Pain with elevation and limited active range of motion suggest shoulder pathology. Pain only from 60 to120 degrees of elevation suggests partial rupture of the supraspinatus tendon, supraspinatus tendinitis, and/or subacromial bursitis. Minimal elevation supporting the arm with the opposite hand point to fracture, dislocation, or complete supraspinatus rupture; in the latter case, passive motions are normal. Pain throughout elevation indicates arthritis. Descriptions of these conditions follow.

Painful arc and impingement sign—rotator cuff injury. See page 602.

Minimal arm elevation—complete supraspinatus tendon rupture, torn rotator cuff. See Page 603.

Frozen shoulder, adhesive capsulitis. See page 603.

Painful trigger points in shoulder muscles. Pain is usually present on arising and after inactivity, diminishing or resolving with exercise. Small nodules may be palpated on the surface of the trapezius or other muscles. Pressure on the nodule reproduces the pain, often with radiation to the neck and upper arm.

Shoulder-pad sign—amyloidosis. Bilateral anterolateral swelling of the shoulder joints is a conspicuous, although uncommon, sign of amyloid disease. The periarticular swelling feels hard and rubbery.

Winged scapula—long thoracic nerve paralysis. Serratus anterior paralysis permits the scapula to separate from the thoracic wall posteriorly, a winged scapula. Have the patient stand and push the hands against a wall while observing the scapulae (Fig. 13-33A). Nerve injury is caused by stretching during heavy lifting or surgical trauma.

Hip, buttock, and thigh signs
Femoral triangle mass. Psoas abscess. A conical mass appears beneath the inguinal ligament (Fig. 13-34B). Painful abscess suggests purulent infection within the abdomen. A painless abscess is usually an extension of spinal tuberculosis. *DDX:* Similar swelling in the iliac fossa distinguishes abscess from psoas bursa effusion. Abscess must be distinguished from fluctuant lymphadenopathy.

Psoas bursitis. A painless effusion in the psoas bursa, occasionally associated with OA of the hip, produces tense, nonfluctuant, immobile conical swelling

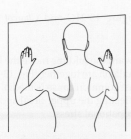 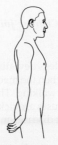 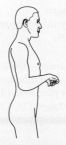

A. Winged scapula   B. Flail arm   C. Spastic arm

FIG. 13-33 Disorders of the Intact Shoulder. A. Winged scapula. When pushing the hands against a wall, the involved scapula protrudes posteriorly, forming a winged scapula. **B. Flail arm.** The arm hangs limply at the side with palm posterior and fingers partially flexed. **C. Spastic arm.** The arm flexes at the elbow, wrist, and fingers, with slight adduction of the humerus; the forearm is pronated.

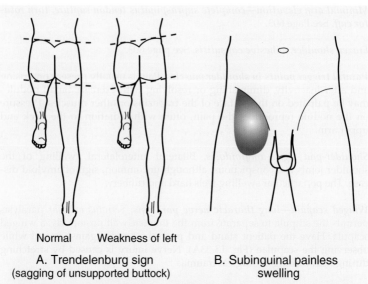

Normal   Weakness of left

A. Trendelenburg sign   B. Subinguinal painless
(sagging of unsupported buttock)   swelling

FIG. 13-34 **Lesions of the Hip and Groin. A. Trendelenburg sign.** When the patient stands on one foot, the contralateral buttock falls. **B. Subinguinal painless swelling.** Swelling below the inguinal ligament may be either a psoas abscess or an effusion in the psoas bursa.

beneath the inguinal ligament (Fig. 13-34B). The absence of a mass in the iliac fossa excludes psoas abscess.

Lymphadenopathy. See Chapter 5, page 83.

Femoral hernia. See Chapter 9, page 462 and Figure 9-37, page 463.

Knee signs
Neurogenic arthropathy—Charcot joint. Figure 13-21C and *Charcot Joint,* page 584.

Genu varum—bowleg. The legs deviating toward the midline move the knees farther apart than normal when the medial malleoli are together (Fig. 13-10C). The feet turn inward when walking. The most common cause is medial knee compartment OA. Other causes are rickets affecting the upper tibial and lower femoral epiphyses, Paget disease, and occupational stress.

Genu valgum—knock-knee. The legs deviate away from the midline, often bilaterally (Fig. 13-10C). The most common cause is narrowing of the lateral knee compartment in OA.

Knee swelling—fluid in the joint. Excess synovial fluid in the knee joint is an *effusion.* Blood in the joint space is *hemarthrosis.* Pus indicates suppurative arthritis. Fluid signs are independent of fluid type, so specific diagnosis is made by aspiration. Effusion is commonly caused by trauma, RA, reactive arthritis, OA, gout, other crystalline arthritides (calcium pyrophosphate, basic calcium phosphate), or intermittent hydrarthrosis. Traumatic hemarthrosis suggests intracapsular fracture or ligament disruption. Nontraumatic hemarthrosis occurs with hemophilia and neoplasms.

Anterior knee swelling. *Prepatellar bursitis.* A fluctuant subcutaneous swelling appears anterior to the lower patella and patellar ligament in the distribution of the prepatellar bursa (Fig. 13-21D). It is often associated with occupational trauma to the tissue overlying the patella. *DDX:* Fluid in the joint cavity produces swelling beside the patella.

Infrapatellar bursitis. Swelling appears in a bursa on both sides of the patellar ligament near the tibial tuberosity (Fig. 13-21E). Fluctuance is demonstrable from one side of the ligament to the other. This often results from occupations requiring kneeling, such as roofing and laying floors.

Infrapatellar fat pad. The infrapatellar fat pad becomes inflamed causing tenderness and swelling on both sides of the patellar ligament. Tenderness and lack of fluctuance distinguish it from bursitis and synovitis.

Popliteal swelling—semimembranosus bursitis. Fluid accumulates in the bursa between the head of the gastrocnemius and the semimembranosus tendon forming the upper medial border of the diamond-shaped popliteal fossa (Fig. 13-35). Knee extension causes painful tensing of the bursa, while flexion relaxes it. Fluctuance is difficult to demonstrate.

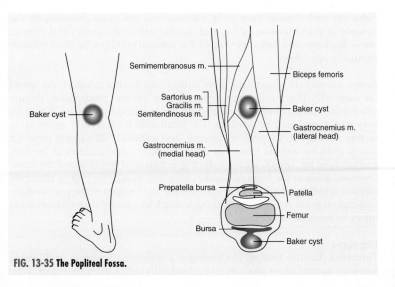

FIG. 13-35 The Popliteal Fossa.

Popliteal swelling—Baker cyst. The cyst is a pressure diverticulum of the synovial sac protruding through the posterior joint capsule of the knee. Sometimes, dull pain is present. The cyst is best seen by inspecting the fossa when the patient is standing. In contrast to semimembranosus bursitis, the swelling is in the midline at or below the tibiofemoral junction (Fig. 13-35). The cyst is not visible with flexion, unless it is very large, but protrudes when the knee is extended. When the cyst freely communicates with the joint, gradual, steady pressure forces some fluid back into the joint cavity, temporarily reducing the swelling. The swelling may be translucent. Baker cysts often complicate RA and OA. Large cysts can compress the popliteal vessels. If the artery is compressed, forced extension of the knee or strong dorsiflexion of the foot may obliterate the pedal pulse.

Popliteal mass—popliteal aneurysm. This feels like a cyst and only a conscious effort to detect pulsation identifies it.

Medial knee swelling—medial meniscus cyst. This is a developmental anomaly of the medial meniscus felt as a fluctuant joint line swelling. Dull pain may be present on standing. The oval, transversely elongated cyst protrudes either anterior or posterior to the MCL. Knee flexion makes it more prominent.

Lateral knee swelling—lateral meniscus cyst. This congenital cyst occurs at the tibiofemoral junction, posterior to the fibular collateral ligament. Flexion accentuates the transverse fluctuant swelling. It may be painful and, occasionally, protrudes into the popliteal fossa.

Knee pain and recurrent locking. A history of intermittent joint pain with recurrent effusion or locking suggests a loose body in the joint or a torn meniscus. Crepitus may be present; rarely, the examiner may palpate a mass. Loose bodies are usually a chip of bone from previous injury.

Subacute and chronic knee pain. *Osteonecrosis and stress fractures.* In the absence of direct trauma or signs of disease within the joint, tibial plateau stress fractures and osteonecrosis of the femoral condyles or tibial plateau should be considered.

Remote injury. Pain occurring acutely with or shortly after trauma is discussed on page 552. The more common scenario is chronic progressive, though often intermittent, knee pain frequently made worse by exercise. The pain may be accompanied by swelling. The location of the pain and aggravating factors are helpful. Crepitation, locking, and instability all suggest previous injury. With no specific history of injury consider abnormalities of the feet, gait, and/or leg length, each producing unbalanced forces about the knee. Overuse, often in the form of sudden increases in activity from a relatively inactive baseline, should also be considered. The location of the pain and the findings on exam will be similar though much less severe than with an acute injury to the same structure.

Leg signs
Thickened Achilles tendon. Thickening is a response to overuse or ill-fitting footwear putting direct pressure on the tendon inducing an injury-repair cycle.

Thickening is most easily detected by inspection and palpation with the foot dorsiflexed. Several conditions produce inflammation, e.g., seronegative spondyloarthropathies, or deposits in the tendon, e.g., xanthomas.

Ankle signs

Ankle swelling—joint effusion. The foot is held in slight dorsiflexion and inversion. The distended joint bulges beneath the extensor tendons near the talotibial junction and in front of the lateral and medial malleolar ligaments.

Pain or click during ankle dorsiflexion with eversion—slipping of peroneal tendons. The *tendons* of the *peroneus longus* and *brevis* curve behind and under the lateral malleolus, held in a groove by the *superior peroneal retinaculum*. Relaxation of the retinaculum permits slipping of the tendons during dorsi-flexion with eversion accompanied by pain or a click. Physical exam at rest is normal but active motion may produce palpable tendon subluxation.

Pain on inversion of the foot—chronic peroneal tendon sheath stenosing tenosynovitis. This causes pain only on inverting the foot. Tenderness and swelling occur in the sheath behind and below the lateral malleolus.

Foot signs

Foot nodules—fibroma. Fibromas are benign growths of fibrous tissue that occur anywhere on the foot, or elsewhere, usually following minor soft tis-sue trauma. They are frequently painful, especially on the sole or if impinged upon by footwear. They are firm, discrete, rubbery, and occasionally tender nodules usually fixed to the underlying soft tissues, not to bone.

Talipes, clubfoot. Most common are *talipes varus* (inversion), *talipes valgus* (eversion), *talipes equinus* (plantar flexion), *talipes calcaneus* (dorsiflexion), and *talipes* or *pes cavus* (hollowing the instep) (Fig. 13-36). Combined deformities are *talipes equinovarus* (clubfoot), *talipes equinovalgus*, *talipes calcaneovarus*, and *talipes calcaneovalgus*. The diagnosis is usually made by inspection.

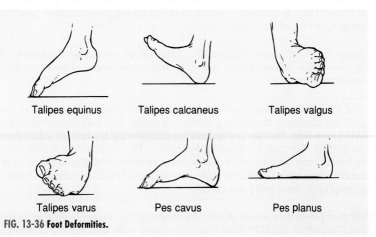

Talipes equinus   Talipes calcaneus   Talipes valgus

Talipes varus   Pes cavus   Pes planus

FIG. 13-36 Foot Deformities.

Pes planus (flatfoot). One or more pedal arch is flattened (Fig. 13-36). Functional classification identifies *relaxed flatfoot*, in which the arch is lowered only while bearing weight; *rigid flatfoot*, caused by bony or fibrous ankylosis; *spasmodic flatfoot*, from contraction of the peronei; and, *transverse flatfoot*, from flattening of the transverse arch.

Heel pain—retrocalcaneal bursitis. The bursa between the Achilles tendon and the calcaneus is inflamed causing pain, swelling, and tenderness near its insertion (Fig. 13-37B). This is caused by pressure from footwear, especially high-heeled shoes and stiff-backed boots.

Plantar heel pain. *Plantar fasciitis.* The plantar fascia is a thick fibrous band arising from the medial tuberosity of the calcaneus and spreading like a fan across the sole to insert on the proximal phalanges of the toes. Unusual or prolonged weight-bearing activity leads to microtrauma, which is concentrated at the calcaneal insertion. Pain is present in the plantar aspect of the heel and is usually worst with the first steps in the morning. Pain improves with activity, only to recur after rest. Tenderness is elicited at the insertion of the plantar fascia on the distal calcaneus somewhat medially.

Calcaneal fat pad inflammation. Fibrous bands extend from the calcaneal periosteum to the skin; their interstices are filled with fat. Infection or inflammation is compartmentalized by the fibrous bands leading to increased tissue pressure and intense pain. The region is too tender to permit weight bearing. Usually edema accumulates around the ankle; fluctuance is occasionally present.

Localized dorsal swelling—ganglion. The cyst arises from a tarsal joint capsule or an extensor tendon.

Instep pain—deep fascial space infection. The central plantar space has four compartments between the sole and the pedal arch (Fig. 13-37D). The spaces are infected from direct puncture or extension backward from an interdigital space. There is tenderness in the instep (midfoot), dorsal edema, and the instep's curve is obliterated.

Plantar fascia contracture. Unilateral or bilateral asymptomatic thickening of the plantar fascia is associated with Dupuytren contracture of the palms and Peyronie syndrome.

Great toe lateral deviation—hallux valgus. Lateral deviation and rotation of the great toe produces abnormal prominence of the first metatarsophalangeal (MTP) joint (Fig. 13-37E). The second toe may overlap the first, or it may be a hammertoe. The great toe retains good motion. Pain is caused by accompanying hammertoe, an inflamed bursa over the prominent MTP joint (*bunion*), or metatarsalgia from transverse flatfoot (*splay foot*). The most common causes are improper shoes and primary OA.

Stiff great toe—hallux rigidus. A prominent osteophyte is usually present on the dorsal aspect of the MTP joint. Pain may occur with walking and climbing.

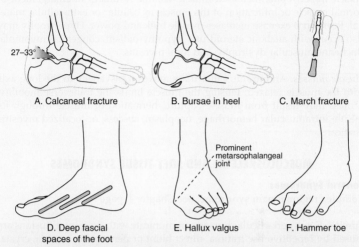

27–33°

A. Calcaneal fracture
B. Bursae in heel
C. March fracture

Prominent
metatarsophalangeal
joint

D. Deep fascial
spaces of the foot
E. Hallux valgus
F. Hammer toe

FIG. 13-37 Lesions of the Foot. A. Calcaneal fracture. B. Bursae in the heel. C. March fracture of a metatarsal bone. D. Deep fascial spaces of the foot. E. Hallux valgus. This deformity shows lateral great toe deviation with a prominent MTP joint. **F. Hammer toe.** The second toe is always affected with fixed PIP flexion.

MTP extension is severely limited and flexion occurs mainly in the interphalangeal joint.

Hammer toes. The second through fourth toes can be involved. The MTP is fixed in dorsiflexion and the PIP is fixed in plantarflexion, whereas the DIP is freely movable (Fig. 13-37F). A corn or inflamed bursa frequently occurs over the PIP joint. Hammer toes are usually bilateral involving several toes on each foot. It often accompanies hallux valgus.

Painful toe swelling—fractured phalanx. No matter how trivial the trauma seems, consider the possibility that the bone has been fractured.

Painful first MTP swelling—gout. This is the classic lesion (podagra) of early gout, described on page 583.

Toenail signs. See Chapter 6, *The Skin and Nails*, page 126.

Muscle signs
Muscular wasting. Loss of muscle mass is the result of disuse or damage to muscle or motor nerves. Fasciculation indicates denervation; the history reveals injury or disuse.

Muscle contracture. Prolonged disuse, immobilization, ischemia leading to muscle necrosis, or inflammation result in muscle fibrosis, muscle with inelastic shortening. The shortened muscle does not permit full range of movement. The joints, however, are normal, a distinction from joint contracture. The muscle is firm to hard and atrophic.

Muscle hypertrophy. Increased muscle volume results from enlargement of normal muscle or infiltration of the muscle by cellular or extracellular material. Resistance exercise increases muscle bulk and power. Hypertrophy may also occur with anabolic steroid use, hypothyroidism, congenital myotonia, Duchenne muscular dystrophy, and focal myositis.

Muscle masses. An intramuscular mass moves transversely to the long axis with the muscle relaxed; tensing the muscle limits the transverse mobility. A mass may result from muscle rupture, herniation of muscle through its sheath, intramuscular hemorrhage, neoplasm, abscess, or localized myositis ossificans.

MUSCULOSKELETAL AND SOFT TISSUE SYNDROMES

General Syndromes

Complex regional pain syndrome. See Chapter 4, page 75.

Bursitis. Some periarticular bursae communicate with the joint. Effusions are caused by repetitive use trauma, direct blunt or penetrating trauma, crystal deposition, and infection. Knowing the anatomy is a prerequisite for interpreting the history and exam.

Hypertrophic osteoarthropathy (HOA). This is a periostitis of unknown cause with: (1) clubbing of the fingers, (2) new subperiosteal bone in the long bones, (3) swelling and pains in the joints, and (4) autonomic disturbances of the hands and feet, such as flushing, sweating, and blanching. The earliest sign is clubbing (see page 564). With progression, bone pain occurs while joint swelling and pain may become severe. Palpating the distal forearms and legs elicits tenderness. When advanced, sweating and flushing of the hands and feet can alternate with Raynaud phenomenon. HOA is congenital, appearing in childhood, or acquired. Primary hereditary HOA (*Marie-Bamberger syndrome*) is an autosomal dominant syndrome expressed more commonly in males. It has clubbing, greasy skin thickening, especially noticeable on the face, and hyperhidrosis of the hands and feet. Acquired HOA is caused by systemic disease.

CLINICAL OCCURRENCE: *Congenital:* Familial, cyanotic congenital heart disease, cystic fibrosis; *Endocrine:* Graves disease, pregnancy; *Degenerative/ Idiopathic:* Emphysema, cirrhosis; *Infectious:* Lung or liver abscess, bronchiectasis, tuberculosis, bacterial endocarditis, dysentery; *Inflammatory/Immune:* Ulcerative colitis, Crohn disease, chronic interstitial pneumonitis, sarcoidosis, dysproteinemia; *Metabolic/Toxic:* Malabsorption, chronic hypoxemia; *Neoplastic:* Lung, pleural, and gastrointestinal cancer, metastatic disease to lung; *Vascular:* Aortic aneurysm.

- **Necrotizing soft-tissue infection.** Rapid expansion of infection in subcutaneous tissue planes produces local vascular thrombosis leading to ischemia of fat, connective tissue, skin and underlying muscle. Infection and necrosis spread proximally and distally along tissue planes and invade deeper structures along neurovascular bundles penetrating these planes. When there is muscle fascia involvement it is *necrotizing fasciitis*. Pain and fever accompany signs of inflammation (erythema, warmth, tenderness) resulting from infection with group A streptococci or polymicrobial soft-tissue infections (mixed aerobic/anaerobic). Systemic hypotension, tachycardia, and delirium develop rapidly, and outcome is fatal without complete surgical debridement. Predisposing factors include diabetes mellitus, immunosuppression, and puncture wounds. Urgent surgical debridement is mandatory to save limb and life [Hoadley DJ, Mark EJ. Weekly clinicopathological exercises: Case 28–2002: a 35-year-old long-term traveler to the Caribbean with a rapidly progressive soft-tissue infection. *N Engl J Med*. 2002;347:831–837].

Acromegaly and gigantism. Excess growth hormone, usually from an anterior pituitary adenoma, stimulates bone and soft tissue overgrowth. Onset before the epiphyses close enlarges the entire skeleton so the body is well proportioned, known as *gigantism*. When overgrowth occurs after epiphyseal closure, the skeletal pattern is called *acromegaly*, in which the hands, feet, face, head, and soft tissues are thickened. Patients often have diffuse muscle or joint stiffness and may complain of headaches and back pain. Exam shows soft tissue thickening, particularly apparent in the face, hands, and feet. The bones widen without lengthening leading to a prominent jaw, wide spacing of the teeth, prominent supraorbital ridge, and enlarged hands and feet. OA is common. Suprasellar extension of the tumor produces signs of hypopituitarism and bitemporal hemianopsia.

Marfan syndrome. This congenital disorder results from mutations in the fibrillin-1 gene, frequently inherited as autosomal dominant. Sporadic cases also occur. It affects the development of bone, ligaments, tendons, arterial walls, and supporting structures in the heart and eyes. Although the complete syndrome is striking, many persons show only a few signs. The long, slender phalanges (*spider fingers*) are known as *arachnodactyly* (Fig. 13-31); some patients lack this sign. The skull is long and narrow and the palate is high and arched. The long bones are thin and elongated, so the outspread armspan exceeds body height. Thoracic deformities are either *pectus excavatum* (funnel breast) or *pectus carinatum* (pigeon breast). The spine may exhibit fused vertebrae or spina bifida. Joint laxity permits hyperextension (double-jointedness), dislocations, kyphoscoliosis, pes planus, or pes cavus. The ears may be long and pointed, *satyr ear*. Weak supporting structures in the eye produce globe elongation (myopia), retinal detachment, lens dislocation, and blue sclerae. Vascular elastic media degeneration leads to aneurysmal dilatation of the aorta and/or pulmonary artery. Aortic dissection and rupture are common causes of early death. Deformed cardiac valves are sites for bacterial endocarditis. The foramen ovale may remain patent.

Syndromes Primarily Affecting Joints

Arthritis—inflammatory and noninflammatory joint disease. The diagnosis of *arthritis* requires signs of acute or chronic joint inflammation: redness, warmth, tenderness, synovial thickening, effusion, bony enlargement, or erosive changes on X-ray. Careful examination distinguishes joint involvement (synovium and articular cartilage: arthritis) from inflammation of the periarticular tendon and ligament insertions into bone (the enthesis: enthesitis), the tendons and their sheaths (tendonitis and tenosynovitis) or the underlying bone (osteitis). When tendon inflammation is suspected, listen with the stethoscope for a rub over the painful site.

The most diagnostically useful descriptive classification of joint diseases is based upon the history and physical findings. First, the number of joints actively involved is assessed as *monarticular* (1 joint), *oligoarticular* (2–4 joints), or *polyarticular* (>4 joints). For patients with oligo- or polyarthritis, note the pattern of joint involvement: (1) *large more proximal joints or distal small joints*, (2) *axial joints and/or peripheral joints*, and (3) whether involvement is *symmetric* or *asymmetric*. Widespread and symmetrical joint involvement increases the likelihood of a systemic inflammatory disease primarily involving the joints, e.g., rheumatoid arthritis.

A second group of arthritis syndromes are classified as *spondyloarthritis*. These disorders have in common prominent enthesopathy, involvement of the sacroiliac joints and spine, variable large joint disease (oligoarthritis), and associations with inflammatory and infectious diseases in other organs (gastrointestinal tract, genitourinary tract, skin, and eye).

No classification system is perfect, and the examiner must always be alert to the evolving pattern over days, weeks, or years. Remember, polyarthritic diseases may initially present with single joint involvement. Correct rheumatologic diagnosis requires patience and an open mind.

Monarticular arthritis. Arthritis involving a single joint is likely caused by local mechanical, inflammatory, or infectious factors. Less commonly, it is the initial manifestation of a systemic process that will involve other joints. Sequential involvement of single joints with intervening remissions suggests an underlying systemic disorder (congenital or acquired) with superimposed local precipitating events, for example, trauma in hemophilia.

CLINICAL OCCURRENCE: *Congenital:* Hemophilia; *Endocrine:* Hyperparathyroidism, hypothyroidism; *Degenerative/Idiopathic:* Osteoarthritis; *Inflammatory/Immune:* Postinfectious reactive arthritis, psoriasis, RA (initial presentation), SLE, amyloidosis; *Infectious:* Acute septic arthritis (*Staphylococcus aureus*, gonococcemia, others), Lyme disease, syphilis, mycobacteria, osteomyelitis, viral (e.g., HIV, parvovirus, others); *Mechanical/Traumatic:* Blunt trauma, hemarthrosis, fracture, repetitive use/overuse; *Metabolic/Toxic:* Crystal-induced diseases (e.g., gout, calcium pyrophosphate deposition, calcium hydroxyapatite, calcium oxalate), scurvy; *Neoplastic:* Sarcoma (bone, synovium, or cartilage), metastases to bone, benign tumors (e.g., osteochondroma, osteoid osteoma, pigmented villonodular synovitis), leukemia; *Neurologic:* Neuropathy producing a Charcot joint; *Vascular:* Osteonecrosis.

Septic arthritis. Direct extension of a bacterial infection (most commonly with *S. aureus*) from skin, soft tissue, or periarticular bone or hematogenous spread (e.g., bacterial endocarditis, gonorrhea bacteremia) produces infection within the joint. Release of lysosomal enzymes can rapidly destroy the joint. Usually one joint is involved, often the knee, but in gonococcal arthritis, three-fourths of the patients have an initial transient (2–4 days) migratory oligoarthritis and/or tenosynovitis. Symptoms often begin suddenly with chills and fever. The joint swells rapidly, the overlying skin is red and warm, and the joint is painful and tender to touch. The swelling becomes fluctuant, indicating effusion. Signs of inflammation are frequently absent in immunosuppressed patients. Joint aspiration discloses purulent fluid that must be cultured to identify the causative organism. In addition to *S. aureus* and gonorrhea, less-common organisms to consider are streptococci, meningococci, *Haemophilus influenzae* (especially in unimmunized infants and children), and, rarely, brucellosis, typhoid fever, glanders, blastomycosis, granuloma inguinale, tuberculosis, fungi, and others.

Gout. Genetic (primary gout) or acquired (secondary gout) causes of uric acid overproduction or decreased excretion result in uric acid accumulation in tissues and extracellular fluids. When the fluid becomes supersaturated, crystals form. Crystals shed into joint fluid and phagocytosed by polymorphonuclear neutrophils induce acute inflammation. Because a history of recurrent stereotypic episodes is very suggestive of gout, the initial attack presents the chief diagnostic challenge. Frequently, the patient is awakened from sleep by severe burning pain, tingling, numbness, or warmth in a joint. The joint rapidly swells and becomes excruciatingly tender, intolerant to the pressure of the bedclothes. Typically, the overlying skin becomes red or violaceous. There may be malaise, headache, fever, and tachycardia. Untreated, the attack lasts for 1–2 weeks. In more than half the cases, the MTP joint of the great toe is affected initially (*podagra*) (Fig. 13-38). Other sites are the midfoot (instep), ankle, knee, elbow, or wrist. Acute gout in the midfoot resembles cellulitis. Attacks may be triggered by trauma, surgery, acidosis, infection, cold exposure, changes in atmospheric pressure, overindulgence in alcoholic beverages, or any acute illness. Large tissue deposits of uric acid (*tophi*) occurring around joints over bony prominences are not usually inflamed.

Calcium pyrophosphate dihydrate deposition disease (CPPDD)–pseudogout, chondrocalcinosis. Calcium pyrophosphate dihydrate, shed from articular cartilage, forms small, rhomboidal, weakly positive birefringent crystals that trigger inflammation. Articular fibrocartilage may calcify and be detected by X-ray (*chondrocalcinosis*) in the knee, pelvis (hip joints and symphysis pubis)

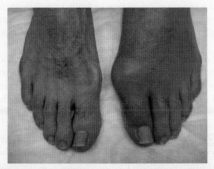

FIG. 13-38 Podagra: Gout. The left first MTP joint is swollen and exquisitely tender; the entire forefoot is erythematous and warm. Note also the bunions (L > R).

or wrist. CPPDD is like gout in both its acute and chronic forms. The attack begins abruptly with painful swelling and heat, usually in a single joint, occasionally in two or more joints. The knee, ankle, and wrist are most commonly affected. Untreated, the pain and tenderness are intense for 2–4 days, then gradually subside during the next 1–2 weeks. It is associated with increasing age, OA, hyperparathyroidism, and hemochromatosis (~5% of CPPDD).

Charcot joint. Loss of pain sensation or proprioception leads to joint instability. Repeated injuries cause three successive stages of articular damage: swelling, joint degeneration, and new bone formation. Erythema and swelling are the first signs. The course is progressive with hypermobility, traumatic osteophyte formation, and subluxation leading to painless deformity and crepitus on movement. The absence of pain with movement and loss of pain sensation and proprioception in the involved limb are diagnostic. A single joint may be affected, or, commonly, all the joints in an anatomic region (e.g., the midfoot joints) are involved. Determine if the neuropathy is a local or systemic neuropathic process. Classic clinical conditions causing Charcot joints include tabes dorsalis (knee most commonly involved; hip, ankle, lower spine, less frequently involved, Fig. 13-21C), diabetes mellitus (tarsal and metatarsal joints most commonly, ankle occasionally, knee rarely), syringomyelia (usually upper limb joints), and leprosy.

Trauma. Mechanical trauma causes bleeding (*hemarthrosis*) or effusion with pain from damage to the joint capsule, intra- or periarticular ligaments, cartilage, or bone. The knee and ankle are commonly affected. The exact mechanism of injury, time course of pain (immediate versus delayed), and physical exam suggest the type and degree of injury.

Tuberculosis. There is chronic swelling of a single joint with only moderate pain. Joint effusion and synovial thickening may be present. The hips, knees, and spine are most frequently affected. Previous intraarticular or oral corticosteroids and immunosuppressive drugs are major risk factors. Cultures of aspirated joint fluid or synovial biopsy yield *Mycobacterium tuberculosis*.

Recurrent painless knee effusion. The patient experiences episodes of painless swelling and joint effusion in one or both knees, with no constitutional symptoms over years, with an average duration of 3–5 days. The cause is unknown, though, occasionally, the condition presages rheumatoid arthritis.

Oligoarthritis and polyarthritis. Arthritis involving several joints, simultaneously or sequentially, is oligoarthritis (2–4 joints) or polyarthritis (>4 joints). The pattern helps make the exact diagnosis. Generally, oligoarthritis involves larger joints and is *asymmetric* whereas the classic polyarthritis syndromes (RA, SLE) involve *symmetric* joints, including the small joints of the hands and feet. These are not hard-and-fast rules.

CLINICAL OCCURRENCE: *Congenital:* Hemophilia, familial Mediterranean fever, hemochromatosis, sickle cell disease, alkaptonuria/ochronosis; *Endocrine:* Hyperparathyroidism, hypothyroidism, acromegaly; *Degenerative/ Idiopathic:* Inflammatory and noninflammatory OA; *Infectious:* Septic arthritis, Lyme disease, viral (e.g., HIV, parvovirus, rubella, mumps, others), Whipple disease, mycoses (coccidioidomycosis, histoplasmosis, blastomycosis, cryptococcosis), actinomycosis, secondary syphilis, brucellosis, typhoid fever; *Inflammatory/Immune:* Reactive arthritis, psoriasis, RA, systemic erythematosus, rheumatic fever, ankylosing spondylitis, systemic sclerosis (scleroderma), polymyositis/dermatomyositis, antisynthetase syndrome, Still disease, Behçet syndrome, relapsing polychondritis, amyloidosis, sarcoidosis, erythema multiforme, erythema nodosum, drug reactions, serum sickness; *Metabolic/Toxic:* Crystal-induced diseases (e.g., gout, calcium pyrophosphate deposition, calcium hydroxyapatite, calcium oxalate), ochronosis, scurvy; *Neoplastic:* Sarcoma (bone, synovium, or cartilage), metastases to bone, benign tumors (e.g., osteochondroma, osteoid osteoma, pigmented villonodular synovitis); *Vascular:* Osteonecrosis, systemic vasculitis, HOA.

Rheumatoid arthritis (RA)—deforming symmetrical distal polyarthritis. RA is characterized by proliferation of inflamed synovial tissue (*pannus*) that enters the joint cavity in tongue-like projections. The pannus erodes cartilage, periarticular bone, and soft tissues, including tendons and ligaments. Untreated, the result is destruction of the joint surfaces and supporting structures producing subluxation, deformity, and loss of joint function. The onset may be insidious with morning stiffness and pain followed by swelling and tenderness of the joints, proceeding over weeks to months into a small and large joint polyarthritis. Less commonly, the onset is sudden with pain and swelling occurring simultaneously in several joints accompanied by fever and prostration. Smaller joints of the hands (MCP, PIP), feet (MTP), wrists, and ankles are typically involved early and symmetrically; onset in a single larger joint, usually a knee, is not rare. Interphalangeal joints become fusiform from joint effusion (fluctuant) or thickening of the joint capsule (nonfluctuant). DIP joints are invariably spared. Tenderness is confined to the region of the capsule. Joint motion is initially limited by pain or effusion, later by fibrosis and/or muscle shortening. Muscle weakness and wasting may be rapid and disproportionate to the amount of disuse. Although remissions may occur, the disease is usually progressive over a period of years. If RA is left untreated or very difficult to control, joint contracture and subluxations are frequent, with subluxation of the MCP joints producing characteristic ulnar deviation of the fingers. Tenosynovitis is manifest as swelling of the tendon sheaths. In 20%–35% of cases, subcutaneous rheumatoid nodules develop over bony prominences and tendon sheaths. They are painless, firm, and freely movable over bones, like those in RF. A serious late complication is cervical spine instability from subluxation of C1 on C2 that may present as neck pain or upper motor neuron signs. Diagnosis is based upon clinical and laboratory criteria. Frequently, the patient must be observed for many months before the diagnosis is secure. *RA Variants. Felty Syndrome* is the triad of RA, splenomegaly, and leukopenia. *Palindromic Rheumatism* presents as multiple afebrile attacks of mono or oligoarthritis lasting for only 2–3 days, leaving no residua. *Secondary Sjögren Syndrome* is diagnosed when keratoconjunctivitis sicca and xerostomia accompany RA. *Vasculitis* may accompany RA and involve the skin (necrosis and nodules), nervous system, and lung. *Juvenile Idiopathic Arthritis* is a group of disorders which may overlap with the adult disease. See pediatric texts for descriptions and details. *DDX:* RA frequently involves the temporomandibular joint unlike RF. In RF, arthritis is migratory, whereas it is persistent in RA. Reactive arthritis is usually oligoarticular and mainly affects large joints, especially ankles and knees. An initial monarthritis may suggest an infectious or crystalline arthritis; however, joint aspiration excludes these possibilities.

Systemic lupus erythematosus (SLE)—nondeforming symmetrical distal polyarthritis. The cause is unknown. Inflammation of multiple tissues and organs is accompanied by antibodies to specific nuclear antigens usually degraded in the nucleosome. These autoantibodies are the hallmark of SLE, but their role in its pathogenesis is unclear. SLE is a chronic inflammatory multisystem disease, more common in women than men. No one symptom or sign is pathognomonic of SLE; rather, the diagnosis is established by clinical criteria. The most common symptoms and signs are fatigue, malaise, or fever (90%), arthritis or arthralgias (90%), and skin rashes (50%–60%). The arthralgias, myalgias, and joint inflammation resemble mild RA, but deformities usually do not develop. The malar ("butterfly") rash is a macular to maculopapular, sometimes scaly, erythematous dermatitis forming the "wings" of the butterfly on each malar prominence, with the "trunk" on the bridge of the nose. It may be more intense after sunlight exposure. In addition, there may be skin atrophy, telangiectasia, and mucosal ulcers. Serositis is common, presenting as pleurisy (with effusion and/or pleural rubs), abdominal pain, and/or pericarditis. Nonbacterial endocarditis with valvular insufficiency (usually mitral), central nervous system disease (with personality change, psychosis, or seizures), and glomerulonephritis can occur at any time and may be the presenting syndrome. Other signs are recurrent urticaria, mononeuritis multiplex and lymphadenopathy. Fetal wastage and thromboembolic disease are associated with antiphospholipid antibodies.

Rheumatic Fever (RF)—migratory polyarthritis. RF is a delayed inflammatory reaction following infection with specific Lancefield groups of group A beta-hemolytic streptococci. Tissues affected include the heart, joints, skin, and central nervous system. Its clinical manifestations are protean. The classic presentation, beginning from 1 to 4 weeks after streptococcal pharyngitis, is gradual onset of malaise, fatigue, anorexia, and fever. A single large joint becomes painful, tender, and swollen, with red and hot overlying skin and a turbid sterile effusion. Although the fever and other signs of illness persist, the joint inflammation spontaneously subsides in a few days, only to reappear in another joint, and later in another joint—a *migratory polyarthritis*. Joint involvement may be so mild that pain is not accompanied by signs of inflammation. Months of observation may be required to distinguish it from RA; involvement of the temporomandibular joint often occurs in RA, practically never in RF. RF leaves no residual joint deformity. At onset, the inflammation of a single joint with effusion requires distinction from suppurative arthritis. *Carditis* manifests as tachycardia, muffled heart sounds, heart enlargement, valvular insufficiency murmurs, pericardial friction rub, and/or gallop rhythm. The electrocardiogram may show PR prolongation. Two skin lesions are associated with RF, although neither is pathognomonic. *Erythema marginatum* or *circinatum* is characterized by coalescing migratory and transitory, circular erythematous lesions over the trunk and extremities that change within an hour. With chronic disease, subcutaneous *rheumatic nodules* appear as firm, nontender masses over joint prominences and tendon sheaths of the limbs, scalp, and spine. They are loosely attached to the underlying tissue. When numerous, their distribution tends to be symmetrical. *Sydenham chorea* may appear several months after onset. There are no diagnostic laboratory tests, but the full clinical picture is distinctive. Diagnosis is based upon the Jones criteria of major and minor manifestations.

Tophaceous gout. See page 583. Tophi are masses of monosodium urate crystals deposited in the tissues often over bony prominences and around joints where they erode bone. Acting as foreign bodies, they stimulate low-grade inflammation that may extrude the tophi through the skin. The asymmetrical nodular swellings and cartilage degeneration may impair joint function. Clinical signs of inflammation are variable, from mild to moderately severe. The olecranon, and prepatellar bursae, and hands are most frequently affected.

Osteoarthritis (OA), degenerative joint disease (DJD)—noninflammatory polyarthritis of large and small joints. This disease of articular cartilage is produced by proteoglycan matrix degradation leading to fissuring, thinning, and loss of articular cartilage with secondary thickening of subchondral bone. In late stages, the bone ends rub directly on each other, so their surfaces become worn and polished. The joint capsules are little affected, so adhesions are not formed, and although joint motion is restricted, ankylosis does not occur. The bony joint margins proliferate forming spurs, lipping, and exostoses. Genetic and acquired factors (trauma, surgery, obesity, excessive use) contribute to the pathogenesis. Symptoms are usually first noticed in the weight-bearing joints after age 40 and signs of inflammation are relatively slight. Symptoms correlate poorly with the objective extent of joint disease. The most common symptom is pain with use that disappears with rest. The patient may note grating during motion. Initially, the range of motion is normal, but gradually decreases as the disease progresses. Enlargement of the DIP and PIP joints of the fingers (Heberden and Bouchard nodes, respectively), is frequent. Painless knee effusion is frequent as is asymmetric loss of knee cartilage leading to valgus or varus deformity.

Gonococcal arthritis—migratory oligoarthritis. Neisseria gonorrhoeae infects the urethra or uterine cervix and then disseminates hematogenously to synovial membranes and skin, causing local inflammation. Infectious arthritis, tenosynovitis, and skin lesions are the most common extragenital complications of gonorrhea. One to four weeks after the onset of urethritis, inflammation suddenly develops in the knees, wrists, and ankles, although other joints may be affected. The most common pattern is a migratory oligoarthritis and tenosynovitis. Small thin effusions may accumulate in joint cavities. In other cases, suppurative arthritis develops, with inflammation of a single joint with purulent effusion. Tenosynovitis in the hands, wrists, or ankle is more common in gonorrhea than in arthritis from any other cause. The diagnosis may not be easy since the gonococcus is difficult to culture from the joints. Pustular skin lesions on an erythematous base are seen with gonococcal bacteremia helping to distinguish gonococcal arthritis from other conditions. Genital, rectal, and throat specimens for culture and polymerase chain reaction testing of urine for gonococcus and chlamydia should be obtained.

DDX: Reactive arthritis following nongonococcal urethritis may be misdiagnosed because conjunctival infection is present in up to 10% of patients with gonorrhea.

Hemochromatosis. The second and third MCP joints and the radiocarpal joint of the wrist are most commonly affected. *Chondrocalcinosis* is often present. Symmetric noninflammatory arthritis of the MCP joints should initiate a search for an iron-storage disorder.

Relapsing symmetrical seronegative synovitis with pitting edema (RS3PE). This condition of unknown cause presents with recurrent episodes of symmetrical synovitis of the hands and wrists with pitting edema and erythema of the dorsum of the hands. Pain is relatively mild, and the condition usually remits after several days to a couple of weeks. When RS3PE occurs as a paraneoplastic condition, it may be more chronic.

Spondyloarthritis. Inflammation at the insertion of ligaments and tendons into bone (*the enthesis, enthesitis*) leads to joint and tendon sheath effusions and ossification of periarticular structures. Genes (HLA-B27) and acquired illness (inflammatory bowel disease, infectious colitis, nongonococcal urethritis, and psoriasis) predispose to these disorders. Asymmetric oligoarthritides of the large joints with prominent involvement of the spine and SI joints and negative tests for rheumatoid factor are typical of *seronegative spondyloarthritides*. Patients present with back pain and stiffness, and occasionally with fever, malaise, and weight loss. Look for extraarticular disease such as genitourinary or gut symptoms, eye involvement (*uveitis*), and skin disease.

Known associations include ankylosing spondylitis, enteropathic arthritis (inflammatory bowel disease), psoriasis, reactive arthritis after diarrheal and genitourinary infections, and. *DDX:* Degenerative intervertebral disk disease, diffuse idiopathic skeletal hyperostosis (DISH), and ochronosis are noninflammatory conditions with similar spinal manifestations.

Ankylosing spondylitis. Inflammation of the ligament attachments to the vertebrae (*enthesitis*), the sacroiliac (SI) joints, and the junction of the annulus fibrosis and the vertebral end plates leads to new bone formation and bridging resulting in ankylosis. This chronic, progressive arthritis begins with SI involvement and progresses proximally often leading to severe ankylosis. Nonspecific symptoms, often beginning in adolescence, occur intermittently for 5–10 years. Pain and morning stiffness are felt in the lumbar region, buttocks, and SI region. Fatigue, fever, and weight loss may occur. Decreased lumbar spinal motion is an early sign with the normal lumbar lordosis straightened, diminished anterior flexion, and impaired spinal rotation and lateral bending. The process slowly ascends the lumbar and thoracic spine sometimes reaching the cervical spine. Episodes of acute or subacute arthritis involve hip, shoulder, sternoclavicular, or manubriosternal joints. The involved joints are tender. *Iridocyclitis* occurs in one-fifth of the cases. *Aortic regurgitation* is a late complication in 3% of patients. Idiopathic ankylosing spondylitis needs to be distinguished from psoriatic arthritis and enteropathic associated spondyloarthritis (Crohn disease and ulcerative colitis), Whipple disease, and DISH.

Reactive arthritis. Following infection of the urethra (chlamydia) or gut (*Shigella, Salmonella, Yersinia,* and *Campylobacter*) an oligoarthritis, predominately of the lower extremities, develops. It may be accompanied by enthesitis of the hands, ankles, and feet, conjunctivitis, urethritis, and rash on the glans penis (*circinate balanitis*) and feet (*keratoderma blenorrhagica*). Sacroiliitis and spine involvement may occur. Eighty-five percent of patients are HLA-B27-positive.

Enteropathic arthritis. Inflammatory asymmetric arthritis predominately of the ankles and knees occurs in association with inflammatory bowel disease (ulcerative colitis or Crohn disease). Enthesitis is common, especially at the Achilles tendon insertion, and symmetrical SI and spinal involvement occurs. The arthritis may precede clinical manifestations of the inflammatory bowel disease.

Psoriatic arthritis. The joint disease is usually an asymmetrical oligo- or polyarthritis of small and large joints. It is occasionally a symmetrical polyarthritis resembling RA. Destructive arthritis of the DIP joints is seen in psoriatic arthritis but not in RA. Spondylitis and sacroiliitis occur in up to 25% of patients with psoriatic arthritis, especially those with HLA-B27. Enthesitis predominates in some patients. The arthritis may precede, accompany, or follow onset of the skin lesions. Physical exam should include a careful skin examination, especially of the scalp (the rash may be hidden by hair or dismissed as seborrhea) and fingernails (looking for pits and onycholysis).

Conditions Primarily Affecting Bone

Osteoporosis. Bone resorption exceeds bone formation, leading to decreased bone mass and decreased mechanical strength. Trabecular bone is affected more than cortical bone. Increased bone resorption results from immobilization, inflammation, multiple myeloma, and hyperparathyroidism. Decreased bone formation results from gonadal hormone deficiency, glucocorticoid steroid excess, and advanced age. Trabecular bone deficiency is especially important in the vertebrae and pelvic bones, whereas cortical bone loss is predominant in long bones. Osteoporosis is asymptomatic until insufficiency fractures occur, usually in the thoracic or lumbar spine and pelvis. Thoracic kyphosis results from anterior wedging of thoracic vertebrae. Bone mineral density is assessed by dual energy X-ray absorptiometry (DEXA) scan. The bones are much more susceptible to fracture with minor trauma; hip and wrist fractures from falls should initiate evaluation for osteoporosis in both men and women.

CLINICAL OCCURRENCE: *Congenital:* Vitamin D-resistant rickets, Marfan syndrome, hemochromatosis, Ehlers–Danlos syndrome, hemophilia, thalassemia, positive family history; *Endocrine:* Postmenopausal estrogen deficiency, premature menopause, hypogonadism, hyperthyroidism, hyperparathyroidism, Cushing syndrome, glucocorticoid use, diabetes mellitus, pregnancy, adrenal insufficiency, acromegaly, hyperprolactinemia; *Degenerative/ Idiopathic:* Advanced age; *Inflammatory/Immune:* Sarcoidosis, amyloidosis,

RA, ankylosing spondylitis; *Mechanical/Traumatic:* Immobilization, disuse, and nonweightbearing; *Metabolic/Toxic:* Vitamin D deficiency, malnutrition, chronic renal insufficiency, heparin, cirrhosis, postgastrectomy, parenteral nutrition, cigarette smoking, low body weight; *Neoplastic:* Multiple myeloma, paraneoplastic (parathyroid hormone (PTH)-related protein secretion), lymphoma, prolactinoma; *Neurologic:* Paralysis, stroke, multiple sclerosis; *Psychosocial:* Anorexia nervosa; *Vascular:* Hyperemia of bone.

Osteomalacia. Vitamin D deficiency, hypocalcemia, or hypophosphatemia after the epiphyses are closed prevents calcification of newly formed bony matrix. Early there are no symptoms or signs, whereas later, bone pain and tenderness occur. Low back pain and striking muscle weakness are common. Low serum calcium levels produce spontaneous carpopedal spasm with the Chvostek and Trousseau signs. Insufficiency (stress) fractures are common and pseudofractures may be seen by X-ray.

    CLINICAL OCCURRENCE: *Congenital:* Vitamin D-resistant rickets; *Endocrine:* Hyperparathyroidism, rapid tissue deposition of calcium and phosphorus after parathyroid ablation in osteitis fibrosa cystica, hypoparathyroidism; *Inflammatory/Immune:* Celiac disease; *Metabolic/Toxic:* Vitamin D deficiency, hypocalcemia, hypophosphatemia, malabsorption, pancreatic insufficiency, malnutrition, chronic renal insufficiency, renal tubular acidosis, Fanconi syndrome, ureterosigmoidostomy, essential hypercalciuria, drugs (anticonvulsants, e.g., phenytoin, glucocorticoids, etidronate), fluoride and aluminum intoxication.

Rickets. Vitamin D deficiency in childhood, before epiphyseal closure, results in inadequate calcification of cartilage forming new bone. See Chapter 8, Figure 8-29, page 299. Softening of bone produces widened cranial sutures and fontanelles (craniotabes), Parrot bosses, rachitic rosary, Harrison grooves, thoracic kyphosis or lordosis, genu valgum or varum, and a contracted pelvis. With the sole exception of the rosary, all deformities are permanent stigmas of childhood disease.

Paget disease. Increased bone resorption combines with rapid new bone growth with disordered architecture and decreased mechanical strength. The cause is unknown. Bone pain may occur but is seldom severe. Except for the hands and feet, any bone may be involved. The skin over affected bones may be warm. The classic osseous deformities are increased girth of the calvarium, thoracic kyphosis, genu varum, and shortening of the spine by flattening of the vertebrae, giving the appearance of disproportionately long arms (Fig. 13-39). Spontaneous or stress fractures occur, and osteogenic sarcoma develops rarely. Increased blood flow through the spongy bone may produce an arteriovenous fistula leading to high-output cardiac failure.

Hyperparathyroidism, primary—osteitis fibrosa cystica. Increased PTH production causes bone resorption to exceed new bone formation, leading to hypercalcemia, hypercalciuria, hyperphosphaturia, and hypophosphatemia. The disease may be asymptomatic, although many patients have diffuse musculoskeletal aching and fatigue. Late findings are bone tenderness, muscle weakness, and waddling gait. Subperiosteal cysts in the skull and long bones

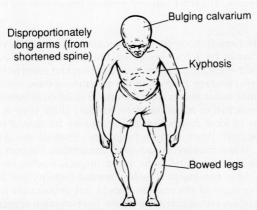

Disproportionately long arms (from shortened spine)

Bulging calvarium

Kyphosis

Bowed legs

FIG. 13-39 Bony Signs of Osteitis Deformans (Paget Disease of Bone). The chief features of Paget disease are the enlarged calvarium (contrasting with the normal-sized face underneath), kyphosis and shortening of the spine so the arms look proportionally longer than the trunk, and bowed legs. The figure represents a collection of features, which are unlikely to occur together in the same person.

cause visible and palpable swellings. Peptic ulcer and urolithiasis should prompt a search for hyperparathyroidism.

Hyperparathyroidism, secondary, and tertiary. Hyperphosphatemia and hypocalcemia combined with disordered vitamin D metabolism in chronic renal failure (renal osteodystrophy), or osteomalacia from other causes, leads to increased production of PTH, parathyroid gland hyperplasia, and progressive bone disease. Combinations of dietary, hormonal, and renal replacement therapies can help control the disorder. When PTH production is not suppressible with appropriate treatment, it is termed tertiary hyperparathyroidism.

Multiple myeloma. This malignant clonal proliferation of immunoglobulin-producing plasma cells (terminally differentiated B cells) in the bone marrow causes destruction of bone by activating osteoclasts leading to hypercalcemia. Normal immunoglobulin production is suppressed, there is production of monoclonal plasma proteins (heavy chains, light chains, and intact immunoglobulin), and anemia and thrombocytopenia develop. Renal insufficiency results from tubular toxicity of light chains (Bence Jones proteins), hyperuricemia, and hypercalcemia. This is the most common malignant tumor primarily affecting bone. The presenting complaints may be referable to anemia, renal failure, or a pathologic fracture. Fatigue or generalized aching may be the only early symptoms. The most common specific symptom is bone pain. Spinal compression fractures cause localized pain in the back with radicular distribution. Multiple myeloma should be considered in patients more than 45 years of age with back pain and anemia.

Bone metastases. Metastatic disease presents as a localized swelling or pain in a bone, a pathologic fracture, or is found incidentally on radiographs taken for another reason. The most frequent primary carcinomas are breast, lung, and prostate.

Fractures. Mechanical disruption of mineralized bone and its collagenous matrix are caused by forces exceeding the tensile and/or compressive strength of the bone. This occurs from a single forceful event or from repetitive less forceful loading. Fracture of the mineralized bone leaving the collagenous matrix intact results from trauma in children (*greenstick fracture*) and repetitive activities in adults (*stress fracture*). If the bone is inherently weak because of local destructive disease, it may fracture at usual loads (*pathologic fracture*). When fracture fragments penetrate the skin, it is an *open fracture*. When fracture is suspected, immobilize the part and assess neurovascular function distal to the injury. Inspection often reveals deformity. Unavoidable movement reveals abnormal mobility and bone crepitus, distinctive signs of fracture one should not deliberately try to elicit. Muscle contraction attempting to splint the fracture often aggravates pain. Localized bone tenderness indicates the fracture site. Shortening of a long bone is the sign of an impacted fracture.

Spontaneous or pathologic fracture. This is a fracture that occurs with trauma insufficient to break a normal bone. Judging the amount of trauma is difficult, hence spontaneous fractures are easily mistaken for traumatic fractures; a high index of suspicion is warranted. X-ray signs of generalized or local bone disease should be sought if a pathologic fracture is suspected. Sometimes spontaneous fractures are less painful than those of healthy bone. Osteomalacia, osteoporosis, Paget disease, hyperparathyroidism, multiple myeloma, osteogenesis imperfecta, and primary and metastatic neoplasms in bone are common underlying conditions.

Osteomyelitis, acute. Blood-borne bacteria are carried to the terminal capillary loops of the metaphyseal cortex, causing a necrosing infection that erodes to the periosteum. The initial infection is in the metaphysis, near but not involving the epiphysis. *S. aureus* is the most common organism. Osteomyelitis is most common in children. The onset is usually sudden, with fever and pain. Older children may be able to point to the painful site, although the pain may be referred to the nearest joint where sympathetic effusion may be noted. Localized swelling and redness of the overlying skin with increased warmth may be seen. Light bone percussion frequently discloses tenderness; localize the site with finger pressure on the bone moving toward the suspected site until the point of maximum tenderness is located. The proximal femoral metaphysis is within the hip joint in children, so they present with a septic hip. Sometimes deep cellulitis cannot be distinguished clinically from osteomyelitis.

Osteomyelitis, chronic. After the acute phase, the purulent discharge from the necrosing bone breaks through the periosteum and drains through sinuses in the skin. The circulation of the cortex becomes impaired, producing islands of dead bone, *sequestra*. A sequestrum may be absorbed, discharged through the sinus, or surrounded by new bone, the *involucrum*. Continuing bone necrosis and retention of sequestra support persistent infection.

Osteogenesis imperfecta. These inherited disorders of type I collagen decrease the mechanical strength of all bones leading to pathologic fractures during the first decade of life. Autosomal dominant inheritance occurs in 60% of cases; several forms of the disorder are recognized. The bones are harder and more brittle than normal, so spontaneous or pathologic fractures are common. The fractures are sometimes painless. Blue sclerae may be observed. Short stature is usual and skull deformity is often present. Joint hypermobility is common.

Fibrous dysplasia of bone. The cause is unknown. The architecture of one or more bones is distorted by fibrosis; the cranium and long bones are especially involved. There is asymptomatic bowing of affected long bones. The skin often contains melanotic spots with jagged borders. Girls may have precocious puberty.

Hereditary multiple exostoses—osteochondromatosis. The autosomal dominant condition is characterized by exostoses arising from the bony cortex deforming the metaphyseal region of some long bones. Involvement is usually bilateral but not symmetrical. The ulna may be shortened, producing ulnar deviation of the hand. Valgus deformities of the ankle are common. The only symptom may be mechanical interference with joint function.

Neck, Spine, and Pelvis Syndromes
Neck, shoulder, and arm pain
Cervical spondylosis and radiculopathy. Spondylosis results from intervertebral disk degeneration. Cervical root impingement in the neural foramen produces severe pain in the nerve's distribution. Commonly, the cause is narrowing of intervertebral foramina or compression of nerve roots by osteophytes. Uncommonly, the lesion is caused by protrusion of an intervertebral disk or by C1–C2 instability from RA. Usually, minor trauma precedes the pain. Painful muscle spasms of the neck muscles cause temporary torticollis, with the head tilted away from the painful side. Sharp, shooting pain spreads slowly down the shoulder, lateral arm, and radial forearm, to the wrist. The neck muscles are rigid on the affected side. With a C5 or C6 radiculopathy the biceps tendon reflex is frequently diminished or absent. The triceps reflex is decreased with a C7 radiculopathy. There may be tingling and numbness in the thumb, index, and middle fingers, but muscle wasting is rare. Pain on extending and laterally rotating the neck is *Spurling sign*. Active and passive neck movements are restricted and may be painless, but often produce subjective and objective crepitus. Coughing with the head held in extension may reproduce the pain. *DDX:* Other causes, such as incomplete rupture of the supraspinatus, Pancoast tumor, and peripheral neuropathy must be excluded. Symptoms remit gradually over days to weeks.

Pancoast tumor, superior sulcus syndrome. Locally invasive lung cancer at the thoracic apex involves the pleura, thoracic muscles, and neurovascular bundles, including the brachial plexus and cervical sympathetic chain. Pain is felt in local structures and is referred in the distribution of the involved nerves. Severe pain is present in the posterior shoulder and axilla, often shooting down the arm, with paresthesia in the arm and hand. Paresis or wasting of arm muscles may occur. In addition to neck and shoulder pain, the complete syndrome includes *Horner syndrome* (unilateral miosis, ptosis, and ipsilateral absence of sweating on the face and neck). It may be confused with supraspinatus tendon rupture, cervical spondylosis, and peripheral neuritis.

Back pain

- **Epidural spinal cord compression.** A mass in the closed epidural space may erode bone, compress spinal nerves, and/or compress the spinal cord. Most epidural masses extend from an adjacent vertebra or from a retroperitoneal malignancy and compress the anterior or anterolateral cord. Progressive back pain, unrelieved by recumbency, should prompt an immediate evaluation for spinal cord compression. Pain is the most common presenting symptom followed by leg weakness, constipation, incontinence, and sensory disturbances. The latter indicate advancing cord compression with less chance for complete recovery. Paraplegia may occur in a matter of hours after the onset of neurologic signs. The pain may occur at any level and is increased by straight-leg raising, Valsalva maneuver, neck flexion, and movement. MRI of the entire vertebral column and cord is the most sensitive and specific test. Breast, prostate, and lung cancer are the most frequent causes. Other cancers in adults include multiple myeloma, malignant lymphoma, renal carcinoma, sarcoma, and melanoma. In children, consider lymphoma, sarcoma, and neuroblastoma. Epidural abscess complicates infectious spondylitis.

Back pain and stiffness
Infectious spondylitis. Spinal infection most commonly starts in the disks (*diskitis*) and anterior vertebral endplates leading to vertebral erosion and collapse. Infection may extend anteriorly into the psoas or posteriorly into the epidural space leading to spinal cord compression. Pain and tenderness of the vertebral spinous processes are usually present over the site of infection, often with spasm of the sacrospinalis. The pain may be referred along a spinal nerve to be mistaken for appendicitis, pleurisy, or sciatica. Collapse of the vertebral body causes a gibbus deformity and paraplegia may result. Psoas abscess may form along the psoas sheath and point beneath the inguinal ligament. Spine pain is localized by the heel-drop test: have the patient rise onto tiptoes, and then drop onto the heels eliciting pain at the site of infection. Infections with pyogenic organisms (*S. aureus*) are most common. Tuberculosis, Salmonella, brucellosis, fungi, and actinomycosis are less common.

Tuberculous spondylitis (Pott disease). Spinal tuberculosis is an indolent osteomyelitis of the anterior vertebral endplates often extending to the paravertebral soft tissues. Patients present with fever, night sweats, and pain. With cervical infection, the neck is held stiffly, spontaneous rotation of the head is absent, and, when seated, the patient may support the head with the hands (*Rust sign*). A cervical vertebral abscess may track to the retropharyngeal space. Patients with epidural extension can develop spinal cord compression. Vertebral collapse in the thoracic or lumbar spine produces a gibbus deformity and instability. Rarely, prevertebral extension along the psoas sheath presents as a cold abscess under the inguinal ligament.

Diffuse idiopathic skeletal hyperostosis (DISH). Asymmetric osteophytes at multiple levels of the spine bridge intervertebral spaces producing irregular ankylosis with decreased spinal motion, especially in the cervical and lumbar regions. The disk spaces are preserved. Men are affected more often than women.

Rigid spine syndrome. The clinical syndrome of rigid spine, proximal muscle weakness, scoliosis, and joint contractures can have several different etiologies. The combination of restrictive chest disease and muscle weakness can lead to respiratory failure.

Low back pain
Lumbosacral strain. Mechanical forces applied to the back are concentrated where the mobile lumbar spine meets the fixed sacrum. Injury commonly occurs to the soft tissues (muscles, tendons, and ligaments) of the low back at the transition zone. Injury is the result of a single, large loading force or of repetitive loading with lesser forces. Usually the patient complains of aching pain near L5 and S1. The pain may radiate laterally or to the lateral thigh. The lumbar lordosis is increased and spine flexion is limited and painful due to muscle spasm. The patient cannot lie flat without flexing the knees and hips to reduce pain. The straight-leg-raising test produces non-radiating lumbosacral pain at extreme hip flexion. Have the patient lie prone with the pelvis resting on four pillows to separate the spinous processes. In this position, palpation of the spines and supraspinous ligament may reveal tenderness above or below the spine of L5; sometimes a depression is found indicating spondylolisthesis.

Sciatica. Compression or direct injury to the sciatic nerve produces pain, altered sensation (dermatomes L4–S2), loss of muscle reflexes (ankle jerk), and, if severe, muscle power in the distribution of the nerve (e.g., ankle flexion, extension, inversion and eversion, great toe extension). Sciatica is pain in the distribution of the sciatic nerve. Pain is initially felt in the buttock and posterior thigh and may extend to the posterolateral leg, the lateral dorsum of the foot, and the entire sole. When nerve function is compromised, paresthesias are felt in the same distribution. Pain and paresthesias are intensified by coughing or straining. The nerve trunk is tender when palpated at the sciatic notch or stretched when the leg is extended while the thigh is flexed (*Lasègue sign*) and/or with straight-leg raising. Rectal exam should always be done to looking for a pelvic mass; pulsating rectal mass associated with sciatica suggests internal iliac or common iliac artery aneurysm. Most cases are caused by herniated intervertebral disk.

Herniated intervertebral disk. Herniation of a desiccated nucleus pulposus through tears in the annulus fibrosa produces pressure on nerve roots in the neural foramina laterally or directly on the cauda equina, conus or spinal cord if the extrusion is directly posterior (Fig. 13-26B, page 563). The onset of pain is gradual or sudden and is partially relieved in recumbency. Sciatica is often the presenting symptom with buttock pain radiating to the thigh. When severe, the pain involves the leg, usually the lateral aspect, and toes (dermatomes L4–S2). Coughing, sneezing, and/or Valsalva accentuate the pain.

Chronic herniated disk is attended by symptom-free periods; continuous pain is usually caused by something else. On exam, the spine may be flexed, frequently deviating laterally toward the affected side. Active spine flexion and extension are more limited than lateral bending and rotation. Muscle spasm is most severe over the ipsilateral sacrospinalis with rigidity and tenderness, most pronounced on the affected side 5 cm lateral to the midline. Palpate for muscle rigidity, and other areas of tenderness including trigger points and fibrositis tender points. Have the patient heel-and-toe walk and extend the great toe against resistance. Pain with the straight leg test often occurs at <40 degrees with a prolapsed disk. If the straight-leg-raising test is positive, test for sciatic nerve irritability by sharply dorsiflexing the foot to stretch the sciatic nerve as the painful angle is again approached. Check sensation noting the affected dermatome.

Spinal stenosis. Overgrowth of bone, congenital narrowing, or degenerative disk disease narrows the spinal canal compressing lower lumbar and sacral roots. Pain in the buttocks, bilateral posterior thighs, and calves while standing or walking upright, that is relieved by sitting or bending forward (reversing the lumbar lordosis and decreasing the degree of stenosis) is *pseudoclaudication*. *DDX:* Unlike intermittent claudication from vascular insufficiency, pain occurs while standing without walking. Sitting gives relief, in contrast to lumbar disk disease. Osteoporosis, spondylolisthesis, trauma, laminectomy, spinal fusion, spondylosis, scoliosis, acromegaly, and Paget disease are all potential contributors. Congenital narrowing of the canal is not uncommon. Characteristically, patients shop leaning forward onto a shopping cart.

Sacral pain
Cauda equina lesions. Compression of the cauda equina ("horse's tail": the spinal roots below the level of the spinal cord termination, or conus) compromises nerve function in one or more lumbar or spinal nerves, often accompanied by pain. Pain is localized to the sacrum and inner thigh, and the skin may be anesthetic. Bladder symptoms (including decreased urinary stream, hesitancy, and urinary retention), anal sphincter laxity, absent anal wink, and impotence are common. Compression occurs from a herniated intervertebral disk with posterior protrusion, epidural hematoma or abscess, and neoplasms.

Sacroiliac pain
Sacroiliac arthritis. There is painful stiffness in the upper medial buttocks on arising, that improves with exercise. Pain may be referred to the upper outer quadrant of the buttock, or the posterolateral thigh. Sometimes there is a limp. Spinal rotation accentuates pain. The joint is tender to palpation or percussion. SI arthritis is characteristic of spondyloarthritis.

Sacroiliac strain. Mechanical strain or postpartum relaxation of the ligaments about the joint is followed by inflammation. The patient complains of pain in the joint or upper inner quadrant of the buttock or the posterolateral thigh (dermatomes L4, L5, S1). The joint is tender. The pain is accentuated by compressing the anterior iliac crests while the patient lies supine. The tendon reflexes in the legs are normal.

Ischial tuberosity pain

Ischiogluteal bursitis. When standing, the gluteal muscles cover the ischial tuberosities. With thigh flexion, such as sitting, the muscles slide upward exposing the tuberosities and their tendon insertions to pressure, protected only by intervening skin, subcutaneous tissue, and the ischiogluteal bursa. Irritation of the bursa and/or tendon insertions leads to secondary sciatic nerve irritation. This is most common with occupations characterized by sitting on a poorly cushioned seat. The pain is aggravated by sitting, coughing, walking, and standing on tiptoe. When standing and walking the patient lists to the affected side, the stride is shortened, and the foot circumducts. The patient sits with the affected buttock elevated and, on lying, supports the pelvis on that side. There is point tenderness on the ischial tuberosity. Straight-leg-raising causes pain. The *FABER sign* is present. On rectal exam a region of tender, bulging, doughy tissue may be palpable in the lateral rectal wall. *DDX:* Patients with herniated disk and lumbosacral disease lie quietly and lack the FABER sign. This bursa may also be affected by gout. Pain is referred to the tuberosity from intramedullary lesions of the femoral head.

Upper Extremity Syndromes

Finger snapping or locking—trigger finger. Inflammation or repetitive trauma induces nodular thickening of a long flexor tendon just proximal to the metacarpal head. with the finger extended, the nodule lies within the flexor tendon sheath; during flexion, it is easily pulled from the proximal end of the sheath. The constricted mouth of the sheath resists reentry of the nodule during extension until it is suddenly achieved with a noticeable click. The middle or ring finger is usually involved (Fig. 13-28D). Flexion of the finger feels normal, but extension is accompanied by a snap that the patient sometimes refers to the region of the PIP joint. The palpable nodule moves with the tendon on active and passive flexion–extension. Triggering may or may not be painful.

Finger infections. It is essential to distinguish superficial infections from deep infections that are initially limited to a specific tissue compartment giving characteristic signs.

Paronychia. The skin over the nail matrix and the lateral nail folds is swollen, reddened, painful, and tender (Fig. 13-40A). When infection is over the nail root, light palpation provokes exquisite pain. Pain from pressure on the nail plate indicates *subungual abscess*, between the nail plate and periosteum.

Chronic paronychia. *Candida* paronychia is minimally tender and does not drain. Chronic ulceration of the nail mantle and lateral folds occurs in occupations requiring frequent immersion of the hands in water or contaminated oil. The ulcers are indolent; abscess formation is rare.

Apical space abscess. Symptoms follow a puncture wound beneath the nail. The distal nail bed becomes red and extremely painful with little swelling (Fig. 13-40B). Maximum tenderness is proximal to the nail plate's free edge, unlike a felon, which produces tenderness at the fingertip. When the abscess ruptures, it drains at the free edge of the nail plate.

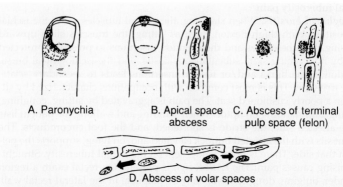

A. Paronychia B. Apical space abscess C. Abscess of terminal pulp space (felon)

D. Abscess of volar spaces

FIG. 13-40 Common Locations for Finger Abscesses. A. Paronychia. B. Apical space abscess. The apical space is in the nail bed near the free margin of the nail plate. **C. Terminal pulp space abscess (felon).** The stippled region on the volar surface is where it ruptures through the skin. **D. Volar space abscesses.** The stippled regions are the sites of abscesses; the arrows point in the direction of burrowing to reach the flexor creases of the finger.

Terminal pulp space abscess (Felon). Finger pad infection is confined within small fascial compartments attached to the periosteum (Fig. 13-40C). The fingertip is swollen with dull pain that becomes intense and throbbing with exquisite tenderness. Induration indicates the presence of pus. The abscess may drain through the volar surface of the finger pad; osteomyelitis can occur.

Middle volar pulp space abscess. The finger is held in partial flexion to reduce the pain. There is tender swelling on the volar aspect of the finger between the PIP and DIP joints (Fig. 13-40D). The symptoms resemble those of a felon. Osteomyelitis may occur. The abscess may drain after burrowing to the distal flexor crease.

Proximal volar pulp space abscess. An abscess forms on the volar aspect between the MCP and PIP joints (Fig. 13-40D). The symptoms and signs are like those in the middle space, except the infection burrows proximally to involve the web space.

Barber's pilonidal sinus. Short hair shafts penetrate the soft skin in the finger webs producing inflammation. One or more palpable nodules are drained by sinuses seen as black dots between the fingers.

Localized thickening of palmar fascia—Dupuytren contracture. There is a painless nodular thickening of the palmar aponeurosis from hyaliniza-tion of collagen fibers beginning near the base of the digit. It extends to form a plaque or band adhering to the palmar fascia producing retraction and dimpling of the palmar skin and flexion contracture of the fingers. The condition occurs exclusively in Caucasians, predominately men, and 40% have a positive family history. It is more common in patients with alcoholism, epilepsy, or diabetes mellitus; the cause for these associations is unknown. It usually begins after age 40 years as an inconspicuous hard nodule fixed to the skin in the distal palm. Both hands may be involved. The ring finger is more often affected than the little, long, index or thumb. Fascial retraction pulls the finger(s) into partial flexion (Fig. 13-30I). Palpation reveals a hard cord over the tendon that is raised in extension, making it readily seen. With progression, painless contracture of the digit(s) requires surgical correction. Other fibrosing conditions may be part of the same diathesis, occurring singly or in combination, including plantar fibrosis (*Lederhosen syndrome*) and fibrosis of the corpus cavernosum (*Peyronie disease*).

Hand infections. Infections in the hand can be trivial or tragic depending upon the site of infection and organism. Care must be taken to identify deep space infections resulting from puncture or bite wounds that can rapidly destroy hand function.

Web space infection. Fever, malaise, and diffuse pain in the hand and dorsal edema occur early. The two involved fingers are separated at their bases by a tender erythematous swelling; tenderness is maximal on the palmar surface (Fig. 13-41A).

Thenar space infection. The thenar eminence is swollen, tender, and may have erythema and warmth. *DDX:* Deep hematoma gives similar symptoms and signs but with a history of blunt trauma. Extension at the IP joint is not painful as it is with flexor pollicis longus tenosynovitis.

Deep palm abscess. There is usually a history of penetrating trauma, often minor. There is pain, swelling and limited motion. In addition to severe dorsal edema, the concavity of the palm is obliterated, or even elevated; the raised area is tender and erythematous, the erythema may extend *under* the flexor retinaculum to the volar wrist. This is a surgical emergency.

Ulnar bursa infection. There is dorsal edema and fullness on the ulnar side of the palm (Fig. 13-41A). Maximum tenderness is halfway between the lunate and the fifth MCP joint.

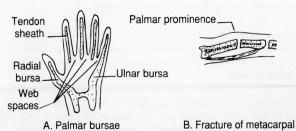

FIG. 13-41 Swellings of the Hand. A. Palmar bursae. The bursae locations are indicated by stippling. Note the tendon sheaths ending proximally near the palmar crease; there is a connection between the radial and ulnar bursae. The radial bursa is continuous from the thumb to the region of the thenar eminence. The web spaces are sites of abscesses. **B. Metacarpal fracture.** The fragments may displace into the palm producing a prominence.

Radial bursa infection. The IP joint of the thumb is flexed; passive extension produces pain. There is tenderness and swelling over the flexor pollicis longus sheath.

Metacarpal fracture. In a transverse fracture, the metacarpal bone fragments bow into the palm producing a painful prominence (Fig. 13-41B). The prominence may be obscured by soft-tissue swelling, but dorsal palpation localizes tenderness at the fracture site. In a spiral fracture, proximal slippage of the distal fragment produces shortening revealed by loss of prominence in the corresponding knuckle when the fist is closed. The distal fragment is rotated if the affected finger does not align with the unaffected fingers when the tips are flexed onto the base of the thenar eminence. *Bennett fracture* is an oblique break through the base of the first metacarpal, frequently with subluxation of the carpal-metacarpal joint. The thumb is semiflexed and cannot be opposed to the ring or little finger and the fist cannot be clenched.

Tenosynovitis
Acute suppurative flexor tenosynovitis–painful palm and finger swelling.
Throbbing pain, beginning in a finger, progresses toward the palm. The finger and dorsum of the hand are swollen. The finger is held slightly flexed; the patient resists movement. Passively extending adjacent fingers is painful, of the affected finger, exquisitely so. Find the point of maximum tenderness by gently palpating the palm and flexor surface of the finger with the blunt end of an applicator or tongue depressor. If it is located at the proximal end of the tendon sheath of the index, middle, or ring finger, involvement of the sheath is certain. If there is no localization, the sheath may have ruptured.

Thumb extensor tenosynovitis—painful swelling in the anatomic snuffbox.
Inflammation in the tendon sheaths of the *extensor pollicis longus and brevis* as they pass under a fibrous band near the radial styloid causes pain and tenderness. Pain is felt in the region of the snuffbox. The patient has pain with pinching, thumb extension, and wrist ulnar deviation. When the fist is clenched over the flexed thumb, gentle but firm ulnar deviation of the hand by the examiner elicits pain at the radial styloid process, *Finkelstein test* (Fig. 13-42B). The pain may transmit down the thumb or toward the elbow. Passive thumb extension is painless. Crepitus may be felt or auscultated over the tendon sheath during thumb flexion–extension.

Acute tenosynovitis. A sausage-like swelling ~4 cm long (Fig. 13-42C), involves the tendon sheaths at the radial border of the snuffbox. The cause is usually trauma, although gout, pseudogout, and gonococcal infection can produce inflammation.

Chronic stenosing tenosynovitis—de Quervain tenosynovitis. The symptoms are like the acute process and are frequently chronic and recurrent, exacerbated by repetitive movements of the wrist and thumb. Chronic inflammation involves all layers of the tendon sheath.

Flexor compartment syndrome and Volkmann ischemic contracture—forearm pain and weakness. See compartment syndrome, page 608). In

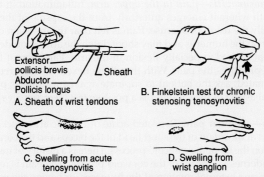

Extensor pollicis brevis
Abductor Pollicis longus
Sheath
A. Sheath of wrist tendons

B. Finkelstein test for chronic stenosing tenosynovitis

C. Swelling from acute tenosynovitis

D. Swelling from wrist ganglion

FIG. 13-42 Some Disorders of the Wrist. A. Tendon sheaths of on the radial wrist. In chronic stenosing tenosynovitis swelling limits motion of the extensor pollicis brevis and abductor pollicis longus tendons. **B. Finkelstein test for tenosynovitis.** The thumb is clenched in the fist while the examiner pushes the fist toward the ulna. A positive test elicits pain at the radial styloid process. **C. Swelling from acute nonsuppurative tenosynovitis. D. Frequent site of ganglion of the wrist.** The swelling is painless and sometimes translucent.

acute forearm compartment syndrome, the fingers are often edematous and may be cyanotic, passive finger extension produces forearm pain, the radial pulse is absent, the skin over the hands is cool, and median nerve sensation is diminished. Emergent surgical consultation is required. Volkmann contracture is a late finding in which the fingers are fixed in flexion by shortening of the fibrotic bellies of the digital flexors in the forearm. Because the flexor tendons are free to move in their sheaths, slight extension of the fingers is permitted with the wrist in flexion distinguishing it from adhesions of flexor tendons to their sheaths. Precipitating events are forearm and supracondylar fractures and circumferential bandages or casts applied shortly after trauma.

Elbow pain
Lateral and medial epicondylitis, tennis elbow. Repetitive forceful wrist and/ or finger flexion and extension focus tension on the common proximal tendon insertions at the lateral (extensors) and medial (flexors) humeral epicondyles. *Lateral Epicondylitis* causes pain in the lateral aspect of the elbow, accentuated by use of the hand during a power grip (when the wrist extensors are also contracting), as in lifting objects. Palpation discloses tenderness over the lateral epicondyle and 1 cm distally. Having the patient hold the long finger in full extension against resistance reliably reproduces the pain. In the *Cozen test* (resisted wrist extension), the patient is asked to keep the fist clenched while extending the wrist against resistance reproducing the patient's lateral epicondylar pain. In the *Mill maneuver*, the elbow is held in extension with the wrist flexed; when you pronate the forearm against the patient's resistance, epicondylar pain is elicited. *Medial Epicondylitis* is less common. The pain is located just distal to the medial epicondyle in the flexor tendons and is reproduced by maneuvers requiring wrist and finger flexion or arm pronation against resistance.

Bicipital tenosynovitis—pain in the upper arm. Inflammation in the biceps tendon sheath where it emerges anteriorly from the capsule of the shoulder joint is usually the result of overuse. Pain is felt near the insertion of the pectoralis major on the humerus and may shoot down the arm. Shoulder motions are somewhat limited, especially flexion of the arm. Palpation of the bicipital groove reproduces the pain. With the elbow flexed to 90 degrees and the forearm pronated, ask the patient to supinate against resistance; pain in the anteromedial aspect of the shoulder is a positive test (*Yergason Sign*).

Coracoiditis—shoulder pain. Repeated acute or chronic arm work produces inflammation at the origin of the short head of the biceps and the coracobrachialis muscles on the tip of the coracoid process. There is a history of trauma with pain and tenderness at the tip of the coracoid process. The pain is reproduced by adduction and external rotation of the humerus, or having the patient perform against resistance either supination of the forearm with the elbow flexed, forward flexion of the shoulder, or adduction of the flexed shoulder.

Rotator cuff injury—painful arc and impingement sign. During arm abduction the supraspinatus tendon and its insertion on the proximal greater humeral tuberosity pass beneath the acromion. The subacromial bursa is positioned to decrease friction or impingement with this motion. Repetitive forceful motion causes mechanical irritation to the tissues eliciting inflammation of the tendon and bursa. Sudden or severe loading of the shoulder may result in incomplete or complete tears of the tendon. Three conditions present with similar signs and symptoms. A history of sudden onset favors partial tear of the tendon, whereas repetitive shoulder motion and subacute or chronic symptoms favor tendonitis or bursitis. All have painful abduction between 60 and 120 degrees, often prohibiting full active range of motion. Less painful passive range of motion is preserved (Fig. 13-43). *Precise distinction between the three is not possible by physical exam.*

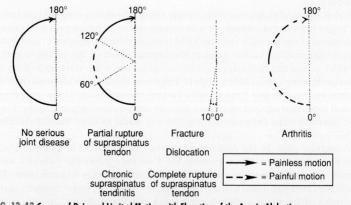

FIG. 13-43 Causes of Pain and Limited Motion with Elevation of the Arm in Abduction.

Partial supraspinatus tendon rupture. When the tendon is incompletely torn, the rotator cuff is intact. Pain is referred to the humeral insertion of the deltoid muscle, but there is no tenderness at that point. Sometimes the pain extends down the arm to the elbow or beyond. Tenderness is elicited just beneath the acromial tip or in the notch between greater and lesser humeral tubercles. *DDX:* If supraspinatus weakness, weak external rotation, and impingement signs are all present, a rotator cuff tear is likely.

Acute supraspinatus tendinitis. This usually occurs in a person 25–45 years of age, with a dull ache developing in the shoulder without antecedent trauma. The pain steadily worsens and may be excruciating. The diagnostic test is abduction to 90 degrees and then full internal rotation, reproducing the pain. Tenderness beneath the acromial tip is pronounced.

Chronic supraspinatus tendinitis. Dull shoulder pain develops in a patient who is usually 45–60 years old without preceding trauma. Abduction is painless to 60 degrees, where the patient feels a jerk with pain in the region of the deltoid muscle. Pronounced tenderness can be elicited in the notch between the greater and lesser tubercles of the humeral head or beneath the acromial tip. Crepitus may also be present. Lying on the shoulder produces pain that prevents sleeping on the affected side for months.

Subacromial bursitis. This can be acute or chronic and often accompanies supraspinatus tendonitis. The pain is constant and aggravated by elevation in abduction. There is often a history of heavy arm use.

Complete supraspinatus tendon rupture, torn rotator cuff—minimal arm elevation. The supraspinatus muscle initiates arm abduction from 0 to 45 degrees, where the deltoid engages. Inability to initiate elevation in 90 degrees abduction indicates complete supraspinatus tendon rupture. This usually occurs after age 40. The patient cannot elevate the arm against minimal resistance at 30 degrees elevation and 90 degrees abduction, but passive motion is free and painless. Initial shoulder motion is mostly with the scapula. There is resistance to external rotation when the arm is held at the side with elbow flexed. As the arm is moved forward, one may palpate a jerk, fine crepitus, or an indentation in the subacromial region between the greater and lesser humeral tubercles (Fig. 13-18D, page 545). Wasting of the supraspinatus and infraspinatus occurs after 3 weeks.

Adhesive capsulitis—frozen shoulder. Chronic inflammation of the rotator cuff and joint capsule leads to shortening of the usually loose tendinous cuff with progressive loss of motion. All types of arthritis may involve the shoulder. In early inflammatory processes, motions are inhibited by pain; later, adhesions restrict motion, often following unresolved subacromial bursitis or supraspinatus tendinitis. At onset, pain is that of the original injury. Progressive limitation of motion ensues until capsular contraction and fibrosis abate the pain. Chronically limited motion is associated muscle wasting. *DDX:* OA may be associated with crepitus in the joint, but effusions are relatively rare. Joint effusion suggests rheumatoid arthritis, crystal arthritis, or less-common disorders such as villonodular synovitis.

Conditions of the Entire Upper Limb

Flail arm. Lower motor neuron or peripheral nerve injuries denervate muscles with flaccid paralysis and muscle wasting. After injuries to the brachial plexus or poliomyelitis, the arm may hang limply at the side with the flexed palm facing backward (Fig. 13-33B).

Spastic arm. Injury to upper motor neurons leads to tonic muscle contraction with the antigravity flexors overpowering the weaker extensors. With hemiplegia, the arm is carried with flexion at the elbow, wrist, and fingers (Fig. 13-33C).

Lower Extremity Syndromes

Painless limp–Osteonecrosis, aseptic hip necrosis. Ischemia of the femoral head leads to bone necrosis with femoral head collapse and mushrooming. It can be unilateral or bilateral. Although the cause may be unknown, corticosteroid use, diabetes, obesity, *SLE*, and alcohol each associated with increased risk. Osteonecrosis of the epiphysis in childhood (*Legg–Calvé–Perthes disease*) is relatively painless, whereas osteonecrosis in adults may be painful. Usually it begins with a painless limp and all hip motions are slightly impaired. Later, there is severely limited abduction and rotation. Muscle wasting and limb shortening are common. *Trendelenburg gait* suggests hip dislocation.

Painful hip

Osteoarthritis. Boring pain in the groin and buttocks, sometimes with referral to the knee is frequent. Initially, stiffness on arising disappears with exercise, but later walking is limited by pain. The thigh is held in adduction. Passive motion is restricted in internal rotation and abduction and may be painful. Palpable and audible crepitus may be present.

Septic arthritis. Usually, there is groin pain, fever, leukocytosis, and prostration. The thigh is held in slight abduction and external rotation to best accommodate the joint effusion. All hip motion is painful. Fluctuance is rarely felt. By referral, pain may only be felt in the knee, so knee pain should always prompt hip examination. Diagnosis is urgent; joint cartilage may be irreparably damaged within hours without drainage and antibiotics. Tuberculous arthritis is more insidious, often presenting with a limp and pain only after exertion.

Slipped capital femoral epiphysis. The femoral head dislocates on the femoral neck at the relatively weak growth plate during rapid growth in adolescence. Patients walk with a limp accompanied by pain. The distinguishing feature is painful limitation of internal rotation with the thigh and knee flexed. This may be succeeded by shortening and external rotation from anterosuperior femoral neck displacement.

Torn labrum. There is a traumatic tear in the acetabular labrum. Patients are usually young men with persistent hip pain but full motion. There may be no history of injury, or only of injury thought to be minor. The hip is less stable. *DDX:* Hip impingement syndrome is should be considered in the differential diagnosis.

Chronic hip dislocation. Hip dislocation is congenital or acquired. Weakness of the supporting muscles (from nerve or muscle injury), joint infections, and trauma lead to dislocation in adults. Prosthetic hips are especially susceptible to dislocation with flexion and external rotation. For congenital hip dislocation, consult pediatric texts. In adults, *Trendelenburg gait* (page 548) is present. With the patient supine and the hips and knees flexed, the knee of the affected leg is lower when observed from the foot of the bed. When standing on one, the pelvis normally tilts upwards on the nonweight-bearing side (Fig. 13-34A). With dislocation, when standing on the affected leg, the pelvis tilts downward on the nonweightbearing side (*Trendelenburg sign*); the muscles cannot support the pelvis when the femoral head does not engage the acetabulum. The sign is also positive with disease of the glutei, femoral head fracture, and severe coxa vara. In adults, there is hip pain and premature OA of the joint.

Medial knee pain–anserine bursitis. The anserine bursa is superficial to the tibial collateral ligament and deep to the *pes anserina* (goose foot) formed by the sartorius, gracilis, and semitendinosus tendons (Fig. 13-35). Pain and tenderness without swelling are located in the anterior medial knee 2–3 cm distal to the joint line. Pain is aggravated by walking, especially climbing stairs.

Anterior knee pain
Chondromalacia patellae. The articular surface of the patella degenerates from unknown cause, more commonly in women than men. Pain, aggravated by prolonged sitting and descending stairs, is felt anteriorly. A small effusion may be present. Passive joint motion is painless. Rocking the patella in the femoral groove frequently elicits pain, often with palpable crepitation.

Quadriceps and patellar tendonitis. Pain in the anterior knee either above (quadriceps) or below (patellar) the patella follows an unusual level of activity, e.g., running, lifting, climbing, and up-down squatting and/or from chronic overuse. Pain localizes to the involved tendon and is reproduced by direct pressure and resisted knee extension.

Tibial tubercle osteochondritis (Osgood–Schlatter disease). Before closure of the tibial tubercle epiphysis during adolescence, vigorous exercise produces chronic traction injury partially avulsing the tubercle. Pain is after exercise and a tender hard swelling is seen and felt at the attachment of the patellar tendon.

Exertional leg pain
Intermittent claudication. See Chapter 8, page 297.

Tibial stress fracture. Repeated strenuous leg use induces an incomplete cortical fracture. Dull aching pain, persisting for hours, begins gradually and with progressively shorter intervals after exercise. There is localized tenderness over the tibia, frequently along the medial border. Pain at the fracture site may be elicited by springing the tibia: with the patient supine, place one hand on the knee and the other on the heel; pull the tibia laterally against your knee as a fulcrum.

Tibial compartment syndrome. See page 608. Several hours after unusually strenuous leg exercise, there is stiffness followed by severe pain in the anterior tibial muscle compartment. The compartment becomes swollen, tense, tender, and warm. Ischemic necrosis of the muscles may occur if the pressure is not relieved by fasciotomy.

Foot pain–tarsal tunnel syndrome. The tarsal tunnel is behind and inferior to the medial malleolus. Its bony floor is roofed by the *flexor retinaculum* extending from the medial malleolus to the calcaneus. Through the tunnel pass several tendons and the *posterior tibial nerve*, which divides into the *calcaneal nerve* to the skin of the heel, the *medial plantar nerve* to the skin and muscles of the medial sole, and the *lateral plantar nerve* to the lateral sole. Nerve compression in the tunnel causes numbness, burning pain, or paresthesias in portions of the sole. Paresis or paralysis of some small foot muscles can occur. Occasionally, a tender area is palpated at the posterior margin of the medial malleolus. Confirmation is by nerve conduction studies. Precipitating conditions include fracture or dislocation of the bones near the tunnel, traumatic edema, tenosynovitis, chronic stasis of the posterior tibial vein, and foot strain.

Forefoot pain
Metatarsalgia. Loss of the normal transverse metatarsal arch from the first to the fifth metatarsal heads leads to abnormal weight bearing on the insufficiently cushioned second to fourth metatarsal heads. Pain is around the distal metatarsal heads. Exam may show callus under the second to fourth metatarsal heads and decreased callus under the first and fifth. Pressure on the callus reproduces the pain. Symmetrical bilateral metatarsalgia may be an early symptom of rheumatoid arthritis. DDX: Fibroneuroma gives similar pain reproduced by squeezing the foot transversely.

Metatarsal stress fracture. Excessive walking or standing can cause a metatarsal shaft stress fracture (Fig. 13-37C) with pain developing gradually. Muscle cramps and slight swelling can occur. Moving the corresponding toe is painful. Pain usually localizes several centimeters proximal to the metatarsal head.

Interdigital space infection. Puncture of the sole infect one of the four interdigital subcutaneous spaces. The abscess points between two metatarsals causing dorsal swelling on the foot. Walking produces pain between the metatarsals. Tenderness is localized to the interdigital space.

Chronic painless leg enlargement. Several causes must be distinguished. Although some *obesity* is present elsewhere in the body, adipose tissue about the ankles may be disproportionately great, while sparing the feet. The tissue has the consistency of fat and doesn't pit. *Chronic deep vein obstruction* usually is preceded by a history suggesting thrombophlebitis. Venous insufficiency may produce pain in the legs. Some pitting edema is usually present, although it may be obscured by skin thickening from chronic inflammation. The skin is hemosiderin stained and may be cyanotic. Superficial veins may be dilated. *Postphlebitic syndrome* results from previous deep vein occlusion without recanalization or from destruction of the valves with persistent venous incompetence. One-third of patients with acute deep vein thrombosis will develop postphlebitic syndrome (Chapter 8, page 378). The leg is persistently enlarged, usually with pitting edema. Sensations of fullness and pain occur with prolonged sitting or standing, and chronic stasis changes are common. *Varicose veins* are readily recognized when they are associated with edema. Chronic edema from any cause leads to subcutaneous and cutaneous fibrosis with nonpitting woody induration (*dermatoliposclerosis*). *Lymphedema* causes firm, uniform, nonpitting swelling extending to the feet without venous engorgement or cyanosis.

Muscle Syndromes

Fibromyalgia. See *Tender Points*, page 561. Fibromyalgia is at the extreme end of an ill-defined group of disorders variously described as polysomatic distress or functional somatic disorders. It is characterized by chronic widespread pain (CWP) involving both sides of the body above and below the waist, and the axial skeleton. The pain is described as diffuse aching and accompanied by stiffness, nonrestorative sleep, and fatigue. To make the diagnosis, symptoms must be unexplained by another disorder and have been present >3 months. Fibromyalgia is more common in women than men. The 1990 American College of Rheumatology (ACR) diagnostic criteria included at least 11 of 18 paired, bilateral tender points elicited on physical exam (Fig. 13-44). In 2010, new ACR criteria eliminated the tender points. The criteria are now based on a Symptom Severity (SS) scale and the Widespread Pain Index (WPI). Each symptom (fatigue, waking unrefreshed, and cognitive symptoms), and the

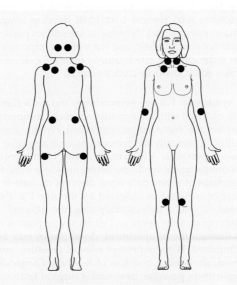

Tender points of fibromyalgia
in at least 11 of 18 sites

FIG. 13-44 The Tender Points of Fibromyalgia. See text page 561.

widespread somatic symptoms are scored 0–3. The combined WPI and SS replace the dichotomous classification with a continuous polysymptomatic distress scale.

Myofascial pain syndrome. Afferent signals from trigger areas are thought to remodel spinal and possibly thalamic pain pathways causing reflex muscle spasm and diminishing blood flow, which, in turn, increase the sensitivity of the trigger area. See *Trigger Points*, page 561. Chronic recurrent pain is experienced roughly in the distribution of one or more muscles and their area(s) of referred pain. The pain is lancinating, aching, boring, or there may be only muscle stiffness. The onset is often related to a specific injury or activity. The distinguishing feature is the presence of one or more trigger points, with or without palpable muscle spasm. Carefully palpate the entire region applying firm pressure with the fingertips. Often, the trigger point is some distance from the area of referred pain. The diagnosis is confirmed if the pain is relieved by injecting the primary trigger point with a local anesthetic.

Polymyalgia rheumatic. This inflammatory disorder of unknown cause is characterized by pain in proximal muscle groups, with inflammation demonstrable by MRI in the shoulder girdle tendon sheaths and bursae, and less commonly the shoulder joint itself. It usually occurs after the sixth decade and is most common in women. Pronounced morning stiffness of the neck, shoulder, and upper back muscles usually begins gradually. Some patients have sudden onset and can note the day and time of their first symptoms. Muscles of the low back, pelvic girdle, and thighs are less prominently involved and/or may develop later. It is common in patients with temporal arteritis, but only 15% of patients who present with PMR develop temporal arteritis. Although spontaneously painful, the muscles are seldom particularly tender, trigger points are not characteristic, and the stiffness improves with activity. The erythrocyte sedimentation rate is usually markedly elevated; symptoms are promptly relieved by low-dose corticosteroids.

Compartment syndrome. Edema, hemorrhage, and/or inflammation from injury to muscle enclosed within a constricting fascial compartment increase the pressure within the compartment occluding venous drainage, further increasing swelling. Eventually the pressure exceeds arteriolar pressure and ischemic necrosis supervenes. A high index of suspicion is required to diagnose and treat a compartment syndrome before muscle is irreversibly injured. The patient complains of severe pain often disproportionate to the apparent injury. The onset of ischemia is indicated by the five P's: Pain, Puffiness, Pallor, Pulselessness, and Paralysis. Palpating the affected compartment reveals tense distention of the fascia and elicits severe pain. If major arteries or nerves pass through the compartment, distal pulses may be diminished and sensation impaired. Without prompt relief of pressure, muscles necrose leading to fibrosis, shortening, and loss of function. Diagnosis is made by measuring compartment pressure; treatment is surgical fasciotomy.

Trichinosis. Heavy infection with *Trichinella spiralis* after ingestion of incompletely cooked infected meat (pork, bear meat) causes severe illness, and infrequently, death. The organisms localize in muscle. One to four days after ingestion, the patient complains of nausea and vomiting, diarrhea, and abdominal pain. Within 10 days, there is fever, dyspnea, anorexia, myalgia, and asthenia. Physical findings include periorbital edema, scarlatiniform rash, splinter hemorrhages under nails, tremors, and involuntary movements.

MUSCULOSKELETAL TRAUMA SYNDROMES

STOP: Fractures are discussed in this section only to illustrate relatively common physical findings. This text should not be used as a guide for the definitive diagnosis of traumatic musculoskeletal injuries. Orthopedic texts should be consulted for details, differential diagnosis, and as a guide to diagnosis and management.

- **Fat embolism.** After trauma to large bones, and especially after fractures, fat globules embolize to the lungs, brain, and other tissues. The pathogenesis remains controversial. Symptom onset is sudden with restlessness and vague chest pain. Symptoms reach a maximum in ~48 hours. Dyspnea and cyanosis are common and purulent sputum, occasionally containing diagnostic fat droplets, may be produced. Fever is accompanied by a disproportionately high pulse rate. Cerebral symptoms and signs are extremely variable; delirium and coma indicate a grave prognosis. Fat droplets may be seen in retinal or conjunctival vessels. On the second or third day, petechiae may appear over the shoulders and chest as well as in the conjunctivae and retinae. Fat embolism should be considered in acutely ill patients with trauma to long bones or skull, insertion of prosthetic joints, chronic alcoholism, diabetes mellitus, and sickle cell disease.

STOP: Following trauma with suspected spine injury, the spine must ALWAYS be immediately IMMOBILIZED. Place the neck in a rigid collar and the patient on a back board PRIOR TO ANY MOVEMENT or examination.

Traumatic Neck Pain

- **Fracture of the atlas (C1) or odontoid process (C2).** Disruption of the bony-ligamentous ring restraining the odontoid process and fracture at the odontoid's base produce instability of C1 on C2 and cervical spinal cord compression is immanent. If not immediately fatal, the patient supports the head with the hands and is unwilling to nod the head. There is severe occipital headache. The patient cannot rotate the head. If not diagnosed immediately and the neck completely immobilized, sudden death may ensue. In rheumatoid arthritis pannus can erode the transverse ligament of C1 supporting the posterior odontoid leading to C1–C2 dislocation from trivial trauma. A high index of suspicion is required to make these diagnoses.

Neck flexion fracture. When the neck is forcefully hyperflexed, e.g., a diver striking his head on the bottom, the C5 vertebral body is the most frequently fractured. The patient who escapes immediate death or quadriplegia may be unable to walk without supporting his head with his hands. Pain restricts all neck motion. The spinous process of the affected vertebra is tender and may be more prominent.

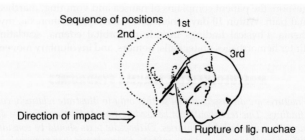

FIG. 13-45 Cervical Spine Extension Injury (Whiplash). Violent impact from behind rapidly extends the neck followed by rebound flexion rupturing the ligamentum nuchae.

Partial dislocation from hyperextension. A fall or blow on the forehead, hyperextending the neck, ruptures the anterior longitudinal ligament. There is intense neck pain. One spinous process may be more prominent. Paraplegia is frequent.

Whiplash cervical injury. When an automobile is struck from behind, passengers experience sudden forceful neck hyperextension with recoil flexion (Fig. 13-45). Posterior neck pain develops over hours or days. Nerve-root irritation produces muscle spasm and torticollis. Occipital headache develops, sometimes with blurring of vision. The chin turns toward the painful side. Palpation over the lower cervical spinous processes elicits tenderness. An effusion with soft crepitus can sometimes be felt over the lowest part of the ligamentum nuchae. The biceps reflex may be diminished or absent on one or both sides. Occasionally, the pupil dilates on the affected side.

Spinous process fracture. A direct blow or violent muscle contraction, such as lifting a heavy load with a shovel, can break the long, thin, spinous process of a vertebrae near the cervicothoracic junction. Sudden, severe pain extending from the neck to the shoulder is accentuated by neck flexion and rotation. Tenderness is exquisite over the fractures spinous process. Sometimes the fractured process is mobile laterally and crepitus can be felt.

Traumatic Back Pain
Stable vertebral compression fracture with intact spinal ligaments. The thoracic or lumbar vertebrae are fractured by trauma that crushes their bodies, e.g., forceful spine hyperflexion, a fall landing on the feet or buttocks, or a downward blow on the shoulders (Fig. 13-26C). Pain and tenderness can be mild or even absent for weeks, so fracture may not be suspected until a radiograph is obtained. Occasionally, slight kyphosis is present.

Unstable vertebral compression fracture with torn spinal ligaments. Interspinal and supraspinal ligament rupture accompanying a compression fracture permits the articular facets of two adjacent vertebrae to slide apart; on recoil, they may interlock (Fig. 13-26E). Suspect this dangerous condition when a gap is palpated between two spinous processes (Fig. 13-26D).

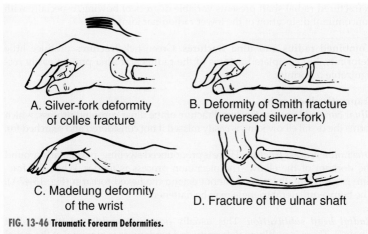

A. Silver-fork deformity
of colles fracture

B. Deformity of Smith fracture
(reversed silver-fork)

C. Madelung deformity
of the wrist

D. Fracture of the ulnar shaft

FIG. 13-46 Traumatic Forearm Deformities.

Vertebral dislocation. Violent spine hyperflexion, in addition to fracturing the vertebrae, may tear the supporting ligaments, permitting vertebral dislocation and consequent spinal cord damage. This potentially unstable condition requires immediate immobilization and evaluation. Suspect this when the palpating finger finds a gap between two spinous processes.

Transverse process fracture. A vertebral transverse process, usually lumbar, fractures from violent contraction of the attached muscles. There is severe pain in the lumbar region, with intense muscle spasm. The spinous processes are not tender. If caused by a direct blow, hematuria signifies a concomitant kidney injury.

Traumatic Wrist, Arm, and Shoulder Pain

Colles fracture—wrist silver-fork deformity. The most common cause is a fall on the outstretched hand. The radius is fractured within 2.5 cm of its distal end (Fig. 13-46A). The ulnar styloid is fractured half the time. The pronated arm's profile resembles a dinner fork lying horizontally with the tines pointing downward, the base of the tines curving upward. Dorsal displacement of the distal radius fragment produces a corresponding hump in the fractured arm.

Smith fracture, reversed Colles fracture—reversed silver-fork deformity. Like the Colles fracture, the distal end of the radius is broken, but the distal fragment displaces volarward, making a deformity resembling the silver fork with its tines pointing upward (Fig. 13-46B). The fracture usually results from a blow or fall on the hyperflexed hand.

Radius and ulna fractures. Ulnar shaft fractures are well splinted by the radius, so displacement and deformity are rare (Fig. 13-46D). The only physical signs are localized tenderness and swelling. Ulnar fractures accompanied by volar dislocation of the radial head (*Monteggia fracture/dislocation*), especially common in children, permit considerable bowing of the fractured ulna.

A fractured radial shaft presents variable degrees of bowing, especially with concomitant dislocation of the lower radioulnar joint.

Combined radius and ulna fractures. Greenstick fractures produce little deformity, but complete fractures of the radius and ulna present easily recognizable deformity.

Traumatic elbow pain
Ulnar coronoid process fracture. Fracture of the ulnar coronoid process, which forms the distal elbow joint, is easily missed if not considered and searched for.

Olecranon process fracture. There is pronounced swelling, particularly around the dorsum of the elbow. The olecranon process is tender. When the fracture is complete, the patient cannot extend the flexed forearm (Fig. 13-47A). The bony equilateral triangle may be flattened.

Radial head subluxation. This usually occurs in childhood (the "pulled elbow"). There is no elbow deformity and tenderness is maximal at the radial head. Flexion–extension is painful; pronation and supination are not.

Radial head fracture. This usually follows a fall on the outstretched hand. Swelling is minimal and there is no deformity; the bony equilateral triangle is normal. Flexion and extension are painless, but there is severe restriction of pronation-supination and the radial head is tender.

Traumatic painful shoulder immobility
Humeral shaft fracture. Transverse fracture is usually caused by a direct blow and there is unmistakable deformity. Spiral fracture, commonly from falling on the hand, may not cause deformity. These are painful injuries. The arm is

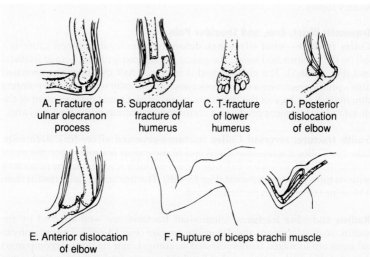

A. Fracture of ulnar olecranon process   B. Supracondylar fracture of humerus   C. T-fracture of lower humerus   D. Posterior dislocation of elbow

E. Anterior dislocation of elbow   F. Rupture of biceps brachii muscle

FIG. 13-47 Fractures and Dislocations about the Elbow.

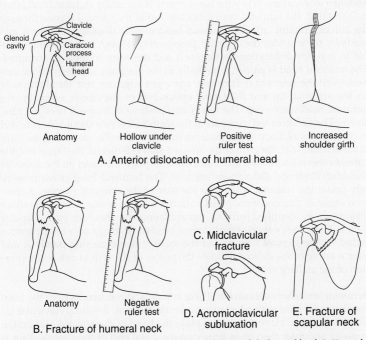

FIG. 13-48 Traumatic Shoulder Disorders. **A.** Anterior dislocation of the humeral head. **B.** Humeral neck fracture. **C.** Midclavicular fracture. **D.** Acromioclavicular subluxation. **E.** Scapular neck fracture.

held in the opposite hand and is useless. Lacking deformity, gently palpate the lateral and medial aspects of the humerus for local tenderness and swelling. Shaft fractures can lacerate the radial nerve and distal brachial artery where they are in contact with the posterior upper third of the humerus. In all humeral fractures, feel the radial artery pulse and test for radial nerve injury. Test the nerve's motor function by looking for wrist-drop when the patient flexes the elbow with the forearm pronated. Radial nerve sensory loss produces anesthesia on the radial dorsum of the hand.

Humeral neck fracture. Commonly the result of a fall on the outstretched hand. There is pain in the shoulder, and the arm is supported by the opposite hand. Viewed from the side there may be an anterior angular deformity (Fig. 13-48B). The axillary aspect of the arm and the chest wall may be ecchymotic. Rotate the arm gently while palpating the humeral head; if the fracture is not impacted, the head does not move with the shaft, confirming the diagnosis. When displacement is present, the ruler test of Hamilton (see Shoulder Dislocation below) may be positive. If a break is not obvious, consider impacted fracture. Measure the distance from acromial tip to epicondyle on both sides, the impacted side is shorter. Bony disruption impairs bone transmission of sound. Tap the olecranon while listening over the manubrium with a stethoscope; compare side to side.

Shoulder dislocation. When the hand or arm is forcefully abducted and externally rotated, the humeral head dislocates out of the glenoid tearing through
the anterior rotator cuff. The humeral head usually displaces anteriorly and
medially to lie under the coracoid process (Fig. 13-48A). The shoulder profile in anterior dislocations is flattened and the bony triangle is disrupted.
The humeral head is palpated medially in the normally soft belly of the deltoid. With the *ruler test of Hamilton*, a straight edge can rest simultaneously
on the acromial tip and the lateral epicondyle of the elbow; normally, the
humeral head intervenes. The test is also positive in humeral neck fracture,
above. The *Calloway test*, comparing the girth of the two shoulders, is useful
in obese patients. Loop a tape measure through the axilla measuring the girth
at the acromial tip; the girth of the affected joint is larger. In the *Dugas test*, the
patient cannot adduct the arm sufficiently to place the hand on the opposite
shoulder. Posterior dislocations are rare. The humeral head is felt posteriorly under the scapular spine near the base of the acromial process. A common cause of this uncommon dislocation is a major motor seizure. Shoulder
dislocation is identified without manipulating the shoulder by a scapular
Y-view X-ray. Dislocation of the humeral head can damage adjacent structures
including the glenoid labrum and the axillary nerve causing paralysis and
later wasting of the deltoid. Palpate the pulses of the arm to detect compression of the axillary vessels.

Acromioclavicular subluxation. There is pain and tenderness over the acromioclavicular joint with reluctance to elevate the arm; the distal clavicular tip
is often elevated. Have the patient place the hand of the affected side on the
opposite shoulder then press firmly on the distal end of the clavicle. Pain is
elicited and the end of the clavicle moves downward (Fig. 13-48D). When the
patient holds weights in both hands, the end of the clavicle on the affected
side becomes more prominent.

Clavicle fracture. Fractures at the center of the shaft are most common.
Because the fragments are usually displaced, diagnosis is made by inspection
and palpation (Fig. 13-48C). Greenstick or impacted fractures are detected by
tenderness and swelling.

Scapula fracture. There is pain in the shoulder preventing elevation of the
arm (Fig. 13-48E). Sit at the patient's affected side supporting the forearm
while palpating the shoulder. Abduct the forearm to 90 degrees; when the
clavicle is intact, crepitus in the joint strongly suggests scapular neck fracture.

Traumatic painful shoulder motion
Sternoclavicular subluxation. The more common injury is forward subluxation, arm elevation in abduction producing painful clicking in the joint. The
deformity is usually obvious. The rarer backward dislocation produces a
hollow where the normal clavicular head protrudes. If the mediastinum is
invaded and trachea compressed, dyspnea and cyanosis can occur.

Traumatic Hip Pain
Hip dislocation. A blow on the knee while sitting drives the femoral head
posteriorly out of its socket, frequently fracturing the rim of the acetabulum
(Fig. 13-49A). The rare anterior traumatic dislocation results from landing on

the feet in a fall. When a prosthetic hip is placed into abduction and external rotation, dislocation with minimal force is common. *Anterior Dislocation:* The joint is fixed in abduction, outward rotation, and slight flexion (Fig. 13-49C-1). There is no limb shortening because the head is impaled anteriorly in the iliofemoral ligament. *Posterior Dislocation:* Inguinal and thigh pain is severe and constant. The thigh lies in extreme internal rotation, adduction, and slight flexion (Fig. 13-49C-2) and only the foot can be actively moved without pain. The greater trochanter is abnormally prominent, while palpating for the femoral head beneath the inguinal ligament reveals an indentation. The limb is shortened, and passive rotation of the femur is absent.

Femoral neck fracture. The femoral neck can fracture below the capsule, a *low fracture,* or within the capsule, a *high fracture* (Fig. 13-49A). In the *extracapsular fracture*, the femur is shortened and externally rotated in the supine position (Fig. 13-49C-1). With an *intracapsular fracture*, the tense joint capsule restrains rotation and swelling of the upper thigh is considerable. If the patient can lift the foot off the bed, the fracture is impacted. In *impacted fractures*, the patient can sometimes walk with little pain, so a fracture may not be suspected. However, passive thigh rotation is usually painful.

Femoral shaft fracture. This can lead to shock from blood loss, so careful observation is required. The thigh is rotated externally, often with obvious deformity and shortening from muscle spasm and overlap of the proximal and distal femur.

Traumatic Knee Pain: Once femur and tibia fractures have been excluded, other etiologies need to be explored. The evaluation of patients with knee injuries starts with a detailed history emphasizing the mechanism of injury. A complete knee examination should be attempted but may be limited by pain. See page 552.

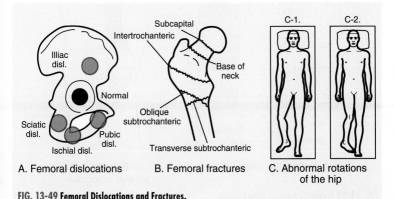

FIG. 13-49 Femoral Dislocations and Fractures.

Traumatic pain proximal to the patella

Rectus femoris muscle rupture. The rectus femoris muscle fibers attach to the tendon well above the patella. Traumatic muscular tears often occur at the musculotendinous junction. The injury is painful, and the knee is held in semiflexion. Retraction of the torn fibers may form a lump that enlarges on contracting the thigh muscles and the normal muscle mass is not felt distal to the lump above the patella.

Quadriceps tendon tear. This occurs from a direct blow or during sudden forceful quadriceps contraction with the knee bent and the foot fixed. The knee is held in extension and the torn tendon is tender to palpation. Complete tears lead to proximal retraction of the muscle forming a hump in the distal thigh. Partial tears are often more painful than complete rupture.

Traumatic knee pain

Patella fracture. This is the result of a direct blow to the patella, usually from falling onto the flexed knee. Stellate fractures are often not displaced and are easily missed without proper imaging. With nondisplaced fractures, active extension is preserved but painful. Transverse fractures are most likely to be displaced. If the bone fragments are separated, the joint is semiflexed and active extension is impossible (Fig. 13-50A). To identify separation, palpate for a crevice down the surface of the patella. Displaced fractures always produce hemarthrosis.

Patellar tendon tear. The mechanism of injury is the same as quadriceps tendon tears. The tear is partial or complete. There is swelling distal to the patella and the knee is held in extension. After the swelling subsides, the ruptured tendon may be palpated (Fig. 13-50A) and a defect felt. The pathognomonic sign of a complete tear is the proximal shift of the patella. Tenderness at the tibial tuberosity suggests concomitant avulsion of the tuberosity.

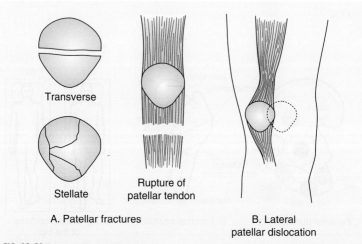

Transverse

Stellate

Rupture of
patellar tendon

A. Patellar fractures

B. Lateral
patellar dislocation

FIG. 13-50 Traumatic Anterior Knee Injuries.

Dislocated patella. This frequently recurrent problem may be diagnosed from the history. The knee abruptly gives way with pain and subsequent swelling. Acutely, the patella displaces laterally (Fig. 13-50B). Between episodes, the patella has increased lateral mobility and quadriceps wasting may be seen.

Medial collateral ligament injury. MCL injuries occur from valgus stress on the knee, such as a blow to the lateral side of the knee during weight bearing. Usually the femoral attachment is torn. The ligament is tender and somewhat swollen. The medial meniscus attaches to the midportion of the ligament and MCL injury often accompanies medial meniscus injury. With incomplete tears medial stability is present and function is not completely lost. The medial knee is tender and valgus stress elicits severe pain. When complete rupture occurs, there is medial instability palpated as separation of the tibia from the medial femoral condyle with valgus stress. Always compare the injured to the uninjured side, as there is considerable individual variation in baseline joint stability.

Medial meniscus injury. The meniscus is usually injured when the femur rotates medially while the knee is flexed, and the foot and tibia are fixed by bearing weight. The cartilage may split longitudinally, or either the anterior or posterior horn is torn. Most common is a bucket-handle tear, the horns remaining attached while the curved portion is torn. Locking may occur. The most consistent sign is joint line tenderness over the MCL with the knee flexed. Tearing the posterior horn causes tenderness posterior to the MCL. *McMurray* and *Apley tests* may be positive. MCL injuries often coexist.

Lateral collateral ligament injury. With the femur externally rotated on the fixed tibia, a varus force on the knee tears the ligament's fibular attachment; the head of the fibula can be avulsed. The knee between the lateral femoral epicondyle and the fibular head is tender. With a complete tear, the defect in the ligament may be palpable. Crepitus indicates avulsion of the fibular head. Test stability by placing a varus stress on the knee while palpating for opening of the lateral joint line. The common peroneal nerve may be injured simultaneously, so test strength of the anterior and lateral leg muscles and the short toe extensors.

Lateral meniscus injury. The trauma may be so slight as to escape attention. Pain is felt laterally or medially. The lateral joint line is tender. *McMurray* and *Apley tests* may be positive. Locking is uncommon.

Anterior cruciate ligament (ACL) injury. Partial ACL tear and complete rupture result from high-impact injuries where the tibia is driven anteriorly relative to the femur. There is severe pain and the joint is held in slight flexion. Because of pain and limited mobility secondary to tense hemarthrosis, acutely testing the ligament is difficult or impossible . After aspiration or resolution of the hemarthrosis, anterior instability, complete tears are demonstrated by a positive *Lachman test*.

Posterior cruciate ligament (PCL) injury. PCL injury results from a direct blow on the head of the tibia while the knee is flexed. With both knees flexed at 90 degrees, the tibia may sag posteriorly. The acute and late signs are like ACL injury except that there is a positive *posterior* drawer sign elicited by pushing the tibial head backward on the femoral condyles with the knee flexed at 90 degrees. With the knee flexed 90 degrees, hold the heel and have the patient attempt to resist active knee extension. This is much weaker or impossible on the injured side. Lastly, with the knee in 90 degrees of flexion, a sharp blow to the proximal anterior tibia elicits pain.

Traumatic Calf Pain

Gastrocnemius and soleus injury. Both muscles insert into the Achilles tendon powering ankle plantar flexion. Foot dorsiflexion loads both muscles and knee extension additionally loads the gastrics, since it originates on the femoral condyles. The most common injury is a strain of one or both felt as pain in the distal belly of the calf at the musculotendinous junction. Gastrocnemius Tear: A forceful combination of knee extension and ankle dorsiflexion is felt like a blow to the posterior calf, sometimes with an audible snap. Walking is immediately intensely painful in the posteromedial mid-calf and there is tenderness and a palpable defect in the medial belly of the gastrocnemius. After a few hours, swelling obscures the defect for a few days. The power of plantar flexion is diminished and ecchymoses develops over days extending from the calf to the heel, ankle, and foot. Soleus Tear: Trauma causing extreme foot dorsiflexion tears the soleus producing severe pain and tenderness in the mid-calf.

Achilles tendon rupture. The most common scenario is a man, more than 45 years of age, attempting unusual and vigorous activities requiring sudden accelerations or jumping. Complete rupture is usually ~5 cm above the calcaneal insertion. There is sudden excruciating pain and walking is impossible. In the prone position with the feet hanging over the end of the table (Fig. 13-23B, page 553), the affected foot is less plantar flexed and passive dorsiflexion is excessive. With incomplete rupture, squeezing the calf muscles transversely produces plantar flexion of the foot (*Simmonds test*). When the tendon is completely severed no motion occurs, a gap is felt in the tendon, the distal tendon is thicker and less taut, and the calf muscles shorten into a visible lump.

Traumatic Anterior Leg Pain

Fibula shaft fracture. A direct blow on the anterolateral leg is most common. Fracture proximal to the ankle may also accompany severe inversion ankle injuries. There is pain at the fracture site, but the patient can usually walk. Squeezing the tibia and fibula together elicits pain at the fracture site.

Traumatic Ankle Pain: Ankle trauma is common, and a practical approach to the evaluation is needed. The most common mechanism of injury is inversion of the flexed ankle. Ligament injuries are expected, but fractures can occur, thus the diagnostic dilemma. Ankle X-ray is necessary only if there is pain near the malleoli, the patient is older than 55 years of age, is unable to bear weight immediately after the injury or take four steps at the time of exam, or has bone tenderness at the posterior edge or tip of either malleolus. If these conditions are not met, fracture is very unlikely.

Calcaneofibular ligament rupture, common ankle sprain. This results from forced inversion of the foot. The tenderness is anterior and inferior to the lateral malleolus. With complete rupture, careful passive inversion of the foot tilts the talus. When the lateral malleolus is fractured, the posterior-lateral malleolus itself is tender.

Calcaneofibular ligament—deltoid ligament rupture. This ligament is rarely injured in isolation. It occurs as part of severe ankle fracture-dislocation.

Joint capsule rupture. Forceful plantarflexion with foot eversion disrupts the anterolateral articular capsule. Pain and tenderness are just anterior to the calcaneofibular and talofibular ligaments. A hematoma develops rapidly, accompanied by some edema.

Traumatic Heel Pain
Calcaneus fracture. Falling and landing on the heel fractures the calcaneus (Fig. 13-37A). From the back, the heel appears broader than normal and the hollows beneath the malleoli are obliterated. Tenderness is maximal in the calcaneus near the Achilles tendon insertion. The sides of the calcaneus palpated below the malleoli, rather than being indented, feel flush with the malleolus. Pain restricts all ankle movement. A hematoma forms in the sole of the heel. Signs of fracture may be subtle, so a high index of suspicion is needed.

CLINICAL VIGNETTES AND QUESTIONS

CASE 13-1

A 19-year-old woman presents with an acute knee injury. While playing volleyball she jumped, came down twisting her knee, and heard a "pop." She has pain with weight bearing and a sense that it may give out when she attempts to walk. The knee is swollen and she has difficulty bearing weight. She has had no previous injury to her knee.

QUESTIONS:
1. How do you test for integrity of the collateral ligaments?
2. How do you test the integrity of the cruciate ligaments?
3. What is a common mechanism of injury for an ACL tear?

CASE 13-2

A 19-year-old man presents with a knee injury. He was out for his daily run and stepped in a hole with his knee fully extended causing him to hyperextend the knee. He did not have any twist associated with the injury. He noted a popping sensation. It has been painful to walk and he has catching and locking of the knee. His cruciate and collateral ligaments are intact with no laxity.

QUESTIONS:
1. How do you perform a McMurray's test and what does it tell you?
2. How do you perform an Apley's grinding test and what does it tell you?
3. When should the Duck Waddle test be used?

CASE 13-3

A 54-year-old man complains of right shoulder pain. Over the years he has occasionally had shoulder pain after activities such as playing softball. Over-the-counter NSAIDs have given relief in the past. Last weekend he painted the ceiling in his living room. The pain worsened throughout the day causing increasing difficulty reaching over his head. He had to start using his left hand to paint to relieve the pain.

QUESTIONS:
1. What is your differential diagnosis for the shoulder pain?
2. What physical examination findings do you expect with a supraspinatus tendon tear?
3. What examination findings do you expect with subacromial bursitis, supraspinatus tendonitis, or a partial tear of the supraspinatus tendon?

CASE 13-4

A 65-year-old man presents for a health maintenance examination. He has not seen a physician in over 20 years and comes at his daughter's urging. She had recently visited and thought his fingers looked different and should be checked. He has no complaints. He has a smoker's cough and some shortness of breath that he attributes to his over 100 pack-years of smoking. He is a pipe fitter and has worked with asbestos. He drinks a 6 pack of beer daily and on occasion has used intravenous heroin.

QUESTIONS:

1. How do you assess for clubbing?
2. What is the differential diagnosis if he is found to have clubbing?

CASE 13-5

A 48-year-old woman presents with numbness of her dominant left hand that has been occurring for more than 6 months and awakens her from sleep. Over the last month she has developed weakness in the hand causing her to drop objects. She works as an office assistant in a local bank. The numbness is worst in the thumb, index, and middle finger.

QUESTIONS:

1. What will you look for specifically on physical examination of the hand and why?
2. What findings would you expect on examination if the patient had an ulnar neuropathy?

CASE 13-6

A 45-year-old woman presents with diffuse soreness that has been going on for at least 9 months. She describes it as a severe deep ache involving the hips, neck, shoulders, and back. It makes it difficult for her to sleep. When she gets up in the morning she feels stiffness that lasts all day. She feels fatigued and finds it a struggle to work at her daycare. She has not had swollen or reddened joints. She has gained 5 lb which she attributes to decreased activity. She has tried acetaminophen and ibuprofen without relief.

QUESTIONS:

1. What is your differential diagnosis for this presentation?
2. What findings will you look for on physical examination?
3. What are the risk factors for developing fibromyalgia?

CASE 13-7

A 72-year-old woman presents with a very painful, red, swollen knee that started yesterday. She denies an injury. She has never had previous episodes like this. She has not had fevers, chills, or sweats and she does not felt ill. She has osteoarthritis and hypertension and takes acetaminophen and hydrochlorothiazide. Physical examination reveals a red swollen knee with an effusion that is tender to palpation and painful with any motion.

QUESTIONS:
1. What is your differential diagnosis of this presentation?
2. What disease or risk factors are associated with the development of pseudogout?
3. What joints are most commonly affected by gout and by pseudogout?

CHAPTER 14

The Nervous System

The diagnostic exam of the nervous system evaluates specific functions, many while taking the history and examining the body by regions. When nervous system malfunction is encountered, a complete, systematic neurologic examination is required. The first objective is to identify all cognitive, sensory, motor, and coordination deficits. From this inventory, the site(s) and mechanism(s) of injury are hypothesized using the following general principles:

1. *Deficits of intellect, memory, and/or higher brain function* imply lesions of the cerebral hemispheres.
2. *Deficits of consciousness* indicate a brainstem reticular activating system lesion or bilateral cerebral damage.
3. *Paralysis with loss of deep tendon reflexes* indicates a lower motor neuron (LMN) lesion interrupting the reflex arc at the spinal cord, spinal root, plexus or peripheral nerve level. Acute upper motor neuron (UMN) lesions can be associated with decreased reflexes initially but increased reflexes after hours to days.
4. *Paralysis with accentuated deep tendon reflexes* (spasticity) indicates an UMN lesion in the cerebral hemisphere, brainstem, or spinal cord.
5. *Unilateral loss of touch and position sensation and contralateral loss of temperature and pain sensation* indicate a unilateral spinal cord lesion ipsilateral to the sensory loss. This happens because the ascending tracts for touch and position decussate in the medulla, whereas the ascending tracts for pain and temperature sensation cross near their entry into the spinal cord.
6. *Paralysis is contralateral to lesions above the medulla and ipsilateral below* because the descending motor tracts, like the tracts for discriminative sense, decussate in the medulla.
7. *Lower motor neuron paralysis accompanied by anesthesia in an appropriate distribution usually indicates a peripheral nerve lesion*, many nerves carrying both motor and sensory fibers. Spinal root and segmental cord lesions sometimes produce similar signs.
8. *Muscle wasting with fasciculation indicates a lower motor neuron lesion.* Without fasciculation, wasting is often attributable to intrinsic muscle disease.

OVERVIEW OF THE NERVOUS SYSTEM

A comprehensive understanding of the anatomy and functional organization of the nervous system is required to interpret neurologic exam findings. The reader should consult anatomy and neurology texts for detailed discussions of neuroanatomy and functional physiology.

Anatomic Organization of the Nervous System: For diagnostic purposes, the nervous system is divided anatomically into the brain, spinal cord, spinal roots, and peripheral nerves. The brain is encased within the rigid skull and the spinal cord within the spinal canal of the vertebral column. The ganglia, plexuses, and nerve trunks are inaccessible to physical exam since they lie deep to the muscles and bones of the spine, chest, abdomen, and pelvis. The peripheral nerves, however, course with their corresponding arteries and veins in neurovascular bundles and may be palpable where they exit the trunk and in the extremities.

Central nervous system (CNS). The brain consists of the cerebrum, brainstem, and cerebellum. The *cerebrum* performs cognitive functions, is the site of emotion and mood formation, and determines personality and behavior. The deep cerebral structures modulate motor and sensory function and control endocrine and appetitive functions. The *brainstem* consists of the midbrain, the pons, and the medulla and contains nuclei of CN III to CN XII. The *cerebellum* is involved in many motor and sensory pathways and coordinates complex motor functions.

Spinal cord. The ascending sensory tracts, descending motor and autonomic tracts, and LMNs which activate skeletal muscles reside within the spinal cord. The *dorsal and ventral spinal roots* contain the sensory and motor tracts, respectively. The *dorsal root ganglia* contain the cell bodies of afferent sensory nerves.

The Peripheral Nervous System: The peripheral nervous system is equally complex. *Cranial and spinal nerves* come together to form *ganglia* and *plexuses* (brachial, lumbar, sacral) where the sensory and motor components of the cranial and spinal segments are redistributed into *peripheral nerves* directed to specific peripheral anatomic structures.

Functional Organization of the Nervous System: It is necessary to understand the functional organization of the nervous system. Function is systematically categorized as cognition (intellect, language, registration, memory, attention, orientation, spatial discrimination), mood and affect, special sensation (sight, hearing, balance, taste, smell), somatic and visceral sensation (touch, position, pain, temperature, vibration, pressure, two-point discrimination), motor function (pyramidal tracts and extrapyramidal system), posture, balance, and coordination (cerebellar, vestibular, and basal ganglia function), and autonomic function. The autonomic nervous system is divided into the *parasympathetic* and *sympathetic* systems. Parasympathetic outflow is from the cranial, cervical, and sacral roots, with ganglia close to the organs they innervate. The sympathetic outflow is from thoracic and lumbar roots via the sympathetic spinal ganglia.

THE NEUROLOGIC EXAMINATION

Mental Status Screening Examination: The patient's mental status is evaluated during the history and physical exam. In addition, supplemental screening tests like the SLUMS, Mini-Cog, and Mini-Mental State Examination can be used. These are described in Chapter 15, page 713. The mental status components of most interest for neurologic disease are the level of consciousness, memory, and language.

Cranial Nerve (CN) Exam: The 12 paired cranial nerves emerge from the brain and exit through foramina in the skull base. They are designated by Roman numerals I–XII according to their position from forebrain to brainstem. The evaluation of several cranial nerves is discussed with the head and neck in Chapter 7.

Olfactory nerve (CN-I). The olfactory mucosa lining the upper third of the nasal septum and the superior nasal concha contains the receptors and ganglion cells. Their fibers converge into ~20 branches that pierce the cribriform plate of the ethmoid bone and consolidate forming the olfactory tract.

Testing smell. Evaluate the nasal passages for patency. With the eyes closed, test each nostril, while the other is occluded, with familiar odors, e.g., coffee, cloves, or peppermint.

Optic nerve (CN-II). The optic nerve is a tract of the CNS, not a true cranial nerve. It carries afferent impulses from the retina to the Edinger–Westphal nucleus and the visual cortex in the occipital lobes.

Testing for gross visual fields defects by confrontation. Use the following tests to detect visual field defects. Finger, face, and hand confrontation readily detect temporal field cuts. *To detect nasal field cuts, each eye must be tested independently.*

Finger confrontation. Fingers are presented simultaneously in the same quadrant on each side of the midline, testing all quadrants sequentially. The gaze is kept straight ahead at the examiner's nose allowing the examiner to use their visual field as a control. The patient sums the number of fingers seen. Because it is difficult to differentiate three fingers from four, it is best to use one, two, or five fingers. This test reveals an absolute defect in one quadrant. Sensitivity is increased by decreasing the presentation time and increasing the distance from the patient.

Face and hand confrontation. For *face confrontation*, the patient looks at the examiner's face, first with one eye and then the other, and is asked if the face is clear with each eye and if the images are the same. Lack of clarity in one eye or a difference between the eyes suggests a field defect. With *hand confrontation*, the patient fixes on the examiner's nose and the examiner's hands are held on either side of the vertical midline first above then below the plane of gaze. The patient is asked if the hands appear the same. A cloudy or a faded-color appearing hand represents a relative and subtle defect along the vertical plane.

Color confrontation. This test is traditionally done with red caps of mydriatic bottles. (1) *Color comparison* about the vertical midline is performed as hand comparison above. This is a very sensitive test for relative hemianopic defects. (2) For *central scotoma testing* of each eye, the subject is asked to cover the opposite eye and fix their gaze on one red cap just lateral to the usual axis of gaze, whereas the other is held in their nasal visual field. Ask which cap is redder or brighter. If the peripheral cap appears brighter, when in fact they are the same, there is a central scotoma. Do not hold the peripheral cap in the temporal field as a cecocentral defect may confound interpretation; likewise, you might place the cap in the patient's blind spot.

Kinetic boundary test. This technique is more time consuming and less sensitive and specific than the first three; it is not recommended. Face the patient ~1 m (40 in) away at the same eye level. Have the patient cover the left eye (Fig. 14-1). Ask the patient to fix constantly on your left eye. Cover your right eye fixing your gaze on the patient's right eye. Hold your left hand off to the side in the midplane between your faces. With a flicking finger or penlight for a target, bring it slowly toward the midline between you (Fig. 14-1). Ask the patient to indicate when the target first appears comparing that with your perception. Also, test vertical and oblique runs. Test the nasal field with your right hand. Test the second eye similarly.

Technique for uncooperative patients. In obtunded adults, watch for eye movements to novel targets or a blink in response to a threat by an abrupt movement toward the head in each field. If the movement pushes air over the cornea, it will stimulate a corneal reflex that can be misinterpreted as a visual response.

Oculomotor (CN-III), trochlear (CN-IV), and abducens nerves (CN-VI). CN-III is the motor nerve to five extrinsic eye muscles: the levator palpebrae superioris, medial rectus, superior rectus, inferior rectus, and inferior

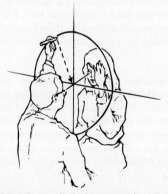

FIG. 14-1 Test for Tunnel Vision. The patient fixes on the examiner's left eye. The examiner imagines a line of sight extending between the patient's open eye and the examiner's own eye. The examiner imagines radii that are perpendicular to the line of sight and center at a point equidistant between the two opposing eyes. A target on any point of such a radius will be equidistant between the opposing eyes at all locations. The examiner slowly moves a flicking finger or a penlight target along a radius from the periphery toward the center until the patient can see it comparing that with his perception.

oblique. Its nucleus in the posterior midbrain has a locus for each muscle. CN-IV innervates the superior oblique muscle and CN-VI innervates the lateral rectus. These cranial nerves are tested together because they work together to move the eyes.

The optical globe's axis passes from the cornea's midpoint to the fovea. The globe is suspended from the orbital rim by a fascia continuous with the orbital septum and orbital periosteum. This floating suspension allows the globe to rotate about three axes intersecting perpendicularly at the center of rotation. The gaze can therefore be directed to any anterior location combining any of these planes. Rotation about the vertical axis through the equatorial plane of the globe permits *abduction* and *adduction*; rotation about the horizontal axis through the equator produces *elevation* and *depression*; and, rotation about the optic axis allows *intorsion* (toward the nose) and *extorsion* (away from the nose).

Six muscles rotate the globe around the three axes. The *four recti* originate in a fibrous ring around the optic foramen at the orbital apex (Fig. 14-2) and insert slightly anterior to the global equator, spaced 90 degrees apart: the *superior* and *inferior recti* attach to the superior and inferior meridian; the *lateral* (external) and *medial* (internal) recti are opposed on the horizontal meridians. The lateral rectus muscles, pulling toward the orbital apex, are longer than the medial recti. The *superior oblique* muscle, originating above the four recti at the optic foramen, run anteriorly and medially to the trochlea, a fibrous pulley in the medial side of the anterior orbit, from which it runs laterally and posteriorly under the superior rectus inserting behind the equator in the upper lateral quadrant of the posterior globe. Its physiologic point of action is at the pulley. The *inferior oblique muscle* originates anteriorly near the medial lacrimal groove, passes posteriorly and laterally between the inferior rectus and orbital floor to its insertion in the posterior lower lateral quadrant.

In the primary position, the globes are suspended with their optic axes horizontal in the sagittal plane. The superior and inferior recti do not pull exactly in the direction of the optic axis in the primary position (Fig. 14-3A). Study Figure 14-3 to visualize the movement imparted by each of the six muscles starting from the primary position. Medial rectus contraction, with

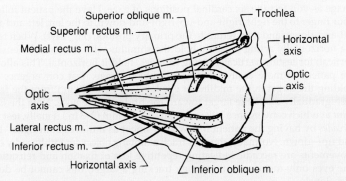

FIG. 14-2 The Extraocular Ocular Muscles. The right orbit viewed through the lateral wall.

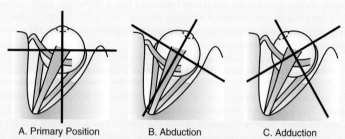

A. Primary Position   B. Abduction   C. Adduction

FIG. 14-3 Positions of the Right Globe in Relation to the Ocular Muscles. In all positions, the lateral rectus produces abduction and the medial rectus causes adduction. **A. With the optic axis in the primary position**, the superior rectus elevates and intorts, the inferior oblique elevates and extorts, the inferior rectus depresses and extorts, and the superior oblique depresses and intorts. **B. With the globe abducted**, so the optic axis coincides with the pull of the superior and inferior recti, these muscles produce elevation or depression without extorsion or intorsion. **C. In adduction**, the optic axis coincides with the pull of the oblique muscles along the equator producing elevation and depression without intorsion or extorsion.

the opposed lateral rectus relaxed, produces adduction; lateral rectus contraction and medial rectus relaxation results in abduction. Superior rectus contraction elevates and intorts the globe, the angular pull producing some rotation about the optic axis. Similarly, the inferior rectus causes depression and extorsion. The superior oblique depresses and intorts, assisting the depression while countering the extorsion of the inferior rectus. The inferior oblique assists the superior rectus in elevation, whereas its extorsion counters the intorting action of the superior rectus. When the eyes deviates from the primary position, the relative effects of the muscles change. When the eye is abducted (Fig. 14-3B), the pull of the superior and inferior recti coincides with the optic axis, the recti producing pure elevation and depression, respectively. Similarly, adduction can produce a position where the oblique muscles pull along the equator producing pure elevation and depression without intorsion or extorsion (Fig. 14-3C). Convergence is accomplished by contracting the two medial recti.

Testing extraocular movements. Have the patient indicate if they see a double image as you test the six cardinal positions of gaze. Have the patient follow your finger to the right, right-and-up, right-and-down, to the left, left-and-up, left-and-down, and then return to the primary position (Fig. 14-4). When testing horizontally acting muscles, hold the stimulus with the long dimension vertical; for testing vertically acting muscles, hold it horizontal. This allows the patient to more easily identify a doubled image. Test convergence by holding the target in the midline at eye level, ~50 cm (20 in.) from the face, then gradually move the target toward the bridge of the nose. Note the *near point* at which convergence fails, normally, 50–75 mm (2–3 in.). Finally, test for *saccades* by having the patient follow your finger as it moves both right↔left and up↔down. Normally, the eyes track a moving object smoothly; jerky eye movements are saccadic indicating repetitive loss of fixation and refixation. The eyes only move smoothly when tracking a target; this cannot be done consciously.

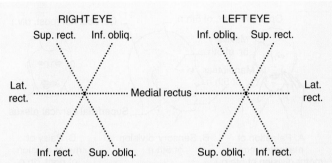

FIG. 14-4 The Cardinal Positions of Gaze. Each of the six positions is the result of synergists and antagonists acting with a specific muscle. Paralysis of the specific muscle prevents the eye from attaining the cardinal position for the muscle.

Trigeminal nerve (CN-V). CN-V, the largest CN has three divisions. Its sensory root supplies the superficial and deep structures of the face and the deep structures of the head; its motor root innervates the muscles of mastication. The *first division, or ophthalmic branch* (CN-V1), contains sensory fibers from the cornea, ciliary body, conjunctiva, nasal cavity and sinuses, and skin of the eyebrows, forehead, and nose. The *second division, or maxillary branch* (CN-V2), contains sensory fibers from the skin on the side of the nose, the upper and lower eyelids, the palate, and maxillary gums. The *third division, or mandibular branch* (CN-V3) is a mixed nerve with sensory and motor fibers: its sensory fibers are from the temporal region, the external ears, lower lip, lower face, mucosa of anterior two-thirds of the tongue, mandibular gums, and teeth. The motor root supplies the muscles of mastication: masseter, temporalis, and internal and external pterygoid.

Testing the trigeminal nerve. Motor Division: Inspect for muscle wasting in the temporal region, jaw tremor, and trismus (spasm of the masticatory muscles). Palpate the temporal and masseter muscles comparing muscle bulk and tension on the two sides with the teeth clenched (Fig. 14-5A). If the incisors are misaligned when the mouth is opened, the weak side pterygoid muscle is affected. Sensory Division: With the eyes closed, test light touch, pain, and temperature in each division comparing the two sides (Fig. 14-5B). The *jaw jerk* tests both motor and sensory function. Test the *corneal reflex* by having the patient look upward while gently touching the cornea (not the sclera) with a small shred of sterile gauze. This normally induces a blink. The corneal reflex is a bilateral reflex testing the CN-V and CN-VII on the side stimulated and CN-VII consensually.

Facial nerve (CN-VII). The facial nerve contains motor, autonomic, and sensory fibers. It supplies motor fibers to the muscles of the scalp, face, and auricula as well as to the buccinator, platysma, stapedius, stylohyoideus, and the posterior belly of the digastricus. Autonomic motor fibers in the *chorda tympani* nerve, a branch of CN-VII, supply the submandibular and sublingual salivary glands. CN-VII carries sensation from the ear canal and behind the ear and taste on the anterior two-thirds of the tongue.

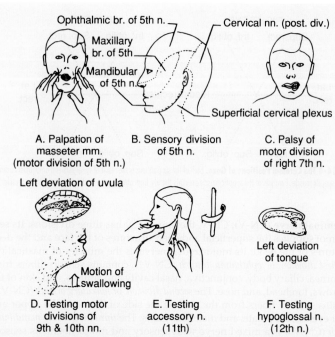

FIG. 14-5 Testing Some CNs. A. Motor division of the trigeminal nerve (CN-V). See text. **B. Sensory division of the trigeminal nerve (CN-V).** The three branches of the sensory trigeminal are ophthalmic, maxillary, and mandibular, as indicated by the areas. **C. Motor division of the facial nerve (CN-VII).** When the patient opens the mouth to show clenched teeth, only the unparalyzed side of the face retracts. The cheek muscles form creases on the normal side and the eyelid fissures are increased. The paralyzed side remains smooth with eyelid open. **D. Motor division of the glossopharyngeal and vagus nerves (CNs-IX and X).** When the patient opens the mouth and says "ah," the uvula deviates toward the strong side. Upon swallowing, the larynx normally elevates, as indicated by the motion of the thyroid cartilage in the neck (Adam's apple); it does not rise in bilateral paralysis. **E. The accessory nerve (CN-XI).** The patient is asked to rotate the head toward the midline against resistance of the examiner's hand, the other hand palpating sternocleidomastoid muscle tension. The trapezius can likewise be tested for paralysis. **F. The twelfth hypoglossal nerve (CN-XII).** The protruding tongue deviates to the paralyzed side; muscle atrophy may also be present.

Testing the facial nerve. **Motor:** Inspect the face in repose for paralysis or spasm. Have the patient perform the tasks below to detect asymmetry indicating unilateral paralysis and to determine whether the cause is an LMN or an UMN lesion: (1) inspect the face in repose noting the palpebral fissures, nasolabial folds, and corners of the mouth; (2) elevate the eyebrows and wrinkle the forehead or have them look up inspecting the forehead wrinkles; (3) frown; (4) tightly close the eyes; (5) show the teeth; (6) whistle and puff the cheeks; and (7) smile. **Sensory:** Test taste on the anterior two-thirds of the tongue with sugar, vinegar (dilute acetic acid), quinineand table salt. Write the words sweet, sour, bitter, and salty on a piece of paper and have the patient identify the sensation. Holding the tongue in gauze, touch the anterior two-thirds successively on one side then the other with an applicator saturated with the test substance. Remember, sweet receptors are located on the tip of the tongue. Get the patient's response before testing the other side. Have the patient rinse the mouth with water between tests.

Acoustic nerve (CN-VIII). The eighth nerve is a relatively short trunk consisting of the *cochlear* and *vestibular sensory nerves*. They are morphologically and functionally distinct. The cochlear nerve supplies the *organ of Corti*, whereas the vestibular nerve furnishes sensory endings for the semicircular ducts.

Testing the cochlear portion (hearing). See Chapter 7, page 173.

Testing vestibular function (balance). See Chapter 7, page 173.

Glossopharyngeal nerve (CN-IX). CN-IX contains sensory, motor, and autonomic fibers. The sensory nerves are for pain, touch, and temperature from the mucosa of the pharynx, fauces, and palatine tonsil, and taste from the posterior third of the tongue. Somatic motor fibers travel through both the glossopharyngeal and vagus, CN-X, to innervate the pharyngeal muscles.

Testing the glossopharyngeal nerve. This is tested with the vagus nerve, below.

Vagus nerve (CN-X). The vagus carries motor, sensory, and autonomic fibers to and from the neck, thorax, and abdomen. It exits the skull in the jugular fossa. Its *cervical branches* are the pharyngeal, superior laryngeal, recurrent laryngeal, and superior cardiac nerves. The *thoracic branches* are the inferior cardiac, anterior and posterior bronchial, and esophageal nerves. The major *abdominal branches* are the gastric and hepatic nerves, and the celiac and superior mesenteric ganglia.

Testing glossopharyngeal and vagus nerves. Listen for voice quality and normal variations of tone. Pharynx: While inspecting the pharynx, have the patient say "ah," noting elevation of the uvula and whether the faucial pillars converge equally. Test the gag reflex by touching the back of the tongue with a tongue blade. Test the pharyngeal mucosa for anesthesia by touching it with an applicator. Larynx: Watch the laryngeal contours in the neck seeing if they rise with swallowing (Fig. 14-5D). Have the patient swallow water observing for coughing or reflux into the posterior nose. Vocal cord exam is described in Chapter 7 on page 184.

Accessory nerve (CN-XI). The accessory nerve is the motor nerve to the trapezius and sternocleidomastoid muscles.

Testing the accessory nerve. Palpate the upper borders of the trapezii while the patient raises the shoulders against resistance. Look for scapular "winging" as the patient leans against a wall with palms and arms extended. Test the strength and the bulk of the sternocleidomastoid by having the patient turn his head to one side then attempt to bring his chin back to the midline against resistance (Fig. 14-5E).

Hypoglossal nerve (CN-XII). The hypoglossal is the motor nerve to the tongue.

Testing the hypoglossal nerve. Inspect for fasciculations and wasting with the tongue at rest in the floor of the mouth. Fasciculations can be normal when the muscles contract to protrude the tongue. When one side is paralyzed, the tongue protrudes toward the weak side (Fig. 14-5F). Test muscle strength by pushing the tongue against the cheek, your finger resisting from the outside. Test lingual speech by having the patient repeat "La, La, La."

K, L, M test for dysarthria. To parse cranial nerve deficits causing dysarthria, have the patient say: "Ka, Ka, Ka" (gutturals, CN IX and CN X); "La, La, La" (linguals, CN XII); and "Me, Me, Me" (labials, CN VII).

Motor Examination: Normal motor function requires that the skeleton, muscles, and motor nerves (pyramidal and extrapyramidal) are intact. Assessing muscle movements requires joint motion; hence the orthopedic, rheumatologic, and neurologic examinations are interdependent.

Inspecting for muscle wasting. Compare the muscle masses side to side and the relative masses in different regions.

Evaluating muscle tone. With the patient relaxed, assess muscle tone by resistance to passive range of motion. You may need to divert the patient's attention to relax the muscles. Gently rocking or lifting a limb and letting it fall reveals the tone. When the patient sits on the exam table the freedom of dangling leg swing indicates their tone.

Testing muscle strength. Have the patient actively move the joint through its range of motion. Then have the patient try moving against resistance while palpating the contracting muscle (Fig. 14-6). If the limb cannot move against gravity, position it to move unaffected by gravity. An arbitrary scale is used for grading muscle strength.

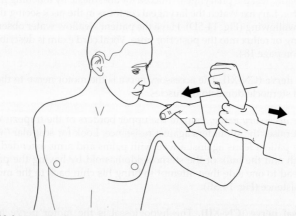

FIG. 14-6 Testing Muscle Strength. The patient is required to act against the resistance of the examiner.

Grading muscle strength (Oxford Scale)

> Grade 0—No muscle movement.
> Grade 1—Muscle movement without joint motion.
> Grade 2—Moves with gravity eliminated.
> Grade 3—Moves against gravity but not resistance.
> Grade 4—Moves against gravity and light resistance.
> Grade 5—Normal strength.

Lower extremity muscle strength usually exceeds an examiner's arm strength, so mild leg weakness is easily missed with resisted motion. Therefore, the following tests are useful. (1) Watch the patient get up after sitting on the floor. Use of both arms and raising the buttocks first by working the hands on the floor toward the feet and then up the legs, indicates proximal muscle weakness (*Gowers sign*). (2) Ask the sitting patient to stand without using their arms for assistance; if they do this easily, see if it can be done one leg at a time using the hands only for balance. (3) Have the patient hop on the balls of the feet, then on each foot individually. Normally, the heel will not strike the ground. Having the patient hop on a piece of paper accentuates the sound of a heel strike (creating a "gallop" rhythm), indicating gastrocnemius and soleus muscle weakness.

Examining Reflexes: In the screening examination, the clinician usually tests a few reflex arcs, representative of various spinal cord and brainstem levels. A normal reflex confirms the integrity of each element in the reflex arc and proper descending motor tract function. When an abnormality is found, localize the lesion by mapping the normal and abnormal reflexes to their spinal cord and brainstem levels.

Brainstem reflexes. These are tested during the cranial nerve examination. The CN innervation of the afferent and efferent limbs are shown in parentheses.

Direct pupillary reaction to light. The iris constricts when bright light is shone on the retina (afferent CN-II; efferent ipsilateral CN-III).

Consensual pupillary reaction to light. Light stimulating of one retina produces contralateral pupil constriction (afferent CN-II; efferent contralateral CN-III).

Ciliospinal reflex. Pinching the skin on the back of the neck causes the pupils to dilatate (afferent cervical somatic nerves; efferent cervical sympathetic chain).

Corneal reflex. Touching the cornea causes blinking (afferent CN-V; efferent CN-VII).

Jaw reflex. With the mouth partially open and the muscles relaxed, tapping the chin closes the jaw. The reflex center is in the mid-pons (afferent CN-V; efferent CN-V).

Gag reflex. Gagging is precipitated when the pharynx is stroked. The reflex center is in the medulla (afferent CN-IX, CN-X; efferent CN-IX, CN-X).

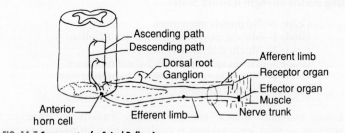

FIG. 14-7 Components of a Spinal Reflex Arc.

Muscle stretch reflexes. Muscle stretch reflexes, often misnamed "tendon" reflexes, are elicited by stretching the muscle by a brisk tap on its taut tendon of insertion. These are simple reflex arcs containing a muscle cell, a sensory, and a motor neuron (Fig. 14-7). A diminished or absent reflex indicates a break in the arc. When the descending motor pathway (the pyramidal tract) in the spinal cord is injured above the level of the reflex arc, normal cortical inhibition is lost, producing a hyperactive or spastic reflex.

General principles for eliciting muscle stretch reflexes. The limb should be relaxed. Identify the tendon of the muscle to be tested. Position the limb so that the muscle is slightly stretched. Strike a brisk blow on the tendon with the finger or reflex hammer. If the tendon cannot be struck directly, strike a thumb placed on the tendon. Use reinforcement if no reflex is identified by having the patient concentrate on a voluntary act such as pulling on interlocked fingers or clenching the fists while the reflex is again tested.

There is considerable variability in normal reflexes, from absent to brisk. Significant right-left asymmetry is abnormal. *Clonus*, the sustained repetitive firing of the reflex arc with tonic stretch of the muscle, is always abnormal. A four-point scale, denoted by numbers or pluses, is used to grade the reflex response.

0, 0	No response
1, +	Detectable only with reinforcement
2, + +	Easily detectable
3, + + +	Brisk with at most a few beats of clonus
4, + + + +	Sustained clonus

The reflexes below are listed by descending level of the spinal reflex center. The peripheral nerves carrying the afferent and efferent signals are in parentheses.

Reflex center at C5–T1: pectoralis reflex (medial and lateral anterior thoracic nerves). Support the arm in 10 degrees of elevation at 90 degrees of abduction (Fig. 14-8A). Place the fingers of your left hand on the patient's shoulder with your thumb extended downward pressing firmly on the tendon of the

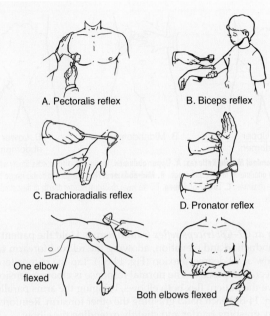

A. Pectoralis reflex

B. Biceps reflex

C. Brachioradialis reflex

D. Pronator reflex

One elbow flexed

Both elbows flexed

E. Triceps reflex (alternative positions)

FIG. 14-8 Deep Reflexes I. A. Pectoralis reflex. B. Biceps reflex. C. Brachioradialis reflex. D. Pronator reflex. E. Triceps reflex. There are two positions: 1. hold the patient's arm at 90 degrees abduction, allowing the relaxed forearm to dangle with the elbow at flexion; and 2. have the patient fold the arms and grasping the forearms with the hands (tighten the grip for reinforcement).

pectoralis major. Strike a blow directed upward toward the axilla. The muscle contraction can be seen and/or felt.

Reflex center at C5–C6: biceps reflex (musculocutaneous nerve). Flex the elbow at 90 degrees with the arm slightly pronated. Grasp the elbow with your left hand so that the fingers are behind, and your thumb presses the biceps tendon (Fig. 14-8B). Strike a series of blows on your thumb varying the thumb pressure with each blow until the best response is obtained. The normal reflex is elbow flexion.

Reflex center at C5–C6: brachioradialis reflex (radial nerve). Hold the patient's wrist with your left hand with the forearm relaxed in pronation (Fig. 14-8C). With a vertical stroke, tap the forearm directly, just above the radial styloid process. The normal response is elbow flexion and forearm supination.

Reflex center at C6–C7: pronator reflex (median nerve). Hold the patient's hand vertically so the wrist is suspended (Fig. 14-8D). From the medial side, strike the distal end of the radius directly with a horizontal blow. The normal response is pronation of the forearm. Alternatively, strike the distal end of the ulna directly with a blow in the opposite direction.

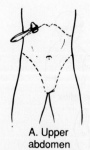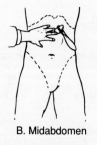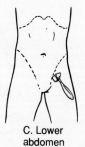

A. Upper abdomen   B. Midabdomen   C. Lower abdomen

FIG. 14-9 Abdominal Muscle Reflexes. A. Upper abdomen. Tap the abdominal muscles directly with the reflex hammer near their attachments to the costal margin. **B. Mid-abdomen.** Place a finger or a double-tongue blade on the muscle and tap the pleximeter. **C. Lower abdomen.** Tap the lower abdominal muscles directly at their attachments near the symphysis pubis.

Reflex center at C7–C8: triceps reflex (radial nerve). Hold the patient's arm at 90 degrees abduction and elevation, allowing the relaxed forearm to dangle with the elbow at 90 degrees flexion (Fig. 14-8E). Tap the triceps tendon just above the olecranon process. The normal response is elbow extension. Alternatively, have the patient flex both elbows, bringing the arms parallel across the chest (Fig. 14-8E) each hand grasping the other forearm. Reinforcement is performed by grasping harder and slightly extending the elbow.

Reflex center at T8–T9: upper abdominal muscle reflex. Tap the muscles directly near their insertions on the costal margins and xiphoid process (Fig. 14-9A).

Reflex center at T9–T10: middle abdominal muscle reflex. Stimulate the muscles of the mid-abdomen by tapping an overlaid finger or doubled-tongue blades (Fig. 14-9B).

Reflex center at T11–T12: lower abdominal muscles. Tap the muscle insertions directly, near the symphysis pubis (Fig. 14-9C).

Reflex center at L2–L4: quadriceps reflex (femoral nerve). Several methods are available. The normal response is knee extension and palpable quadriceps contraction. *Legs Dangling* (Fig. 14-10A): Grasp the lower thigh with your left hand, then tap the patellar tendon. *Sitting, Feet on the Floor* (Fig. 14-10B): The patient sits on a chair or low bed with the toes curled in plantar flexion and knee slightly extended from a right angle. Tap the patellar tendon directly. *Lying Supine (Three Methods): Method 1*—With your hand under the popliteal fossa, lift the patient's knee from the table. Tap the patellar tendon directly (Fig. 14-10C). *Method 2*—Grasp the patient's foot, flexing the hip and knee, and rotate the knee outward and dorsiflex the foot. Tap the patellar tendon directly (Fig. 14-10D). *Method 3*—With the knee extended and the leg lying on the table and your index finger on the quadriceps tendon insertion, push the patella distally. Tap downward on the index finger (Fig. 14-10E). The contracting muscle pulls the patella proximally.

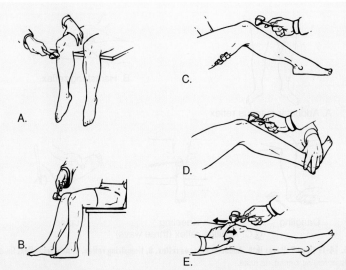

FIG. 14-10 Knee Jerk (Alternative Positions). **A.** With the patient's legs dangling. **B.** Sitting. **C.** With the patient supine, Method 1. **D.** With the patient supine, Method 2. **E.** With the patient supine and knee extended, Method 3.

Reflex center at L2–L4: adductor reflex (obturator nerve). With the patient supine, place the limb in slight abduction (Fig. 14-11A). Directly tap the adductor magnus tendon just proximal to its insertion on the medial epicondyle of the femur. Normally, the thigh adducts. An absent quadriceps reflex and normal adductor reflex indicates a femoral nerve lesion.

Reflex center at L4–S2: hamstring reflex (sciatic nerve). Have the patient supine with hips and knees flexed at about 90 degrees and the thighs rotated slightly outward. Place your left hand under the popliteal fossa so the index finger compresses the medial hamstring tendon (a bundle of tendons from semitendinosus, semimembranosus, gracilis, sartorius) (Fig. 14-11B). Tap your finger. The normal response is knee flexion and contraction of the medial hamstring muscles. Test the lateral hamstrings in an equivalent manner with your finger compressing the lateral hamstring tendon just proximal to the fibular head and tapping your finger. The normal response is contraction of the lateral hamstring (biceps femoris) and knee flexion.

Reflex center at L5–S2: Achilles reflex (tibial nerve). Assess both muscle contraction and relaxation. The normal response is gastrocnemius contraction and plantar flexion of the foot. Delayed relaxation (hung-up reflex) is characteristic of hypothyroidism. *Legs Dangling* (Fig. 14-11C): With your left hand, grasp the patient's foot pulling it into dorsiflexion to find the amount of Achilles stretch that produces the best response. Tap the tendon directly. *Kneeling* (Fig. 14-11C): The patient kneels with the feet hanging over the edge of a chair, table, or bed and your left hand dorsiflexing the foot. Tap the

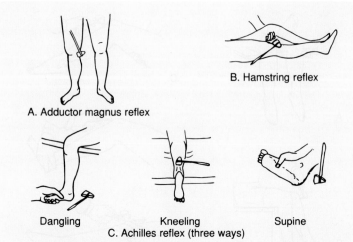

A. Adductor magnus reflex

B. Hamstring reflex

Dangling   Kneeling   Supine

C. Achilles reflex (three ways)

FIG. 14-11 Deep Reflexes II. A. Adductor magnus reflex. B. Hamstring reflex. C. Achilles reflex. Three ways: leg dangling, kneeling, and supine.

tendon directly. *Supine* (Fig. 14-11C): Partially flex the hip and knee while rotating the knee outward as far as comfort permits. With your left hand, grasp the foot pulling it into dorsiflexion, then tap the Achilles tendon directly.

Superficial (skin) reflexes. These reflex arcs have receptors in the skin. Their adequate stimulus is stroking, scratching, or touching. If there is no response, a painful stimulus can be tried. The superficial reflexes are lost in pyramidal tract disease.

Reflex center at T5–T8: upper abdominal skin reflex. Have the patient supine and relaxed, with the arms at the sides and knees slightly flexed. Stroke the skin over the lower thorax from the midaxillary line toward the midline (Fig. 14-12A) watching for ipsilateral muscle contraction in the epigastric abdominal wall. If contractions are not seen, look for the umbilicus deviating toward the stimulated side. In very obese persons, retract the umbilicus toward the opposite side to feel it pull toward the stimulated side.

Reflex center at T9–T11: mid-abdominal skin reflex. Stroke the skin from the flank toward the midline at the umbilical level.

Reflex center at T11–T12: lower abdominal skin reflex. Stroke the skin from the iliac crests toward the hypogastric midline.

Reflex center at L1–L2: cremasteric reflex. In males, stroking the inner thigh from the inguinal crease downward (Fig. 14-12B) elicits cremaster contraction, promptly elevating the ipsilateral testis. A slow irregular rise results from dartos tunic contraction and is not the reflex response.

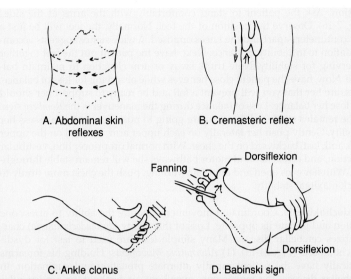

A. Abdominal skin reflexes

B. Cremasteric reflex

Dorsiflexion

Fanning

C. Ankle clonus

Dorsiflexion

D. Babinski sign

FIG. 14-12 Skin Reflexes and Pyramidal Tract Signs. A. Abdominal skin reflexes. B. Cremasteric reflex. C. Ankle clonus. With the patient supine, lift the knee in slight flexion with the muscles relaxed. Grasp the foot jerking it into dorsiflexion then hold it under slight tension. The foot reacting with cycles of alternating dorsiflexion and plantarflexion is a positive response. The motion may stop after a few cycles (unsustained clonus) or it may persist while the tension is held (sustained clonus). **D. Babinski sign.**

Reflex center at L4–S2: plantar reflex. Grasping the ankle with your left hand, with a blunt point and moderate pressure, stroke the sole near its lateral border from the heel toward the metatarsal heads then curve medially following the bases of the toes (Fig. 14-12D). For the blunt point, use a wooden-tip applicator, the end of a split wooden tongue blade, or the dull handle end on a reflex hammer. If no response is observed, a pin should be used as this is a nociceptive reflex. The expected response is plantar flexion of the toes and, often, the entire foot. With pyramidal tract disease some or all four components of the abnormal reflex are seen: great toe dorsiflexion (extension), fanning of all toes, ankle dorsiflexion, and knee and thigh flexion. This is *Babinski sign*, recorded as present or absent.

Reflex center at S1–S2: superficial anal reflex (anal wink). Stroking the perianal skin elicits anal sphincters contraction.

Posture, Balance, and Coordination—The Cerebellar Exam: Precise voluntary movement requires graded contraction of the agonist, or prime mover, with a corresponding graded relaxation of the antagonist about each joint, other muscles acting to fix the joint. The complete integration of these movements, *coordination*, is partially mediated through efferent and afferent cerebellar tracts, the vestibular apparatus and cerebral cortex also participating. Maintaining posture and balance requires sensory inputs from joints, muscles, tendons, and vestibular system, and coordinated motor outputs mediated by the cerebral cortex and basal ganglia.

Station. Ask the patient to stand comfortably with the arms at the sides (Fig. 7-16). Observe the position of the feet. Normally, the feet will be just a few centimeters apart and the knees opposed. A wide stance suggests accommodation to instability of stance. Next, have the patient put the feet together observing for stability. Note trunk sway or arm elevation to maintain balance. Now, have the patient close her eyes while observing for loss of balance. Reassure her that you will prevent a fall and be ready to support her should she lose her balance. Loss of balance during the maneuver is the *Romberg sign.* If she remains stable, tell her you are going to push her gently to assess her stability. Gently push her laterally on each upper arm, forward on the upper back and, last, backward on the chest. With normal proprioception, vestibular function, and cerebellar and motor pathways she will remain stable throughout. With her eyes open and after fair warning, push the chest more firmly to check maximal stability.

Diadochokinesia. Coordinated movements require the ability to arrest one motion and initiate its opposite. Loss of this ability (*dysdiadochokinesia*) characterizes cerebellar disease. Many simple tests are used to test for dysdiadochokinesis (Fig. 14-13). (1) *Alternating Movements:* Holding his forearms vertically have the patient rapidly alternate pronation and supination. In cerebellar disease, the movements overshoot, undershoot, or are irregular and inaccurate. Movement may be slowed or incomplete in pyramidal tract disease. Alternatively, have the patient rapidly tap his fingers on the table, or close and open the fists. (2) Holding the arms at 90 degrees elevation and

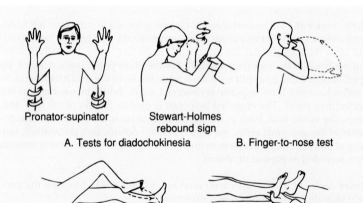

Pronator-supinator   Stewart-Holmes
                            rebound sign

A. Tests for diadochokinesia   **B. Finger-to-nose test**

C. Heel-to-knee test   D. Hoover sign of hysteria

FIG. 14-13 Test for Cerebellar Disease. See text for full descriptions. **A. Tests for diadochokinesia.** The ability to perform alternating movements is tested by having the patient hold the forearms vertically while quickly alternating pronation and supination. Another method is the *Stewart–Holmes rebound test.* The patient is attempting to flex the biceps against resistance. While at full strength, the examiner suddenly releases the wrist observing for control of the rebound. **B. Finger-to-nose test. C. Heel-to-shin test. D. Hoover sign of hysteria.** This distinguishes hysterical paralysis of the lower limb from paralysis with an organic cause. From the foot of the exam table, cradle each heel in a palm while resting your hands on the table. Have the patient attempt to raise the affected limb. In organic disease, the unaffected heel to presses downward (a *synkinesis*); in hysteria, the synkinesis is absent.

0-degree abduction may show the affected arm deviating in abduction. (4) While the patient clenches his fist with elbow flexed and forearm pronated, grasp his fist from above and pull strongly attempting to extend his elbow against his resistance; suddenly release your grip observing for rapid control of rebound (*Stewart–Holmes Rebound Sign*); the patient may strike himself if not guarded. With cerebellar disease, the forearm may rebound in several extension-flexion cycles.

Dyssynergia and dysmetria. Finger-to-Nose Test: With the eyes open, have the patient fully extend his elbow and, in a wide arc, rapidly bring the index fingertip to the tip of his nose (Fig. 14-13B). In cerebellar disease, this is attended by an action tremor. With the eyes closed, this evaluates shoulder and elbow position sense. In a variation the patient makes wide arcs with both arms to touch his index fingertips in front of him. Heel-to-Shin Test: With the patient supine and the lower limbs resting in extension, ask the patient to raise one heel and place it on the opposite knee, then slide the heel down the shin (Fig. 14-13C). The foot should be dorsiflexed, and the motion should be slow and accurate. In cerebellar disease, the arc of the heel to the knee is jerky and wavering, the knee is frequently overshot, and the slide down the shin is accompanied by an action tremor. With the eyes closed, the motions are inaccurate in posterior spinal column disease. Frequently, the heel slides off the shin, but action tremor is absent.

Gait. Gait is influenced by the rate, rhythm, and character of the individual walking movements. Before assessing the neurologic contribution to gait, exclude painful and/or restrictive conditions of the joints, muscles, and other structures. Observe the patient's gait in a well-lighted hallway. Note head, neck and trunk posture, swing of each arm, leg swing, width of stance, step size, and clearance of the toes from the floor. Observe all three phases of gait: *touch-down*, which should occur with the lateral heel; *stance*, which should be centered; and *push-off* which should come off the great toe. Foot strikes are normally in a nearly straight line. Also, observe a turn for loss of balance or multiple small steps to get turned around. Next, have the patient walk away from you on the toes, observing from behind, turn and walk toward you on the heels observing from the front; note how far the heels and toes, respectively, are held off the ground. Examine wear on the patient's shoes; abnormal wear patterns are a reliable clue to disorders of the foot and gait.

Past pointing. Have the patient sit facing you, pointing his index fingers toward you with his eyes closed (Chapter 7, Fig. 7-15). Hold your index fingers lightly under his. Ask the patient to raise his arms and hands, and then return his fingers to yours. Normally, this maneuver can be performed accurately. Past pointing indicates either loss of position sense or labyrinthine stimulation. Other tests of labyrinth function are described in Chapter 7, page 173.

Skilled acts. To inspect handwriting ask the patient to write a sentence. Test facility at buttoning and unbuttoning a coat or shirt or picking up pins or threading a needle. Test his skill at cutting figures out of paper with scissors.

Sensory Examination: A complete assessment of sensory modalities is not made during the routine physical examination. A history of diabetes, localized pain, numbness, or tingling, or the finding of motor deficits, calls for a detailed sensory examination. The patient must be lucid and have adequate attention to cooperate with the examination. The clinician must have a detailed knowledge of segmental and peripheral nerve distribution in the skin (refer to Figs. 14-14 and 14-15) and make a drawing of the distribution of sensory deficits. The diagram may be used for immediate comparison on retesting; abnormal sensory examinations should be repeated for consistency, progression or resolution. Disparities between examinations may indicate factitious findings.

The detailed cranial nerve exam includes testing the special senses and the cutaneous sensation of the head. For the remainder of the body, the distribution of sensibility for cutaneous pain, touch, pressure, position, and vibration should be evaluated. If a deficit in pain sensation is detected, temperature sensation must be tested. When an area of altered cutaneous sensibility is found, the borders should be marked with a skin pencil, and a diagram recorded in the patient's record.

Superficial pain—sharp-dull. Sensibility to pain may be increased (*hyperalgesia*), normal, reduced (*hypalgesia*) or absent (*analgesia*). Have the patient close his eyes. The skin is stroked lightly with the point of a sterile pin asking if the sensation is painful (Fig. 14-16A). Observe the patient's facial expression for signs of discomfort. If there is doubt about the response, mix sharp and dull stimuli from the point and head of the pin. Compare side-to-side with the same pressure; it is better for the patient to report differences than for you suggest them. In mapping deficit borders, slowly stimulate the skin from nonsensitive to sensitive skin, having the patient indicate where the sensation changes.

Deep pain. Test for deep or protopathic pain by pressure on nerve trunks, and tendons. For example, in the *Abadie sign* for tabes dorsalis, the normal pressure tenderness of the Achilles tendon is lost.

Temperature sense. When pain sense is impaired, test for the closely associated temperature sensibility asking the patient to distinguish between warm and cold. With the eyes closed, touch the skin with glass tubes of hot and cold water. Alternatively, test cold perception with a tuning fork and warm perception by exhaling on the skin through your widespread lips.

Tactile sense. With the eyes closed, compare sensation right to left by stroking the skin with a shred of sterile gauze. Have the patient indicate when and where you touch him. If you suspect that he is using his eyes, make sham tests near but without touching the skin. Grade the results as *hyperesthetic, normal, hypesthetic,* or *anesthetic.*

Proprioception (position sense). With the patient's eyes closed, grasp a finger on the sides (avoid grasping on the top and bottom or touching adjacent fingers because that provides touch cues). Extend or flex the finger at one joint and ask the patient its position (Fig. 14-16B). Similarly, test position

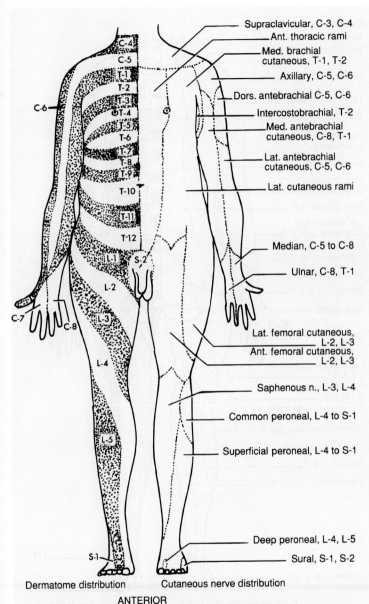

Supraclavicular, C-3, C-4
Ant. thoracic rami
Med. brachial cutaneous, T-1, T-2
Axillary, C-5, C-6
Dors. antebrachial C-5, C-6
Intercostobrachial, T-2
Med. antebrachial cutaneous, C-8, T-1
Lat. antebrachial cutaneous, C-5, C-6
Lat. cutaneous rami
Median, C-5 to C-8
Ulnar, C-8, T-1
Lat. femoral cutaneous, L-2, L-3
Ant. femoral cutaneous, L-2, L-3
Saphenous n., L-3, L-4
Common peroneal, L-4 to S-1
Superficial peroneal, L-4 to S-1
Deep peroneal, L-4, L-5
Sural, S-1, S-2

Dermatome distribution   Cutaneous nerve distribution

ANTERIOR

FIG. 14-14 Cutaneous Sensation in the Anterior Aspect of the Body.

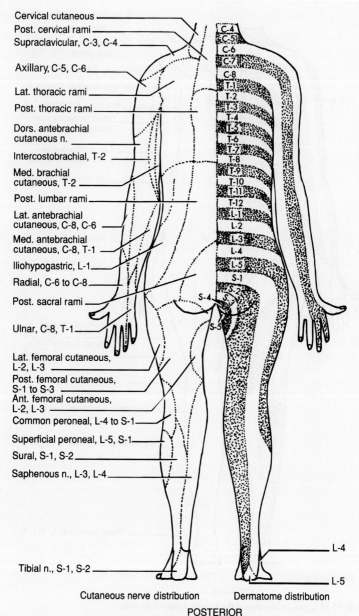

Cervical cutaneous
Post. cervical rami
Supraclavicular, C-3, C-4

Axillary, C-5, C-6

Lat. thoracic rami

Post. thoracic rami

Dors. antebrachial
cutaneous n.

Intercostobrachial, T-2

Med. brachial
cutaneous, T-2

Post. lumbar rami

Lat. antebrachial
cutaneous, C-8, C-6

Med. antebrachial
cutaneous, C-8, T-1

Iliohypogastric, L-1

Radial, C-6 to C-8

Post. sacral rami

Ulnar, C-8, T-1

Lat. femoral cutaneous,
L-2, L-3

Post. femoral cutaneous,
S-1 to S-3

Ant. femoral cutaneous,
L-2, L-3

Common peroneal, L-4 to S-1

Superficial peroneal, L-5, S-1

Sural, S-1, S-2

Saphenous n., L-3, L-4

Tibial n., S-1, S-2

C-4
C-5
C-6
C-7
C-8
T-1
T-2
T-3
T-4
T-5
T-6
T-7
T-8
T-9
T-10
T-11
T-12
L-1
L-2
L-3
L-4
L-5
S-1
S-2
S-3
S-4
S-5

L-4

L-5

Cutaneous nerve distribution   Dermatome distribution

POSTERIOR

FIG. 14-15 Cutaneous Sensation in the Posterior Aspect of the Body.

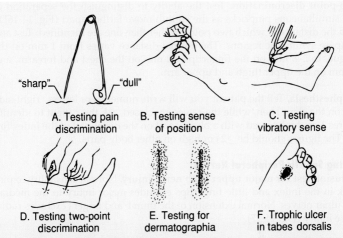

"sharp" "dull"

A. Testing pain discrimination

B. Testing sense of position

C. Testing vibratory sense

D. Testing two-point discrimination

E. Testing for dermatographia

F. Trophic ulcer in tabes dorsalis

FIG. 14-16 Sensory Testing and Other Phenomena. See text for descriptions. **A. Testing "sharp-dull" with a safety pin. B. Testing position sense in the toes. C. Testing vibratory sense. D. Testing** two-point **discrimination. E. Testing for dermatographism.** Stroke the skin with a blunt object. The normal response is a pale line. The abnormal responses is a faint red that becomes bright red then extends with red mottling, and, with more exaggerated response, a raised, edematous, and pale wheal develops. **F. Trophic plantar ulcer** advanced diabetic neuropathy or tabes dorsalis.

sensation in the metatarsophalangeal joint of the great toe. Normal young patients discriminate 1–2 degrees of movement in their distal finger joints and 3–5 degrees of the great toe. Test position sense in the leg or arm with the eyes closed by place one limb in a position asking the patient to place its counterpart in a symmetrical position.

Vibration sense (pallesthesia). Place the handle of a vibrating 128-Hz tuning fork over bony prominences, such as the radial styloid, the subcutaneous aspects of the tibiae, the ankle malleoli, or the great toe interphalangeal joint (Fig. 14-16C). Compare symmetrical points. When the patient indicates that the fork's vibration has ceased, place the handle on your own wrist to detect any persistent vibration. Make sham tests by setting the fork in vibration then unobtrusively stopping it with your finger before applying the handle to the patient.

Pressure sense. Standardized monofilaments precisely check for protective pressure sensation. Anesthesia to a 10-g monofilament is sensitive for loss of protective sensation to pressure injury. All diabetics should be tested at least once a year. Test the ability to discriminate objects of different weight in their palms. Test the ability to distinguish between pressures from the head of a pin and the tip of your finger. Press over the joints and subcutaneous aspects of bones for pressure perception.

Testing Higher Integrative Functions
Stereognosis. Simple sensory perception must be normal. With the eyes closed, test the ability to identify objects placed in the hands. Use coins, pencils, glass, wood, metal, cloth, and other familiar articles.

Two-point discrimination. Test the ability to distinguish the separation of two simultaneous pinpricks as the stimuli move farther apart (Fig. 14-16D). Find the distance at which two points rather than one are identified. Test and compare symmetric regions. The normal distance varies from 1 mm on the tongue, to 2–8 mm on the fingertips, 40 mm on the chest and forearm, and 75 mm on the upper thigh and upper arm.

Graphesthesia. Tell the patient you will write numerals or letters "right-side up" on the skin. Then, while their eyes are closed, ask the patient to identify figures 1 cm high traced with a blunt point on the distal pad of the index finger. The figures should be ≥2 cm high on other body parts.

Testing Specific Peripheral Nerves
Exclusion test for major upper limb nerve injury. Normal sensibility to pinprick in the index and little fingertips excludes major injury to the median and ulnar nerves. Normal extension of the thumb and fingers excludes radial nerve injury (Fig. 14-17).

Median nerve. Motor Function: Ochsner Test, Fig. 14-18A: The patient clasps the hands firmly together; the index finger cannot flex when the innervation of the *flexor digitorum sublimis* is injured below the antecubital fossa. Thumb Flexion, (Fig. 14-18B): Hold the first metacarpophalangeal joint with your thumb and index finger extending the metacarpal then ask the patient to bend the interphalangeal joint. Failure to do so indicates *flexor pollicis longus* paralysis, innervated by median nerve volar interosseous branches originating in the middle third of the forearm. Thumb Abduction: Testing the *abductor pollicis brevis*, innervated exclusively by the median nerve, distinguishes median from low-level ulnar nerve paralysis. (1) Wartenberg Oriental Prayer Position, (Fig. 14-18C): The patient extends and adducts the four fingers of each hand, with thumbs extended, then raise the two hands in front of the face so they are side by side in the same plane, with thumbs and index fingers touching tip to tip. Abductor pollicis brevis paralysis prevents full thumb abduction, so thumbs do not come together when index fingers touch. (2) Pen-Touching Test (Fig. 14-18D): The patient rests the supinated hand on a table holding the fingers flat. Ask the patient to raise his thumb straight up off the table to touch a pen or pencil held horizontally above it. **Sensory Function:** Test touch, two-point, and sharp-dull on the thumb, index, middle, and fourth fingers, and palm comparing right to left (Fig. 14-18E). Decreased or absent sensation indicates a median nerve lesion.

Ulnar nerve. Motor Function: *Interosseus palmaris* paralysis causes weak finger adduction. Demonstrate this by pulling a sheet of paper from between the patient's extended and adducted fingers revealing inability to apply pressure by the sides of the fingers (Fig. 14-19A). Paralysis of the *adductor pollicis* is tested by pinching each end of a folded paper between thumbs on top and index fingers underneath, then pulling the hands apart while gripping the paper. The thumb with an inadequate adductor flexes at its interphalangeal joint from involuntary use of the *flexor pollicis longus*, innervated by the median nerve (Fig. 14-19B). With lesions at or below the elbow, test for paralysis of the *flexor carpi ulnaris*. Lay the supinated hand on the table

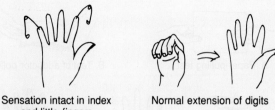

FIG. 14-17 Exclusion Test for Major Nerve Injury in the Upper Limb. Sensation is intact in the palmar tips of the index and little fingers; extension of the digits of the hand is unimpaired.

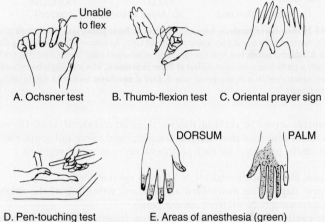

FIG. 14-18 Median Nerve Injury. See text for descriptions. **A. Ochsner test.** The patient cannot flex the index finger on the paralyzed side. **B. Thumb flexion test.** The patient cannot flex the IP joint of the thumb. **C. Wartenberg-oriental prayer sign.** Paralysis prevents thumb extension so its tip cannot reach its mate. **D. Pen-touching test.** The thumb cannot abduct to touch the object when the median nerve is paralyzed. **E. The area of anesthesia.** This includes the radial three digits of the palmar aspect and folds over the tips to the dorsal aspect where it covers the distal phalanges of the same digits (green).

holding all but the little finger flat against the table. Have the patient maximally abduct the little finger; the tensed tendon should be seen or palpated at the wrist (Fig. 14-19C). **Sensory Function:** With sensory loss, the ulnar digits, the corresponding region of the palm, and back of the hand are anesthetic (Fig. 14-19D). When the nerve lesion is at the wrist, anesthesia is only on the distal half of the little finger.

Specific Muscle and Nerve Movements: It is useful to identify the muscles and nerves implicated in a movement deficit. The following is list of the principal movements, the muscles involved, and their innervation (in parentheses). This survey starts with CN and precedes distally sequentially identifying

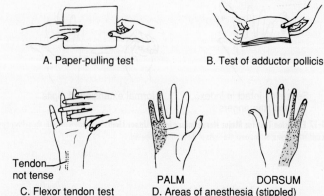

A. Paper-pulling test

B. Test of adductor pollicis

Tendon not tense

C. Flexor tendon test

PALM

DORSUM

D. Areas of anesthesia (stippled)

FIG. 14-19 Ulnar Nerve Paralysis. See text for descriptions. **A. Paper-pulling test.** Tests the finger adductors by having the patient hold a piece of paper between two adducted fingers. The examiner pulls the paper testing adductor strength. **B. Adductor pollicis test.** In ulnar paralysis, the thumb cannot exert enough pressure in adduction, so it flexes involuntarily to use the flexor pollicis longus. **C. Test of flexor carpi ulnaris.** While attempting to flex the free finger, the paralyzed muscle's tendon in the wrist does not tense. **D. Area of anesthesia.** The ulnar 1.5 digits on both aspects of the hand (green).

movements served by cervical, thoracic, lumbar, and sacral roots. The reader can trace an abnormal movement to the peripheral nerve and spinal root or a deficit can be predicted for each peripheral nerve or spinal segment.

Eyebrow, elevation. Frontalis (CN-VII from inferior pons).
Eyebrow, depression downward and inward, wrinkling of the forehead. Corrugator (CN-VII from inferior pons).
Upper eyelid, elevation. Levator palpebrae superioris (CN-III from upper midbrain).
Eyelid closing, forehead wrinkling, lacrimal sac compression. Orbicularis oculi (CN-VII from inferior pons).
Eyeball.
  Elevation and adduction. Superior rectus (CN-III from upper midbrain).[1]
  *Elevation and outward rotation. Inferior oblique (CN-III from upper midbrain).
  *Depression and rotation downward and inward. Inferior rectus (CN-III from upper midbrain).
  *Depression and rotation downward and outward. Superior oblique (CN-IV from midbrain) or primary downward rotation, secondary inward (intorsion) rotation, and tertiary weak outward rotation.

---

[1]***Ophthalmologic Interpretation of Muscle Action.** The items marked with asterisks constitute the actions of the oculorotatory muscles, as assigned by the anatomists and some neurologists. Sharply divergent interpretations are furnished by the ophthalmologists on the basis of clinical findings. The direction of movement of the eyes is a result of the actions of synergists and antagonists producing six cardinal positions of gaze, corresponding to the six extraocular muscles. Paralysis of a single muscle results in the inability of the eye to attain its cardinal position, which, in four of the six muscles, does not correspond to the prediction of the anatomists.

Adduction. Medial rectus (CN-III from upper midbrain).

Abduction. Lateral rectus (CN-VI from inferior pons).

Pupil constriction. Ciliary (CN-III and parasympathetic from upper midbrain).

Lips.

Retraction. Zygomatic (CN-VII from inferior pons).

Protrusion. Orbicularis oris (CN-VII from inferior pons).

Mouth opening. Mylohyoid (CN-V from pons), digastricus (CN-VII from pons).

Mandible.

Elevation and retraction. Masseter and temporalis (CN-V from mid-pons).

Elevation and protrusion. Pterygoid (CN-V from mid-pons).

Pharynx, palate elevation, and pharynx constriction. Levator veli palatini and pharyngeal constrictor (CN-IX and CN-X from medulla).

Tongue depression and protrusion. Genioglossus (CN-XII from medulla).

Neck.

Head rotation. Sternocleidomastoid and trapezius (CN-XI from medulla and upper cervical cord).

Flexion. Rectus capitis anterior (C1 to C3).

Extension and head rotation. Splenius capitis et cervicis (C1 to C4).

Lateral bending. Rectus capitis lateralis (C1to C4 and suboccipital nerve).

Spine.

Flexion. Rectus abdominis (T8 to T12).

Extension. Thoracic and lumbar intercostals (thoracic nerves from T2 to L1).

Extension and rotation. Semispinalis (thoracic nerves from T2 to T12).

Extension and lateral bending. Quadratus lumborum (lumbar plexus from T10 to L2).

Ribs.

Elevation and depression. Scaleni and intercostal (cervical and thoracic nerves from C4 to T12).

Elevation. Serratus posterior superior (from T1 to T4).

Diaphragm, elevation and depression. The diaphragmatic muscles (phrenic nerve from C3 to C5).

Scapula.

Rotation and extension of neck. Upper trapezius (CN-XI from C3 to C4).

Retraction with shoulder elevation. Middle and lower trapezius (CN-XI from C3 to C4).

Elevation and retraction. Rhomboids (dorsal scapular nerve from C5).

Arm.

Elevation. Supraspinatus (suprascapular nerve from C5 to C6), upper trapezius (CN-XI from C3 to C4).

Elevation and rotation. Deltoid (axillary nerve from C5 to C6).

Depression and adduction. Middle pectoralis major (anterior thoracic nerve from C5 to T1).

Depression and medial rotation. Subscapularis (subscapular nerve from C5 to C7), teres major (thoracodorsal nerves from C5 to C7).

Depression and lateral rotation. Infraspinatus (suprascapular nerve from C5 to C6).

Elbow.

Flexion. Biceps brachii, brachialis (musculocutaneous nerve from C5 to C6).

Extension. Triceps brachii (radial nerve from C7 to T1).

Supination. Biceps brachii (musculocutaneous nerve from C5 to C6), brachioradialis (radial nerve from C5 to C6).

Supination and flexion. Brachioradialis (radial nerve from C5 to C6).

Pronation. Pronator teres (median nerve from C6 to C7).

Wrist.

Extension and adduction. Extensor carpi ulnaris (radial nerve from C7 to C8).

Extension and abduction of hand. Extensor carpi radialis longus (radial nerve from C6 to C7).

Extension of the hand. Extensor digitorum communis (radial nerve from C7 to C8).

Flexion and abduction. Flexor carpi radialis (median nerve from C7 to C8).

Flexion and adduction. Flexor carpi ulnaris (ulnar nerve from C7 to C8).

Thumb.

Adduction and opposition. Adductor pollicis longus (ulnar nerve C8 to T1).

Abduction and extension. Abductor pollicis longus and brevis (median and radial [and posterior interosseous nerves] from C7 to C8).

Extension of distal phalanx. Extensor pollicis longus (radial nerve from C7 to C8).

Extension of proximal phalanx. Extensor pollicis brevis (radial nerve from C7 to C8).

Flexion of distal phalanx. Flexor pollicis longus (median nerve from C7 to T1).

Flexion of proximal phalanx. Flexor pollicis longus and brevis (median nerve from C7 to T1).

Flexion and opposition. Opponens pollicis (median nerve from C8 to T1).

Fingers.

Flexion and adduction of little finger. Opponens digiti minimi (ulnar nerve from C8 to T1).

Adduction of four fingers. Palmar interossei (ulnar nerve from C8 to T1).

Abduction of four fingers. Dorsal interossei (ulnar nerve from C8 to T1).

Extension of hand. Extensor digitorum communis (radial nerve from C7 to C8).

Flexion of hand. Palmar interossei (interosseous nerves from C7 to T1), lumbricales (ulnar and median nerves from C7 to T1).

Extension of interphalangeal joints. Interossei palmaris and lumbricales (interosseous nerve; median and ulnar nerves from C7 to T1).

Flexion of the distal phalanges. Flexor digitorum profundus (median and ulnar nerves from C7 to T1).

Flexion of middle phalanges. Flexor digitorum sublimis (median nerve from C7 to T1).

Abdomen.

Compression with trunk flexion. Rectus abdominis (lower thoracic nerves from T6 to L1).

Flexion of abdominal wall obliquely. Obliquus abdominis externus (lower thoracic nerves from T6 to L1).

Hip.

Flexion. Iliacus (femoral nerve), psoas (L2 to L3), sartorius (femoral nerve from L2 to L3).

Extension. Gluteus maximus (inferior gluteal nerve from L4 to S2), adductor magnus (sciatic nerve and obturator nerve from L5 to S2).

Abduction. Gluteus medius (superior gluteal nerve from L4 to S1), gluteus maximus (inferior gluteal nerve from L4 to S2).

Adduction. Adductor magnus (sciatic and obturator nerves from L5 to S2).

Outward rotation. Gluteus maximus (inferior gluteal nerve from L4 to S2), obturator internus (branches from S1 to S3).

Inward rotation. Psoas (branches from L2 to L3).

Knee.

Flexion. Biceps femoris, semitendinosus, semimembranosus, gastrocnemius (all through sciatic nerve from L5 to S2).

Extension. Quadriceps femoris (femoral nerve from L2 to L4).

Ankle.

Plantar flexion. Gastrocnemius and soleus (tibial nerve from L5 to S2).

Dorsiflexion. Anterior tibial (deep peroneal nerve from L4 to S1).

Inversion. Posterior tibial (tibial nerve from L5 to S1).

Eversion. Peroneus longus (superficial peroneal nerve from L4 to S1).

Great toe, dorsiflexion. Extensor hallucis longus and brevis (superficial peroneal nerve from L4 to S1).

NEUROLOGIC SYMPTOMS

General Symptoms

Headache. The head contains many pain-sensitive structures, most innervated by the trigeminal nerve (CN-V). Mechanisms of headache include inflammation, infection, arterial dilation, hemorrhage, pressure changes within closed spaces, expanding mass lesions producing traction or compressing structures, trauma, ischemia, and tissue destruction. The common extracranial cause of headache is sustained contraction of the head, neck, and shoulders muscles. Headache refers to more than momentary pain in the cranial vault, orbits or nape; pain in the face is not included. An urgent search for serious pathology is required when a severe headache is unlike any experienced in the past.

CLINICAL OCCURRENCE: *Congenital:* Arteriovenous malformations, hydrocephalus; *Endocrine:* Pheochromocytoma; *Degenerative/Idiopathic:* Idiopathic intracranial hypertension; *Infectious:* Meningitis, encephalitis, rickettsia infections, sinusitis, otitis, mastoiditis, non-CNS viral infections (e.g., influenza, cytomegalovirus, varicella), parasites (e.g., malaria, neurocysticercosis), protozoa (e.g., toxoplasmosis); *Inflammatory/Immune:* Giant cell arteritis, sarcoidosis; *Mechanical/Traumatic:* Accelerated and malignant hypertension, trauma (concussion), muscle tension, TMJ disease, increased intracranial pressure, glaucoma, decreased intracranial pressure (CSF leak); *Metabolic/Toxic:* Analgesic rebound headache, hypoxia, hypercapnia, hypoglycemia, alcohol and illicit drug withdrawal, carbon monoxide poisoning, caffeine abstinence; *Neoplastic:* Primary and metastatic brain tumors; *Neurologic:* Migraine, cluster headache, paroxysmal hemicrania, trigeminal neuralgia, occipital neuralgia; *Psychosocial:* Stress; *Vascular:* migraine, intracranial aneurysm, hemorrhage (intracerebral, subdural, epidural, and subarachnoid), venous sinus thrombosis, stroke, cerebral vasculitis. For specific headache syndromes see page 680.

Clinical Examination for headache. **History:** Inquire carefully for the attributes of pain (PQRST); *Provocative and Palliative Factors:* Trauma, medications, substance abuse, head and body position, coughing, straining, emotional state, relief with massage, and resolution with sleep; *Quality:* Whether burning, aching, deep or superficial, lancinating, throbbing, or continuous; *Region Involved and Radiation:* Cranial, facial, orbital, unilateral, bilateral; *Severity:* Use the 1–10 scale; and *Timing:* when headaches began, frequency, time of day, duration, pattern of intensity. Inquire about family members with a headache history. Identify associated symptoms, e.g., fever, stiff neck, nausea and vomiting, constipation or diarrhea, diuresis, rhinorrhea, visual disturbances (photophobia, scotomata, tearing, diplopia), cerebral symptoms (confusion, slurred speech, aura, paresthesias, anesthesias, motor paralysis, vertigo, mood, and sleep disturbances). **Physical Exam:** Inspect the skin and scalp for bulges and areas of erythema. With deep pressure palpate and percuss the bones of the cranium and face for tenderness and irregularities. Palpate the neck muscles and the upper borders of the trapezii for tenderness. Palpate the carotid and temporal arteries for pulsations and tenderness. Examine the eyes for pupil contour and response to light and near point, conjunctival injection or abnormal extraocular motion; use confrontation testing (page 625) to detect gross visual field defects . Examine the fundus for choked disks and retinal hemorrhages. Auscultate the cranium for bruits. Perform a thorough neurologic exam with special attention to the CN and the deep tendon reflexes.

Memory loss. Four components of memory are distinguished by function and location in the brain. *Episodic memory* records episodic events in the medial temporal and frontal cortex (cingulate gyrus). *Semantic memory* records names, general knowledge and information in the lateral temporal lobes. *Procedural memory* retains the ability to perform complex behaviors and tasks in the frontal lobes, basal ganglia and cerebellum. *Working memory* stores immediately useful information at which attention is directed in the frontal lobes, amygdala and parietal cortex. Information from working memory is either stored or deleted if not recalled or used. Patients often complain of forgetfulness, especially of names. Paradoxically, the patient concerned about memory loss rarely has a significant problem. Changes in behavior, failure to complete expected tasks, difficulty with instrumental activities of daily living, especially managing finances, are better clues to significant memory and/or cognitive impairment. Always formally screen for cognitive impairment if there is any concern.

Spells. The patient experiences one or more episodes of altered perception or behavior, usually lasting seconds or minutes. When multiple, they are usually described as stereotypic. The spell may have only subjective symptoms or be associated with behavioral changes observed by others. The patient may be aware throughout the spell or be amnestic for the episode. When accompanied by changes in consciousness, behaviors, or motor events, the reports of observers are often key to making the diagnosis. Inquire about triggering events or sensations, associated symptoms and signs (e.g., loss of muscle tone with falling, injury, and/or incontinence), the spells' duration, and the patient's responsiveness during and after the spell. Spells generally indicate a primary or secondary brain event. Common considerations include seizures (especially complex partial and absence seizures), transient ischemic events, stroke, nonconvulsive seizures, tics, conversion disorder, panic attacks, hyperventilation, narcolepsy, delirium, drug toxicity, and intoxication.

Insomnia. Disorders of sleep are common, especially in shift workers and following long distance air travel. A careful history of the onset and pattern of disrupted sleep with close attention to sleep hygiene often discloses the source of sleep disruption. Two common patterns are *initial insomnia*, the inability to get to sleep at the usual time, and *terminal insomnia*, early awakening producing deficits in rapid eye movement sleep. Common considerations include poor sleep hygiene, medications, illicit drug and alcohol use, depression, anxiety disorder, panic disorder, obstructive sleep apnea, and hypomania or mania.

Loss of balance and falling. Maintaining balance requires normal proprioceptive sensory nerves and tracts, vestibular system, motor tracts and nerves, muscles, cerebellum, and basal ganglia. Major abnormalities in any of these pathways results in falls. More commonly, there are less severe impairments in several systems. Falls are common, especially with advancing age. Many patients do not volunteer information about falls, so asking is appropriate. When proprioceptive function is impaired, patients locate themselves in space using their eyes. Hence, visual impairment (including use of bi- and trifocal lenses) and low-light conditions frequently contribute to falling. Skeletal abnormalities, especially of the joints, are a common precipitant. Decreased mentation and reaction times because of drugs (e.g., benzodiazepines, anticholinergics) and/or aging increase the risk of falling. A complete neurologic examination identifies all contributing abnormalities. Fall prevention is a major focus of a geriatric assessment. Losing control of the center of mass during standing and transferring, rather than poor base support, causes most falls. The major risk for future falls is a history of previous falls.

Cranial Nerve Symptoms
Vision loss. See Chapter 7, page 189.

Absent or abnormal taste and smell—ageusia, dysgeusia, anosmia. See Chapter 7, pages 190 and 218.

Ringing in the ears—tinnitus. See Chapter 7, page 188.

Hearing loss. See Chapter 7, page 245.

Vertigo. See Chapter 7, page 245.

Double vision—diplopia. Perception of two visual images results from abnormal refraction or, less commonly, nonconjugative gaze. A careful history will determine the pattern of diplopia (e.g., vertical or horizontal), precipitating activities, the direction of gaze where diplopia is apparent, and the head position and/or direction of gaze that relieves the diplopia. If the patient reports *monocular diplopia* or diplopia when one eye is covered, the cause is nearly always refractive. *Binocular diplopia* results from impairment of the CN III, IV, and/or VI, damage to or weakness of the extraocular muscles, or globe displacement. Careful physical exam differentiates between these causes. Important diagnostic considerations are myasthenia gravis, Graves ophthalmopathy, and ophthalmoplegias.

Difficulty swallowing—dysphagia. See Chapter 7, pages 190 and 251.

Difficulty speaking
Dysarthria. See page 666.

Aphasia. See page 704.

Facial pain, trigeminal neuralgia/tic douloureux. A common cause is an artery compressing CN-V as it exits the brainstem. A nonpainful stimulus provokes a paroxysm of "hot" lancinating pain, always unilateral, and initially limited to one trigeminal nerve (CN-V) division. The intense pain causes grimacing resembling a tic. Each patient has a unique, adequate stimulus in the trigger area: a light touch, chewing, sneezing, a draft, or tickling the skin. The maxillary division is most commonly involved giving pain in the maxilla, upper teeth and lip, and lower eyelid. Uncommonly, the mandibular division is involved with pain in the lower teeth and lip, the oral portion of the tongue, and the external acoustic meatus. The ophthalmic branch is rarely affected. There are no motor or sensory changes. *DDX:* The initial stage of herpes zoster may suggest tic douloureux.

Asymmetrical face or smile. See page 665, Facial Nerve Signs.

Hoarseness. See Chapter 7, page 232.

Motor Symptoms
Weakness. See page 667. Weakness results from an abnormality in the brain, spinal cord, peripheral nerves, motor endplate, and/or muscle. Either primary neuromuscular disease or a generalized metabolic abnormality can be the cause. A common complaint, weakness requires a complete evaluation. A careful history identifies the specific activities that are impaired. Difficulty with rising from a chair or climbing stairs suggests proximal muscle weakness, whereas difficulty writing, opening jars and doors, and catching the toes while walking suggests distal weakness. Global weakness is seen with generalized muscle diseases, myasthenia gravis, and polyneuropathies (e.g., Guillain–Barré syndrome). During the physical exam observe for fasciculations, assess muscle mass, tone, and strength, and evaluate the reflexes. Hysterical weakness and malingering are not rare, but these diagnoses are only made after organic disease is excluded by a thorough evaluation.

Acute episodic weakness—cataplexy. Episodic loss of motor and postural control is precipitated by laughter or strong emotions. There is momentary loss of voluntary motor power including speech, without loss of consciousness or postural tone. Cataplexy is associated with narcolepsy.

Muscle pain—myalgia. See also Chapter 13, page 557. This is a common, though nonspecific, complaint. Generalized myalgias, especially in the back and proximal limb muscles, frequently accompany febrile illnesses of any cause. Severe myalgias are especially common in several infectious diseases (e.g., Lyme disease, trichinosis, and dengue), but other elements of the history are of more use than the presence of myalgia in making a specific diagnosis. Drugs (e.g., statins) also cause myalgias so a complete medication and herbal therapy history is mandatory. In persons above age 50, abrupt onset of myalgias in the proximal muscles (shoulders > pelvic girdle) suggests polymyalgia rheumatica.

Muscle stiffness. Overuse of skeletal muscle induces a damage–repair cycle felt as pain and stiffness. Underuse leads to muscle wasting, which may be accompanied by stiffness. The deconditioned patient often complains of sore, stiff muscles 1–2 days following unaccustomed exercise (weekend athlete syndrome). Examination shows no abnormalities other than tenderness and occasionally mild spasm in the affected muscles. Patients with inherited disorders of muscle metabolism or electrolyte disorders can develop severe myonecrosis with exercise. *DDX:* Abrupt onset of proximal muscles stiffness in a person over age 50 without a clear-cut precipitating event suggests polymyalgia rheumatica. Generalized cramps with tetany are seen with hypocalcemia. The bradykinesia and increased muscle tone of Parkinsonian syndromes is often described by the patient as stiffness. Rare causes are stiff person syndrome, myotonia, and hypocalcemia.

Twitches and tics. See page 674.

Irresistible leg movements—restless legs syndrome. See page 707.

Muscle spasm—cramps, dystonias. See page 703.

Posture, Balance, and Coordination Symptoms
Loss of balance—falling. See page 653.

Difficulty walking. See page 672.

Vertigo. See Chapter 7, page 245.

Tremors. See page 673.

Sensory Symptoms
Altered sensation—tingling and numbness, paresthesias. Tingling or numbness of a body part indicates impaired pressure, pain, and/or touch sensation. Numbness, a negative symptom, implies nerve damage while tingling, a positive symptom, suggests nerve stimulation. The symptom pattern reliably indicates the anatomic level of injury: symptoms on one side of the entire body indicate a problem in the thalamus or cortex; loss on one side of the body below a specific level suggests spinal cord injury; symptoms in a peripheral nerve distribution implies injury to that nerve; and symmetrical distal paresthesia (stocking-glove distribution) suggests a generalized sensory (with or without motor) axonal neuropathy. Testing the specific sensory modalities is required. Unilateral loss of touch and position sensation with contralateral loss of temperature and pain sensation indicates a unilateral spinal cord lesion ipsilateral to the touch and position loss.

Pain with nonpainful stimuli—allodynia. See page 675.

NEUROLOGIC SIGNS

Cranial Nerve Signs: The signs of CN dysfunction are mimicked by non-neurologic end-organ diseases, so consider these during the head and neck exam. These conditions are fully discussed in Chapter 7. Once end-organ disease is excluded, decide whether the neurologic lesion is central (brain) or peripheral (nerve). The following is a brief list of *some* specific cranial nerve signs.

Anosmia—olfactory nerve (CNI). Lesions of CN-I, often shearing of the nerve ending passing through the cribriform plate, or nasal obstruction produce loss of smell. Anosmia is invariably accompanied by a perceived change in the taste of food, which seems bland and unpalatable. The most common identified cause is closed head trauma.

Visual field signs
Monocular field defects—optic nerve or retina. Monocular visual field loss occurs from disease isolated to that eye including retina or optic nerve disease. The optic nerve is damaged to variable degrees by ischemia (giant cell arteritis, Anterior Ischemic Optic Neuropathy (AION, Chapter 7, page 207), increased intraocular pressure (glaucoma), demyelinating disease (optic neuritis), trauma, and increased intracranial pressure. Destructive retinal lesions also result in monocular field defects. Retinal ischemia from emboli, arteritis, or ipsilateral internal carotid artery stenosis produces transient monocular blindness (amaurosis fugax). Retinal ischemia also results from ophthalmic artery or vein occlusion.

Bilateral visual field defects—hemianopsia (hemianopia). Hemianopsia means that half of a visual field is not perceived. Hemianopsia involves nerves projecting from both eyes, so it is caused by a lesion in the optic chiasm, optic tracts, or brain. The optic nerves carry all the nerve fibers from the ipsilateral retina. At the optic chiasm the fibers from the nasal retinas cross the midline (decussate) joining the fibers of the lateral retina from the opposite side forming the optic tracts. The right optic tract carries all fibers to the right side of the brain, projecting the left visual field (Fig. 14-20). The left side of the brain receives the right nasal and left temporal retinal fibers, projecting the right visual field of each eye.

Homonymous hemianopsia. The same side of each *field* contains a defect (Fig. 14-21A). A left homonymous hemianopsia results from a lesion in the right optic tract or the right side of the brain. With a tract lesion, the pupillary reflex is absent when light is only projected from the blind hemifield; the pupil reacts when the lesion is in the optic radiations or occipital lobe posterior to the geniculate body. Transient homonymous hemianopsia may occur with migraine.

Crossed hemianopsia. Signals from both temporal or both nasal retinae are blocked, so the defect is *bitemporal or binasal.* A lesion of the decussating fibers

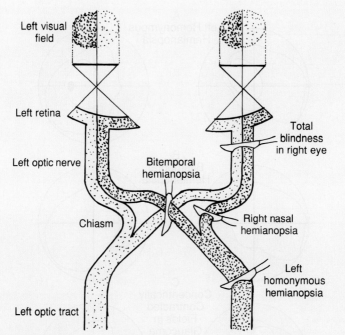

FIG. 14-20 Neural Pathways from Retina to Brain. The cutting knives indicate lesions. Above are the resultant visual field defects.

in the chiasm causes *bitemporal hemianopsia* (Fig. 14-21B) by injuring the fibers from both nasal retinae, commonly a pituitary macroadenoma. *Binasal hemianopsia* is uncommon because it requires injury to both lateral halves of the optic nerves or tracts. When only a quadrant of each field is lost, it is a *quadrantanopsia*.

Eye movement signs. Abnormal eye movements are caused by either primary extraocular muscle disease or by disease of the CNS and/or cranial nerves. It is more important for the generalist to identify neurologic disease than primary muscle disease. Therefore, these signs are discussed with the neurologic examination.

Nystagmus. One or both eyes cannot maintain fixation so the eye(s) drifting slowly to one side return to the original position by a quick correcting movement. This is the normal eye movement maintaining fixation when the head is in motion. Nystagmus results from damage to the labyrinth, its cerebellar connections, or the cerebellum. The patient is unstable standing with the eyes open. Nystagmus is named by the direction of the quick component. It may be horizontal, vertical, rotatory, oblique, or mixed. When both eyes participate, the nystagmus is *associated*; movement of one eye only is *dissociated*. Fewer than 40 jerks per minute is "slow"; more than 100 jerks per minute is

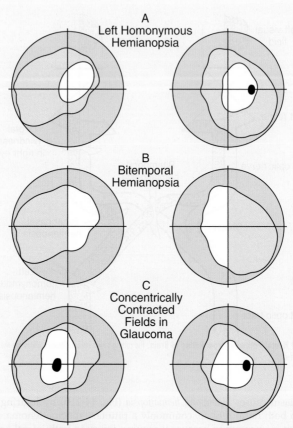

FIG. 14-21 Pathologic Visual Fields. The normal left and right normal visual fields are gray and white in the green background. Areas in gray are obscured by the respective pathologic condition while vision is retained in the white areas.

"fast." Amplitudes <1 mm are *fine*; amplitudes >3 mm are *coarse*. *DDX:* There are several varieties of nystagmus. Ocular instabilities resembling nystagmus include ocular flutter, opsoclonus, and ocular bobbing.

Congenital nystagmus is characterized by unsystematic wandering movements, with various frequencies and amplitudes.

End-position nystagmus occurs only with fixation far to the side, so it is always in the direction of fixation (Fig. 14-22A).

Labyrinthine end-position nystagmus usually occurs in disease of the semicircular canals. It is horizontal-rotatory initiated by fixation in the end position, but it persists for some time after resuming the primary position.

Fixation nystagmus occurs in many normal persons when they are required to fix to one side or the other; it is horizontal or horizontal-rotatory, moderate to coarse.

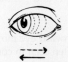

A. End-position nystagmus   B. Nystagmus in primary position

FIG. 14-22 Nystagmus. A slow drift of the eyes away from the position of fixation (broken arrows) is corrected by a quick corrective movement (solid arrow). The direction of the nystagmus is named from the quick component. Nystagmus from the primary position is more likely to be of serious import than that from the end position.

Muscle-paretic nystagmus presents as a dissociated movement of an eye with a paretic muscle when visual fixation is directed in the direction of action of the paretic muscle and the muscle attempts to maintain fixation.

Gaze-paretic nystagmus appears in paralysis of conjugate movements. Both eyes show more nystagmus to one end position than to the other.

Primary position nystagmus occurs with fixation in the primary position or at a point away from the direction of the quick component (Fig. 14-22B).

Peripheral labyrinthine nystagmus is horizontal-rotatory, with medium frequency and amplitude, commonly seen in Ménière syndrome, benign paroxysmal positional vertigo, labyrinthitis, perilymphatic or labyrinthine fistula, and vestibular neuritis.

Central nystagmus may be horizontal, rotatory, vertical, or mixed, usually in the direction of the diseased side. It is found in multiple sclerosis, encephalitis, brain tumors, and with transient or permanent vascular insufficiency involving the vestibular nuclei or medial longitudinal fasciculus.

Vertical nystagmus usually indicates a midbrain lesion.

Three types of nystagmus identify more localized lesions.

Convergence–retraction nystagmus occurs in the dorsal midbrain syndrome with lid retraction (*Collier sign*), limited up-gaze, and light-near dissociation.

Seesaw nystagmus is found with parasellar lesions and is characterized by rising and intorting of one eye while the other falls and extorts.

Downbeat nystagmus typically signifies lesions at the foramen magnum such as the Arnold–Chiari malformation, but may be seen with other disorders, including magnesium depletion, Wernicke encephalopathy, and lithium intoxication.

Saccadic intrusions. Saccadic movements are rapid start-stop movements when the eyes are fixed on a moving object, as opposed to the normal smooth pursuit movements. Voluntary eye movements are saccadic; you cannot move your eyes smoothly without fixing on a moving object. Inappropriate saccadic eye movements suggest cerebellar disease. The quick component of nystagmus is a saccadic movement.

Ocular flutter. This is arrhythmic and rapid horizontal eye movement. When there are both horizontal and vertical components, it is *opsoclonus*. These

conditions are associated with vascular, immune, neoplastic, and paraneoplastic processes.

Ocular bobbing. This is intermittent, conjugate, rapid, downward eye movement followed by a slow return to primary position. It is often seen in coma
from a pontine lesion.

Gaze abnormalities
Oculomotor (CN-III), trochlear (CN-IV), and/or abducens (CN-VI) nerve. See
Figure 14-23. Unilateral complete paralysis is usually caused by direct pressure
from tumor, aneurysm, or herniating brain. Less common are cavernous sinus
thrombosis and granulomatous process at the base of the brain, e.g., tuberculous
meningitis and Tolosa–Hunt syndrome. Transient pupillary-sparing oculomotor and abducens nerve palsies may complicate diabetes mellitus.

Comitant strabismus (nonparalytic heterophoria)—constant squint angle.
The muscles are normal; the disorder probably results from abnormal cranial
nerve nuclei because the squint angle disappears during general anesthesia.
The word *comitant*, when applied to strabismus, indicates that the angle
between the two optic axes, the *squint angle*, remains constant in all positions
assumed by the globes, no matter which eye fixates. Neither eye has limited
motion (Fig. 14-23). Because comitant strabismus occurs in the very young,
children learn to suppress the image from one eye and do not have diplopia.
In most cases, the optic axes converge, which is termed *comitant convergent
strabismus* or *esotropia*. When hypermetropia causes excessive convergence,
the condition is called *accommodative squint*. Occasionally the optic axes
diverge, which is termed *comitant divergent strabismus* or *exotropia*.

Failure of convergence. The lesion is in the frontopontine pathway. All movements are normal except convergence (Fig. 14-24E). Normal abduction of
both globes to the right and left indicates that the medial recti are normal.

Varying squint angle—noncomitant strabismus (paralytic heterotropia). This
is caused by paralysis of one or more eye muscles: *ophthalmoplegia.* The squint
angle changes with the direction of fixation. As opposed to comitant strabismus, the motions of the paralyzed eye are limited. To avoid diplopia, the head
is positioned to limit the action of the paralyzed muscle. The squint angle
is greatest when the unaffected eye is fixed in the visual field requiring the
action of the paralyzed muscle, *secondary deviation*. When paralysis is acquired
during maturity, diplopia occurs at the onset, frequently accompanied by vertigo. *To avoid confusion, only paralyses of the right eye muscles are used as examples.
In the figures, only the deficient eye movements are illustrated; all others are normal.*

Right lateral rectus paralysis. In the primary position, the optic axes are parallel or the right eye converges slightly (Fig. 14-23B). The right eye cannot
move laterally. The lateral rectus muscles most frequently develop isolated
paralysis. The abducens nerve (CN VI) is damaged by ischemia, inflammation, infectious diseases, orbital periostitis, petrous fracture of the temporal
bone, carotid artery aneurysm within the cavernous sinus, and lesions of the
posterior pons near the midline.

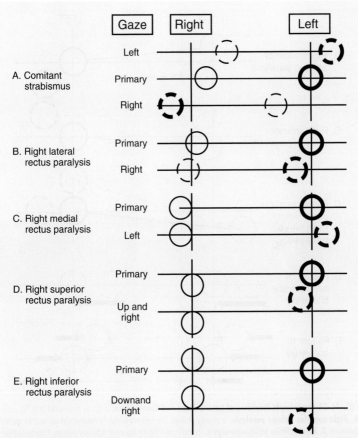

FIG. 14-23 Strabismus (Squint). Squint refers to disorders in which the optic axes are not parallel. The diagrams illustrate positions of the patient's eyes as they appear to the observer. The unbroken circles connected by the unbroken lines show pairs in the primary position with the normal or fixing eye represented in heavier lines. Pairs with broken lines are in secondary positions with the heavier lines for the fixing eye. **A. Comitant strabismus.** The squint-angle between the two optic axes is constant in all positions regardless of which eye fixates. **B. Right lateral rectus paralysis.** The right eye is unable to move laterally. **C. Right medial rectus paralysis.** The right eye is lateral in the primary position; it fails to move medially. **D. Right superior rectus paralysis.** The right eye is slightly depressed in primary position and fails to move farther upward. **E. Right inferior rectus paralysis.** The right eye is elevated slightly in primary position; it cannot move downward.

Right medial rectus paralysis. In the primary position, the right eye deviates laterally; it cannot move medially (Fig. 14-23C). The head turns to the left to avoid diplopia.

Right superior rectus paralysis. In the primary position, the right eye deviates downward; it cannot move upward to the right (Fig. 14-23D). The squint angle and diplopia increase by fixing the left eye upward to the right.

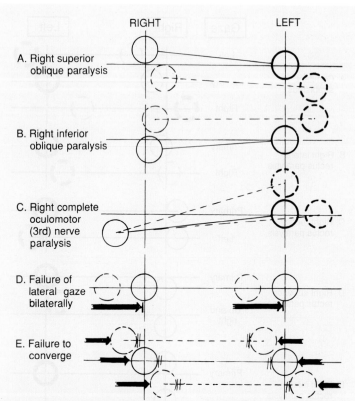

FIG. 14-24 Strabismus: Disorders of Lateral Gaze and Convergence. Diagrams constructed as in Fig. 7-35.
A. Right superior oblique paralysis. In primary position, the right eye is slightly elevated and can only be slightly depressed. **B. Right inferior oblique paralysis.** The right eye is slightly depressed in primary position; it can be elevated only slightly. **C. Right complete oculomotor nerve paralysis.** The right eye is fixed in depressed and lateral position. **D. Failure of lateral gaze.** Both eyes cannot be moved beyond the median to the left or right, as the case may be. **E. Failure of convergence.** In no position can the two eyes converge.

Right inferior rectus paralysis. In the primary position, the right eye deviates upward; it cannot move down to the right (Fig. 14-23E). Fixing the left eye downward and to the right increases the squint angle and diplopia.

Right superior oblique paralysis. In the primary position, the right eye deviates upward; movement is limited down and to the left (Fig. 14-24A). The squint angle increases when the left eye is fixed downward and to the left. A characteristic head tilt toward the left shoulder compensates for the pronounced extorsion (*ocular torticollis*). In this position the normal intorsion of the left eye corrects the torsional diplopia. Tilting the head to the right side rotates the right eye upward.

Right inferior oblique paralysis. In the primary position, the right eye deviates downward; its movement upward and to the left is limited (Fig. 14-24B). Fixing the gaze upward and to the left increases the squint angle.

Paralysis of two or more ocular muscles. Only the oculomotor nerve (CN-III) supplies more than one muscle, so partial ophthalmoplegia only involves CN-III. Involvement of all the nerves in the superior orbital fissure or the cavernous sinus causes unilateral total ophthalmoplegia; a bilateral lesion could result only from a focus in the base of the brain.

Varying squint angle—complete right oculomotor (CN-III) nerve paralysis. This produces paralysis of the levator, the superior, medial, and inferior recti, the inferior oblique muscles, and the pupillary sphincter (Fig. 14-24C). Only the superior oblique and the lateral rectus muscles are functioning. In the primary position, the right eye deviates downward and outward to the right. Motion to the left and upward is absent. The squint angle and diplopia increase when the left eye fixes to the left. Levator paralysis cause ptosis. The most frequent causes are a circle of Willis aneurysm and acute diabetic neuropathy, the latter usually sparing the pupil.

Internuclear ophthalmoplegia. Internuclear ophthalmoplegia is caused by lesions of the medial longitudinal fasciculus interconnecting the CN III, IV, and VI nuclei to coordinate conjugate eye movements. There is failure of adduction in horizontal lateral gaze, but convergence is normal. Common causes are multiple sclerosis and stroke.

Conjugate failure of lateral gaze. There is a lesion in the frontopontine pathway (Fig. 14-24D). When the lesion is on the right, there is constant conjugate deviation to the right; the patient turns the head to the left to fixate in front. The optic axes are parallel in all positions, so there is no diplopia. Neither eye can move to the left of the midline. In partial failure of lateral gaze, the patient can *will* the gaze to the left, but cannot fix it, so there is bilateral nystagmus to the left. *DDX:* This is distinguished from combined paralysis of the left lateral rectus and the right medial rectus by retention of convergence.

Conjugate failure of vertical gaze. This is a supranuclear disorder thought to be in the rostral midbrain. The patient is unable to gaze upward since the eyes cannot move above the horizontal. The head tilts backward to compensate. There is no diplopia. When failure is incomplete, there is slight upward movement with upward nystagmus. Rarely, upward failure is combined with downward failure, or failure of downward gaze may be present alone. *DDX:* Bilateral paralyses of the superior recti and the inferior obliques (innervated by CN-III) produces similar findings, but vertical gaze palsy is distinguished by retention of the normal *Bell phenomenon:* reflex elevation of the globes when the lids close. This reflex is mediated by fibers between the nuclei of CN-III and CN-VII in the medial longitudinal fasciculus, CN-III suppling the superior rectus and inferior oblique and CN-VII innervating the orbicularis. Persistence of the reflex, proving that both nuclei are intact, means the lesion must be supranuclear.

Pupil signs

Normal pupil reaction. Parasympathetic stimulation of the sphincter contracts the pupil; the dilator widens the pupil with sympathetic stimuli. The sphincter pupillae is a circular muscle embedded in the iris near the margin of the pupil. It is innervated by parasympathetic fibers from the Edinger–Westphal nucleus near the oculomotor nerve (CN-III) nucleus (Fig. 14-25). The fibers enter the orbit in the third nerve and accompany the motor branch to the inferior oblique muscle, where the parasympathetic fibers synapse in the ciliary ganglion; from there, other fibers enter the eye through the short ciliary nerves. The dilator pupillae is arranged radially in the peripheral two-thirds of the iris. It receives sympathetic fibers arising in the cortex, descending to the hypothalamus and ciliospinal center; postsynaptic fibers go to the cervical sympathetic chain and ascend to the superior cervical ganglion. They synapse with third-order neurons running to the carotid plexus and then to the first division of the trigeminal nerve (CN-V) into the eye. Pupil size fluctuates with changes in tone of these muscles. Exaggerated wavering is *hippus* or *physiologic pupillary unrest*; it is of little clinical significance. *Mydriasis* is dilatation; *miosis* is pupil constriction. Bright light causes constriction, accompanied by a consensual constriction in the unexposed eye, the pupils remaining equal in size. In older persons, the pupils may react sluggishly to light; the reaction is hastened after several stimulations. Near point miosis, associated with lens accommodation, occurs when the eye is fixed on a near object. The pupils of patients with Cheyne–Stokes respirations may dilate during the hyperventilation phase and constrict with apnea.

Unequal pupils—anisocoria. Unequal pupils result from constriction or dilation of one pupil. Anisocoria is often unimportant and beware the artificial eye. To determine whether one pupil is too small or the other too large, measure them in bright and dim light. If one pupil cannot contract the discrepancy is exaggerated in bright light. If one pupil cannot dilate, the difference is greater in darkness. *Physiologic anisocoria*, a constant difference in pupil size in light and dark, is a normal finding in 20% of normal persons. Miosis of one pupil with a large size disparity suggests sympathetic nerve damage (*Horner Syndrome*), iris sphincter inflammation (iritis), or use of a miotic drug (e.g., pilocarpine). Dilatation of one pupil can result from parasympathetic nerve damage (CN-III paralysis from posterior communicating artery

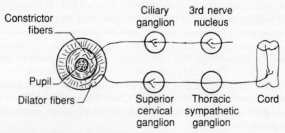

FIG. 14-25 Innervation of the Pupillary Muscles.

aneurysm), iris ischemia from acute, severe increase in intraocular pressure (angle closure glaucoma), damage to the ciliary ganglion (Adie tonic pupil), or a mydriatic drug (e.g., atropine). Artificial eyes are painted with a pupil midway between constricted and dilated resulting in apparent anisocoria.

Relative afferent pupillary defect (RAPD, Marcus–Gunn pupil). There is an asymmetrical decrease in light detection by the retina or in signal transmission through the optic nerve and tract to the geniculate ganglia and Edinger–Westphal nuclei. In the swinging light test (Chapter 7, page 177), both pupils constrict less when light is directed into the pupil of the affected eye than when directed into the unaffected eye.

Argyll Robertson pupil. There is no agreement on the site of the lesion. The classic signs are severely miotic pupils with weak or absent contraction to light that does not improve with dark adaptation but have normal or exaggerated contraction to near point (often and inaccurately referred to as accommodation). The pupils may be irregular and unequal in size. The fully developed Argyll Robertson pupil is almost pathognomonic of tabes dorsalis or taboparesis.

Tonic pupil (Adie pupil). Adie tonic pupil is in the differential diagnosis of anisocoria from a dilated pupil. Reaction to light and near focus are present but extremely sluggish with a prolonged latent period prior to constricting. Response to light may be absent, with a full but tonic response to near point focus. Classically there are sectoral or vermiform movements of both the pupillary border and the related sector of iris stroma, demonstrating the partial parasympathetic denervation of the pupil. It is usually unilateral but can be bilateral. *DDX:* Tonic pupil is most frequent in young women with normal-sized pupils in contrast to the requisite miosis of Argyll Robertson pupils whose response is prompt if minimal.

Unreactive pupil—internal ophthalmoplegia. The pupil does not constrict to either light or near. It is generally dilated and never miotic. Topical mydriatics are the most common cause. Less-common causes are syphilitic meningitis, vasculitis, viral encephalitis, diphtheria or tetanus toxin, lead poisoning, midbrain lesions, bilateral CN III lesions, Adie pupils, iris dysfunction from trauma, and systemic anticholinergic medications, e.g., scopolamine patches, benztropine mesylate.

Unilateral miosis—horner syndrome. This is caused by a lesion in the sympathetic pathway. The complete syndrome is miosis, ptosis, and anhydrosis on the affected side. See page 708.

Other cranial nerve signs
Jaw weakness and spasm—CN-V, trigeminal nerve. Jaw closure is weak and/or asymmetric. The jaw jerk can be absent or hyperreflexic. Irritative lesions of the motor root may cause spasm or trismus.

Facial weakness and paralysis—CN-VII, facial nerve. Because the LMN of the upper lids and forehead are innervated bilaterally by UMN, UMN lesions do not affect the upper lid or forehead. The following observations help localize the lesion from the functional impairments. (1) Face in repose: shallow nasolabial folds in both UMN and LMN; palpebral fissure widens in LMN. (2) Eyebrow elevation and forehead wrinkling: absent in LMN; present in UMN. (3) Frowning: eyebrow lowering is absent in LMN, present in UMN. (4) Tight closing of an eyelid: absent in LMN associated with upturning of the unclosed eye (*Bell phenomenon*); the lids close normally in UMN. When the eyes are tightly closed, weakness of one upper lid is detected by forcing the lids open with the thumb. Irritation of the cornea (*keratitis*) and conjunctivae (*keratoconjunctivitis sicca*) results from inadequate lid closure. (5) Showing teeth: the lips do not retract fully in either UMN or LMN (Fig. 14-5C). (6) Whistling and puffing cheeks: absent or diminished in both UMN and LMN. Weakness causes pocketing of food in the cheeks and difficulty with mastication. (7) A natural smile: the lips and corners of the mouth do not fully elevate with LMN lesions. The paralysis is overcome by movements responding to emotion, so a symmetrical smile may occur in UMN disease. Abnormalities of taste accompany LMN lesions. Facial spasm (clonic facial muscle contractions) may occur following partial facial muscle denervation. The cause of peripheral facial nerve palsies is usually not established. It occasionally occurs in sarcoidosis, tumors of the temporal bone and cerebellopontine angle, poliomyelitis and post-polio syndrome, neoplasms, infectious polyneuritis (Guillain–Barré syndrome), Lyme disease, herpes simplex, AIDS, and syphilis. In the *Ramsay–Hunt syndrome*, varicella-zoster virus infects the geniculate ganglion of the sensory branch of the facial nerve producing a facial palsy, loss of taste on the anterior two-thirds of the tongue, and pain and vesicles in the ipsilateral external auditory canal. Herpetic lesions in the ear canal is the clue to diagnosis. Idiopathic facial nerve paralysis is *Bell palsy*.

Abnormal corneal reflex—CN-V and CN-VII. The bilateral corneal reflex tests CN-V and CN-VII on the side stimulated and CN-VII consensually. With an afferent (CN-V) lesion, the response from both sides is depressed. With an ipsilateral efferent (CN-VII) lesion, the direct reflex is lost, but the consensual is preserved.

Abnormal hearing—auditory nerve (CN-VIII). See Chapter 7, page 245.

Abnormal balance—auditory nerve (CN-VIII). See Chapter 7, page 245.

Dysarthria—glossopharyngeal (CN-IX) and/or vagus (CN-X) nerve. Patients have difficulty with articulation and the pharyngeal phase of swallowing. Exam shows poor and/or asymmetric soft palate and uvula elevation. Absent elevation indicates bilateral paralysis. Unilateral injury causes the uvula to deviate toward the strong side (see Fig. 14-5D).

Dysphagia—glossopharyngeal (CN-IX) and/or vagus (CN-X) nerve. See Chapter 7, page 251. Laryngeal paralysis (CN-X, recurrent laryngeal nerve) can result in coughing or reflux into the posterior nose when swallowing liquids.

Hoarseness—vagus nerve (CN-X). See Chapter 7, page 232. Hoarseness may indicate unilateral vocal cord paralysis, whereas dyspnea and inspiratory stridor are associated with bilateral paralysis.

Weak head rotation and shoulder shrug—CN-XI, accessory nerve. Sternoclei-domastoid and trapezius weakness produce weak head rotation and shoulder shrug.

Tongue deviation and wasting—CN-XII, hypoglossal nerve. The tongue protrudes by tensing the two lateral muscle bundles; paralysis of one bundle causes the tongue to deviate to the paralyzed side (see Chapter 7, Fig. 7-62, page 228). With longstanding lesions, the two halves of the tongue are of unequal size because of muscle atrophy.

Motor Signs: Most abnormal movements reflect normal muscles responding to abnormal uncoordinated neural control signals.

Weakness—muscle paralysis, paresis, and palsy. *Paralysis* is complete loss and *paresis* is diminished muscle power from abnormalities of the UMN, LMN, peripheral nerve, or muscle fibers. *Palsy* is a nonspecific descriptive term indicating varying degrees of paralysis and/or paresis. Increased tone and uninhibited reflexes (spasticity) occur with UMN lesions, whereas LMN and peripheral nerve lesions result in flaccid paralysis and muscle atrophy. Primary muscle disease is associated with flaccid paralysis and variable changes in muscle bulk. Take a careful history delineating the onset of paralysis: acute, subacute, or chronic. Muscle wasting results from disuse; muscle atrophy, indicated by fasciculations, from LMN denervation.

CLINICAL OCCURRENCE: *Congenital:* Porphyria, muscular dystrophy, familial periodic paralysis, paramyotonia congenita, cerebral palsy; *Endocrine:* Hyperthyroidism; *Degenerative/Idiopathic:* Noninflammatory myopathies; *Infectious:* Poliomyelitis, post-polio syndrome, West Nile virus; *Inflammatory/ Immune:* Guillain–Barré syndrome, chronic idiopathic demyelinating polyneuropathy, myasthenia gravis, polymyositis, dermatomyositis, multiple sclerosis (MS), vasculitis; *Mechanical/Traumatic:* Brain and spinal cord trauma, peripheral nerve trauma; *Metabolic/Toxic:* Electrolyte disturbances (high or low potassium, magnesium, calcium, low copper), drugs (muscle relaxants, anesthetics, aminoglycosides rarely), heavy metal poisoning, beriberi, anemia, pernicious anemia, amyloidosis; *Neoplastic:* Epidural metastases; *Neurologic:* Polyneuropathy, transverse myelitis; *Psychosocial:* Hysteria, malingering; *Vascular:* Stroke, spinal cord infarction, subdural and epidural bleeding, vasculitis.

Muscle wasting. Loss of the trophic effect of motor nerves on muscle fibers results in the severe muscle wasting typical of LMN lesions. Less wasting results from peripheral nerve injury and much less with UMN lesions. Wasting becomes apparent weeks to months following the nerve injury. *Fasciculations* are seen with LMN lesions but not with UMN lesions. Generalized weakness and wasting accompanied by fasciculations, often most evident in the tongue and small hand muscles, along with UMN signs, suggest primary motor neuron disease, e.g., amyotrophic lateral sclerosis. Segmental disease is characteristic of poliomyelitis, West Nile virus, and diseases of the spinal cord and nerve plexuses.

Decreased muscle tone—hypotonia. Decreased resting muscle tone occurs with LMN injury, such as poliomyelitis, a root syndrome, and peripheral neuropathy. It is also encountered with cerebellar and other central lesions.

Increased muscle tone—hypertonia. Extrapyramidal lesions, such as parkinsonism, produce increased resting muscle tone. Three types are common. *Cogwheel rigidity:* On passive limb motion muscular resistance is felt as a series of stepwise relaxation–arrest cycles, rather than a smooth giving way. It disappears during sleep. *Lead pipe rigidity:* There is constant resistance to passive movement throughout the range of motion. *Clasp knife rigidity:* Initial resistance to passive movement suddenly gives way, like shutting a clasp knife. All can be seen with Parkinsonism; cogwheeling is an early sign.

Myoclonus. A single sudden jerk, or a short series occurring in succession, may be so powerful as to throw the patient to the floor. Unlike tremor, myoclonus may not disappear with sleep and is frequent at sleep onset. It is a common complication of chronic meperidine use and other metabolic encephalopathies.

Myotonia. The muscles continue in contraction after a voluntary or reflex action has ceased. Relaxation of a contraction induced by tapping a muscle belly with a reflex hammer is prolonged. After shaking hands, the fingers are slow to relax. When the fingers are flexed on the supinated palm, attempted extension is slow and difficult. Myotonia is typical of myotonia congenita and myotonic dystrophy.

Tetany. The threshold for muscular excitability is lowered such that involuntary painless or painful sustained contractions occur. Any cause of a low ionized serum calcium can result in tetany, including hypoparathyroidism, acute hyperventilation, and hypomagnesemia. The contracting muscles feel rigid and unyielding. Spasm may be preceded by numbness and tingling in the lips and limbs. Contractions of the hands and feet are collectively termed *carpopedal spasm*. In carpal spasm, the wrist is flexed and flexion at the metacarpophalangeal joints is combined with extension of the interphalangeal joints. The hyperextended fingers are also adducted to form a cone with the thumb flexed on the palm. In *latent tetany*, carpal spasm may be induced by occluding the brachial artery for 3 minutes with an inflated blood pressure cuff, the *Trousseau sign*. Tapping the facial nerve against the bone just anterior to the ear produces ipsilateral contraction of facial muscles, *Chvostek sign*. It is uniformly present in latent tetany but also occurs in some normal persons.

Fasciculation and fibrillation. Damage to the nerve supplying a muscle leads to spontaneous motor unit firing visible as *fasciculations*. *Fibrillations* are invisible twitches of individual muscle fibers detected by electromyography. Coarse twitches are often caused by cold exposure, fatigue, or other conditions, and are not serious. Fasciculations are not powerful enough to move a joint or a part, so the muscle must be at rest to see them. When associated with muscle wasting and/or weakness, fasciculations indicate muscle denervation.

Reflex Signs
Clonus and spasticity. Normal central spinal cord inhibition limits stretch reflexes to a single beat. Without this inhibition the reflex becomes self-perpetuating. *Spasticity* occurs with complete loss of cortical inhibition and

leads to sustained contraction of opposing muscle groups, the flexors dominating in the arms, and the extensors in the back and legs. A hyperactive reflex can produce *clonus*, rhythmic muscle contraction triggered by stretching. During the acute stage after injury, as in spinal shock, stretch reflexes are absent. When a spastic limb is moved the resistance may suddenly cease, giving a *clasp-knife* effect. Chronic spasticity results in a shortened fibrotic muscle, a contracture. Clonus may be unsustained, just a few jerks, or sustained, persisting as long as stretch is applied. Pyramidal tract lesions almost invariably cause complete suppression of the superficial skin reflexes caudal to the level of the lesion.

Ankle clonus. With the patient's knee flexed, grasp the foot and briskly dorsiflex it. Rhythmic gastrocnemius and soleus contractions make the foot alternate between dorsiflexion and plantar flexion (Fig. 14-12C).

Patellar clonus. With the patient supine and the relaxed lower limb extended, grasp the patella and push it quickly distal. The patella will jerk up and down from the rhythmic quadriceps femoris contractions.

Wrist clonus. Grasp the patient's fingers forcibly hyperextending the wrist, the wrist alternates rhythmically between flexion and extension because of the contracting wrist flexors.

Hoffmann sign—finger flexor reflex. This uninhibited muscle stretch reflex, by itself, has low sensitivity and specificity for cervical spinal cord compression. Hold the patient's pronated hand in your left hand, with fingers extended and relaxed. Support the patient's extended middle finger by your right index finger held transversely under the distal interphalangeal joint crease (Fig. 14-26B). Flick the patient's fingernail with your right thumb to quickly flex distal IP joint. Thumb flexion and adduction is abnormal, Hoffmann's sign is present. The other fingers may also flex. When present bilaterally, it may be a normal variant.

Babinski sign. See Plantar Reflex, page 639. Babinski sign is a pathologic response to noxious stimuli in or spreading to the S1 dermatome resulting

 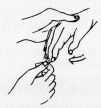

A. Grasp reflex   B. Hoffman sign   C. Mayer reflex

FIG. 14-26 Some Pathologic Reflexes. See text for descriptions. **A. Grasp reflex.** With lesions in the premotor cortex, the patient may be unable to release their grip. **B. Hoffmann sign.** With pyramidal tract disease, the patient's thumb may flex and adduct asymmetrically. **C. Mayer reflex.** The hand is relaxed and supinated hand. Firmly flex the ring finger at the metacarpophalangeal joint. The normal response is adduction and flexion of the thumb which is absent in pyramidal tract disease.

from loss of central spinal cord inhibition. Partial responses include only great toe dorsiflexion, failure of the small toes to abduct or fan, and fanning of small toes without great toe dorsiflexion. Complete and partial responses indicate differing degrees of pyramidal tract disease, so record the details of each response. Alternate methods of eliciting this reflex include *Oppenheim sign,* great toe dorsiflexion elicited with pressure applied by the thumb and index finger or knuckles to the anterior tibia beginning at the proximal third and continuing to the ankle, and *Chaddock sign* in which a dull point scratches a curve around the lateral malleolus then along the dorsolateral foot.

Primitive reflexes, release signs. Each sign, though sometimes present in normal individuals, may indicate diffuse cerebral disease.

Grasp reflex. Though normal in infants, it indicates a premotor cortex lesion in adults. Lay your index and middle fingers across the patient's palm between the thumb and index finger. Gently pull them across the palm with a stroking motion. Grasping with the thumb and index finger is a positive response (Fig. 14-26A). The patient cannot release the fingers at will.

Palmomental reflex. Scratching or pricking the thenar eminence causes ipsilateral contraction of the chin muscles.

Snout/suck reflexes. Scratching or gentle percussion on the upper lip induces puckering or a sucking movement.

Spinal automatisms. Spinal automatisms occur in severe brain or spinal cord disease when central reflex inhibition is lost.

Mass flexion reflex. In extensive cord and midbrain lesions painful stimulation of a limb produces ipsilateral flexion of both upper and lower extremities, called ipsilateral mass flexion reflex, spinal withdrawal, or shortening reflex.

Mass reflex. A transverse cord lesion produces flexion followed by extension of the limbs below the level of lesion. In complete transection, only flexion occurs, accompanied by contractions of the abdominal wall, incontinence of urine and feces, and autonomic responses including sweating, flushing, and/or piloerection. This complex is a *mass reflex.* Involuntary urination may be stimulated by stroking the skin on the thighs and abdomen, an *automatic bladder.* Priapism and seminal ejaculation may be induced as well.

Other spinal automatisms. Flexion of one limb triggers extension of its counterpart, the *crossed extensor reflex.* Pressure on the sole causes leg extension, the *extensor thrust reaction.* When the leg is placed in flexion, scratching the skin on the thigh induces leg extension. Painful stimulation of the arm or chest may cause arm abduction and outward rotation of the shoulder.

Signs of meningeal irritation. Meninges irritated by meningitis, subarachnoid hemorrhage, drugs, or increased intracranial pressure induce involuntary coordinated muscle contraction to splint the meninges when movement would aggravate the painful inflammation. *Nuchal Rigidity:* The patient

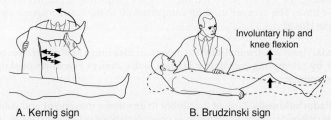

FIG. 14-27 Two Signs of Meningeal Irritation. A. Kernig sign. With the patient supine, flex the hip and knee, each to ~90 degrees. With the hip immobile, attempt to extend the knee. In meningeal irritation, this attempt is resisted and causes pain in the hamstring muscles. **B. Brudzinski sign.** Place the patient supine holding the thorax down on the bed. Attempt to flex the neck. With meningeal irritation this causes involuntary flexion of the hips.

cannot place the chin on the chest. Passive flexion of the neck is limited by involuntary muscle spasm, whereas passive extension and rotation are normal. *Kernig Sign:* With the patient supine, passively flex the hip to 90 degrees while the knee is flexed at about 90 degrees (Fig. 14-27A). Attempts to extend the knee while keeping the hip in flexion produce pain in the hamstrings and resistance to further extension. *Brudzinski Sign:* With the patient supine and the limbs extended, passively flex the neck. Hip flexion is a positive Brudzinski sign (Fig. 14-27B).

Opisthotonos. In extreme cases the spinal muscles go into tetanic contraction, producing rigid hyperextension of the entire spine with the head forced backward and the trunk thrust forward, *opisthotonos.*

POSTURE, BALANCE, AND COORDINATION SIGNS

Cerebellar Signs

Ataxia. Disorders involving the cerebellum, proprioception, labyrinth, and vision can result in poorly coordinated movements. Uncoordinated movement or maintenance of posture is *ataxia*. If present lying down, it is *static ataxia*. If the ataxia is only evident on standing or moving, it is *kinetic ataxia*. Cerebellar ataxia is not ameliorated by visual orientation. Ataxia from posterior column disease involves disordered proprioception; it is partially compensated by a wide stance and worsens when the eyes are closed. Proprioceptive ataxia may only appear when the eyes are closed, e.g., Romberg sign.

Cerebellar ataxia. The gait is staggering, wavering, and lurching, and uncompensated by vision. A lesion in the mid-cerebellum or vermis produces instability in all directions. When one lateral lobe is involved, staggering and falling are toward the affected side, and partially compensated by a wide base gait. Ataxia secondary to vestibular disease can be similar.

Impaired proprioception. A lesion in peripheral sensory nerves (e.g., diabetes) or posterior column of the spinal cord (e.g., vitamin B_{12} and copper deficiency, tabes dorsalis) impairs proprioception. The gait and stance are wide-based.

In walking, the feet are lifted too high and are frequently set down with excessive force. The eyes are used for compensation so the ataxia increases with the eyes closed.

Apraxia. *Apraxia* is the inability to convert an idea into a skilled act. It is best tested by attempting previously learned skills. Perfect execution of skilled acts is *eupraxia*.

Dysdiadochokinesis. Loss of the ability to arrest one movement and substitute its opposite, *dysdiadochokinesia*, is characteristic of cerebellar disease (see page 640).

Dyssynergia and dysmetria. Failure to coordinate the contraction of synergistic muscles during a movement is *dyssynergia*. Inability to control the distance, power, and speed of a movement is *dysmetria*. Finger-to-Nose Test: In cerebellar disease, this action is attended by an action tremor. Performing the maneuver with the eyes closed tests the position sense in the shoulder and elbow. Heel-to-Shin Test: In cerebellar disease, the arc of the heel to the knee is jerky and wavering, the knee is frequently overshot, and an action tremor accompanies the slide down the shin. In posterior column disease, the heel may have difficulty finding the knee, and the ride down the shin weaves side-to-side, or the heel falls off altogether.

Romberg sign. Stable standing with the eyes closed requires normal labyrinthine function, position sense, cerebellar function, and strength. Persistent labyrinthine stimulation or loss of position sense leads to unsteadiness, arm elevation for balance, or a fall. With labyrinthine stimulation, the patient falls in the direction of endolymph flow. Inability to maintain balance with the eyes open suggests an abnormality of the labyrinth, cerebellum, or sight. Record the sign as Romberg present or absent.

Positive past pointing test. Deviation to the right or left of the target fingers, *past pointing*, indicates either labyrinthine stimulation or loss of position sense. The endolymph flow is in the direction of the past pointing.

Gait Disorders

Foot drop—steppage gait. The foot slaps onto the floor due to paralyzed dorsiflexors. Compensating for the toe drop, the thigh is raised higher, as if walking upstairs. Unilateral foot drop is usually the result of peroneal nerve injury. Polyneuropathies, poliomyelitis, cauda equina lesions, and Charcot–Marie–Tooth disease cause bilateral dorsiflexor weakness.

Hemiplegic gait. The affected leg is extended at the hip, knee, and ankle, and the foot inverted. The thigh swings in an arc laterally (*circumduction*) or the inverted foot is pushed along the floor.

Spastic gait, scissors gait. With paraparesis, increased adductor tone pulls the knees together and the trunk leans away from the stepping limb so the foot can clear the floor. The feet may alternately overstep each other laterally, crossing the line of travel with each step.

Festinating gait—Parkinson gait. See page 697. The trunk and neck are rigidly flexed and arm swing is diminished or absent, on one or both sides. To avoid falling forward, the short shuffling steps become faster chasing the center of gravity, *festination*. Turns are slow and in-block, without the head rotating on the trunk or the trunk on the pelvis.

Magnetic gait. The stance is wide, and the steps are short and shuffling. The feet are not lifted from the floor, as if held down by magnets. This indicates diffuse cerebral disease or multisystem damage.

Waddling gait—muscular dystrophy. The patient walks with a broad base. To compensate for quadriceps weakness, the thighs are thrown forward by rotating the pelvis. Bilateral hip dislocations create a similar gait.

Gait ataxia and dementia. Gait ataxia in patients without dementia is associated with a significantly increased risk for developing non-Alzheimer dementia over several years.

Movement Disorders

Tremors. Poorly coordinated contractions of opposing muscle groups are unable to maintain stable posture and/or smooth movement resulting in oscillating movements at one or more joints. The amplitude is either fine or coarse, and the rate rapid or slow. Movements are rhythmic or irregular. All tremors disappear during sleep. Examine the affected part in repose with the muscles relaxed, while maintaining a posture against gravity, and with movement.

Essential tremor. This is an accentuation of the normal fine motor movements made to maintain posture. It is accentuated with increased adrenergic stimulation of muscle and may be a familial trait. The tremor is rapid and fine, absent is repose, and accentuated by trying to maintain a posture. Everyone has this tremor, but usually at an amplitude not apparent by inspection. The tremor is accentuated by anxiety and is characteristic of hyperthyroidism and alcohol withdrawal.

Parkinson tremor. See Parkinson Disease, page 697. The tremor is present at rest and diminished or absent with movement. It is slow and coarse, often described as "pill-rolling" from the characteristic finger and wrist movements. Parkinson disease tremor always starts unilaterally.

Cerebellar tremor, action or intention tremor. Poor coordination of movement-associated muscle contractions leads to limb oscillation, often accentuated when attempting fine control. Voluntary movements initiate and sustain a slow oscillation of wide amplitude. Action or intention tremor occurs in multiple sclerosis and cerebellar disease.

Tics. Normal movements of muscle groups, such as grimacing, winking, or shoulder shrugging, are repeated at inappropriate times. Each patient's tics are stereotypic. Tics are acquired behavioral habits or a sign of organic disease, e.g., Tourette syndrome. They may be abolished by diverting the patient's attention and they disappear during sleep.

Dyskinesia. Dyskinesias are complex abnormalities of muscle movement mediated centrally. Several characteristic patterns are recognized.

Chorea. Rapid, purposeless, jerky, asynchronous movements involve various body parts. Although some are spontaneous, many are initiated by a voluntary movement. All are accentuated by voluntary acts, such as extending the arms or walking. They disappear with sleep. Sydenham chorea is associated with rheumatic fever. Huntington disease is hereditary, and the chorea is more coarse and bizarre than in Sydenham chorea.

Athetosis. Athetosis is slower than chorea and writhing, resembling the movements of a worm or snake. They disappear with sleep. The distal parts of the limb are more active than proximal parts. Grimaces are more deliberate than in chorea. The grotesque athetoid hand is produced by flexion of some digits with others extended. The mechanism is not understood. Athetosis is associated with basal ganglia disease and is induced by levodopa treatment for Parkinson disease.

Hemiballismus. One side of the body manifests sustained, violent, involuntary flinging movements of the limbs. These result from a lesion in the contralateral *subthalamic nucleus of Luys,* usually secondary to stroke. They disappear with sleep.

Asterixis. When the arms are held straight forward from the shoulders with the fingers and wrists extended and fingers spread, there is sudden loss of wrist and interphalangeal extensor tone. The loss and regaining of tone results in a flapping motion. The fingers deviate laterally and exhibit a fine tremor. A similar flap occurs at the ankle when the leg is elevated and the foot dorsiflexed. Ask the obtunded patient to squeeze two of the examiner's fingers; asterixis is felt as an alternately clenching and unclenching grip. Asterixis occurs in any form of metabolic encephalopathy including liver failure, uremia, and hypercapnia.

Muscle cramps—dystonias. See page 703.

Synkinesias. *Synkinesias* are complex involuntary muscle activations that normally accompany voluntary acts. Examples include swinging the arms while walking, facial movements of expression, and motions accompanying coughing and yawning. Frequently, these are lost in disease of the pyramidal tract or basal ganglia. For example, the patient with parkinsonism walks without swinging the arms. An early sign of corticospinal tract damage may be loss of synkinetic movements. Knowledge of normal and abnormal patterns of synkinesis can assist in the identification of the patient with factitious neurologic illness. The detailed testing of synkinesis is beyond the scope of this text. The reader should consult textbooks of neurologic diagnosis.

Sensory Signs: Peripheral and/or central nervous system injury can cause loss of normal sensory modalities. The distribution of the sensory loss, the modalities affected, and the presence or absence of motor involvement distinguish peripheral nerve from plexus, root, and central injury.

Pain and temperature sensory loss. Pain and temperature fibers cross near their entry into the cord. Disruption of the crossing fibers leads to loss of these modalities with preservation of other regional sensation. Ask the patient to distinguish between hot and cold. Temperature and pain discrimination is lost in syringomyelia whereas tactile sense is retained.

Tactile extinction. In parietal lobe disease, the patient accurately perceives touch applied to the right and left consecutively, but extinguishes the perception on the affected side when the stimulus is applied simultaneously to both sides.

Position and vibration sensory loss. Damage to the posterior columns of the spinal cord results in impaired proprioception leading to abnormalities in stance and gait. Posterior column diseases include vitamin B_{12} or copper deficiency and tabes dorsalis.

Analgesia and hypalgesia. Decreased (*hypalgesia*) or absent (*analgesia*) pain sensation indicates damage to the peripheral or central pain pathways. The distribution of lost sensation (e.g., peripheral nerve vs dermatome) indicates the level of the lesion. Look for loss of other modalities, especially temperature and touch.

Hysterical anesthesia. Hysteria may be revealed by marking the borders of an area of anesthesia. Stimulate from the center to the border in a zigzagging line and then in the opposite direction. Repeat after examining other areas. A disparity between successive tests supports this diagnosis.

Hyperesthesia. *Hyperesthesia* is increased sensitivity to a sensory stimulus. Stroke the skin lightly with a pin or, alternatively, gently lift a skin fold off the underlying tissue without squeezing it. The sensation is more intense, but not painful in areas of cutaneous hyperesthesia.

Hyperalgesia. *Hyperalgesia* is increased sensitivity to a painful stimulus disproportionate to the strength of the stimulus.

Allodynia. Allodynia indicates damage to the sensory pathways, usually in the dorsal root or spinal cord; it is not a sign of peripheral nerve injury. *Allodynia* (*allo* = differing from normal; *dynia* = pain) is the perception of pain with stimuli that are normally not painful such as light touch or vibration. Patients complain of pain with the touch of clothing or bedding and in the feet with weight bearing. To elicit allodynia, lightly touch and stroke the skin and apply a vibrating tuning fork to the suspected area. *DDX:* Allodynia is common with post-herpetic neuralgia, diabetic radiculopathy, and complex regional pain syndrome.

Astereognosis— loss of integrative function. Inability to recognize familiar objects by touch is *astereognosis*. If the primary sensory modalities are intact, it is a sign of cortical disease, an inability to integrate the multiple inputs.

Autonomic Nervous System Signs

Temperature regulation. See Chapter 4, page 46. Some instances of hyperthermia occur from hypothalamic or high cervical cord lesions. Hypothermia is encountered in insulin shock and myxedema, although the role of the autonomic system in the latter condition is doubtful.

Perspiration. Localized areas of sweating may occur in syringomyelia, peripheral nerve injury, or neuropathy. *Anhidrosis* is a component of Horner syndrome, autonomic insufficiency (severe combined degeneration), and anticholinergic medications or poisoning. Increased perspiration can be seen with use of β-blockers.

Trophic disturbances. Loss of autonomic innervation leads to functional deficiencies of the skin's sweat and oil glands. The skin becomes shiny, smooth, thin, and dry. The skin is more vulnerable to injury and infection, especially when combined with decreased protective pressure and pain sensation. Painless ulcers may develop over bony prominences of the feet in peripheral neuropathy from diabetes or tabes dorsalis, and syringomyelia (Fig. 14-16F).

Pilomotor reactions. Scratching the midaxillary skin produces pilomotor erection (gooseflesh). The normal response is abolished below the level of a transverse cord lesion. An exaggerated reaction may occur on the affected side in hemiplegia.

Blood pressure regulation. See Chapter 4, page 67. Orthostatic hypotension without tachycardia is common with autonomic nervous system diseases.

Bladder and bowel function. Patients with autonomic nervous system diseases often lose control of bladder and bowel function producing incontinence and/or urinary and fecal retention.

Some Peripheral Nerve Signs

Weak ankle plantar flexion—tibial nerve palsy (sciatic component). The tibial nerve is the motor nerve to the *gastrocnemius* group and *intrinsic muscles in the sole of the foot*. Paralysis causes a calcaneovalgus deformity from the unopposed action of the dorsiflexors and evertors (Fig. 14-19A); plantar flexion and inversion of the foot are weak, and the ankle jerk is absent. Since the nerve is sensory to the skin of the sole, damage results in an anesthetic sole vulnerable to pressure ulcers.

Weak ankle dorsiflexion—common peroneal nerve palsy (sciatic component). The common peroneal nerve is the motor nerve to the muscles of the anterior and lateral compartments of the leg and the short toe extensors, and it is sensory to the dorsum of the foot and ankle. Peroneal paralysis causes an equinovarus deformity with inability to dorsiflex the foot and toes, a foot drop (Fig. 14-28B). Anesthesia covers the dorsum of the foot, sometimes extending up the lateral side of the leg. The nerve is susceptible to pressure injury where it winds around the fibular head.

Lack of knee extension—femoral nerve palsy. The femoral nerve is the motor nerve for the *quadriceps femoris*. When the nerve is injured, patients cannot walk, and standing is unstable. Knee extension is impossible (Fig. 14-19C). Anesthesia is widespread over the anteromedial aspect of the thigh, knee, leg, and the medial foot.

Shoulder weakness—dorsal scapular nerve paralysis. The nerve supplies the *rhomboids* that elevate and retract the scapula. These muscles ascend obliquely from the medial border of the scapula to the spinous processes of the upper thoracic vertebrae. Although covered by the trapezius, they can be palpated when the shoulders are drawn backward.

Winged scapula—long thoracic nerve paralysis. The nerve supplies the *serratus anterior* that holds the scapula to the thorax. Paralysis produces a

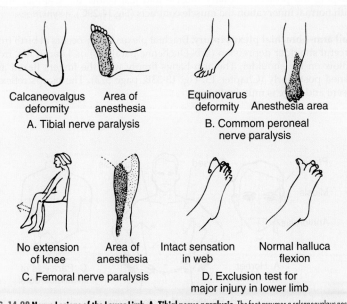

Calcaneovalgus deformity   Area of anesthesia

A. Tibial nerve paralysis

Equinovarus deformity   Anesthesia area

B. Commom peroneal nerve paralysis

No extension of knee   Area of anesthesia

C. Femoral nerve paralysis

Intact sensation in web   Normal halluca flexion

D. Exclusion test for major injury in lower limb

FIG. 14-28 Nerve Lesions of the Lower Limb. A. Tibial nerve paralysis. The foot assumes a calcaneovalgus posture from paralysis of the plantar flexors. The sole of the foot is anesthetic (green). **B. Common peroneal nerve paralysis.** The foot assumes an equinovarus position; it cannot be dorsiflexed—a foot drop. The dorsum of the foot and frequently the lateral aspect of the leg, are anesthetic (green). **C. Femoral nerve paralysis.** The knee cannot be extended when sitting. The region of anesthesia covers the major portion of the anterior thigh and medial aspect of the leg. **D. Exclusion test for major nerve injury in lower limb.** Sensation is intact in the web between the great toe and second toe; great toe extension (dorsiflexion) is normal.

winged scapula when the patient pushes forward against a wall (Chapter 13, Fig. 13-33A, page 573).

Inability to initiate arm elevation in abduction—suprascapular nerve paralysis. The nerve supplies the *supraspinatus* and the *infraspinatus*. Paralysis results in weakness in the first 30 degrees of shoulder abduction and of external rotation. Wasting of these muscles is appreciated as depressions above and below the scapular spine.

Weak arm elevation in abduction—axillary nerve paralysis. The *deltoid* is paralyzed and atrophied. Elevation of the arm above 30 degrees in 90 degrees of abduction is impossible. A patch of sensory loss on the lateral aspect of the shoulder is often found. This injury can result from humeral neck fracture, shoulder dislocation, or scapula fracture.

Weak adduction and depression of the arm—anterior thoracic nerve paralysis. This nerve supplies the *pectoralis major and minor*. Paralysis is demonstrated when the patient presses the hands down on the hips (Fig. 14-29B).

Weak adduction and depression of the arm—thoracodorsal nerve paralysis. This nerve innervates the *latissimus dorsi*. Ask the patient to cough while grasping the posterior axillary muscle fold just below the scapular angle. With normal innervation the muscle contracts (Fig.14-29C), a *synkinesis*.

Flail arm—brachial plexus injury. Brachial plexus injury occurs at birth from forceful shoulder depression (Erb–Duchenne paralysis) or, later in life, from a blow on the shoulder. The arm hangs limply with the fingers flexed and turned posteriorly (Chapter 13, Fig. 13-33B, page 573). The biceps reflex is absent and there is muscle wasting.

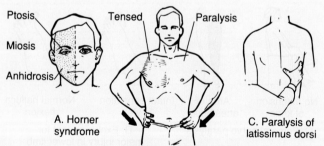

FIG. 14-29 Nerve Lesions of the Upper Trunk. A. Horner syndrome. Injury to the superior cervical sympathetic ganglion on one side causes ipsilateral eyelid ptosis, miosis, and anhidrosis of the face. **B. Paralysis of the pectoralis major muscle.** Injury to the anterior thoracic nerve causes paralysis of the pectoralis major and minor muscles. When the patient presses the hands down on the hips, the normal pectoralis muscle tenses but not the paralyzed one. **C. Paralysis of the latissimus dorsi muscle.** The examiner grasps the latissimus muscles and asks the patient to cough. A paralyzed muscle does not tense with coughing.

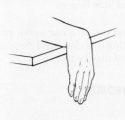
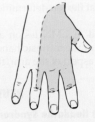

Wrist drop   Area of anesthesia

FIG. 14-30 Radial Nerve Paralysis. The wrist extensors are paralyzed the hand drooping when placed at the end of a table with no support, a wrist-drop. The region of anesthesia includes the dorsal aspect of the radial three digits (green shading).

Weak elbow flexion—musculocutaneous nerve paralysis. The *biceps brachii* and *brachialis* are supplied by this nerve. Paralysis can usually be demonstrated by inspecting the arm while the elbow is flexing against resistance. A small area of anesthesia occurs on the volar forearm.

Weak arm, wrist, and finger extension—radial nerve paralysis. Motor deficits depend upon the level of injury. Injury in the axilla causes paralysis of the *triceps brachii, anconeus, brachioradialis,* and *extensor carpi radialis longus.* A lesion at the upper third of the humerus spares the triceps whereas damage between the upper third and 5 cm above the elbow also spares the brachioradialis. Innervation of the wrist extensors may be injured at a lower level. Any lesion involving the *extensor carpi radialis longus* prevents fixation at the wrist in grasping, producing a wrist-drop (Fig. 14-30A). Paralysis of the *extensor digitorum communis* prevents extension of the wrist and fingers with thumb and finger drop. When the deep branch of the radial nerve is injured, radial deviation of the wrist may occur without wrist-drop. Sensory loss on the dorsum of the hand is quite irregular, but it usually includes the dorsum of thumb to first phalanx and web (Fig. 14-30B). Injury results from external pressure on the nerve in the spiral groove of the humerus (*Saturday night palsy*) or from fracture of the humerus.

Weak flexion of thumb and fingers—median nerve paralysis. The nerve is exposed to trauma in the antecubital fossa. It supplies the flexors of the wrists, digits, and forearm pronators, all innervated below the elbow: *pronator teres, pronator quadratus, flexor carpi radialis, flexor digitorum sublimis, flexor digitorum profundus* (except the fourth and fifth digits), *flexor pollicis brevis, flexor pollicis longus, opponens pollicis, lumbricals, abductor pollicis longus,* and *abductor pollicis longus brevis.* The most common site of median nerve entrapment is at the carpal tunnel (Carpal Tunnel Syndrome, page 702).

Weak finger adduction—ulnar nerve paralysis. The ulnar nerve is most vulnerable near the elbow where it curves posteriorly around the medial epicondyle. The chief motor disability is loss of the finer intrinsic hand motions. Inspection shows an abduction deformity of the little finger from paralysis of the interossei, interosseous muscle wasting, and partial clawhand from inter-phalangeal flexion deformities of the ring and little fingers.

Clawhand. A LMN lesion at the brachial plexus or ulnar nerve produces paralysis of the intrinsic hand muscles resulting in a clawhand. Sensation on the ulnar aspect of the arm, forearm, and hand may be lost.

NEUROLOGIC SYNDROMES

Recurrent Headache Syndromes

Migraine. The pathogenesis is uncertain, but genetic factors are important. Some patterns have a defined genetic basis, for example, 50% of patients with familial hemiplegic migraine have an identified genetic abnormality. Spreading cortical depression is characteristic, perhaps initiated in the trigeminal projection system of the brainstem. Vascular constriction and dilation occur in many, but not all patients; constriction can rarely lead to ischemic cerebral events. Release of substance P and neurogenic inflammation may play a role. Serotonin, dopamine, and noradrenaline are all important in migraine and blocking their receptors is used in treatment. It is a heritable disorder, more common in women than in men, with periodic unilateral headache frequently preceded by an aura (*classic migraine*). Generalized throbbing headache is associated with nausea, light and sound sensitivity, and frequently allodynia ipsilateral to the headache. The prevalence of migraine is estimated to be up to 25% in the United States. Patients with migraine have an increased incidence of Raynaud phenomenon. Onset is usually in adolescence but may occur at any age; many have experienced motion sickness in childhood. The attacks occur from a few times a year to several times per week. Periods of frequent attacks may be separated by periods of no or few attacks. Often, migraine is coincident with some phase of the menstrual cycle. The clinical pattern varies so much among individuals that everyone must be considered separately. Persons with recurrent "sick" or "sinus" headaches, without definite documentation of infection, most likely have migraine.

Migraine with aura (classic migraine). Migraine with aura has four phases. **Prodrome:** An attack is often triggered or preceded by a period of anxiety, tension, or sluggishness. Triggers include bright lights, loud noise, strong odors, skipped meals, various foods and beverages, and inadequate sleep. **Aura:** A day or so before the attack, the patient may feel depressed or feel a sense of unusual well-being; occasionally, hunger is noted. Migrainous phenomena are typically unilateral but are occasionally bilateral; the side may vary in different attacks. Patients tend to repeat their distinctive aura in successive attacks. A *scintillating scotoma*, usually involving both visual fields, presents as flashing lights; sometimes there are black and white wavy lines, like the shimmering made by heat waves rising from pavement. *Fortification spectra* may be exhibited, with zigzag colored patterns with dark centers moving slowly across the visual field. Distinct patterns of the aura are associated with migraine variant syndromes (see *Migraine Variants*, below). Some patients experience a typical aura without a succeeding headache. Other neurologic symptoms occurring during the aura define special migraine syndromes discussed below. **Headache:** The attack may begin any time of the day or night; it is frequently present on awakening. Usually, as the aura diminishes, unilateral headache appears on the side opposite to unilateral visual or somatosensory symptoms during the aura. The pain may start above one orbit and spread over the entire side of the head to the occiput and neck, or it may begin in the back of the head and move forward. Rarely, the site of pain is below the eye, in front of the ear, behind the mandibular angle, in the nape, or in the shoulders. Over an hour, the pain spreads and intensifies to a severe throbbing, boring, aching headache. Constant nonthrobbing pain occurs in 50% of patients. The pain is often augmented by reclining and lessened by sitting or standing. Shaking the head, coughing, or straining at stool intensifies the pain. Although the pain may be severe, it usually does not disrupt sleep. The pain is usually lessened by lying in a dark, quiet room. Nausea and, less commonly, vomiting often accompany the headache. *Photophobia, phonophobia,* and annoyance from odors (*hyperosmia*) are common during the headache. During the headache the patient may appear normal or be incapacitated with cold limbs and pale skin. Lacrimation, conjunctival injection, nasal congestion, and rhinorrhea are not rare, leading to the misattribution of "sinus headache." The duration of the paroxysm is usually from 2 to 6 hours. It is relieved by sleep. **Recovery:** When an attack terminates with sleep, the patient awakens without headache experiencing a sense of buoyancy and well-being. **DDX:** The diagnosis is easy in a long-established case with relatively typical symptoms. When the onset is recent and the symptoms unusual, other intracranial disorders must be excluded. *Ophthalmoplegic migraine* can simulate an aneurysm in the circle of Willis. Although hemiplegia can be a migrainous phenomenon, more serious causes should be sought.

Migraine variants. These variant forms of migraine are distinguished by the pattern of the aura.

Migraine without aura (common migraine). The onset is slower than classic migraine and the duration is often longer, 4–72 hours. It may persist through sleep. The headache is unilateral or bilateral. In other respects, common and classic migraines are similar. There is considerable overlap of common migraine and tension type headache.

Ophthalmic migraine. This rare disorder may have scotomata that are succeeded by momentary blindness, *anopsia*, in the entire field, or in the lower or upper quadrants; or the pattern may be bitemporal or homonymous hemianopsia.

Ophthalmoplegic migraine. Transient unilateral oculomotor nerve paralysis (CN-III) produces lateral deviation and ptosis. This occurs in young girls.

Basilar artery migraine. The scotomata and anesthesia of the face and limbs are bilateral, and vertigo or CN palsies may be present from ischemic brainstem nuclei. The transition from aura to headache may be accompanied by momentary loss of consciousness or light sleep.

Hemiplegic migraine. This is spectacular but rare. Paralysis is most likely to occur in migraine patients who experience paresthesias. The right side is more often involved. The patient complains of numbness or woodenness of the affected limbs. Although weakness may be the complaint, it may only be manifest by exaggerated muscle stretch reflexes and Babinski sign. The paralysis lasts 10–40 minutes but may persist for 2–3 days. Usually there are no permanent sequelae. The diagnosis is strongly supported by a family history of hemiplegic migraine.

Cluster headache. The headache is produced by dilatation of branches of the internal carotid artery innervated by the trigeminal nerve, especially those supplying the meninges. Although the syndrome can be simulated by the injection of histamine into the internal carotid artery, there is no conclusive evidence that histamine plays a role in the natural disorder. Cluster headache is five to six times more common in men than women with onset typically in the third or fourth decade of life. A family history of migraine or cluster headaches is not uncommon. Cluster headache is most commonly episodic occurring several times a day or week for several weeks, with long intermissions between episodes. However, it may be chronic with the cluster persisting for more than a year without intermission. The headache begins without aura and lasts 15–120 minutes (average 40 minutes). It is unilateral, severe, boring, and throbbing. It recurs consistently on the same side. It is usually maximal just inferior to the medial canthus of the orbit but may occur in the temple or side of the face, and it may spread to the neck and shoulder. Flushing, edema and sweating of the skin, lacrimation, conjunctival injection, nasal congestion, rhinorrhea, partial Horner syndrome, and temporal artery dilatation may occur on the affected side. *DDX:* Paroxysmal hemicrania is briefer and more common in women. In Raeder syndrome, the pain is identical in quality but is persistent without discreet attacks. Trigeminal neuralgia is much briefer lancinating pain, though overlap syndromes exist.

Paroxysmal hemicrania. The cause is unknown; women are more commonly affected than men. It is more often chronic than episodic. The headache is indistinguishable from cluster headache, but the pattern is distinct. Headaches are short, lasting on average 15 minutes, more frequent, up to 40 times per day, and uniformly abolished by indomethacin.

Tension-type headache. Though pain is traditionally attributed to sustained contraction of the neck, head, and shoulder muscles, this is unsubstantiated. Chronic intermittent headaches occur in the occiput and temporal regions, often with tenderness in the neck and trapezii. Usually the pain has recurred irregularly for many years, without periodicity. The sensation is described as mild or moderate discomfort, vise-like, a heavy feeling, a sense of pressure, a tight band, cramping, aching, or soreness; it is steady rather than throbbing. The pain is not augmented by coughing, straining at stool, or shaking the head. It usually begins in the occiput extending upward to the temporal regions and down the nape to the shoulders. It may last for a few hours, with intensification near the day's end; or it may persist for many days, waxing and waning throughout. The onset of an episode is often related to emotional strain or to occupational activity. The pain is relieved by external support of the head, the application of hot packs or massage to the neck and mild analgesics. Tenderness may be found in the upper border of the trapezii or the intrinsic neck muscles. *DDX:* The symptoms and signs are characteristic. Tension-type headaches are the only type not intensified by coughing or straining at stool; they are also the only type ameliorated by shaking the head. It is common to have features of both tension type and migraine headache.

Chronic daily headache—transformed migraine, rebound headache. Long-term analgesic use leads to rebound headaches when use is interrupted for a few hours. This common cause of chronic daily headache occurs in patients with a history of tension-type or migraine headache who have developed daily persistent headache relieved only temporarily by medication. A history of regular daily use of prescription or over-the-counter analgesics and the absence of aura, neurologic findings, or other causes of headache are the keys to diagnosis. Overuse of caffeine in migraineurs will also precipitate chronic daily, rebound headaches. The treatment is complete abstinence from analgesics for 2 weeks. Migraineurs should not use analgesics more than 2 days a week.

Ice cream headache. See Chapter 7, page 240.

Intracranial Traction, Displacement, and Inflammation Causing Headache: The pain-sensitive intracranial structures are the dura and arteries at the base of the brain, the cerebral arteries in the same region, the great venous sinuses, and certain nerves (CNS-V, IX, X, and C1–C3). The greater portion of the dura and cranium is insensitive. Mechanisms producing intracranial headaches include: (1) traction on superficial cerebral veins and venous sinuses, (2) traction on the middle meningeal arteries, (3) traction on the basilar arteries and their branches, (4) distention and dilatation of intracranial arteries, (5) inflammation near any pain-sensitive region, and (6) direct pressure or traction by tumors on cranial and cervical nerves. The resulting headaches may be throbbing when arteries are involved; otherwise the pain is steady. Headaches are often intensified by head movements, certain postures, and rapid changes in CSF pressure.

Brain tumor. Benign and malignant intracranial neoplasms compress and place traction on surrounding structures. Headache may be the first symptom. It can be intermittent or constant. The pain may be mild or excruciating and occur anywhere in the cranium. The headaches are not characteristic of any defined headache syndrome. *Pulse synchronous tinnitus* identifies raised intracranial pressure. *DDX:* Brain tumor should be considered with new headaches, especially with persistent and worsening rather than episodic pain, a recent change in a customary headache pattern, or an apparent migraine aura persisting after the headache subsides.

- **Meningitis.** See CNS Infections, page 697.
- **Brain abscess.** See CNS Infections, page 698.

Lumbar puncture headache. CSF leaks out through the lumbar puncture hole in the dura, decreasing the CSF volume suspending the brain. A few hours or days after a lumbar puncture, a constant or throbbing, usually bifrontal or suboccipital, deep headache begins. Moderate neck stiffness may occur. The pain is intensified when standing, shaking the head, or with bilateral jugular vein compression. It is lessened by lying down and flexing or extending the neck.

Idiopathic intracranial hypertension. Symptoms resemble those of a brain tumor. CSF pressure is elevated with no structural abnormality. The typical patient is a young obese woman with recent rapid weight gain. Papilledema is present and, if longstanding, the disks may be pale. Transient *visual obscurations* are common. Prompt diagnosis and therapy are necessary to prevent permanent vision loss. The headache is like common migraine, except often daily. *Pulse synchronous tinnitus* is commonly present indicating increased intracranial pressure.

Intracranial Bleeding Headaches

Epidural hematoma. In a young person, trauma lacerates the middle meningeal artery before the dura is firmly attached to the skull. The resulting lenticular hematoma, expanding between the skull and the dura, compresses the brain. This is always the result of trauma. Pain is from the temporal parietal skull fracture. Loss of consciousness, progressive mental clouding, or focal motor and/or sensory defects suggests epidural hemorrhage; urgent head CT is mandatory.

Subdural hematoma. This is most common in older adults. Decreasing brain volume with aging increases traction on the veins spanning the space between the mobile arachnoid and brain and the dural sinuses which, at this age, are fixed to the skull. Trauma tears these small veins producing low-pressure bleeding and a slowly accumulating hematoma. After a severe head injury, the immediate accumulation of blood in the subdural space is not unexpected and offers no diagnostic difficulty. However, minor head trauma may be followed by a latent period of days, weeks, or months before the appearance of headaches or other neurologic symptoms. The progression, timing, and attributes of the pain are like a brain tumor with relatively rapid expansion. Often no physical signs are present initially; later, there are localizing signs of an expanding intracranial mass. Drowsiness, confusion, or coma may appear without headache or other signs, especially with bilateral frontal subdural hematomas. The diagnosis is confirmed by CT or MRI imaging.

- **Intracerebral hemorrhage.** Hypertensive intracerebral bleeding is usually from deep striatal vessels, rarely is it subarachnoid. Cerebral amyloid angiopathy, weakening vessel walls, is associated with intracerebral hemorrhage without preceding hypertension. In half the patients, onset is marked by a sudden, severe, generalized headache, followed by rapidly evolving neurologic signs. Frequently, the patient vomits; often, there is nuchal rigidity. Seizures and/or coma may supervene. The sequence of events and neurologic manifestations vary with the site and volume of hemorrhage. Putamen: A sensation of intracranial discomfort is followed in 30 minutes by dysphagia, hemiplegia, and sometimes anesthesias. Thalamus: Hemiplegia and hemianesthesias with dysphasia, homonymous hemianopsia, and extraocular paralyses are common.

Cerebellum: Slowly developing occipital headache with repeated vomiting, vertigo, paralysis of conjugate lateral gaze, and other ocular disorders. Pons: Prompt unconsciousness and death within a few hours. Contributing conditions to consider are hypertension, aneurysm (traumatic, inflammatory, saccular or mycotic), angiomas, cerebral amyloid angiopathy, eroding neoplasm, cerebral infarction (embolism, thrombosis), hemorrhagic disorders, primary CNS lymphoma, and coagulation defects.

- **Subarachnoid hemorrhage.** Subarachnoid hemorrhage usually results from rupture of a saccular (berry) aneurysm of the circle of Willis. Often, rupture is preceded by leakage, in contrast to arteria; rupture from hypertension. New onset of severe headache between age 14 and 50 suggests a ruptured aneurysm; prompt diagnosis and therapy can be lifesaving. If seen, CN-III signs always suggest a ruptured aneurysm. The neck may be stiff, but a supple neck does not exclude a ruptured aneurysm. The patient usually reports having the worst headache of his life. Excruciating generalized headache may be succeeded by nuchal rigidity, coma, and often death. Small hemorrhages may be missed, especially in patients with normal mental status, leading to adverse clinical outcomes.

Other Headaches

Thunderclap headache. Thunderclap headache is a severe excruciating headache of sudden onset maximally intense within seconds. A first severe headache meeting this description requires urgent evaluation. If accompanied by altered level of consciousness, nausea, visual changes, vertigo, paralysis, or paresthesias, a serious intracranial problem is likely. Classically attributed to subarachnoid hemorrhage, it occurs with intracerebral hemorrhage, migraine, cluster headache, stroke, with intercourse (*coital headache*), cerebral venous thrombosis, or cerebral vasoconstriction syndromes.

Hypertensive headache. The evidence points to segmental dilatation of external carotid artery branches. With mild to moderate hypertension, headache types and incidence are no different than in normotensive persons. The diastolic pressure must be >120 mm Hg to cause headache. In accelerated hypertension without encephalopathy, half of the patients experience headache. The headaches are often occipital and there is no aura.

Headache present on awakening. Headaches present on awakening suggest migraine, carbon monoxide poisoning, sleep apnea, and analgesic rebound headache. Tension headaches are not present on first awakening.

- *Carbon monoxide poisoning.* Elevated carboxyhemoglobin levels from inhaling carbon monoxide gas decrease tissue oxygenation. Products of combustion are inhaled in poorly ventilated spaces, e.g., cars with malfunctioning exhaust systems, homes with malfunctioning gas furnaces or wood stoves, and burning charcoal in an enclosed space. Symptoms are headache, dizziness, nausea and vomiting, confusion, and visual disturbances progressing to obtundation, coma, and death. The skin and mucosa are cherry-red, the pulse is bounding, and hypertension, muscle twitches, stertorous breathing, and dilated pupils are common.

Giant cell arteritis. See Chapter 8, page 361.

Paranasal sinusitis. See Chapter 7, page 248. There is considerable debate as to the incidence of headache related to sinusitis. Many experts believe that many, if not most of the conditions labeled "sinus headache," are migraine. Sinus and nasal symptoms are common in association with both migraine and cluster headache. No consensus has been reached.

Seizures: Seizures are caused by paroxysmal disordered electrical activity in the brain that may be focal, focal in onset with generalization, or generalized at the onset. Seizures are classified as generalized or partial. Partial seizures are those with a focal onset, regardless of whether they eventually generalize.

    CLINICAL OCCURRENCE: *Congenital:* Congenital brain injury; *Endocrine:* Hypoglycemia; *Degenerative/Idiopathic:* Idiopathic epilepsy; *Infectious:* Meningitis, encephalitis, brain abscess, neurocysticercosis; *Inflammatory/ Immune:* Vasculitis; *Mechanical/Traumatic:* Head trauma; *Metabolic/Toxic:* Fever, drug withdrawal (alcohol, barbiturates, benzodiazepines, anticonvulsant medications), amphetamines, cocaine, phencyclidine, theophylline, hypoglycemia, hypocalcemia, uremia, liver failure, hypoxia, penicillins and other β-lactams; *Neoplastic:* Primary or metastatic cancer, insulinoma; *Neurologic:* Epilepsy, degenerative CNS diseases; *Psychosocial:* Drug abuse, physical abuse; *Vascular:* Stroke, vasculitis, hemorrhage.

Evaluating a patient with seizure. When a person seizes, the immediate concern is to prevent injury and support cardiorespiratory function if necessary. A thorough history and examination are essential to exclude other causes of impaired consciousness. In a patient treated for seizures, look for causes of relapse and evaluate adequacy of therapy. For patients with new onset seizures, seek the cause, supplementing the neurologic exam with appropriate imaging and laboratory studies.

Partial seizures. Partial seizures begin within a specific brain region identified by the initial symptoms. They may remain localized, spread to a larger but limited area of the cortex, or progress to a generalized seizure involving both hemispheres. Partial seizures are classified as *simple* if the event is limited to a small portion of one cortex and consciousness is not altered. *Complex* partial seizures involve larger areas of the cortex and consciousness is impaired, although not lost.

Partial motor seizure. The seizures are caused by a focal lesion in the motor cortex. The seizure begins with muscle twitching in a single body region that becomes more violent with increasing amplitude. It may spread to contiguous muscle groups until the entire ipsilateral side develops clonic contractions. The seizure may stop at any stage of spread, or the contralateral cortex may be affected producing a generalized motor seizure. Consciousness is retained unless the attack is generalized.

Partial-complex seizure. The seizure often begins in the temporal lobe producing complex psychomotor symptoms, hence the old term temporal lobe seizures. They are often accompanied by an aura of an abnormal psychic event that can be olfactory, visual, or gustatory disturbances, or déjà vu. The attack lasts from a few minutes to a few hours. Sudden but subtle loss of higher levels of consciousness occurs. The patient becomes unaware of what happens while retaining motor functions and the ability to react in an automatic fashion. The patient may respond to questions, but the answers disclose lack of understanding. This may be the only objective clue. Repetitive movements, which are often stereotyped, may be reported. Patients generally do not become violent or assaultive during an attack. Only occasionally are there tonic muscle spasms of the limbs. Amnesia for the attack is partial or complete. Search for a focal lesion in the temporal lobe.

Secondary generalized seizure. Most major motor seizures begin from a unilateral small focus in one hemisphere then progress to involve the ipsilateral hemisphere and cross the corpus callosum to involve the contralateral hemisphere, producing a secondary generalized seizure. There may or may not be a warning or aura. Several hours or days before the attack a prodrome may be noted, with feelings of strangeness, dreamy states, increased irritability, lethargy or euphoria, ravenous appetite, feeling of impending disaster, headaches, or other symptoms. The prodrome is a partial seizure, and the patient learns its significance. The patient may experience vague epigastric sensations such as nausea or hunger and palpitation, vertigo, or sensations in the head. Any aura or focal seizure reflects focal brain disease. Consciousness is lost suddenly and simultaneously with the epileptic cry from suddenly expelling air through the glottis. The patient is helpless and falls, often incurring injuries. Tonic spasm of all muscles occurs which may be so violent as to fracture bones. Breathing ceases from spasm of the thoracic muscles and cyanosis may be deep. Suddenly, the tonic state subsides, followed by clonic movements that increase in strength with repetition then cease. Foaming at the mouth is the result of forced expulsion of air and saliva. Clonic jaw movements cause biting of the tongue, cheeks, and lips. There may be involuntary defecation and urination. Unconsciousness usually lasts a few minutes but may last hours. On return of consciousness, the patient is confused and amnestic for the seizure and preceding events, and complains of headache, stiffness, and sore muscles. Seizures are frequently followed by a deep sleep.

Generalized seizure. Generalized seizures involve the entire cerebral cortex at onset so they do not have an aura. History from bystanders is critical to determine whether a seizure's onset was generalized or focal.

Absence seizure—petit mal. There is a sudden decrease in or loss of consciousness lasting up to 90 seconds, with no abnormal muscle movements. The patient's eyes are wide open and staring. Full consciousness rapidly and completely returns. During the momentary lapse the patient may be injured, but, since postural tone is not lost, he does not fall to the ground. Subsequently, the patient is vaguely aware of having "missed something."

Major motor seizure—grand mal. Consciousness is lost without warning and the patient is amnestic for the event. Except for the absence of any evidence of focal onset, the seizure is identical to a secondary generalized seizure.

Sudden Unexplained Death in Epilepsy (SUDEP). Patients with epilepsy have an increased risk of sudden death. The causes are not certain but may be linked to centrally triggered cardiac arrhythmias. Traumatic deaths including drowning are also increased.

Transiently Impaired Consciousness: Disturbances of consciousness are classified according to severity. *Lethargy* is drowsiness caused by a condition other than normal sleep. *Stupor* is a somnolent state from which the patient may be momentarily aroused by questions or painful stimuli. *Coma* is the deepest state of unconsciousness in which the patient is motionless and unresponsive to stimuli. *Syncope* is a brief loss of consciousness that is a distinct diagnostic problem. *Confusion* denotes decreased attentiveness and may be present with any level of consciousness. The hallmark of confusional states is impaired perception, memory, and awareness of surrounding. *Delirium* is confusion accompanied by hallucinations. Although delirium is sometimes accompanied by agitation and violent emotional responses, the patient may be quiet and withdrawn.

Narcolepsy. Narcolepsy is idiopathic or secondary to brain injury. There is impaired ability to voluntarily maintain wakefulness associated with immediate onset of rapid eye movement sleep. The idiopathic form usually occurs in young adults and may be associated with sudden loss of motor tone without loss of consciousness (*cataplexy*), inability to move upon awakening (*sleep paralysis*), and visual or auditory hallucinations at sleep onset (*hypnagogic hallucinations*) or on awakening (*hypnopompic hallucinations*). The patient experiences unexpected, inappropriate, and irresistible short spells of sleep. There may be several attacks per day with no deterioration of mentation.

Syncope. Syncope results from transient arrest of cerebral or brainstem functions. This usually results from momentary arrest of effective cerebral or brainstem perfusion. Impaired brain perfusion is caused by ineffective cardiac contraction (myocardial insufficiency or dysrhythmias), peripheral vasodilation producing hypotension, or from vascular reflexes. In the erect position, consciousness is lost when the mean arterial pressure declines to 20–30 mm Hg or when the heart stops for 4–5 seconds. In the horizontal position, more extreme conditions can be tolerated. The patient complains of weak spells, light-headedness, or blackouts. A careful history must be obtained from both the patient and witnesses. The history and initial physical exam are of the greatest usefulness in establishing a specific etiology. Extensive investigations are unlikely to be useful, unless the history or exam direct attention to a specific diagnosis. The most common cause of syncope is the vasovagal or vasodepressor faint. Other considerations are cardiac dysrhythmias (Adams–Stokes attacks—either tachy- or bradycardia), seizure, or autonomic dysfunction with orthostatic hypotension, pulmonary embolism, aortic stenosis, and cerebrovascular disease. Neurogenic causes can nearly always be differentiated with a good history or eyewitness report.

Neurocardiogenic syncope (vasovagal syncope, fainting). Sudden vasodilation leads to cardiac underfilling and forceful myocardial contraction on the underfilled ventricle. This triggers myocardial receptors that reflexively cause strong vagal outflow, leading to bradycardia, further hypotension, and syncope. With recumbency, the venous return improves, and recovery ensues. The attack is induced in healthy persons by fear, anxiety, or pain. A hot environment, fatigue, illness, alcohol consumption, and hunger increase susceptibility. The attack usually has a prodrome that is brief, often beginning with feeling light-headed and unsteady. Yawning, dimming of vision (intraocular pressure collapsing arterioles), nausea and vomiting, and sweating are common. The face becomes pale or ashen. If the patient reclines promptly, the attack may be aborted. The syncopal stage consists of loss of postural tone and impaired consciousness. The patient falls to the floor either slowly or abruptly, usually avoiding injury. The patient may be confused but still hear voices and dimly see the surroundings. Complete unconsciousness lasts for a few seconds to at most a few minutes. Usually the muscles are utterly flaccid and motionless, although sometimes there are a few clonic jerks of arms and legs, but seldom a full tonic–clonic convulsion. Urinary or fecal incontinence is rare. Recovery follows assumption of the horizontal position. During recovery the patient remains weak, but is awake and lucid, the face gradually suffuses with pink, the blood pressure rises, the pulse becomes palpable and accelerated, the breathing deepens and quickens, the eyelids may flutter. The patient awakens with immediate awareness of the surroundings and memory for the prodrome. The muscle weakness persists for some time, so attempts to rise prematurely may induce another attack.

Orthostatic syncope. See Chapter 4, page 67. In the erect position, blood-pooling in the legs is prevented by vasoconstriction mediated through the autonomic nervous system. When there is decreased intravascular volume, or the compensatory mechanism is blocked, blood pools in the legs resulting in arterial hypotension. Distinctive features of autonomic insufficiency are normal heart rate and absence of pallor and sweating. Recovery occurs in the horizontal position.

Adams-Stokes syndrome. Attacks of unconsciousness occur when effective cardiac contractions are absent for >5 seconds in the vertical position or 10 seconds when horizontal. Usually, asystole results during the transition from a partial to a complete heart block or from the onset of paroxysmal tachycardia or ventricular fibrillation. When the heart rhythm is regular and the rate less than 40 per minute, heart block is suggested by variable intensity of the first heart sounds. An ECG is required for confirmation. This form of syncope occurs in any position without a prodrome.

Valvular heart disease. In patients with a fixed cardiac output, vasodilation in muscle with exercise leads to cerebral hypoperfusion and syncope. Exertion induces syncope in severe aortic stenosis or, less commonly, aortic regurgitation or pulmonary hypertension.

Carotid sinus syncope. This occurs most commonly in patients aged >60 years with hypertension or occlusion of one carotid artery. Rotation of the head or a tight collar puts pressure on the carotid bulb, inducing vagal stimulation that results in one of three responses: (1) sinoatrial block, (2) hypotension without bradycardia, or (3) syncope with normal pulse rate and blood pressure.

Syncope related to specific neck movements suggests carotid sinus syncope. Carotid sinus massage is dangerous and should not be used to test the diagnosis as cerebral infarction and death have resulted from this maneuver. Never palpate both carotids simultaneously. *DDX:* Neck rotation may precipitate syncope in patients with severely impaired vertebrobasilar circulation.

Hyperventilation. Hyperventilation results in hypocapnea that decreases cerebral blood flow. Before the attack, the patient is usually anxious or emotionally upset. The patient feels chest tightness or suffocation accompanied by numbness and tingling of hands and face, sometimes with carpopedal spasm. Loss of consciousness may be prolonged compared with most other types of syncope. The symptoms are reproduced by having the patient overventilate. Rebreathing into a paper bag arrests the attack and demonstrates a method of self-treatment.

Cough syncope. Severe paroxysms of coughing, laughing, or vomiting can induce syncope; this is rare in women. The history is usually diagnostic. The mechanism is disputed.

Micturition syncope. Voiding a large volume, particularly after arising from a warm bed, can precipitate syncope. Similarly, rapid decompression of an overfilled bladder by catheterization or the removal of large volumes of ascitic fluid may also cause syncope.

Akinetic epilepsy. Common features in akinetic epilepsy, but rare in syncope, are lack of pallor, sudden onset without prodrome, injury from falling, tonic convulsions with upturned eyes, urinary or fecal incontinence, and postictal confusion with headache and drowsiness.

Hysterical syncope. This is the swoon of Victorian novels. It occurs in the presence of witnesses. The fall is graceful and harmless. The skin color, heart rate, and blood pressure are all normal. The patient lies motionless or makes resisting movements.

Persistently Impaired Consciousness

- **Coma.** Coma results from disruption of the reticular activating system. Coma is a state of prolonged unconsciousness. Since the patient cannot cooperate, evaluation requires a special approach. In most cases, the correct diagnosis is rapidly established by structured physical and neurologic exams combined with imaging and laboratory tests keeping two axioms in mind. (1) Finding one cause for coma is not sufficient. For example, a comatose patient with alcohol on the breath may have sustained a head injury while intoxicated; a person injured in an automobile accident may have had an antecedent stroke leading to the accident; or, an unconscious patient with a few sedative tablets at the bedside may have taken the drug for symptoms of meningitis or brain tumor. (2) A complete neurologic examination is necessary but not sufficient. All other systems must also be assessed. For instance, finding atrial fibrillation raises the possibility of cerebral embolism; the retinae may contain signs of diabetes; consolidated lung suggests lobar pneumonia and pneumococcal meningitis; or, a distended bladder leads to a diagnosis of uremia from bladder outlet obstruction. The differential diagnosis and management of coma is beyond the scope of this text. The reader should consult textbooks of medicine, neurology, and emergency medicine.

History of the comatose patient. Interview the relatives, acquaintances, attendants, or police officers who discovered the patient. Circumstances of Discovery: How was the patient found? Were there any drugs or poisons near-by? Do the surroundings suggest poisoning from carbon monoxide or other fumes? Was there evidence of trauma? What was known about the patient's antecedent intake of food and fluids? Who prepared the food? What were the symptoms and actions before the onset of coma? Did the patient have pain, diarrhea, or vomiting? Past History: Is the patient known to have epilepsy, diabetes, hypertension, or alcohol or drug addiction? Did the patient have suicidal thoughts? Is there a history of mental illness? Is the patient known to be taking medication? Is there a history of malignancy? Is there a history of previous coma?

Examining the comatose patient. Assess airway patency, respirations, and pulse, the ABC's. Vital Signs: Note any abnormalities. General Inspection: Note posture, tremors, and muscle jerks; inspect the respiratory pattern for bradypnea, tachypnea, and Kussmaul or Cheyne–Stokes breathing. Color: Look for pallor, icterus, the cyanosis of methemoglobinemia, the cherry-red color of carboxyhemoglobin. Scalp and Skull: Look for contusions, lacerations, gunshot wounds; palpate for depressed skull fractures and inspect the mastoid for hematoma of basilar skull fracture (*Battle sign*). Eyes: Inspect for periorbital bruising (*raccoon sign*) of basilar skull fracture. Lift the eyelids and let them close; lagging of one lid suggests hemiplegia. The hysterical patient closes the lids tighter resisting opening. In coma, the eyes remain fixed or oscillate slowly side-to-side; in hysteria the don't oscillate but may wander, fixing momentarily. Conjugate deviation of the eyes is toward the side of destructive frontal lobe lesions and away from irritative lesions. Extraocular muscle palsies assist localization of an intracranial lesion. After confirming a normal cervical spine, open the eyelids and quickly turn the head side-to-side. With cerebral damage the eyes turn conjugately in the opposite direction if the brainstem is intact (*doll's eyes*). This *oculocephalic reflex* is lost with pons or midbrain lesions. *Caloric testing* provides similar information: irrigate the ear canal with 30–50 mL of ice water; with cerebral dysfunction and an intact brainstem, tonic conjugate deviation of the eyes lasting 30–120 seconds is toward the cold ear. The bilateral pupils are widely dilated in profound posttraumatic shock, massive cerebral hemorrhage, encephalitis, anticholinergic poisoning, and the end stages of brain tumor. Bilateral pinpoint pupils suggest opiate poisoning or pontine hemorrhage. A unilateral unreactive pupil indicates a rapidly expanding lesion on the ipsilateral side, as in subdural or middle meningeal epidural hemorrhage or brain tumor. Examine the fundi for the exudates and hemorrhages and the choked disks of increased intracranial pressure. Facial Muscles: Facial asymmetry, a drooping mouth and a cheek puffing out with each expiration, may indicate hemiplegia on the affected side. Painful supraorbital notch pressure causes an asymmetric grimace, revealing the weak side. Oral Cavity: Tongue lacerations suggest biting during a seizure. Look for a diphtheritic membrane, pharyngitis, and ulceration or discoloration from poisons. Breath: Smell the breath for acetone, ammonia, alcohol or its successor aldehydes, paraldehyde, and other odors. Ears: Look for pus, spinal fluid, or blood emerging from the external acoustic meatus or blood behind the drum from basilar skull fracture. Neck: Test for signs of meningeal irritation: nuchal rigidity and Kernig and Brudzinski signs. Chest: Percuss and auscultate the chest for pneumothorax, consolidation, wheezing, or crepitation. Heart: Auscultate for rhythm, rate, strength of the heart sounds, and abnormal sounds. Abdomen: Auscultate for bruits and palpate for masses or rigidity suggesting peritonitis or fluid. Limbs: Test each limb successively for flaccidity by lifting it and letting it fall to the bed. If muscle tone is retained, a difference in the two sides indicates a hemiplegia. Reflexes: The reflexes on the paralyzed side are absent during the stage of spinal shock, but in deep coma all reflexes are lost. In deep coma, the Babinski reflex is present bilaterally, so it cannot localize a lesion. If some reflexes are retained, a difference in the two sides is significant. Sensory Examination: Only response to painful stimuli can be evaluated. The patient shows defensive reactions when pricked in sensitive areas, but no response is forthcoming when analgesic regions are stimulated. If the stimulated region is sensitive but paralyzed, a defense or withdrawal movement may occur on the opposite side and the facial expression indicates pain. Deep pressure sense is tested by compressing the Achilles tendon, testis, and supraorbital notch.

The Glasgow Coma Scale (Table 14-1) measures the degree of cerebral dysfunction: 13–15 points is mild, 9–12 is moderate, and 3–8 is severe. Patients with scores <8 are in coma. An alternative coma scoring system has been proposed and validated by one group, the Full Outline of UnResponsiveness (FOUR) Score (Table 14-2). It is used in patients on ventilators and has high interobserver reliability.

Differential diagnosis of coma. The multiple etiologies of coma are conveniently divided into three categories:

Metabolic encephalopathy. Metabolic derangements or toxin exposure impairs cerebral function leading to coma. Coma occurs with normal pupillary responses, normal brainstem reflexes, and no focal neurologic deficits. Asterixis, myoclonus, and Cheyne–Stokes respiration are seen. Examples are hypoglycemia, hypoxia, hypercarbia, hyponatremia, intoxications (e.g., alcohol, benzodiazepines, barbiturates, opiates), hepatic insufficiency, advanced kidney failure, and severe hypothyroidism; there are many others.

Hypoglycemic coma. The prodrome resembles a vasovagal spell but with prominent confusion. The syncopal stage is frequently prolonged, and loss of consciousness is usually incomplete. Instead, there is muscle weakness with mental confusion. The blood sugar is usually <30 mg/100 mL; the symptoms are relieved by the intravenous glucose or glucagon injection.

Transtentorial herniation. A supratentorial mass expands herniating the uncus of the temporal lobe. Typically, the uncus compresses the third nerve and then the midbrain initially producing focal deficits. Progression from the focal

TABLE 14-1 Glasgow Coma Scale

Response		Score
Eyes Open		
_____	Spontaneous	4
_____	To speech	3
_____	To pain	2
_____	Absent	1
Verbal		
_____	Converses/oriented	5
_____	Converses/disoriented	4
_____	Inappropriate	3
_____	Incomprehensible	2
_____	Absent	1
Motor		
_____	Obeys	6
_____	Localizes pain	5
_____	Withdraws (flexion)	4
_____	Decorticate (flexion) rigidity	3
_____	Decerebrate (extension) rigidity	2
_____	Absent	1

deficits to coma and death can be rapid. Commonly encountered etiologies are brain tumor (primary or metastatic), bleeding (intracerebral, subdural, epidural), cerebral edema associated with infarction (arterial or venous), abscess, encephalitis, and massive liver necrosis.

Brainstem injury. The brainstem reticular activating system running from the upper pons to the lower diencephalon is responsible for maintaining consciousness; damage, results in coma. The onset is usually abrupt, either following trauma or acute severe headache. Emergent neuroimaging is required. Trauma and spontaneous hemorrhage are the most common etiologies.

Chronic vegetative state. This condition results from severe injury to the cortex, thalamus, and/or white matter of the brain. The clinical syndrome is wakefulness and sleep without awareness or responsiveness to the environment. The cycling of wakefulness and sleep is distinct from coma.

Minimally conscious state. These patients show some awareness behaviors and imaging suggests that some have considerable awareness without the ability to respond, akin to the locked-in state. Clinicians should always assume comatose patients are able to perceive what is done to them and hear

TABLE 14-2 FOUR Score Coma Scale

Response	Points				
	0	1	2	3	4
Eyes	Eyelids open, tracking and blinking on command	Eyelids open, but not tracking	Eyelids closed but open to loud voice	Eyelids closed but open to pain	Eyelids remain closed to pain
Motor	Thumbs up, fist or peace sign to command	Localizing to pain	Flexion response to pain	Extensor posturing to pain	No response to pain or generalized myoclonus; status epilepticus
Brainstem Reflexes	Pupillary and corneal reflexes present	One puli wide and fixed	Pupillary or corneal reflexes absent	Pupillary and corneal reflexes absent	Absent pupillary, corneal and cough reflexes
Respirations	Not intubated, regular breathing	Not intubated, Cheyne-Stokes pattern	Not intubated, irregular breathing pattern	Breathing above ventilator rate	Breathing at ventilator rate or apnea

Reprinted from Wolf CA, Wijdicks EF, Bamlet WR, McClelland RL. Further Validation of the FOUR Score Coma Scale by Intensive Care Nurses. *Mayo Clin Proc.* 2007;82(4):435-8. Copyright 2007, with permission from Elsevier.

and comprehend what is said at the bedside. The prognosis is very difficult to predict.

Ischemic Cerebrovascular Disease

Transient ischemic attack. Transient ischemic attack (TIA) is the result of decreased perfusion usually from altered hemodynamics or microembolism. Less common causes are in situ arterial thrombosis, arterial dissection, and venous sinus thrombosis. The symptoms reflect the area of ischemia. TIA is, by definition, the acute onset of a focal neurologic deficit in a specific vascular distribution with full recovery within 24 hours. Neurologic signs are absent between attacks. The correct diagnosis and prompt evaluation are important because TIA signals possible impending cerebral infarction: up to 25% of patients with a new TIA will have a stroke within 24 hours. The risk for stroke within 7 days of a TIA is predicted by the $ABCD^2$ score derived from age, blood pressure, clinical features, duration, and the presence or absence of diabetes. *DDX:* Diplopia, syncope, transient confusion, and paraparesis are uncommon symptoms of TIA. The differential diagnosis of TIA includes convulsions, syncope, migraine, focal cerebral masses (e.g., subdural hematoma), cardiac disease, and labyrinthine disorders.

Carotid artery TIA. Symptoms and signs are related to the ipsilateral cerebral hemisphere and/or retina. Findings include contralateral weakness, clumsiness, numbness of the hand, hand and face, or the entire half of the body, dysarthria, aphasia, and ipsilateral *amaurosis fugax* with monocular visual loss, usually described as a shade coming down. Visual loss may be complete blindness or sector visual loss. Carotid bruits or retinal emboli may be found.

Vertebrobasilar artery TIA. Symptoms and signs are related to the posterior circulation and may affect vision and cranial nerve functions. Frequent complaints are combinations of binocular visual disturbance or loss, vertigo, dysarthria, ataxia, unilateral or bilateral weakness, or numbness and drop attacks (sudden loss of postural tone and collapse, without loss of consciousness).

Ischemic stroke. Arterial obstruction by thrombosis, embolism, or dissection produces ischemia and infarction. The area of infarction is surrounded by a penumbra of ischemic tissue which is salvageable with prompt restoration of perfusion. Ischemic stroke is painless, and the patient remains conscious. Symptom onset may be abrupt or stuttering (see TIA). The specific symptoms reflect the functional loci within the distribution of the affected vessel. The *middle cerebral artery* is most commonly affected, the arm being more severely affected than the leg. With *anterior cerebral artery* stroke, the leg is more affected than the arm. *Posterior cerebral* strokes result in homonymous hemianopsia. *Basilar artery* strokes are frequently associated with vertigo, diplopia, dysarthria, or Horner syndrome; hemiparesis is not a feature. *Cerebral venous sinus* thrombosis presents with symptoms and signs of cerebral vascular disease with less discrete evidence of focal lesions. The National Institutes of Health Stroke Scale (Table 14-3) is the preferred tool for evaluating the severity of initial stroke symptoms and signs and response to therapy.

Middle cerebral artery—hemiparesis. Paresis of either the right or left side indicates contralateral disease of the brain or ipsilateral high spinal disease. The most common cause is vascular occlusion of the middle cerebral artery. Paralysis is partial or complete. Sensory loss occurs in the same distribution. Consciousness is not impaired. With right-sided infarcts, the patient may not be aware of the deficit. Lesions in the left hemisphere often affect Broca's area disrupting fluent speech while comprehension remains intact. If the visual pathways are affected, a homonymous hemianopsia is found. *DDX: Conversion Reaction:* In patients with complaints of unilateral weakness or paralysis of the legs but confusing findings, try to elicit the *Hoover sign*, which depends on the absence of a normal associated movement (*synkinesia*). Place the patient supine, stand at the foot of the table, and place a palm under each heel. Ask the patient to raise the affected limb (Fig. 14-13D). In organic disease, the unaffected limb presses downward with the effort to raise the affected limb; this does not occur in conversion reaction. The sign is helpful only when the patient has, or claims to have, paralysis of one leg. Paraplegia must be excluded. Hysterical arm paralysis is identified by dropping the flaccid arm onto the face. With organic paralysis, the arm strikes the face; in hysteria, it always misses.

- **Cavernous sinus thrombosis.** Thrombosis of the cavernous sinus results from bacterial infection of the upper lip, tooth socket, eyes, or face. Patients present with pain in the eye and forehead, chills, fever, and impaired vision. Physical findings include chemosis, edema of the eyelids, exophthalmos, hyperemia, papilledema, orbital tenderness, and palsies of CNs-III, IV, and VI. Progression leads to leptomeningitis, blindness, intracerebral abscess, septicemia, and death.

TABLE 14-3 National Institutes of Health Stroke Scale

Domain	Score					
	0	1	2	3	4	5
Level of consciousness (LOC)	Alert	Drowsy	Stuporous	Coma		
LOC questions: ask month and age	Both correct	One correct	None correct			
LOC commands: close eyes, make fist	Both correct	One correct	None correct			
Best gaze	Normal	Partial gaze palsy	Forced deviation			
Visual fields	No loss	Partial hemianopsia	Complete hemianopsia	Bilateral hemianopsia		
Facial palsy	Normal	Minor	Partial	Complete		
Right arm	No drift	Drift but does not hit the bed	Drifts down to the bed	No effort against gravity	No movement	Amputation or joint fusion
Left arm	No drift	Drift but does not hit the bed	Drifts down to the bed	No effort against gravity	No movement	Amputation or joint fusion
Right leg	No drift	Drift but does not hit the bed	Drifts down to the bed	No effort against gravity	No movement	Amputation or joint fusion
Left leg	No drift	Drift but does not hit the bed	Drifts down to the bed	No effort against gravity	No movement	Amputation or joint fusion
Limb ataxia	Absent	Present in one limb	Present in two limbs			
Sensation to pin	Normal	Partial loss	Severe loss			
Best language	No aphasia	Mild-moderate aphasia	Severe aphasia	Mute		
Dysarthria	None	Mild-moderate	Near to unintelligible or worse	Intubated or other barrier		
Extinction and inattention	No neglect	Partial neglect	Complete neglect			

Reproduced from Lewis SL, Ende J, et al. MKSAP 14: Neurology. 2006, American College of Physicians. www.ninds.nih.gov/doctors/NIH_Stroke_Scale_Booklet.pdf.

Degenerative and Autoimmune CNS Diseases

Parkinson disease and Parkinsonism. Parkinson disease is caused by loss of dopaminergic neurons in the substantia nigra decreasing dopamine delivery to the striatum; some variants are familial. Parkinson disease is one of a family of extrapyramidal motor system conditions presenting with posture and movement abnormalities. The onset of Parkinson disease is asymmetric and gradual. Familial forms exist. Two-thirds of patients have a slow (~6 Hz) repose tremor, usually beginning in one hand, that disappears with movement and sleep. Other classic features are slow voluntary movements (*bradykinesia*), *rigidity, masked face, postural instability*, and a small-stepped gait (*marche au petit pas*) with minimal foot lift, absent arm swing, difficulty turning smoothly, and a tendency to fall forward (*festinating gait*). Other early features include *micrographia*, decreased blink rate, and *anosmia*. Cognitive and emotional disturbances are late findings. **DDX:** Absence of tremor, though not rare, raises the likelihood of another Parkinsonian syndrome. Early cognitive or emotional instability, fluctuating mental status, and hallucinations suggest *Lewy body disease*. Symmetrical onset without tremor but with eye findings, particularly paralysis of upward gaze, and falls suggests *progressive supranuclear palsy*. Orthostatic hypotension, urinary incontinence, and dysarthria, also without tremor, suggests *multisystem atrophy* (Shy–Drager syndrome). Parkinsonism induced by drugs affecting the dopaminergic system (e.g., metoclopramide, antipsychotics, and others) is not uncommon.

Multiple sclerosis. Multifocal demyelination in the nervous system is presumed to be mediated by autoimmunity. The onset is usually abrupt over hours to a few days, with remissions occurring over weeks, if at all. *Optic neuritis* with transient visual loss lasting weeks to months is a common presenting symptom. Other signs, depending upon the location of the demyelinating lesion(s), include incoordination, paresthesias, weakness, loss of sphincter control, ataxia, dysarthria, intention tremor, ocular palsies, visual loss, hyperactive stretch reflexes, diminished abdominal reflexes, and trophic skin changes. The *Charcot triad* is intention tremor, nystagmus, and scanning speech. The disease may be progressive from onset with inexorable loss of function, or relapsing–remitting with complete resolution of the symptoms and signs between relapses. Many patients with initially relapsing–remitting disease progress to chronic progressive disease with incomplete remissions after each relapse.

Neuromyelitis optica—devic syndrome. IgG antibodies to a unique class of CNS membrane aquaporin is thought to be the cause. Symptoms are vision loss, paresthesias, and painful spasticity and weakness in the arms and legs.

CNS Infections

- **Bacterial meningitis.** A generalized, throbbing or constant headache is a prominent early symptom accompanied by fever and stiff neck. The headache may be accompanied or followed by drowsiness or coma. Because the meninges are inflamed, the headache is intensified by sudden head movements. Other signs of meningeal irritation are nuchal rigidity and Kernig and Brudzinski signs. Although many febrile illnesses are accompanied by headache, the headache of meningitis is especially severe. When headache is associated with stiff neck, a lumbar puncture is indicated. Viral meningitis causes headache that is generally less severe and more gradual in onset; *the distinction cannot be made clinically.*

- **Brain abscess.** An encapsulated infection of the brain parenchyma, consisting of liquefied brain and pus, is either hematogenously seeded or extends from a local source. Symptoms and signs of brain mass appear coincident with or after infection in the ears, paranasal sinuses, lungs or, rarely, osteomyelitis, or another source. If the primary infection has not been recognized, the distinction from brain tumor may not be evident until imaging is obtained. Less than half the patients with brain abscess exhibit the classic triad of fever, headache, and focal deficit.

CLINICAL OCCURRENCE: *Direct Extension:* From otitis, sinusitis, and mastoiditis; *Hematogenous:* Pneumonia, endocarditis (especially *Staphylococcus aureus*), osteomyelitis, other bacteremias (patients with cyanotic congenital heart disease and right-to-left shunts are particularly susceptible), systemic arteriovenous malformations; *Penetrating Trauma:* After neurosurgery, gunshot wounds, open skull fractures.

Neurosyphilis. Chronic, tertiary *Treponema pallidum* infection causes degeneration of the spinal-cord's posterior columns, dorsal roots, and dorsal root ganglia. Brain infection produces degenerative brain disease. The patient is often unaware of having been infected and, with many years intervening, the history of a chancre may be lost. Other signs of tertiary syphilis may be present, such as aortitis with aortic insufficiency, and gumma formation. Two CNS syndromes are recognized:

Tabes dorsalis. Spinal cord involvement produces lightning-like pains in the trunk and lower limbs, paresthesias, urinary incontinence, and impotence. There is loss of position sense, ataxic wide-based gait, footdrop, and loss of reflexes. Loss of position sense leads to joint destruction with Charcot deformities. *Tabetic crisis* is abdominal pain and vomiting with a relaxed abdominal wall.

General paresis. Use the pneumonic *PARE-SIS* to remember findings: Personality, *A*ffect, loss of *R*eflexes, *E*ye findings (Argyll Robertson pupil), *S*ensory changes, *I*ntellectual deterioration (*dementia precox*), and *S*peech changes.

- **Rabies.** This neurotropic virus is transmitted by the bite of infected mammals. Onset is marked by local dysesthesia radiating from the entry site, malaise, nausea, and sore throat. Later, restlessness and hallucinations appear. There is hyperesthesia of the wound and later, dysarthria, dysphagia for liquids, convulsions, delirium, and opisthotonos stimulated by lights or noises. Breathing becomes shallow and irregular with hoarseness or aphonia. The stretch reflexes are hyperactive. Nuchal rigidity and Babinski sign are followed by flaccid paralysis and death. A high index of suspicion is required for early diagnosis to prevent contact with body fluids. Many patients diagnosed in the United States do not have an identified source of infection; bats are the most commonly identified source.

Spinal Cord Disorders

Paraparesis. Loss of UMN innervation to both legs indicates a transverse spinal cord lesion. The level is determined by the sensory findings. Frequent causes of paraparesis are trauma and transverse myelitis following viral infection. Extrinsic cord compression by herniated disk, epidural abscess, or neoplasm are less common but potentially treatable. Dural arteriovenous malformations cause venous congestion and spinal cord ischemia without infarction; the deficits are fully reversible if the diagnosis is made and the malformation closed.

Spinal cord hemisection—Brown-Sequard syndrome. Hemisection of the cord damages the ipsilateral descending motor pathways and ascending proprioceptive pathways that cross in the brainstem, and the contralateral sensory pathways for pain and temperature that cross at their spinal root levels. Patients have motor paralysis with spasticity and loss of proprioception on the side of the lesion and absent pain and temperature sensation below the level of the injury on the opposite side.

Quadriparesis. Paresis or paralysis of all limbs without changes in consciousness indicates impairment of the descending corticospinal (pyramidal) tracts. The most common cause is traumatic injury to the cervical spine sparing the bulbar muscles. Less common causes, usually with some bulbar involvement, are multiple sclerosis, primary motor system disease, and botulism. Onset of nontraumatic generalized weakness or paralysis over a few hours or days suggests an electrolyte disturbance (most commonly severe hypokalemia). In the hospital, other causes to be considered are inadvertently high spinal anesthesia, paralytic drugs, and the polyneuropathy of severe illness.

Syringomyelia and Chiari malformations. A cavity expanding within the cervical spinal cord damages centrally crossing sensory and pyramidal tracts. The cause is unknown. Syringomyelia is frequently associated with herniation of the cerebellar tonsils through the foramen magnum (Chiari type-1). Patients present with decreased pain and temperature sensation in the arms and shoulders, LMN weakness in the arms, and UMN weakness with spasticity in the legs. Chiari type-2 malformation (incomplete closure of the spinal canal) is always accompanied by myelomeningocele.

Amyotrophic lateral sclerosis. UMN and LMN degeneration leads to progressive weakness and muscle wasting. The disease begins gradually, proceeds progressively, and ends fatally, usually in 2–3 years. Muscle aches and cramps are accompanied by weak distal upper limbs, spreading to the lower limbs. Dysarthria, dysphagia, and drooling indicate bulbar involvement. Muscle fasciculation and severe wasting are seen, especially in upper limbs. Fasciculations may be evident in the tongue. Hyperreflexia and spasticity of lower limbs indicate UMN involvement [O'Neill GN, Gonzalez RG, Cros DP, Ackerman RH, Brown RH Jr, Stemmer-Rachamimov A. Case records of the Massachusetts General Hospital. Case 22–2006: a 77-year-old man with rapidly progressive gait disorder. *N Engl J Med*. 2006;355:296–304].

Posterior column disease. Deficiencies of vitamin B_{12} and copper and neurosyphilis (tabes dorsalis) lead to degeneration of the posterior columns with loss of proprioception in the lower extremities producing abnormalities of gait and balance. Nitrous oxide anesthesia may precipitate severe B_{12} deficiency in patients with minimal stores. *DDX:* Glossitis, macrocytic anemia, and dementia accompany severe B_{12} deficiency; a spastic gait disorder may accompany copper deficiency.

Peripheral Neuropathies: Neuropathies are classified as *axonal* if the nerve cell axon is primarily involved or *demyelinating* if the lesion is in the nerve's myelin sheath. Single nerve trunk lesions are traumatic, ischemic, or inflammatory. Peripheral nerve dysfunction in the absence of CNS disease is common. Patients present with numbness, burning, unsteadiness (often described as dizziness), falling, or weakness. Physical exam may show sensory impairment (pressure, vibration, position, pain, and temperature or simple touch depending on the size of nerves involved), muscle weakness and wasting with fasciculations, and/or diminished reflexes. Release signs are not present and plantar response is flexor. *Demyelinating neuropathies* present acutely or more slowly with involvement of both motor and sensory nerves; often the motor component dominates with weakness and areflexia. They can involve any nerve at any level from root distally so the pattern is usually asymmetrical involving proximal as well as distal muscles. *Axonal neuropathies* are diffuse, symmetrical, slowly progressive and usually sensory at onset with later involvement of motor nerves; they are primarily distal and progress proximally affecting the feet before the hands. Isolated nontraumatic involvement of all components of a single nerve is called *mononeuritis multiplex*, usually resulting from an inflammatory lesion causing ischemia; recovery is common and complete.

CLINICAL OCCURRENCE: *Congenital:* Charcot–Marie–Tooth disease, porphyria, Fabry disease, familial neuropathy; *Endocrine:* Diabetes; *Degenerative/Idiopathic:* ICU polyneuropathy, idiopathic polyneuropathy; *Infectious:* Leprosy, rabies (early at inoculation site), postherpetic neuralgia; *Inflammatory/Immune:* Acute and chronic inflammatory demyelinating polyneuropathy, vasculitis, SLE, amyloidosis, celiac disease, monoclonal gammopathy; *Mechanical/Traumatic:* Contusion and laceration, repetitive use, vibration (e.g., jackhammers, pneumatic drills), cold injury (chilblains and frostbite), electrical injury; *Metabolic/Toxic:* Amyloidosis, porphyria, diabetes, Fabry disease, poisoning (arsenic, other heavy metals, pyridoxine), drugs (e.g., vincristine), nutritional deficiency (vitamins B_{12}, copper, and B_6); *Neoplastic:* Paraneoplastic syndromes, metastatic invasion of nerves; *Psychosocial:* Substance abuse producing unconsciousness with pressure-induced ischemia; *Vascular:* Vasculitis.

Diabetic neuropathies. Diabetes types-1 and 2 are associated with peripheral nerve injury with a latency of ~15 years from onset for type-1. Damage is thought to be metabolic in most forms and ischemic in the acute reversible forms. Several forms of diabetic neuropathy are recognized.

Distal sensorimotor axonal neuropathy. This is most common, presenting as numbness or burning pain in the feet progressing proximally with loss of protective sensation, trophic skin changes, pressure-induced ischemic ulceration, and infection leading to amputation, if preventive measures are not taken. Limbs at risk are insensitive to 10-g monofilament testing. In severe forms, muscle wasting, and Charcot joints occur.

Autonomic neuropathy. This late onset neuropathy frequently involves the stomach with gastroparesis and delayed gastric emptying which make blood sugar control difficult. Sudomotor injury contributes to skin fragility and ulceration. Impotence is common and colon and bladder dysfunction not rare. The sensorimotor and autonomic neuropathies are delayed or prevented by tight blood glucose control.

Diabetic amyotrophy or polyradiculopathy. This is an acute, painful, inflammatory, or ischemic injury to one or more spinal roots. Patients present with severe back, chest, abdominal or proximal leg pain, and progressive weakness and may have bowel and bladder dysfunction. It is usually acute in onset and asymmetric. Most people recover over months.

Cranial nerve paralysis. This is not uncommon and often mistaken for much more serious intracranial pathology. CNs-III, IV, and VI are most often involved. The pupil is spared in CN-III lesions. Diabetic amyotrophy and CN lesions are not clearly related to the duration of diabetes or degree of blood sugar control.

Acute inflammatory demyelinating polyneuropathy (AIDP)—Guillain–Barre syndrome. This is an immune-mediated demyelinating disorder occurring 1–3 weeks after viral infection, *Campylobacter jejuni* gastroenteritis, or, rarely, after surgery or with malignant lymphoma. There is usually rapidly progressive ascending flaccid paralysis with pain in the back and limbs. Nausea and vomiting can occur. There are diminished deep and superficial reflexes and distal numbness and tingling. CN involvement causes dysphasia, dysphagia, and dysarthria. With chest wall involvement, respiratory failure supervenes.

Chronic inflammatory demyelinating polyneuropathy (CIDP). There is chronic immune-mediated demyelination of nerve roots, plexuses, and peripheral nerves. Multiple nerves may be involved often asymmetrically. Onset is sudden or gradual with motor and sensory symptoms and signs referable to a spinal root, plexus or peripheral nerve. Symptoms may progress gradually or remit and relapse. Weakness and areflexia accompany sensory findings indicating involvement of mixed nerves.

Numb chin syndrome. Malignant cells, most commonly from an aggressive lymphoma, infiltrate the mental or inferior alveolar nerve(s) branches of CN-IX. The patient is usually a young adult presenting with a numb lower lip and chin, no other complaints and the physical exam is normal other than decreased sensation on the chin. The patient should *not* be reassured; further evaluation is indicated.

Compression neuropathies. Nerves are vulnerable to compression injury at sites of frequent motion, trauma, external pressure, or excessive traction. Symptoms are usually pain and dysesthesia initially but may progress to weakness if the nerve is a mixed motor and sensory nerve. Knowledge of the distribution and exact anatomic locations of vulnerable portions of the peripheral nerves greatly assists diagnosis. Reproduction of the symptoms by *gently* tapping the nerve at the sight of compression (*Tinnel sign*) supports the diagnosis; however, all sensory nerves are positive if struck hard enough (e.g., the ulnar nerve "funny bone"). Some common examples are listed below.

Carpal tunnel syndrome. The median nerve is compressed beneath the volar transverse carpal ligament at the wrist (Fig. 14-31) producing dysesthesia and pain, then loss of fine (two-point) sensation, and, finally, thenar muscle atrophy and weakness. The patient complains of numbness and tingling in the hand, particularly at night. There may be associated pain, limited to the hand or running up the forearm. Ultimately, there is progressive weakness and awkwardness in the finer finger movements. It is unilateral or bilateral. Although patients frequently describe tingling of the entire hand, hypoesthesia is distributed on the palmar aspects of the 3.5 radial digits and the distal two-thirds of the dorsal aspects of the same fingers. Light percussion on the radial side of the palmaris longus tendon may produce a tingling sensation (*Tinel sign*, Fig. 14-31). Flexion of the wrists at 90 degrees apposing the dorsal surfaces of the hands for 60 seconds (*Phalen test*) may reproduce the pain (Fig. 14-31). Neither maneuver is particularly sensitive nor specific as measured against nerve conduction studies. The condition is most common with repetitive use injury, e.g., meat-packing workers, grocery clerks, and keyboard operators. Contributing factors to consider are congenitally small carpal tunnel, hypothyroidism, diabetes, acromegaly, pregnancy, osteoarthritis, rheumatoid arthritis, amyloidosis, sarcoidosis, gout, Paget disease, repetitive wrist flexion and extension, posttraumatic arthritis, multiple myeloma, and monoclonal gammopathy of unknown significance (MGUS).

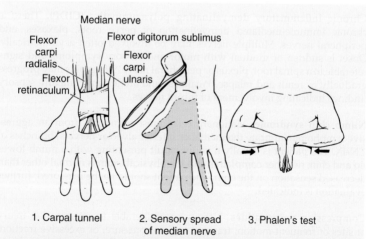

1. Carpal tunnel   2. Sensory spread   3. Phalen's test
                               of median nerve

FIG. 14-31 Carpal Tunnel Syndrome. 1. The carpal tunnel. The flexor retinaculum compresses the median nerve producing hyperesthesia in the radial digits. **2. Tinel sign.** Percussion on the radial side of the palmaris longus tendon produces tingling in the digital region. Tinel sign also applies to tingling induced by tapping any peripheral nerve; it may be normal, e.g., tapping the ulnar nerve at the elbow ("funny bone"). **3. Phalen test.** Hyperflexion of the wrist for 60 seconds produces pain in the median nerve distribution, which is relieved by wrist extension.

Lateral femoral cutaneous nerve—meralgia paresthetica. The lateral femoral cutaneous nerve is entrapped under the anterior superior iliac spine and inguinal ligament or directly compressed by tight fitting belts resulting in lateral thigh numbness. Since it is a pure sensory nerve, there are no motor signs. It frequently occurs with obesity, rapid weight loss, and pregnancy.

Tarsal tunnel syndrome. The posterior tibial nerve is entrapped in the tarsal tunnel under the medial malleolus causing pain and tingling on the sole of the foot and toes aggravated by standing.

Cubital tunnel syndrome. The ulnar nerve is entrapped behind the medial humeral condyle at the elbow. It is aggravated when elbow flexion stretches the nerve. Symptoms are fourth and fifth fingers numbness progressing to weakness of the intrinsic hand muscles.

Radial nerve. The radial nerve is compressed where it wraps around the upper third of the humerus. This is often associated with prolonged unconsciousness because of injury or overdose with the arm weight resting on a hard object. Numbness of the dorsum of the arm and hand is associated with weak finger and wrist extensors.

Common peroneal nerve. The common peroneal nerve wraps around the lateral fibular head where it can be compressed by casts, crossed legs, or pressure during unconsciousness. There is a foot drop and there may be numbness on the lateral calf and dorsum of the foot.

Other Motor and Sensory Syndromes

Dystonia. Dystonias are abnormally prolonged tonic muscle or muscle group contractions. Dystonias are often associated with specific activities and can become disabling. The patient refers to them as cramps. Examples are writer's cramp, torticollis, and dystonias associated with playing musical instruments.

Autonomic neuropathy. Damage to the subcortical autonomic control systems in the hypothalamus and brainstem and/or peripheral nerve damage results in loss of normal autonomic regulation. Patients present with abnormalities of cardiovascular, gastrointestinal, urogenital, and sudomotor function. Decreased functions is more common than overactivity. *Orthostatic hypotension*, not accompanied by a rise in pulse, and not infrequently combined with hypertension when supine, is the most frequent presenting sign. Heart rate and blood pressure responses to Valsalva and carotid massage are blunted. The heart rate does not vary with deep breathing. Other frequent symptoms are constipation or diarrhea, absent or excessive sweating, problems with bladder function (difficulty voiding or incontinence), and erectile and ejaculatory dysfunction. Patients with anhydrosis are susceptible to overheating in warm, especially humid, environments. Longstanding diabetes is the most common association, but multisystem atrophy, subacute combined degeneration, Parkinson disease, Fabry disease, syringomyelia, porphyrias, paraneoplastic neuropathies, and amyloidosis, among others, must be considered.

Myasthenia gravis. An autoantibody binding to the acetylcholine receptor at the neuromuscular junction blocks neuromuscular transmission, especially with repetitive excitation. There is an association with thymoma. Affected individuals complain of increased fatigability, transient muscle weakness, diplopia, ptosis, easy fatigue with chewing and talking, regurgitation, and dysphagia. During an exacerbation there may be lack of facial expression, abnormal speech or aphonia, and disconjugate gaze. In extreme cases, the patient cannot lift his head from the pillow. Acetylcholine is stored while asleep so muscle function is normal, and diplopia absent on awaking. The levator and, to a lesser extent, the other ocular muscles recover after rest. Ptosis is quickly relieved by neostigmine, but the other paralyses do not respond as dramatically.

Lambert–Eton syndrome. Antineuronal antibodies are associated with an occult malignancy. Weakness improves with repetitive action, just the opposite to myasthenia gravis. Nonsmall cell lung cancer is the most common association.

Botulism. Neurotoxins produced by *Clostridium botulinum* are ingested or absorbed from contaminated wounds. Symptoms appear over hours with variable combinations of weakness, headache, dizziness, dysphagia, abdominal pain, nausea and vomiting, diarrhea, and diplopia. Physical findings include fixed and dilated pupils, nystagmus, ptosis, irregular respiration, swollen tongue, hyporeflexia, and incoordination. Improperly home canned foods and wound and skin infections are the most common causes.

Tetanus. Tetanus is caused by the toxin of *Clostridium tetani* acting on the myoneural junctions. A single muscle or many groups become rigid with sustained tonic spasm. The masseter is frequently involved early, hence the term lockjaw (*trismus*). Loud noises, bright lights, or pain induce superimposed violent generalized spasms. The condition should not be confused with tetany, which it resembles only in name.

Disorders of Language and Speech

Aphasia. Language is instantiated in the dominant hemisphere, which is the left hemisphere in >99% of right- and left-handed people. Damage to specific language-processing areas produces distinct aphasias. Language is the symbolic representation and interpretation of meaning in voice sounds and written symbols (*symbolization*). It is a far more complex activity than speech, requiring extensive central interconnectivity. Aphasia is an acquired brain disorder causing inability to use language correctly. Congenital or developmental language disorders are *dysphasias*. Language is evaluated during history taking and with mental status exam. Six domains are assessed: (1) speech expression, both spontaneous and automatic sequences (e.g., singing, nursery rhymes, and cursing); (2) naming; (3) speech comprehension; (4) repetition; (5) reading; and (6) writing.

Broca aphasia. Broca area of the left frontal lobe is damaged. Speech is not fluent; pronouns, prepositions, and the like are often left out. Reading and writing are also affected. Patients are aware of their difficulty and become frustrated. They appear to know what they want to say. Speech comprehension for simple communications is relatively spared.

Wernicke aphasia. Speech is fluent, but words are jumbled and substituted, obscuring all meaning (*paraphasia*). Writing is similarly affected. Reading and verbal comprehension are poor. The patient is unaware of the deficit and may become angry when not understood.

Global aphasia. This is a combination of Broca and Wernicke aphasia.

Alexia, dyslexia and agraphia. Alexia is the inability to read. Dyslexia is an impairment of reading ability. Agraphia is the inability to write.

Other aphasias. See neurology texts for discussion of conduction, anomic, transcortical, and subcortical aphasias.

Speech disorders—dysarthria, dysphonia, ataxia, and apraxia. Normal speech has many qualities, each of which may be specific to an individual, allowing recognition of individual voices. Specific qualities are articulation, phonation, fluency, and repetition.

Dysarthria and dyslalia—articulation. Articulation is the production of sounds and their combinations into syllables. Brain disorders produce *dysarthria*; specific dysarthrias are identified by the sounds which are improperly formed (page 666). *Dyslalia* is impaired articulation from nonneurologic structural defects or hearing loss.

Dysphonia—voice. Dysphonia is disturbance in coordination and control of the larynx and the resonating qualities of the pharynx affecting pitch, quality, and volume. *Hypernasality* and *hyponasality* refer to nasal resonance.

Ataxia—rhythm. This deals with the timing and sequence of syllables. Irregular, slow speech with pauses and bursts of sounds is called *scanning speech* indicating a cerebellar disorder, e.g., MS. Faltering or interruptions in speech are termed *stuttering*; this is frequently inherited or may be a developmental disorder.

Apraxia—sound selection. This is the inability to properly and consistently program a correct sequence of sounds, especially consonants. Have the patient repeat the word "artillery" five times; each sound is formed correctly, but they are misplaced and no two attempts may be alike. The problem is evident with writing as well.

Delirium
Hepatic encephalopathy. Severe hepatocellular dysfunction and/or portal hypertension with portal-systemic shunting allows toxic metabolites to accumulate leading to cerebral dysfunction. This presents four features—only the last two are distinctive: (1) Altered mental state varying from slight memory loss to confusion, slurred speech, sedation, and coma; (2) Asterixis, also present in cerebrovascular disease, uremia, and severe pulmonary insufficiency; (3) Signs of abnormal liver function such as jaundice, palmar erythema, spider angiomata, hepatomegaly, and ascites; (4) When present, *fetor hepaticus*, smelling something like old wine, acetone, or new-mown hay, is distinctive of hepatic coma.

Wernicke–Korsakoff syndrome. Thiamine deficiency is common with alcoholism and symptoms may occur when glucose administration precipitates acute thiamine deficiency (*Wernicke encephalopathy*) leading to chronic brain injury (*Korsakoff syndrome*). Wernicke syndrome presents with confusion, nystagmus, ataxia, ophthalmoplegia, impaired memory, and decreased attention. Immediate recognition and treatment with parenteral thiamine prevents Korsakoff syndrome, an irreversible chronic encephalopathy with antegrade and retrograde amnesia and confabulation. Thiamine deficiency can be a late complication of bariatric surgery.

Impaired Cognition Syndromes

Mild cognitive impairment. Cognitive function is below normal for age but does not significantly impair daily life. Memory is the most frequently observed abnormality. More than half of patients with mild cognitive impairment progress to dementia within five years, others remaining stable for variable lengths of time.

Dementia. Dementia is a decline in cognitive function sufficient to impair function. It includes memory loss (recent more than remote, e.g., loss of orientation) and at least one of the following: aphasia, apraxia, agnosia, or abnormal executive function. It is chronic and usually progressive, although the rate of progression is quite variable. Personality changes and loss of normal social inhibitions are often late findings. Dementia is easily missed early in its course if not specifically sought. There are no early physical findings, the release signs being late manifestations of advanced disease. Screening with the clock drawing task, SLUMS tool (Chapter 15, Fig. 15-1, page 714), or Mini-Cog is useful. *The Folstein MMSE is proprietary, and fees must be paid to use it, so its use is discouraged.* Medical illness can present as dementia, so it is essential to exclude the many potentially reversible medical conditions, e.g., hypothyroidism, other endocrinopathies, medication side effects, and vitamin B_{12} deficiency. There are many causes of dementia, but Alzheimer disease is most common. Most reversible causes are accompanied by some blunting of consciousness.

CLINICAL OCCURRENCE: *Congenital:* Familial Alzheimer disease, adrenoleukodystrophy, Huntington disease, lipopolysaccharidoses, Wilson disease, mitochondrial disease, porphyria, Down syndrome (trisomy 21); *Endocrine:* Hypothyroidism, Addison disease, Cushing syndrome, hyper- and hypoparathyroidism; *Degenerative/Idiopathic:* Alzheimer disease, Pick disease, Lewy body disease, progressive supranuclear palsy, frontotemporal dementias, limbic encephalitis; *Infectious:* HIV infection, syphilis, prion disease (Creutzfeldt–Jacob disease [CJD], bovine spongiform encephalopathy [variant CJD (vCJD)], and others), progressive multifocal leukoencephalopathy (papovavirus), Whipple disease, postencephalitis; *Inflammatory/Immune:* Vasculitis, subacute sclerosing panencephalitis, sarcoidosis; *Metabolic/Toxic:* Chronic alcoholism, vitamin B_{12}, thiamine, and nicotinic acid deficiency, uremia, liver failure, aluminum toxicity (dialysis dementia), postanoxia, drug intoxication; *Mechanical/Traumatic:* Acute and chronic head trauma, normal pressure hydrocephalus, chronic subdural hematoma; *Neoplastic:* Paraneoplastic limbic encephalitis, brain tumors, and metastatic cancer; *Neurologic:* Nonconvulsive seizures, Parkinson disease; *Psychosocial:* Depression (*pseudodementia*), schizophrenia; *Vascular:* Vascular dementias (multi-infarct, Binswanger disease).

Alzheimer disease. Neurofibrillatory tangles and plaques, with extracellular amyloid precursor protein deposition, accumulate in the brain. The cause is partly genetic and possibly partly environmental. Slowly progressive dementia usually begins in the seventh or eighth decade of life; it may occur at younger ages, especially in the hereditary syndromes. The identical syndrome occurs uniformly in patients with trisomy-21 (Down syndrome) at an earlier age, usually in the fourth decade of life. The mental deterioration begins insidiously with memory loss, depression, anxiety, suspicion, and later amnesia, agnosia, aphasia, shuffling gait, and rigidity. The diagnosis is clinical, after excluding treatable forms of dementia. Imaging reveals diffuse atrophy of the cerebral cortex with symmetrical enlargement of the lateral and third ventricles. *DDX:* If severe psychiatric symptoms are present (e.g., hallucinations, psychosis), consider Lewy body disease. If the dementia is rapidly progressive, consider CJD or bovine spongiform encephalopathy (vCJD).

Dementia with lewy bodies. This accounts for ~20% of diagnosed dementias. It is accompanied by fluctuating mental status with periods of delirium separated by more clear times, visual hallucinations and Parkinsonism. Fluctuation is defined as any three of the following: sleeping for >2 hours during the day; daytime sleepiness not related to inadequate nighttime sleep; prolonged staring episodes; and garbled speech with clear words but unorganized content. Patients have more visual spatial problems than Alzheimer patients. Syncope, frequent falls, difficulty sleeping, and depression are common as well. When you feel the need for both a neurologist and a psychiatrist you may be dealing with Lewy body disease.

Normal pressure hydrocephalus. Enlargement of the ventricular system at normal CSF pressure is accompanied by dementia, gait apraxia, and urinary incontinence. The symptoms and signs are reversible with appropriate treatment, so a high index of suspicion should be maintained.

Psychosis. See Chapter 15, page 728.

Other Syndromes
Tourette syndrome. This neurodevelopmental disorder presents in childhood. Patients have a complex array of vocal and facial tics, echolalia, and coprolalia often impairing social function. With conscious effort, the patient can suppress the tics. Obsessive–compulsive disorder and attention-deficit hyperactivity disorder occur in association with Tourette syndrome.

Restless legs syndrome. The cause is unknown but has been reported with iron and folate deficiency and uremia. Familial forms occur. The patient complains of leg discomfort at rest, often prior to sleep. The sensation may be aching, drawing, pulling, prickling, restlessness, formication, or completely nondescript. Always bilateral, the sensations are relieved by walking or massage. There are no pertinent physical findings. Many patients also have periodic limb movements of sleep. Diagnosis is based upon four criteria: onset of symptoms at rest, urge to move, symptoms relieved by movement, and symptoms worse in the evening. Most patients obtain some relief with dopamine agonists.

Horner syndrome. This is caused by a lesion of the cervical sympathetic chain. The following signs are seen on the ipsilateral side: (1) Partial ptosis of the upper eyelid (weakness of Mueller muscle) and some elevation of the lower lid ("inverse ptosis"); (2) Constriction of the pupil, miosis, accompanied by pupil dilation or delay after a light reflex (dilation lag); (3) Absence of sweating on the forehead and face of the affected side (Fig. 14-29A, page 678). If the damage occurs early in life, pigmentation of the iris may be affected; for example, the affected iris may remain blue when the other changes to brown if the patient is brown-eyed. Horner syndrome occurs with an ipsilateral mediastinal tumor and has been reported with spontaneous pneumothorax and brainstem stroke.

Complex regional pain syndrome—reflex sympathetic dystrophy, causalgia. See Chapter 4, page 75.

Repeated bell palsy—Melkersson syndrome. This is a triad of scrotal tongue (*Lingua plicata*) with repeated attacks of Bell palsy and painless, nonpitting, facial edema. The cause is unknown.

Death. Death is an obvious fact of life. Most adults can make a reasonably accurate diagnosis of death, but occasional cases prove complicated. One of the horror stories in medical history is a probably apocryphal episode in the life of Vesalius. In 1564, during the height of his European fame as an anatomist, he was appointed physician to Philip II of Spain. He is said to have conducted an autopsy in Madrid on a young nobleman who had been his patient. According to the custom of the time, this was carried out before a large crowd of citizens. When the thorax of the body was opened, the heart was seen to be beating, and the anatomist was compelled to leave Spain hastily. Such experiences have made it necessary to have a physician or other trained person pronounce death. Biological death is the cessation of function of all bodily tissues. In the process of dying, tissues and organ functions deteriorate at varying rates, so a precise time of death is difficult to define. For ordinary purposes, it is conclusive to recognize the irreversible cessation of circulatory, respiratory, brain, or brainstem functions. This is partially assessed by unconsciousness and absence of vital signs (cardiac activity, respirations, and maintained body temperature). However, these indicators have proved inadequate in victims of cold-water drowning, when unconsciousness, apnea, and imperceptible heartbeat are still compatible with resuscitation and full recovery. Different criteria are also required for patients receiving mechanical respiration and cardiac pacing.

Death examination for most patients. Examine for evidence of heart contraction by palpating for pulsations in the carotid arteries and auscultating the precordium for heart sounds. An ECG will determine if cardiac electrical activity is present in the absence of mechanical contraction. Search for respiratory activity by placing the diaphragm of your stethoscope over the patient's mouth listening for breath sounds. Also, holding a cold mirror at the nostrils and mouth can detect exhaled water vapor. Several tests assess neurologic function: call to the patient to test responsiveness; retract the eyelids observing the pupillary reaction to light (fixed dilated pupils are seen with death and some drug intoxications); with the lids retracted, rotate the head side-to-side observing whether the eyes remain fixed in their orbits or move in conjugate (doll's eyes), indicating an intact brainstem; if there are no eye movements, perform ice water caloric stimulation; press the sternum and squeeze the Achilles tendons looking for a deep pain response; lift and let the limbs fall testing muscle tone; check for gag and corneal reflexes.

Supplementary death examination, especially for near-drowning and patients on mechanical ventilation, and/or pacemakers. Victims of cold-water immersion drowning experience rapid total body cooling (severe hypothermia) and may meet all the preceding criteria of death yet still be capable of resuscitation with excellent neurologic function after immersion of up to 1 hour. A reasonable practical guideline is that such patients are not dead until they are warm (core temperature >35°C) and dead. Other patients needing special consideration are those sustained by mechanical ventilation and pacemakers who fail to meet the cardiac and respiratory criteria for death, but who may be dead by irreversible loss of brain function. The clinician should always seek consultation from a neurologist in these complicated clinical situations.

CLINICAL VIGNETTES AND QUESTIONS

CASE 14-1

A 37-year-old woman is brought to the ER with inability to stand because of leg weakness. She had been recovering from an upper respiratory tract infection. Her neurological examination reveals bilateral grade 2/5 muscle strength in proximal and distal leg muscles. Leg muscle stretch reflexes are absent and passive leg movement shows marked hypotonia.

QUESTIONS:
1. What is the most likely diagnosis?
2. What is a functional anatomic approach to a patient with muscle weakness?
3. What symptoms differentiate proximal from distal weakness?
4. How do you distinguish between upper and lower motor neuron lesions?

CASE 14-2

A healthy 45-year-old man notices a right facial droop. On examination facial asymmetry is evident and some saliva has accumulated at the right corner of the mouth. When he attempts to close his eyes, his right eye does not close, although it rolls upward. He is unable to show his teeth or inflate his cheek on the right. The remainder of the neurologic examination is normal.

QUESTIONS:
1. What is the most likely diagnosis?
2. How do you test for facial weakness?
3. What differentiates an upper motor neuron (central weakness) from a lower motor neuron lesion (peripheral weakness) as the cause of this presentation?
4. What is Ramsay Hunt syndrome?

CASE 14-3

A 24-year-old man presents to the emergency department after experiencing a syncopal episode while running a marathon. He has been healthy. While taking the family history he tells you that his grandfather died of unknown cause at the age of 30.

QUESTIONS:
1. Describe the pathophysiology of syncope?
2. What is the differential diagnosis of a syncopal episode which occurs with exertion?
3. What is the most likely cause of this patient's syncopal episode?
4. Which pathophysiological states can result in cardiac syncope?

CASE 14-4

A 56-year-old man on long-term haloperidol for schizoaffective disorder presents with oral, facial, and lingual dyskinesia including protruding and twisting movements of the tongue, pouting, and puckering of the lips.

QUESTIONS:

1. What is this movement disorder called?
2. What are the risk factors for developing this movement disorder?
3. What is the underlying pathophysiology for this movement disorder?
4. What is tardive dystonia?

CASE 14-5

You are seeing a 45-year-old man with leg weakness, paresthesias, ataxia, and loss of vibration and position sense. His hemogram last year showed a macrocytic anemia.

QUESTIONS:

1. What causes loss of position and vibration sense?
2. What conditions specifically affect position and vibration sense?
3. Clinically, how might you differentiate between B12 deficiency and copper deficiency?

CASE 14-6

You are evaluating a 50-year-old man for a sudden onset headache with nausea which started 30 minutes ago and reached its maximal intensity within a few seconds. He has never experienced a headache like this before.

QUESTIONS:

1. What is this type of headache called?
2. What is the most urgent diagnostic consideration?
3. What are other potential etiologies for this presentation?

CHAPTER 15

The Mental Status, Psychiatric, and Social Evaluations

Psychiatric and social disorders frequently confound patient evaluation in medical settings. A psychiatric diagnosis in no way decreases the probability of organic disease in a patient with appropriate signs and symptoms. We must strive to simultaneously, not sequentially, diagnose and appropriately treat coexisting psychiatric and medical illnesses. Delayed diagnosis of organic disease in patients with psychiatric illness is all too common; clinicians must take extra care evaluating these complicated patients. Consult with a psychiatric colleague whenever there is concern for a confounding psychiatric disorder.

The distinction between neurologic and psychiatric illness is likely an artifact of our limited understanding of brain physiology and pathophysiology. Disorders with identifiable structural, genetic, physiological, or biochemical disorders are considered neurologic and those without psychiatric. Many psychiatric syndromes show genetic predispositions and respond to medications that alter brain function. Functional imaging studies are increasingly identifying localized abnormalities of brain function in some psychiatric disorders. For the practitioner, it is sufficient to recognize that psychiatric syndromes are recognized by abnormalities of thought, mood, affect, and behavior rather than specific tests of brain structure or clinical laboratory testing.

Behavior disorders, including violence, are also common problems in American society. To properly evaluate and care for patients, clinicians must know each patient's social situation, which can influence their physical and psychiatric complaints. All patients deserve a complete social and psychiatric history with attention to current living arrangement, past or current abuse (e.g., physical, sexual, emotional, and/or financial), current safety, education and literacy, and social resources.

This chapter introduces common psychiatric syndromes encountered in clinical practice and provides guidance for recognizing them. The *Diagnostic and Statistical Manual of Mental Disorders,* Fifth Edition (*DSM-V*), published by the American Psychiatric Association, is a particularly valuable resource [American Psychiatric Association. *Diagnostic and Statistical Manual of Mental Disorders.* 5th ed. Washington, DC: American Psychiatric Association; 2013]. In addition to diagnostic criteria, the DSM reviews the epidemiology and presentations of mental disorders.

SECTION 1
The Mental Status
and Psychiatric Evaluation

THE MENTAL STATUS EVALUATION

Psychiatric diagnosis relies on the interview and exclusion of medical illness. Psychiatric interviews require time, patience, and experience. Standardized screening questionnaires assist when evaluating psychological symptoms. Useful screening tools include the Mini-Cog, SLUMS test, the Folstein Mini-Mental State Examination (MMSE), clock drawing test, Beck Depression Inventory, Hamilton Depression Scale, and the Prime MD instruments. None is perfect, but each helps categorize patients by standardized criteria.

The clinician assesses the mental status throughout the history and physical exam. When problems are suspected, formal testing is indicated. The MMSE has been used most often, but *the authors charge for its use.* A validated open source alternative is the SLUMS tool (Fig. 15-1), developed at Saint Louis University. The Mini-Cog, another validated screening tool, combines the MMSE registration and recall questions with clock drawing. The latter is performed by drawing a circle placing the numeral "12" in its proper clock position, then asking the patient to fill in the remaining numerals followed by placing the hour and minute hands at a particular time, e.g., "4:35." An error in either task indicates the need for detailed cognitive evaluation.

The psychiatric evaluation addresses the following dimensions of mental processes:

Level of Consciousness (LOC): Patients are alert, lethargic, stuporous, or in coma. These are arbitrary categories on a continuum and the LOC may fluctuate. Although patients may be lethargic from medications or intoxications, all patients who are less than fully alert must be assumed to have an organic neurologic disorder until proven otherwise.

Orientation: This has four dimensions: person, place, time, and situation. Does the patient know who he and others in the room are? Does he know their names and roles? Does he know where he is—the place, city, state, country? Does he know the year, season, day, and date?

Attention: This is the ability to stay on task, avoiding distractions, during a conversation or interview. Attention deficits are the hallmark of confusional states, including delirium, and suggest a possible metabolic disorder. Decreased attention is too frequently attributed to a lack of cooperativeness when, in fact, the patient is unable to cooperate. Digit span recall is a good test of attention. Have the patient repeat random sequences of digits starting with two and working up. Seven is normal whereas four or less is definitely abnormal. Tests of serial 7s, serial 3s (subtract 3 sequentially, starting at 20), and attempting to spell "world" backward also test attention. A nonverbal task is the tap-no-tap test. Have the patient tap his or her hand twice when you tap

Saint Louis University
Mental Status (SLUMS) Examination

Name _____   Age _____
Is patient alert? _____   Level of education _____

① 1. What day of the week is it?

① 2. What is the year?

① 3. What state are we in?

4. Please remember these five objects. I will ask you what they are later.
       Apple   Pen   Tie   House   Car

① 5. You have $100 and you go to the store and buy a dozen apples for $3 and a tricycle for $20.
How much did you spend?
② How much do you have left?

6. Please name as many animals as you can in one minute.

⓪ 0–5 animals   **①** 5–10 animals   **②** 10–15 animals   **③** 15+ animals

⑤ 7. What were the five objects I asked you to remember? 1 point for each one correct.

8. I am going to give you a series of numbers and I would like you to give them to me backwards.
For example, if I say 42, you would say 24.

⓪ 87   **①** 649   **①** 8537

9. This is a clock face. Please put in the hour markers and the time at
10 minutes to 11 o'clock.

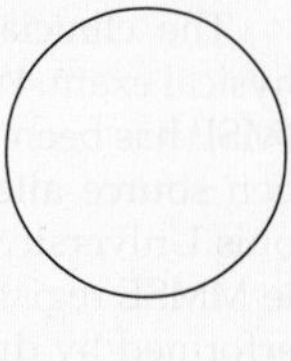

② Hour markers okay
② Time correct

① 10. Please place an X in the triangle.

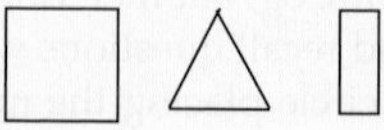

① Which of the above figures is largest?

11. I am going to tell you a story. Please listen carefully because afterwards, I am going to ask you
some questions about it.

Jill was a very successful stockbroker. She made a lot of money on the stock market. She then met Jack, a
devastatingly handsome man. She married him and had three children. They lived in Chicago. She then
stopped work and stayed at home to bring up her children. When they were teenagers, she went back to
work. She and Jack lived happily ever after.

② What was the female's name?   **②** What work did she do?
② When did she go back to work?   **②** What state did she live in?

Scoring		
High School Education		**Less than High School Education**
27–30 ••••••••••••••••	Normal	•••••••••••••••• 20–30
20–27 ••••••••••••••••	MCI	•••••••••••••••• 14–19
1–19 ••••••••••••••••	Dementia	•••••••••••••••• 1–14

Questions? FAX: (314) 771-8575 • email: agingsuccess@slu.edu   Aging Successfully, Vol. XII, No. 1   **1**

FIG. 15-1 St Louis University Mental Status (SLUMS) Tool. A validated tool for assessing mental status.

once; if you tap twice, they are not to tap. Always consider the patient's level
of education in interpreting these tasks.

Memory: This is the ability to register and retain material from previous
experience. Memory is a complex phenomenon. It is usefully classified as
immediate recall (registration), short- and long-term memories.

Immediate recall. This is the ability to *register* items presented.

Short-term memory. Registered items recalled within 5–10 minutes are stored in short-term memory.

Long-term memory. Events from the distant past, from days to years, are recalled from long-term memory.

The SLUMS and MMSE include tests of immediate recall and short-term memory. Short- and long-term memories are evaluated while taking the history. Identify the patient's interests, e.g., politics, sports, cooking, etc., then ask them detailed questions about their interests, questions that demand specific quantitative memories, rather than vague qualitative answers.

Thought: This is how the brain consciously communicates with itself. Thought has several dimensions.

Content. What the patient is thinking about? Is it appropriate to his or her situation and a reasonable perception of the world?

Sequence. How are thoughts linked one to the next? Can the patient digress and get back to the original point?

Logic. How are events connected and explained? What is the nature of cause and effect in his or her life? What reasons are given for seeking care?

Insight. The ability to look at one's self and situation with comprehension and understanding demonstrates insight. Lack of insight into the nature or consequences of behaviors or thoughts is a clue to mental illness.

Judgment. The ability to make reasonable assessments of the external world and effective choices between alternative actions requires judgment. How are decisions made? How does the patient evaluate alternatives? How are potential benefits and risks considered?

Perception: This is a global term for the sensory experiencing the world through the senses of sight, touch, hearing, smell, and taste. Distorted perceptions suggest neurologic and/or psychiatric disease. *Structural perception,* the ability to place objects and shapes in relation to one another, is tested by copying interlocked pentagons or performing clock drawing.

Intellect: Intellect is generally held to be an innate brain faculty, though may be difficult to separate intellectual from educational deficits. To properly evaluate the clinician must know the patient's *educational and literacy levels.* Culture greatly influences tests of intellect so making assessments across cultures is hazardous. Intellect has several dimensions:

Information. Does he know about important local, national, or international events? What are his or her sources of information?

Calculation. The ability to manipulate numbers, is tested first by simple and then gradually more complex arithmetic tasks.

Abstraction. The ability to see general principles in concrete statements tests abstraction. Ask the patient to interpret proverbs, e.g., "people in glass houses shouldn't throw stones" = "don't criticize others for things you have probably done yourself." Interpretation at the simplest level, "they would break the windows," is indicative of a concrete thinking and a deficit in abstract thinking. Remember that proverbs are culturally bound and may not be recognizable to people from diverse cultural backgrounds.

Reasoning. Solving problems involving simple logical sequences test reasoning.

Language. Brains use language to communicate with each other. Evaluate it during the interview and by having the patient follow both written and verbal instructions and by writing a sentence. Assess the patient's vocabulary and the complexity of the patient's spoken language. Other dimensions of language are fluency of speech, body language, facial expression, and other nonverbal forms of communication; all should be thought of as language.

Mood: Mood is a sustained affective state, how a person feels. It is more like the tidal flow of emotion than the waves of affect. Mood is classified as normal, depressed, or elevated. Mood should be assessed, by asking the patient, how his or her mood has been over the last 2 weeks. Also ask how the patient feels about his or her life, their thoughts of the future, their confidence in their abilities, and their hopes, and the intensity of these feelings. If depression is suspected, inquire about suicidal thoughts or plans. Depressed patients may have blunted affect with little range.

Affect: This is a more transient emotional state varying from minute-to-minute and day-to-day with the setting and types of social and personal interactions in which the person is engaged. Affect is the clinician's assessment of emotion assessed by facial expression, tone, and modulation of voice and specific questions about how the patient feels. Affect is also reflected by the intensity and range of expression. Affective states include happy, sad, angry, fearful, worried, and wary.

Appearance and Behavior: Closely observe the patient during the interview. How is he dressed and groomed? How is his personal hygiene? Does he make and sustain eye contact? Does he answer questions promptly and fully? Are there areas of questioning that he avoids or tries to deflect? What is his body language? Is he fidgeting or unusually still? What is his tone of voice, volume, and speech rhythm?

PSYCHIATRIC SYMPTOMS AND SIGNS

In psychiatric illness, the symptoms and signs are the patient's behaviors and the patient's perception and description of those behaviors. Therefore, this chapter discusses symptoms and signs together.

Abnormal Perception: We perceive the world through our senses, which we take as reliable and valid reflections of the external environment. Sensory perceptions are distorted by injury to the sensory organs or pathways, from abnormal processing of these signals, or from false perceptions arising within the brain. Injuries to the sensory organs and pathways cause loss of perception (*negative* change) or exaggeration or distortion of the normal sensory signal (*positive* change, e.g., tinnitus, paresthesia, hyperalgesia, allodynia). Altered perception from the processing centers and cortex are more complex.

Hallucinations. Hallucinations are abnormal sensory perceptions (auditory, visual, olfactory, tactile/somatic, or gustatory) perceived only by the patient, not by an observer, without external cues. The patient may or may not recognize them as unreal. Auditory hallucinations are common in schizophrenia; visual hallucinations are more typical of delirium. Olfactory and gustatory hallucinations suggest partial seizure disorders (temporal lobe epilepsy).

Illusions. Illusions are misinterpretations of real sensory events experienced by the patient and an observer. They are particularly common with sensory impairment such as visual loss. Poor attentiveness in delirium leads to false attribution of sensory phenomena such as misidentifying people and misinterpreting behaviors.

Confusion—Delirium. See page 721 and Chapter 14, page 705.

Parasomnias: Parasomnias are perceptual and behavioral disorders associated with sleep. The most common parasomnias are *nightmares* and *sleep terrors*. Auditory hallucinations commonly occurring while falling asleep (*hypnogogic*) and awakening (*hypnopompic*) do not indicate pathology without other hypnagogic symptoms.

Sleepwalking. The patient performs complex activities while asleep awakening with no recollection. Hypnotic drugs, by inducing antegrade amnesia, increase risk for sleepwalking.

Periodic limb movements of sleep. Arousals in obstructive and central sleep apneas are associated with frequent leg movements during sleep. Though often quite disturbing to the bed partner, the patient is unaware of a problem except for finding disrupted bedding and the partner absent. In contrast, a complaint of being unable to hold the legs still on going to bed suggests *restless legs syndrome*.

Abnormal Affect and Mood: Feelings are emotional reactions to perceptions and events. Normally, feelings of varying intensity are experienced throughout the day. Abnormally extreme feelings, in degree and/or duration, may indicate a psychiatric disorder.

Behavior and mood changes. Significant behavior changes raise concern for a medical or psychiatric illness. Changes in school or job performance and withdrawal from social activities are frequent in thought and mood disorders and with substance abuse.

Elevated Affect and Mood. Elevated affect is a normal transient response to positive events. *Mania* is an abnormally elevated, expansive, and/or irritable mood lasting ≥1 week combined with three or more of the following: inflated self-esteem or grandiosity, decreased need for sleep, increased talkativeness, flight of ideas, distractibility, increase in goal-directed activity, or excessive involvement in pleasurable activities with a high potential for adverse consequences (physical, sexual, or financial). *Hypomania* is similar the symptoms being milder and of shorter duration.

Depressed affect and mood. *Depressed affect* is a normal brief response to negative events and feelings. *Mood depression* is more persistent. It may be accompanied by loss of interest in activities or pleasure, anorexia, weight loss, insomnia or somnolence, psychomotor agitation or retardation, fatigue, inappropriate guilt and/or a sense of worthlessness, decreased concentration, thoughts of death, and suicidal ideation. Persistence >2 weeks accompanied by changes in sleep, eating, and/or behavior indicates *major depression*. *Dysthymia* is a persistent, usually lifelong, mildly depressed affect not meeting criteria for a major depression.

Anxiety. Anxiety is a state of apprehension or fear accompanied by increased sympathetic nervous system activity. It is a normal response to physical or psychological threats that resolves when the threat is resolved. Onset in the absence of real danger, or persistence after the danger is resolved, is abnormal.

Phobias. These are irrational fears of situations, events, or objects producing uncontrollable fear and anxiety. Pathological phobias alter social and/or psychological function.

Anhedonia. This is the absence of pleasure from normally emotionally rewarding activities including eating, sexual stimulation, social activities, and personal or business success. It is characteristic of depression.

Depersonalization. This is a feeling of being outside the body, an observer of oneself and one's surroundings. It is accompanied by a loss of affective connection with the people and events in one's environment. It is normal during highly stressful, traumatic events, but abnormal in other situations or if persistent or recurrent. Depersonalization may occur with anxiety disorders.

Abnormal Thinking: Thinking is the process by which we connect and explain events to ourselves and subsequently to others. It is a relational activity of great complexity. Patients with thought disorders manifest verbal symptoms or unusual behaviors resulting from the disordered thoughts.

Paranoia. This is the belief that one is being systematically threatened or persecuted by a person, persons, or organizations. It is pathological when the result of a fixed delusion or when it significantly alters activities. Paranoia can be a relatively mild personality trait or a manifestation of psychosis.

Disordered thinking. Thinking is usually logical and linked to an explicit rational system of cause and effect. The train of thought connecting each sequential idea is either apparent to an observer or readily explained by the patient and comprehensible to the observer. Disordered thinking is unconnected from thought-to-thought or connected by irrational or incomprehensible explanations. It is a sign of *schizophrenia*.

Delusions. Delusions are fixed, false beliefs about the causal relations between perceptions, events, and people and are pathological when they continue to be believed despite strong, otherwise persuasive, evidence to the contrary. Though based on real sensory perceptions and events, the linkages are illusory. Delusions are characteristic of *schizophrenia*, *manic psychosis*, and *delirium*.

Obsessions. Obsessions are recurrent intrusive thoughts or fears that cannot be suppressed or controlled despite knowing they are unreasonable. When function is impaired it becomes *obsessive–compulsive disorder*.

Compulsions. Compulsive activities are repetitive stereotypic behaviors that the person feels compelled to perform to reduce distress or fear of an unavoidable outcome should they stop. When function is impaired it becomes *obsessive–compulsive disorder*.

Abnormal Memory: The hippocampus and temporal lobes are essential for forming and storing memories. Abnormal memory reflects failure to register, retain, or recall information. Memory for names is frequently impaired with normal aging and is not a cause for concern. Short-term memory loss, or the inability to make new memories, leads to disorientation and behavior changes severely impairing function. Memory loss is the most common characteristic of *dementia* and may be the only finding in *mild cognitive dysfunction*.

Amnesia. Amnesia is a loss of memory. It can be retrograde for events of the past, or antegrade, the inability to form new memories. It is global or selective for specific events or memory domains. It is indicative of brain injury or a psychological disorder.

Confabulation. Confabulation occurs in the setting of severe memory loss. The patient constructs fabulous explanations for events and behaviors, the correct explanation having been lost. This is typical of *Korsakoff syndrome*.

Abnormal Behaviors: How we behave, our actions in private and public, is the result of how we feel, how we think, and how we perceive the constraints and rewards of the social environment. Behavior is culturally bound such that behaviors appropriate in one culture or setting may be quite inappropriate in another. Normative evaluations of private thoughts, feelings, and behaviors are problematic at best; however, public behaviors are reasonably and readily subject to normative evaluation. Behaviors which are consistently abnormal or unacceptable are indicative of personality or psychiatric disorders.

Suicidal Behavior. See Suicide, page 723.

Stereotypic behaviors. Activities, movements, or vocalizations that are repeated stereotypically without precipitants or explanation suggest tics, compulsions, or possibly complex partial seizures.

Catatonia. Catatonic patients often exhibit a profound retardation in motor activity, retaining postures, expressing negativism, and repeating the phrases or motions of other persons (*echolalia*, *echopraxia*). However, patients can have excessive apparently purposeless motor activity not influenced by external stimuli. Most common in affective disorders, catatonia is also seen in psychosis.

Abnormal sexual feelings and behaviors—paraphilias. Paraphilias are abnormal and/or unusually intense feelings of sexual arousal toward inappropriate sexual objects such as children, animals, or nonhuman objects, or the need for inappropriate behaviors such as sadism or masochism during sexual activity. Paraphilic thoughts are not necessarily abnormal, but, when acted upon with nonconsenting partners or children, they indicate psychiatric illness.

Bulimia. Bulimia is alternating binge eating and purging with either induced vomiting or other cathartic activity. When the pattern is sustained and secretive, it is a major eating disorder.

Anorexia nervosa. See Anorexia Nervosa and Bulimia Nervosa, page 726.

Dyssomnias. These sleep disorders include difficulty getting to or maintaining sleep (*insomnia*), abnormal daytime sleepiness, sudden sleep onset (*narcolepsy*), sleep-disorder breathing, and other circadian sleep cycle disorders, e.g., jet lag. Ask about sleep quality and disruption. Abnormal sleep patterns can result from or lead to psychiatric disorders. Terminal insomnia is associated with major depression, whereas initial insomnia characterizes atypical depressive disorder.

PSYCHIATRIC SYNDROMES

The disorders below need to be recognized by clinicians to initiate treatment or psychiatric referral. Indications for psychiatric consultation include suicidal or homicidal ideation, psychotic symptoms, severe anxiety or depression, mania, dissociative symptoms, and failure to respond to therapy.

    To facilitate research, the American Psychiatric Association developed criteria for the diagnosis and classification of mental disorders. These have proved reliable and have improved diagnosis and therapy. Practitioners should consult the *DSM-V*. There are few, if any specific signs or laboratory findings of psychiatric disease, so diagnosis depends upon an experienced observer obtaining a complete history from the patient and collateral informants.

Multiaxial Assessment: The *DSM-V* uses multiaxial assessment, a method enabling a systematic approach to these disorders. Every clinician needs to be familiar with this system.

Axis I: Clinical disorders; other conditions that may be a focus of clinical attention. These are the major psychiatric and behavior syndromes addressed in the DSM-V. If more than one disorder is present, list the principle disorder or reason for the current visit first.

Axis II: Personality disorders; mental retardation. These are listed separately from Axis I disorders because they may coexist and complicate the diagnosis and management of Axis I problems.

Axis III: General medical conditions. Here are listed medical conditions, by system, which may be important for understanding and management of the Axis I and II disorders.

Axis IV: Psychosocial and environmental problems. List problems in the patient's psychosocial and physical environment which influence the diagnosis, management, or prognosis of the Axis I, II, and III problems.

Axis V: Global assessment of functioning. Record the patient's global level of function using the Global Assessment of Functioning Scale, a 0–100 scale descriptive of the functional impairment from the psychiatric (Axis I and II) disorders. The full scale is in the DSM-V.

Acute and Subacute Confusion

Delirium. Metabolic abnormalities (including prescription and nonprescription drugs), pain, restraints, or sleep deprivation impair cognitive function, particularly attention, judgment, and perception. This is usually a metabolic encephalopathy. Failure to recognize and treat delirium is associated with a high incidence of long-term morbidity and increased mortality. Delirium is frequently confused with a primary psychiatric disorder, especially by examiners who have not known the patient in the premorbid state. Delirium is characterized by inattentiveness, fluctuating mental status, progressive loss of orientation, and confusion. Persons at highest risk are the older adults, especially those on multiple medications. The chief features are *decreased attentiveness* (distractibility, loss of train of thought), *alteration of consciousness* (from hypervigilance and agitation to lethargy or coma), *disorientation* (for time and place), *illusions* (misinterpreted sensory impressions), *hallucinations* (mostly visual), *wandering, fragmented thoughts, delusions, recent memory loss*, and *affective changes*. The patient may be restless or picking at the bedclothes. Hypoactive delirium occurs as well. Myoclonus may be present. Some forms of delirium, e.g., alcohol withdrawal, produce prominent autonomic dysfunction with fever, tachycardia, and hypertension (*delirium tremens*). Common causes of delirium include drug intoxication or withdrawal (e.g., narcotics, sedatives, tranquilizers, alcohol, steroids, salicylates, digitalis, alkaloids), liver disease, uremia, hypoxia, hypoventilation, congestive heart failure, electrolyte abnormalities, urinary retention, fever, and infection. In hospitalized patients, sensory deficits, restraints, urinary catheters, and invasive procedures are associated with an increased incidence of delirium.

Anxiety Disorders

Generalized anxiety disorder. Anxiety is an experienced emotional state caused by activity in the deep cortical structures of the limbic system. In addition to the subjective feelings, anxiety triggers stress responses via the autonomic nervous system that, being felt by the patient, may heighten the anxiety. Most persons experience some anxiety in response to stress, but excessive or continuous unfocused anxiety may be debilitating and require therapy. The causes of anxiety may be real, potential, or imagined. Symptoms and signs mediated by the autonomic system include palpitations, tachycardia, tremor, chest pain, hyperventilation with paresthesia and dizziness, faintness, fatigue, diaphoresis, nausea, vomiting, diarrhea, and abdominal distress. The Hamilton Anxiety Rating Scale measures severity. Significant impairment of social, occupational, or other functioning is required for diagnosis.

Panic attack. Sudden intense fear or discomfort occurs without an evident external cue. Symptoms include palpitations, sweating, tremor, shortness of breath, choking, chest pain, nausea, faintness or dizziness, paresthesias, and / or flushing accompanied by overwhelming cognitive turmoil, as in fear of dying, losing control, or going crazy. Symptoms peak within 10 minutes and rarely last more than 30 minutes, leaving the patient feeling exhausted.

Panic disorder. Recurrent panic attacks accompanied by ongoing apprehension of further attacks, worry about the prognostic implications of the attacks (their physical and psychological meaning), or significant behavior change resulting from the attacks constitute panic disorder.

Agoraphobia. This is a persistent fear of situations which might cause embarrassment or discomfort or which might precipitate a panic attack. These are often social situations involving groups of people, particularly within confined surroundings such as classrooms, churches, and stores. Agoraphobia commonly accompanies panic disorder.

Social phobia. A compelling desire to avoid social contact, fearing embarrassment or humiliation, is social phobia.

Specific phobias. Phobia may develop to almost any type of event or interaction. To qualify as a phobia the anxiety must be consistently produced by the exposure, the fear must be excessive and unreasonable, and recognized as such by the patient who alters usual behavior patterns to avoid the situation leading to social disruption or extreme distress.

Acute and post-traumatic stress disorders. Persons experiencing an event involving threatened or actual injury or death to themselves or others may develop severe anxiety either soon afterward (*acute stress disorder*) or later with recurrences (*posttraumatic stress disorder*). Flashbacks, depersonalization, denial, avoidance of stimuli inducing the memories, and enhanced arousal are manifestations of post-traumatic stress disorder (PTSD).

Obsessive–compulsive disorder. Obsessive thoughts and compulsive behaviors occur in any combination. The patient recognizes that the connection between the behavior and the feared event or outcome is unreasonable. The obsessive and compulsive behaviors (e.g., hand washing, door locking or checking, cleaning or arranging possessions) consume more than one hour a day and interfere with social functioning.

Mood Disorders: Mood is the person's sustained affective state. Depressed and elevated moods are part of normal life. Abnormal mood is depressed or elevated or cycles between depression and elevation. Ascertain both the amplitude of the swings (the severity of the depression or elevation) and the cycling rate.

Dysthymia. This is a persistent, often lifelong, mildly depressed mood not meeting criteria for major depression. Depression is episodic while dysthymia is chronic, more a trait rather than a state.

Depression. Depression is daily sustained low mood or loss of interest or pleasure. Depression accompanies many serious medical illnesses or the medications prescribed for treatment. Eliminate this possibility before making a diagnosis of major depression. Depression occurs at all ages, but first episodes are most common in the fourth and fifth decades. Depression has psychological, behavioral, and somatic manifestations: loss of appetite and change in weight (up or down); sleep disturbances, most frequently terminal insomnia, although increased sleep can be seen; decreased energy for activities; decreased interest in usual activities and decreased pleasure from usually pleasurable activities; restlessness or listlessness; feelings of guilt and worthlessness; inability to concentrate, initiate activities or make decisions; and thoughts of death or suicide, either passive or active. If depressed mood is sustained >2 weeks and accompanied by four or more of these symptoms, depression is present.

Hypomania, mania, bipolar disorder, and mixed episodes. Mania is characterized by episodes of abnormally elevated mood lasting for at least 1 week. Hypomania is less extreme and patients are functionally successful, as opposed to the destructive consequences of mania. Mania or depression may occur alone (*unipolar*), or the patient may cycle between mania and depression within a single day (*mixed episode*) or over weeks, months, or years (*bipolar*).

Suicide. Suicide attempts are a common and frequently fatal manifestation of psychiatric illness. Expressed suicidal ideation, threats, gestures, and attempts are progressively more serious signs of a potentially life-threatening situation. Persons at highest risk include older men and adolescents, those with a specific plan, those intending to use firearms already in their possession, those who use substances (especially alcohol), and those with previous aborted attempts. All threats of suicide and expressions of suicidal ideation or intent must be taken seriously and immediate psychiatric consultation should be obtained. The practitioner's first obligation is to ensure the patient's safety pending psychiatric evaluation.

Personality Disorders and Abnormal Behaviors: Personality is a global description of how we think, feel, and interact with the world around us. Acceptable feelings and behaviors are culturally determined. Personality disorders are persistent, rather than episodic, lifelong patterns of maladaptive feelings, thoughts, and behaviors with two or more of the following: *abnormal cognition*, that is, how they perceive other people, actions, and themselves; *abnormal feelings* about themselves, people, and events in type, intensity, or duration; *difficulty functioning* with other people socially, educationally, or occupationally; and, *difficulty with impulse control* leading to inappropriate behaviors. Personality traits are consistent over time regardless of social surroundings producing significant stress and disrupting patients' lives. These disorders are pervasive and inflexible not changing over time, with or without therapy. Treatment aims to improve function within the bounds of the disorder. Underlying medical disorders and substance abuse must be excluded before the diagnosis can be made.

Personality disorder clusters. Personality disorders divide into three clusters. Understanding these clusters and the specific personality types within each helps to effectively manage the medical problems. Everyone has some of these traits; *it is the disruption of global function that separates a disorder from a trait.* Many clinicians avoid people with personality disorders. Use the normal emotional responses engendered by these interactions to assist in recognizing the specific disorders and dealing effectively with them. Remember, patients do not choose their personalities and the personality disorders stand between the clinician and effective management of medical problems.

Cluster A: the odd and eccentric. Generally, people with these disorders avoid the medical profession. When they do present, they frequently have somatic complaints such as chronic fatigue and pain.

Paranoid. There is a pervasive suspiciousness of others. They are always questioning the motivations of those around them and suspect that they are not being dealt with honestly.

Schizoid. These individuals are detached and do not form personal or social relationships. They only come to physicians for specific indications or services and otherwise prefer to be socially and personally isolated. The range of their emotional responses is restricted.

Schizotypal. These people are recognized by their eccentric behaviors and often eccentric dress. They have social deficits and unusual cognitive and perceptual experiences, but otherwise function appropriately. These are the people who have been abducted by aliens.

Cluster B: the dramatic, emotional, and erratic. This is the group we often think about when discussing personality disorders. These patients consume an inordinate amount of physician time and emotion without ever getting better, the folks you fear to see on your clinic schedule. Learning to deal with them effectively will help both you and your staff. These patients usually bring more pain and suffering to others than to themselves. Cluster B patients present with somatic complaints and may seek disability or drugs. They often have a history of reactions to multiple medications or feel that their metabolism is different than others.

Antisocial. There is a disregard for the rights of others and a lifelong pattern of difficulty with social and legal limits on behavior. They do not seem to have a conscience nor display regret or guilt for violating the rights of others.

Borderline. Borderline patients are emotionally labile and never happy or satisfied. Life is a constantly dysphoric experience. Their relationships are unstable, and they are given to impulsive actions, not infrequently with self-harm. The emotional lability and intensity of their experiences often makes their caregivers uncomfortable.

Histrionic. These patients have excessive emotionality, often acting out their feelings. They can be sexually provocative and attention seeking. They may be inappropriately dressed (e.g., revealing clothing, excessive make up and jewelry, overly formal or casual, etc.) and have provocative attention-seeking behaviors when alone with the clinician.

Narcissistic. These individuals need to be admired and recognized as exceptional in some, if not all their activities. They are often grandiose and disclose their close relationships with the rich and famous. They are self-centered and lack empathy or insight into the feelings of others.

Cluster C: The anxious and fearful. These people are never satisfied. They have constant fears that produce avoidant, dependent, or obsessive behaviors that disrupt their lives bringing more suffering on themselves than those around them. They manifest anxiety, seeking second opinions and needing reassurance. They often have somatic complaints and/or sensitivities to many medications or environmental exposures.

Avoidant. Feeling inadequate in personal and social interactions, they tend to avoid social situations. They are overly sensitive to negative evaluations which are interpreted as judgments of personal weakness not as improvement opportunities. No amount of reassurance overcomes this pervasive feeling.

Dependent. These patients need to be cared for. They are submissive and clinging and are fearful of separation from others. They can become dependent upon their providers if given an opportunity. They do not take responsibility for their care, shifting the responsibility to others.

Obsessive–Compulsive. These are the perfectionists. They must always be in control of their environment and relationships. They are orderly in the extreme.

Somatoform and related disorders—hysteria, hypochondriasis, Briquet syndrome. Persons with somatoform disorders have multiple physical complaints without medical explanation. They have usually visited several physicians, "who can't seem to find out what's wrong." The diagnosis should not be made until organic causes for the complaints are excluded by thorough evaluation. They have often had extensive prior evaluations so, absent serious abnormalities on the screening physical exam or laboratory tests, the clinician should obtain complete records of all previous workups before initiating expensive or invasive evaluations.

Somatization disorder. This is more common in women, begins before age 30, and leads to frequent visits for medical evaluation and treatment. Symptoms impair social, school, and job performance. Diagnostic criteria include pain in ≥ 4 sites, two or more painless gastrointestinal symptoms, at least one painless sexual or reproductive symptom, and one pseudo-neurologic symptom. The symptoms are not the result of medication, alcohol, or illicit drug abuse or explained by a known medical condition. Unlike factitious disorder, the patient is not fabricating the symptoms or causing self-injury.

Hypochondriasis. Hypochondriacs persistently express fear of a serious illness despite the reassurance of concerned physicians who have searched thoroughly for evidence of organic disease without success.

Factitious disorders. These patients consciously and intentionally produce symptoms and/or signs of disease to gratify psychological needs.

Munchausen syndrome. Munchausen syndrome is dramatic or dangerous behavior resulting in frequent hospitalizations for presumed severe illness. The most common symptoms and signs simulated are urinary or gastrointestinal bleeding, diarrhea, fever, seizures, and hypoglycemia.

Malingering. This is intentionally deceptive behavior. Patients claim to have symptoms or signs of a disease which will benefit them in some way, e.g., by obtaining narcotics or financial support for disability.

Eating Disorders: Marked changes in food selection and abnormal eating behaviors can indicate either organic disease or psychiatric disease.

Anorexia nervosa. Anorexia nervosa is most common in adolescent and young women with overwhelming concern about body image and weight. It is accompanied by a distorted body image—the patient seeing an overweight person where observers see normal body form or emaciation. Patients may be obsessed with food, preparing meals for others but not eating themselves. Excessive exercise may accompany the anorexia as a means of achieving the desired body image. Appetite is severely suppressed or absent. Patients become severely malnourished with retarded secondary sexual maturation, absent menses, and osteoporosis. They risk death from complications of malnutrition. Early recognition and intensive treatment are essential.

Bulimia nervosa. Bulimia is recurrent, secretive, binge eating. Patients feel unable to control the compulsive eating resorting to induced vomiting, purging with laxatives, and/or abuse of diuretics to avoid weight gain. Clues include eroded tooth enamel from acid emesis, abrasions on the roof of the mouth and callus on the backs of the fingers from inducing vomiting, and electrolyte disorders from using laxatives and diuretics. Nutrient deficiencies and malnutrition are uncommon.

Binge eating syndrome. Large meals are eaten rapidly followed by guilt and discomfort. Patients often eat alone and/or secretively despite feeling full and not being hungry. They often express self-disgust at their eating habits. Depression may be increased. They do not vomit or increase exercise to compensate for their increased intake. If the symptoms and behaviors are present for >2 days per week for >6 months, a binge eating syndrome is present.

Night eating syndrome. These patients consume >50% of their total daily energy intake after the evening meal. They snack continuously after the meal and awaken frequently to eat. They feel tension and anxiety that is relieved by eating. They are not hungry on awakening and tend to eat refined sugars and high carbohydrate snacks at other times.

Alcohol-Related Illness: Alcoholic beverages are ubiquitous and commonly used social lubricants. Alcohol intake should not exceed two drinks per day for males and one for females. Individuals vary greatly in their alcohol tolerance which increases with increased use. Problems related to alcohol use have biological, social, and psychological roots. Each person lies somewhere on the continuum from abstinence to alcoholism. The clinician's task is to identify each person's alcohol use, now and in the past, and their risk for addiction and social disruption. All patients should be asked about the frequency, amount, and type of beverages consumed; whether their use is in a social context or if they drink alone; whether they drink to become intoxicated; and whether they have memory losses or driving or other infractions of the law related to alcohol. The AUDIT-C and CAGE questionnaires are validated tools for identifying patients at risk for alcohol abuse disorders. CAGE is an acronym for recalling questions on *cutting* down, *annoyance* by criticism, *guilty* feelings, and *eye openers* (early morning drinks). Positive responses to the CAGE questions or high AUDIT-C score raise suspicion for chronic alcohol abuse. Alcohol abuse is commonly associated with other forms of substance abuse, including tobacco.

Problem drinking. More than the recommended amount of alcohol is consumed but without dependence or social, legal, or occupational issues. Binge drinking in young adults is a form of problem drinking.

Alcohol abuse. Alcohol abuse is defined as regular alcohol use, without dependence, exceeding recommended limits and causing impairments in social functioning, interpersonal and relationship conflicts, legal issues, occupational difficulty, or repeated risky behaviors such as driving while intoxicated.

Alcohol dependence. This compulsive behavioral disorder consists of repeated ethyl alcohol ingestion in quantities sufficient to create biologic and social harm. Two key elements are increasing *tolerance* so that escalating amounts are consumed and *withdrawal symptoms* when attempts are made to discontinue or moderate drinking. The diagnosis is certain when behaviors damaging to the drinker's health and reputation occur repeatedly. Such behavior is socially stigmatized, so the patient often is reluctant to admit to it and may use subterfuges and untruths to conceal the truth. To uncover the facts, the clinician must gain the patient's confidence and be persistent, often using oblique rather than blunt questions to reveal diagnostically pertinent information unrecognized by the patient as being associated with alcoholism, e.g., injury without explanation, unexplained seizures, and job loss. Always inquire about previous treatment for alcoholism and arrests for driving under the influence. Physical signs consistent with chronic alcoholism include cutaneous vascular spiders, hepatomegaly, wrist drop, peripheral sensorimotor neuropathy, cerebellar ataxia, and alcohol or aldehyde on the breath.

Impulse Control Disorders: This group of disorders includes repetitive behaviors that range from the relatively minor (hair twisting and pulling, *trichotillomania*) to the socially disruptive (compulsive gambling, explosive disorder) and to the criminal (kleptomania, pyromania). Repetitive impulsive socially disruptive behaviors may be the result of psychiatric disorders, epilepsy, or tics (Tourette syndrome).

Adjustment Disorders: Sudden, especially unwanted, disruptions of the social environment can produce profound changes in mood and behavior. Failure to restore normal mood in a reasonable time or persistent maladaptive or self-destructive behaviors indicates an adjustment disorder, with or without accompanying anxiety or depression. Common events requiring adjustment are ending an intimate relationship, divorcing, changing school or community, losing employment, getting married, and becoming a parent.

Grieving

Normal grieving. Grieving the loss of a loved one is a normal event, an adjustment to a new type of life. The form and pattern of appropriate grieving is both individually and culturally determined. Normal grieving is a gradual process resolving the acute loss while developing a new appreciation for the lost person. With this resolution a sense of purpose and the ability to find joy in life is restored. Normal grieving for a lost spouse or loved one may last for several months but does not impair global function.

Prolonged grieving. Grieving associated with social withdrawal and depression disrupting normal activities and relationships and persisting for more than 2 months may indicate transition from normal grief to a psychiatric disorder.

Thought Disorders

Psychosis. Serious medical illness and severe mood disorders are frequently associated with disordered thinking and altered perceptions. These secondary psychoses must be differentiated from psychosis arising in an otherwise healthy person.

Schizophrenia. Schizophrenia comprises a group of disorders that are probably etiologically distinct. Primary psychotic disorders occur in adolescence or young adult life. Onset of psychotic symptoms at an older age raises concern for organic brain disease, drug intoxication or withdrawal, or psychosis complicating major depressive or bipolar disease. Schizophrenia involves problems in thinking, affect, socializing, action, language, and perception. *Positive symptoms* represent an exaggeration or distortion of normal functions, including delusions and hallucinations, especially auditory. *Negative symptoms* are losses of normal functions such as affective flattening, alogia, anhedonia, and avolition. *Disorganizational symptoms* include disorganized speech or behavior and short or absent attention span. Several subtypes are recognized. *Catatonic* patients exhibit a profound change in motor activity, retaining postures, expressing negativism, and repeating the phrases or motions of other persons (*echolalia, echopraxia*). *Paranoid* patients are preoccupied with at least one systematized delusion or auditory hallucination related to a single subject. *Disorganized* schizophrenic patients have disorganized speech and behavior and a superficial or inappropriate affect.

Other Disorders: Other major categories of psychiatric syndromes which we do not have space to present inclusively include substance-related disorders; disorders usually first diagnosed in infancy, childhood, or adolescence (including intellectual disability, learning disorders, autism, attention-deficit and disruptive behavioral disorders, and tic disorders); dissociative disorders; sexual and gender identity disorders; sleep disorders; impulse-control disorders; adjustment disorders; relational problems (e.g., parent to child, siblings); and problems related to abuse or neglect. The reader should consult the DSM-V for detailed discussion of these diagnoses.

SECTION 2
The Social Evaluation

Evaluating Social Function and Risk: Health status is strongly correlated with socioeconomic factors including family income, community of residence, education, social connectedness (the number and strength of interpersonal relationships), marital status, and employment status. In addition to any role the social environment plays in the incidence of ill health, it often places significant limitations on the ability of an individual and family to cope with the financial and social demands of illness. The result is a vicious spiral of unmet needs.

Evaluation of the patient's social environment should be part of a global patient assessment. The clinician should inquire about marital status, living arrangements, financial limitations and concerns, health insurance, education, literacy (do not assume that several years of elementary and secondary education equates to the ability to read or write), interpersonal relationships and personal support system, use of community social support systems, and sense of personal safety and security. For older adults and the chronically ill, inquire about the availability of heat in the winter and air conditioning in the summer.

When questions arise or problems are identified consultation with local social service agencies is strongly advised. They are often able to assist patients with medications, transportation, and a wide variety of other services. *Identification of abuse or neglect is especially important, and caregivers are required to report to the appropriate social agency children (<18 years of age), elders (older than age 64 years), or dependent adults of any age who may be victims of abuse or neglect.* The priority in these situations is securing the patient's safety, which may require hospitalization.

A description of a complete social evaluation is beyond the scope of this text. Axis IV of the DSM-V lists the following specific areas of psychosocial and environmental problems. This list is an excellent organizational scheme for identifying and classifying these problems:

1. Problems with primary support group.
2. Problems related to the social environment.
3. Educational problems.
4. Occupational problems.
5. Housing problems.
6. Economic problems.
7. Problems with access to health care services.
8. Problems related to interaction with the legal system/crime.
9. Other psychosocial and environmental problems.

COMMON SOCIAL SYNDROMES AND PROBLEMS

Common Social Syndromes and Problems

Abuse and neglect. Abuse is common and can affect persons of any age and either sex. Child and elder abuse effects both males and females, whereas women are much more commonly affected in midlife. Abuse can be physical, sexual, emotional, or financial. The examiner should first inquire whether the patient has ever felt unsafe in a relationship, then whether there are concerns about current safety, and last whether they wish help in dealing with the current problems. The patient's safety, not the identification of a perpetrator, is the first and most important goal of the interview. Remember that reporting of child, elder, and dependent adult abuse and neglect are mandatory.

Domestic violence. Violence in the home or between intimate sexual partners is common and often difficult to assess. In surveys of ambulatory practice, >20% of women have been abused at one time and 5% of women have been abused within the last year.

Elder abuse. This is an increasingly recognized problem. It can take many forms, and because many elders are dependent upon others for their personal needs, they may be unwilling to volunteer a complaint. This is further complicated when family members are the offending individuals. Abuse may take place in the home or in an institutional setting. An empathetic nonjudgmental approach to the evaluation including questions designed to elicit the patient's feelings (Do you feel safe?) may identify problematic situations.

Illiteracy. Inability to read and/or write is not uncommon. The patient is often embarrassed by the problem and will not volunteer this information. Learn to inquire tactfully and nonjudgmentally about the patient's educational and literacy skills. Illiteracy should be suspected when there is poor adherence to therapy plans and follow-up.

Homelessness. Homeless persons are at increased risk for medical illness and abuse and have high rates of serious psychiatric illness.

Isolation. Social isolation is common, especially in the older adults, in those with impaired motor or communication skills, and in those with limited financial resources. Isolation makes dealing with chronic illness more difficult and may increase the rate of cognitive decline in the older adults.

Institutionalization. A sizable proportion of our society spends time living in various institutional settings from the relatively benign, such as boarding schools, to the punitive, such as prisons. Other institutional settings that may impact on health status are nursing homes and homes for the developmentally disabled. It is important to know the stresses and limitations each of these environments place on our patients.

CLINICAL VIGNETTES AND QUESTIONS

CASE 15-1

A 78-year-old woman is admitted with community-acquired pneumonia. She is responding to antibiotics, but becomes agitated on day 3 of hospitalization. She has pulled out her IV twice, tries to get out of bed without assistance, is calling out frequently, and is not eating. She has angry outbursts and claims the staff is trying to harm her. On one occasion she was found in another patient's room. At other times she is drowsy. On examination she is lethargic; it takes several attempts to gain her attention. Once focused on a question she rambles incoherently. There are no focal neurological deficits and her examination is otherwise unchanged.

QUESTIONS:
1. What is her condition called?
2. What are its distinguishing features?
3. What are some baseline characteristics of patients predisposed to this syndrome?
4. What are some hospital acquired factors that increase the risk for this syndrome?

CASE 15-2

A 56-year-old woman with type 2 diabetes and diabetic nephropathy experiences twitching and deep pressure in her legs when she goes to bed, accompanied by an urge to move her legs. The symptoms improve if she gets up and walks.

QUESTIONS:
1. What is the most likely diagnosis?
2. What are the four criteria to diagnose this disorder?
3. What is a common and treatable condition that can contribute to this disorder?

CASE 15-3

A 35-year-old male bank executive presents with shortness of breath, rapid heart rate, sweaty palms, dizziness, and chest pain. He has been having similar episodes for quite some time, commonly before business presentations. He has been to the emergency room three times over the last 8 months. Each time he had a thorough evaluation that was negative for heart disease.

QUESTIONS:
1. What is the differential diagnosis of this patient's presentation?
2. What is the most likely diagnosis?
3. What is agoraphobia?

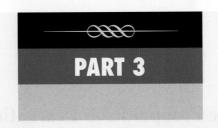

PART 3

Preoperative Evaluation

... I will follow that system of regimen which, according to my ability and judgment, I consider for the benefit of my patients, and abstain from whatever is deleterious and mischievous ...

    —from The Hippocratic Oath

Primum non nocere–First do no harm

    — ATTRIBUTION UNCERTAIN

CHAPTER 16

The Preoperative Evaluation

INTRODUCTION TO PREOPERATIVE SCREENING

The purpose of the preoperative exam is to provide a thorough preoperative risk assessment, optimize medical comorbidities, and detect any unrecognized disease that may lead to a poor surgical outcome. The extent of the evaluation must balance the morbidity and cost of preoperative testing against the potential for meaningfully reducing surgical morbidity. To appropriately counsel the surgeon and patient the history, physical exam, and other studies should assess the risks for cardiovascular, neurological, venous thromboembolic, renal, pulmonary, infectious, and endocrine complications. In addition, patient-specific perioperative management strategies may be pertinent. The consultant, surgeon, and patient must balance the risks of proceeding directly to surgery against the risks of delaying a necessary procedure.

THE HISTORY

First, determine the type and urgency of the proposed surgery. Even high-risk patients undergoing low-risk procedures do not need evaluation beyond a brief screening history and exam. Emergency surgeries should not be delayed for medical consultation. For all other surgeries, the clinician should assess the patient for active heart conditions that could delay surgery. These include decompensated congestive heart failure (CHF), unstable coronary syndromes (myocardial infarction [MI] within 30 days, unstable or severe angina), significant arrhythmias, and severe valvular disease (severe aortic or mitral stenosis).

If no "red flag" features are found, the patient's functional status should be assessed. Patients who have symptoms with activities of <4 metabolic equivalents (METs) have poor functional capacity and an increased risk for perioperative cardiovascular events. One MET is defined as the energy expenditure for sitting quietly. For the average adult this is equivalent to oxygen consumption of 3.5 mL/kg body weight per minute. Activities that correlate with 4–5 METs of activity include mopping floors, cleaning windows, painting walls, pushing a power lawnmower, raking leaves, weeding a garden, or walking up one flight of stairs. One validated tool to help determine level of activity is the Duke Activity Status Index (DASI). If the patient cannot perform activities consistent with 4 METs, then it is important to determine if they are limited by dyspnea or cardiovascular disease requiring further workup. The ability to accomplish these activities without symptoms correlates with a lower perioperative risk.

Find out if complications have occurred with previous operations. Then focus the history and physical exam upon the specific areas of concern outlined below.

Assessing Cardiovascular and Pulmonary Risk from History: The most frequent cause of nonsurgical perioperative morbidity and mortality is acute myocardial infarction. The history is the best method of risk assessment. The American College of Cardiology and the American Heart Association have published guidelines for perioperative cardiovascular evaluation based upon three factors: clinical predictors, functional capacity, and surgery-specific risks.

Ischemic heart disease. Determine whether the patient has angina and if so the frequency, precipitating factors, and response to rest and nitroglycerin. Especially worrisome are increasing occurrence at lower levels of provocation and slower response to nitroglycerin. Examine the electrocardiogram (ECG) for evidence of prior MI or ongoing ischemia. If prior cardiac catheterizations or coronary revascularizations have been performed, obtain the reports. Successful revascularization within 3 years lowers risk. The presence of drug-eluting stents presents unique challenges as described below.

Heart failure. Inquire for CHF symptoms now or in the past, e.g., exertional dyspnea, orthopnea, paroxysmal nocturnal dyspnea, cough, or peripheral edema. Obtain the results of prior cardiopulmonary evaluations, e.g., cardiac catheterization or echocardiography.

Dysrhythmias and cardiac devices. Ask about palpitations, syncope, and other symptoms of arrhythmias, and whether arrhythmias have been documented on prior ECGs or ambulatory monitoring. Examine current and old ECGs for high-grade atrioventricular block, symptomatic ventricular arrhythmias associated with structural heart disease, or supraventricular tachycardias at uncontrolled rates. If the patient has a pacemaker or defibrillator, determine the type and model, date of implantation, and when the battery life and performance were last interrogated.

Valvular and congenital heart disease. The presence of intracardiac shunts or valve abnormalities may require endocarditis prophylaxis. Obtain the results of the most recent echocardiogram, if one has been done. Look especially for evidence of severe valvular heart disease (e.g., aortic stenosis) that might require intervention before proceeding with elective noncardiac surgery.

Cerebrovascular disease. The presence of symptomatic cerebrovascular disease (transient ischemic attack or stroke) is associated with an increased risk for perioperative cardiovascular morbidity including stroke. Ask if there have been prior evaluations or interventions performed on the carotid or peripheral arteries and obtain the results if these tests have been performed.

Pulmonary disease. Record any symptoms of current pulmonary disease; ask if there have been pulmonary complications after previous surgeries. Ask patients with known lung disease if they have had pulmonary function testing (PFT) and if so obtain the results. Record the use of inhaled corticosteroids and bronchodilators for asthma or obstructive lung disease including the strength, frequency of use, and response to rescue inhalers. Postoperative pneumonia, the third most common complication among surgical patients, leads to increased length of stay, costs, and morbidity. A postoperative pneumonia risk index indicates that the type of surgery, age, functional status, weight loss, chronic obstructive pulmonary disease, general anesthesia, impaired sensorium, cerebral vascular accident, blood urea nitrogen level, transfusion, emergency surgery, long-term steroid use, smoking, and alcohol use are additive risk factors for developing postoperative pneumonia. The risk for postoperative respiratory failure can be estimated. Postoperative lung expansion, selective postop nasogastric tube use, and use of short-acting neuromuscular blockade may help reduce pulmonary risk.

Venous thromboembolism. A history of deep vein thrombosis or pulmonary embolism perioperatively or without provocation is associated with an increased risk for perioperative deep vein thrombosis/PE. Inquire whether studies for thrombophilia (e.g., factor V Leiden mutation, lupus anticoagulant, or deficiency of antithrombin III, and protein C or S) were performed and obtain the results if possible.

Assessing Bleeding Risk from History: The best predictor of bleeding is a history of prior postoperative bleeding. Prior surgery without bleeding assures you that the patient is not at increased risk for bleeding in the absence of antiplatelet and/or antithrombotic medications. If concerns arise from the history, a laboratory evaluation may be indicated. Screening tests (e.g., Protime/International Normalized Ratio, Partial thromboplastin time (PT/INR, PTT), platelet count) in a patient with a negative history are not helpful; these tests do not predict bleeding risk.

Personal and familial coagulation disorders. Ask about excessive bleeding with dental extractions, surgery, or childbirth or if there is a family history of excessive bleeding in those circumstances. Ask about heparin-induced thrombocytopenia or other heparin allergies.

Platelet and vessel disorders. Determine whether the patient experiences gingival bleeding, epistaxis, menorrhagia, hematuria, melena, or excessive bleeding or bruising at venipuncture sites or from minor cuts and whether they have noticed petechiae, spontaneous bruising, or large bruises with minor trauma.

Transfusion history. Has the patient ever had a blood transfusion or received procoagulant factor replacement at surgery? If so, determine when, which blood product, and the approximate volume of transfusion. Remember that patients confuse reinfusion of autologous blood and allogenic transfusion.

Assessing Metabolic Risk—Diabetes, Renal, and Hepatic Insufficiency: Assess metabolic abnormalities so they can be controlled preoperatively and managed through the perioperative period.

Glucose intolerance, hyperglycemia, and diabetes. Screen for symptoms of diabetes by asking about polyuria, polydipsia, or weight loss. Ask about a personal history of diabetes mellitus and ask women about gestational diabetes. If the patient is known to have diabetes, assess the use of oral hypoglycemic agents and control. If the patient uses insulin, record the types, schedule, and doses. Determine the frequency and severity of hypoglycemia and whether hypoglycemia unawareness is likely.

Kidney disease. Ask about any history of kidney disease and, if present, determine the stage and whether dialysis has ever been required.

Liver disease. Inquire about a history of liver disease, the etiology, and severity. Determine whether the liver disease is compensated or decompensated. Look for signs of advanced disease such as ascites, encephalopathy, portal hypertension, or GI bleeding. Assess hepatic synthetic function with albumin, bilirubin, and PT/INR only if liver disease is suspected from history.

Age: Biologic capacity declines with age, but it has been difficult to identify age as an independent risk factor for surgery. Comorbidities contribute to adverse surgical outcomes in the elderly, and operative mortality among octogenarians is substantially higher than patients aged 65–69.

Family History: Ask about a family history of adverse reaction to anesthesia (e.g., malignant hyperthermia), deep venous thrombosis or PE, bleeding problems, diabetes mellitus, elevated cholesterol, hypertension, or heart disease.

Medications: Most chronic medications can be continued through the perioperative period. Exceptions are nonsteroidal anti-inflammatory drugs and oral hypoglycemic agents which should be held prior to surgery. All unnecessary medications (including dietary supplements) should be discontinued. The risks and benefits of perioperative use of aspirin, thienopyridines, and warfarin need to be individually assessed balancing the risks of thrombosis and bleeding. When the decision is made to hold these medications prior to surgery, thienopyridines and aspirin are typically stopped 7–10 days prior to surgery while warfarin held 5 days prior to surgery.

Cardiovascular drugs. Review the patient's medications, to see if they are taking cardiac, antiarrhythmic, or antihypertensive medications. Except for diuretics and angiotensin converting enzyme (ACE) inhibitors, most drugs may be continued. Beta blockers should be continued in patients who are already receiving them. Beta blockers titrated to heart rate and blood pressure are recommended for patients undergoing vascular surgery who are at high cardiac risk and for patients whose preoperative assessment identifies coronary artery disease (CAD) or high cardiac risk (more than one clinical risk factor) who are undergoing intermediate risk surgery. Statin use also has been associated with decreased perioperative cardiac events and can be considered in patients with clinical risk factors.

Drugs affecting hemostasis. Ask specifically about the drugs affecting hemostasis or increasing the risk for thromboembolism, e.g., nonsteroidal anti-inflammatory drugs, antiplatelet agents, anticoagulations (warfarin, anti-Xa, and direct thrombin inhibitors), oral contraceptives, and estrogens. Patients receiving coronary stents are prescribed dual antiplatelet therapy. Chest guidelines recommend deferring surgery for at least 6 weeks after placing a bare metal stent and 6 months after placing a drug-eluting stent whenever possible. For those requiring surgery sooner, dual antiplatelet therapy should be continued perioperatively. For patients with a drug-eluting stent who must have procedures that mandate stopping thienopyridine therapy, aspirin should be continued if possible, and the thienopyridine should be restarted as soon as possible after the procedure.

Corticosteroids. Determine when, how much, for what reason, and for how long the patient took the corticosteroid. Steroid-induced adrenal suppression persists for up to a year after even short courses of corticosteroids in doses ≥10 mg/d. If this has occurred, start stress doses of steroids just before surgery and continue for 48–72 hours.

Social History
Substance use and abuse. If the patient uses alcohol or illicit or addicting drugs, identify the drugs and when they were last used. Anticipate drug withdrawal in the postoperative period if addicting drugs, including alcohol, were used recently.

Tobacco. If the patient smokes, quantify how many cigarettes are smoked daily. Quitting smoking for at least 8 weeks prior to surgery is optimal. Preoperative smoking cessation reduces postoperative complications.

Mechanical and Positioning Risks
Musculoskeletal conditions. Patients with rheumatoid arthritis may have cervical spine instability that can result in serious or fatal injury during endotracheal intubation. Also, determine if the patient requires special positioning to avoid excessive pressure on deformed limbs.

THE PHYSICAL EXAM

Focus on identifying active problems in key organ systems that will increase surgical risk or change perioperative management.

Vital signs. Determine blood pressure, heart rate and regularity of rhythm, rate and ease of respiration, and temperature. Hypotension with clinical evidence of hypoperfusion or shock, tachycardia/bradycardia, and fever should be stabilized before proceeding to nonurgent surgery. Systolic blood pressure >180 mm Hg and diastolic pressure >110 mm Hg are not independent risk factors for perioperative cardiovascular events so the potential benefits of optimizing treatment need to be weighed against the risks of delaying surgery.

Heart. Look for significant heart murmurs, extra sounds (S3, S4), signs of CHF, elevated central venous pressure, and peripheral edema.

Circulation. Examine for carotid, abdominal, and femoral bruits.

Lungs. Examine for crackles, wheezes, decreased breath sounds, prolonged expiratory phase, effusions, and estimate pulmonary reserve. Flattened diaphragms limiting inspiratory reserve is suggested by finding the top of the thyroid cartilage <4 cm above the suprasternal notch and depressing <2 cm with deep inspiration.

Hemostasis. Examine for skin integrity, petechiae, and unusual bruising.

Mental status. Cognitive dysfunction greatly increases the risk for postoperative delirium and is easily missed without specific testing. The Mini-Cog tool (three word recall and clock drawing test) is a validated screening tool.

LABORATORY TESTING

Select appropriate laboratory studies based on the history and exam to confirm and quantify abnormalities. Routine laboratory tests are not useful without a specific medical indication.

Electrocardiogram. An ECG is not indicated for asymptomatic subjects undergoing low-risk procedures including endoscopic procedures, superficial procedures, transurethral prostate resection, cataract surgery, and breast surgery. Obtain a 12-lead resting ECG for intermediate or high-risk patients scheduled for intermediate or high-risk procedures, and anyone with diabetes or a recent episode of chest pain or an ischemia equivalent (e.g., shortness of breath). Most experts recommend an ECG on all patients with prior coronary revascularization procedures, patients with prior hospitalization for heart disease, and on asymptomatic males older than 45 years of age or females older than 55 years of age with two or more clinical risk factors (see below).

Echocardiogram. Routine preoperative evaluation of left ventricular function is not recommended. Transthoracic echocardiogram may be indicated in patients with signs/symptoms of valvular heart disease or left ventricular dysfunction.

Myocardial perfusion imaging. *Surgery is not an independent indication for invasive coronary diagnostic or therapeutic procedures.* Coronary revascularization prior to surgery in asymptomatic patients by either coronary artery bypass grafting or coronary angioplasty with or without stenting does not reduce the perioperative cardiac morbidity or mortality risk. The indications for perfusion imaging are the same as for that patient independent of the planned surgery. Clinical risk factors for coronary artery disease include a history of CAD, CHF, or CVA and insulin-treated diabetes, creatinine >2, and high-risk surgery. For patients with ≥3 risk factors undergoing vascular procedures or ≥1 risk factor undergoing intermediate risk surgery noninvasive stress testing can be considered but only *if symptoms dictate.*

Chest x-ray. A chest x-ray is indicated for patients with new respiratory symptoms or suspected congestive heart failure, valvular heart disease, or intracardiac shunts. For patients aged >50 having upper abdominal, thoracic or abdominal aortic surgery, consider obtaining a preoperative chest radiograph even without evidence of pulmonary disease.

Pulmonary function tests. PFTs are unnecessary unless the patient is undergoing lung resection surgery, the etiology of shortness of breath is unclear (cardiac vs. pulmonary vs. deconditioning), or it is uncertain whether a patient's asthma or COPD is optimized prior to elective surgery.

Serum chemistries and CBC. Serum chemistries are not required for low-risk procedures. For intermediate- and high-risk procedures, patients aged

>40 or with DM, HTN, cardiac, or renal disease should, at minimum, have preoperative blood urea nitrogen, serum creatinine, blood glucose, and a complete blood cell count given the risk of asymptomatic renal dysfunction and perioperative blood loss. Serum electrolytes should be included for patients taking medications likely to alter renal function or electrolyte balance.

Hemoglobin and hematocrit. Anemia and red blood cell transfusion are associated with an increased risk of perioperative complications and longer hospital stays. When blood loss of >500 mL is anticipated, an H&H should be obtained at least 4 weeks prior to elective surgery. Anemia (Hb < 12.0 g/dL) should be investigated, the etiology identified and treated, and the H&H corrected prior to elective surgery.

Coagulation studies. Obtain coagulation studies only for patients with a personal or family history suggesting a bleeding diathesis or thrombophilia.

SUMMATIVE RISK ASSESSMENT

The preoperative evaluation estimates the risk of medical morbidity and mortality so that the surgeon and patient can make reasonable choices regarding the appropriateness and timing of the planned procedure. It is not the task of the medical consultant to "clear" a patient for surgery. The decisions of if and when to operate are made by the patient and surgeon after discussing the medical risks and benefits attendant to the surgery. Lee et al.'s Revised Cardiac Risk Index (RCRI) is a validated tool for estimating risk using six independent risk factors: high-risk surgery, a history of ischemic heart disease, congestive heart failure (current or by history), cerebrovascular disease, insulin-treated diabetes, and a creatinine ≥2.0. The risk for complications if 0–1 risk factor was present was <1.0%; for two risk factors, 1.3%; for three risk factors, 4%; and for more than three risk factors, 9%. A retrospective validation study showed that the RCRI discriminated moderately well between patients at low and high risk for cardiac events after mixed noncardiac surgery. This is a simple and easy to use index, but the clinician still must combine this with an assessment of noncardiac risks.

CLINICAL VIGNETTES AND QUESTIONS

CASE 16-1

Myocardial infarction is the most serious medical complication in the perioperative period and it accounts for a large proportion of perioperative morbidity. Several tools have been developed to help estimate the perioperative risk for acute coronary events.

QUESTIONS:
1. Name some of the conditions contributing to increased perioperative risk for acute coronary events.
2. What operative procedures are considered to be high risk for cardiovascular complications?
3. Name some procedures that are considered to be intermediate risk for cardiovascular complications.

CASE 16-2

Functional aerobic capacity is a predictor of a patient's ability to tolerate a major surgical procedure.

QUESTIONS:
1. What is the scale that is used to measure the level of aerobic function?
2. What is the baseline for this metric and how is the scale derived?
3. What is the minimum aerobic capacity for a patient to consider an elective major surgical procedure?
4. Name some activities requiring this minimum level of exertion.

CLINICAL VIGNETTES AND QUESTIONS

CASE 16-1

Myocardial dysfunction is the most serious medical complication in the perioperative period and accounts for a large proportion of perioperative morbidity. Several tools have been developed to help estimate the perioperative risk for acute coronary events.

QUESTIONS:

1. Name some of the conditions contributing to increased perioperative risk for acute coronary events.
2. What operative procedures are considered to be high risk for intravascular complications?
3. Name some procedures that are considered to be high risk for intra- and postoperative complications.

CASE 16-2

Functional capacity is an indicator of a patient's ability to tolerate a major surgical procedure.

QUESTIONS:

1. What is the scale that is used to measure the level of activity function?
2. What is the baseline for this scale and how is the scale developed?
3. What is the minimum score that a surgical patient is required to tolerate an elective major surgical procedure?
4. Name some activities that require this minimum level of function.

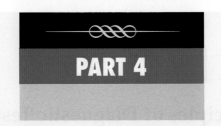

PART 4

Use of the Laboratory and Diagnostic Imaging

Where is the wisdom we have lost in knowledge?

Where is the knowledge we have lost in information?

– T.S. ELIOT
Choruses from "The Rock"

CHAPTER 17

Principles of Diagnostic Testing

Sensitive and specific laboratory tests and imaging studies are essential to accurate diagnosis in many clinical settings. Proper use of the laboratory and imaging requires accurate clinical hypotheses generated at the bedside. Laboratory tests and imaging provide reliable and valid answers to well-conceived clinical questions. They are also liable to overinterpretation and can be quite misleading if not interpreted in the clinical context as answers to specific questions. Beyond a few screening tests, these studies should be used to test the physiologic and diagnostic hypotheses generated during the history and physical exam. The laboratory and the radiology suite are not the places to look for ideas; they are the places to test hypotheses. If you are unable to generate testable hypotheses after the history, physical exam, and screening tests, it will be more useful to seek consultation than to begin an undirected series of laboratory and radiologic studies. A full discussion of the proper use of diagnostic tests is beyond the scope of this text.

PRINCIPLES OF LABORATORY TESTING

Laboratory testing is principally done for two reasons: (1) to obtain information that cannot be determined clinically, but which is often important in forming hypotheses and (2) to test hypotheses. Tests in the first category are commonly described as "routine" testing and include serum electrolytes, blood urea nitrogen, creatinine, complete blood counts, urinalysis, and, less commonly, transaminases and erythrocyte sedimentation rate or C-reactive protein. Some, or all, of these tests are performed in patients with significant illness to help the clinician identify significant abnormalities in major organ function or laboratory signs of inflammation or infection. Tests in the second category are innumerable. They are used to identify specific abnormalities and diseases. The diagnostic performance of these tests is dependent upon the patient population tested. Tests in this category are most useful when the diagnosis in question is in the mid-range of probability, roughly 20%–80%. To understand why this is so, it is necessary to understand the measures of test performance and how interpretation is dependent on both the diagnostic criteria for a disease or condition and the pretest probability that the disease is present.

Principles of Testing for Disease
Disease present or absent. How do we determine who has the disease and who does not? This is done with an independent test or set of criteria accepted as establishing "the diagnosis." The assumption is that a disease is either present or absent. Although this may seem obvious for diseases such as cancer or an infection where a tissue biopsy or culture are the diagnostic standards,

most biologic measurements are continuous variables, not either/or determinations; it is often difficult to say whether rheumatoid arthritis is present or not, or which level of creatinine determines renal failure. Most diseases have variable clinical severity; hence the diagnostic standard used to establish the disease can be either very inclusive (sensitive) or more exclusive (specific). A good example is the American Rheumatologic Association criteria for the diagnosis of rheumatic syndromes. These criteria were developed because laboratory tests have insufficient accuracy to identify these patients. The goal was to identify persons eligible for inclusion in research studies of each specific disease. Hence, the criteria for diagnosis of these syndromes is set to be quite specific, i.e., patients meeting the criteria are very likely to have the syndrome. However, it cannot be concluded that patients not meeting the criteria, who have many of the features and no other explanation, do not have the syndrome.

Test positive or negative. The definition of normal for continuous variables is a statistical determination (see the discussion of cholesterol in Chapter 18 for an exception). At what point abnormal becomes an illness or disease is a judgment based upon the desire to identify those with disease (*true-positives*), but not include a significant portion of patients without the disease (*false-positives*). Furthermore, most tests are not positive in all the patients with a given disease, so there will be patients with the disease who are missed by the test (*false-negatives*). Finally, we want to be sure that a very high proportion of patients who do not have the disease, have a negative test (*true-negatives*). A cut-point is selected by comparing the distribution of the test results in patients with the disease (determined as above) and in those without the disease (Fig. 17-1). When the two populations overlap in part of their range, a cut point is chosen to minimize the misallocation of patients (false-positives and false-negatives). Note, however, that much of the information is lost by looking at tests of continuous variables as positive or negative: very abnormal tests are more likely to be associated with disease than mildly abnormal tests. As discussed below likelihood ratios (LR) capture this information for making diagnostic decisions.

Probability and odds. *Probability* is a ratio or proportion of one part of a population to the whole population. A racehorse that wins 1 race in 20 has a 5% probability of winning ($1/20 = 0.05$). Odds is the ratio of two probabilities. Because most events are uncommon (otherwise we would not need to make all these calculations), odds are customarily expressed as the odds against an event. For our horse, the probability of losing is 0.95 the probability of winning is 0.05 and the odds are 19:1; that it will lose. Odds and probabilities can be derived from one another:

$$\text{Odds} = \text{Probability} / (1 - \text{Probability})$$

$$\text{Probability} = \text{Odds} / (1 + \text{Odds}).$$

Pretest probability and prior odds. Generate physiologic and etiologic hypotheses and a differential diagnosis at the bedside (see Chapter 1). Estimate the probability of each disease in the differential. If 100 patients

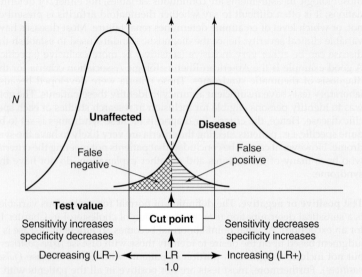

FIG. 17-1 Interpretation of Test Results. A population of unaffected patients is compared with a population of diseased patients. The cut point for determining normal-abnormal is the value with the best compromise between sensitivity and specificity. Likelihood Ratio (LR) can be calculated for test values above and below the usual cut point.

exactly like this patient—same age, sex, comorbidities, presenting symptoms, and physical signs—how many would have each condition? This estimate is the *pretest probability*. Expressed as odds (the probability of having the disease over the probability of not having the disease) this is the *prior odds*.

2 × 2 tables. Tests are evaluated in 2-cell by 2-cell tables (2 × 2 tables) whose parameters, by predetermined criteria, are disease-present, disease-absent, test-positive, and test-negative (Fig. 17-2). The four cells represent the true-positives (disease-present and test-positive), the false-positives (disease-absent but test-positive), the false-negatives (disease-present but test-negative), and the true-negatives (disease-absent and test-negative), respectively conventionally labeled *a, b, c,* and *d*.

Disease prevalence. The first column contains all the patients with the disease $(a + c)$ and the second column all the patients who are disease free $(b + d)$. The ratio of the first column to the sum of the two columns is the disease's prevalence *in the population from which the data in the table is derived*:

$$\text{Prevalence} = (a + c) / (a + b + c + d).$$

To interpret the data we need to know how the persons (diseased and disease-free) were selected for inclusion in each column. If this was a randomly selected, population-based sample, then the prevalence is that of the disease in the population, often a useful number. On the other hand, the

		DISEASE	
		Present	Absent
TEST	Positive	*a* ***True positives***	*b* ***False positives***
	Negative	*c* ***False negatives***	*d* ***True negatives***

$$\text{Sensitivity (Sn)} = \frac{a}{a+c} \qquad \text{Specifity (Sp)} = \frac{d}{b+d}$$

$$\text{Positive predictive value (PPV)} = \frac{a}{a+b} \qquad \text{Negative predictive value (NPV)} = \frac{d}{a+d}$$

FIG. 17-2 The 2 × 2 Table: Sensitivity, Specificity, and Positive Predictive value (PPV) and Negative Predictive Value (NPV).

investigators may have selected a group of patients with the disease and another group known not to have the disease in a predetermined ratio or by some nonrandom method. In this case, the "prevalence" is essentially meaningless for understanding disease prevalence in any useful clinical sense.

Selecting and Interpreting Tests

Sensitivity (Sn). Sensitivity is the number of patients with the disease who have a positive test, divided by the total number with the disease: *sensitivity* = $a/(a+c)$, a probability. *With highly sensitive tests, most patients with the disease have a positive test (very few false negatives).* Tests with high sensitivity (>0.95) are most useful when *negative*, thereby making the diagnosis less likely. Note that the sensitivity of a test, because it is calculated only in those with the disease, is independent of disease prevalence. Sensitivity is increased by changing the cutoff for defining a positive test to a less abnormal value (see Fig. 17-1). Because sensitivity is independent of prevalence, it is susceptible to overinterpretation when disease prevalence is very low (see Example 1). In this case, the false-positive tests (*b*) may significantly outnumber the true positives (*a*). Sensitive tests are used to avoid missing a serious disease. A negative result makes the disease unlikely reassuring the patient and clinician and narrowing the diagnostic possibilities. A positive test needs confirmation with more specific tests before a diagnosis can be established.

Specificity (Sp). Specificity is the proportion of disease-free patients with a negative test: *specificity* $= d/(b + d)$, a probability. *With highly specific tests, most patients without the disease have negative tests (very few false positives).* However, the test may also be negative in those with the disease. Note that patients with the disease are not included in the determination of specificity; it, like sensitivity, is independent of disease prevalence. Specificity can also be improved by changing the cut point for defining abnormal to a more abnormal value (see Fig. 17-1). Because specificity is independent of prevalence, it is susceptible to overinterpretation when disease prevalence (pretest probability) is high (see Example 4). In this case, the false-negative tests (c) may significantly outnumber the true-negatives (d). Highly specific tests are used to confirm a diagnosis. This is especially important when there are serious consequences of the diagnosis for the patient, either for prognosis or therapy.

Setting the positive/negative cut point. The clinical laboratory supplies a reference range for most diagnostic tests (see Chapter 18). This range is determined by testing hundreds of samples from unselected patients, patients with the disease, and patients known to be disease-free. The data generates graphs such as Figure 17-1. The data are analyzed to determine the best statistical fit for distinguishing diseased from disease-free populations. For many clinical tests, such as treadmill exercise tests, interpretation of imaging studies, and application of diagnostic tests, the clinician must decide, based upon the clinical scenario and the diagnostic question (screening, case finding, hypothesis testing), what cut point will best serve to answer the question. Consultation with specialists in laboratory medicine and with experts in the diseases in the differential diagnosis can assist in determining what should be regarded as a positive or negative test in each clinical situation.

Predictive values. When we order a test we are not really interested in the test (sensitivity and specificity), but in how it helps us in understanding our patient's problem: does the presence of a positive test predict that the patient has the disease (*positive predictive value [PPV]*) and does a negative test predict the absence of the disease (*negative predictive value [NPV]*). Predictive values are calculated from 2 × 2 tables (see Fig. 17-2). The predictive values for a test are dependent upon the population used to generate the data in the 2 × 2 table; different populations have different prevalence of disease. To generate meaningful predictive values, the patients generating the data must be chosen randomly from a clinical population that is relevant to the question and patient.

Positive predictive value. The PPV, calculated from the 2 × 2 table, is the proportion of test-positive patients with the disease: $PPV = a/(a + b)$, a probability. Tests with a high PPV have few false-positives, therefore a positive test supports the diagnosis. Note, however, that if the disease is rare in the population (therefore $(b + d) >> (a + c)$, the test will have to be extremely specific (low false-positives, b) for the true-positives to be greater than the false-positives (see Examples). Therefore, when the prevalence of disease is low (low pretest probability), even seemingly good tests (sensitivity, specificity) may perform poorly for predicting the presence of disease.

Negative predictive value. The NPV is the proportion of test-negative patients who are disease-free: NPV $= d/(c + d)$, a probability. Tests with a high NPV have few false-negatives, therefore a negative test argues against the disease. When the condition is prevalent in the population a negative test may not be very helpful; that is, the NPV may be low and the disease may be present despite a negative test.

Using PPV and NPV requires the clinician to know, or have a good estimate of, the disease prevalence in the population which the patient represents. Most clinicians do not have this data. Instead use a clinical estimate of the probability of disease is generated from the history and physical exam.

Likelihood ratios (LR). Another expression of a test's usefulness LR. *A positive likelihood ratio (LR+)* is the ratio of the probability of a positive test in people with the disease (the sensitivity) to the probability of a positive test in people without the disease: LR+ $= [a/(a + c)] \div [b/(b + d)]$. *A negative likelihood ratio (LR−)* is the probability of a negative test in patients with the disease divided by the probability of a negative test in people without the disease (the specificity): LR− $= [c/(a + c)] \div [d/(b + d)]$ (Fig. 17-3). LRs, the ratio of two probabilities, are *odds*.

TEST	DISEASE Present	DISEASE Absent
Positive	***a*** **True positives**	***b*** **False positives**
Negative	***c*** **False negatives**	***d*** **True negatives**

Positive likelihood ratio (LR+)
LR+ $= [c/(a + c)] \div [b/(b + d)]$

Negative likelihood ratio (LR−)
LR− $= [c/(a + c)] \div [d/(b + d)]$

FIG. 17-3 Positive and Negative LR.

LR shows how well a result more abnormal (LR+) or less abnormal (LR−) than a given value (the cut point for test-positive in the 2 × 2 table) discriminates between those with and without the disease. They are a function of the defined parameters of the test and are independent of the prevalence of the disease (see the Examples). LR contains all the sensitivity and specificity information and expresses the relationship between sensitivity and specificity for positive and negative results. A big advantage of LR is that they can be calculated for a range of test values, rather than the single *normal-abnormal* cut point used for sensitivity and specificity. Thus, *LR allows uses all the information rather than the limited information in a single normal-abnormal cut point.* As the LR+ becomes larger, the likelihood of the disease increases; as the LR− approaches zero, the disease becomes much less likely. Generally, LRs 0.5–3.0 are not useful while those 0.3–0.5 and 3.0–5.0 are suggestive but not conclusive. LRs >5 argue for the disease whereas LRs <0.2 argue against the disease.

Post-test probability and posterior odds. LR includes information from each cell of the 2 × 2 table. They are not susceptible to the errors inherent in applying predictive values to conditions of low and high prevalence as discussed above. Therefore, they are diagnostically more useful. Because LR is a ratio of probabilities, they are an expression of odds. Use them to derive a new probability for the disease based upon the test result. Because this new probability is determined after the test, it is the *post-test probability* (PP). To calculate the post-test probability, convert the pretest probability to pretest odds and then multiply by the LR to get the post-test odds (*posterior odds*). Then, convert the post-test odds back to the post-test probability (see Example 1). The post-test probability can be calculated for both a positive test and a negative test.

Clinicians should learn to think in terms of the LR for the parameter ranges of the tests they use. This is the implicit reasoning that experienced and efficient clinicians use in selecting and interpreting their laboratory tests. It is useful to make this process explicit allowing us to do the calculations in the occasional situation where it will be useful, but also helps us to understand and dissect our decision-making processes and to avoid misinterpretation of normal or abnormal laboratory results.

EXAMPLES

Four examples of clinical testing scenarios are presented each with a different estimated disease prevalence. For each example the test is assumed to have 95% sensitivity and 95% specificity. These examples should facilitate an understanding of the concepts discussed above.

Example 1: **Disease prevalence 1%.** Of 10,000 patients, only 100 have the disease (99:1 odds-against) (Fig. 17-4). False-positives are five times more common than true-positives. The calculations are only be shown for this example.

		DISEASE	
		Present	Absent
TEST	Positive	***a*** **True positives** *N* = 95	***b*** **False positives** *N* = 500
	Negative	***c*** **False negatives** *N* = 5	***d*** **True negatives** *N* = 9400
		PPV = 0.16 NPV = 0.999	LR+ = 19 LR− = 0.05

FIG. 17-4 Example 1: Disease Prevalence 1%. The test has a sensitivity of 0.95 and a specificity of 0.95.

Calculation of positive and NPVs:

$$\text{PPV} = \frac{a}{(a+b)} = \frac{95}{(95+500)} = 0.16$$

$$\text{NPV} = \frac{c}{(c+d)} = \frac{5}{(5+9400)} = 0.999$$

Calculation of positive and Negative LR

$$\begin{aligned}\text{LR+} &= [a\,/\,(a+c)] \div [b\,/\,(b+d)]\\ &= [95\,/\,(95+5)] \div [500\,/\,(500+9400)] = 19\\ \text{LR}- &= [c\,/\,(a+c)] \div [d\,/\,(b+d)]\\ &= [5\,/\,(95+5)] \div [9400\,/\,(500+9400)] = 0.05.\end{aligned}$$

The PPV (0.16) is better than the baseline risk (0.01), but is still quite low; so, a positive test does not make the diagnosis very probable. The NPV

		DISEASE Present	DISEASE Absent
TEST	Positive	a ***True positives*** $N = 95$	b ***False positives*** $N = 45$
	Negative	c ***False negatives*** $N = 5$	d ***True negatives*** $N = 855$

PPV = 0.65 LR+ = 19
NPV = 0.999 LR− = 0.05

FIG. 17-5 Example 2: Disease Prevalence 10%. The test has a sensitivity of 0.95 and a specificity of 0.95.

is 0.999 (1 in 10,000), which sounds good, but is not much better than the already low baseline risk of 0.01 (1 in 100).

Has this highly sensitive and specific test helped in this situation? Not much. Although the likelihood of disease is much higher with a positive test (from 99:1 to 16:1), still most positive tests are false-positives requiring further evaluation. This example is typical of screening for an uncommon disease in an asymptomatic population. The test must be very sensitive *and* very specific to be useful. An example of such a test is HIV testing in pregnant women. However, most clinical tests have neither the sensitivity nor specificity required to be effective when disease prevalence is low.

Example 2: **Disease prevalence 10%.** Of 1,000 patients, 100 have the disease (9:1 odds-against) (Fig. 17-5).

$$\text{NPV} = 0.65 \quad \text{LR+} = 19$$

$$\text{NPV} = 0.999 \quad \text{LR−} = 0.05.$$

In this scenario, 65% of the patients with a positive test have the disease; a definite improvement over the 10% at baseline. A positive test is twice as likely to be a true-positive as a false-positive. The NPV is quite low so a negative test reduces the likelihood of disease.

		DISEASE	
		Present	Absent
TEST	Positive	*a* ***True positives*** *N* = 95	*b* ***False positives*** *N* = 5
	Negative	*c* ***False negatives*** *N* = 5	*d* ***True negatives*** *N* = 95

PPV = 0.95 LR+ = 19
NPV = 0.95 LR− = 0.05

FIG. 17-6 Example 3: Disease Prevalence 50%. For these examples, the test has a sensitivity of 0.95 and a specificity of 0.95.

Are either the positive or negative results likely to be enough for diagnosis? A negative test reduces the post-test probability of the disease below any reasonable clinical threshold. A positive test needs to be followed by more specific testing to confirm the diagnosis (raise the probability of disease above the level needed for clinical certainty). This is especially true for diseases with an adverse prognosis or for which therapies are potentially toxic.

This scenario is representative of a case finding strategy in an at-risk population. A test with 95% sensitivity and specificity could be used to separate the population into a low-risk pool and a high-risk pool, the latter to undergo further testing.

Example 3: **Disease prevalence 50%.** You have worked up a patient and your clinical impression is that the patient has a 50% chance (1:1 odds) of having the disease (disease prevalence of 0.5) (Fig. 17-6). You construct a 2×2 table with what you know.

$$\text{NPV} = 0.95 \quad \text{LR+} = 19$$

$$\text{NPV} = 0.95 \quad \text{LR}- = 0.05.$$

The PPV and NPV are both significant improvements over the baseline risk of 0.5. There are relatively few false positives or false negatives.

DISEASE

	Present	Absent
Positive	**a** **True positives** N = 855	**b** **False positives** N = 5
Negative	**c** **False negatives** N = 45	**d** **True negatives** N = 95

TEST

PPV = 0.95   LR+ = 19
NPV = 0.73   LR− = 0.05

FIG. 17-7 Example 4: Disease Prevalence 90%. The test has a sensitivity of 0.95 and a specificity of 0.95.

Does the test help in this clinical situation? The test is clinically useful regardless of the result. Both positive and negative results substantially change the disease probability, and both probably exceed the level of certainty required in most clinical situations.

This example is representative of the situation in which laboratory testing is most useful, that is, true uncertainty, with even odds for and against the disease. Selecting tests with good LR in this setting will profoundly impact your diagnostic process.

Example 4: **Disease prevalence 90%.** You have worked up a patient and your clinical impression is that the patient has a 90% chance (9:1 odds in favor) of having the disease (disease prevalence of 0.9) (Fig. 17-7). You construct a 2 × 2 table with what you know.

$$NPV = 0.95 \quad LR+ = 19$$
$$NPV = 0.73 \quad LR- = 0.05.$$

Based on your clinical assessment it is quite likely the patient has the disease. A positive test (PPV) only minimally improves your accuracy. A negative test (NPV) reduces the probability, but it is still the most likely diagnosis, and one-third of those with a negative test will be misclassified (false-negatives).

Has the test helped you reach the predetermined level of certainty required to either diagnose the disease or exclude it from further consideration? No, a positive result adds nothing, and a third of negative results are false-negatives.

This scenario is representative of a situation when too high a level of certainty is expected for the clinical situation. Neither a positive nor a negative test is helpful.

Comment: Note that our test has excellent LR, and the LR is the same regardless of the prevalence of disease. Like sensitivity and specificity, LR is a function of the value of the test chosen as the cut point. This confirms that the LR tells how well a positive and negative test discriminate the population into higher and lower risk groups. However, the interpretation and usefulness of the test still depends upon the baseline probability of disease (pretest probability): a 20-times improvement in very long odds is still long odds (999:1 to 49:1), and a 20-times decrease in very short odds is still an almost even proposition (1:24 to 20:24).

The reader is encouraged to construct their own examples and vary the prevalence of disease and the sensitivity and specificity of the test to familiarize themselves with these concepts. The formal calculations are rarely done in clinical practice, but the principles and concepts are used every day by skilled clinicians in deciding how to evaluate their differential diagnoses.

As demonstrated in Example 3, diagnostic testing is most useful when true uncertainty exists with nearly even odds for and against the condition. The purpose of a probabilistic differential diagnosis is to identify true uncertainty (approximately even odds) where testing improves the probability assessment. Most physical findings do not have positive LR of sufficient magnitude to be useful for testing hypotheses; they do not establish a diagnosis. The history and physical exam are for generating hypotheses and estimating pretest probabilities (prior odds). Many laboratory tests have LR that allow accurate diagnostic discrimination: the laboratory is the best place to test your specific hypotheses. When clinical probability estimates are either very high or very low, further testing is not useful and is often misleading.

2 × 2 Tables Revisited: Caveat Emptor: If you plan to use the sensitivity, specificity, or LR generated from a 2×2 table, it is necessary to understand the methods used for selection of the test sample that produced the data. Each of these parameters is dependent upon the inclusion criteria for the categories disease-present and disease-absent and the method for identifying the population(s) that were tested.

Severity of disease. Most diseases have a broad spectrum of severity that is generally reflected in the amount of aberration in the tests characteristic of the disease: more-severe disease, more-abnormal tests; less-severe disease, less-abnormal or even normal test results. As can be seen from Figure 17-1 and the preceding discussion, if the investigators choose to define the presence of disease as those with more-severe disease (cut point moved to the right), the test will appear more specific and less sensitive, and the positive LR will improve, whereas the negative LR becomes less useful. If they choose an inclusive definition to reflect the broad range of those with the disease (cut point moved to the left), the test will be more sensitive and less specific, and the negative LR will improve, whereas the positive LR becomes less useful. In addition, if the 2 × 2 table was constructed using patients with unusually severe disease (as may be seen in an academic referral practice), the sensitivity and specificity calculated may be inappropriately high if applied to a more representative patient population.

Sampling. Broadly speaking there are three methods of selecting patients to generate data for a 2 × 2 table.

By far the easiest method is to take patients from a known diseased group (e.g., patients with known systemic lupus erythematosus, attending a rheumatology clinic) and another group of patients from a disease-free population (e.g., blood donors) and apply the test (e.g., an antinuclear antibody test) to both groups. This will generate a 2×2 table weighted to more severe disease because the patients are already diagnosed and attending a clinic (see Severity of Disease). The apparent prevalence is not a real population prevalence; it is an a priori choice of the investigators as to the number of people they want in each group. The sensitivity, specificity, and LR of tests evaluated by this method often appear very good. But, because there are really two independent populations being used to generate the table, the PPV and NPV have no meaning. The clinical usefulness of information generated by this sampling method is marginal at best when the clinician attempts to apply the test parameters to an unselected population.

The second, far more difficult method, is to select a population representing the community at large (e.g., a random sample of adults), test all of them, and evaluate them all by the gold-standard criteria for the disease. When diseases have a low prevalence in the population (e.g., systemic lupus erythematosus), huge numbers of patients would need very thorough evaluations at tremendous expense to identify enough cases to produce meaningful data. Hence, this method is only applied to the evaluation of screening tests proposed for large populations (e.g., fecal immunohistochemical test for colon cancer). This method also does not generate clinically useful data for the clinician outside of the screening paradigm.

The most clinically useful information is generated by selecting patients from a population that presents with the challenge faced by the physician: patients who might have the disease based upon history and physical exam (an intermediate pretest probability, near even odds). A consecutive series of such patients is identified, and the test and diagnostic gold standard are applied to all. The data generated in this way is far more useful to the clinician when faced with a diagnostic challenge. The test parameters (LR, sensitivity, and specificity), the prevalence of disease, and the PPV and NPV are much more likely to be applicable to clinical decision making. The clinician still must assess whether the gender, ethnic mix, ages, and comorbidities of the test population are representative of their patient population.

Rule-In; Rule-Out: The phrases rule-in and rule-out are commonplace in the clinical vernacular but are discouraged. Some diagnoses can be *confirmed* by specific pathologic tests (e.g., neoplasms, vasculitis), by laboratory tests (e.g., HIV infection, myocardial injury, sickle cell disease), or by microbiologic tests (e.g., cultures and polymerase chain reaction [PCR] identification of specific organisms). It is impossible, short of necropsy, to rule-out a diagnosis. When tests with highly negative LR are negative in patients with intermediate or low pretest probability for the disease, the *probability* of the disease becomes very small, but never zero. In each clinical case, we empirically set a clinical level of certainty required to confirm a diagnosis, as discussed in Chapter 1. We also determine a level of clinical certainty needed to effectively exclude a diagnosis from further consideration. This depends upon the patient, the clinical scenario, and the risk associated with drawing a false-negative conclusion. When we have assured ourselves that the diagnosis is less probable than our threshold, we can say it is excluded clinically, but it is never ruled-out. Furthermore, many clinical conditions, especially syndromes (e.g., rheumatoid arthritis), have no gold-standard diagnostic test or exclusion criteria.

Summary: The skilled clinician uses a patient's history and physical exam to generate pathophysiologic and diagnostic hypotheses. The differential diagnosis includes those diseases with the highest estimated probability of being present *in this patient*, and less likely diseases associated with severe morbidity if not promptly diagnosed. An explicit estimation of the probability for each is made. Tests are selected for which the result (positive, negative, or a specific value or finding) will generate a post-test probability (applying the LR) of a clinically significant high or low level. On the basis of the first round of test results and repeat evaluation of the patient, a refined differential diagnosis is constructed and a second round of tests may be ordered. This process is repeated until the post-test probability for the diagnosis exceeds the threshold required by the clinical situation. At that point, a working diagnosis is established.

PRINCIPLES OF DIAGNOSTIC IMAGING

Imaging techniques include standard radiography and computed axial tomography using X-rays with or without contrast, magnetic resonance imaging, ultrasonography (including Doppler flow measurements), and radioisotope imaging (standard nuclear medicine and positron emission tomography [PET]). The amount of information contained in an imaging study is enormous, especially with computed axial tomography and magnetic resonance imaging technologies. This increase in information may be essential for the care of patients, or it may be a distraction in the diagnostic process. Imaging techniques are rapidly evolving, so it is essential to work closely with your radiologist to select the appropriate imaging studies to answer the clinical questions.

Static images reveal body structure; the questions they answer are anatomic, not physiologic questions. Images tell us where anatomy is altered and suggest how it is altered. Images cannot make pathologic, microbiologic or physiologic diagnoses. Be sure that your radiologist describes the images and the anatomic abnormalities using descriptive language rather than conclusions. Radiologists cannot diagnose granulomas, tuberculosis, cancer, or infection. They can describe lesions with characteristics suggestive of these diagnoses.

Dynamic imaging allows accurate evaluation of the mechanical properties of certain organs, such as arterial and venous blood flow and heart muscle and valve function. They also allow reasonably good estimates of intravascular pressure gradients from the Bernoulli equation, which relates flow to the pressure gradient across areas of restricted flow.

As with all tests, beyond the most standard laboratory evaluation discussed above, each imaging study must be ordered to answer a specific clinical question. Ordering imaging studies without a hypothesis or specific question is a bad practice often identifying incidental findings (anatomic variants, degenerative conditions, benign neoplasms, cysts, and hemangiomas) that distract attention even when they have no plausible bearing on the patient's presenting complaints. It is easy to begin evaluating the imaging studies (and the laboratory abnormalities) rather than the patient.

The conclusions drawn from an imaging study need to be drawn by clinicians familiar with the patient. The diagnostic and physiologic hypotheses of the radiologists should follow their description of the images. Again, an easily made mistake is to let the imaging specialist begin to direct the evaluation, often of incidental findings or clinically irrelevant questions. Clinically important questions relevant to the presenting problem should drive the imaging evaluation. Incidental findings can be followed up later if needed. It is extremely uncommon for incidental findings to have major significance for the patient.

CHAPTER 18

Common Laboratory Tests

This chapter discusses normal and pathologic values for commonly ordered tests of the blood (cells and chemistries), urine, cerebrospinal fluid (CSF), and serous fluids. The tests discussed are commonly used in formulating physiologic and diagnostic hypotheses. The much more numerous specific tests used for confirming the diagnosis of a specific disease should not be used until a narrow differential diagnosis has been established. These more specific tests are not discussed here.

Laboratory tests are ordered for one of the four reasons:

1. **Screening.** A small number of tests identify silent disease in patients without symptoms, signs, or specific risk factors for the disease, e.g., testing for hemochromatosis with iron studies and lipids for hypercholesterolemia.
2. **Case finding.** Some tests identify affected asymptomatic individuals within an at-risk population. This differs from screening because a high-risk population, rather than the general population, is selected for testing, e.g., testing the children of BRCA-related breast cancer patients for the genetic abnormality.
3. **Diagnosis.** Tests assist in making (or excluding) a diagnosis suggested by the patient's symptoms and signs. See the discussion in Chapter 17 for a summary of the proper approach to diagnostic testing.
4. **Monitoring.** Tests are often used to monitor the progress of disease, response to therapy, or concentration of medication.

Many laboratory tests are used for more than one, or even for all, of these reasons, depending on the clinical situation. For example, blood glucose is used to screen for diabetes mellitus, to identify cases amongst obese patients with a family history of diabetes who are at high risk for diabetes, to confirm the diagnosis, and to monitor treatment in diabetic patients.

Which tests, if any, to obtain routinely is debated interminably. Certainly, the prevalence of the disease in the population of which your patient is a member should affect test selection. In addition to assisting diagnosis, quantitative tests reflect the severity of physiologic abnormalities. Tests and their usefulness continually change, so the clinician must keep abreast of current indications for and uses of clinical laboratory tests. Consult with the pathologist in charge of the clinical laboratory when questions arise.

Reference ranges are only illustrative; each clinical laboratory determines its own reference ranges.

Many organizations, including the American Medical Association, have supported the proposal of the American National Metric Council to convert result reporting to Système International d'Unités (SI) units introduced in the mid-1980s. US physicians, laboratory staffs, and hospitals have been reluctant to convert to SI units. Indeed, excellent medical journals have chosen to use conventional units, or both. For the non-American reader's convenience, we have included values with SI units in parentheses following the conventional units. Most of the laboratory reference values were adopted from *Harrison's Principles of Internal Medicine*.

Each test is followed by a list of diseases and disorders associated with abnormal values. The lists of associated diseases, syndromes, and conditions highlight the more prevalent conditions and some important rarer diseases. The lists do not include all possibilities but serve as a guide for thinking. Consult textbooks of laboratory medicine for more complete discussions.

BLOOD CHEMISTRIES

Albumin: See Proteins, page 773.

Alkaline Phosphatase, Serum: This includes several cellular enzymes that hydrolyze phosphate esters. They are named from their optimum activity in alkaline media. High blood enzyme concentrations occur during rapid growth, either physiologic or pathologic, and from cellular injury. The enzymes are normally plentiful in hepatic parenchyma, osteoblasts, intestinal mucosa, placental cells, and renal epithelium. Abnormally rapid growth or cell destruction raises their concentration.

Normal alkaline phosphatase: 30–120 U/L (SI units: 0.5–2.0 nkat/L). It is high in newborns, declining until puberty and then rising every decade after 60 years of age.

Increased alkaline phosphatase. This is usually associated with disorders of bone, liver, or the biliary tract.
CLINICAL OCCURRENCE: *Technical Error:* Dehydration of blood specimen; *Endocrine:* Hyperparathyroidism (osteitis fibrosa cystica), acromegaly, hyperthyroidism (effect on bone), subacute thyroiditis, last half of pregnancy; *Degenerative/Idiopathic:* Paget disease, benign transient hyperphosphatasemia; *Infectious:* Liver infections (hepatitis, abscesses, parasitic infestations and infectious: mononucleosis), chronic osteomyelitis; *Inflammatory/Immune:* Primary biliary cirrhosis, sarcoidosis; *Mechanical/Traumatic:* Healing fractures, common bile duct obstruction from stone or carcinoma, intrahepatic cholestasis, passive congestion of the liver; *Metabolic/Toxic:* Osteomalacia, rickets, drug reactions (intrahepatic cholestasis), chlorpropamide, ergosterol, sometimes intravenous injection of albumin, pernicious anemia, hyperphosphatasia, dehydration, rapid loss of weight; *Neoplastic:* Osteoblastic bone tumors, metastatic carcinoma in bone, myeloma, liver metastases, cholangiocarcinoma; *Neurologic:* Cerebral damage; *Psychosocial:* Abuse with skeletal trauma; *Vascular:* Myocardial, renal, and sometimes pulmonary infarction.

Decreased alkaline phosphatase. **CLINICAL OCCURRENCE:** *Technical Errors:* Use of oxalate in blood collection; *Endocrine:* Hypothyroidism; *Degenerative/Idiopathic:* Osteoporosis; *Inflammatory/Immune:* Celiac disease; *Metabolic/Toxic:* Vitamin D toxicity, scurvy (vitamin C deficiency), milk-alkali syndrome, pernicious anemia/B_{12} deficiency.

Anion Gap, Serum: The anion gap is the difference between the concentrations of measured cations and the measured anions in the blood, measured in milliequivalents per liter, mEq/L: $AG = [Na^+] - ([Cl^-] + [HCO_3^-])$. The anion gap accounts for phosphates, sulfates, amino acids, and albumin.

Normal anion gap: 12 ± 2.

Increased anion gap. An increased anion gap indicates accumulation of organic acids and an *anion gap metabolic acidosis.*
CLINICAL OCCURRENCE: Ketoacidosis (diabetes, alcoholism, starvation), intoxication with salicylates, methanol, ethylene glycol, propylene glycol, lactic acidosis, or renal failure.

Decreased anion gap. This is uncommon and suggests the accumulation of positively charged proteins in the blood.
CLINICAL OCCURRENCE: Multiple myeloma and Lithium toxicity.

Alanine Aminotransferase (ALT), Serum: This enzyme occurs mostly in hepatocytes with smaller quantities in skeletal and heart muscle. It is released into the circulation with cellular damage or necrosis.

Normal concentration: 0–35 U/L (SI units: 0–0.58 mkat/L).

Increased ALT. Increased ALT usually indicates liver damage, although severe skeletal muscle damage produces significant elevations.
CLINICAL OCCURRENCE: *Infectious:* Viral hepatitis, mononucleosis, liver abscess; *Mechanical/Traumatic:* Passive liver congestion, extrahepatic biliary obstruction; *Metabolic/Toxic:* Drug-induced liver disease, alcohol; *Neoplastic:* Hepatocellular carcinoma, liver metastases.

Aspartate Aminotransferase (AST), Serum: This enzyme is concentrated in heart, liver, muscle, and kidney cells with lesser amounts in pancreas, spleen, lung, brain, and erythrocytes. Tissue injury releases the enzyme into the extracellular fluids but not necessarily in amounts proportionate to the injury.

Normal AST: 9–40 U/L.

Increased AST. This usually reflects damage to the liver, the muscles, including the heart, and, less commonly, to other organs. It usually rises in concert with the ALT. When the AST is ≥2.0 times the ALT, alcohol abuse with cirrhosis or alcoholic hepatitis should be suspected.
CLINICAL OCCURRENCE: *Technical Error:* False-positive from opiates and erythromycin, dehydration of blood specimen; *Congenital:* Muscular dystrophy; *Endocrine:* Diabetes mellitus; *Degenerative/Idiopathic:* Paget disease, cholecystitis; *Infectious:* Viral hepatitis, pulmonary infections; *Inflammatory/Immune:* Hemolytic diseases, polymyositis, pancreatitis, regional ileitis, ulcerative colitis; *Mechanical/Traumatic:* Severe exercise, clonic and tonic seizures, crushing or burning or necrosis of muscle, inflammation from intramuscular injections, rhabdomyolysis, peptic ulcer, extrahepatic biliary obstruction; *Metabolic/Toxic:* Hepatic necrosis and drug-induced hepatitis, uremia,

myoglobinemia, pernicious anemia, drugs (salicylates, alcohol), dehydration; *Neoplastic:* Bone metastasis, myeloma; *Vascular:* Myocardial, renal, and cerebral infarction.

Decreased AST. **CLINICAL OCCURRENCE:** *Endocrine:* Pregnancy; *Metabolic/ Toxic:* Chronic dialysis, uremia, pyridoxine deficiency, ketoacidosis, beriberi, severe liver disease.

Bicarbonate, Total Serum (HCO_3^-), CO_2 Content: Bicarbonate (HCO_3^-) is formed in the kidney by carbonic anhydrase and distributed through the body fluids as ionized bicarbonate in association with sodium. Bicarbonate is the major buffer consumed when protons (H^+) are produced by metabolizing amino acids or by increased organic acid production or ingestion. Renal bicarbonate production buffers respiratory acidosis (increased $PaCO_2$). Respiratory alkalosis lowers $PaCO_2$. The kidney responds by excreting bicarbonate thus decreasing the bicarbonate concentration, to maintain blood pH.

Normal serum bicarbonate: 22–26 mEq/L (SI: 22–26 mmol/L).

Increased bicarbonate. This indicates a metabolic alkalosis, either primary or secondary to a respiratory acidosis.
CLINICAL OCCURRENCE: *Endocrine:* Hyperaldosteronism, Cushing disease, severe hypothyroidism; *Metabolic/Toxic:* Primary metabolic alkalosis (diarrhea, gastric suction, nausea, and vomiting), diuretics (especially loop diuretics), hypercapnia; *Psychosocial:* Bulimia, purging.

Decreased bicarbonate. A decreased bicarbonate concentration indicates a metabolic acidosis, further classified by the anion gap, see page 761.
CLINICAL OCCURRENCE: *Endocrine:* Addison disease; *Metabolic/Toxic:* Hypocapnia from hyperventilation, metabolic acidosis, for example, renal failure, ketoacidosis (diabetic, alcoholic, and starvation), lactic acidosis, salicylate intoxication, methanol or ethylene glycol intoxication, renal tubular acidosis.

Bilirubin, Total Serum: See Jaundice, Chapter 9, page 414. Four-fifths or more is derived from the catabolism of the heme from aging erythrocytes. Bilirubin is insoluble in water and is bound to plasma proteins until conjugated with glucuronic acid in the liver. Water-soluble conjugated bilirubin is normally excreted in the bile. If the serum level exceeds 0.4 mg/dL, the water-soluble form appears in the urine.

Normal serum bilirubin: 0.3–1.0 mg/dL (SI units: 5.1–17 mmol/L).

Increased bilirubin, hyperbilirubinemia. Increased bilirubin indicates destruction of red blood cells (RBCs) or failure of hepatic excretion.
CLINICAL OCCURRENCE: See Jaundice, Chapter 9, page 414. *Unconjugated hyperbilirubinemia:* Hemolysis, ineffective erythropoiesis, decreased hepatic uptake of unconjugated bilirubin (Gilbert syndrome), or impaired hepatic conjugation (neonatal jaundice, drugs or Crigler–Najjar syndrome; *Conjugated hyperbilirubinemia:* Decreased excretion from hepatocytes (Dubin–Johnson syndrome, Rotor syndrome), intrahepatic cholestasis (hepatitis, drugs, granulomatous disease), and bile duct obstruction.

Decreased bilirubin, hypobilirubinemia. Nonhemolytic anemias and hypoalbuminemia.

Blood Urea Nitrogen (BUN): Molecular weight 60. Urea is synthesized in the liver from ammonia derived from proteins metabolized in the body and gut. It is filtered and reabsorbed by the kidney; reabsorption is inversely related to the rate of urine flow.

Normal serum blood urea nitrogen (BUN): 10–20 mg/dL (SI units: 3.6–7.1 mmol/L).

Increased BUN. An increase indicates decreased glomerular filtration and/or increased tubular reabsorption, or increased production in the gut from ingested protein or blood.
     CLINICAL OCCURRENCE: *Prerenal:* Hypotension, hemorrhage, dehydration (vomiting, diarrhea, excessive sweating), Addison disease, hyperthyroidism, heart failure, sepsis, upper gastrointestinal hemorrhage, increased protein ingestion; *Renal:* Any cause of acute or chronic kidney disease; *Postrenal:* Obstruction of the ureters, bladder, or urethra.

Decreased BUN. CLINICAL OCCURRENCE: Low-protein diets, muscle wasting, starvation, cirrhosis, cachexia, high urine flow.

BUN: creatinine ratio >10:1. This indicates relatively preserved glomerular filtration with either increased urea production or decreased urine flow.
     CLINICAL OCCURRENCE: Excessive protein intake, blood in the gut, excessive tissue destruction (cachexia, burns, fever, corticosteroid therapy); postrenal obstruction, inadequate renal circulation (heart failure, dehydration, shock).

BUN: creatinine ratio <10:1. This indicates decreased urea production.
     CLINICAL OCCURRENCE: Low protein intake, multiple dialyses, severe diarrhea or vomiting, hepatic insufficiency.

B-Type Natriuretic Peptide: Both systolic and diastolic heart failure are accompanied by increased ventricular and atrial wall tension leading to release of natriuretic peptides types A and B. This test is used to distinguish patients with dyspnea and pulmonary infiltrates who have heart failure from those with primary pulmonary disorders.

Normal concentration: <50 pg/mL.

Increased B-type natriuretic peptide. Systolic and diastolic right and left ventricular failure.

Calcium, Serum (Ca^{2+}). Ninety-nine percent of total body calcium is bound to phosphate and carbonate as insoluble salts within the bone matrix, in equilibrium with a small amount in the extracellular fluid. The plasma level varies with the rate of Ca^{2+} absorption from the small intestine and the proximal renal tubular reabsorption rate, under the control of parathyroid hormone (PTH). Calcium is present in the three forms: *ionized or free Ca^{2+}* that is physiologically active; *protein-bound or non-diffusible* Ca^{2+}, most of which is loosely bound to plasma albumin; and *complexed or complex-bound* Ca^{2+}, which forms relatively soluble fractions complexed with carbonates, citrates, or phosphates. PTH accelerates release of Ca^{2+} and PO_4^{3-} from bone and promotes renal excretion of PO_4^{3+} and reabsorption of Ca^{2+}. PTH stimulates renal conversion of vitamin D_3 to the active $1,25\text{-}(OH)_2$ form. *Calcitonin* inhibits bone resorption decreasing serum and extracellular Ca^{2+}.

Normal serum calcium: 9.0–10.5 mg/dL (SI units: 2.2–2.6 mmol/L).

Increased calcium, hypercalcemia. Hypercalcemia indicates increased bone breakdown, decreased renal excretion, and/or vitamin D intoxication.
CLINICAL OCCURRENCE: *Endocrine:* Primary hyperparathyroidism, hyperthyroidism, hypothyroidism, Cushing disease, Addison disease; *Degenerative/Idiopathic:* Osteoporosis, Paget disease; *Inflammatory/Immune:* Sarcoidosis; *Mechanical/Traumatic:* Immobilization; *Metabolic/Toxic:* Vitamin D intoxication, milk-alkali syndrome, hyperproteinemia (sarcoidosis, multiple myeloma), drugs (thiazide diuretics), poisons (berylliosis); *Neoplastic:* Tumor metastatic to bone, lymphoma, multiple myeloma, leukemia, release of PTH-like peptide.

Decreased calcium: hypocalcemia. A low serum calcium is caused by decreased binding proteins, vitamin D deficiency or resistance, precipitation of calcium phosphate salts or calcium soaps, or PTH deficiency.
CLINICAL OCCURRENCE: *Endocrine:* Hypoparathyroidism (post thyroidectomy, idiopathic, or pseudohypoparathyroidism), hypothyroidism, late pregnancy; *Inflammatory/Immune:* Acute pancreatitis with fat necrosis; *Metabolic/Toxic:* Renal insufficiency, excessive fluid intake, malabsorption of calcium and vitamin D or dietary vitamin D deficiency (osteomalacia and rickets), hypoproteinemia (cachexia, nephrosis, celiac disease, cystic fibrosis of the pancreas), drugs (antacids), corticosteroids.

Chloride, Serum (Cl^-): Chloride is the principal anion in extracellular fluids. In intracellular fluid the chief anions are phosphate and sulfate. The serum Cl^- is usually proportionate to Na (see discussion of anion gap, page 761).

Normal serum chloride: 98–106 mEq/L (SI units: 98–106 mmol/L).

Increased chloride, hyperchloremia. **CLINICAL OCCURRENCE:** *Technical Error:* Bromide in blood gives false test for Cl; *Endocrine:* Hyperparathyroidism, diabetes mellitus, diabetes insipidus; *Metabolic/Toxic:* Renal tubular acidosis, acute renal failure, respiratory alkalosis, nonanion gap metabolic acidosis, drugs (acetazolamide, ammonium salts, salicylates), dehydration.

Decreased chloride, hypochloremia. The chloride concentration is low when organic acids accumulate in anion gap metabolic acidosis or bicarbonate replaces chloride in metabolic alkalosis.
CLINICAL OCCURRENCE: *Endocrine:* Diabetic ketoacidosis, Addison disease, primary aldosteronism; *Mechanical/Traumatic:* Congestive cardiac failure, pyloric obstruction; *Metabolic/Toxic:* Anion gap metabolic acidosis, metabolic alkalosis, pulmonary emphysema, excessive sweating, diarrhea, malabsorption, drugs (diuretics).

Cholesterol, Serum: Cholesterol, insoluble in water, circulates associated with lipoproteins. The low-density lipoproteins (LDLs) have the highest cholesterol concentration. Cholesterol is ingested and synthesized by the liver. Cholesterol is essential to every cell and it is a precursor to adrenal steroids, gonadal steroids, and bile salts. Elevated cholesterol, particularly LDL cholesterol, is associated with accelerated atherogenesis. In contrast, elevated high-density lipoprotein (HDL) cholesterol is protective.

Normal concentrations. See Tables 18-1 to 18-3. Note that cholesterol and triglycerides are the only serum chemistries reported as socially determined "desirable" and "undesirable" levels, rather than biologically determined population-based normal ranges.

Increased cholesterol, hypercholesterolemia. **CLINICAL OCCURRENCE:** *Congenital:* Familial hypercholesterolemia and combined hyperlipidemia; *Endocrine:* Hypothyroidism, diabetes mellitus; *Inflammatory/Immune:* Chronic nephritis, amyloidosis, SLE, polyarteritis; *Mechanical/Traumatic:* Biliary obstruction (gallstone, carcinoma, biliary cirrhosis); *Metabolic/Toxic:* Obesity, metabolic syndrome, nephrotic syndrome, maldigestion and malabsorption, cirrhosis, lipodystrophy, alcohol; *Vascular:* Renal vein thrombosis.

Decreased cholesterol: hypocholesterolemia. **CLINICAL OCCURRENCE:** *Congenital:* Tangier disease; *Infectious:* Chronic infections; *Inflammatory/ Immune:* Cirrhosis, severe hepatitis; *Metabolic/Toxic:* Malnutrition, alcohol, starvation, uremia, steatorrhea, pernicious anemia, drugs (lipid-lowering agents, cortisone, adrenocorticotropic hormone [ACTH]).

C-Reactive Protein (CRP): This acute-phase reactant has a short half-life, so it rises rapidly within 4–6 hours of the onset of inflammation or tissue injury and declines relatively rapidly (half-time 5–7 h) with resolution.

Normal CRP: consult local labs.

Elevated CRP. CRP rises with any acute or chronic inflammation, infection, and tissue damage. Levels tend to correlate with the erythrocyte sedimentation rate (ESR, page 780) but respond more rapidly to changes in the patient's status.

Highly sensitive CRP. Highly sensitive CRP (hs-CRP) levels correlate positively in prospective studies with the likelihood for developing an acute coronary event. The strength of the association is equivalent to and additive to LDL-cholesterol elevations. The mechanism is unknown but implies an IL-6 driven inflammatory process.

TABLE 18-1 ATP III Classification of Total Cholesterol and Triglycerides

	Total Cholesterol		Triglycerides	
	mg/dL	*In SI, mmol/L*	*mg/dL*	*In SI, mmol/L*
Desirable	<200	<5.2	<150	<1.69
Borderline	200–239	5.20–6.18	150–199	1.69–2.25
High	≥240	≥6.21	≥200	≥2.26

TABLE 18-2 ATP III Classification of LDL Cholesterol

	LDL Cholesterol	
	mg/dL	In SI, mmol/L
Optimal	<100	<2.59
Desirable	<130	<3.36
Borderline high	130–159	3.36–4.11
High	160–189	4.14–4.89
Very high	≥190	≥4.91

TABLE 18-3 ATP III Classification of HDL Cholesterol

	HDL Cholesterol	
	mg/dL	In SI, mmol/L
High	≥60	≥1.55
Low	≤39	≤1.01

Creatine Kinase (CK), Serum: CK catalyzes high-energy phosphate transfer between creatine and phosphocreatine and between adenosine diphosphate and adenosine triphosphate (ATP). Major concentrations are found in cardiac and skeletal muscle and in the brain. Erythrocytes lack this enzyme, so autolyzed serum specimens are acceptable for testing.

Normal CK: Males: 25–90 mU/mL (SI units: 0.42–1.50 μkat/L); Females: 10–70 mU/mL (SI Units: 0.17–1.17 μkat/L). African Americans may have significantly higher normal levels.

Increased creatine kinase. Increased CK suggests muscle or brain damage. The isoenzyme pattern (CK-MM from skeletal muscle, CK-MB from cardiac muscle, CK-BB from brain) indicates the likely source.
CLINICAL OCCURRENCE: *Congenital:* Progressive muscular dystrophy; *Endocrine:* Hypothyroidism, last few weeks of pregnancy; *Infectious:* Pyomyositis; *Inflammatory/Immune:* Polymyositis, dermatomyositis, inclusion-body myositis, pancreatitis; *Mechanical/Traumatic:* Severe exercise, muscle spasms, clonic and tonic seizures, muscle trauma (crush syndrome, postoperatively for about 5 days), electroshock for defibrillation, muscle necrosis and atrophy, intramuscular injections for 48 hours, dissecting aneurysm; *Metabolic/Toxic:* Megaloblastic anemia, drugs (statins, salicylates, alcohol); *Vascular:* Myocardial and cerebral infarctions.

Decreased creatine kinase. **CLINICAL OCCURRENCE:** *Technical Error:* Drug interference; *Endocrine:* Early pregnancy; *Inflammatory/Immune:* Pancreatitis; *Metabolic/Toxic:* Decreased muscle mass.

Creatinine, Serum: Creatinine, an organic acid product of creatine metabolism in muscle, is distributed throughout the body water. Creatine is synthesized by the liver and pancreas from arginine and glycine and taken up by muscle where it is converted to creatine phosphate, catalyzed by the CK enzyme. Creatine decomposes to creatinine at a rate of 1%–2% per day. The amount of creatinine produced increases with muscle mass and decreases with muscle wasting. Creatinine is cleared by the glomerular filtration (75%) and tubular secretion (25%), without reabsorption. The rate of urinary creatinine excretion is an indicator of glomerular filtration.

Normal serum creatinine: <1.5 mg/dL (SI units: 133 μmol/L).

Increased creatinine. Elevated creatinine indicates decreased renal function, particularly glomerular filtration, from prerenal, renal, or postrenal causes. Because creatinine is dependent upon muscle mass, decreased renal function may be masked in patients with decreasing muscle mass, especially in women and the elderly. See Chapter 10, Table 10-1, page 477, for staging of clinical kidney disease.

CLINICAL OCCURRENCE: *Technical Error:* Drug interference with the assay (cephalosporins, ketones); *Endocrine:* Acromegaly; *Degenerative/Idiopathic:* Renal insufficiency of any cause; *Mechanical/Traumatic:* Burns, crush injury; *Metabolic/Toxic:* Increased muscle mass, ingestion of red meat, excessive intake of protein, dehydration, ureterocolostomy with urinary resorption, medications (cimetidine, probenecid, trimethoprim); *Vascular:* Inadequate blood flow to the kidneys, renal failure, heart failure.

Decreased creatinine. **CLINICAL OCCURRENCE:** Cachexia, decreased muscle mass, and increased glomerular filtration (e.g., the osmotic diuresis of early diabetes).

Creatinine Clearance: Creatinine is filtered by the glomerulus and secreted by the proximal tubule. The clearance of creatinine from the blood, measured in mL/min, is an estimate of glomerular filtration rate (GFR). Creatinine clearance is measured directly with 24-hour urine collections. This is cumbersome and the collections are often incomplete. An estimate of creatinine clearance is most commonly obtained by the 4-variable MDRD study equation (Modification of Diet in Renal Disease Study Group: variables are serum creatinine, age, race and gender) or CKD-EPI study equation (Chronic Kidney Disease Epidemiology Collaboration: variables are serum creatinine, gender, age, and race). Creatinine clearance is also calculated with the Cockcroft–Gault formula though this is not as accurate as the first two:

$$\text{Creatinine Clearance (mL / min)} = [(140 - \text{age}) \times (\text{lean body weight in kg})]$$
$$\div [\text{plasma creatinine (mg / dL)} 72]$$

Multiply by 0.85, for estimating creatinine clearance in women.

Normal creatinine clearance: Females: 100–110 mL/min per 1.73 m^2; Males: 120–130 mL/min per 1.73 m^2.

Increased creatinine clearance. See Increased GFR, below.

Decreased creatinine clearance. See Decreased GFR below and Acute and Chronic Kidney Failure, Chapter 10, page 475.

Ferritin, Serum: Ferritin is the major iron-storage protein in the body. Ferritin is an acute-phase reactant and is, therefore, best interpreted with a test of the acute-phase reaction such as the CRP or ESR.

Normal ferritin: Females: 10–200 ng/mL (SI 10–200 μg/L); Males:15–400 ng/mL (SI units: 15–400 μg/L).

Increased serum ferritin. CLINICAL OCCURRENCE: Increased iron stores (from transfusion hemosiderosis, anemia of chronic disease, leukemias, Hodgkin disease), excess dietary iron, hemochromatosis (usually >400 ng/dL, often >1,000 ng/dL), inflammation, infection, or cancer. Ferritin >10,000 occurs more commonly with Still disease and hemophagocytic syndromes.

Decreased serum ferritin. CLINICAL OCCURRENCE: Iron deficiency.

Glomerular Filtration Rate (GFR): The GFR is determined by the filtration pressure gradient between the glomerular capillary and Bowman space, the glomerular capillary filtration area, and the state of the glomerular endothelium, basement membrane, and epithelial cells. GFR is the most reliable measure of functioning nephron mass as it is independent of tubular absorption and secretion. Direct measurement of GFR is difficult, so various clinical formulae are utilized to estimate GFR. The creatinine clearance is an estimate of GFR, but since creatinine is both reabsorbed and secreted and these mechanisms are enhanced or impaired by drugs, it is not an accurate measure of GFR, especially in advanced kidney disease. An estimate of creatinine clearance is most commonly obtained by 4-variable MDRD study equation (Modification of Diet in Renal Disease Study Group: variables are serum creatinine, age, race and gender) or CKD-EPI study equation (Chronic Kidney Disease Epidemiology Collaboration: variables are serum creatinine, gender, age, and race). The CKD-EPI equation generally performs better and is more accurate than the MDRD equation when the actual GFR is >60 mL/min per 1.73 m². The MDRD formula is more accurate in chronic kidney disease.

Normal GFR: Females: 100–110 mL/min per 1.73 m²; Males: 120–130 mL/min per 1.73 m².

Increased GFR. Osmotic diuresis and efferent arteriolar constriction increase the GFR. GFR increases with hyperglycemia in early diabetic nephropathy.

Decreased GFR. Loss of nephron mass, damaged glomerular capillary loops with vasculitis and glomerulopathies, damaged glomerular basement membrane, and obstructed urine flow each decrease GFR producing renal insufficiency.
CLINICAL OCCURRENCE: See Acute and Chronic Kidney Failure, Chapter 10, page 475.

Glucose, Serum: This six-carbon monosaccharide is a primary energy source for metabolism. The serum level remains constant during fasting and there is a moderate rise after ingesting food. Hepatocytes convert other carbohydrates to glucose. Surplus glucose is converted to glycogen in the liver and muscle or to fat that is deposited throughout the body, predominately in adipocytes. Glucose uptake by the liver, muscle, and adipocytes is insulin-dependent. After an average meal, the blood sugar normally rises to ~180 mg/dL serum, returning to fasting levels within 2 hours. Higher blood glucose levels result from excessively rapid absorption or impaired peripheral disposition, usually related to insulin insufficiency or resistance. When blood glucose concentrations exceed the renal tubular reabsorption threshold, glucose is excreted in the urine (*glycosuria*). The normal renal threshold is a serum glucose of 160–190 mg/dL.

Normal serum glucose: 75–110 mg/dL (SI units: 4.2–6.4 mmol/L).

Diagnostic criteria for diabetes:

1. A fasting glucose of $\geq$126 mg/dL (SI units: $\geq$7.0 mmol/L).
2. Symptoms of diabetes plus a random glucose of $\geq$200 mg/dL (SI Units: $\geq$11.1 mmol/L).
3. A plasma glucose $\geq$200 mg/dL (SI units: $\geq$11.1 mmol/L) 2 hours following a 75-g oral glucose load.

The abnormal test must be confirmed on another day.

Diagnosis of impaired fasting glucose (IFG). A fasting glucose of 110–125 mg/dL (SI units: 6.1–7.0 mmol/L).

Diagnosis of impaired glucose tolerance (IGT). A blood glucose of 140–199 mg/dL (SI units: 7.8–11.0 mmol/L) 2 hours after a 75-g oral glucose load.

Increased glucose, hyperglycemia. Hyperglycemia indicates insulin resistance, diabetes, or release of stress-associated hormones (epinephrine, cortisol, growth hormone).

CLINICAL OCCURRENCE: *Endocrine:* Diabetes mellitus, impaired glucose tolerance, acromegaly, hyperthyroidism, Cushing disease, increased adrenalin, ACTH, pheochromocytoma, pregnancy, toxemia of pregnancy; *Infectious:* Any acute severe infection, for example, pneumonia; *Inflammatory/Immune:* Systemic inflammatory response syndrome, regional enteritis, ulcerative colitis; *Metabolic/Toxic:* Drugs (corticosteroids, diazoxide, epinephrine), poisoning (streptozotocin); *Neurologic:* Wernicke syndrome, subarachnoid hemorrhage, hypothalamic lesions, convulsions; *Vascular:* Myocardial infarction, pulmonary embolism, hemorrhage.

Decreased glucose, hypoglycemia. Inability to maintain a normal blood glucose indicates excessive insulin secretion or administration, or severely impaired hepatic gluconeogenesis.

CLINICAL OCCURRENCE: *Congenital:* Galactosuria, maple syrup urine disease, hepatic glycogenoses; *Endocrine:* Hypopituitarism, hypothalamic lesions, hypothyroidism, Addison disease; *Infectious:* Sepsis; *Inflammatory/Immune:* Pancreatitis; *Mechanical/Traumatic:* Postgastrectomy dumping syndrome, gastroenterostomy; *Metabolic/Toxic:* Insulin administration, oral hypoglycemics, glycogen deficiency, hepatitis, cirrhosis, malnutrition; *Neoplastic:* Insulinoma, some sarcomas.

Hemoglobin A$_{1C}$, Glycohemoglobin: Glycosylation of cellular and extracellular proteins occurs at a rate dependent upon the ambient plasma glucose concentration. The concentration of hemoglobin glycosylated is an accurate measure of the average blood sugar over the average life of the circulating erythrocytes, approximately 6 weeks. Measurement of one glycosylated form of hemoglobin, hemoglobin A$_{1C}$, is used to estimate the average blood sugar, a determinate of diabetes control.

Normal hemoglobin A1C: 3.8%–6.4% (SI units: 0.038–0.064).

Iron, Serum (Fe^{2+}): The body contains ~3–4 g of iron. Iron is a component of hemoglobin, the cytochromes, and other cellular metalloproteins. Approximately 1 mg of iron is absorbed and excreted each day. Most of the iron circulates in erythrocyte hemoglobin (1.0 mg/1.0 mL packed erythrocytes), some is in myoglobin, and a small fraction is in respiratory enzymes. The remainder is stored bound to ferritin. Iron is absorbed in the duodenum by a complex pathway regulated at the level of the enterocyte. Most ingested iron is either not absorbed or is sloughed with the enterocytes, never entering the plasma. Absorbed iron is bound to transferrin. Iron is cleared from the plasma with a half-time of 60–120 minutes, and 80%–90% is incorporated into new circulating erythrocytes over the subsequent 2 weeks. The serum iron concentration decreases by 50–100 mg/dL with the diurnal acceleration of erythropoiesis in the afternoon, so the time of day the specimen is drawn and its relationship to meals should be known. Iron deficiency is very common.

Normal serum iron: 50–100 μg/dL (SI units: 9–27 μmol/L).

Increased serum iron, hyperferremia. An increase in serum iron is seen following a high-iron meal and with hemochromatosis and liver disease.
    CLINICAL OCCURRENCE: *Congenital:* Hemochromatosis, thalassemia; *Inflammatory/Immune:* Acute hepatic necrosis, aplastic anemia, hemolytic anemia; *Metabolic/Toxic:* Excessive absorption (iron therapy, dietary excess), cirrhosis, pernicious anemia.

Decreased serum iron, hypoferremia. Low serum iron results from inadequate dietary intake, excessive blood loss (both with increased iron-binding capacity), or chronic inflammation (decreased iron-binding capacity).
    CLINICAL OCCURRENCE: *Endocrine:* Iron loss to the fetus during gestation; *Infectious:* Tuberculosis, osteomyelitis, hookworm; *Inflammatory/Immune:* Celiac disease, rheumatoid arthritis (RA), SLE; *Mechanical/Traumatic:* Intravascular: hemolysis with hemoglobinuria (paroxysmal nocturnal hemoglobinuria, march hemoglobinuria, prosthetic heart valves); *Metabolic/Toxic:* Iron deficiency, repeated phlebotomy, diminished absorption (decreased ingestion, celiac disease, pica, postgastrectomy); *Neoplastic:* Gastrointestinal cancers, loss of transferrin in nephrotic syndrome; *Psychosocial:* Poverty; *Vascular:* Intrapulmonary hemorrhage (e.g., Idiopathic: pulmonary hemosiderosis), chronic bleeding (e.g., menorrhagia, hematuria, peptic ulcer disease, gastritis, polyps, ulcerative colitis, colon carcinoma).

Iron-Binding Capacity, Serum Total: The total iron-binding capacity mainly reflects transferrin and, with the serum iron, helps distinguish iron deficiency anemia from the anemia of chronic inflammation.

Normal iron-binding capacity: 250–370 μg/dL (SI units: 45–66 μmol/L).

Increased iron-binding capacity. This generally reflects a response to iron deficiency.
     CLINICAL OCCURRENCE: Iron deficiency, acute or chronic blood loss, hepatitis, late pregnancy.

Decreased iron-binding capacity. Transferrin falls with chronic inflammation.
     CLINICAL OCCURRENCE: Anemias of chronic disorders (infections, inflammations, and cancer), thalassemia, cirrhosis, nephrotic syndrome.

Lactate Dehydrogenase (LDH), Serum: LDH catalyzes the reversible oxidation of lactate to pyruvate. It is found in all tissues, so an elevated serum level is a nonspecific indicator of tissue damage.

Normal LDH: 100–190 U/L (SI units: 1.7–3.2 mkat/L).

Increased LDH. LDH elevations suggest injury to and/or liver, hemolysis, or rapid cell division as in lymphomas.
     CLINICAL OCCURRENCE: *Congenital:* Muscular dystrophy in 10% of cases, progressive muscular dystrophy, myotonic dystrophy (CK is more specific for muscle than LDH); *Endocrine:* Hypothyroidism; *Infectious:* Hepatitis with jaundice, mononucleosis; *Inflammatory/Immune:* Polymyositis in 25% of cases, dermatomyositis, hemolytic anemias; *Mechanical/Traumatic:* Cardiovascular surgery, common bile duct obstruction, intestinal obstruction; *Metabolic/ Toxic:* Muscle necrosis, celiac disease, untreated pernicious anemia, alcohol; *Neoplastic:* 50% of lymphoma and leukemia cases; *Vascular:* Acute myocardial infarction, pulmonary embolism or infarction.

Decreased LDH. **CLINICAL OCCURRENCE:** Irradiation, ingestion of clofibrate.

Phosphate, Serum Inorganic: Serum phosphate measures the inorganic phosphorus of ionized PO_4^{2-} and H_2PO_4 which are in equilibrium in the serum; 10%–20% is protein bound. Phosphorus is necessary for synthesizing nucleotides, phospholipids, and high-energy ATP. Phosphates are excreted by the kidney. PTH increases phosphate excretion. When glycolytic energy demands increase, the serum inorganic P decreases.

Normal phosphate: 3.0–4.5 mg/dL (SI units: 1.0–1.4 mmol/L).

Increased phosphate, hyperphosphatemia. Increased phosphate results from defects in vitamin D metabolism, bone breakdown, tissue damage releasing intracellular stores, and/or failure of renal excretion.
     CLINICAL OCCURRENCE: *Congenital:* Fanconi disease; *Endocrine:* Acromegaly, hyperparathyroidism; *Degenerative/Idiopathic:* Paget disease; *Infectious:* Sepsis; *Inflammatory/Immune:* Sarcoidosis; *Mechanical/Traumatic:*

Healing fractures, crush injury, high intestinal obstruction; *Metabolic/Toxic:* Acute and chronic renal failure, vitamin D deficiency (rickets, osteomalacia), muscle necrosis, milk-alkali syndrome, respiratory alkalosis, excess of vitamin D; *Neoplastic:* Multiple myelomas, osteolytic metastases, myelocytic leukemia.

Decreased phosphate, hypophosphatemia. Low serum phosphate results from dietary insufficiency, failure to absorb dietary phosphate, excessive bone uptake, or renal phosphate wasting.
    CLINICAL OCCURRENCE: *Congenital:* Primary hypophosphatemia; *Endocrine:* Hyperparathyroidism, diabetes mellitus; *Metabolic/Toxic:* Renal tubular defects (Fanconi syndrome), anorexia, vomiting, diarrhea, lack of vitamin D, in refeeding after starvation, malnutrition, gout, ketoacidosis, respiratory alkalosis, hypokalemia, hypomagnesemia, primary hypophosphatemia, drugs (intravenous glucose, anabolic steroids, androgens, epinephrine, glucagon, insulin, salicylates, phosphorus-binding antacids, diuretic drugs, alcohol).

Potassium, Serum (K^+): Potassium is the predominant intracellular cation, whereas sodium predominates in the extracellular fluids. Approximately 90% of exchangeable K^+ is within cells; <1% is in the serum. Small shifts of K^+ out of cells causes large changes in serum $[K^+]$. Intracellular acidosis causes an extracellular shift of K^+ buffering the increased intracellular H^+. Plasma K^+ level is tightly regulated by the kidney. Hyperkalemia stimulates aldosterone secretion and potassium excretion. Hypokalemia leads to excretion of urine nearly devoid of potassium. Changes in serum K^+ concentration profoundly affect nerve excitation, muscle contraction, and cardiac conduction. Because the K^+ concentration in the erythrocytes is ~18 times greater than in the serum, hemolysis during sample collection falsely elevates the reported serum K^+.

Normal potassium: 3.5–5.0 mEq/L (SI units: 3.5–5.0 mmol/L).

Increased potassium, hyperkalemia. High serum K^+ can produce cardiac arrest. The risk is greatest with a rapid increase as compared with chronic elevation as in CKD.
    CLINICAL OCCURRENCE: *Technical Error:* Hemolysis in performing venipuncture or intentional clotting in collecting blood specimens, especially with thrombocytosis; *Congenital:* Hyperkalemic periodic paralysis; *Endocrine:* Primary and secondary hypoaldosteronism, adrenal insufficiency (Addison disease, adrenal hemorrhage); *Mechanical/Traumatic:* Rhabdomyolysis, crush injury, hemolysis of transfused blood, urinary obstruction; *Metabolic/ Toxic:* Acute and chronic renal failure, acidosis (metabolic or respiratory), muscle necrosis, drugs (amiloride, spironolactone, triamterene, angiotensin-converting enzyme inhibitors), foods (fruit juices, soft drinks, oranges, peaches, bananas, tomatoes, high-protein diet), dehydration; *Neurologic:* Status epilepticus; *Vascular:* Gastrointestinal hemorrhage, hemorrhage into tissues.

Decreased potassium, hypokalemia. Persistent hypokalemia is almost always associated with low total body K^+.
    CLINICAL OCCURRENCE: *Endocrine:* Diabetes mellitus, Cushing syndrome, hyperaldosteronism; *Mechanical/Traumatic:* Ureterosigmoidostomy

with urinary reabsorption, adynamic ileus; *Metabolic/Toxic:* Vomiting, gastric suction, postgastrectomy dumping syndrome, gastric atony, laxative abuse, polyuria, renal injury, salt-losing nephritis, metabolic alkalosis (from diuresis, primary aldosteronism, pseudoaldosteronism), metabolic acidosis (from renal tubular acidosis, diuresis phase of tubular necrosis, chronic pyelonephritis, diuresis after release of urinary obstruction), malabsorption and malnutrition, drugs (diuretics, estrogens, salicylates, corticosteroids); *Neoplastic:* Aldosteronoma, villous adenoma, colonic cancer, Zollinger–Ellison syndrome.

Protein, Total Serum: Most serum proteins are synthesized in the liver (albumin and many others) or by mature plasma cells (immunoglobulins). Increases or decreases in serum proteins represent an altered balance between synthesis and catabolism or loss into third spaces or the urine. Total protein is the sum of serum albumin and globulins; the fibrinogen was discarded in the clot that separated from the plasma to form the serum specimen. The total serum protein minus the albumin is an estimate of the serum globulins.

Normal total protein: 5.5–8.0 g/dL (SI units: 55–80 g/L).

Increased total protein, hyperproteinemia. The concentration of normal proteins is increased or there is excess immunoglobulins production.
   CLINICAL OCCURRENCE: Water depletion, multiple myeloma, macroglobulinemia, and sarcoidosis.

Decreased total protein, hypoproteinemia. Synthesis is decreased, catabolism is increased by malnutrition, or there is loss into third spaces or the urine (nephrotic syndrome).
   CLINICAL OCCURRENCE: Congestive cardiac failure, ulcerative colitis, nephrotic syndrome, chronic glomerulonephritis, cirrhosis, viral hepatitis, burns, malnutrition.

Protein: Albumin, Serum: Albumin normally comprises more than half the total serum protein. Its molecular weight (~65,000) is low compared to that of the globulins (MW 44,000–435,000). Albumin's smaller molecules account for 80% of the plasma osmotic pressure. Albumin is metabolized during starvation, so low levels may indicate protein malnutrition. It is also a solvent for fatty acids and bile salts and a transport vehicle loosely binding calcium, hormones, amino acids, drugs, and metals. The albumin level must be taken into account when interpreting the serum concentrations of these substances.

Normal albumin: 3.5–5.5 g/dL (SI units: 35–55 g/L).

Increased albumin, hyperalbuminemia. No significant correlation with diseases.

Decreased albumin, hypoalbuminemia. This can only be caused by decreased production (liver), increased metabolism, or loss into third spaces or urine.
   CLINICAL OCCURRENCE: *Congenital:* Analbuminemia; *Endocrine:* Diabetes mellitus; *Infectious:* Viral hepatitis; *Inflammatory/Immune:* Ulcerative colitis,

protein-losing enteropathies, chronic glomerulonephritis, lupus erythematosus, polyarteritis, rheumatoid arthritis, rheumatic fever; *Mechanical/Traumatic:*
Peptic ulcer; *Metabolic/Toxic:* Congestive cardiac failure, cirrhosis, nephrotic
syndrome, malnutrition, drugs (estrogens); *Neoplastic:* Multiple myeloma,
Hodgkin disease, lymphocytic leukemia, macroglobulinemia.

Protein: Globulins, Serum: Subtracting the albumin from the total serum
protein yields the serum globulin fraction. Elevated globulins should be frac-
tionated by serum protein electrophoresis (SPEP) to identify each component.

Serum protein electrophoresis. The proteins are separated by electrophoresis; the proteins migrate, each at its own rate, dependent on its charge and
molecular weight. A serum specimen contains proteins that separate into
several zones according to their mobility. The proteins are named for the
zone in which they are found (named with Greek lowercase letters): alpha 0
(for albumin), alpha 1 (α_1), alpha 2 (α_2), beta (β), gamma (γ), and phi (ϕ) (for
fibrinogen).

Protein: α_1-Globulins: α_1-Globulins include α_1-antitrypsin, α_1-antichymotrypsin,
amyloid A, orosomucoid, α_1-lipoprotein, and some cortisol-binding globulin.

Increased α_1-globulins. Hodgkin disease, peptic ulcer, ulcerative colitis, cirrhosis, metastatic carcinoma, protein-losing enteropathy.

Decreased α_1-globulins. Viral hepatitis.

Protein: α_2-Globulins: α_2-globulins include macroglobulins, haptoglobin, HS
glycoprotein, ceruloplasmin, and some immunoglobulins.

Increased α_2-globulins. Hodgkin disease, peptic ulcer, ulcerative colitis,
cirrhosis, nephrotic syndrome, chronic glomerulonephritis, systemic lupus
erythematosus (SLE), polyarteritis nodosa, rheumatoid arthritis, metastatic
carcinoma, protein-losing enteropathies.

Decreased α_2-globulins. Cirrhosis, viral hepatitis.

Protein: β-Globulins: β-Globulins include transferrin, hemopexin, and some
immunoglobulins.

Increased β-globulins. Rheumatoid arthritis, rheumatic fever, analbuminemia.

Decreased β-globulins. Nephrotic syndrome, lymphocytic leukemia, metastatic carcinoma.

Protein: γ-Globulins: γ-Globulins are predominately immunoglobulins of
the IgG class. Increases in γ-globulins can be *monoclonal*, arising from clonal
proliferation of plasma cells or lymphocytes, or *polyclonal* reflecting an
inflammatory response. Polyclonal γ-globulins produce a *broad-based pattern*
in the gamma zone indicating the presence of proteins from many cell lines.
Plasma immunoglobulins are increased by acute and chronic inflammatory

conditions (polyclonal) or neoplastic (benign or malignant) expansion of a single clone of cells (monoclonal).

Increased polyclonal γ-globulins. Cirrhosis, myelocytic leukemia, lupus erythematosus, RA, analbuminemia.

Decreased polyclonal γ-globulins. Nephrotic syndrome, lymphocytic leukemia, common variable immunodeficiency, hypogammaglobulinemia, protein-losing enteropathies.

Protein: Immunoglobulin IgG: This is the smallest immunoglobulin (MW 160,000) and the only one that crosses the placenta protecting the fetus and newborn until the child's own immunoglobulins are generated. IgG is synthesized after IgM in response to a new antigen. IgG producing plasma cells are the major humoral effector of chronic inflammation.

Normal IgG: 800–1500 mg/dL (SI units: 8.0–15.00 g/L).

Increased IgG. CLINICAL OCCURRENCE: *Infectious:* Pulmonary tuberculosis, hepatitis, osteomyelitis; *Inflammatory/Immune:* SLE, rheumatoid arthritis, vasculitis; *Metabolic/Toxic:* Cirrhosis; *Neoplastic:* Myeloma, monoclonal gammopathy of undetermined significance.

Decreased IgG. CLINICAL OCCURRENCE: *Congenital:* Lymphoid aplasia, agammaglobulinemia; *Inflammatory/Immune:* Common variable immunodeficiency, nephrotic syndrome; *Neoplastic:* Heavy-chain disease, IgA myeloma, macroglobulinemia, CLL.

Protein: Immunoglobulin IgA: Molecular weight 170,000. IgA is especially protective against viral infections. The *excretory form* (molecular weight 400,000) is found in colostrum, saliva, tears, bronchial secretions, gastrointestinal secretions, and nasal discharges. It has a special action against viruses of influenza, poliomyelitis, adenoviral diseases, and rhinoviruses.

Normal IgA: 90–325 mg/dL (SI units: 0.90–3.2 g/L).

Increased IgA. CLINICAL OCCURRENCE: *Congenital:* Wiskott–Aldrich syndrome; *Inflammatory/Immune:* SLE, rheumatoid arthritis, sarcoidosis; *Metabolic/Toxic:* Cirrhosis; *Neoplastic:* IgA myeloma.

Decreased IgA. CLINICAL OCCURRENCE: *Congenital:* Absent in 3 per 1,000 population, hereditary telangiectasia, lymphoid aplasia; *Inflammatory/Immune:* Nephrotic syndrome, Still disease, SLE, common variable immunodeficiency, agammaglobulinemia; *Metabolic/Toxic:* Cirrhosis; *Neoplastic:* Heavy-chain disease, ALL, CLL, CML.

Protein: Immunoglobulin IgM: This is the largest of the immunoglobulins (MW 900,000). It synthesized during a primary antibody response. The rheumatoid factor and the blood group isoantibodies anti-A and anti-B are of this class.

Normal IgM: 45–150 mg/dL (SI units: 0.45–1.5 g/L).

Increased IgM. CLINICAL OCCURRENCE: *Infectious:* Hepatitis, trypanosomiasis; *Inflammatory/Immune:* Biliary cirrhosis, RA, SLE; *Neoplastic:* Macroglobulinemia.

Protein: Immunoglobulin IgD: Molecular weight 185,000. There is no known specific activity for this protein.

Normal IgD: 0–8 mg/dL (SI units: 0–0.08 g/L).

Increased IgD. Chronic infections, IgD myeloma.

Protein: Immunoglobulin IgE: Molecular weight 200,000. IgE binds to mast cell membranes. Specific antigen (allergen) binding to the bound IgE causes mast cell degranulation and an allergic or anaphylactic response. IgE is essential for allergic and atopic reactions.

Normal IgE: 0.025 mg/dL (SI units: 0.00025 g/L).

Increased IgE. Allergic asthma (60%), hay fever (30%), atopic eczema, parasitic infestations, IgE myeloma, hyper-IgE syndromes.

Protein: Monoclonal γ-Globulins: The SPEP has a narrow sharp spike (*M-spike*) in the gamma region indicating a monoclonal protein. The exact nature of the immunoglobulin is determined by immunoelectrophoresis. Monoclonal gammopathies are characterized by a marked elevation of one of the five human immunoglobulins normally present in human serum: IgG, IgA, IgM, IgD, and IgE. Each contains a specific heavy chain (H chain) coupled to one of two types of light chains (L chains). The heavy chains are named with lowercase Greek letters, corresponding to the capital letters designating immunoglobulin type: IgA (α), IgG (γ), IgM (μ), IgD (δ), IgE (ε). The light chains are kappa (κ) and lambda (λ). The five immunoglobulins are identified by immunofixation electrophoresis using specific antibodies to identify the H and L chains.

Monoclonal immunoglobulin. CLINICAL OCCURRENCE: Multiple myeloma, macroglobulinemia, malignant lymphoma, amyloidosis, monoclonal gammopathy of undetermined significance (MGUS).

Sodium, Serum (Na$^+$): Molecular weight 23. This is the predominant cation in the extracellular fluid. Together with Cl$^-$, it makes the major contribution to the plasma osmotic pressure. Loss of Na$^+$ is frequently accompanied by an equivalent amount of water (as an isotonic solution), so normal levels of serum Na$^+$ do not exclude total body loss of Na$^+$. Assessment of total body Na$^+$ status is done by assessing extracellular volume. To maintain extracellular volume, the kidney retains sodium and enough water to maintain normal osmolarity. Because water moves between the intracellular and extracellular compartments maintaining iso-osmolarity between the two, an increase or decrease in the serum [Na$^+$] represents an inverse change in the total body water, i.e., increased serum Na$^+$ indicates a water deficit and decreased serum Na$^+$ indicates water excess.

Normal sodium: 136–145 mEq/L (136–145 mmol/L).

Increased serum sodium, hypernatremia. This always indicates a relative total body water deficit, regardless of the extracellular volume status.
CLINICAL OCCURRENCE: *Endocrine:* Diabetes insipidus, diabetes mellitus, hyperparathyroidism, hyperaldosteronism; *Metabolic/Toxic:* Water loss greater than Na⁺ loss (vomiting, sweating, hyperpnea, diarrhea), drugs (corticosteroids, diuretics), diuretic phase of acute tubular necrosis, diuresis after relief of urinary obstruction, excessive sodium intake, hypercalcemia, hypokalemic nephropathy; *Neurologic:* Thalamic lesions.

Decreased serum sodium, hyponatremia. This always indicates a relative total body water excess, from excess water ingestion or inability of the kidney to excrete a sufficiently dilute urine, regardless of the extracellular volume status.
CLINICAL OCCURRENCE: *Technical Error:* Spuriously normal serum osmolality (hyperlipidemia, hyperglycemia); *Endocrine:* Addison disease; *Infectious:* Pneumonia, meningitis, brain abscess (all cause syndrome of inappropriate antidiuretic hormone secretion); *Metabolic/Toxic:* Congestive heart failure (CHF), salt-losing nephropathy, cirrhosis with ascites, fluid and electrolyte loss (vomiting, sweating, diarrhea, diuresis) with replacement by hypotonic fluids, malnutrition, syndrome of inappropriate antidiuretic hormone secretion (SIADH); *Neoplastic:* Antidiuretic hormone-secreting tumors, especially lung cancers; *Psychosocial:* Anorexia nervosa, psychogenic polydipsia.

Triglycerides: Triglycerides are absorbed from the gut following ingestion of a fatty meal. They are transported in chylomicrons to the adipose tissue where they are cleaved by lipoprotein lipase, leading to the formation of less-triglyceride-enriched very low density (VLDL) and intermediate density (IDL) lipoproteins. Triglycerides are the major form of energy storage, mostly in adipose tissue. They are broken down to free fatty acids which are a highly efficient cellular energy source.

Normal triglycerides: See Table 18-1, page 765.

Increased triglycerides, hypertriglyceridemia. **CLINICAL OCCURRENCE:**
Congenital: Lipoprotein lipase deficiency, familial combined hyperlipidemia; familial hypertriglyceridemia, dysbetalipoproteinemia; *Endocrine:* Diabetes, hypothyroidism; *Metabolic/Toxic:* Alcohol ingestion, high fat diets, metabolic syndrome, drugs (oral contraceptives).

Urea Nitrogen: See *Blood Urea Nitrogen*, page 763.

Uric Acid, Serum: Molecular weight 169. Uric acid is the end-product of purine metabolism. In a normal healthy adult uric acid is produced at the rate of 10 mg/kg per day. The body pool is about 1,200 mg, distributed in the body water. Increased nucleic acid breakdown increases uric acid production. Uric acid leaves the body through renal excretion and by bacterial catabolism in the gut. Renal uric acid excretion is increased by expansion of body fluids (salt or osmotic diuresis). Dehydration and diuretics decrease uric acid excretion.

Normal uric acid: Males: 2.5–8.0 mg/dL (SI units: 150–480 mmol/L); Females: 1.5–6.0 mg/dL (SI units: 90–360 mmol/L).

Increased uric acid, hyperuricemia. High values for uric acid are among the most common abnormalities encountered in routine testing. This probably accounts for the much-too-frequent diagnosis of gout. The serum uric acid is elevated in only two-thirds of patients with gouty arthritis and 25% of acute nongouty arthritis patients have elevated uric acid. A quarter of the relatives of gout patients have elevated uric acid.

CLINICAL OCCURRENCE: *Congenital:* Polycystic kidneys, sickle cell anemia, Wilson disease, Fanconi disease, von Gierke disease, Down syndrome, certain normal populations (Blackfeet and Pima Indians, Filipinos, New Zealand Maoris); *Endocrine:* Hypothyroidism, hypoparathyroidism, primary hyperparathyroidism, toxemia of pregnancy; *Infectious:* Resolving pneumonia; *Inflammatory/Immune:* Psoriasis, hemolytic anemias, sarcoidosis; *Metabolic/Toxic:* Renal failure, drugs (diuretics, small doses of salicylates), high-protein low-calorie diet, high-purine diet (sweetbreads, liver), starvation, gout, relatives of gouty patients, poisons (acute alcoholism, lead poisoning, berylliosis), hypertension, metabolic syndrome; *Neoplastic:* Leukemia, multiple myeloma, polycythemia vera, lymphoma, other disseminated cancers.

Decreased uric acid, hypouricemia. **CLINICAL OCCURRENCE:** *Congenital:* Xanthinuria, Fanconi syndrome, Wilson disease, healthy adults with Dalmatian-dog mutation (isolated defect in tubular transport of uric acid); *Endocrine:* Acromegaly; *Inflammatory/Immune:* Celiac disease; *Metabolic/Toxic:* Drugs (uricosuric medication, allopurinol, ACTH, glyceryl guaiacolate, X-ray contrast media); *Neoplastic:* Carcinomas, Hodgkin disease.

HEMATOLOGIC DATA

Blood Cells: Consult standard hematology textbooks for comprehensive treatment of these subjects. The stained blood film allows examination of the red blood cells (RBC), white blood cells [WBC], and platelets. Cellular morphology depends on the preparation technique, stain, and part of the smear you examine, ideally where the erythrocytes are close but not touching.

Erythrocyte morphology. Evaluate color, size, shape, and contents. *Macrocytes:* Reticulocytosis, liver disease, megaloblastic anemia. *Hypochromic microcytes:* Defects in hemoglobin synthesis (iron deficiency, thalassemias, sickle cell disease, and other hemoglobinopathies); *Spherocytes:* Hereditary spherocytosis, immune hemolysis, *Schistocytes:* Microangiopathic hemolytic anemias (disseminated intravascular coagulation [DIC], thrombotic thrombocytopenic purpura, hemolytic uremic syndrome, vasculitis, thrombotic microangiopathy, prosthetic heart valves, malignant hypertension, scleroderma renal crisis). *Teardrops (dacryocytes):* Marrow damage, e.g., extramedullary hemopoiesis, myelophthisic anemia. *Erythroblasts:* Extramedullary hemopoiesis, myelophthisic anemia, severe hemolytic anemia, erythroleukemia. *Howell–Jolly bodies:* Postsplenectomy, megaloblastic anemia. *Basophilic stippling:* Lead poisoning, hemolytic disease. *Infectious agents: Malaria, Babesia, Borrellia, and Bartonella infection.*

Leukocyte morphology. Confirm the automated differential leukocyte count. *Toxic granulation of neutrophils and metamyelocytes:* Bacterial infections.

Giant cytoplasmic granules: Chediak–Higashi syndrome; *Bilobed neutrophils:* Hereditary Pelger–Huet anomaly or pseudo-Pelger–Huet anomaly in acute leukemia. *Hypersegmented neutrophils:* Nuclear maturation defect, e.g., pernicious anemia, vitamin deficiency, folate deficiency, myeloproliferative diseases. *Neutrophil inclusions:* Granulocytic ehrlichiosis and anaplasmosis. *Myeloblasts, promyelocytes, myelocytes:* Consider AML, acute promyelocytic leukemia, CML, myelofibrosis, polycythemia vera. *Atypical lymphocytes:* Viral infections, especially Ebstein–Barr virus (acute infectious mononucleosis) and cytomegalovirus (CMV). *Large granular lymphocytes:* Natural killer cells of T-gamma lymphoproliferative disease. *Lymphoblasts:* Acute lymphoblastic leukemia, prolymphocytic leukemia, malignant lymphoma, chronic lymphocytic leukemia, infectious mononucleosis. *Monocyte inclusions:* Monocytic ehrlichiosis. *Plasma Cells:* Multiple myeloma.

Platelet morphology. Confirm the automated platelet count. In oil immersion fields at 1,000 magnification, where the erythrocytes are close but not touching, the number of platelets in an average field multiplied by 15×10^3 is approximately equal to the platelet count per mm³. Scan the sides of the smear for clumped platelets that may have been counted inaccurately by instrument. *Megathrombocytes:* Platelets >2 μm in diameter may be increased with accelerated platelet production compensating for increased destruction (e.g., immune thrombocytopenic purpura), B_{12} deficiency, folate deficiency, myeloproliferative diseases, Bernard–Soulier syndrome.

Erythrocyte Measurements

Counts, hemoglobin content, and hematocrit. The hematocrit expresses the relative volume of erythrocytes as a percent of the blood volume in a centrifuged specimen. The hemoglobin measures the grams of hemoglobin per deciliter of whole blood. The total number of erythrocytes per mm³ is counted by machine or a hemocytometer.

Normal values: Hematocrit—Males: 42%–52%; Females: 37%–48%; Hemoglobin: Males: 13–18 g/dL; Females: 12–16 g/dL; Erythrocyte count: 4.15–4.903 $\times 10^6$ per mm³.

Erythrocytic indices. These are all calculated from the RBC counts, hemoglobin content, and hematocrit.

Normal values: Mean corpuscular hemoglobin: 28–33 pg/cell; mean corpuscular volume: 86–98 fL; mean corpuscular hemoglobin concentration: 32–36 g/dL.

High RBC count: erythrocytosis. This usually represents intravascular and extracellular fluid volume loss, chronic hypoxia, iatrogenic or endogenous erythropoietin excess, or polycythemia vera.

CLINICAL OCCURRENCE: *Endocrine:* Diabetic ketoacidosis, third to ninth month of pregnancy and to third week postpartum; *Inflammatory/Immune:* Chronic obstructive and restrictive lung disease with hypoxia; *Mechanical/Traumatic:* Burns (contracted plasma volume), high-altitude hypoxia; *Metabolic/Toxic:* Contracted plasma volume (dehydration, diarrhea, burns,

shock), carboxyhemoglobinemia, sulfhemoglobinemia, secondary polycythemia, drugs (erythropoietin, androgens, diuretics); *Neoplastic:* Polycythemia
vera, renal cyst or carcinoma; *Vascular:* Venous-arterial shunt (right-to-left
shunt), endothelial damage with diffuse capillary leak.

Low RBC count: anemia. See also Chapter 5, Anemia, page 91. Anemia results
from decreased RBC production, hemorrhage, increased RBC destruction (hemolysis), dilution or sequestration in hypersplenism.
   CLINICAL OCCURRENCE: *Congenital:* Thalassemia; *Degenerative/Idiopathic:*
Bone marrow failure; *Inflammatory/Immune:* Hemolysis; *Mechanical/Traumatic:*
Hemolysis or bleeding; *Metabolic/Toxic:* Renal failure, oliguria, macrocytic
anemia (pernicious anemia, vitamin B_{12} deficiency), folate deficiency, myelodysplasia, normocytic normochromic anemias (hemolysis, chronic disease,
infections, renal failure, liver disease), microcytic hypochromic anemias (iron
deficiency, pyridoxine responsive anemia, hemoglobinopathies); *Neoplastic:*
Refractory anemia; *Vascular:* CHF, acute hemorrhage.

Reticulocyte count. Reticulocytes are immature erythrocytes just released
from the bone marrow and retaining some ribosomal RNA seen as basophilic stippling with supravital stain. Normally this staining disappears
within 24–48 hours. When erythropoiesis is accelerated RBCs are released 1–2
days earlier than usual and stain as reticulocytes for 2–2.5 days. Values are
expressed as a percent of erythrocytes or as an absolute number. Increased
absolute numbers of reticulocytes reflect accelerated erythropoiesis.

Normal reticulocytes: 0.5%–1.8%; $29–87 \times 10^9$/L.

Increased reticulocytes: accelerated erythropoiesis. Note: There must be
adequate iron, folate, and protein.
   CLINICAL OCCURRENCE: Hemorrhage or hemolysis, response to erythropoietin from tissue hypoxia or from its therapeutic administration, and
response to therapy of nutrient deprivation (iron, folate, protein).

Decreased reticulocytes: decreased effective erythropoiesis. **CLINICAL OCCUR-
RENCE:** *Nutrient deprivation:* Iron deficiency, pernicious anemia, B_{12} deficiency,
folate deficiency, starvation; *Anemia of chronic disease:* Inflammation, infection,
cancer; *Bone marrow failure:* Alcohol abuse, idiosyncratic drug reactions, cancer chemotherapy, total body irradiation, aplastic anemia, leukemia, lymphoma, multiple myeloma, and other cancers invading bone marrow.

Erythrocyte sedimentation rate. Erythrocytes sediment by gravity. Increased
plasma proteins (especially fibrinogen, other acute-phase reactants, and
immunoglobulins) decrease the repulsive force between erythrocytes allowing larger clumps of cells to form (seen on the smear as rouleaux formation)
which accelerate sedimentation.

Normal ESR: Males: 1–17 mm/h; Females: 0–25 mm/h.

Increased ESR. This nonspecific finding indicates inflammation associated
with infection, inflammatory diseases, and some cancers.

CLINICAL OCCURRENCE: *Endocrine:* Hyperthyroidism, hypothyroidism, normal pregnancy from third month to termination plus 3 weeks postpartum, menstruation; *Infectious:* Many, but especially tuberculosis, endocarditis, osteomyelitis, and pelvic inflammation; *Inflammatory/Immune:* RA, SLE, PMR, giant cell arteritis, vasculitis; *Metabolic/Toxic:* Hyperglobulinemia, hypoalbuminemia, dextran or polyvinyl plasma substitutes; *Neoplastic:* Many cancers; *Vascular:* Vasculitis.

Leukocytes (WBC)

WBC count. This cellular blood compartment includes neutrophils, eosinophils, basophils, lymphocytes, and monocytes.

Normal WBC: $4.3–10.83 \times 10^3/mm^3$.
Normal neutrophil count: 45%–74% of total.

Increase in all blood cells (erythrocytes, leukocytes, platelets), pancytosis.
CLINICAL OCCURRENCE: *Metabolic/Toxic:* Dehydration; *Neoplastic:* Polycythemia vera, the myeloproliferative syndromes.

Decrease in all cellular elements of the blood (erythrocytes, leukocytes, platelets), pancytopenia. **CLINICAL OCCURRENCE:** *Degenerative/Idiopathic:* Marrow failure (aplastic anemia), paroxysmal nocturnal hemoglobinuria; *Infectious:* Bacterial (tuberculosis); viral (hepatitis); *Inflammatory/Immune:* SLE; *Mechanical/Traumatic:* Irradiation; *Metabolic/Toxic:* Pernicious anemia or folate deficiency, drugs (cancer chemotherapy, chloramphenicol), poisons (benzene); *Neoplastic:* Multiple myeloma, carcinomatous invasion, lymphoma, myelodysplasia, acute leukemia, myelofibrosis.

Increased neutrophils, leukocytosis, neutrophilia. Leukocytosis usually represents a response to tissue injury or invasion by pathologic organisms. Always inspect the peripheral smear to detect band forms and toxic granulation.
CLINICAL OCCURRENCE: *Endocrine:* Eclampsia; *Degenerative/Idiopathic:* Leukemoid reactions; *Infectious:* Acute pyogenic infections including pneumonia, meningitis, pyelonephritis, pelvic inflammatory disease, deep abscesses, endocarditis; *Inflammatory/Immune:* Acute necrotizing vasculitis; *Mechanical/Traumatic:* Burns, acute hemolysis; *Metabolic/Toxic:* Exercise, uremia, diabetic acidosis, gout, drugs (granulocyte colony-stimulating factor, granulocyte-macrophage colony-stimulating factor, epinephrine, corticosteroids, lithium carbonate, parenteral foreign proteins, vaccines), poisons (venoms, mercury, black widow spider venom); *Neoplastic:* Myeloproliferative diseases (polycythemia vera, CML, myelofibrosis, Idiopathic: thrombocythemia); *Neurologic:* Seizures *Vascular:* Tissue necrosis, myocardial infarction, acute hemorrhage.

Decreased neutrophils, leukopenia, or neutropenia. Decreases in WBC or specific cells reflects decreased production or increased consumption.
CLINICAL OCCURRENCE: *Congenital:* Gaucher disease; *Degenerative/Idiopathic:* Bone marrow failure (aplastic anemia), cyclic neutropenia; *Infectious:* Viral (Infectious: mononucleosis, hepatitis, HIV, influenza, rubeola, psittacosis), bacterial (streptococcal, staphylococcal diseases, sepsis,

tularemia, brucellosis, tuberculosis), rickettsial disease (scrub typhus, sandfly fever); protozoa (malaria, kala-azar); *Inflammatory/Immune:* Hypersplenism, Felty syndrome, autoimmune neutropenia, SLE; *Mechanical/Traumatic:* Portal hypertension; *Metabolic/Toxic:* Uremia, pernicious anemia/B_{12} deficiency, folate deficiency, cirrhosis, cachexia, drugs and therapy (cancer chemotherapy, sulfonamides, antibiotics, analgesics, antidepressants, arsenicals, antithyroid drugs, radiation), poisons (benzene); *Neoplastic:* Aleukemic leukemia, acute myeloblastic leukemia.

Eosinophil count. Eosinophils are important in the defense against multicellular parasite infections.

Normal eosinophil count: 0%–7% of WBCs.

Increased eosinophils, eosinophilia. **CLINICAL OCCURRENCE:** *Endocrine:* Adrenal insufficiency (Addison disease); *Degenerative/Idiopathic:* Loeffler endocarditis, hypereosinophilic syndrome; *Infectious:* Scarlet fever, parasitic infestations (e.g., trichinosis, echinococcosis); *Inflammatory/Immune:* Asthma, hay fever, urticaria, drug reactions, erythema multiforme, pemphigus, dermatitis herpetiformis, eosinophilic gastroenteritis, ulcerative colitis, regional enteritis, polyarteritis nodosa, Churg–Strauss sarcoidosis pernicious anemia, eosinophilic fasciitis; *Mechanical/Traumatic:* Postsplenectomy, black widow spider bite; *Metabolic/Toxic:* Poisons (phosphorus); *Neoplastic:* Metastatic carcinoma to bone, chronic myelocytic leukemia, polycythemia vera, Hodgkin disease; *Vascular:* Vasculitis (polyarteritis nodosa, Churg–Strauss).

Decreased eosinophils, eosinopenia. Bone marrow failure, corticosteroid treatment.

Basophil count. The function of basophils is uncertain. They are similar to tissue mast cells.

Normal basophil count: 0%–2.0% of WBCs.

Increased basophils, basophilia. **CLINICAL OCCURRENCE:** *Endocrine:* Hypothyroidism (myxedema); *Infectious:* Varicella, variola; *Inflammatory/Immune:* Chronic hemolytic anemias; *Mechanical/Traumatic:* Postsplenectomy; *Metabolic/Toxic:* Nephrotic syndrome; *Neoplastic:* Chronic myelocytic leukemia, polycythemia vera, myeloid metaplasia, Hodgkin disease.

Decreased basophils. **CLINICAL OCCURRENCE:** *Endocrine:* Hyperthyroidism, pregnancy; *Degenerative/Idiopathic:* Bone marrow failure, aplastic anemia; *Metabolic/Toxic:* Drugs (chemotherapy, glucocorticoids).

Lymphocyte count. Most circulating lymphocytes are T cells trafficking continuously between the blood, tissues, and lymph nodes until activated by exposure to specific antigen on antigen-presenting cells.

Normal lymphocyte count: 16%–45% of WBCs.

Increased lymphocytes, lymphocytosis. **CLINICAL OCCURRENCE:** *Infectious:* Infectious mononucleosis, tuberculosis, viral pneumonia, viral hepatitis, cholera, rubella, brucellosis, syphilis, toxoplasmosis, pertussis; *Neoplastic:* Lymphocytic leukemia, malignant lymphoma.

Decreased lymphocytes, lymphopenia. **CLINICAL OCCURRENCE:** *Degenerative/Idiopathic:* Idiopathic: lymphopenia; *Infectious:* Acute infections (viral, HIV), chronic HIV; *Metabolic/Toxic:* Drugs (corticosteroids, irradiation therapy, cancer chemotherapy); *Neoplastic:* Carcinoma, lymphoma.

Monocyte count. Monocytes circulate before entering the tissue to terminally differentiate into antigen-presenting tissue macrophages.

Normal monocyte count: 4%–10% of WBCs.

Increased monocytes, monocytosis. **CLINICAL OCCURRENCE:** *Congenital:* Gaucher disease; *Infectious:* Protozoal (malaria, kala-azar, trypanosomiasis), rickettsial (rocky mountain spotted fever, typhus), bacterial (subacute bacterial endocarditis, tuberculosis, brucellosis, syphilis); *Inflammatory/Immune:* Ulcerative colitis, regional enteritis, SLE, sarcoidosis; myeloproliferative diseases (polycythemia vera, essential thrombocythemia, CML, myeloid metaplasia), monocytic leukemia, recovery from agranulocytosis.

Platelet count. Platelets are primarily responsible for initial hemostasis by adhesion and aggregation at the sites of endothelial damage. The platelet plug is then stabilized by fibrin deposition from activated coagulation.

Normal platelet count: 130,000–400,000/mm^3.

Increased platelet count, thrombocytosis or thrombocythemia. Platelets respond like an acute-phase reactant to tissue injury and many acute infections.
CLINICAL OCCURRENCE: *Infectious:* Acute infections; *Inflammatory/Immune:* Rheumatoid arthritis; *Mechanical/Traumatic:* Burns, postsplenectomy; *Metabolic/Toxic:* Exercise, cirrhosis, iron deficiency; *Neoplastic:* Myeloproliferative diseases (polycythemia vera, essential thrombocythemia, CML, myeloid metaplasia); *Vascular:* Hemorrhage.

Decreased platelet count, thrombocytopenia. The cause is decreased production, increased consumption and/or sequestration in the spleen.
CLINICAL OCCURRENCE: *Congenital:* May–Hegglin anomaly, Gaucher disease, Kasabach–Merritt syndrome; *Degenerative/Idiopathic:* Aplastic anemia, marrow failure; *Infectious:* Subacute bacterial endocarditis, sepsis, AIDS, typhus; *Inflammatory/Immune:* Autoimmune thrombocytopenic purpura), hemolytic uremic syndrome, acquired hemolytic anemia, thrombotic thrombocytopenic purpura, DIC; *Mechanical/Traumatic:* Hypersplenism (congestive splenomegaly, sarcoidosis, splenomegaly, Felty syndrome), massive blood transfusions, irradiation, heat stroke; *Metabolic/Toxic:* Uremia, pernicious anemia, folate deficiency, drugs (cancer chemotherapy, chloramphenicol, heparin induced thrombocytopenia, tranquilizers, antipyretics, heavy metals), poisons (benzol, snake bite, insect bites); *Neoplastic:* Polycythemia vera, myelocytic leukemia.

Coagulation

Normal coagulation. Coagulation is a complex process involving many blood proteins, platelets, calcium, and tissue factors. Normally, a balance between coagulation activators and coagulation inhibitors protects against inappropriate coagulation while allowing clot formation at sites of vessel injury. Two functional tests of coagulation pathways are commonly used.

Prothrombin time (PT). The PT is standardized by the International Normalized Ratio (INR) which adjusts the raw clotting time for the International Sensitivity Index (ISI) of the each thromboplastin. It tests factors VII, V, X, thrombin (II), and fibrinogen (I) involved in the *extrinsic coagulation pathway*. The PT/INR is particularly sensitive to decreases in vitamin K-dependent coagulation factors (II, VII, IX, and X).

Normal PT: 11–15 seconds, highly dependent upon the thromboplastin used to initiate coagulation.
Normal INR: 1.0–1.2.

Prolonged PT/NR. Deficiencies in factors I, II, V, VII, or X, liver disease, DIC, vitamin K deficiency, steatorrhea, hemodilution, warfarin administration, abnormal fibrinogen, and technical errors especially incomplete filling of the Vacutainer tube during the blood draw.

Activated partial thromboplastin time (aPTT). The aPTT assesses the *intrinsic coagulation pathway* which uses factors XII, XI, IX, VIII, V, X, II, and I.

Normal aPTT: 22–39 seconds.

Prolonged aPTT. Deficiency of any of the clotting factors—I, II, V, VIII, IX, X, XI, or XII; DIC, heparin, SLE (lupus anticoagulant), antiphospholipid syndrome, and antibody-mediated inhibitors of clotting factor activity.

Fibrinogen. The conversion of fibrinogen to fibrin by thrombin is the final step in clot formation. Abnormal fibrinogen levels indicate decreased synthesis or, more commonly, increased consumption because of diffusely activated clotting.

Normal fibrinogen: 200–400 mg/dL.

Increased fibrinogen. As an acute-phase reactant fibrinogen levels are higher during menstruation and pregnancy, infections, inflammation, and hyperthyroidism.

Decreased fibrinogen. Afibrinogenemia, DIC, hemodilution, fibrinolysis.

URINALYSIS

Midstream urine is optimally collected from the first morning voiding and examined within 30 minutes to assess renal-concentrating ability and permit identification of casts before they disintegrate. Experience is required for microscopic interpretation so clinicians should establish the habit of person-ally examining the urine, especially in challenging cases.

Color: The urine is usually yellow to amber. Other colors provide clues to the presence of abnormal substances for which chemical tests should be performed. Normal urine is clear or cloudy from precipitation of normally excreted urates, phosphates, or sulfates.

Abnormal colored urine. Dark yellow to green (bilirubin); red to black (erythrocytes, hemoglobin, myoglobin); purple to brown on standing in the sunlight from porphyrins.

Acidity: Normally the urine is acid and the urine pH can reach 5.0 with an acid load. High urine pH suggests either an alkali load or inability to fully acidify the urine by distal tubular H^+ excretion. Interpretation of the urine pH is interpreted in reference to the serum or plasma acid-base status. Urinary pH monitoring is necessary when attempting to alkalinize or acidify the urine to enhance the solubility and excretion of certain substances and drugs.

Normal range of pH: 4.6–6.0.

Increased urine pH. Infection with urea-splitting organisms (e.g., Proteus), systemic alkalosis, renal tubular acidosis, carbonic anhydrase inhibitors.

Specific Gravity: An index of weight per unit volume, the specific gravity measures the kidney's ability to concentrate urine in response to antidiuretic hormone and to dilute the urine after a water load. Fasting during 8 hours of sleep should produce a first morning urine with a specific gravity >1.018.

Normal urine specific gravity range: 1.003–1.030, achieved with forced water drinking and fasting, respectively.

Increased urine specific gravity. Fasting and dehydration, glycosuria, pro-teinuria, radiographic contrast media.

Decreased urine specific gravity. Compulsive water drinking, diabetes insipidus.

Fixed specific gravity, isosthenuria (1.010). This reflects inability to concen-trate or dilute the urine indicating damage to the renal medulla.
CLINICAL OCCURRENCE: Severe renal parenchymal damage from many causes, e.g., gout, prolonged potassium deficiency, hypercalcemia, myeloma kidney, sickle cell disease.

Protein: Normally, only the smallest protein molecules pass the filtration barrier of the glomerulus and most of those are reabsorbed by the tubules. Glomerular disease produces measurable proteinuria by allowing filtration of more and larger molecules. Because of its low molecular weight, increased urinary albumin excretion is an early sign of glomerular injury. Tubular injury limits reabsorption of filtered proteins.

Normal urine protein: 5–15 mg/dL; Males: 0–60 mg/d; Females: 0–90 mg/d.

Elevated urine protein, proteinuria. **CLINICAL OCCURRENCE:** *Mild Elevations:* Pyelonephritis, fever, benign orthostatic proteinuria, focal glomerulonephritis. *Severe Proteinuria:* Nephrotic syndrome (defined as >3.5 g/d of proteinuria) in glomerulonephritis, diabetes mellitus, SLE, renal vein thrombosis, amyloidosis, and others.

Glucose: Glucose is filtered in the glomerulus and completely re-absorbed, mostly in the proximal tubule. Glucose should be undetectable in randomly collected fresh urine specimens. When the serum glucose is >200 mg/dL, the filtered load exceeds the tubular reabsorption capacity and glucose appears in the urine. Dipsticks impregnated with glucose oxidase and a color provide a convenient, rapid, and semiquantitative estimate of glucosuria.

Normal glucose excretion: 3–25 mg/dL; 50–300 mg/d.

Increased urine glucose, glucosuria. **CLINICAL OCCURRENCE:** Hyperglycemia in diabetes mellitus; infrequently with renal abnormalities, including acute tubular damage, hereditary renal glycosuria, and proximal tubular dysfunction as in the Fanconi syndrome.

Ketones

Increased urinary ketones, ketonuria. Fatty acid metabolism produces ketones, ketonuria indicating that cells are using fatty acids rather than glucose for energy. Progressively diminished glucose utilization in uncontrolled diabetes mellitus leads to lipolysis with increasing plasma and urinary concentrations of acetoacetic acid, β-hydroxybutyric acid, and ketones.
CLINICAL OCCURRENCE: Diabetic acidosis, fasting, starvation, alcoholic ketoacidosis, isopropyl alcohol intoxication (the clue is an obtunded patient with normal glucose and acid–base status, and urine tests positive for ketones and an osmolar gap).

Urine Sediment: Erythrocytes, leukocytes, hyaline casts, and crystals (urate, phosphate, oxalate) are found in the sediment of a fresh urine specimen collected after a night's fast.

Examining the urinary sediment. Centrifuge 10 mL of urine in a conical tube for 5 minutes, decant the supernatant, flick the tube to disperse formed elements in the remaining drop, and place it on a slide under a cover slip to be examined with the high-power field (hpf) objective of a microscope. Abnormal cell numbers, casts, and bacteria suggest disease.

Erythrocytes, hematuria. Normal: 0–5 RBCs/hpf
CLINICAL OCCURRENCE: Microscopic hematuria occurs with fever and exercise and many urinary tract lesions from the glomerulus to the urethral meatus. Causes of gross hematuria include coagulation defects, renal papillary necrosis, renal infarction, sickle cell disease, glomerulonephritis, Goodpasture syndrome, kidney stone or carcinoma, hemorrhagic cystitis, bladder stone or carcinoma, and prostatitis.

Leukocytes, pyuria. Normal: 0–10 WBCs/hpf

CLINICAL OCCURRENCE: In addition to neutrophils excreted into the urine from the same anatomic sites as erythrocytes, leukocytes from vaginal exudates frequently contaminate routine specimens collected from women. Suspect infection or inflammation in the urinary tract if >10 WBCs/hpf are found in an uncontaminated specimen.

Casts

Hyalin casts. Arising from mucoproteins normally secreted from renal tubules these are occasionally seen in fresh concentrated urine specimens.

Granular casts. Finding many broad, fine, or coarse granular casts (composed of serum proteins like albumin, IgG, transferrin, haptoglobin) in urine containing excessive protein indicates renal parenchymal disease.

Red cell casts. Generally these indicate glomerular disease with RBCs passing the damaged glomeruli in large quantities. Red cell casts containing 10–50 distinct erythrocytes and doubly refractile fat bodies, indicate glomerular disease (glomerulonephritis).

Fatty casts. The urine of patients with the nephrotic syndrome exhibiting glomerular proteinuria and hyperlipoproteinemia contains fatty casts with *doubly refractile fat bodies*, and *Maltese crosses* when examined in polarized light.

White cell and/or renal tubular epithelial cell casts. These are found in the urinary sediment of patients with pyelonephritis, polyarteritis, exudative glomerulonephritis, and renal infarction. *Bacteria* accompanying white cell casts indicate urinary tract infection. Broad orange or brown *hematin* casts occur in acute tubular injury and chronic renal failure.

CEREBROSPINAL FLUID (CSF)

The brain and spinal cord are surrounded by, and suspended in, clear, colorless CSF. Patients with acute CNS symptoms often require CSF analysis. Below are the most commonly ordered tests, their reference ranges, and the more frequent causes of abnormality.

Protein. Normal CSF Protein: 20–50 mg/dL

Increased CSF Protein: Traumatic tap, infection, hemorrhage, metabolic and demyelinating disorders.

Decreased CSF Protein: Young children, CSF leakage, water intoxication, CSF removal, hyperthyroidism.

Glucose. Normal CSF Glucose: 40–70 mg/dL (SI Units: 2.2–3/9 mmol/L).

Elevated CSF Glucose: Hyperglycemia.

Decreased CSF Glucose: Hypoglycemia, infection (especially bacterial or mycobacterial), meningeal malignancy.

Cell Count and Differential: Normal CSF Cell Count: adult, 0–5 mononuclear cells per microliter; neonates, 0–30 mononuclear cells per microliter.

Increased CSF Leukocytes: *Mononuclear cells* increase in CNS infection (viral and early bacterial meningitis, meningoencephalitis, or abscess), neurologic disorders, and hematologic malignancies. *Neutrophils* increase in bacterial infection, hemorrhage, and meningeal malignancy. *Eosinophils* increase in shunt, parasitic infection, and allergic reactions.

SEROUS BODY FLUIDS

Normally, the pleural, pericardial and peritoneal contain a small amount of fluid to wet their surfaces. Any clinically detectable fluid accumulation (effusion or ascites) in the cavity is caused by a pathologic condition. Effusions should be examined microscopically to determine the differential count of cells and to detect malignant cells (cytology). Cell counts are useful in peritoneal fluid but are less helpful in pleural fluid. Increased inflammatory cells have the same implications as those in other locations: *Neutrophils* (infection, neoplasm, leukemia); *lymphocytes* (infection, infarction, lymphoma, leukemia, neoplasm, rheumatologic serositis); *eosinophils* (air in cavity, infection, infarction, neoplasm, rheumatologic disease, CHF). Microbiologic examination, stains, and culture are indicated in exudates. Cytology identifies abnormal/malignant cells. Effusions are generally classified as *transudate* (low protein) or *exudate* (high protein).

Transudates: Transudates, commonly bilateral in the pleural cavities, are secondary to heart failure or medical conditions causing a low serum albumin, e.g., cirrhosis or nephrotic syndrome. Clear and pale, straw-colored fluids are usually transudates, and additional information is rarely provided by testing beyond that required to confirm that the fluid is a transudate. The few cells found in transudates are mesothelial cells and mononuclear cells (lymphocytes and monocytes) with very few neutrophils.

Exudates: Exudates are more frequently unilateral in the pleural cavities and secondary to localized disorders such as infection or neoplasm. Exudates can be cloudy from increased cellularity (leukocytes), red or pink from hemorrhage or trauma, green white from purulence, or milky from increased lipids.

Pleural effusion: See Chapter 8, page 308. Tests frequently useful in pleural effusions include gross appearance, fluid/serum protein ratios (<0.5, transudate; >0.5, exudate), fluid/serum LDH ratios (<0.6, transudate; >0.6, exudate), fluid/serum cholesterol ratio (<0.3, transudate; >0.3, exudate), morphologic examination (hematology and cytology), and pH (<7.20 with WBC count >1,000/mm^3 and low glucose suggests empyema). *Note:* If the protein and LDH ratios are equivocal, the cholesterol ratios may help identify transudate/exudate. Transudates rarely benefit from further testing. Cell counts are rarely useful.

Peritoneal Effusion, Ascites: See Chapter 9, page 416. Tests frequently useful in peritoneal effusion include gross appearance, serum/ascites albumin concentration gradient, cell count and differential, cytology and cultures for bacteria and mycobacteria.

Serum/ascites Albumin Gradient: Subtracting peritoneal albumin from simultaneously determined serum albumin determines the *serum/ascites albumin gradient (SAAG)*. Values <1.1 indicate an exudate (bacterial peritonitis, neoplasm, nephrotic syndrome, pancreatitis, vasculitis); values >1.1 indicate a transudate (portal hypertension caused by cirrhosis, hepatic vein thrombosis, portal vein thrombosis, CHF). *Note:* Protein and LDH ratios described above for pleural fluid are not reliable in peritoneal fluid to separate transudates from exudates.

WBC Counts: Detection of spontaneous bacterial peritonitis in patients with transudative ascites is important. Neutrophil counts of >250/mm³ indicate infection and the need for treatment and long-term prophylaxis. High leukocyte counts (>500/mm³), mostly mononuclear cells, are also seen in malignancy.

APPENDIX

Case Answers and Clinical Pearls

CASE 4-1 ANSWERS

1. The differential diagnosis includes meningitis or encephalitis, neuroleptic malignant syndrome, serotonin syndrome, heat exhaustion, anticholinergic drug use, and toxin exposure.
2. Neuroleptic malignant syndrome
3.

	Temp	Heart Rate	Blood Pressure	Mental Status	Rigidity	Tremor	Clonus
NMS	>38°C	Tachycardia	Hypertensive or labile	Agitated, delirium, confusion, catatonia	Yes	Yes	No
Serotonin Syndrome	>38°C	Tachycardia	Hypertension may progress to shock	From mild agitation to agitated delirium	Yes	Yes	Yes

CLINICAL PEARL. Serotonin Syndrome will cause inducible clonus and ocular clonus; neuroleptic malignant syndrome does not cause clonus.

CASE 4-2 ANSWERS

1. You should anticipate hyperpnea (Kussmaul breathing). This is deep regular respiration, it occurs in response to the metabolic acidosis. It increases alveolar ventilation creating a respiratory alkalosis by increased CO_2 excretion to compensate for the metabolic acidosis.
2. Kussmaul breathing is seen with any severe metabolic acidosis and it is a direct effect of salicylate toxicity. It may also be seen with decreased tissue oxygen delivery from severe anemia or hemorrhage.
3. The Cheyne–Stokes respiratory pattern is cyclic hyperventilation followed by compensatory apnea.
4. The periodic Cheyne–Stokes breathing is caused by a phase delay in the feedback controls attempting to maintain a constant $PaCO_2$. This is the most common periodic breathing pattern. In each cycle, the rate and amplitude of successive breaths increase to a maximum,

then progressively diminish into the next apneic period. Pallor may accompany the apnea. The patient is frequently unaware of the irregular breathing. Patients may be somnolent during the apneic periods and then arouse and become restless during the hyperventilation phase.

5. It may be seen during sleep in normal children and the aged. Other causes are disorders of the cerebral circulation (stroke, atherosclerosis), heart failure and low cardiac output of any cause, increased intracranial pressure (meningitis, hydrocephalus, brain tumor, subarachnoid hemorrhage, intracerebral hemorrhage), head injury, drugs (opiates, barbiturates, alcohol), and at high altitude during sleep before acclimatization.

CLINICAL PEARL. Irregular breathing—Biot breathing. This is an uncommon variant of Cheyne–Stokes respiration in which periods of apnea alternate irregularly with a series of breaths of equal depth that terminate abruptly. It is most often seen in meningitis.

CASE 4-3 ANSWERS

1. The blood pressure drops without a corresponding increase in pulse. This indicates autonomic insufficiency.
2. Causes include decreased intravascular volume (hemorrhage, dehydration), loss of vascular tone (autonomic insufficiency-multisystem atrophy), deconditioning after a prolonged illness, peripheral neuropathies (diabetes, tabes dorsalis, alcoholism), medications (tricyclic antidepressants, vasodilators, ganglion blockers), and impaired venous return (ascites, pregnancy, venous insufficiency, inferior vena cava obstruction or hemangiomas of the legs).
3. Multiple system atrophy.
4. Parkinsonism type: patients have slow movement, rigidity, and tremor. Cerebellar type: patients have difficulties with coordination and speech. Combined type: patients will have Parkinsonism and cerebellar dysfunction.

CLINICAL PEARL. When the drop in BP is not accompanied by a rise in pulse rate, autonomic insufficiency is suggested. Patients with chronic orthostatic hypotension frequently have postprandial hypotension and reversal of the normal circadian BP pattern, that is, higher BP at night than during the day.

CASE 4-4 ANSWERS

1. Wide pulse pressure. A pulse pressure of >65 mm Hg is abnormal.
2. Pulse pressure increases when the peak systolic pressure is increased (increased stroke volume, increased rate of ventricular contraction,

decreased aortic elasticity) and/or there is decreased diastolic pressure (aortic insufficiency, decreased peripheral resistance as in sepsis and arteriovenous shunts).

3. <u>Increased systolic pressure</u>: Systolic hypertension, atherosclerosis, increased stroke volume (aortic regurgitation, hyperthyroidism, anxiety, bradycardia, heart block, pregnancy, fever, systemic arteriovenous fistulas, post-PVC, after a long pause in atrial fibrillation); <u>increased diastolic runoff</u>: aortic regurgitation, sepsis, vasodilators, patent ductus arteriosus, hyperthyroidism, arteriovenous fistulas, beriberi.

4. <u>Aortic regurgitation</u> may produce a diastolic decrescendo murmur heard best at the left sternal border, "water-hammer" pulses, head bobbing, booming systolic and diastolic sounds auscultated over the femoral artery, and visible systolic pulsations of the uvula, retinal arterioles, and the fingernail bed visible with light compression of the fingernail.

CLINICAL PEARL. Persistent ductus arteriosus is a congenital heart defect that can cause a widened pulse pressure. It is more common in females and premature infants.

CASE 5-1 ANSWERS

1. <u>Acute HIV infection.</u> Many symptoms and signs are possible in *acute retroviral syndrome*. The most common are fever, lymphadenopathy, sore throat, rash, myalgia/arthralgia, and headache.

2. <u>Acute HIV infection.</u> Nontender adenopathy primarily involving the axillary, cervical, and occipital nodes, mostly observed during the second week acute retroviral syndrome.

> <u>Infectious mononucleosis.</u> Moderate to high fever, pharyngitis, and lymphadenopathy are common with involvement of the posterior cervical chain more than the anterior chain.
> <u>Mycobacterial infection.</u> Miliary tuberculosis is an important consideration in patients with generalized lymphadenopathy. *Mycobacterium tuberculosis* is the usual cause in adults.
> <u>Systemic lupus erythematosus.</u> Lymphadenopathy occurs in about 50% of patients.
> <u>Lymphoma.</u> Hodgkin's and non-Hodgkin's lymphoma
> <u>Medications.</u> Many medications (e.g., phenytoin) cause serum sickness characterized by fever, arthralgias, rash, and generalized lymphadenopathy.
> <u>Uncommon causes.</u> Secondary syphilis, Castleman's disease (angiofollicular lymph node hyperplasia), Kikuchi's disease (histiocytic necrotizing lymphadenitis), and angioimmunoblastic T-cell lymphoma.

CLINICAL PEARL. Infectious causes of <u>heterophile-negative mononucleosis-like illnesses</u> include cytomegalovirus, human herpesvirus 6, human immunodeficiency virus, adenovirus, herpes simplex virus, and *Toxoplasma gondii*.

CASE 5-2 ANSWERS

1. <u>Anterior cervical lymphadenopathy.</u> Infections of the head and neck, infectious mononucleosis (Epstein–Barr virus, cytomegalovirus infection, or toxoplasmosis). <u>Posterior cervical lymphadenopathy.</u> EBV infection, mycobacterial infection, lymphoma, Kikuchi's disease, head and neck malignancy (lymphomas or metastatic squamous cell carcinoma).

2. *Mycobacterium tuberculosis* or atypical mycobacteria infection is suggested when multiple enlarged cervical nodes develop over weeks to months and become fluctuant or matted without significant inflammation or tenderness.

3. <u>Infectious mononucleosis syndrome</u> (triad of moderate to high fever, pharyngitis, and lymphadenopathy). Lymph node involvement is typically symmetric and involves the posterior cervical more than the anterior chain. Lymphadenopathy may also be present in the axillary and inguinal areas, which helps to distinguish infectious mononucleosis from other causes of pharyngitis.

CLINICAL PEARL. Hard cervical lymph nodes, particularly in older patients and smokers, suggest metastatic head and neck cancer. These patients should be referred to an otolaryngologist for fiberoptic examination of the oropharynx or possibly triple endoscopy (oro/nasopharynx-laryngeal, esophageal, bronchoscopic). <u>Never do an excisional biopsy before consultation</u>; cutting through tissue planes may preclude curative surgery.

CASE 5-3 ANSWERS

1. Hypoglycemia
2. (1) Symptoms of hypoglycemia. (2) Documented hypoglycemia at the time of symptoms. (3) Correction of symptoms with glucose. The Whipple triad is the classic presentation of an insulinoma.
3. The history is consistent with an insulinoma.
4. The most common cause of symptomatic hypoglycemia is use of sulfonylureas or insulin. Insulinoma is very rare.

CLINICAL PEARL. Patients with insulinomas must be evaluated for MEN-I to exclude hyperprolactinemia from a pituitary adenoma, hyperparathyroidism from parathyroid hyperplasia, and hypergastrinemia from a gastrinoma.

CASE 5-4 ANSWERS

1. The axillary nodes receive drainage from the <u>arm, chest wall, and breast</u>.
2. <u>Infections</u> including cat scratch disease, <u>malignancy</u>, and <u>silicone breast implants</u> can cause supraclavicular and axillary lymphadenopathy.

3. <u>Breast cancer</u>. In the absence of upper extremity lesions, cancer is often found. In one series of 31 patients with isolated axillary masses, 9 had breast cancer (5 in the contralateral breast) and 9 had metastases from other sites.

CLINICAL PEARL. The epitrochlear nodes are not normally palpable. Palpable epitrochlear nodes are always pathologic. The differential diagnosis includes infections of the forearm or hand, lymphoma, sarcoidosis, tularemia, and secondary syphilis.

CASE 5-5 ANSWER

1. Palpation of the lymph nodes provides information suggesting whether the process is localized or systemic and the likelihood of a malignant versus an inflammatory process.

- <u>Location</u>: generalized adenopathy is usually a manifestation of systemic disease.
- <u>Size:</u> insignificant if less than 2 cm, except in the supraclavicular fossa where >1 cm is significant.
- <u>Consistency:</u> soft (insignificant), rubbery (classically lymphoma), hard (classically malignancy and granulomatous infection).
- <u>Fixation:</u> normal lymph nodes are freely movable in the subcutaneous space. Abnormal nodes can become fixed to adjacent tissues (invading cancers or inflammation) or they can become fixed to each other ("matted") by the same processes.
- <u>Tenderness:</u> tenderness suggests recent, rapid enlargement that has put pain receptors in the capsule under tension and this typically occurs with an inflammatory processes, most often infection. Nontender nodes suggest either malignancy or chronic infection with more indolent organisms (e.g., mycobacteria, fungi).

CLINICAL PEARL. Enlarged inguinal lymph nodes are very common. Usually, they are often small and hard ("shotty"—feels like buck shot) that are of no clinical concern. Splenomegaly associated with lymphadenopathy suggests lymphoma, chronic lymphocytic leukemia, acute leukemia, or infectious mononucleosis.

CASE 6-1 ANSWERS

1. Generalized erythroderma results from diffuse dilation of the cutaneous capillaries as a result of systemic inflammation, fever, or release of bacterial toxins.
2. Differential diagnosis includes staphylococcal or streptococcal toxic shock syndrome, staphylococcal scalded-skin syndrome, scarlet fever, drug eruptions (exfoliative dermatitis), Steven-Johnson

syndrome, toxic epidermal necrolysis (TEN), psoriasis, SLE, and cutaneous T-cell lymphoma.

3. Erythema multiforme manifests as iris and/or target-shaped lesions typically on the extremities (especially palms and soles) and mucous membranes. Mouth lesions are painful and tender.

4. Common etiologies are medications (sulfonamides, phenytoin, barbiturates, penicillin, allopurinol) and infections (HSV and mycoplasma).

CLINICAL PEARL. Steven-Johnson syndrome (skin sloughing is limited to less than 10% of the body surface) and toxic epidermal necrolysis (skin sloughing of greater than 30% of the body surface area) are characterized by fever and mucocutaneous lesions leading to necrosis and sloughing of the epidermis. They are severe idiosyncratic reactions, most commonly triggered by medications.

CASE 6-2 ANSWERS

1. Bullous pemphigoid. Tense bullae arise from erythematous macules or urticarial lesions. Bullae are intact (subepidermal) and intertriginous areas are commonly affected. Up to one-third of cases have oral lesions; there is no association with malignancy.

2. Pemphigus vulgaris. Flaccid intradermal bullae on noninflamed skin rupture forming large erosions; Nikolsky sign is present. Oral lesions are present in the majority of patients. It is associated with an increased incidence of lymphoreticular malignancy.

3. Nikolsky sign: slight lateral pressure on the skin may cause blistering and a subsequent erosion.

CLINICAL PEARL. Bullous diabetic dermopathy. The cause is not known. The lesions are sterile noninflamed bullae that occur without trauma on the lateral aspects of the fingers in patients with poorly controlled diabetes. The blisters are tense and nontender.

CASE 6-3 ANSWERS

1. Herpes simplex. The vesicle is often preceded by pain or tingling. The most common locations are the vermilion border (herpes labialis) and genital area; they can occur anywhere. Herpes simplex remains dormant in spinal ganglia; reactivation produces recurrent disease in the area of primary infection.

2. Herpes simplex, herpes zoster (grouped vesicles in a dermatomal distribution), and dermatitis herpetiformis (chronic recurrent, intensely pruritic symmetrical papulovesicular lesions appear on extensor surfaces, nearly always associated with gluten intolerance).

CLINICAL PEARL. Herpes zoster lesions appearing on the tip of the nose represent infection of the nasociliary nerve and may predict corneal infection via the ophthalmic branch of the trigeminal nerve. Immediate ophthalmology consultation is required.

CASE 6-4 ANSWER

1. **Terry's nails** have proximal paleness extending halfway up the nail, often eliminating the lunula, and a darker distal band. They are encountered in states of stress (e.g., advanced age, liver disease/cirrhosis, CHF, DM2).

   Lindsay's nails (half-and-half nails) have a distal brown transverse band caused by increased pigment deposition. They are seen in kidney disease.

   Beau's lines are transverse depressed ridges produced by severe infection, MI, hypotension/shock, hypocalcemia, surgery, malnutrition, and some chemotherapy.

   Muehrcke's lines (leukonychia striata) are narrow white transverse lines that are not depressed like Beau's lines. They are associated with hypoalbuminemia (usually <2.2 g/dL) resulting from decreased protein synthesis or increased protein loss, as occurs with certain chemotherapy and nephrotic syndrome.

   Mees' lines are transverse white lines (usually one per nail, no depressions) that often disappear if pressure is placed over the line. It is strongly associated with arsenic poisoning, thallium poisoning, and to a lesser extent other heavy metal poisoning.

CLINICAL PEARL. Finger nails grow at a rate of about 0.8 to 1.0 mm per week. Using this, you can approximate when the clinical scenario causing the nail finding occurred. Nail pitting is a nonspecific sign for psoriasis (additional signs include onycholysis, thickening, and "oilspot" lesions which are yellow patches on the nail).

CASE 6-5 ANSWERS

1. Lung cancer. COPD is not a cause of clubbing: if you see clubbing in a COPD patient, think lung cancer. Remember "beware of the yellow clubbed digit" (yellow from tobacco tars and clubbed from cancer).

2. Lungs. Cancer, pus in the lung (bronchiectasis as in cystic fibrosis, but also lung abscess and empyema), pulmonary fibrosis. Heart. Right to left shunts, endocarditis, and pericarditis. Gastrointestinal. Inflammatory bowel disease, cirrhosis.

CLINICAL PEARL. If a patient complains of painful wrists and/or ankles and you miss the clubbing, you will likely go down the wrong path looking for causes of arthritis and arthralgia when the likely diagnosis is hypertrophic pulmonary osteoarthropathy (HPOA). The causes of HPOA are the same as those of clubbing.

CASE 6-6 ANSWERS

1. Tularemia, plague, syphilis, anthrax, rat-bite fever, rickettsial pox, cat-scratch disease, mycobacterium marinum, scrub typhus, sporotrichosis, nocardia, lymphogranuloma venereum, herpes simplex, cowpox, and trypanosomiasis.
2. A detailed travel and exposure history is critical to developing a focused differential.
3. <u>Syphilis.</u> The chancre is the primary lesion of syphilis. A painless, shallow ulcer developing at the site of inoculation is associated with nontender, nonsuppurating swelling of regional lymph nodes.

<u>Tularemia.</u> *Francisella tularensis* is inoculated by fly or tick bites or skin contact with an infected rabbit. The incubation period is 1 to 10 days followed by lassitude, headache, chills, nausea and vomiting, and myalgia accompanied by a rather benign-looking ulcer at the inoculation site with surrounding erythema, but little pain. Regional fluctuant painful lymphadenopathy develops, that may suppurate.

<u>Anthrax.</u> Malaise and a painless pruritic pustule on the skin may be followed by dyspnea and hemoptysis during dissemination. The painless "malignant pustule" begins on an exposed surface as an erythematous papule which then vesiculates, ulcerates, and is surrounded by characteristic nontender brawny edema. Despite the name, it is not pustular unless superinfected. A black eschar may form. Regional lymphadenopathy is occasionally present.

CLINICAL PEARL. Nodular lymphangitis manifests as erythema, induration, and nodular thickening of the cutaneous and subcutaneous lymphatics. Causative organisms include sporotrichosis, *Mycobacteria marinum*, nocardia, leishmaniasis, tularemia, coccidioidosis, histoplasmosis, blastomycosis, cryptococcosis, *Pseudomonas pseudomallei*, and anthrax. Failure of the skin lesions to resolve with an appropriate course of antibiotics for *Staph.* and *Strep.* should raise clinical suspicion for one of these less common pathogens.

CASE 6-7 ANSWERS

1. <u>Basal cell cancer.</u>
2. <u>Basal cell cancer</u> is the most common type of skin cancer. It arises without a precursor lesion on sun-exposed skin, most commonly the face and upper back. The lesions are pearly papules, often with surface telangiectasias. They slowly enlarge and may ulcerate. They may have considerable local extension and tissue destruction, but do not metastasize. *Superficial basal cell cancers* are flat, indurated, pink plaques with a rolled border.

<u>Squamous cell cancer</u> arises in areas of sun damage from pre-existing actinic keratoses or in the genital region as a result of human

papillomavirus infection. When limited to the epidermis (*squamous cell carcinoma in situ*, *Bowen disease*), they present as sharply demarcated, slightly scaling plaques that may be several centimeters in diameter. *Invasive squamous cell carcinoma* may present as an ulcerated area of indurated skin (common on the lip) or as an eroded exophytic growth. These cancers invade the dermis and metastasize to regional lymph nodes.

CLINICAL PEARL. The primary approach to the prevention of BCCs is protection from sun exposure. Although these tumors have a low metastatic potential, they are locally invasive and can be destructive of skin and the surrounding structures.

CASE 6-8 ANSWERS

1. Osler nodes are painful, palpable red lesions usually on fingers/toes. They are caused by the inflammatory response to immune complexes deposited in the capillary walls.
2. Janeway lesions are painless macules, usually on palms/soles. They are caused by septic emboli, most commonly seen in acute *Staphylococcus aureus* endocarditis.

CLINICAL PEARL. Osler and Janeway lesions are indicative of a subacute or chronic infection and will not be found with acute bacterial endocarditis. When they are found, look for evidence of an immune complex glomerulopathy. Splinter hemorrhages which appear as red to black small thin longitudinal lines under the nail plate can be seen with infective endocarditis. Splinter hemorrhages are seen more commonly with trauma and nail psoriasis (the two most common causes) rather than systemic illnesses like infective endocarditis or connective tissue disorders.

CASE 7-1 ANSWERS

1. The differential diagnosis includes optic neuritis, neuromyelitis optica (Devic's syndrome), nutritional optic neuropathies, retinal artery occlusion, and herpes simplex keratitis.
2. The most likely diagnosis is optic neuritis based on the central scotoma, and painful movement of the eye. Optic neuritis is more common in females, approximately 3:1 compared to males.
3. Findings may include an afferent pupillary defect (Marcus Gunn pupil), the optic disc may be hyperemic with indistinct margins from edema in the peripapillary nerve fiber layer, and the disk surface maybe elevated above the surrounding retina. Decreased color distinction may also be seen using Ishihara plates or other tests for chromagraphic distinction.

CLINICAL PEARL. The probability that optic neuritis is a manifestation of multiple sclerosis increases further the patient is from the equator.

CASE 7-2 ANSWERS

1. Cavernous sinus thrombosis, periorbital cellulitis, orbital cellulitis, acute angle closure glaucoma, sinusitis, and epidural and subdural infections.
2. Cavernous sinus thrombosis.
3. Based on her complaints of diplopia in the setting of presumed cavernous sinus thrombosis, the most likely nerve to be affected is CN-VI as it is located within the sinus whereas CN-III and CN-IV are located within the lateral wall.
4. Facial infections, sinusitis, or an infected furuncle involving the nose or upper lip (especially after manipulation by squeezing or incision) are predisposing factors.

CLINICAL PEARL. Bilateral findings are highly suggestive of cavernous sinus thrombosis.

CASE 7-3 ANSWERS

1. The differential diagnosis includes Behçet's disease, inflammatory bowel disease, amyloidosis, HIV, SLE, and polyarteritis nodosa.
2. Behçet's disease.
3. The International Study Group on Behçet's disease criteria are at least three episodes of aphthous or herpetiform ulcers in a 12-month time period (reported or observed), and at least two of the following:

   A. Genital ulcers that heal with scarring;
   B. Eye pathology including uveitis, retinal vasculitis, or hypopyon;
   C. Skin lesions including erythema nodosum-like lesions, pseudofolliculitis, or papulopustular/acneiform lesions;
   D. Positive pathergy skin test.

4. Pathergy is present when a pustule develops at the site of minor skin trauma like a needle stick.

CLINICAL PEARL. A history of recurrent aphthous ulcers should raise the possibility of Behçet's or Crohn's disease.

CASE 7-4 ANSWERS

1. The differential diagnosis includes a retropharyngeal abscess, epiglottitis, peritonsillar abscess, bacterial tracheitis, EBV infection, diphtheria, measles, and croup. Based on the history a foreign body or burn seems unlikely.
2. Epiglottitis.
3. Likely pathogens are *Haemophilus influenzae* type b (Hib) and *Streptococcus pneumoniae*. Hib vaccination has reduced the incidence of epiglottitis.

4. Causes of stridor in adults include mass lesions such as carcinoma that impair vocal cord mobility or reduce the glottic aperture, vocal cord paralysis which limits the effective glottis opening, a swollen epiglottis due to epiglottitis, and inhalation or thermal injury. Neck trauma can also cause stridor.

CLINICAL PEARL. Examination of the oral pharynx in the setting of presumed epiglottis should be performed with caution since this can increase the work of breathing further compromising the airway. Securing the airway is the top priority.

CASE 7-5 ANSWERS

1. Differential diagnosis includes Lemierre's syndrome (septic thrombophlebitis of the internal jugular vein), retropharyngeal abscess, peritonsillar abscess, pneumonia, and mononucleosis syndrome.
2. Lemierre's syndrome (septic thrombophlebitis of the internal jugular vein). Patients typically present with a history of recent oral infection (pharyngitis) and have fevers, rigors, and neck pain and swelling. Lymphadenopathy may be present; a palpable venous cord may also be present.
3. *Fusobacterium necrophorum.*

CLINICAL PEARL. Patients with Lemierre's syndrome may have pulmonary symptoms related to septic emboli. They may develop multiple pulmonary abscesses.

CASE 7-6 ANSWERS

1. Peripheral vertigo may cause nausea and vomiting. Symptoms are often improved with fixation of the gaze, and they are able to walk, though it may be uncomfortable due to increased vertigo. With central vertigo the patient often cannot stand without falling.
2. **1: Bidirectional nystagmus.** A change in the direction of the nystagmus with alteration of gaze without changing head position always has a central etiology. **2: Head impulse test.** With the patient fixing his gaze on your nose, quickly turn his head to the right and then left about 45 degrees. If the eyes move to restore fixation, indicating an abnormal vestibular ocular reflex, the cause is peripheral. **3: Vertical squint.** Perform the cover–uncover test with the gaze directed first upward then downward. Movement of either eye to restore fixation on uncover indicates a central cause. **4: The Dix–Hallpike maneuver.** A positive test indicates a labyrinthine disorder. **5: The Fukuda stepping test.** Have the patient stand upright with the eyes closed and the arms outstretched. Ask the standing patient to march in place with the eyes closed; rotation of >30 degrees is a positive test indicating asymmetric inner ear function.
3. Peripheral vertigo, probably labyrinthitis.

CLINICAL PEARL. In benign positional vertigo otolith repositioning is often curative, but recurrences do happen.

CASE 7-7 ANSWERS

1. <u>Acute angle closure glaucoma.</u>
2. A sudden dilation of the pupil such as dim lighting can precipitate angle closure.
3. This is more common in women, Asians, Eskimos, the elderly, and those with hyperopia. Predisposing anatomic variations include a narrow angle, hollow anterior chamber, short axial eye length, anterior lens, thick iris, and an overdeveloped iris dilator muscle.
4. Medications that can precipitate acute angle closure include anticholinergics, sympathomimetics, cocaine, selective serotonin reuptake inhibitors, tricyclic antidepressants, and sulfonamides.

CLINICAL PEARL. Acute angle closure glaucoma is an emergency. Without prompt treatment permanent vision loss will ensue.

CASE 8-1 ANSWERS

1. Pulsus paradoxus is an exaggerated decrease in systolic blood pressure during inspiration (greater than 10 mm Hg).
2. Inflate the cuff beyond the point where you hear any Korotkoff sounds. Very slowly deflate the cuff until you hear the first beats, which will be in expiration. The rate of deflation must allow for several heart beats and at least one respiratory cycle with each 2 mm Hg decrease in the pressure. Keep slowly deflating the cuff to find the pressure at which you hear every beat. The difference between the two is the *pulsus paradoxus*. Greater than 10 mm Hg is considered significant.
3. Inspiration lowers intrathoracic pressure, expanding the lungs *and* the pulmonary venous capacity. The expanded lungs are filled with incoming air; the increase in pulmonary circulatory capacity decreases LV filling. The intrathoracic pressure drop is also transmitted to the heart causing a larger gradient between the extrathoracic great veins and the right atrium and ventricle therefore increasing venous return to the right heart. When there is restricted right + left ventricular volume expansion, the inspiratory increase in RV volume and further decrease in LV volume results in bulging of the interventricular septum into the left ventricle. Both the bulging of the interventricular septum and the reduction in left ventricular filling contribute to a large decrease in LV stroke volume during inspiration producing the pulsus paradoxus. This is the direct consequence of the <u>ventricular interdependence</u>.

CLINICAL PEARL. Differential diagnosis of pulsus paradoxus includes (1) moderate to severe cardiac tamponade; (2) constrictive pericarditis; (3) COPD exacerbations; and (4) asthma attacks.

CASE 8-2 ANSWERS

1. <u>Mitral stenosis.</u> In the great majority of cases mitral stenosis is caused by rheumatic mitral valve disease.
2. <u>First heart sound.</u> As a result of the elevated left atrial pressure and slow LV filling, the stenotic mitral leaflets are still ballooning into the LV at the onset of ventricular contraction. The increased excursion of the leaflets leads to the loud S1. <u>Opening snap (OS).</u> An OS is heard at the apex when the leaflets are still mobile. Fusion of the leaflet tips leads to the abrupt halt of leaflet motion after rapid initial rapid filling in early diastole. It is best heard at the apex and lower left sternal border. <u>Diastolic murmur.</u> The murmur in MS is a low-pitched diastolic rumble most prominent at the apex. It is heard best in a quiet room using the bell of the stethoscope with the patient lying on the left side holding full expiration.
3. S1 becomes softer as the leaflets become more, fibrotic, thickened, and calcified limiting their motion. P2 increases in intensity with the development of pulmonary hypertension. As PA pressure increases further, splitting of S2 is reduced and ultimately S2 becomes a single sound. The murmur becomes softer as the stenosis becomes severe and it may be inaudible or absent when MS is very severe. As the MS progresses and left atrial pressure increases, the OS occurs earlier after S2. Thus, shorter A2–OS interval indicates more severe mitral stenosis.
4. Pathologic pulmonic regurgitation secondary to pulmonary hypertension results in the Graham Steell murmur, a high-pitched decrescendo diastolic murmur audible at the upper sternal border. This can be heard with severe mitral stenosis.

CLINICAL PEARL. With the marked decline in the incidence of acute rheumatic fever in developed countries, mitral stenosis is becoming a rare condition.

CASE 8-3 ANSWERS

1. <u>Aortic regurgitation/insufficiency.</u>
2. <u>Aortic regurgitation/insufficiency murmur</u> is heard in early diastole beginning immediately after A2. It is high pitched, often with a blowing quality, and may have sustained intensity or decrescendo. The <u>apical impulse</u> is displaced laterally and inferiorly and is diffuse and hyperdynamic. The increased stroke volume results in abrupt distension of the peripheral arteries and an elevated systolic pressure while regurgitation into the LV with quick collapse of the arteries rapidly decreases arterial pressure; this is noted as the <u>wide pulse pressure (water hammer or Corrigan's pulse).</u> This can produce multiple other signs associated with each heartbeat: head bobbing *(de Musset's sign)*; a pistol shot heard over the femoral arteries *(Traube's sign)*; systolic and diastolic bruits when the femoral artery is partially compressed

(Duroziez's sign); capillary pulsations in the fingernails, fingertips, or lips *(Quincke's pulses)*; systolic pulsations of the uvula *(Mueller's sign)*; visible pulsations of the retinal arteries and pupils *(Becker's sign)*; popliteal cuff systolic pressure exceeding brachial pressure by more than 60 mm Hg *(Hill's sign)*; systolic pulsations of the liver *(Rosenbach's sign)*; systolic pulsations of the spleen *(Gerhard's sign)*.

3. Severe acute aortic regurgitation (AR) commonly presents catastrophically with sudden cardiovascular collapse. Endocarditis, aortic dissection, or rupture of the valve leaflets are some of the underlying causes of acute aortic regurgitation.

4. Aortic root dilation (Marfan syndrome, familial cystic medial necrosis, Ehlers–Danlos, ankylosing spondylitis, aortitis from giant cell arteritis or syphilis), congenital bicuspid aortic valve, subacute endocarditis, and rheumatic heart disease.

CLINICAL PEARL. Bicuspid aortic valve is associated with aortic root and/or ascending aorta dilatation that can lead to aneurysm formation or dissection.

CASE 8-4 ANSWERS

1. S3 and S4 are associated with ventricular filling and increasing ventricular volume. S3 is heard during early diastolic rapid filling and S4 is heard in late diastole during ventricular filling associated with atrial contraction.

2. S3 and S4 are best heard with the bell of the stethoscope over the apex. The left lateral decubitus position is preferable for appreciating a left ventricular S3 and S4. Right ventricular S3 and S4 are best heard along the lower left sternal border.

3. S3 can occur in healthy young adult, but it is usually abnormal in patients over the age of 40 years. The S3 suggests an enlarged ventricular chamber and is specific for systolic ventricular failure. Due to decreased ventricular compliance with age S4 can be heard in many healthy older adults without heart disease. A pathologic S4 is most frequently associated with decreased left ventricular compliance. Left ventricular hypertrophy in hypertensive heart disease, aortic stenosis, and hypertrophic cardiomyopathy leads to decreased left ventricular distensibility. S4 is usually abnormal in young adults and children. Right ventricular S3 and S4 usually increase in intensity during inspiration, while left ventricular S3 and S4 remain unchanged.

CLINICAL PEARL. S3 and S4 may be confused with a split S2 and split S1, respectively. When split, the two parts of S1 or S2 typically have a similar pitch, while S3 and S4 are lower pitched than S2 and S1. This difference in pitch is identified by listening alternately with the bell and the diaphragm of the stethoscope. The lower-pitched S3 and S4 are more pronounced with the bell applied lightly to the skin; the higher-pitched split S1 and S2 are more pronounced using the diaphragm or when pressing the bell more firmly to the skin.

CASE 8-5 ANSWERS

1. This patient has the classic murmur of <u>aortic stenosis</u>. The murmur is best heard at the right upper sternal border and will radiate into the carotid arteries. Bicuspid aortic valves usually become calcified and stenotic between the ages of 50 and 70 years.
2. The carotid arterial pulse in aortic stenosis (AS) reflects the obstruction to blood flow across the aortic valve. The upstroke is delayed and reduced in amplitude. It has been described as "parvus and tardus," that is, weak and slowly rising.
3. With fixed valvular AS the initial upstroke and peak of the carotid pulse are delayed and the volume may be reduced. With obstructive hypertrophic cardiomyopathy (HCM) the initial upstroke is usually sharp and the volume is normal, but a second upstroke may be felt, the bifid pulse of hypertrophic cardiomyopathy. During the straining phase of a Valsalva maneuver venous return and LV volume decrease leading to a louder murmur with HCM, while the AS murmur will become softer. The same changes occur when standing from a squatting position.

CLINICAL PEARL. Most midsystolic murmurs are benign (innocent) flow murmurs. They are short and soft systolic ejection murmurs, with normal S1 and S2, normal cardiac impulse, and no evidence of any hemodynamic abnormality.

CASE 8-6 ANSWERS

1. <u>Elevated "a" wave.</u> Resistance to right atrial emptying at or beyond the tricuspid valve including pulmonary hypertension, rheumatic tricuspid stenosis, and right atrial mass or thrombus.
2. <u>Cannon "a" wave.</u> Large positive "a" wave occurs when the atrium contracts against a closed tricuspid valve during AV dissociation. This is seen with premature atrial, junctional, or ventricular beats, complete AV block, and ventricular tachycardia.
3. <u>Absent "a" wave.</u> This occurs when the atrium is not contracting as in atrial fibrillation.
4. <u>Elevated "v" wave.</u> The regurgitant jet associated with tricuspid regurgitation is the most common cause (Lancisi's sign). Severe tricuspid regurgitation may be accompanied by a pulsatile liver felt at the lower costal margin.

CLINICAL PEARL. *Friedrich's sign* is an exaggerated diastolic collapse of the neck veins (x-wave) in constrictive pericarditis.

CASE 8-7 ANSWERS

1. So-called <u>typical organisms</u> are *Streptococcus pneumoniae, Haemophilus influenzae, Moraxella catarrhalis,* and less commonly *Staphylococcus*

aureus, Group A streptococci, anaerobes, and aerobic gram-negative bacteria. Atypical pneumonia refers to pneumonia caused by *Legionella spp, Mycoplasma pneumoniae, Chlamydophila* (formerly *Chlamydia*) *pneumoniae,* and *C. psittaci.* Although imprecise, these terms are used because of their acceptance amongst clinicians. In the individual patient, there are no findings from history, physical examination, or routine laboratory studies that allow the clinician to distinguish pneumonia caused by atypical versus typical organisms.

2. Legionnaires' disease. Respiratory symptoms are not prominent initially and at first the cough is mild and only slightly productive. Diarrhea, nausea, vomiting, and abdominal pain can be prominent symptoms. Laboratory abnormalities commonly encountered with Legionnaires' disease include renal and hepatic dysfunction, thrombocytopenia, leukocytosis, hyponatremia, and hypophosphatemia.

3. Extrapulmonary manifestations include hemolysis (rarely clinically significant), skin rash (including Stevens–Johnson syndrome), carditis, and, more commonly in children, encephalitis and other central nervous system complications.

CLINICAL PEARL. Pontiac fever is a mild self-limited form of Legionella infection characterized by fever, malaise, chills, fatigue, and headache, without respiratory complaints.

CASE 8-8 ANSWERS

1. Pneumothorax.
2. There is usually sudden severe chest pain, often unilateral, and rarely localized, followed immediately by increasing dyspnea. With a large pneumothorax, the physical signs are distinctive: hyperresonant percussion, decreased fremitus, voice transmission, and breath sounds on the affected side, and tracheal deviation away from the affected side. Respiratory movements of the ribs are decreased with persistent expiratory distention of the hemithorax.
3. The visceral pleura adheres to the parietal pleura and chest wall due to the negative pressure in the potential space between the two layers. When air enters the pleural space the lung separates from the chest wall leading to failure of respiratory mechanics and lung collapse. The severity of the symptoms is primarily related to the volume of air in the pleural space, with dyspnea being more prominent if the pneumothorax is large.
4. In the absence of trauma, rupture of a subpleural bleb is most likely. Blebs are associated with pulmonary emphysema, and, occasionally, from nonsuppurative lung disease, such as sarcoidosis, fibrosis, or silicosis. In women pulmonary lymphangioleiomyomatosis is a consideration.

CLINICAL PEARL. Labored breathing and hemodynamic compromise suggests a tension pneumothorax, which necessitates emergency decompression. The sudden pain of a spontaneous pneumothorax must be distinguished from pulmonary embolism, myocardial infarction, and acute pericarditis.

CASE 8-9 ANSWERS

1. Stridor is a high-pitched, musical sound produced as turbulent flow passes through a narrowed segment of the extrathoracic respiratory tract. It is often clearly heard without the aid of a stethoscope. Although stridor is usually inspiratory, it can also be expiratory or biphasic.

2. Extrathoracic airway obstruction can be due to acute epiglottitis, airway edema after device removal, anaphylaxis, vocal-cord dysfunction, inhalation of a foreign body, laryngeal tumors, or tracheal neoplasm.

3. Vocal-cord dysfunction, also called paradoxical vocal-cord motion, is characterized by the inappropriate vocal-cord adduction resulting in airflow limitation at the level of the larynx, accompanied by stridorous breathing. It has been associated with psychosocial disorders, stress, exercise, perioperative airway and neurologic injury, gastroesophageal reflux, and irritant inhalational exposures.

CLINICAL PEARL. Vocal-cord dysfunction can be easily misdiagnosed as asthma. The diagnosis is confirmed by laryngoscopy (sometimes following exercise) showing abnormal adduction of the true cords (during inspiration, throughout the respiratory cycle, or rarely just during expiration).

CASE 8-10 ANSWERS

1. Air is interposed between the lung and the chest wall.

2. The findings of thoracic inspection, palpation, percussion, and auscultation must be synthesized to suggest a pathophysiologic process or diagnosis. The signs of altered lung density (in this case markedly reduced density within the chest suggesting air) serve as a starting point for the differential diagnosis. It is especially useful to draw a chest diagram to help synthesize your findings and hypotheses.

3. Tension pneumothorax. A one-way tissue valve permits air to enter the pleural space during inspiration, but prevents its expulsion during expiration. Thus, the intraplueral pressure builds up to exceed atmospheric pressure. The increasing intrapleural and intrathoracic pressure collapses the affected lung, causes tracheal deviation, compression of the unaffected lung, and decreased venous return to the heart.

CLINICAL PEARL. Decreased respiratory excursion of a distended tympanitic hemithorax combined with tracheal deviation away from the immobile side is diagnostic of pneumothorax with tension. This is accompanied by deep cyanosis, severe dyspnea, and shock that demands aspiration of air from the cavity as a lifesaving measure.

CASE 9-1 ANSWERS

1. Differential diagnosis includes acute viral hepatitis (A, B, E, less likely C), accidental medication overdose (acetaminophen), medication toxicity (statins and certain antibiotics), alcoholic hepatitis, autoimmune hepatitis, Budd–Chiari, and chemical exposure (carbon tetrachloride and others).
2. Additional history should focus on ill contacts, risk factors for the different causes, a detailed social history (alcohol and illicit drug use, sexual history, avocations), travel history, medication use including OTC and herbals, occupational history, diet, and sources of foods (e.g., mushrooms). Ask about immunization history/status for hepatitis A and B.
3. Look for signs of chronic liver disease including muscle wasting, ascites, spider angiomas, palmar erythema, splenomegaly, and liver size which may be large, normal, or small. If all are absent, then an acute process indicated by liver tenderness is more likely. Also, look for signs of injection drug use.

CLINICAL PEARL. Hepatitis A infection usually occurs before age 5 in developing countries. In developed countries hepatitis A outbreaks usually occur in older age groups.

CASE 9-2 ANSWERS

1. <u>Diverticulitis.</u>
2. The patient may present with fever, tenderness, and guarding in the left lower quadrant. Diverticulitis most often occurs in the sigmoid colon, but can occur on the right side of the colon. In more severe cases an inflammatory mass (*phlegmon*) or abscess may be felt. Frank peritonitis indicates perforation into the peritoneal cavity.
3. *Psoas and obturator signs* should be performed in patients with abdominal pain. *Psoas sign* indicates inflammation of the psoas muscle or the overlying peritoneum. The *obturator sign* suggests inflammation of the obturator muscle or pelvic peritoneum.

CLINICAL PEARL. Bleeding from a diverticulum is usually painless presenting as dark red blood or clots; it usually stops without specific therapy.

CASE 9-3 ANSWERS

1. He is presenting with an upper GI bleed. The differential includes gastritis, peptic ulcer disease, esophagitis, esophageal varices, Dieulafoy's lesion, malignancy (esophagus or stomach), Mallory–Weiss tear, and arteriovenous malformations.
2. It will be important to assess volume status by evaluating the heart rate, blood pressure, orthostatic vital signs, skin turgor, capillary refill,

and mucous membranes. Given his long history of alcohol abuse, it is important to assess for signs of end-stage liver disease that would increase the likelihood of esophageal varices. These include palmar erythema, caput medusa, ascites, spider angiomas, Dupuytren's contracture, jaundice, gynecomastia, hemorrhoids, and hypogonadism.

3. A Mallory-Weiss tear is a linear tear in the gastroesophageal junction. The tear is preceded by violent retching or vomiting leading to hematemesis.

CLINICAL PEARL. Patients with gastrointestinal bleeding should have two large bore IVs immediately placed for volume resuscitation.

CASE 9-4 ANSWERS

1. The direction of venous flow can help elucidate the underlying cause in patients with ascites:

   - Flow away from the umbilicus is seen in portal hypertension.
   - Flow upward from the pelvic brim is seen in IVC obstruction.
   - Flow to the umbilicus is rare and may be seen with portal vein thrombosis.

2. Hepatic vein thrombosis (Budd–Chiari syndrome).
3. Most patients have an underlying hypercoagulable state predisposing them to thrombosis in low flow major veins. A pro-thrombotic state is present with oral contraceptive use, pregnancy, malignancies, inherited hypercoagulable states, TPN, chronic inflammatory diseases, and chronic infections.

CLINICAL PEARL. Approximately one-third of all cases of Budd–Chiari do not have an identifiable underlying cause.

CASE 9-5 ANSWERS

1. A direct inguinal hernia enters the inguinal canal through the posterior wall at Hesselbach's triangle that lies directly behind the external inguinal ring. Its surface landmarks are the inferior epigastric artery, lateral border of the rectus muscle, and the inguinal ligament. Indirect inguinal hernias follow the course of the spermatic cord or round ligament starting at the internal inguinal ring and extending into the inguinal canal. Inguinal hernias may extend for only a short distance in the canal or extend into the scrotum or labia majora.

2. Insert the fingertip inserted into the inguinal canal through the external inguinal ring, then ask the patient to cough or strain. A direct hernia is felt as an impulse on the pad of the distal phalanx. With an indirect hernia the impulse is felt on the fingertip. A large hernia may feel like a mass in the canal.

3. A femoral hernia will be felt below the inguinal ligament medial to the neurovascular bundle when the patient coughs or strains.

CLINICAL PEARL. Direct inguinal hernias occur almost exclusively in males; they are acquired. In both men and women a small indirect hernia often produces a small bulge over the internal inguinal ring at the midpoint of the inguinal ligament.

CASE 9-6 ANSWERS

1. Painless jaundice is often associated with common bile duct obstruction by a malignant mass in the head of the pancreas, either a pancreatic adenocarcinoma or cholangiocarcinoma. Nonbiliary causes of painless jaundice include hemolysis, ineffective erythropoiesis, and ineffective clearance of unconjugated bilirubin due to congenital defects such as Gilbert's syndrome or Crigler–Najjar.
2. Painless jaundice, anorexia, and weight loss in this age group is most likely <u>pancreatic cancer</u> causing biliary obstruction.
3. Patients with pancreatic cancer may present with migrating superficial thrombophlebitis, recurrent deep vein thrombosis (Trousseau's syndrome), nonbacterial thrombotic endocarditis (NBTE, marantic endocarditis), and depression. NBTE presents with multiple systemic arterial emboli.

CLINICAL PEARL. Pancreatic cancer in the head of the pancreas typically presents as painless jaundice. If the tumor enlarges into the retroperitoneal structures and the nerves of the celiac plexus, the patient will develop dull, poorly localized pain in the mid-epigastrium, flank, or back.

CASE 9-7 ANSWERS

1. His presentation is consistent with steatorrhea which is a sign of malabsorption. This can occur in a number of conditions including pancreatic insufficiency, celiac disease, short-gut syndrome, bacterial overgrowth in the small intestine, giardiasis, or Whipple's disease.
2. Though uncommon, the most likely diagnosis is <u>Whipple's disease</u>. In addition to steatorrhea and weight loss, he has fever, fatigue, large joint arthralgia/arthritis, generalized lymphadenopathy, and graying of the skin, all of which may occur in Whipple's disease. Other findings can include anemia, pericarditis, endocarditis, heart failure, neurologic symptoms including frontal release signs, dementia, headache, facial numbness, ataxia, and visual problems such as uveitis.
3. The intestinal mucosa and lamina propria are invaded by *Tropheryma whippelii* which are ingested by gut phagocytes, producing foamy macrophages filled with glycoprotein that can obstruct the lymphatics and cause malabsorption.

CLINICAL PEARL. Whipple disease predominately affects white males. It may be more prevalent in areas with poor sanitation, but the exact mode of transmission is not known.

CASE 10-1 ANSWERS

1. Acute loss of kidney function is classified as **prerenal** (caused by under perfusion from true loss of volume or decreased effective arterial volume), **renal** (problem with the glomeruli, tubules, interstitium or vessels), or **postrenal** (obstruction within the urinary system).
2. The physical examination must include assessment of intravascular volume, cardiac output, and the presence of severe liver disease to identify prerenal causes, and any findings suggesting obstruction (enlarged bladder, prostate hyperplasia, pelvic mass).
3. Urine microscopy helps to distinguish between glomerular causes (microscopic hematuria, red blood cell casts, proteinuria), tubular (muddy brown granular cast on urine microscopy) and interstitial disease (white blood cells and white blood cell cast).
4. The history (diarrhea, orthostatic blood pressure drop), increased BUN/creatinine ratio, urine sodium <20, and concentrated urine all suggest a prerenal state.

CLINICAL PEARL. In prerenal states drugs like angiotensin converting enzyme inhibitors, angiotensin receptor blockers, nonsteroidal anti-inflammatory, cyclosporine, and tacrolimus should be avoided as they interfere with autoregulation in the kidney.

CASE 10-2 ANSWERS

1. Nephrotic syndrome is defined by the presence of heavy proteinuria (protein excretion greater than 3.5 g/24 hours in an adult), hypoalbuminemia (less than 3.0 g/dL), and peripheral edema. Hyperlipidemia and lipiduria may be present.
2. Systemic disease such as diabetes mellitus, amyloidosis, or systemic lupus erythematosus are responsible for about 30% of nephrotic syndrome; the remaining cases are usually due to primary renal disorders such as membranous nephropathy (associated with malignancies), focal segmental glomerulosclerosis (higher incidence in black patients and with HIV), and minimal change disease (associated with lymphoma and NSAID use). Minimal change disease is the predominant cause in children.
3. Membranous nephropathy. The patient presented with nephrotic syndrome which is compatible with minimal change disease, focal segmental glomerulosclerosis, or membranous nephropathy. Membranous nephropathy is associated with malignancies, and thus, the most likely diagnosis.

CLINICAL PEARL. Nephrotic syndrome increases risk for venous thrombosis (particularly deep vein and renal vein thrombosis) and pulmonary emboli. Renal vein thrombosis (flank pain, gross hematuria, and a decline in renal function) is found disproportionately with membranous nephropathy, particularly with more than 10 g of protein per day.

CASE 10-3 ANSWERS

1. Free plasma hemoglobin entering the urine or lysis of red blood cells present in the urine. When hemoglobin enters the plasma by the intravascular hemolysis it binds to haptoglobin; when the binding capacity of haptoglobin is exceeded, free hemoglobin passes through the glomerular basement membrane.

2. Hemoglobin both intracellular and extracellular gives a positive dipstick. It is distinguished from hematuria by the absence of erythrocytes in freshly voided urine.

3. *Congenital:* G-6-PD (glucose-6-phosphate dehydrogenase) deficiency; *Endocrine:* pregnancy and the puerperium; *Idiopathic:* paroxysmal nocturnal hemoglobinuria; *Inflammatory/Immune:* major transfusion reaction, autoimmune hemolytic anemia, hapten-associated hemolysis (quinine, sulfonamides), high-titer cold agglutinin disease; *Infectious:* malaria, blackwater fever, typhus, gas gangrene; *Metabolic/ Toxic:* oxidant drugs or fava beans in persons with G-6-PD deficiency (sulfonamides, sulfones, primaquine), envenomation by snake or spider bites; *Mechanical/Traumatic:* march hemoglobinuria, mechanical heart valves, severe aortic and paraprosthetic mitral regurgitation, extracorporeal circulation, major burns, intravascular devices; *Psychosocial:* injection of distilled water; *Vascular:* microangiopathic hemolytic anemia-thrombotic thrombocytopenic purpura, hemolytic uremic syndrome, and malignant hypertension.

4. Paroxysmal nocturnal hemoglobinuria increases risk for hepatic vein thrombosis.

CLINICAL PEARL. Because hemoglobinuria is a prominent complication of PNH, all patients with PNH should be evaluated for the presence of iron deficiency.

CASE 10-4 ANSWERS

1. Signs of glomerular bleeding include red cell casts, dysmorphic red cells, gross hematuria and , brown " cola-colored" urine. The presence of red cell casts is virtually diagnostic of glomerulonephritis or vasculitis.

2. IgA nephropathy is the most common cause of isolated glomerular hematuria. Thin basement membrane nephropathy (also called thin basement membrane disease) in which gross hematuria is unusual and the family history may be positive. Alport's syndrome (hereditary nephritis) presents as hematuria with a positive family history of renal failure, and sometimes deafness or corneal abnormalities.

3. IgA nephropathy.

4. Postinfectious glomerulonephritis can present a similar picture, with low complement levels (C3 and C4), but 10 to 14 days after the URI. In IgA nephropathy hematuria occurs simultaneously with the infection (synpharyngitic).

CLINICAL PEARL. The two most common causes of apparently idiopathic hematuria (no proteinuria or infection, negative radiologic evaluation) in children are hypercalciuria and hyperuricosuria. Both are often associated with a family history of stone disease.

CASE 10-5 ANSWERS

1. Urine centrifugation is done first to determine if the color is in the sediment or supernatant. If the sediment is red, the patient has true hematuria. If the supernatant is red, and the dipstick is positive for heme, the patient either has hemoglobinuria or myoglobinuria. If the dipstick is negative for heme, the patient most likely has beeturia, phenazopyridine, or porphyria.
2. A positive dipstick test must always be confirmed with microscopic examination of the urine. Causes for false positives are when semen is present, a urine pH >9, contamination with oxidizing agents used to clean the perineum, myoglobinuria, and hemoglobinuria.
3. (1) Age >35 years; (2) smoking history (risk directly related to cumulative exposure); (3) occupational exposure (printers, painters, chemical plant workers) to chemicals or dyes (benzenes or aromatic amines); (4) gross hematuria; (5) pelvic irradiation; (6) exposure to cyclophosphamide; (7) chronic indwelling foreign body; and (8) analgesic abuse.

CLINICAL PEARL. Gross hematuria with clots almost always indicates a lower urinary tract source.

CASE 10-6 ANSWERS

1. Polyuria is defined as <u>urine output exceeding 3 L/day</u> in adults.
2. <u>Primary polydipsia</u>, primarily seen in adults and adolescents; <u>central diabetes insipidus</u>; and <u>nephrogenic diabetes insipidus</u>.
3. <u>Primary polydipsia</u> (sometimes called psychogenic polydipsia) is a primary increase in water intake. It is most often seen in middle-aged women, and in patients with psychiatric illnesses. <u>Central DI (also called neurohypophyseal or neurogenic DI)</u> is associated with deficient antidiuretic hormone (ADH) secretion. It is most often idiopathic (possibly due to autoimmune injury to the ADH-producing cells). It can follow trauma, pituitary surgery, compression or infiltration of the pituitary stalk (sarcoidosis), or hypoxic or ischemic encephalopathy. <u>Nephrogenic DI</u> is characterized by normal ADH secretion but varying degrees of renal resistance to its water-retaining effect. It is most commonly acquired. Causes include chronic lithium use or chronic electrolyte disorders (hypercalcemia, hypokalemia). Nephrogenic DI presenting in childhood is almost always due to an inherited defect, for example, mutations in the AVPR2 gene encoding the ADH receptor V2, or aquaporin-2 water channel gene.
4. <u>Nephrogenic diabetes insipidus from chronic lithium use.</u>

CLINICAL PEARL. Urine osmolarity is low in DI and primary polydipsia whereas it is high in osmotic diuresis. Plasma sodium concentration is low in primary polydipsia whereas it is high normal in diabetes insipidus.

CASE 11-1 ANSWERS

1. Diagnostic possibilities include an ectopic pregnancy, ovarian/adnexal torsion, ruptured ovarian cyst, appendicitis, nephrolithiasis, tubo-ovarian abscess, cystitis, diverticulitis, endometritis, and bleeding associated with ovulation.
2. Physical examination in ovarian torsion can often be nonspecific. Findings may include a tender adnexal mass but failure to find this does not rule out torsion. Purulent cervical discharge is suggestive of infection such as a tubo-ovarian abscess or pelvic inflammatory disease.
3. Typically ovarian torsion occurs around a pathologically enlarged ovary as occurs with functional cysts or benign tumors such as a teratoma. Torsion usually occurs in women of child-bearing age but can occur in younger or postmenopausal women. Women receiving ovulation induction for infertility are at higher risk. Onset is often associated with exercise or other jarring activity.

CLINICAL PEARL. Ultrasound is the imaging modality of choice; it will often show an enlarged adnexa. Doppler examination showing maintained arterial flow does not rule out torsion.

CASE 11-2 ANSWERS

1. Genital ulcers can be seen with syphilis, chancroid, Behçet's disease, herpes, granuloma inguinale, and condyloma.
2. <u>Syphilis</u>. A painless ulcer with a raised border with regional lymphadenopathy and the presumptive incubation period is most likely syphilis.
3. Untreated primary syphilis can progress to secondary syphilis that has a widely varied presentation including mucocutaneous rash and generalized painless lymphadenopathy. Tertiary syphilis presents years to decades later with chronic inflammation of many organs. Findings include cardiovascular involvement with arterial invasion causing aortic aneurysms and aortic insufficiency, CNS involvement causing cranial nerve palsies, tabes dorsalis, and syphilitic meningitis.

CLINICAL PEARL. Patients with genital ulcers are more susceptible to acquisition of HIV infection due to the disruption of mucosal defenses.

CASE 11-3 ANSWERS

1. Bacterial vaginosis caused by *Gardnerella vaginalis*.
2. The normal pH of vaginal secretions is <4.6. Changes in the pH predisposes to overgrowth by pathogens. Factors that can raise the vaginal pH include use of feminine hygiene products (sprays and douches), birth control pills, sexual intercourse, antibiotics, stress, and vaginal medications. Other influences are age, other sexually transmitted disease, immune status, and some skin diseases.
3. The other two most common pathogens are Candida and Trichomoniasis. Candida typically presents with pain, itching, dyspareunia, and a thick odorless white discharge. Trichomoniasis often will have frothy white to green discharge; pruritus and dysuria may occur.

CLINICAL PEARL. Less common noninfectious causes of vaginitis include contact dermatitis (latex, spermicidal lubricants), atrophic vaginitis, lichen sclerosis et atrophica and Bowen's disease.

CASE 11-4 ANSWERS

1. The differential diagnosis is quite broad and includes: *Congenital:* delayed puberty, uterine agenesis, imperforate hymen, ovarian agenesis or dysgenesis (Turner's syndrome), and other disorders of sex chromosomes; *Endocrine:* hypo- and hyperthyroidism, hypopituitarism, androgens; *Metabolic/Toxic:* lead, mercury, morphine, alcohol, malnutrition, chemotherapy, excessive exercise, obesity, debilitating diseases; *Mechanical/Traumatic:* hysterectomy, oophorectomy, pelvic irradiation; *Neoplastic:* androgen-producing tumors, prolactinoma, craniopharyngioma; *Psychosocial:* anorexia nervosa, depression.
2. You may see lower set ears, a short webbed neck, the chest may have widely spaced nipples, the extremities may show lymphedema and the arms may show a wide carrying angle (cubitus valgus). Skin examination may show pigmented nevi, nail hypoplasia, and hyperconvex uplifted nails. Oral examination may reveal abnormal tooth development and morphology, high-arched palate, micrognathic mandible, and distal molar occlusion. Eye examination may reveal epicanthal folds, ptosis, strabismus, and palpebral fissures that have an upward slant.

CLINICAL PEARL. Neck webbing in Turner's syndrome is associated with coarctation of the aorta and bicuspid aortic valve. The apex of the lung extends high into the "web" making it vulnerable to inadvertent puncture during insertion of subclavian or internal jugular venous access.

CASE 12-1 ANSWERS

1. In young sexually active men chlamydia, gonorrhea, and the genital mycoplasmas are the most common pathogens responsible for urethritis. It is usually classified as gonococcal or nongonococcal. In men over age 40 enteric bacteria predominate.

2. The *acute presentation of a frankly purulent urethral discharge* is most suggestive of <u>gonorrhea</u>. *Dysuria alone* is more likely a <u>chlamydial infection</u>. *Dysuria accompanied by painful genital ulcers* is most likely due to <u>genital HSV</u>. Patients with primary HSV infection may also complain of fever, tender local inguinal lymphadenopathy, and headache.

3. <u>Gonococcal urethritis.</u>

4. Urethritis, conjunctivitis, and arthritis are the triad of *reactive arthritis* (Reiter's disease); the urethritis frequently is the presenting sign.

5. *Campylobacter*, *Yersinia*, *Shigella*, and *Salmonella* enterocolitis and sexually transmitted infections, especially *Chlamydia*.

CLINICAL PEARL. Coinfection with two or more sexually transmitted pathogens is common. Up to 30% of men with gonococcal urethritis have concurrent chlamydia infection.

CASE 12-2 ANSWERS

1. <u>HSV</u> and *Haemophilus ducreyi* (<u>chancroid</u>) present as multiple ulcers. <u>HSV</u> typically starts as multiple vesicles on an erythematous base progressing to ulcers that have a clean base. In <u>chancroid,</u> the ulcers begin as papules that go on to ulcerate. The ulcers are characteristically deep and ragged with a purulent, yellow-gray base, and an undermined, violaceous border. <u>Syphilis</u> classically presents as a single, indurated, well-circumscribed painless ulcer. It can, however, be soft, non-indurated, irregular, and occasionally painful. In <u>lymphogranuloma venereum</u> the lesion begins as a single papule or a shallow ulcer. <u>Granuloma inguinale</u> presents as one or more nodular lesions that ulcerate and slowly enlarge. The ulcers are often friable and have raised, rolled margins.

2. Inguinal lymphadenopathy is seen with most infections causing genital ulcers. The nodes are often tender with HSV, chancroid, and LGV. Rubbery nontender nodes are often seen in late primary syphilis. Matting or suppuration of the lymph nodes or the development of a painful "buboes" can occur with chancroid or LGV.

3. <u>Genital herpes simplex.</u> Herpetic lesions begin as one or more grouped vesicles on an erythematous base. These vesicles subsequently open resulting in shallow ulcerations. Under the foreskin and around the labia and rectum vesicles often break prior to being noticed.

CLINICAL PEARL. Significant concomitant inguinal, cervical, and/or axillary lymphadenopathy raises concern for simultaneous HIV infection.

CASE 12-3 ANSWERS

1. (1) Herpes simplex virus (HSV); (2) *Treponema pallidum*, the cause of syphilis; (3) *Haemophilus ducreyi*, the cause of chancroid; (4) *Chlamydia trachomatis* serovars L1–3, cause lymphogranuloma venereum (LGV);

(5) *Klebsiella granulomatis* causes granuloma inguinale, also known as Donovanosis.
2. Noninfectious etiologies include fixed drug reactions, Behçet's disease, neoplasms, and trauma.
3. Recurrent ulcers should suggest HSV infection, and less commonly noninfectious etiologies such as Behçet's disease or fixed drug eruption.

CLINICAL PEARL. Painful ulcers are more typical of HSV and chancroid, while ulcers associated with syphilis, LGV, and granuloma inguinale are usually painless.

CASE 12-4 ANSWERS

1. Varicocele.
2. It is caused by dilatation of the pampiniform plexus of spermatic veins.
3. It occurs predominantly on the left; occasionally it is bilateral and almost never is the right side involved exclusively. The left-sided predominance is explained anatomically. The left spermatic (gonadal) vein is one of the longest veins in the body. It enters the left renal vein at a perpendicular angle. The intravascular pressure in the left renal vein is higher than on the right because it is compressed between the aorta and the superior mesenteric artery above the renal vein, thereby producing a "nutcracker effect."
4. A varicocele, unlike an indirect inguinal hernia containing omentum, should decrease in size or resolve when the patient lies down. Place your gloved finger over the subcutaneous inguinal ring. When the patient stands, with your finger in place, the veins refill but the hernia will be held back.

CLINICAL PEARL. Unilateral right varicoceles are very rare and should alert the clinician to possible inferior vena caval obstruction (renal cell carcinoma with IVC thrombus, right renal vein thrombosis with clot propagation down the IVC, etc.), since the right gonadal vein directly empties into the IVC.

CASE 12-5 ANSWERS

1. Acute epididymitis.
2. The cremasteric reflex is usually absent in patients with testicular torsion in contrast to epididymitis and other causes of scrotal pain, in which the reflex is typically intact.
3. The cremasteric reflex is assessed by stroking or gently pinching the skin of the upper thigh while observing the ipsilateral testis. A normal response is cremasteric muscle contraction with elevation of the testis.

4. *Chlamydia trachomatis* and *Neisseria gonorrhoeae* are the most common organisms responsible for bacterial epididymitis in men under the age of 35. Sexually transmitted organisms are less likely to be the cause of epididymitis in older men, in whom *Escherichia coli*, other coliforms, and *Pseudomonas* species are more common.

CLINICAL PEARL. The most common causes of acute scrotal pain in adults are testicular torsion and epididymitis. Testicular torsion presents with abrupt onset of severe testicular pain. Immediate detorsion is required to maintain viability of the testis.

CASE 13-1 ANSWERS

1. Grasp the calf with one hand while the other hand supports and stabilizes the femur from behind with the thumb and fingertips on opposite joint margins overlying the collateral ligaments. Stress the lateral, then the medial collateral ligaments by exerting a varus, then a valgus force on the calf while palpating over joint margin. Feel for separation of the tibia from the femur and look for medial or lateral displacement of the tibia.
2. Test the anterior cruciate with the *Lachman test*. Have the patient lie supine and flex the affected knee 30 degrees. Sit on the patient's foot to fix it. Grasp the upper part of the leg with your fingers in the popliteal fossa and your thumbs on the anterior joint line. Pull the head of the tibia toward you so it glides on the femoral condyles. Forward movement of more than 1 cm is a positive Lachman test, indicating rupture of the ACL. To test the posterior cruciate, start as in the Lachman test and observe for sagging of the tibia posteriorly. Then push the head of the tibia posteriorly. Displacement should be less than 5 mm.
3. An ACL tear occurs when the tibia is driven forward relative to the femur as in a hyperextension, or a rapid stop and change in direction with a twisting motion. It often occurs without contact with another player.

CLINICAL PEARL. MCL injuries and lateral meniscus injuries often occur at the same time as an ACL injury, especially with a lateral blow or tackle.

CASE 13-2 ANSWERS

1. With the patient supine on the table, grasp the patient's knee with one hand so that your fingers press the medial and lateral aspects of the joint. Grasp the patient's heel with your other hand so that the plantar surface of the foot rests along your wrist and forearm. First, flex the knee until the heel nearly touches the buttock. To test the posterior half of the medial meniscus, rotate the foot laterally, and then slowly fully extend the knee. If a click is felt or heard during the extending motion, and the patient recognizes it as the sensation

preceding pain or locking, the medial meniscus is torn. For the lateral meniscus, repeat the examination with the foot rotated medially.

2. Have the patient lie prone on a low couch, approximately 2 ft (60 cm) high, with the patient's affected limb toward you. Grasp the foot with both your hands, flex the knee to 90 degrees, and rotate the foot laterally. This should cause little discomfort. Now, rest your knee on the patient's hamstrings to fix the femur, and pull the leg to further flexion while the foot is held in lateral rotation; pain indicates a lesion of the MCL. Next, compress the tibial condyles onto the femoral condyles by placing your body weight onto the plantar surface of the foot, still in lateral rotation. Pain from this maneuver indicates tear of the medial meniscus.

3. This test should be reserved for testing athletes for a tear of the posterior horn of the meniscus.

CLINICAL PEARL. It has been shown that in patients with a degenerative medial meniscus tear and no OA there was no benefit to arthroscopic partial menisectomy compared to a sham procedure.

CASE 13-3 ANSWERS

1. Possible causes of this presentation include acute rotator cuff tendonitis, partial- or full-thickness tear of the supraspinatus tendon, partial or complete tear of other rotator cuff tendons, subacromial bursitis, biceps tendonitis, or a muscle strain.

2. Inability to initiate elevation in 90-degree abduction indicates rupture of the supraspinatus tendon. The patient cannot elevate the arm against minimal resistance at 30 degrees elevation and 90 degrees abduction, but passive motion is free and painless. Initial shoulder motion is mostly with the scapula. There is resistance to external rotation when the arm is held at the side with elbow flexed. As the arm is moved forward, one may palpate a jerk, fine crepitus, or an indentation in the subacromial region between the greater and lesser humeral tubercles.

3. All have painful abduction between 60 degrees and 120 degrees, often prohibiting full active range of motion. Less painful passive range of motion is preserved. Precise distinction among the three is not possible by physical examination.

CLINICAL PEARL. Adhesive capsulitis often follows unresolved subacromial bursitis or supraspinatus tendonitis.

CASE 13-4 ANSWERS

1. The three key observations are floating of the nail base, loss of the unguophalangeal angle, and increased longitudinal convexity of the nail plate. Obliteration of the unguophalangeal angle. Inspect the profile of the terminal digit. Normally, the nail makes an angle

of 20 degrees or more with the projected line of the digit. With clubbing, this angle is diminished, may be obliterated, or extend below the projected line of the digit. <u>Floating nail.</u> Palpate the proximal nail with the tip of your finger. You can feel and see the springy softness as the root of the nail is depressed. <u>Convexity of the nail.</u> A month or so after the floating nail and nail angle changes, a transverse ridge appears in the plate from beneath the mantle. The ridge marks the change from the normal distal curve to a new curve of smaller radius in the proximal nail.

2. Clubbing has been seen in a number of conditions that this patient could have including alcoholic cirrhosis, lung cancer, mesothelioma, and endocarditis.

CLINICAL PEARL. Recent evidence suggests that clubbing is a consequence of vascular endothelial growth factor reaching the systemic circulation via arteriovenous shunts either in the lung or by extra pulmonary shunts.

CASE 13-5 ANSWERS

1. Her symptoms are consistent with carpal tunnel syndrome. Given her weakness you will look specifically for thenar wasting. The thenar eminence is formed by the bellies of the opponens pollicis, abductor pollicis brevis, and flexor pollicis brevis, all innervated by the median nerve.

2. Ulnar nerve damage causes decreased sensation in the pinky and ring finger predominately on the palmar aspects. Hypothenar wasting may be seen. The hypothenar eminence is composed of the bellies of the palmaris brevis, abductor digiti quinti and the opponens digiti quinti, all innervated by the ulnar nerve. Wasting of the intrinsic hand muscles can be seen. In severe cases patients can develop a claw hand.

CLINICAL PEARL. If both thenar and hypothenar wasting are seen, cervical myelopathy must be considered.

CASE 13-6 ANSWERS

1. The differential diagnosis includes fibromyalgia, chronic fatigue syndrome, hypothyroidism, depression, primary sleep disorder, Lyme disease, polymyalgia rheumatica, systemic lupus erythematosus, rheumatoid arthritis, statin myopathy, osteomalacia, or chronic idiopathic myalgia.

2. You must evaluate for evidence of hypothyroidism including checking for a goiter, changes in hair or skin, and hung-up reflexes. A thorough musculoskeletal examination looking for tenosynovitis or joint effusions should be performed. The patient should be evaluated for the tender points associated with fibromyalgia.

3. It most often occurs in women in middle adulthood. It is less common in men and in the young or elderly. The cause is not known but is more common in people with depression, anxiety, irritable bowel, osteoarthritis, or rheumatoid arthritis. It may also run in families. The condition is sometimes triggered by emotional or physical stress.

CLINICAL PEARL. Trigger points occur in muscles under frequent tonic contraction and cause firm nodules or bands. Trigger points must be differentiated from fibromyalgia since the treatment is different.

CASE 13-7 ANSWERS

1. The differential diagnosis for a monoarticular arthritis includes gout, pseudogout (calcium pyrophosphate dehydrate deposition disease), and septic arthritis.
2. Pseudogout increases as people age, usually occurring after age 60. If it occurs in younger people, it may be related to hyperparathyroidism, hemochromatosis, Wilson's disease, hypothyroidism, or acromegaly.
3. Over 50% of first gout attacks are podagra (the MTP joint of the great toe); other sites include the midfoot, ankle, knee, elbow, or wrist. CPPD typically affects the knee, ankle, or wrist.

CLINICAL PEARL. Gout of the midfoot is easily misdiagnosed as cellulitis.

CASE 14-1 ANSWERS

1. Acute inflammatory demyelinating polyneuropathy (AIDPN) or Guillain–Barré syndrome (GBS).
2. Muscle weakness may arise from lesions in the brain, spinal cord, peripheral nerves, motor endplate, or muscle.
3. Difficulty rising from a chair or climbing stairs suggest proximal muscle weakness; difficulty writing, opening jars and doors, and catching the toes while walking suggest distal muscle weakness.
4. Weakness/paralysis with loss of deep tendon reflexes, hypotonia, muscle wasting, and fasciculations suggest a LMN lesion. Chronic LMN lesions lead to severe muscle wasting. Weakness/paralysis with hyperreflexia and spasticity without severe wasting suggest a UMN lesion. An extensor plantar response (Babinski's sign) is present with any lesion (UMN or LMN) in the corticospinal motor tract.

CLINICAL PEARL. (1) Severe respiratory muscle weakness necessitating ventilatory support develops in 10% to 30% of patients with GBS; (2) Hysterical weakness is not rare and malingering is perhaps more common. These diagnoses can only be made after organic disease is excluded by a thorough evaluation.

CASE 14-2 ANSWERS

1. <u>Bell's palsy,</u> idiopathic lower motor neuron injury to the facial nerve.
2. Facial weakness is best demonstrated by asking the patient to *"Close your eyes"* (testing the upper face) and *"Show me your teeth"* (testing the lower face). Denervation of the orbicularis oculi muscles results in inability to close the eyelids effectively; denervation of the risorius muscle results in limited retraction of the angle of the mouth.
3. <u>Peripheral.</u> Weakness in both the upper and lower face. The lesion is ipsilateral to the facial weakness and is either in the peripheral nerve or the pons. <u>Central.</u> Weakness only in the lower face, sparing of the upper face. The lesion is contralateral to the lower facial weakness and above the level of facial nucleus in the pons.
4. <u>Ramsay Hunt syndrome.</u> Varicella-zoster virus infects the geniculate ganglion of the sensory branch of the facial nerve leading to facial palsy, loss of taste on the anterior two-thirds of the tongue, pain, and vesicles in the ipsilateral external auditory canal.

CLINICAL PEARL. Some cases of Bell's palsy have been attributed to ischemia from diabetes and arteriosclerosis. However, HSV type 1 probably causes most cases of Bell's palsy.

CASE 14-3 ANSWERS

1. Syncope results from transient arrest of cerebral or brainstem function. This usually results from a momentary arrest of effective cerebral or brainstem perfusion. Impaired brain perfusion may occur from ineffective cardiac contraction (myocardial insufficiency or dysrhythmias), peripheral vasodilation producing hypotension, or from vascular reflexes.
2. Syncope occurring with exertion strongly suggests aortic stenosis, pulmonary hypertension, mitral stenosis, coronary artery disease, or hypertrophic cardiomyopathy with obstruction, all conditions where the increased demand for cardiac output cannot be met due to the underlying condition which limits cardiac output.
3. <u>Hypertrophic obstructive cardiomyopathy.</u>
4. Cardiac syncope due to inadequate cardiac output may be caused by outflow-tract obstruction, tachycardia, or bradycardia.

CLINICAL PEARL. In patients with syncope, structural heart disease is the most important factor predicting the risk of arrhythmias and death. EKG is recommended in almost all patients, despite its low yield, because the findings can affect the immediate management of the underlying condition.

CASE 14-4 ANSWERS

1. <u>Tardive dyskinesia (TD).</u> This is a hyperkinetic movement disorder that appears after prolonged use of dopamine receptor blocking

agents. Most often TD presents with choreiform movements of the mouth, tongue, and lips.

2. Increased risk is associated with advanced age and organic cerebral dysfunction; lower risk is associated with younger age and atypical antipsychotics. Roughly one-third of TD cases resolve within 3 months of discontinuing the offending drug. Most of the rest slowly improve over a course of years.

3. The ability of antipsychotic drugs to block postsynaptic dopamine receptors is a potential mechanism for the development of TD. An updated version of the dopamine hypothesis suggests that an imbalance between D1 and D2 receptor-mediated effects in the basal ganglia may be responsible.

4. Tardive dystonia is associated with chronic neuroleptic exposure and is typified by axial muscle involvement and a characteristic rocking motion. Tardive dystonia often persists after the offending medication is discontinued and it is refractory to therapy.

CLINICAL PEARL. Chronic metoclopramide use is a major cause of tardive dyskinesia in adults. Other drugs associated with hyperkinetic movement disorders include phenytoin, carbamazepine, tricyclic antidepressants, fluoxetine, oral contraceptives, buspirone, digoxin, cimetidine, diazoxide, lithium, methadone, and fentanyl.

CASE 14-5 ANSWERS

1. Position and vibration sense are carried in the posterior columns of the spinal cord. Damage to the posterior columns results in impaired proprioception leading to abnormalities in stance and gait.

2. Posterior column injury is common to vitamin B12 or copper deficiency and tabes dorsalis.

3. Glossitis, macrocytic anemia, and dementia accompany severe B12 deficiency; a spastic gait disorder may accompany copper deficiency.

CLINICAL PEARL. Nitrous oxide anesthesia may precipitate severe B12 deficiency in patients with minimal stores.

CASE 14-6 ANSWERS

1. <u>Thunder clap headache</u>. The sudden onset of a severe excruciating headache that reaches maximal intensity within seconds of onset is often termed a thunderclap headache.

2. Subarachnoid hemorrhage should be the first consideration. A first severe headache meeting this description must be evaluated urgently. If accompanied by a change in the level of consciousness, nausea,

visual changes, vertigo, paralysis or paresthesias, the likelihood of a serious intracranial problem is increased.

3. Thunderclap headache may occur with intracerebral hemorrhage, cluster headache, stroke, intercourse (coital headache), cerebral venous thrombosis, or cerebral vasoconstriction.

CLINICAL PEARL. Since the pain from a cluster headache can reach full intensity within minutes, it may be confused with a more serious headache disorder. However, cluster headache is transient (usually lasting less than 1–2 hours) and is associated with characteristic ipsilateral autonomic signs such as tearing or rhinorrhea.

CASE 15-1 ANSWERS

1. Delirium.
2. Delirium is characterized by loss of attentiveness, fluctuating level of consciousness, progressive loss of orientation, and confusion.
3. Advanced age, multiple medications especially sedatives, poor functional status, cognitive impairment, depression, alcohol abuse, drug intoxication, chronic liver and kidney disease, infections and volume depletion are all predisposing factors.
4. Drug withdrawal (e.g., narcotics, sedatives, tranquilizers, alcohol, steroids, salicylates, and digitalis), hypoxia, hypoventilation, acute kidney injury with or without uremia, congestive heart failure, electrolyte abnormalities, and urinary retention.

CLINICAL PEARL. Delirium is usually a metabolic encephalopathy. Failure to recognize and treat delirium is associated with a high incidence of long-term morbidity and increased mortality.

CASE 15-2 ANSWERS

1. Restless leg syndrome. This is characterized by irresistible urge to move the limbs, often to stop unusual or uncomfortable sensations in the legs.
2. (1) An urge to move the legs—with or without associated paresthesias and dysesthesias; (2) symptoms are worse or triggered by rest and relaxation; (3) symptoms worsen in the evening or at night; and (4) symptoms improve with activity.
3. Iron deficiency.

CLINICAL PEARL. Most cases of restless leg syndrome are idiopathic. It is seen in younger patients with family history of this syndrome. Secondary restless leg syndrome is often associated with iron deficiency, pregnancy (third semester), and end-stage kidney disease. The only testing required for secondary causes is a ferritin level.

CASE 15-3 ANSWERS

1. <u>Psychiatric conditions.</u> Panic disorder, somatic symptoms disorder (somatization disorder), and illness anxiety disorder. <u>Stimulant abuse.</u> Overuse of caffeine and abuse of drugs such as cocaine and amphetamines. <u>Medical disorders.</u> Arrhythmias, angina, asthma, pulmonary embolism, hyperthyroidism, pheochromocytoma, recurrent hypoglycemia, and complex partial seizures (temporal lobe epilepsy).

2. <u>Panic disorder.</u> *Panic attacks* are characterized by an abrupt surge of intense fear or intense discomfort that reaches a peak within minutes, accompanied by specific somatic, cognitive, and affective symptoms. *Panic disorder* results when panic attacks lead to persistent concern or anxiety about possible recurrence resulting in changes in behavior, such as agoraphobia, hypochondriacal concerns, and high medical utilization.

3. <u>Agoraphobia</u> is a persistent fear of public or group situations which might precipitate a panic attack causing embarrassment or discomfort without escape. Agoraphobia commonly accompanies panic disorder.

CLINICAL PEARL. Cardiovascular, neurologic, and gastrointestinal symptoms are the most common somatic symptoms of panic disorder.

CASE 16-1 ANSWERS

1. The presence of known coronary artery disease, previous stroke or other cerebrovascular disease, a history of congestive heart failure, insulin-treated diabetes, a creatinine >2.0 mg/dL, and increased age all contribute independently to an increased risk.

2. High-risk procedures include all aortic and major vascular procedures, peripheral vascular procedures, and emergent procedures especially in the elderly.

3. Intermediate risk procedures include carotid endarterectomy, any intrathoracic or intraperitoneal procedure, head and neck procedures, major orthopedic procedures, and prostatectomy.

CLINICAL PEARL. Most low-risk patients and patients requiring emergency surgery do not require preoperative cardiac testing. The indications for assessment for coronary artery disease are identical in the preoperative patient as in a patient who is not having surgery. If you would not order the tests absent the planned surgery do not order them preoperatively.

CASE 16-2 ANSWERS

1. <u>Metabolic equivalents (METS).</u>

2. METS are multiples of the oxygen consumption required to sit comfortably, which is 1 MET, therefore 6 METS is a sixfold increase in oxygen consumption.

3. <u>4 METS.</u>
4. Some activities requiring 4–5 METS are mopping floors, cleaning windows, painting walls, raking leaves, pushing a power lawnmower on the level, and walking up one flight of stairs.

CLINICAL PEARL. Further cardiac testing should be considered in patients with anginal symptoms or those with clinical risk factors and poor exercise tolerance (<4 METS or cannot assess METS), if testing would change perioperative management. Historically surgeons would walk the patient up and down a flight of stairs to assess their surgical risk. It takes a little time but is still a reliable predictor.

3-3.5 METS

4. Some activities requiring 4-5 METs are mopping floors, cleaning windows, painting walls, raking leaves, pushing a power lawnmower on the level, and walking up one flight of stairs.

Further cardiac testing should be considered in patients with atypical symptoms or those with clinical risk factors and poor exercise tolerance (<4 METs or cannot assess METs). If testing would change perioperative management. [Historically, surgeons would walk the patient up and down a flight of stairs to assess their surgical risk. It takes a little time but is still a reliable predictor.]

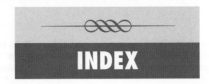

INDEX

Note: Page numbers followed by *f* and *t* represent figures and tables respectively.